OBSTETRIC & GYNECOLOGIC EMERGENCIES

Diagnosis and Management

OBSTETRIC & GYNECOLOGIC EMERGENCIES

Diagnosis and Management

Edited by

Mark D. Pearlman, MD
S. Jan Behrman Professor and Vice Chair
Department of Obstetrics and Gynecology
Professor, Department of Surgery
Associate Chief of Staff
University of Michigan Health System
Ann Arbor, MI

Judith E. Tintinalli, MD, MS
Professor and Chairman
Department of Emergency Medicine
University of North Carolina at Chapel Hill
Chapel Hill, NC

Pamela L. Dyne, MD
Assistant Professor
Department of Emergency Medicine
UCLA Emergency Medical Center
David Geffen School of Medicine at UCLA
Los Angeles, CA

McGraw-Hill
Medical Publishing Division

New York Chicago San Francisco Lisbon London Madrid Mexico City Milan New Delhi San Juan Seoul Singapore Sydney Toronto

Obstetric & Gynecologic Emergencies: Diagnosis and Management

1234567890 DOCDOC 09876543

ISBN 0-07-137937-1

This book was set in Times Roman by TechBooks.
The editors were Andrea Seils and Regina Y. Brown.
The production supervisor was Catherine H. Saggese.
The index was prepared by Jerry Ralya.
RR Donnelly was the printer and binder.

This book was printed on acid-free paper.

Library of Congress Cataloging-in-Publication Data

Obstetric and gynecologic emergencies : diagnosis and n
Judith E. Tintinalli, Pamela Dyne.
p. ; cm.
Includes bibliographical references and index.
ISBN 0-07-137937-1
1. Gynecology—Handbooks, manuals, etc. 2. Obstetri
3. Emergency medicine—Handbooks, manuals, etc. I. Pe
Judith E. III. Dyne, Pamela.
[DNLM: 1. Genital Diseases, Female—Handbooks. 2
3. Pregnancy Complications—Handbooks. WP 39 O141 2
RG103.O24 2003
618.1—dc21 2002035351

CONTENTS

SECTION V Problems in Labor, Delivery, and the Postpartum Period

SECTION VI Pediatric and Adolescent Gynecology

SECTION VII The Reproductive Age and Older Women

Appendices

Contributors

Esam H. Alhamad, MD [13]
Fellow in Pulmonary and Critical Care Medicine
University of Michigan Health System
Ann Arbor, Michigan

Imran I Ali, MD [18]
Associate Professor
Director, Comprehensive Epilepsy Program
Department of Neurology
Medical College of Ohio
Toledo, Ohio

Deirdre Anglin, MD, MPH [34]
Associate Professor of Emergency Medicine
Keck School of Medicine
University Southern California
Los Angeles, California

Mel L. Barclay, MD [2]
Associate Professor
Department of Obstetrics & Gynecology
Division of Maternal-Fetal Medicine
University of Michigan Health System
Ann Arbor, Michigan

Sheela M. Barhan, MD [32]
Assistant Professor
Department of Obstetrics & Gynecology
Wright State University School of Medicine
Dayton, Ohio

Lynn Borgatta, MD [6]
Clinical Associate Professor of Obstetrics & Gynecology
Boston University School of Medicine
Boston, Massachusetts

Emmanuel G. Christodoulou, PhD [App. 1]
Senior Allied Health Technical Specialist
Department of Radiology
University of Michigan Health System
Ann Arbor, Michigan

Reb Close, MD [28]
Chief Resident
Department of Emergency Medicine
Community Hospital of the Monterey Peninsula
Monterey, California

Christine H. Comstock, MD [35]
Associate Professor
Department of Obstetrics & Gynecology
Wayne State University
Detroit, Michigan
Clinical Assistant Professor
Department of Obstetrics & Gynecology
University of Michigan Health System
Ann Arbor, Michigan
Head, Division of Fetal Imaging
William Beaumont Hospital
Royal Oak, Michigan

Robert G. Dart, MD [5]
Associate Professor of Emergency Medicine
Boston University School of Medicine
Research Director and Vice Chair
Department of Emergency Medicine
Boston Medical Center
Boston, Massachusetts

John O. L. Delancey, MD [1]
Professor of Gynecology
Department of Obstetrics & Gynecology
University of Michigan Health System
Ann Arbor, Michigan

Diana L. Dell, MD [19]
Assistant Professor
Department of Psychiatry and Behavioral Health
Duke University Medical Center
Durham, North Carolina

Gary A. Dildy, III, MD [8]
Professor of Obstetrics & Gynecology
Division of Maternal-Fetal Medicine
Louisiana State University School of Medicine
New Orleans, Louisiana

Mary S. Dolan, MD, MPH [17]
Assistant Professor
Division Chief, Women's Primary Health
Department of Obstetrics & Gynecology
University of North Carolina at Chapel Hill
Chapel Hill, North Carolina

Pamela L. Dyne, MD [4, 5]
Associate Clinical Professor of Medicine
UCLA Emergency Medicine Center
David Geffen School of Medicine at UCLA
Los Angeles, California

Mary E. Eberst, MD [16]
Assistant Professor
Departments of Emergency Medicine and Medicine
University of North Carolina at Chapel Hill
Chapel Hill, North Carolina

Sebastian Faro, MD, PhD [29, 30]
Attending Physician
The Woman's Hospital of Texas
Houston, Texas
Professor, Volunteer Faculty
Department of Obstetrics, Gynecology, and Reproductive Science
The University of Texas-Houston
Houston, Texas

Keri Gardner, MD [21]
Chief Resident
UCLA Emergency Medicine Center
David Geffen School of Medicine at UCLA
Los Angeles, California

Mitchell M. Goodsitt, MS, PhD [App. 1]
Professor of Radiological Sciences
Department of Radiology
Professor of Environmental and Industrial Health
University of Michigan Health System
Ann Arbor, Michigan

Jennifer Gunter, MD [14]
Assistant Professor
Department of Obstetrics & Gynecology
The University of Colorado Health Sciences Center
Denver, Colorado

Wendy F. Hansen, MD [3]
Assistant Professor
Department of Obstetrics & Gynecology
University of Iowa Hospitals and Clinics
Iowa City, Iowa

William W. Hurd, MD [32]
Nicholas J. Thompson Professor and Chair
Department of Obstetrics & Gynecology
Wright State University School of Medicine
Dayton, Ohio

Jean A. Hurteau, MD [32]
Associate Professor
Director, Division Gynecologic Oncology
Department of Obstetrics & Gynecology
University of Illinois at Chicago
Chicago, Illinois

Timothy R.B. Johnson, MD [10]
Bates Professor of Diseases of Women and Children and Chair, Department of Obstetrics and Gynecology
University of Michigan Health System
Ann Arbor, Michigan

Vern Katz, MD [11]
Center Genetics and Maternal-Fetal Medicine
Medical Director of Prenatal Service
Sacred Heart Medical Center
Eugene, Oregon
Clinical Associate Professor
Oregon Health Sciences University
Portland, Oregon

Raymond H. Kaufman, MD [30]
Professor
Department of Obstetrics & Gynecology
Baylor College of Medicine
Houston, Texas

Robert P. Lorenz, MD [15]
Director, Maternal Fetal Medicine
Vice Chief, Obstetrics
William Beaumont Hospital
Royal Oak, Michigan

Mark J. Lowell, MD [7]
Clinical Assistant Professor, Emergency Medicine
Medical Director, Survival Flight
Director, Chest Pain Center
University of Michigan Health System
Ann Arbor, Michigan

Maurizio L. Maccato, MD [22]
Assistant Professor
Department of Obstetrics & Gynecology
Baylor College of Medicine
Houston, Texas

Ritu Malik, MD [33]
UCLA Emergency Medicine Center
David Geffen School of Medicine at UCLA
Los Angeles, California

Fernando J. Martinez, MD, MS [13]
Professor of Internal Medicine
Division of Pulmonary and Critical Care Medicine
University of Michigan Health System
Ann Arbor, Michigan

Lisa L. May, MD [App. 3]
Biltmore Dermatology Associates
Ashville, North Carolina

Connie Mitchell, MD [34]
Assistant Clinical Professor
Department of Pediatrics
University of California Davis Medical Center
Director, Domestic Violence Education
California Medical Training Center
Sacramento, California

Rona Molodow, MD, JD [25]
Associate Clinical Professor
Department of Pediatrics
Olive View- UCLA Medical Center
David Geffen School of Medicine at UCLA
Sylmar, California

Malcolm G. Munro, MD [27]
David Geffen School of Medicine at UCLA
Los Angeles, California

Linda M. Nicholas, MD, MS [19]
Assistant Professor of Psychiatry
University of North Carolina at Chapel Hill
Chapel Hill, North Carolina

Rita Oregon, MD [27]
Assistant Clinical Professor
Department of Obstetrics & Gynecology
David Geffen School of Medicine at UCLA
UCLA Olive View Medical Center
Sylmar, California

Mark D. Pearlman, MD [9, 22, 29]
S. Jan Behrman Professor and Vice Chair
Department of Obstetrics & Gynecology
Professor, Department of Surgery
Associate Chief of Staff
University of Michigan Health System
Ann Arbor, Michigan

Diana O. Perkins, MD, MPH [19]
Associate Professor
Department of Psychiatry
University of North Carolina at Chapel Hill
Chapel Hill, North Carolina

Carl L. Pierson, PhD [App. 2]
Assistant Professor of Pathology
Director, Clinical Microbiology/Virology Laboratories
University of Michigan Health System
Ann Arbor, Michigan

Elisabeth H. Quint, MD [24]
Clinical Associate Professor
Department of Obstetrics & Gynecology
University of Michigan Health System
Ann Arbor, Michigan

Khurram Rehman, MD [10]
Fellow in Reproductive Endocrinology
Department of Obstetrics & Gynecology
University of Texas
Southwestern Medical Center
Dallas, Texas

David S. Rosen, MD, MPH [23]
Chief, Section of Teenage and Young Adult Health
Clinical Associate Professor
Department of Pediatrics
University of Michigan Health System
Ann Arbor, Michigan

William A. Rutala, PhD, MPH [17]
Professor of Medicine
Director of Hospital Epidemiology and Occupational Health
University of North Carolina at Chapel Hill
Chapel Hill, North Carolina

Carolyn Sachs, MD [33]
Assistant Professor of Medicine
UCLA Emergency Medicine Center
David Geffen School of Medicine at UCLA
Los Angeles, California

Eric Savitsky, MD [11]
Associate Professor of Medicine
UCLA Emergency Medicine Center
David Geffen School of Medicine at UCLA
Los Angeles, California

Monica Sifuentes, MD [24]
Associate Professor and Program Director and Vice Chair of Education
Department of Pediatrics
Harbor-UCLA Medical Center
David Geffen School of Medicine at UCLA
Torrance, California

Jack D. Sobel, MD [31]
Professor of Medicine
Chief, Division of Infectious Diseases
Wayne State University and Harper Hospital
Detroit, Michigan

Shannon Sovndal, MD [20]
Resident
Department of Emergency Medicine
Stanford University, Medical Center
Stanford, California

Phillip G. Stubblefield, MD [6]
Professor and Chair
Department of Obstetrics & Gynecology
Boston University School of Medicine
Director of Obstetrics & Gynecology
Boston Medical Center
Boston, Massachusetts

Jeffrey Tabas, MD [20]
Assistant Clinical Professor of Medicine
Department of Emergency Services
San Francisco General Hospital
San Francisco, California

Brian R. Tiffany, MD, PhD [36]
Chairman
Department of Emergency Medicine
Maricopa Medical Center
Phoenix, Arizona

Judith E. Tintinalli, MD, MS [28]
Professor and Chairman
Steven J. Dresnick, MD Distinguished Professor and Chair in Emergency Medicine
Department of Emergency Medicine
University of North Carolina at Chapel Hill
Chapel Hill, North Carolina

Marc R. Toglia, MD [12]
Assistant Clinical Professor
Department of Obstetrics & Gynecology
Thomas Jefferson School of Medicine
Riddle Memorial Hospital
Media, Pennsylvania

Bradley Vaughn, MD [18]
Associate Professor
Department of Neurology
University of North Carolina at Chapel Hill
Chapel Hill, North Carolina

David J. Weber, MD, MPH [17]
Professor of Medicine, Pediatrics, and Epidemiology
Medical Director of Hospital Epidemiology and Occupational Health
University of North Carolina Health Care Systems
Chapel Hill, North Carolina

Jeannette Wolfe, MD [16]
Assistant Professor
Department of Emergency Medicine
Baystate Medical Center
Tufts University School of Medicine
Springfield, Massachusetts

Daphne Wong, MD [25]
Assistant Clinical Professor
Department of Pediatrics
David Geffen School of Medicine at UCLA
Mattel Children's Hospital
Los Angeles, California

Janet Simmons Young, MD [26]
Assistant Professor
Department of Emergency Medicine
University of North Carolina at Chapel Hill
Chapel Hill, North Carolina

PREFACE

THE PURPOSE OF THIS BOOK is to provide information necessary for emergency gynecologic and obstetric care of women and children. The focus is on emergency conditions in which diagnosis and treatment are specifically gender-based. Emergency conditions of pregnancy are stressed because they have the potential for high morbidity and mortality for mother and/or fetus and because of the unique anatomic and physiologic changes that influence diagnosis and management.

The intended reader is the emergency and acute care provider. The emphasis is on the provision of care in the emergency department, urgent care clinic, or rural setting where there is limited emergency availability of obstetric and gynecologic consultation.

The book is divided into sections:

1. Problems of pregnancy (Sections II to V)
2. Pediatric and adolescent gynecology (Section VI)
3. Problems of the reproductive age and older women

Appendices are provided for areas that need frequent referencing, and include tables of radiation dosage, guidelines for treating common dermatologic problems associated with pregnancy and key information on the collection and transport of common microbiologic specimens from women.

Providing emergency gynecologic and obstetric care requires a knowledge of gynecologic anatomy, an understanding of the most important physiologic and pathologic gynecologic and obstetric processes, differences in presentation and frequency of certain diseases in women, and an appreciation of comorbidities and socioeconomic considerations that affect pregnancy and gynecologic disorders. These points are covered in the text.

There are some common practice patterns should be emphasized in the emergency care of women:

1. *All women of childbearing age are presumed pregnant until demonstrated otherwise*. In general, this includes postpubertal women up to the age of 50 who have not had oophorectomy or hysterectomy. The potential for pregnancy affects diagnostic evaluation (e.g., radiographs, causes of lower abdominal pain and changes in normal values of common laboratory tests) and treatment (e.g., avoidance of drugs that have potential to harm the fetus). Medical conditions that were formerly thought to be incompatible with pregnancy can be associated with unexpected pregnancy and can be managed with successful outcomes. These conditions include disorders such as sickle cell anemia, cancer after chemotherapy treatment, end-stage renal failure, organ transplantation, and cystic fibrosis.
2. *The evaluation of lower abdominal pain in women requires pelvic examination and should be complemented by pelvic ultrasonography and abdominopelvic CT scanning when clinically appropriate*. The pelvic examination is neither sensitive nor specific for many disease processes, and reliability is affected by pain and body habitus. Consequently, ultrasonography and CT scanning have become increasingly important in the evaluation of lower abdominal pain in women, and are often necessary to establish a definitive diagnosis in the emergency department. At the same time, only an appropriately performed pelvic examination can detect pelvic tenderness, visualize abnormal lesions, discharge or ulcerations, and can guide the decision making for the need for additional pelvic imaging.
3. *Documentation of gynecologic and obstetric review of systems (ROS) and family history is necessary* for women with emergency conditions, so the potential effects of gynecologic and obstetric comorbidities on the patient's chief complaint can be assessed. For example, the diagnostic concerns in a woman with abdominal pain become more focused if a maternal history of ovarian carcinoma is elicited. Understanding past gynecologic surgery is important in the assessment of potential pregnancy or pregnancy complications as a cause of acute abdominal pain. Patients who are pregnant as a result of in vitro fertilization have comorbidities for complications that are different from those of women with spontaneous pregnancy.
4. When treating pregnant women for acute medical conditions, *fetal heart tones should be documented* by

ultrasound or by Doppler stethoscope, and recorded as part of the maternal vital signs on the ED record. While the best maternal treatment will provide the best fetal treatment, it is important to ensure fetal well-being during maternal treatment.

5. *Women with a potentially viable fetus (generally over 22 weeks' gestation) who have experienced direct or indirect blunt abdominal trauma require fetal monitoring (cardiotocodynamometry) as soon as possible after ED presentation* in order to identify patients at risk for placental abruption. Coordinating management with an obstetrician is important to allow appropriate interpretation of fetal monitoring and allow for emergency delivery if necessary.
6. *Domestic violence should be considered* when women present with isolated facial injuries, with unexplained assault especially during pregnancy, with implausible explanations for injury, or for failure to obtain timely emergency care or follow-up treatment. Physicians and nurses should be trained in the principles of screening for domestic violence, and should have a system for providing on-site and follow-up counseling. A mechanism for providing safe shelter for the mother and her children should also be available.

SECTION I

GENERAL PRINCIPLES

1

Functional Gynecologic Anatomy

John O.L. DeLancey

KEY POINTS

- Bartholin's Duct abscess points toward the normal duct orifice at 5 and 7 o'clock positions. More lateral drainage will be bloodier and/or deeper.
- In blunt traumatic injuries to the vulva, blood can track up the anterior abdominal wall. Bleeding from the vestibular bulb or clitoris can be massive and requires direct compression and emergent surgical repair.
- Piriformis or obturator internus muscle strain should be considered in the differential diagnosis of pelvic pain. Diagnosis is made by reproducing the pain with direct muscle palpation and thigh abduction with lateral rotation.

INTRODUCTION

This chapter reviews the gross anatomy of the vulva, vagina, perineum, uterus, and adnexae. Anatomic principles are important for clinicians to keep in mind in order to properly consider or exclude disease states. Interestingly, pelvic anatomy is generally described as if it were static in location, however there is individual variation based upon body habitus, age, and physiology. For example, in women of child-bearing age, a full bladder will displace the uterine fundal tip about 2 cm superiorly and .25 cm posteriorly, and the ovaries about 2 cm superiorly and .32 cm anteriorly.[1] Thus, the clinician must recognize these individual variations for proper diagnosis and treatment.

SUBCUTANEOUS TISSUES OF THE VULVA

The structures of the vulva lie on the pubic bones and extend caudally under their arch (Fig. 1-1). They consist of the mons, labia, clitoris, vestibule of the vagina, and associated erectile structures and their muscles. The mons comprises hair-bearing skin over a cushion of adipose tissue that lies on the pubic bones. Extending posteriorly from the mons, the labia majora are composed of similar hair-bearing skin and adipose tissue, which contains the termination of the round ligaments of the uterus and the obliterated processus vaginalis (canal of Nuck). The round ligament may give rise to leiomyomas in this region; the obliterated processus vaginalis can be a dilated embryonic remnant in the adult.

Between the two labia majora, the labia minora, vestibule, and glans clitoris can be seen. The labia minora are hairless skin folds, each of which splits anteriorly to run over and under the glans of the clitoris. The more anterior folds unite to form the hood-shaped prepuce of the clitoris, while the posterior folds insert into the underside of the glans as the frenulum. Preclitoral abscess often arises from an infection beginning under the hood of the clitoris and presents as a fluctuant mass over the glans. The best anatomic point to drain it is in the cleft between the hood and the glans. Incising the hood in the midline carries the risk of permanently exposing the sensitive glans; therefore opening along the normal cleavage plane is preferred.

In the posterior lateral aspect of the vestibule, the duct of the major vestibular gland (Bartholin) can be seen 3 to 4 mm outside the hymenal ring (Fig. 1-1). Abscess arising in the duct of Bartholin's gland is common and presents frequently in the emergency department. The duct abscess points toward the normal duct orifice posteriorly and laterally in the vestibule, lying at the 5 or 7 o'clock position. More lateral drainage will involve a deeper and bloodier dissection, and posterior drainage, if too deep, can injure the rectum.

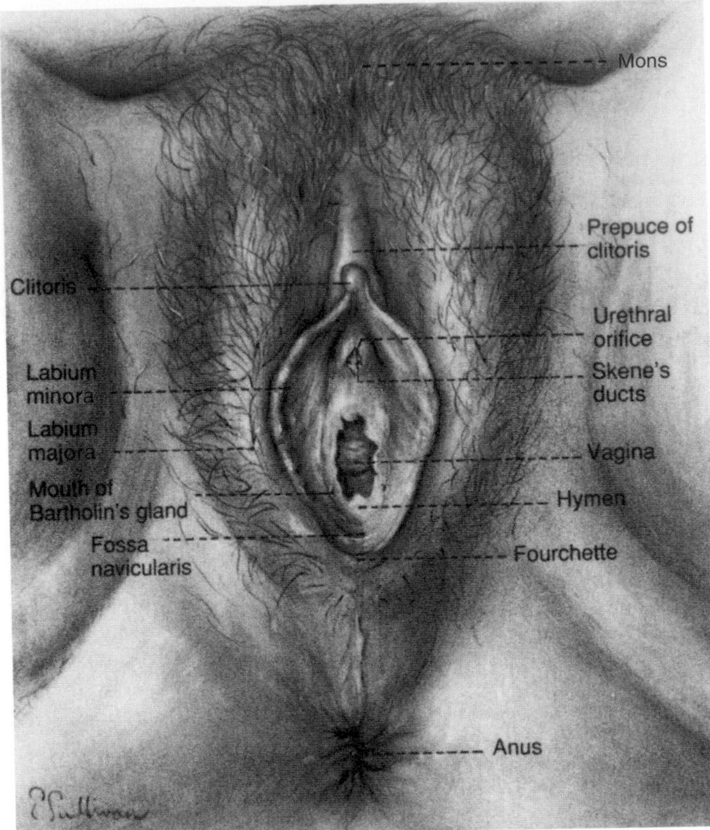

Fig. 1-1. External genitalia. (From Rock JA, Thompson JD (eds): *TeLinde's Operative Gynecology,* 8th ed. Philadelphia: Lippincott-Raven, 1997, with permission.)

The minor vestibular gland (Skene) openings are found along a line extending anteriorly from the site of Bartholin duct, parallel to the hymenal ring and extending toward the urethral orifice. The urethra protrudes slightly through the vestibular skin anterior to the vagina and posterior to the clitoris. Its orifice is flanked on either side by two small labia. Skene ducts open into the inner aspect of these labia and can be cystically dilated in some women; such a duct will present as a fluid-filled mass lateral to the external urethral meatus, usually deviating the external urinary orifice to the side opposite the cyst. These cysts usually do not require drainage unless they are large or symptomatic. These glands can be involved in gonococcal infections and therapy with antibiotics is curative.

Within the skin of the vulva are specialized glands that can become enlarged and thereby require surgical removal. The holocrine sebaceous glands in the labia majora are associated with hair shafts; in the labia minora they are freestanding. They lie close to the surface, and this explains their easy recognition with minimal enlargement. In addition, lateral to the introitus and anus, there are high densities of apocrine sweat glands in addition to the normal eccrine sweat glands. The former structures undergo cyclic change with the menstrual cycle, having increased secretary activity in the premenstrual period. They can become chronically infected as hidradenitis suppurativa or neoplastically enlarged as hidradenomas. The eccrine sweat glands present in the vulvar skin rarely present abnormalities, but can form palpable masses as syringomas.

The hymenal ring lies at the junction of the introitus and vagina. There is tremendous variation in its development and configuration. (see Chapter 25).

Deeper within the vulvar tissues lies the clitoris, whose midline shaft and paired crura lie on the pubic symphysis and extend along the caudal margins of the inferior pubic rami. The paired vestibular bulbs lie beneath the vestibular skin on either side of the introitus and are made up of erectile tissue. The ischiocavernosus muscles cover the crura of the clitoris, while the bulbocavernosus muscles lie on the vestibular bulbs (Fig. 1-2). There are a few muscle

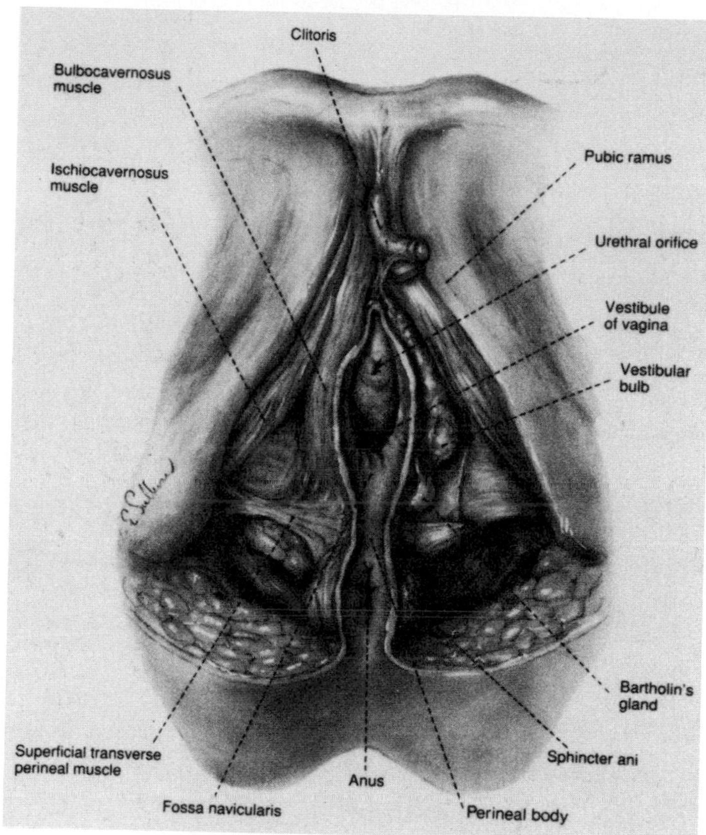

Fig. 1-2. Deep structures within the vulva. (From Rock JA, Thompson JD (eds): *TeLinde's Operative Gynecology,* 8th ed. Philadelphia: Lippincott-Raven, 1997, with permission.)

fibers that originate in common with the ischiocavernosus muscles from the ischial tuberosity and run medially to the perineal body. These are called the superficial transverse perineal muscles. The paired vestibular bulbs lie immediately under the vestibular skin and are composed of erectile tissue. They are covered by the bulbocavernosus muscles, which originate in the perineal body and lie over their lateral surfaces. These muscles, along with the ischiocavernosus muscles, insert into the body of the clitoris and act to pull it downward. In a woman with suspected neurologic damage to the caudal nerves, watching to see if the clitoris is pulled downward during contraction and assessment of its motion following stroking of the perineal skin (the bulbocavernosus reflex) can help test the integrity of the sacral roots.

Traumatic injury to the vulva is common. Straddle injuries occur when a fall brings the vulva into contact with a bike bar or fence rail, tearing the skin over the pubic rami, lacerating the deeper structures, or causing a hematoma to form. Blood collections in the superficial space tend to track anteriorly onto the abdominal wall and are limited by the peripheral attachments of Colles fascia.[2] This subcutaneous fascia has a lateral attachment to the ischiopubic rami and dorsal attachment to the posterior edge of the perineal membrane (or urogenital diaphragm), so that blood in the deep subcutaneous space cannot track beyond these attachments. The open ventral margin, however, allows blood to track into the subcutaneous tissues of the abdominal wall (Fig. 1-3). Trauma to the erectile tissue of the vestibular bulb or clitoris can result in massive bleeding from these erectile bodies and requires immediate direct compression followed by urgent surgical repair.

PUDENDAL NERVE AND VESSELS

The pudendal nerve is the sensory and motor nerve of the perineum. Its course and distribution in the perineum parallel the pudendal artery and veins, which connect with the internal iliac vessels (Fig. 1-4). The nerve arises from the sacral plexus (S2-S4) and the vessels originate from the anterior division of the internal iliac artery.

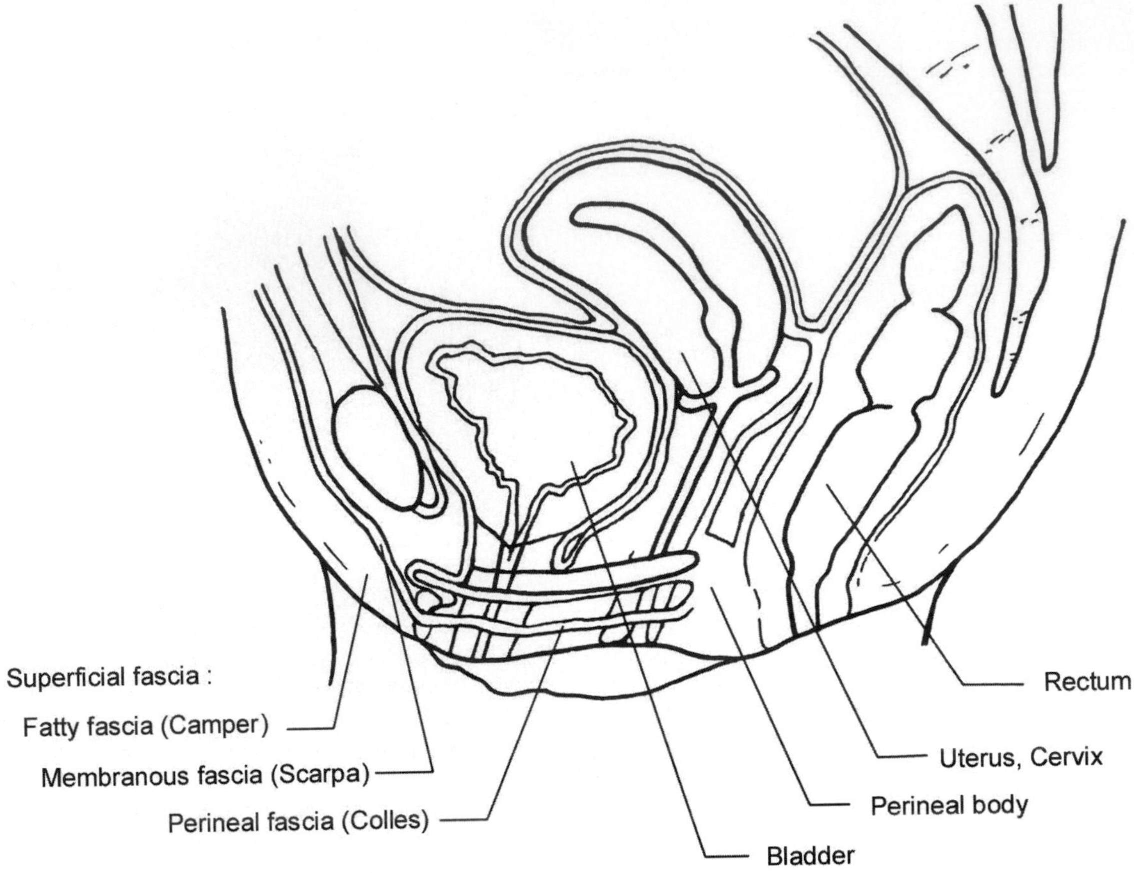

Superficial fascia :
Fatty fascia (Camper)
Membranous fascia (Scarpa)
Perineal fascia (Colles)
Rectum
Uterus, Cervix
Perineal body
Bladder

Fig. 1-3. Sagittal view of female pelvis demonstrating superficial and deep fascial layers.

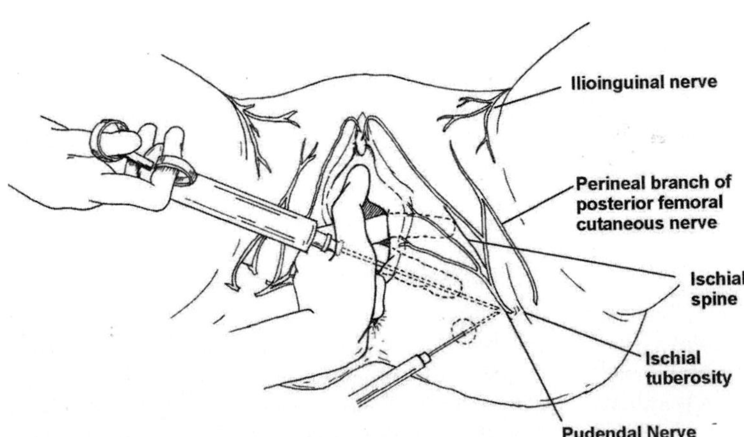

Fig. 1-4. Pudendal block.

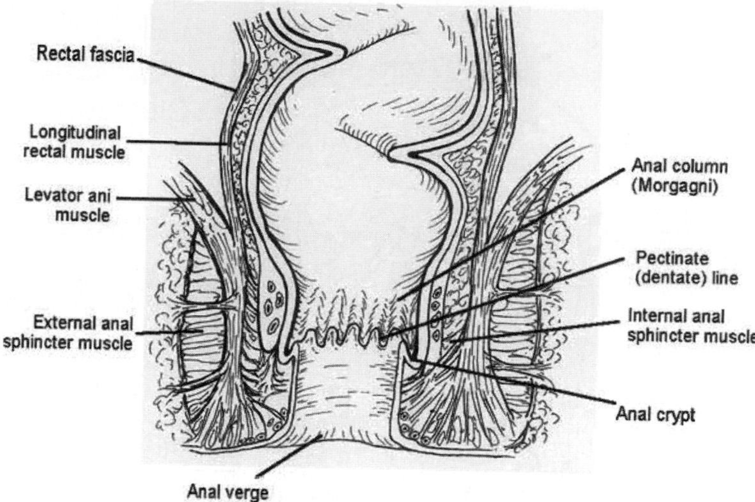

Fig. 1-5. External and internal anal sphincters.

There are three branches of the pudendal nerve and vessels: the clitoral, perineal, and inferior hemorrhoidal (rectal) branches. They supply the clitoris, the subcutaneous tissues of the vulva, and the bulbocavernosus, ischiocavernosus, and transverse perineal muscles. The pudendal nerve and vessels also supply the skin of the inner portions of the labia majora, the labia minora, and the vestibule. The inferior hemorrhoidal branch goes to the external anal sphincter and perianal skin. Pudendal nerve block performed by perforating the sacrospinous ligament at the tip of the ischial spine proves useful not only to decrease pain during vaginal birth, but also for local anesthesia during emergency procedures involving the perineal skin[3] (Fig. 1-4).

PERINEAL BODY AND ANAL SPHINCTERS

Within the area bounded by the lower posterior vaginal wall, the perineal skin, and the anus is a mass of connective tissue called the *perineal body*.[4] The term *central tendon* of the perineum has also been applied to this structure and is quite descriptive, suggesting its role as a central point into which a number of muscles insert.

The perineal body is attached to the inferior pubic rami and ischial tuberosities through the perineal membrane and superficial transverse perineal muscles. Anterolaterally, the perineal body receives the insertion of the bulbocavernosus muscles (Fig. 1-2). The upper portions of the perineal body, on its lateral margins, are connected with some of the fibers of the pelvic diaphragm. Posteriorly, the perineal body is attached to the coccyx by the external anal sphincter, which is embedded in the perineal body anteriorly and is attached at its other end to the coccyx. All of these connections anchor the perineal body and its surrounding structures to the bony pelvis and help keep it in place.

The external anal sphincter lies in the posterior triangle of the perineum. It has a teardrop shape with a point tethered on the coccyx dorsally and the loop extending between the rectum and vagina. The circular external orifice of the anal canal is attributed to a subcutaneous component that does encircle the anal canal, but the majority of the external sphincter is a loop that pulls dorsally on the anal canal.

The internal anal sphincter is a thickening in the circular muscle of the anal wall. It lies just inside the external anal sphincter and is separated from it by a visible intersphincteric groove. It can be identified just beneath the anal submucosa in repair of a chronic fourth-degree laceration of the perineum. The longitudinal rectus muscle of the bowel, along with some fibers of the levator ani, separate the external and internal sphincters (Fig. 1-5).

Lacerations of the perineal body occur frequently at the time of vaginal delivery, during some sexual assaults, or after perineal trauma. An anatomic reconstruction is needed to restore structural continuity and function to this important region. Gynecologic consultation is best for these repairs. The depth of a laceration should be explored to look for a separated anal sphincter muscle, which

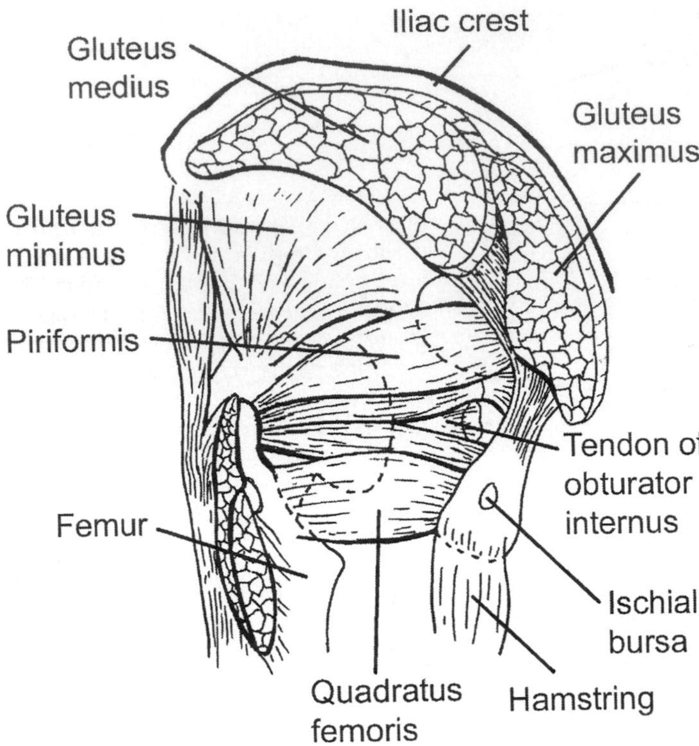

Fig. 1-6. Deep pelvic muscles.

is normally between the vaginal canal and anal canal, just below the perianal skin. If complete transection of the perineal body has occurred, so the anal canal is opened, the internal anal sphincter, which lies between the external sphincter and anal canal, must be repaired.

PELVIC MUSCLES

The obturator internus arises from the inner surface of the obturator foramen and membrane and leaves the pelvis through the lesser sciatic foramen to insert into the medial surface of the greater trochanter (Fig. 1-6). The piriformis takes its origin from the anterior aspect of the sacrum and passes through the greater sciatic foramen to insert into the upper border of the greater trochanter. A muscle strain in either of these muscles can lead to discomfort in the pelvic area and may present to the emergency department as low abdominal, hip, or pelvic pain. Palpating the tender muscle anterolaterally just cephalad to the inferior pubic ramus in the case of the obturator internus, and posterior and superior to the ischial spine and sacrospinous ligament in the case of the piriformis muscle, assists in making this diagnosis. Both of these pelvic wall muscles are lateral rotators and abductors of the thigh, and maneuvers that stretch them may reproduce the pain and confirm the nature of the problem. This muscle pain can pose a diagnostic dilemma when focus is placed on searching for a visceral cause of pelvic pain. Simply entertaining this diagnosis, however, allows the clinician to make the diagnosis easily through reproducing the patient's complaint by palpating the tender muscle.

The opening between the bones and muscles of the pelvic wall is spanned by the muscles of the pelvic diaphragm: the pubococcygeus, the iliococcygeus, the puborectalis, and the coccygeus muscles. The most medial of these muscles is the puborectalis-pubococcygeus complex. The pubococcygeus portion of these muscles has an insertion into the anococcygeal raphe and the superior surface of the coccyx, while the puborectalis represents those inferior fibers that pass behind and also insert into the rectum. Some women develop pain in these muscles from recent vigorous use of Kegel exercises in much the same way that someone beginning a program of running may have sore legs. This can lead a woman to seek care for dyspareunia.[5]

Table 1-1. Vaginal Lacerations and Associated Anatomic Considerations

Location	Consideration
Anterior upper vagina	Bladder, urethral, ureteral injury
Posterior upper vagina	Intraperitoneal or bowel injury
Posterior lower vagina	Rectal injury
Lateral vagina, cervix, or uterine wall	Profuse bleeding

PELVIC ORGANS

Vagina

The vagina is a pliable hollow viscus whose shape is determined by the structures surrounding it and by its attachments to the pelvic wall. These attachments are to the lateral margins of the vagina, so that its lumen is a transverse slit, with the anterior and posterior walls in contact with one another. The lower portion of the vagina is constricted as it passes through the urogenital hiatus in the levator ani. The upper vagina is more capacious. The cervix lies within the anterior vaginal wall, making the vagina shorter anteriorly than posteriorly by approximately 3 cm, with the former being 7 to 9 cm in length. There is, however, great variability in this dimension. The bladder and urethra lie in contact with the anterior vaginal wall, making them accessible to palpation during pelvic examination, while the rectum lies posteriorly and can also be felt through the vaginal wall.

Deep lacerations of the vaginal canal can involve the structures adjacent to the vaginal canal (Table 1-1). In the upper vagina anteriorly, both the bladder and the ureters lie immediately adjacent to the vagina and may be injured along with the vagina (Fig. 1-7). In instances in which

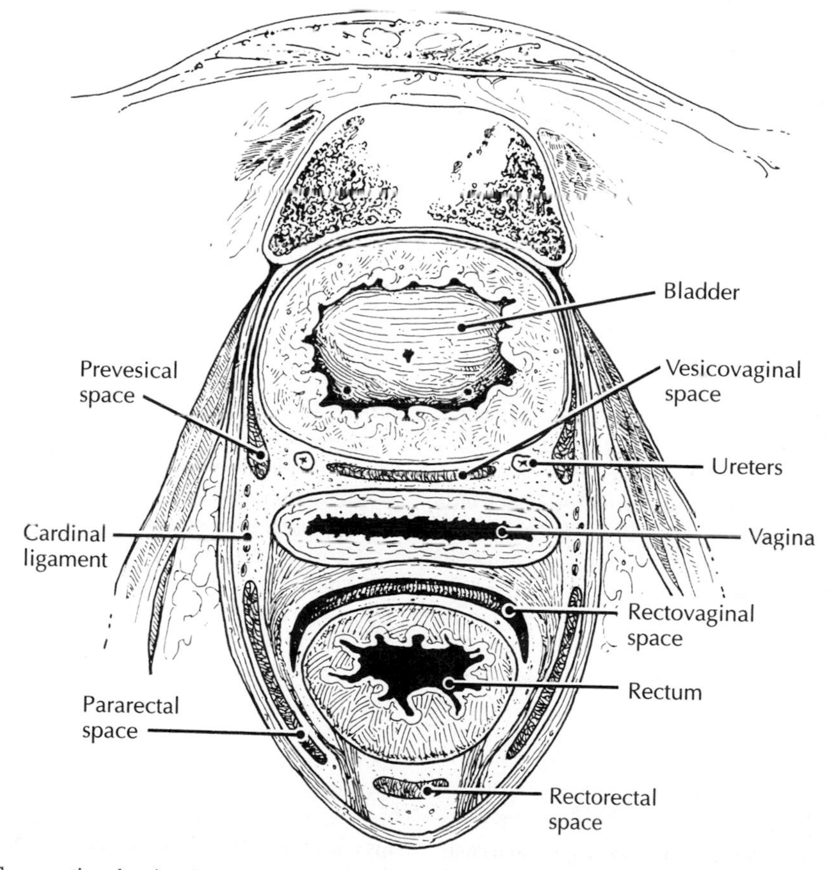

Fig. 1-7. Cross section showing the ureters adjacent to the vagina. (© John O.L. DeLancey and McGraw-Hill, 1996.)

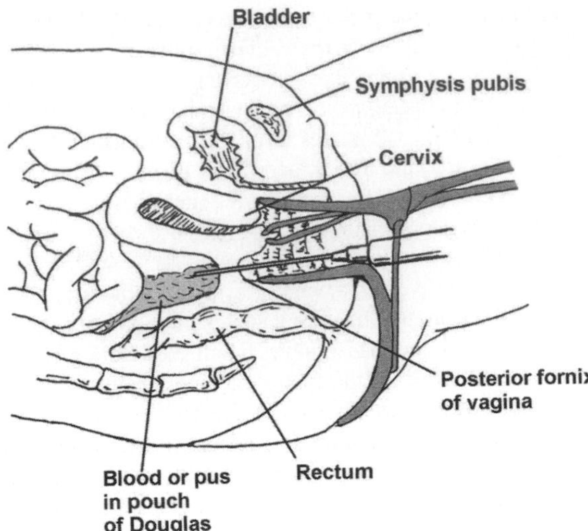

Fig. 1-8. Culdocentesis. Needle entering pouch of Douglas.

there is a deep laceration in the upper vagina, care should be taken to inspect this area to make sure that no injury to the bladder or ureters has occurred. Instillation of a dilute methylene blue solution into the bladder allows recognition of bladder injury when this contrast material is seen in the vagina. Ureteral injury is somewhat more difficult to detect. Visualization of clear fluid coming from the wound in the absence of a bladder laceration implies a ureteral injury, but intravenous pyelography or cystoscopy with retrograde contrast injection would be needed to confirm this. Near the introitus, the urethra causes a bulge in the anterior vaginal wall. Masses present in this area may represent a urethral diverticulum that can be infected, can carry a stone, or may simply be an asymptomatic finding.

The posterior vaginal wall has different anatomic relationships in its upper and lower portions. The upper vagina lies adjacent to the cul de sac of Douglas for the 4 cm below the vaginal-cervical junction (Fig. 1-8). This anatomic relationship allows a needle to be placed transvaginally into the cul de sac (culdocentesis). In women with an upper vaginal laceration, consideration must be given to intestinal injury. The lower portion of the vagina lies immediately adjacent to the rectum. Rectal damage can be assessed simply with a rectal examination, and this should be performed whenever a laceration involves the posterior vaginal wall.

UTERUS: CORPUS AND CERVIX

The uterus is a fibromuscular organ whose shape, weight, and dimensions vary considerably depending on both estrogenic stimulation and previous parturition. It has two portions, an upper muscular corpus and lower fibrous cervix. In the reproductive age woman, the corpus is considerably larger than the cervix; but before menarche and after the menopause, the corpus and cervix are relatively similar in size. Within the corpus there is a triangular-shaped endometrial cavity surrounded by a thick muscular wall. That portion of the corpus which extends above the top of the endometrial cavity (i.e., above the insertions of the fallopian tubes) is called the *uterine fundus.*

The uterus is lined by a unique mucosa, the *endometrium.* It has both a columnar epithelium, which forms glands, and a specialized stroma. The superficial portion of this layer undergoes cyclic change with the menstrual cycle. Spasm of hormonally-sensitive spiral arterioles lying within the endometrium causes shedding of this layer at the end of each cycle, but a deeper basal layer of the endometrium remains to regenerate a new lining. Separate arteries supply the basal endometrium, explaining its preservation at the time of menses (see Chapter 27).

The cervix is divided into two portions: the portio vaginalis, which is that part protruding into the vagina, and the portio supravaginalis, which lies above the vagina and below the corpus. The upper border of the cervical canal is marked by the internal os, where the narrow cervical canal widens out into the endometrial cavity. The cervix contains numerous gland clefts. When the orifice of one of these clefts becomes occluded, cystic dilatation occurs, resulting in the common *nabothian cyst.* These cysts can be small and numerous or single and large. Collections of large numbers of these cysts can substantially enlarge the cervix and give it a hard, firm consistency. Confirmation that this was caused by cystic dilatation can be

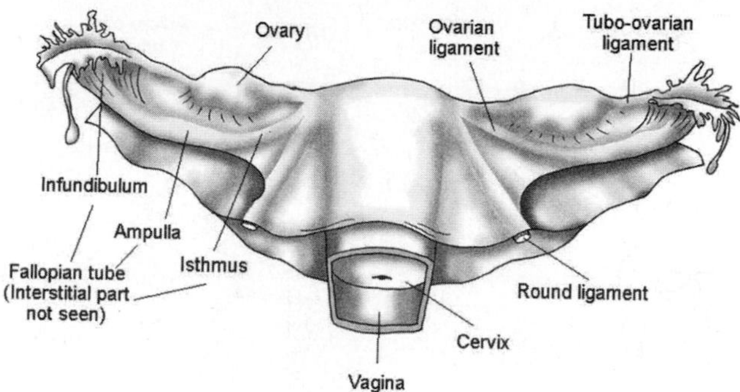

Fig. 1-9. Uterus and adnexae.

made by aspirating one of the cysts with an 18-gauge needle. Return of thick mucus confirms that the enlargement is caused by nabothian cysts. These cysts are rarely if ever the cause of any discomfort and are an incidental finding.

The cervix changes its appearance substantially during pregnancy. It becomes cyanotic and swollen. The bright red glandular tissue of the endocervical canal pushes downward and outward so that it becomes visible at the external orifice of the cervix. This is a normal physiologic ectropion associated with pregnancy. It is also often seen with oral contraceptive use. Unlike cervical cancer, which usually produces a firm and scirrhous distortion of the cervix, this is smooth and soft. If there is concern about cervical cancer, biopsy of the lesion is indicated.

ADNEXAL STRUCTURES AND BROAD LIGAMENT

The fallopian tubes are paired tubular structures 7 to 12 cm in length. Each has four recognizable portions (Fig. 1-9). At the uterus, the tube passes through the corpus as an interstitial portion. Upon emerging from the corpus, a narrow isthmic portion begins with a narrow lumen and thick muscular wall. Proceeding toward the abdominal end, next is the ampulla, which has an expanding lumen and more convoluted mucosa. The fimbriated end of the tube has a great number of frond-like projections to provide a wide surface for ovum pickup. The distal end of the fallopian tube is attached to the ovary by the fimbria ovarica, which is a smooth muscle band responsible for bringing the fimbria and ovary close to one another at the time of ovulation. The outer layer of the tube's muscularis is composed of longitudinal fibers; the inner layer has a circular orientation. Ectopic pregnancy occurs most frequently in the fallopian tube. Because of the varying distensibility of the tube, depending on its varying diameter, there are great variations in the time when tubal pregnancy presents.

The lateral pole of the ovary is attached to the pelvic wall by the infundibulopelvic ligament and the ovarian artery and vein contained therein. Medially it is connected to the uterus through the uteroovarian ligament. During reproductive life, it measures approximately 3 to 5 cm long, 1.5 to 3 cm in thickness, and 0.6 to 1 cm in width, varying with its state of activity or suppression, as with oral contraceptive medications. Functional cysts of the ovary are common and present either as incidental findings on pelvic examination or may cause pain resulting in a visit to the emergency department. The differential diagnosis of adnexal enlargement includes a large hemorrhagic corpus cyst, ovarian torsion, or malignancy.

The round ligaments are extensions of the uterine musculature and represent the homologue of the gubernaculum testis. They begin as broad bands arising on each lateral aspect of the anterior corpus. Pain from muscular spasm in these structures presents as abdominal pain during pregnancy, is usually associated with movement, and is usually not associated with other abdominal symptoms.

BLOOD SUPPLY AND LYMPHATICS OF THE GENITAL TRACT

The blood supply to the genital organs comes from the ovarian arteries and the uterine and vaginal branches of the internal iliac artery (Fig. 1-10).[6] A continuous arterial arcade connects these vessels on the lateral border of the adnexa, uterus, and vagina. The blood supply of the upper adnexal structures comes from the ovarian arteries, which arise from the anterior surface of the aorta just below the level of the renal arteries. The accompanying plexus of veins drains into the vena cava on the right and the renal vein on the left.

The uterine artery originates from the internal iliac artery. It usually arises independently from this source but may have a common origin with either the internal pudendal or vaginal artery. It joins the uterus at approx-

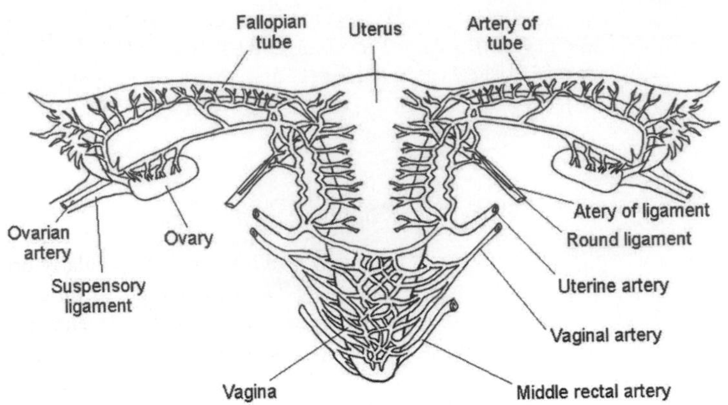

Fig. 1-10. Arterial supply of vagina, uterus, and adnexae.

imately the junction of the corpus and cervix, but this position varies considerably both with the individual and also with the amount of upward or downward traction on the uterus. Accompanying each uterine artery are several large uterine veins that drain the corpus and cervix.

Upon arriving at the lateral border of the uterus (after passing over the ureter and giving off a small branch to this structure), the uterine artery flows into the side of the marginal artery that runs along the side of the uterus. Through this connection it sends blood both upward toward the corpus and downward to the cervix. As the marginal artery continues along the lateral aspect of the cervix, it eventually crosses over the cervicovaginal junction and lies on the side of the vagina.

The vagina receives its blood supply from a downward extension of the uterine artery along the lateral sulci of the vagina and from a vaginal branch of the internal iliac artery. These form an anastomotic arcade along the lateral aspect of the vagina at 3 and 9 o'clock. There are also branches from these vessels that merge along the anterior and posterior vaginal walls. The distal vagina also receives supply from the pudendal vessels, and the posterior wall has a contribution from the middle and inferior hemorrhoidal vessels.

In women presenting to an emergency department after hysterectomy with profuse vaginal bleeding, the source of the bleeding is usually along the lateral margin of the vagina at the vaginal cuff. Lacerations of the lateral portion of the uterus, cervix, and upper vagina cause the most dramatic bleeding. Therefore, in lacerations within this area, the lateral aspect should be searched first for the site of the bleeding vessel. During termination of pregnancy, a lateral laceration of the uterus can cause profound bleeding. This may well be retroperitoneal and not disclosed through the cervix or uterus. Therefore, a woman with a relatively small amount of bleeding who has systemic evidence of more profound blood loss should be evaluated to determine whether blood has accumulated in the retroperitoneal space beside the uterus (see Chapter 6).

The uterus receives its nerve supply from the uterovaginal plexus (Frankenhausers ganglion), which lies in the connective tissue of the cardinal ligament, and through nerves accompanying the ovarian blood vessels. The uterovaginal plexus connects to the central nervous system through the hypogastric nerves and hypogastric plexis. Injection of local anesthetic agents through the lateral vaginal fornix blocks conduction of pain through this region and greatly reduces the discomfort of cervical dilation. It does not, however, blunt perception of pain from the uterine corpus.

REFERENCES

1. Nicholson R, Coucher J, Thornton A, et al: Effect of a full and empty bladder on radiation dose to the uterus, ovaries, and bladder from lumbar spine CT and x-ray examinations. *Br J Radiology* 73(876):1290–6, 2000 Dec.
2. Tobin CE, Benjamin JA: Anatomic and clinical reevaluation of Camper's, Scarpa's and Colles' fasciae. *Surg Gynecol Obstet* 88:545, 1949.
3. Klink EW: Perineal nerve block: An anatomic and clinical study in the female. *Obstet Gynecol* 1:137, 1953.
4. Oh C, Kark E: Anatomy of the perineal body. *Dis Colon Rectum* 16:444, 1973.
5. DeLancey JOL, Sampselle CM, Punch MR: Kegel dyspareunia: Levator ani myalgia caused by overexertion. *Obstet Gynecol* 82:658, 1993.
6. Roberts WH, Krishingner GL: Comparative study of human internal iliac artery based on Adachi classification. *Anat Rec* 158:191, 1967.

2

Critical Physiologic Alterations in Pregnancy

Mel L. Barclay

KEY POINTS

Important Parameters in Pregnancy

- Uterine size and gestation
  - Pelvic brim — 10 weeks
  - Halfway between pubic symphysis and umbilicus — 16 weeks
  - Xiphoid — 38 weeks
- Detection of cardiac activity
  - Transvaginal Ultrasonography — 6 weeks
  - Doppler stethoscope or Abdominal ultrasonography — 10 weeks
  - Fetoscope — 20 weeks
- Left lateral decubitus position
  - In the second half of pregnancy, left lateral decubitus position or manual uterine deflection to the left avoids inferior vena cava compression and maintains cardiac output and blood pressure.
- Fetal Cardiac Activity
  - 6 weeks ultrasonography detects cardiac activity
  - 10 weeks Doppler stethoscope
  - 20 weeks Delee stethoscope

As a result of its special physiologic impact on the mother, pregnancy often alters the presentation of a number of disease processes. Elements of physiology that are normal for pregnancy may easily be mistaken for pathophysiology. On the other hand, the appearance of true pathophysiology may be altered or masked by pregnancy in ways that complicate or delay diagnosis and treatment.

There are three major types of physiologic alterations that occur in pregnancy: (1) increasing levels of circulating steroids, especially progesterone; (2) increased metabolic activity; and (3) increased perfusion requirements of the placental and uterine circulation, causing a hyperdynamic state. These three types of changes help explain how individual body systems are altered in pregnancy.

PROGESTERONE

Levels of circulating steroid hormones, particularly progesterone, are greatly increased and produce a variety of clinical changes. Produced mainly by the placenta, progesterone and its metabolic by-products are increased to levels that are more than 20 times normal in the serum of pregnant women.[1]

Progesterone has many effects, but effects on smooth muscle are most important. Progesterone hyperpolarizes the cell membranes of smooth muscle, thereby increasing the amount of energy necessary to cause depolarization and the subsequent contraction of the smooth muscle fibers.[2–5] The ultimate effect is smooth muscle relaxation. This effect has implications for all of the homeostatic mechanisms that depend on the action of smooth muscle for maintenance of the internal milieu. From the uterus, which must be conditioned to contain the rapidly-growing fetus, to the most distal peripheral arteriole, the impact of progesterone is at least partly responsible for the many changes in the homeostatic mechanisms observed in the pregnant woman.

Changes in the responsiveness of the vascular tree to various stressors, decreased peripheral resistance, and changes in circulatory dynamics are due to the relaxing effects of progesterone on smooth muscle. Changes in gastrointestinal motility, compliance of the bronchial tree, and the changes in the urinary collecting system are also attributable, at least in part, to the effects of circulating serum progesterone. These changes are listed in Table 2-1.

METABOLISM AND HEAT PRODUCTION

The metabolic activity of the fetus and placenta heats the maternal internal milieu. During the course of gestation, there is a net flow of heat energy from the fetus and placenta to the mother.[6–8] In providing a place for growth and sustenance of the intrauterine fetus and placenta, the pregnant woman houses within her a rapidly metabolizing and heat-producing organism. The total energy output for an average-sized pregnant woman at 36 weeks' gestation is approximately 97.72±2.81 W (8443±243 kJ/d).

Table 2-1. Impact of Smooth Muscle Relaxation on Various Systems in Pregnancy

Cardiovascular
- ↓ Mean arterial pressure
- ↑ Venous capacitance
- ↓ Vascular response to postural change
- ↓ Peripheral resistance

Genitourinary
- ↓ Uterine contractile activity
- ↑ Ureteral dilatation
- ↑ Renal collecting system volume

Gastrointestinal
- ↑ Gastric emptying time
- ↓ Bowel motility
- ↑ Gallbladder emptying time
- ↑ Gastroesophageal reflux

Respiratory
- ↑ Inspiratory capacity

A similarly-sized, nonlactating and nonpregnant woman has an energy output of approximately 80.68±1.99 W (6971±172 kJ/day),[9] about 17 percent less.

Homeothermic mammals function within an exceptionally narrow range of temperatures as compared with poikilothermic animals. Being temperature-dependent, the normal function of enzyme systems and the most basic elements of cellular homeostasis require very stable thermal limits. The narrow tolerances of temperature variation permitted in this area of mammalian physiology sometimes necessitate profound adjustments in homeostatic mechanisms to maintain the constancy of internal temperature.[10] Many of the physiologic adjustments observed in the pregnant state bear a close resemblance to those observed in the heat-adapted homeothermic mammal. Changes observed in heat-adapted humans—such as increased plasma volume, heart rate, respiratory rate, and tidal volume—are similar to physiologic alterations commonly seen in pregnancy. The impressive decrease in peripheral circulatory resistance in pregnancy, manifest as warm skin and fingertips, results from the increased blood flow to the extremities and skin, which is an important aspect of pregnancy physiology.[11]

HYPERDYNAMIC VASCULAR STATE

Burwell and colleagues suggested that much of what appears to be maternal adaptation in pregnancy could be the result of alterations in maternal circulatory dynamics in response to the large-scale perfusion requirements of the placental and uterine circulation.[12] In the third trimester in particular, the placental and uterine circulation increases substantially.

Placental and uterine circulation varies linearly with fetal size during the course of gestation. At term, the typical flow rate in normal pregnancy is 600 to 800 mL/min. This amounts to approximately 15 to 20 mL/100 g of fe-

Table 2-2. Important Central Hemodynamic Alterations in Pregnancy[a]

Parameter	Nonpregnant	Pregnant	Units
Cardiac output	4.3±0.9	6.2±1.0	L/min
Heart rate	71±10.0	83±10.0	beats/min
Systemic vascular resistance	1530±520	1210±266	dyn·s·cm^{-5}
Pulmonary vascular resistance	119±47.0	78±22.0	dyn·s·cm^{-5}
Colloid oncotic pressure	20.8±1.0	10.5±2.7	mmHg
Mean arterial pressure	86.4±7.5	90.3±5.8	mmHg
Pulmonary capillary wedge pressure	6.3±2.1	7.5±1.8	mmHg
Left ventricular stroke work index	41±8	48±6	g·min·m^{-2}
Central venous pressure	3.7±2.6	3.6±2.5	mmHg

[a]Measurements between 36 and 38 weeks' gestation and 11 and 13 weeks postpartum in ten normal volunteers.

Source: Adapted from Clark et al,[38] with permission.

tal tissue per minute.[13,14] This level of flow is similar to the flow rates in antecubital arteriovenous (AV) fistulas constructed for purposes of extracorporeal circulation in renal dialysis.[15,16]

Many of the findings associated with AV fistulas of significant size are also seen in pregnancy. These include increased plasma volume, decreased peripheral resistance, increased cardiac output, decreased mean arterial pressure, and Branham's phenomenon (decreased pulse rate and increased blood pressure in response to closure of the fistula; see Table 2-2).

IMPORTANT ANATOMIC ALTERATIONS IN PREGNANCY THAT AFFECT DIAGNOSIS AND TREATMENT

Changes in maternal body habitus are among the most obvious alterations in the pregnant state. Some of these changes have significant impact on diagnosis and treatment. Uterine growth, the most obvious anatomic change in pregnancy, has important effects on the location of peritoneal contents. By altering the position and mobility of adjacent structures or by physically impinging on them, the enlarging pregnant uterus has important effects on the presentation of intraabdominal disease processes as well as on penetrating and blunt abdominal trauma. Women with multiple pregnancies have even greater uterine enlargement and may therefore experience even more profound compression-related physiologic alterations and even disability on the basis of uterine size alone.

During the course of normal gestation, the uterus grows from 50 grams to approximately 1200 grams and the fetus from a few grams to 3 to 4 kilograms. Growth of the uterine fundus is approximately linear in the first trimester. Beginning at 20 weeks' gestation, the number of weeks of pregnancy approximately equals the straight-line length from the superior margin of the symphysis pubis to the uterine fundus in centimeters. As the uterus emerges from the cavity of the pelvis, changes are produced in the relationships and positions of the movable peritoneal contents. The pattern of uterine growth is depicted in Fig. 2-1. Notably, the uterine fundus becomes a palpable abdominal organ at approximately 10 weeks, when the fundus becomes distinct at the pelvic brim just superior to the upper border of the symphysis pubis. At 16 weeks of gestation, the fundus is palpable approximately halfway between the symphysis and the umbilicus. At 20 weeks, it appears at the umbilicus, and at 38 weeks, it is at the xiphoid. At term, because the fetal presenting part descends into the

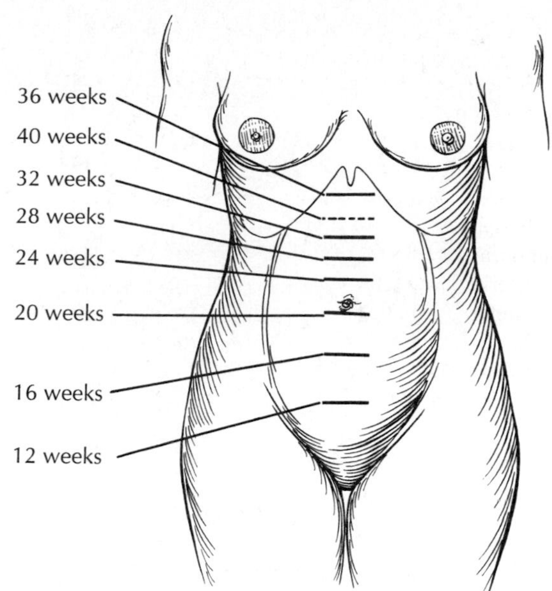

Fig. 2-1. Growth of the pregnant uterus during the course of gestation.

pelvis, the fundus falls to several centimeters below the level of the xiphoid process (Fig. 2-1).

Bowel is displaced laterally, posteriorly, and upwardly because the anterior surface of the uterus glides along the parietal peritoneum of the anterior abdominal wall with growth. As pregnancy progresses and the uterus enlarges, the uterus becomes the most anterior intraperitoneal organ and is therefore more subject to traumatic injuries than in the first 12 weeks of pregnancy, when it is well protected by the pelvic girdle.

Because of these altered anatomic relationships and the dramatically increased blood supply to the pelvic organs, gunshot wounds with and without fetal injury, abdominal stab wounds, and blunt trauma resulting from vehicular accidents have additional implications[17-21] (see Chap. 9).

Uterine growth and the displacement of peritoneal contents alter the ability of the omentum to wall off subsections of the peritoneal cavity. Infectious processes can become more disseminated than they might be in a nonpregnant state. An important aspect of intestinal displacement that potentially complicates the diagnosis of all intraabdominal problems is the change in location of the appendix. As the uterus grows, the appendix is thought to be displaced laterally and upward (Fig. 2-2), although a

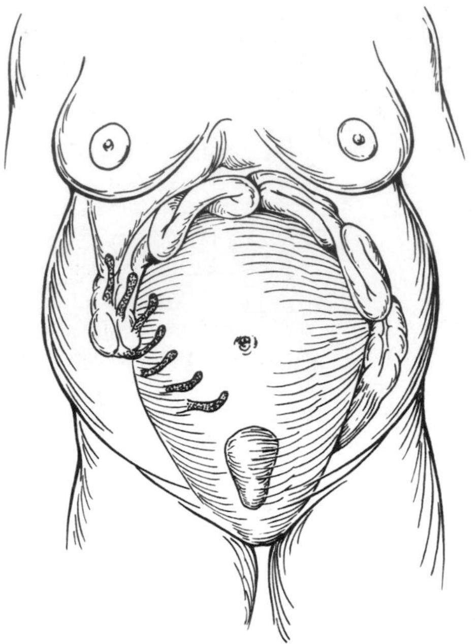

Fig. 2-2. Alterations in the placement of the appendix and bowel with uterine growth in pregnancy.

recent study[22] has challenged that opinion. Clinical presentation of appendicitis can be changed not only by appendiceal location, but also by the altered responses that anatomic changes engender. A leaking, partially-ruptured appendix elevated out of the pelvis by a pregnant uterus may produce greater peritoneal sepsis because of the inability of the omentum to limit infection. Additionally, measures of intraabdominal infection such as elevation of the neutrophil count, which are normal in the pregnant woman, may confuse the diagnostic picture. Table 2-3 demonstrates the changes normally observed in the white blood cell count and other laboratory values during the course of pregnancy. Anorexia, common in early pregnancy with appendicitis, is less pronounced later in gestation, as is rectal and rebound tenderness. Delays in diagnosis and treatment of pregnant women because of the normal physiologic alterations of pregnancy and the variations in natural history and presentation of disease may increase morbidity and mortality for both mother and baby.

Other alterations in the function of the gastrointestinal system in pregnancy include increased gastric emptying time and slowing of peristalsis throughout the entire gut. Common symptoms related to this include constipation and reflux of gastric contents. The major impact of differences in gastrointestinal motility are related clinically to the dangers of aspiration when general anesthesia is needed. In clinical circumstances necessitating the induction of anesthesia emergently for a nonelective procedure in an unprepared pregnant patient, the likelihood of aspiration of stomach contents is increased.

IMPORTANT MILESTONES IN FETAL DEVELOPMENT RELATED TO UTERINE SIZE

Uterine growth is a reflection of fetal growth, and medical and surgical interventions that involve the mother obviously and necessarily involve the fetus. Along with uterine size for estimation of gestational age, a number of fetal parameters are useful. Auscultation of the fetal heart is the most basic means of determining the state of fetal welfare and may also provide a means of assessing gestational age.

Fetal heart tones are typically first audible at 20 weeks of gestation with a Delee auditory-type stethoscope (fetoscope) and at about 10 weeks with a Doppler ultrasound device. The earliest visual confirmation of heart activity is at about 6 weeks with sonographic methods. The detection of heart tones using these various modalities can serve to establish a baseline for estimating fetal age. Quickening, or the occurrence of the first maternally-detectable fetal movements, generally occurs at about 17 to 18 weeks in multiparous women and at 19 to 20 weeks in nulliparas. This information can be useful clinically and may be the only data available when rapid decision-making regarding gestational age is necessary.

With modern-day neonatal intensive care methods, a majority of infants born before term can survive from about 26 weeks onward and sometimes even prior to this. The incidence of serious neurologic problems, such as cerebral palsy, in babies born prematurely is considerable. However, in the face of maternal circumstances that portend serious compromise, the determination of the potential of fetal viability adds to the burden of those caring for the mother under less-than-ideal circumstances.

IMPORTANT CARDIOVASCULAR ALTERATIONS IN PREGNANCY

Anatomic alterations produced by uterine and fetal growth have major implications for cardiovascular function in pregnancy and for the emergency treatment of the preg-

Table 2-3. Important Laboratory Values in Pregnancy

Test	Nonpregnant Range	Pregnant Effect	Gestational Timing
Serum chemistries			
Albumin	3.5–4.8 g/dL	↓1 g/dL	By midpregnancy
Calcium	9.0–10.3 mg/dL	↓10%	Falls gradually
Chloride	95–105 mEq/L	No change	
Cholesterol	200–240 mg/dL	↑50%	Progressive
Creatinine	0.6–1.1 mg/dL	↓0.3 g/dL	By midpregnancy
Fibrinogen	200–400 mg/dL	↑600 mg/dL	By term
Glucose, fasting	65–105 mg/dL	↓10%	Gradual fall
Potassium (plasma)	3.5–4.5 mEq/L	↓0.2–0.3 mEq/L	By midpregnancy
Protein (total)	6.5–8.5 g/dL	↓1 g/dL	By midpregnancy
Sodium	135–145 mEq/L	↓2–4 mEq/L	By midpregnancy
Urea nitrogen	12–30 mg/dL	↓50%	First trimester
Uric acid	3.5–8 mg/dL	↓33%	First trimester
Urine Chemistry			
Creatinine	15–25 mg/kg/d	No change	
Protein	Up to 150 mg/d	Up to 250–300 mg/day	By midpregnancy
Creatinine clearance	90–130 mL/min/1.73 m^2	↑40–50%	By 16 weeks
Serum Enzymes			
Alkaline phosphatase	30–120 U/L	↑3- to 5-fold	By 20 weeks
Amylase	60–180 U/L	Controversial	
Creatinine phosphokinase	26–140 U/L	↑2- to 4-fold	After labor (MB bands as well)
Lipase	10–140 U/L	No change	
Aspartate aminotransferase (AST)	5–35 mU/mL	No change	
alanine aminotransferase (ALT)	5–35 mU/mL	No change	
Formed Elements of Blood			
Hematocrit	36–46%	↓4–7%	Nadir at 30–34 weeks
Hemoglobin	12–16 g/dL	↓1.4–2.0 g/dL	Nadir at 30–34 weeks
Leukocyte count	4.8–10.8 × 10^3/mm^3	↑3.5 x 10^3/mm^3	Gradual increase to term, as high as 25 × 10^3/mm^3 in labor
Platelets	150–400 × 10^3/mm^3	↓ (slight)	

nant woman. From a functional standpoint, pregnancy represents an augmented (but not hyperdynamic) cardiac state.[23] Many parameters traditionally used to assess the state of the cardiovascular system—including pulse rate, stroke volume, and cardiac output—are increased significantly. All of the changes observed are conditioned by the growth needs of the pregnancy and thus change over the duration of the gestation. Parameter values are often different at different stages of gestation. Typical normal values are listed in Table 2-2 and illustrated in Fig. 2-3 as they relate to maternal position and point in gestation.

During the course of normal pregnancy, a number of changes occur in the anatomy of the heart. As noted both

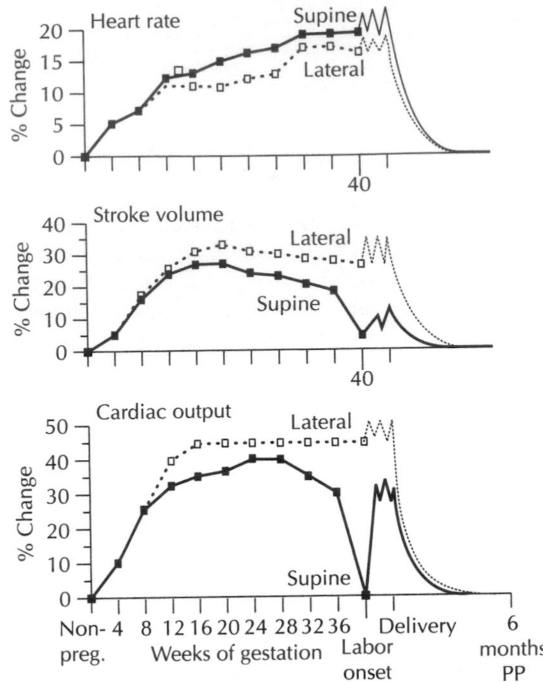

Fig. 2-3. The time pattern of altered cardiovascular dynamics in the course of pregnancy.

by physical examination and using various imaging techniques, the heart is increased in size. Cardiac volume is increased by approximately 12 percent or 70 to 80 mL. Radiologically, images of the pregnant heart show straightening of the upper left cardiac border and simulated left atrial enlargement in the right oblique and lateral views. These features, which are normal for pregnancy and the immediate puerperium, can be mistaken for similar radiographic findings associated with mitral stenosis.[24] Ultrasonic measurements of left atrial and left ventricular end-diastolic dimensions as well as cross-sectional measurements of the aortic, pulmonary, and mitral valves have confirmed these well-established observations. Robson and colleagues reported a 12 to 14 percent increase in the cross-sectional areas of the aortic, pulmonary, and mitral valves during the course of pregnancy, presumably on the basis of increased flow and cardiac output.[25]

Changes in blood flow produce alterations in the auscultatory findings of the pregnant heart. The first heart sound is louder and more widely split than in the nonpregnant state. Systolic murmurs, particularly along the lower portion of the left sternal border and over the pulmonary valvular area, are very common in pregnancy. Typically they are most audible at midsystole and have the diamond-shaped characteristics of ejection-type flow murmurs. A continuous cervical venous hum over the supraclavicular fossa just lateral to the insertion of the sternocleidomastoid muscle may be present. When present, this is more prominent on the right side. Mammary artery souffle is occasionally present and may be mistaken for a pathologic diastolic murmur.[26]

The increased dimensions and work of the heart in pregnancy effect a change in the position of the heart in the thorax; the cardiac apex is moved upward and laterally. This change in position creates alterations in normal physical findings, moving the palpable point of maximal cardiac impulse lateral to the midclavicular line and up several intercostal spaces. Electrocardiographic (ECG) findings may suggest left axis deviation. Oram and Holt,[27] among others, have reported ST-segment depression and T-wave changes in approximately 14 percent of normal pregnant women. T-wave inversions are most commonly seen in V_2. These changes are seen in the ECG of a pregnant woman as pictured in Fig. 2-4. Small Q waves can normally be seen in leads II, III, and aVF. These changes, which are apparently innocent, have recently been reported to occur frequently during operative delivery and during exercise. The major importance of these findings relates to the possibility of confusing these nonserious changes with signs of myocardial ischemia.[27–29]

In addition to the changes noted in the ECGs of normal pregnant women, Abramov and colleagues[30] have stressed the importance of considering the impact of pregnancy and labor on the assessment of laboratory data, with particular regard to the interpretation of results in the area of cardiac diagnosis. In a prospective study, these investigators report a significant elevation of serum creatine phosphokinase and its MB isoenzyme in normal postpartum women without any evidence of myocardial disease.[30]

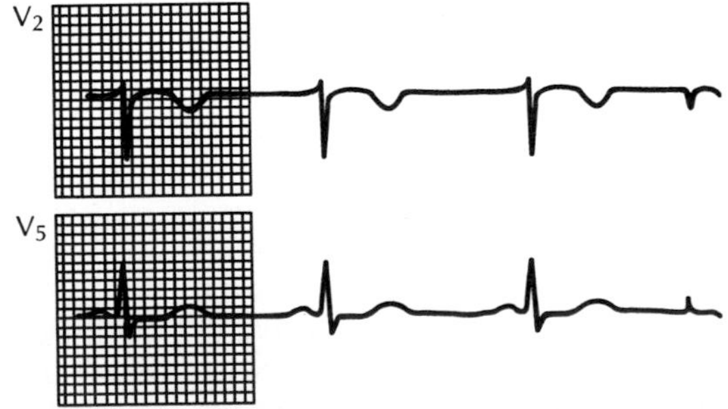

Fig. 2-4. An electrocardiogram showing T-wave inversion in lead V_2 in early pregnancy.

Among the reported changes in the maternal cardiovascular system, there is a unique and important alteration relating cardiac output to the mother's posture. When the pregnant woman who is near term is in the supine position, the enlarged uterus falls onto the inferior vena cava. The resulting compression produces decreased venous return to the right heart and a decrease in cardiac output of between 25 and 30 percent.[31] The anatomic relationships that produce this phenomenon are pictured in Fig. 2-5*A*. As demonstrated in Fig. 2-5*B*, this effect can be minimized by placing the patient in the lateral position or displacing the uterus manually. During spinal or epidural conduction anesthesia, in which sympathectomy accompanies the anesthetic effect, this can be very important. Also, when managing the pregnant trauma victim on a backboard, displacing the uterus off the inferior vena cava and aorta can be critically important in maintaining adequate perfusion.

Caval and aortic compression based on this phenomenon may be of critical importance during cardiopulmonary resuscitation of the pregnant patient. Lee and colleagues[32] and others have written about the special circumstances surrounding cardiopulmonary resuscitation of the pregnant woman and the effect that this particular phenomenon can have. Left uterine deviation of the gravid uterus or placing the woman being resuscitated into some degree of lateral recumbency may make the difference between successful resuscitation and death. The possibility that immediate delivery of the fetus may facilitate both fetal and maternal resuscitation efforts based on these factors is supported by the recent case reports of O'Connor and Sevarino[33] and DePace and associates[34] (see Chap. 29).

During the course of normal gestation, the cardiac output is increased by 30 to 50 percent over levels normal for nonpregnant women. The increase in cardiac output begins as early as the tenth week of gestation and increases steadily until the twentieth to twenty-fourth weeks of pregnancy. This increased level of cardiac output is then sustained at approximately the same level until the time of delivery. Early in the course of pregnancy, this increase in cardiac output seems to be more dependent on increasing stroke volume than on increased heart rate. Later in the course of gestation, the heart rate becomes the more important component of the increase in cardiac output.

In the longitudinal studies done by Mabie and colleagues,[35] total peripheral resistance fell consistently during the course of pregnancy. Duvekot and associates and others have found that most of the fall in total peripheral resistance in pregnancy occurs during the first trimester, at the same time that cardiac output increases most appreciably.[36,37] Systolic blood pressure decreases 10 to 15 mmHg during the middle trimester and gradually increases to prepregnancy levels in the third trimester.

Clark and coworkers reported a significant fall in pulmonary vascular resistance in normal pregnancy that surpasses the decrease in total peripheral resistance.[38] They found no change in pulmonary capillary wedge pressure or central venous pressure during the course of pregnancy. The implications of these findings are that pregnancy is not normally characterized by hyperdynamic left ventricular function. A tabular summary of central cardiovascular measurements made on normal women is given in Table 2-2.

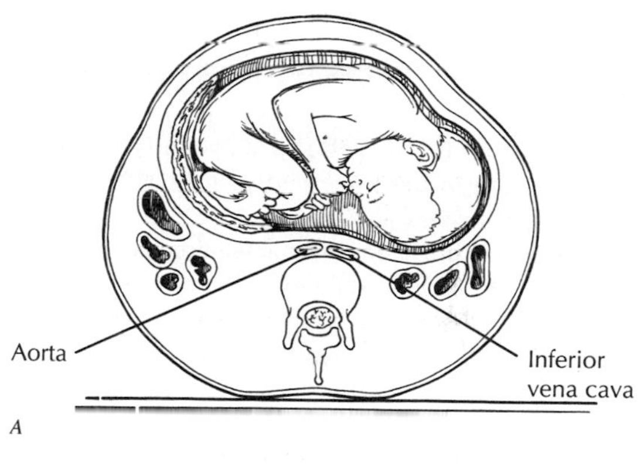

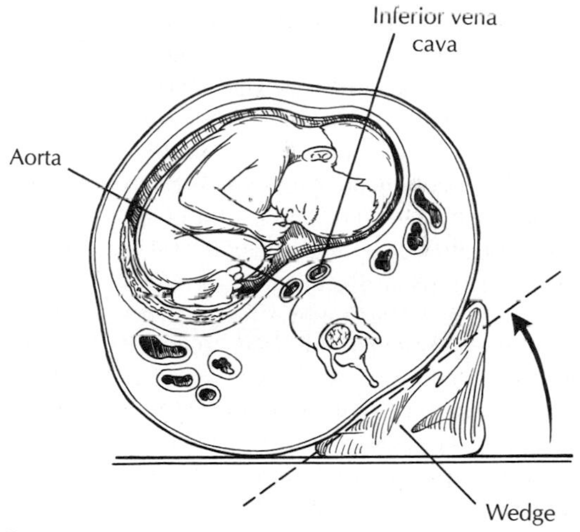

Fig. 2-5. *A*. A transverse section at the umbilicus demonstrating the compression of the aorta and vena cava by the uterus when the mother is completely supine. *B*. The same transverse section with aortic and vena caval compression relieved by left uterine deviation.

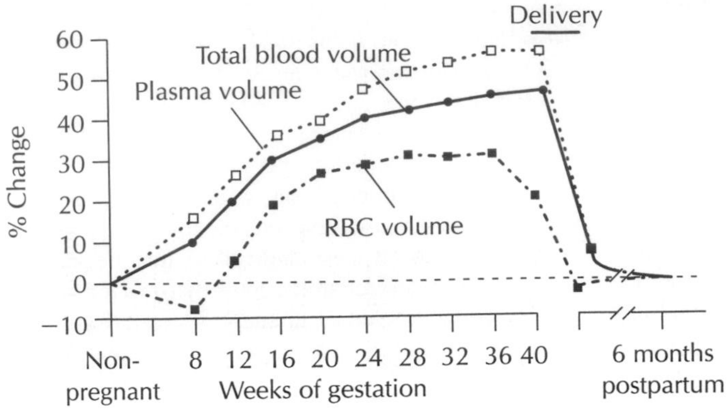

Fig. 2-6. Changes in blood volume, plasma volume, and red cell mass during the course of normal gestation. (From Bonica JJ: *Obstetric Analgesia and Anesthesia,* 2d ed. Amsterdam: World Federation of Societies of Anesthesiologists, 1980, p 2, with permission.)

The expansion of the total blood volume by 45 to 50 percent above nonpregnant levels is probably generated by a number of related factors, including the increase in the size of the vascular tree produced by the addition of the placental circulation, the effects of enormously elevated levels of estrogen and progesterone, and the thermal and metabolic demands of pregnancy.

Changes in total blood volume and red cell mass are illustrated in Fig. 2-6. The clinical impact of expanded blood volume has important ramifications in the dosing of some drugs, as expansion of the intravascular space may effectively dilute the concentration of certain medications, such as anticonvulsants, below therapeutic levels. Expansion of the plasma volume also occurs at a faster rate than the accompanying increase in circulating red cell mass. Early in pregnancy, this produces a dilutional anemia that can be mistaken for an authentic anemia.

Serum proteins are also diluted significantly, creating a decrease in plasma colloid osmotic pressure. This change in serum protein is thought to be partially responsible for the dependent edema often seen in later pregnancy. These notable and important changes in plasma and blood volume have major implications for all forms of drug, fluid, and electrolyte therapy. Changes in body fat content are also important for fat-soluble or fat-stored substances, where uptake by fatty tissues is an important factor in the metabolism or excretion of drugs.

Table 2-3 summarizes how a number of important laboratory tests are altered during the course of pregnancy.

IMPORTANT CHANGES IN THE PULMONARY SYSTEM IN PREGNANCY

Dyspnea occurs during the course of normal, healthy pregnancy in as many as 60 to 70 percent of normal women. This alteration in normal pulmonary function complicates the diagnosis and management of pulmonary difficulties when they do occur. The presence of the pregnant uterus in the abdominal cavity necessitates some changes in pulmonary physiology that are peculiar to pregnancy. As the uterus grows, the diaphragms are elevated. Compensation for this effect is demonstrated by the resulting increased circumference of the maternal thorax and the increased subcostal angle. Somewhat paradoxically, the tidal volume is increased in pregnancy, as are the alveolar and minute ventilation. Although there are mixed data regarding the issue of respiratory rate, there is general agreement that hyperventilation is the normal state of affairs in pregnancy. This results in a decreased $P{CO_2}$, increased pH, and decreased bicarbonate. The pregnant woman is, by most methods of assessment, in a state of partially compensated respiratory alkalosis. The picture can be confusing when one is dealing with other causes of respiratory alkalosis, such as pneumonia or pulmonary embolism.[39] The functional pulmonary changes seen in pregnancy are depicted in Fig. 2-7.

The changes in pulmonary function that occur in pregnancy, particularly the increase in minute ventilation, promote more efficient transfer of gases from the maternal lung to the blood. This implies that changes in maternal respiratory status occur more rapidly than in the nonpregnant state. Hypoxia as well as hyper- and hypocarbia occur more easily with assisted ventilation. During anesthesia with inhalational agents, the patient gets deeper faster and emerges from anesthesia faster. Because of additional fetal oxygen consumption, hypoxia can become more significant sooner when there is hypoventilation or respiratory obstruction. The greater affinity of fetal hemoglobin for oxygen at a lower partial pressure of oxygen in maternal blood may compound maternal hypoxia.

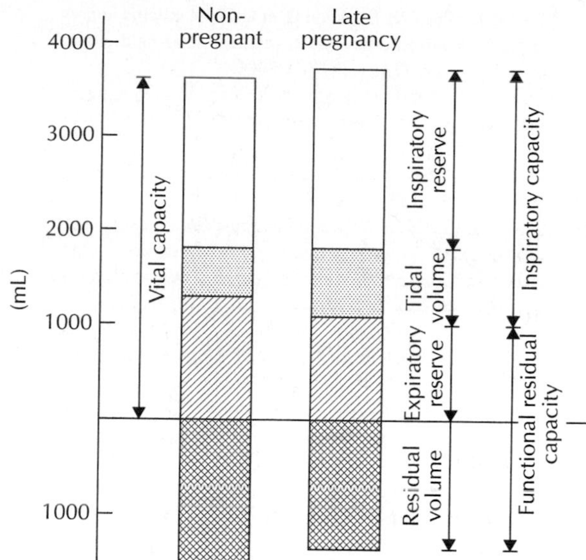

Fig. 2-7. Functional changes in measurements of lung volume during the course of pregnancy as compared with the nonpregnant state.

REFERENCES

1. Pearlman WH: Progesterone metabolism in advanced pregnancy and in oophorectomized-hysterectomized women. *Biochem J* 67:1, 1957.
2. Csapo AI: The molecular basis of myometrial function and its disorders, in *La Prophylaxie en Gynecologie et Ostetrique.* Geneva: Georg, 1954, p 693.
3. Calzada L, Bernal A, Loustaunau E: Effect of steroid hormones and capacitation on membrane potential of human spermatazoa. *Arch Androl* 21:121, 1988.
4. Mahesh VB, Brann DW, Hendry LB: Diverse modes of action of progesterone and its metabolites. *J Steroid Biochem Mol Biol* 56(1–6, special issue):209, 1996.
5. Fu X, Ulsten U, Backstrom T: Interaction of sex steroids and oxytocin on term human myometrial contractile activity in vitro. *Obstet Gynecol* 84:272, 1994.
6. Abrams RM, Caton D, Curet LB, et al: Fetal brain:maternal aorta temperature differences in sheep. *Am JPhysiol* 217:1619, 1969.
7. Walker DW, Wood C: Temperature relationship of the mother and fetus during labor. *Am J Obstet Gynecol* 107:83, 1970.
8. Macaulay JH, Randall NR, Bond K, Steer PJ: Continuous monitoring of fetal temperature by noninvasive probe and its relationship to maternal temperature, fetal heart rate and cord arterial oxygen and pH. *Obstet Gynecol* 79:469, 1992.
9. Heini A, Shutz Y, Jequier E: Twenty-four-hour energy expenditure in pregnant and nonpregnant Gambian women, measured in a whole-body indirect calorimeter. *Am J Clin Nutr* 55:1078, 1992.
10. Kleiber M: Animal temperature regulation, in *The Fire of Life: An Introduction to Animal Energetics.* Huntington, NY: Krieger, 1975, p 150.
11. Nielsen B, Hales JR, Strange S, et al: Human circulatory and thermoregulatory adaptations with heat acclimation and exercise in a hot, dry environment. *J Physiol (Lond)* 460:467, 1993.
12. Burwell CS, Strayhorn WD, Flinkinger D, et al: Circulation during pregnancy. *Arch Intern Med* 62:979, 1938.
13. Assali NS, Rauramo L, Peltonen T: Uterine and fetal blood flow and oxygen consumption in early human pregnancy. *Am J Obstet Gynecol* 79:86, 1960.
14. Romney SL, Reid DE, Metcalfe J, Burwell CS: Oxygen utilization by the human fetus in utero. *Am J Obstet Gynecol* 70:791, 1955.
15. Johnson G, Blythe WB: Hemodynamic effects of arteriovenous shunts used for hemodialysis. *Ann Surg* 171:715, 1970.
16. Oudenhoven LF, Pattynama PM, de Roos A, et al: Magnetic resonance: A new method for measuring blood flow in hemodialysis fistulae. *Kidney Int* 45:884, 1994.
17. Dittrich KC: Rupture of the gravid uterus secondary to motor vehicle trauma. *J Emerg Med* 14:177, 1996.
18. Dahmus MA, Sibai BM: Blunt abdominal trauma: Are there any predictive factors for abruptio placentae or maternal-fetal distress? *Am J Obstet Gynecol* 169:1054, 1993.
19. Neufeld JD: Trauma in pregnancy, what if . . .? *Emerg Med Clin North Am* 11:207, 1993.
20. Awwad JT, Azar GB, Seoud MA, et al: High-velocity penetrating wounds of the gravid uterus: Review of 16 years of civil war. *Obstet Gynecol* 83:259, 1994.
21. Goff BA, Muntz HG: Gunshot wounds to the gravid uterus: A case report. *J Reprod Med* 35:436, 1990.

22. Mourad J, Elliott JP, Erickson L, et al: Appendicitis in pregnancy: New information that contradicts long-held clinical beliefs. *Am J Ob Gyn* 182:1027, 2000.
23. Clark SL, Cotton DB, Lee W, et al: Central hemodynamic assessment of normal term pregnancy. *Am J Obstet Gynecol* 161:1439, 1989.
24. Turner AF: The chest radiograph in pregnancy. *Clin Obstet Gynecol* 18:65, 1975.
25. Robson SC, Dunlop W, Moore M, et al: Combined Doppler and echocardiographic measurement of cardiac output: Theory and application in pregnancy. *Br J Obstet Gynaecol* 94:1014, 1987.
26. Elkayam U, Gleicher N: *Cardiovascular Physiology of Pregnancy in Cardiac Problems in Pregnancy.* New York: Liss, 1982, pp 20–21.
27. Oram S, Holt M: Innocent depression of the ST segment and flattening of the T-wave during pregnancy. *J Obstet Gynaecol Br Commonw* 68:765, 1961.
28. Mathew JP, Fleisher LA, Rinehouse JA, et al: ST segment depression during labor and delivery. *Anesthesiology* 77:635, 1992.
29. Veille JC, Kitzman DW, Bacevice AE: Effects of pregnancy on the electrocardiogram in healthy subjects during strenuous exercise. *Am J Obstet Gynecol* 175:1360, 1996.
30. Abramov Y, Abramov D, Abrahamov A, et al: Elevation of serum creatine phosphokinase and its MB isoenzyme during normal labor and early puerperium. *Acta Obstet Gynecol Scand* 75:255, 1996.
31. Ueland K, Novy MJ, Petersen EN, Metcalfe J: Maternal cardiovascular dynamics: IV. The influence of gestational age on the maternal cardiovascular response to posture and exercise. *Am J Obstet Gynecol* 104:856, 1969.
32. Lee RV, Rodgers BD, White LM, Harvey RC: Cardiopulmonary resuscitation of pregnant women. *Am J Med* 81:311, 1986.
33. O'Connor RL, Sevarino FB: Cardiopulmonary arrest in the pregnant patient: A report of successful resuscitation. *J Clin Anesthesiol* 6:66, 1994.
34. DePace NL, Betesh JS, Kotler MN: Postmortem cesarean section with recovery of both mother and offspring. *JAMA* 248:971, 1982.
35. Mabie WC, DiSessa TG, Crocker LG, et al: A longitudinal study of the cardiac output in normal human pregnancy. *Am J Obstet Gynecol* 170:849, 1994.
36. Metcalfe J, Ueland K: Maternal cardiovascular adjustments to pregnancy. *Prog Cardiovasc Dis* 16:363, 1974.
37. Duvekot JJ, Cheriex EC, Pieters FA, et al: Early pregnancy changes in hemodynamics and volume homeostasis are consecutive adjustments triggered by a primary fall in systemic vascular tone. *American Journal of Obstetrics & Gynecology* 169:1382–92, 1993.
38. Clark SL, Cotton DB, Lee W, et al: Central hemodynamic assessment of normal term pregnancy. *Am J Obstet Gynecol* 161:1439, 1989.
39. Prowse CM, Gaensler EA: Respiratory and acid-base changes during pregnancy. *Anesthesiology* 26:381, 1965.

3

Drug Use in Pregnancy

Wendy Hansen

INTRODUCTION

The emergency physician often needs to prescribe drugs for the various problems encountered in pregnancy or is faced with a woman already on a medication who coincidentally learns she is pregnant. A few key principles should be kept in mind. Virtually all drugs cross the placenta to some degree, with the exception of very large molecules such as heparin and insulin. The decision to give a drug is easy when the drug has been well studied and has no ill effects or when absolutely contraindicated. However, the vast majority of drugs fall somewhere in between, and a risk:benefit analysis must be made. Today many women with complex medical problems such as transplants, epilepsy, congenital heart disease, inflammatory bowel disease (IBD), and systemic lupus erythematosus (SLE) are enjoying successful pregnancies. All require chronic medication use and the acceptance of some risk to the fetus. However, the alternatives of a rejected organ, uncontrolled seizures, arrhythmias, or a flare of IBD or SLE have potentially devastating consequences for both mother and fetus. Although life-threatening encounters are rare in pregnancy, the emergency physician is the most likely to be involved and often the first to be present. In such instances, fetal considerations would not be expected to be paramount in the decision to administer a drug. Perhaps the best example is cardiac resuscitation, when advanced cardiac life support drug management is unaltered by pregnancy.

An effective approach to the use of medication for problems encountered in pregnancy starts with the question "What would I do for this woman if she were not pregnant?" If the answer is to treat with an antibiotic, an antihypertensive, or a pain reliever, the answer is most often unchanged (i.e., to treat the pregnant woman). The next question should be which drug best suits the situation that is safest for mother and fetus. This may be different in the pregnant woman. Therefore, this chapter uses a rating scale that describes the: (1) primary drug of choice; (2) drugs that are recommended if the patient is currently using or if primary agent is contraindicated; (3) drugs for which we have no information and a risk:benefit analysis must be made; and (4) drugs the emergency physician should avoid completely.

Since 1979, the FDA has used a drug classification system of A, B, C, D, and X. Many physicians find this classification cumbersome, confusing, and clinically difficult to use. (e.g., virtually all new drugs are categorized as C). However, because this system is currently, the most commonly used, many of the chapters in this textbook will refer to the FDA classification. Table 3-1 summarizes the categories along with the percentage of drugs in each category. The Teratology Society for Public Affairs Committee recommended that the FDA pregnancy ratings be deleted from drug labels and be replaced by narrative statements. This process is in its infancy and is not yet in place. For purposes of this chapter, the FDA labeling system is not used, but rather each individual drug was researched on the teratology databases using REPRORISK® and a variety of books listed below. There are a few drugs that are generally contraindicated in pregnancy, and those are summarized in Table 3-2. Tables 3-3 to 3-22 give risk factors associated with and comments about the use of various medications in pregnancy. There are unusual exceptions where drugs in Table 3-1 are used during pregnancy (e.g., methotrexate for ectopic pregnancy, indomethacin for preterm labor), however these unusual exceptions should generally only be prescribed in consultation with an obstetriciasm.

KEY REFERENCES

All emergency treatment centers should have ready access to an up-to-date reference for drugs in pregnancy and lactation. In addition to this text, the following is a list of Internet web sites and respected books that give up-to-date information concerning drugs.

- REPRORISK® System: http://www.micromedex.com/products/reprorisk/ (subscription required)
- American Academy of Pediatrics: http://www.aap.org/ (free)
- http://www.perinatology.com/exposures/druglist.htm (free)
- http://www.otispregnancy.org (free)

Databases

MICROMEDEX® Healthcare Series Databases include access to:

REPRORISK System (Reproductive Risk Information).

Table 3-1. Percentage of Drugs in Each U.S. Food and Drug Administration Risk Category as Listed in the *Physicians' Desk Reference*

Category	Percentage
A: Controlled studies show no risk	0.7
B: No evidence of risk in humans	19
C: Risk cannot be ruled out	66
D: Positive evidence of risk	7
X: Contraindicated in pregnancy	7

The REPRORISK System is a collection of reproductive risk information databases. It provides information covering full-range health effects that is helpful when assessing reproductive risk of drugs, chemicals, and physical and environmental agents.

REPRORISK includes the following modules:

- REPROTEXT® Database
- REPROTOX® Reproduction Hazard Information
- Shepard's Catalog of Teratogenic Agents
- TERIS Teratogenic Information System

REPROTOX

Developed by the Reproductive Toxicology Center, Columbia Hospital for Women Medical Center, Washington, D.C.

Shepard's Catalog of Teratogenic Agents

Developed by Dr. Thomas H. Shepard, Professor of Pediatrics, University of Washington

TERIS (Teratogen Information System)

Developed by the University of Washington

Addresses

MICROMEDEX Inc.

6200 South Syracuse Way, Suite 300, Englewood, CO 80111-4740

Telephone 800-525-9083 (in U.S. and Canada)

Website http://www.micromedex.com (subscription required)

Reproductive Toxicology Center (REPROTOX®)

7752 Woodmont Avenue, Suite 213, Bethesda, MD 20814-6030

Telephone 301-657-5984

Website http://www.reprotox.org (subscription required)

Teratogen Information Service (TERIS)

University of Washington, Box 357920, Seattle, WA 98195-7920

Telephone 206-543-2465

Website http://depts.washington.edu/~terisweb (subscription required)

Books

Yankowitz J, Niebyl JR (eds): *Drug Therapy in Pregnancy,* 3d ed. Lippincott Williams & Wilkins: New York, 2001.

Briggs GG, Freeman RK, Yaffe SJ (eds): *Drugs in Pregnancy and Lactation,* 6th ed. Lippincott Williams & Wilkins: New York, 2001.

Rayburn, WF (ed.): Drugs in pregnancy. *Clin Obstet Gynecol* 2002;45:1-169.

Table 3-2. Drugs Contraindicated in Pregnancy

Medication	Comments
Isotretinoin	Highly teratogenic: CNS malformations, microtia/anotia, micrognathia, cleft palate, cardiac, thymic, eye
Misoprostol	Congenital anomalies resulting from vascular disruptions, Möbius syndrome (palsies of 6th cranial nerve), amniotic bands, uterine contractions, abortion
Methotrexate	Embryopathy: craniofacial and skeletal defects; miscarriage rate is high when given in first trimester
Warfarin	Warfarin embryopathy: IUGR, nasal hypoplasia, stippled epiphyses, vertebral abnormalities, fetal bleeding in 2nd and 3rd trimester Only potential indication is that of a mechanical valve in pregnancy
Ergotamines	Congenital anomalies due to vascular disruption. Uterine contractions
Angiotensin-converting enzyme inhibitors	Fetal hypocalvaria, renal failure, oligohydramnios, and fetal and neonatal death, especially after the first trimester
Angiotensin II receptor antagonists	Data is based on that of ACE inhibitors
Nitroprusside sodium	Consider delivery; risk of cyanide poisoning to fetus
Quinolones	High affinity for bone, tissue, and cartilage causing arthropathies in children
Tetracyclines	Firmly bound by chelating to calcium in developing bone and teeth; discoloration effect after 20 weeks
Nonsteroidal antiinflammatory drugs	Associated with third-trimester (after 32 weeks) pregnancy complications: oligohydramnios, premature closure of ductus anteriosus
Antiepileptic drugs	All AEDs prescribed for long-term management have a pattern of similar malformations (orofacial clefts, congenital heart disease, midfacial hypoplasia, open neural tube defects)
Streptomycin, kanamycin	Sensorineural deafness reported
Lindane	Potential neurotoxicity in fetus
Ketoconazole (systemic)	Ketoconazole interferes with steroid hormone production; systemic maternal treatment may affect genital development in male fetuses
Amiodarone	Risk of neonatal thyroid dysfunction or goiter following chronic maternal treatment with amiodarone may be substantial; risk not expected before 10 weeks' gestation; risk likely to depend on dose and duration of maternal treatment

Table 3-3. Use of Analgesics in Pregnancy

Medication	Risk	Comments
Opioids and opioid agonists		
Meperidine	1	Neonatal narcotic withdrawal is seen in women using opioids long term
Morphine	1	
Fentanyl (Sublimaze, Duragesic)	2	Almost all cause respiratory depression in the neonate when used near delivery
Hydrocodone	1	
Oxycodone	2	Used for treatment of acute pain: nephrolithiasis, cholelithiasis, appendicitis, injury, postoperative pain
Propoxyphene	2	
Codeine	1	
Hydromorphone	2	
Methadone	3	
Nonsteroidals		
Diclofenac	4	Associated with third-trimester (after 32 weeks) pregnancy complications: oligohydramnios, premature closure of ductus arteriosus
Etodolac	4	
Ibuprofen	2/4	Both ibuprofen and indomethacin have been used for short courses before 32 weeks gestation without harm; indomethacin is often used to arrest preterm labor
Indomethacin	2/4	
Ketoprofen	4	
Ketorolac	4	
Naproxen	4	
Sulindac	4	
Other		
Full-strength aspirin	4	Full-strength aspirin can cause constriction of ductus arteriosus
Low-dose (baby) aspirin	1	Low-dose (baby) aspirin safe throughout pregnancy
Salicylates		
Acetaminophen	1	Widely used
Salicylates-opioids		
Acetaminophen-codeine	1	Widely used for treatment of acute pain
Acetaminophen-hydrocodone	1	
Acetaminophen-oxycodone	1	
Acetaminophen-propoxyphene	2	

1, Primary recommended agent; 2 recommended if currently using or their primary agent is contraindicated; 3, limited data to support or prescribe use; 4 not recommended.

Table 3-4. Use of Antiasthmatics in Pregnancy

Medication	Risk	Comments
Methylxanthines		
Theophylline, aminophylline	1	
Beta-agonists		Widely used in pregnancy
Albuterol	1	
Metaproterenol sulfate	1	
Salmeterol	1	
Terbutaline	1	
Inhaled corticosteroids		Widely used in pregnancy
Beclomethasone dipropionate	1	
Budesonide	3	
Flunisolide	1	
Fluticasone	2	
Triamcinolone	2	
Leukotriene modifiers		
Zafirlukast	3	
Zileuton	3	
Systemic corticosteroids		Only 5–10% crosses the placenta
Prednisone	1	
Others		
Cromolyn sodium	1	Widely used
Epinephrine	2	
Nedocromil	3	Not as much information

1, Primary recommended agent; 2, recommended if currently using or their primary agent is contraindicated; 3, limited data to support or prescribe use; 4, not recommended.

Table 3-5. Use of Antibiotics in Pregnancy

Medication	Risk	Comments
Aminoglycosides		
Gentamicin	2	Extended interval dosing (EID) for gentamicin not widely studied in pregnancy; controversy exists regarding an idiosyncratic response of the fetus to gentamicin and sensorineural hearing loss; should be used with gram-negative infections resistant to beta-lactam antibiotics; gentamicin is the aminoglycoside of choice during pregnancy
Tobramycin	3	
Kanamycin	4	Congenital deafness reported with kanamycin and streptomycin
Streptomycin	4	
Carbapenems		
Imipenem/cilastatin	3	
Meropenem	2	
Cephalosporins		Widely used in pregnancy
First generation	1	
Cefazolin		
Cephalexin		
Second generation	1	
Cefotetan		
Cefuroxime		
Third generation	1	
Cefepime		
Cefotaxime		
Ceftazidime		
Cefpodoxime		
Ceftriaxone		
Lincosamides		
Clindamycin	1	Widely used in pregnancy
Macrolides		Widely used in pregnancy
Azithromycin	1	
Clarithromycin	1	
Erythromycin	1	
Monobactams		
Aztreonam	2	
Miscellaneous		
Metronidazole	3/1	3 in the first trimester/1 anytime else in pregnancy
Nitrofurantoin	1	
Penicillins		Penicillins have been widely used in pregnancy for many years
Extended Spectrum	1	
Piperacillin		Wide margin of safety for both mother and fetus. Serum levels lower and renal clearance higher compared with nonpregnant state
Piperacillin-tazobactam		
Ticarcillin disodium + clavulanate		

(*Continues*)

Table 3-5. (*Continued*) Use of Antibiotics in Pregnancy

Medication	Risk	Comments
Aminopenicillins	1	
Amoxicillin		
Ampicillin		
ampicillin + clavulanate potassium (Augmentin®)		
Ampicillin sodium/ sulbactam sodium (Unasyn®)		
Penicillinase-resistant	1	
Cloxacillin		
Dicloxacillin		
Methicillin		
Nafcillin		
Oxacillin		
Penicillins G and V	1	
Penicillin G benzathine		
Penicillin G procaine		
Penicillin V potassium		
Quinolones		
Ciprofloxacin	4	All quinolones have high affinity for bone, tissue, and cartilage causing arthropathies in animal studies; generally contraindicated in pregnancy
Levofloxacin	4	
Norfloxacin	4	
Ofloxacin		
Sulfonamides		Often used in treatment of urinary tract infections in pregnancy
Sulfadiazine	1	Theoretical risk only to the newborn; should not be given near delivery or in the last month of pregnancy
Sulfamethoxazole + trimethoprim	3/1	Theoretical risk in first trimester from trimethoprim (folic acid antagonist); 1 anytime else until near delivery.
Tetracyclines		Contraindicated
Doxycycline	4	Firmly bound by chelating to calcium in developing bone and teeth; discoloration; tetracycline worse than doxycycline
Minocycline	4	
Tetracycline	4	

1, Primary recommended agent; 2, recommended if currently using or their primary agent is contraindicated; 3, limited data to support or prescribe use; 4, not recommended.

Table 3-6. Use of Anticoagulants in Pregnancy

Medication	Risk	Comments
Enoxaparin (low molecular weight)	1	Commonly used in acute treatment of thromboembolism
Heparin (unfractionated)	1	Commonly used in acute treatment of thromboembolism
Warfarin	4	Teratogenic in first trimester; potential fetal bleeding in second and third trimesters

1, Primary recommended agent; 2, recommended if currently using or their primary agent is contraindicated; 3, limited data to support or prescribe use; 4, not recommended.

Table 3-7. Use of Antidepressants in Pregnancy

Medication	Risk	Comments
Selective serotonin receptor inhibitors		Fluoxetine is the best studied of the SSRIs; children have been followed through age 6 with no neurobehavioral effects observed Poor transient neonatal adaptation with SSRIs has been reported The other SSRIs have been studied but not to the same extent
Citalopram	2	
Fluoxetine	1	
Fluvoxamine	2	
Paroxetine	2	
Sertraline	2	
Monoamine oxidase inhibitors		
Phenelzine	3	
Tranylcypromine	3	
Tricyclics		Tricyclics have been used the longest during pregnancy Children have been followed to age 6 with no observed neurobehavioral effect
Amitriptyline	1	
Clomipramine	1	
Desipramine	2	
Doxepin	2	
Imipramine	1	
Nortriptyline	2	
Miscellaneous		Information on these agents is increasing: Bupropion Pregancy Registry Glaxo-Smith-Kline, Wilmington, NC 1-800-336-2176
Bupropion	3	
Mirtazapine	3	
Nefazodone	3	
Trazodone	3	
Venlafaxine	3	
Mood stabilizers		
Lithium	1	Lithium has a small risk of Ebstein's anomaly; drug of choice for unstable bipolar disease in pregnancy
Carbamazepine	4	
Valproate	4	

1, Primary recommended agent; 2, recommended if currently using or their primary agent is contraindicated; 3, limited data to support or prescribe use; 4, not recommended.

Table 3-8. Use of Antiemetics in Pregnancy

Medication	Risk	Comments
Pyridoxine B_6	1	Commonly used for nausea of early pregnancy
Antihistamines		These medications are commonly used in the first trimester for control of the nausea and vomiting of pregnancy
Diphenhydramine	1	
Hydroxyzine	2	
Promethazine	1	
Meclizine	2	
Dimenhydrinate	2	
Doxylamine	2	
Doxylamine + vitamin B_6	2	
Antidopaminergics		
Prochlorperazine	1	Both drugs are widely used in the first trimester for control of nausea and vomiting of pregnancy
Metoclopramide	1	
Others		
Trimethobenzamide hydrochloride	3	
Ondansetron hydrochloride	3	

1, Primary recommended agent; 2, recommended if currently using or their primary agent is contraindicated; 3, limited data to support or prescribe use; 4, not recommended.

Table 3-9. Use of Antiepileptic Drugs (AEDs) in Pregnancy

Medication	Risk	Comment
Carbamazepine	4	Similar malformations (orofacial clefts, congenital heart disease) are seen with all AEDs; teratogenic effect is caused by elevated levels of epoxide, which is dependent on the enzyme activity of epoxide hydrolase
Phenobarbital	4	Despite their potential teratogenic effect, continuation is a risk:benefit decision because of the deleterious effect of uncontrolled seizures in pregnancy
Phenytoin	4	Preconception counseling is ideal
Primidone	4	If seizure-free for 2 years, can consider stopping AED; monotherapy has lower risk than polytherapy
Valproic acid	4	All women should be on 4 mg/day folic acid prior to conception if an AED is necessary
Ethosuximide	4	
Clonazepam	3	
New Antiepileptic Drugs		
Felbamate	4	Data is very limited on the new AEDs
Gabapentin	4	Potentially similar teratogenic effects as the older agents
Lamotrigine	4	All women should be on 4 mg/day folic acid prior to conception if an AED is necessary
Levetiracetam	4	
Oxcarbazepine	4	
Tiagabine	4	
Topiramate	4	
Drugs Used for Acute Control of Seizure or Status Epilepticus		
Diazepam	1	Drug of choice in status epilepticus
Magnesium sulfate	1	Drug of choice in seizures secondary to eclampsia

1, Primary recommended agent; 2, recommended if currently using or their primary agent is contraindicated; 3, limited data to support or prescribe use; 4, not recommended.

Table 3-10. Use of Antihypertensives in Pregnancy

Medication	Risk	Comments
Angiotensin-converting enzyme (ACE) inhibitors		Contraindicated in pregnancy Angiotensin-converting enzyme inhibitors have been associated with fetal hypocalvaria, renal failure, oligohydramnios, and fetal and neonatal death, especially in the second and third trimesters
Captopril	4	
Enalapril	4	
Lisinopril	4	
Angiotensin II receptor antagonists		Data extracted from ACE inhibitors
Losartan	4	No role in pregnancy
Beta-blockers		
Atenolol	2	Widely used for the treatment of hypertension in pregnancy
Esmolol	2	May have a *small* effect on fetal growth. Newborns should be observed for signs of beta blockade
Labetalol	2	
Metoprolol	2	Labetalol is the primary drug used in hypertensive emergencies
Propranolol	2	
Timolol	2	
Calcium channel blockers		Not as widely used as beta-blockers
Amlodipine	2	**DO NOT USE WITH MAGNESIUM SULFATE.**
Diltiazem	2	
Felodipine	2	
Nifedipine	2	
Nimodipine	2	
Verapamil	2	
Diuretics		Do not initiate long-term diuretic therapy in pregnancy
Hydrochlorothiazide	3	Many women present on diuretics. It is reasonable to continue
Peripheral vasodilator		
Hydralazine	1	Primary drug in hypertensive emergencies during pregnancy
Minoxidil	3	Hypertrichosis in exposed fetus
Central and adrenergic inhibitors		
Methyldopa	1	Most commonly used; longest studied
Clonidine	3	Use is very limited

1, Primary recommended agent; 2, recommended if currently using or their primary agent is contraindicated; 3, limited data to support or prescribe use; 4, not recommended.

Table 3-11. Drugs Recommended and Not Recommended in Hypertensive Emergencies

Medication	Risk	Comments
Labetalol	1	Commonly used in preeclampsia intravenously
Hydralazine	1	Commonly used in preeclampsia intravenously
Nifedipine	2	Used when labetalol or hydralazine not effective; do not use if a woman is on magnesium sulfate
Nitroprusside sodium	4	Consider delivery; risk of cyanide poisoning to fetus

1, Primary recommended agent; 2, recommended if currently using or their primary agent is contraindicated; 3, limited data to support or prescribe use; 4, not recommended.

Table 3-12. Use of Antiinfectives in Pregnancy

Medication	Risk	Comments
Lindane	3	Small risk of fetal neurotoxicity cannot be excluded; high risk of congenital anomalies unlikely
Permethrin	2	Not well studied; not likely to have an adverse effect
Pyrethrins with piperonyl butoxide	1	Drug of choice in pregnancy
Antifungals		
Amphotericin B	3	
Caspofungin	3	
Fluconazole		
High-dose chronic parenteral	4	
Single low dose	2	
Flucytosine	3	Flucytosine is biotransformed to 5-fluorouracil
Griseofulvin	2	
Itraconazole	2	Itraconazole for a long course has more risk than a short course
Ketoconazole (Nizoral)		Ketoconazole interferes with steroid hormone production;
Topical	2	systemic maternal treatment may affect genital development in male fetuses
Systemic	4	
Nystatin		
Topical	1	
Terbinafine		
Topical	3	
Antivirals		
Acyclovir	1	Acyclovir and valacyclovir are used often for primary and recurrent herpes in pregnancy
Valacyclovir	1	
Famciclovir	3	An acyclovir/valacyclovir registry was closed in 1998; no harmful effect seen
Amantadine	3	Amantadine primary drug of choice for influenza pneumonia in pregnancy
Oseltamivir	3	No data on influenza chemoprophylaxis; avoid in pregnant women who are healthy
Ganciclovir	3	Ganciclovir reserved for liver transplant patients with CMV

1, Primary recommended agent; 2, recommended if currently using or their primary agent is contraindicated; 3, limited data to support or prescribe use; 4, not recommended.

Table 3-13. Use of Antipsychotics and Anxiolytics in Pregnancy

Medication	Risk	Comments
Phenothiazines		
Chlorpromazine	1	
Fluphenazine	3	
Mesoridazine	3	
Perphenazine	3	
Thioridazine	2	
Trifluoperazine	2	
Nonphenothiazines		
Haloperidol	1	
Clozapine	2	
Loxapine	3	
Olanzapine	2/3	
Quetiapine	3	
Risperidone	3	
Thiothixene	3	
Ziprasidone	3	
Anxiolytics		
Alprazolam	1	
Buspirone	3	
Chlordiazepoxide	1	
Diazepam	1	
Hydroxyzine	1	
Lorazepam	3	
Oxazepam	1	

1, Primary recommended agent; 2, recommended if currently using or their primary agent is contraindicated; 3, limited data to support or prescribe use; 4, not recommended.

Table 3-14. Use of Antireflux Agents in Pregnancy

Medication	Risk	Comments
Antacids		
Sucralfate	1	
H_2-receptor antagonists		H_2-receptor antagonists widely used throughout pregnancy
Cimetidine	2	
Famotidine	1	
Ranitidine	1	
Nizatidine	1	
Motility agents		
Metoclopramide	1	
Proton pump inhibitors		
Omeprazole	3	
Lansoprazole	3	
Other		
Misoprostol	4	Absolutely contraindicated unless being used for labor induction or pregnancy termination; congenital anomalies resulting from vascular disruptions, Möbius syndrome (palsies of 6th cranial nerve), amniotic bands, uterine contractions, abortion

1, Primary recommended agent; 2, recommended if currently using or their primary agent is contraindicated; 3, limited data to support or prescribe use; 4, not recommended.

Table 3-15. Use of Antituberculosis Drugs in Pregnancy

Medication	Risk	Comments
Ethambutol	1	
Isoniazid (INH)	1	Administer 50 mg/d of pyridoxine to prevent fetal neurotoxicity with INH
Pyrazinamide	3	
Rifampin	1	
Streptomycin	4	Sensorineural deafness reported with streptomycin

1, Primary recommended agent; 2, recommended if currently using or their primary agent is contraindicated; 3, limited data to support or prescribe use; 4, not recommended.

Table 3-16. Use of Vaginal Antiinfectives in Pregnancy (see also tables 3-8 and 3-12)

Medication	Risk	Comments
Boric acid	3	
Clotrimazole	1	These agents are used commonly in all trimesters
Metronidazole	1	
Nystatin	1	
Povidone-iodine	1	
Terconazole	1	

1, Primary recommended agent; 2, recommended if currently using or their primary agent is contraindicated; 3, limited data to support or prescribe use; 4, not recommended.

Table 3-17. Use of Cardiac Agents in Pregnancy

Medication	Risk	Comments
Adenosine	1	Drug of choice for supraventricular tachycardia in pregnancy.
Cardiac glycoside		
Digoxin[a]	1	
Class I-A		
Quinidine[a]	3	
Procainamide[a]	3	
Disopyramide phosphate	3	This agent has a possible connection with preterm labor
Class I-B		
Lidocaine		
Systemic	3	
Local	1	
Mexiletine	3	
Tocainide	3	
Class I-C		
Flecainide[a]	3	
Propafenone[a]	3	
Beta-Blockers		Chronic use of beta-blockers is associated with a small decrease in fetal growth Newborns need to be observed for hypoglycemia, respiratory distress, and bradycardia
Atenolol	2	
Carvedilol	3	
Esmolol	3	
Labetalol	2	
Metoprolol	2	
Nadolol	3	
Pindolol	2	
Propranolol	2	
Sotalol[a]	2	
Calcium channel blockers		**DO NOT USE WITH MAGNESIUM SULFATE.**
Amlodipine	2	
Diltiazem	2	
Felodipine	2	
Nifedipine	2	
Nimodipine	2	
Verapamil	2	
Amiodarone[a]	4	Risk of neonatal thyroid dysfunction or goiter following chronic maternal treatment with amiodarone may be substantial; risk not expected before 10 weeks' gestation; risk likely to depend on dose and duration of maternal treatment
Bretylium	3	
Dofetilide	3	
Ibutilide	3	

[a]Drugs that have been administered to mother for treatment of fetal tachyarrhythmias.
1, Primary recommended agent; 2, recommended if currently using or their primary agent is contraindicated; 3, limited data to support or prescribe use; 4, not recommended.

Table 3-18. Drugs Used to Treat Colds, Nasal Congestion, and Allergies in Pregnancy

Medication	Risk	Comments
Cetirizine	3	
Chlorpheniramine	1	
Fexofenadine	2	
Loratadine	2	
Triprolidine with pseudoephedrine	1	
Pseudoephedrine	1	

1, Primary recommended agent; 2, recommended if currently using or their primary agent is contraindicated; 3, limited data to support or prescribe use; 4, not recommended.

Table 3-19. Use of Antimigraine Agents in Pregnancy

Medication	Risk	Comments
Acetaminophen, butalbital, and caffeine	1	
Acetaminophen, isometheptene, and dichloralphenazone	4	
Dihydroergotamine	4	
Ergotamine	4	Congenital anomalies due to vascular disruption; uterine contractions
Triptans		
Naratriptan	3	Sumatriptan Pregnancy Registry by Glaxo-Wellcome reported 208 outcomes with exposure in all trimesters; no differences from nonexposed
Sumatriptan	3	

1, Primary recommended agent; 2, recommended if currently using or their primary agent is contraindicated; 3, limited data to support or prescribe use; 4, not recommended.

Table 3-20. Use of Specific Immune Globulins in Pregnancy

Medication	Risk	Comments
Hepatitis A	1	Indications for use of these specific immune globulins are unaltered by pregnancy
Hepatitis B	1	
Measles	1	
Rabies	1	
Tetanus	1	
Varicella	1	

1, Primary recommended agent; 2, recommended if currently using or their primary agent is contraindicated; 3, limited data to support or prescribe use; 4, not recommended.

Table 3-21. Use of Vaccines in Pregnancy

Medication	Risk	Comments
Diphtheria-tetanus	1	Indications for use of all of these vaccines are unaltered by pregnancy
Hepatitis B	1	
Influenza	1	The Centers for Disease Control recommends that all pregnant women who will be in the second or third trimester during influenza season be vaccinated
Measles, mumps, rubella (MMR)	4	Use of live or live attenuated virus should not be administered during pregnancy due to theoretical risk of fetal infection.
Meningococcal	1	
Pneumococcal	1	
Polio	1	
Rabies	1	
Smallpox	4	Smallpox vaccine should not be administered during pregnancy unless patient has been directly exposed to smallpox.
Varicella	4	Pregnancy should be avoided for one month (28 days) following administration of live vaccine.

1, Primary recommended agent; 2, recommended if currently using or their primary agent is contraindicated; 3, limited data to support or prescribe use; 4, not recommended.

Table 3-22. Use of Thyroid and Antithyroid Drugs in Pregnancy

Medication	Risk	Comments
Levothyroxine sodium	1	
Methimazole	2	
Propylthiouracil	1	Drug of choice for hyperthyroidism in pregnancy

1, Primary recommended agent; 2, recommended if currently using or their primary agent is contraindicated; 3, limited data to support or prescribe use; 4, not recommended.

SECTION II
PROBLEMS DURING THE FIRST 20 WEEKS OF PREGNANCY

4

Vaginal Bleeding and Other Common Complaints in Early Pregnancy

Pamela L. Dyne

KEY POINTS

- Retained products of conception are suggested by heavy vaginal bleeding and an open internal cervical os. Fever and/or uterine tenderness suggest concomitant endometritis.
- A falling B-hCG does not necessarily exclude ectopic pregnancy; conversely, an insufficient rise in B-hCG is about 75% sensitive and 93% specific for an abnormal gestation.
- Patients with pregnancy-induced nausea and vomiting present with few physical signs other than those of dehydration. Presence of abdominal pain or tenderness, or fever, imply an alternative diagnosis.
- First time headaches during pregnancy warrant thorough investigation. The diagnosis of migraine for a first-time headache requires the exclusion of more serious causes.

INTRODUCTION

The most common emergency department complaints in pregnancy are vaginal bleeding, abdominal pain, nausea and vomiting, headache, back pain, and dizziness or syncope. The differential diagnosis for vaginal bleeding is relatively short, with ectopic pregnancy being the most serious condition, and threatened abortion being the most common. Threatened abortion occurs in 20 to 30 percent of all pregnancies, and up to 50 percent of those will go on to spontaneously abort.[1] An understanding of the definitions of the different classifications and management options for non-viable gestations is important for effective management in the ED and communication with consultants. Septic abortions and gestational trophoblastic disease are also discussed.

Nausea and vomiting of pregnancy ("morning sickness") and hyperemesis gravidarum are most commonly seen in the first trimester of pregnancy with estimated incidence of 50 to 70 percent of all pregnancies. Given the common nature of this ED complaint, the identification of women who require hospitalization will be the focus of our discussion here.

Headache and back pain are also very common in pregnancy, with some severe and life-threatening etiologies in their differential diagnoses, and will be addressed in this chapter from the emergency department perspective. Ectopic pregnancy is discussed in depth in Chap. 5, abdominal pain is addressed in Chap. 14, and syncope and dizziness are discussed in Chap. 20.

VAGINAL BLEEDING IN EARLY PREGNANCY

The differential diagnosis of bleeding in early pregnancy includes ectopic pregnancy, threatened abortion, abortion in progress, completed abortion, and other causes of vaginal bleeding in the lower genital or GI tract (Table 4-1). ED evaluation requires pelvic examination, urinalysis, CBC, quantitative serum β-hCG, and pelvic ultrasonography. If the patient is hypotensive, tachycardic, or has orthostatic hypotension, begin volume resuscitation with intravenous fluids. Administer type-specific and cross-matched blood if the patient's hemodynamic status does not respond to 2 liters of crystalloid. If the patient is Rh-negative, administer Rh immune globulin. Continuous heavy vaginal bleeding may require immediate gynecologic consultation.

Table 4-1. Differential Diagnosis for Vaginal Bleeding in Pregnancy

Common
Ectopic pregnancy
Spontaneous abortion (see Table 4-2)
Implantation bleeding

Less common
Vaginal wall lesions: neoplasm, foreign body, laceration, ulceration
Benign cervical conditions: polyp, ectropion
Infections: Cervicitis, bacterial vaginosis
Cervical carcinoma
Nonvaginal bleeding source: urinary, bowel

Confirming Pregnancy

While many ED patients presenting with vaginal bleeding know if they are pregnant, many do not. A history of possible or confirmed pregnancy is one of the first questions to ask. In one study, about 60% of women who thought they were pregnant were in fact pregnant; about 11% who denied pregnancy were pregnant, and about 7 percent who report a normal menstrual history and deny sexual contact are pregnant.[2] Therefore, a negative history for pregnancy is unreliable and all women of childbearing age with vaginal bleeding should have a pregnancy test, regardless of menstrual history.

The urine pregnancy test is 99.4 percent sensitive for diagnosing pregnancy at about the same time as when the woman misses her period, or when the serum β-hCG is greater than 25 mIU/mL. False-negative reactions can occur when the serum β-hCG is between 10 and 50 mIU/mL. When positive, the urine bedside pregnancy test establishes the patient as pregnant. False-positive serum pregnancy tests occur with a frequency of 1 in 10,000 to 1 in 100,000 tests. Most of these false-positives are caused by lab interference by non-human chorionic gonadotropin substances, the detection of pituitary human chorionic gonadotropin, and exogenously injected hCG. In all of these cases, the urine pregnancy test will be negative.[3] Given the extremely rare nature of this in the ED setting, the practitioner is advised to assume a positive serum pregnancy test is a true positive.

Pelvic Examination

A pelvic examination involving both a speculum examination and bimanual examination is essential for differentiation of the entities listed in Tables 4-1 and 4-2.

The speculum examination is necessary for visualization of abnormal lesions, discharge, or ulcerations; to obtain cervical cultures; and to confirm that bleeding

Table 4-2. Spontaneous Abortions

Term	Clinical	Ultrasound findings
Threatened abortion	Vaginal bleeding or abdominal pain, os closed	Embryo with cardiac activity, or empty gestational sac (5-6.5 weeks), empty uterus (3-5 weeks), or subchorionic hemorrhage with any of the above
Complete abortion	History of vaginal bleeding, benign exam, os closed, falling β-hCG	Empty uterus
Incomplete abortion	History of vaginal bleeding, benign or tender exam, os open or closed, slowly falling or plateau β-hCG	Thickened, irregular endometrium (>5 mm double stripe)
Abortion in progress/inevitable abortion	Vaginal bleeding, os open	Gestational sac in process of expulsion
Embryonic demise (missed abortion)	Varied, os closed	Embryo lacking cardiac activity with crown-rump length >5 mm
Blighted ovum (anembryonic gestation, embryonic failure)	Varied, os open or closed	Gestational sac too big to not have embryo (>20 mm)
Septic abortion	Varied, os open or closed, tender exam, peritoneal signs, CMT, foul cervical discharge	Thickened endometrium and/or retained products of conception

originates from the cervix or vagina. In the pregnant patient, bleeding can result from causes unrelated to the pregnancy. If the spotting or bleeding does not appear to be from the cervix or vagina, bleeding from the lower gastrointestinal tract should be evaluated by inspection of the anus for hemorrhoids, palpation of the rectal canal, and evaluation for blood in the stool. Avoid cross-contamination of the stool guaiac test from vaginal blood.

Causes of cervical or vaginal bleeding not due to pregnancy itself include cervical carcinoma, vaginitis, cervical polyp, or cervical ectropion.

Cervical carcinomas can cause watery, foul, or bloody discharge, frequently presenting after intercourse. A recent normal Pap smear does not definitively rule out carcinoma, and any suspicious lesion should be referred to a gynecologist for biopsy. However, a lesion on the pregnant cervix should not be biopsied in the emergency department, as profuse bleeding can ensue and may be difficult to control.

Cervicitis from gonorrhea, *Chlamydia Trichomonas,* or bacterial vaginosis can lead to a spectrum of symptoms, ranging from no symptoms, to abnormal discharge, pain, or vaginal spotting. A wet-prep examination may assist in differentiating these diagnoses (see Chaps. 29 and 31). Cervical cultures for chlamydia and gonorrhea should be performed. See Appendix 2 for proper specimen collection and transport techniques.

Cervical ectropion or polyps can cause bleeding, especially postcoital bleeding. *Cervical ectropion* is common in pregnancy and easily recognizable. This is a normal condition, in which the more friable columnar epithelium that lines the endocervical canal is visible on the cervix. It appears as a smooth, reddened ring of tissue surrounding the cervical os. When touched with a cotton swab, it may start to ooze gently or cause a surprisingly steady stream of bleeding.

Cervical polyps are benign, pinkish buds that may protrude from the os. They should not be removed in the emergency department, as profuse bleeding may develop.

The walls of the vagina should also be inspected, as ulcers, small lacerations, and erosions due to infections, trauma, foreign body, or neoplasm can cause vaginal bleeding.

Bimanual Pelvic Examination

The pelvic examination should include an evaluation of the status of the internal os, and an attempt at assessing uterine size and the degree of uterine and/or adnexal tenderness.

Multiparous patients will often have a soft and slightly dilated external os, but it is the internal os that must dilate in order for passage of products of conception to occur. This can be assessed by *gently* passing one's examining finger through the external os into the internal os (but not into the uterus!). Often the cervix has a conical shape, with the closed internal os as the point of the cone. When the internal os is open and the uterus is in the process of expelling its contents, the cervix generally has a more shortened, softer, and cylindrical shape. If the examining finger is able to pass through the end-point of the cone or cylinder, then the internal os is open. If the examining finger is not able to penetrate the point of the cone, then the internal os is closed. One should not aggressively force the examining finger or attempt to pass any object other than the finger through the internal os to determine its integrity; to do so can cause injury to the os itself or potentially cause spontaneous abortion.

The uterus will not be appreciably tender unless products of conception are retained or passing through the cervix at that moment, or unless infection is present. Assessment and reassessment of the internal os and uterine tenderness over time are crucial for clinically differentiating incomplete from complete abortion.

Laboratory Evaluation

Urinalysis, Rh factor determination, CBC, and serum quantitative β-hCG are generally required to assess patients with first-trimester vaginal bleeding. Serum progesterone can also be determined, although it is not clinically useful at this time.

Urinalysis

A urinalysis should be ordered in all pregnant patients with vaginal bleeding to diagnose UTI even if there are no symptoms. UTIs are a risk factor for spontaneous abortion. Asymptomatic bacteriuria and pyuria occur in 2 to 11 percent of pregnant women, and up to one-fourth will develop upper-tract infections[4] (see Chap. 17 for further discussion of UTIs). Given the difficulty in obtaining a truly clean-catch specimen in a woman with vaginal bleeding, an in-and-out catheterized urine specimen is frequently necessary for efficient patient management.

Rh Factor Determination and Rh Immune Globulin Administration

Completed abortion, ectopic pregnancy, antepartum hemorrhage, and trauma are associated with fetomaternal transfusion, and thus raise the potential for Rh isoimmunization if the mother is Rh-negative and the fetus is Rh-positive. The literature support for this concept in patients with threatened abortion is equivocal,[5] but it is the standard of care to administer Rh immune prophylaxis to Rh-negative pregnant women with vaginal bleeding.[6,7] If the gestation is less than 12 weeks, a dose of 50 mcg IM is sufficient. However, as pregnancy dating can be difficult and inaccurate, it is recommended that Rh-negative women with vaginal bleeding in the first or second trimester receive 300 mcg of Rh immune globulin IM. Protection is provided if Rh immune globulin is administered within 72 hours of the onset of bleeding, but because follow-up cannot be certain, it should be given in the ED. It is not necessary to repeat the dosage at subsequent ED or clinic visits for continued or repeated bleeding before 20 weeks gestation. Another 300 mcg dose should be administered in the third trimester or prior to delivery.

Complete Blood Count

A CBC is routinely obtained in bleeding patients to assess blood loss and to establish a baseline.

Serum Quantitative Beta Human Chorionic Gonadotropin (β-hCG)

The quantitative beta human chorionic gonadotropin (β-hCG) is a measure of trophoblastic tissue activity, which is a marker for the volume of living trophoblastic tissue and a function of renal clearance. Both ectopic and intrauterine pregnancies produce β-hCG, though they usually differ in the rate at which the quantitative β-hCG level increases. Patients with ectopic pregnancy tend to have a lower quantitative β-hCG than those with viable intrauterine pregnancies of the same gestational age[8] (see Chap. 5). However, abnormal intrauterine pregnancies (IUPs) may have lower β-hCGs than normal ones. Because of the wide range of β-hCG for each stage of embryonic development, a single β-hCG level is not useful for differentiating between normal IUP, abnormal IUP, and ectopic pregnancy.[9] However, comparisons of at least two serum β-hCG values 48 hours apart are useful for identification of a variation in the expected rate of rise of the β-hCG level.[7] The β-hCG normally doubles in 1.9 ± 0.5 days, and plateaus at a level of about 10,000 mIU/mL or at about 10 weeks' gestational age.[10] Also, an increase of $\geq$66 percent over 48 hours is seen in 85 percent of normal intrauterine pregnancies. An insufficient, abnormal increase is thus <66 percent over 48 hours,[11] and this is 75 percent sensitive and 93 percent specific for an abnormal gestation of some variety.[10] Eighty-five percent of ectopic pregnancies and 15 percent of normal intrauterine pregnancies have abnormal β-hCG dynamics.[12] Declining β-hCG levels indicate nonviability of the pregnancy, either ectopic or intrauterine. The rate of fall of β-hCG has been found to differ significantly between ectopic pregnancy and abortion. The half-life of the β-hCG is >7 days in ectopic pregnancy, whereas it is <1.4 days in aborting IUPs.[12] A falling β-hCG does not exclude the possibility of ectopic pregnancy. A β-hCG of <1000 mIU/mL should not preclude a clinician from obtaining a pelvic ultrasound to rule out ectopic, because 15 percent of these patients will have a diagnostic ultrasound.[13]

Serum Progesterone

There has been a great deal of literature about progesterone, another hormone elevated in pregnancy, and its potential to discriminate between normal gestation, abnormal gestation, and ectopic pregnancy. The progesterone level does not vary with gestational age. A progesterone level >25 ng/mL implies a 97 percent chance of normalcy and a progesterone of <5 ng/mL is nearly 100 percent predictive of abnormal gestation.[14] However, 31 percent of IUPs, 23 percent of abnormal IUPs, and 52 percent of ectopic pregnancies had progesterone values that fell between 10 and 20 ng/mL.[15] Thus there is too much overlap between categories for the progesterone level to be clinically useful.

Pelvic Ultrasonography

Pelvic ultrasonography is essential for identifying viable intrauterine and molar pregnancies, a key component in distinguishing between complete and incomplete abortion, and diagnosing ectopic pregnancy. If the cervical os is closed, bleeding is not heavy, and there is little uterine tenderness on pelvic examination, ultrasound can confirm the clinical diagnosis of complete abortion based on the presence of an empty uterus.[16] Ultrasound is also useful in evaluating the prognosis for a gestation that is threatened clinically. There are sonographic findings consistent

Table 4-3. Sonographic Landmarks of Early Pregnancy

	Est. Gestational Age (weeks)	Serum Quantitative β-hCG (mIU/mL)
Gestational sac	4.5	>1500
Yolk sac	5.5	1000-7500
Embryo with cardiac activity	6.5	7000-23,000

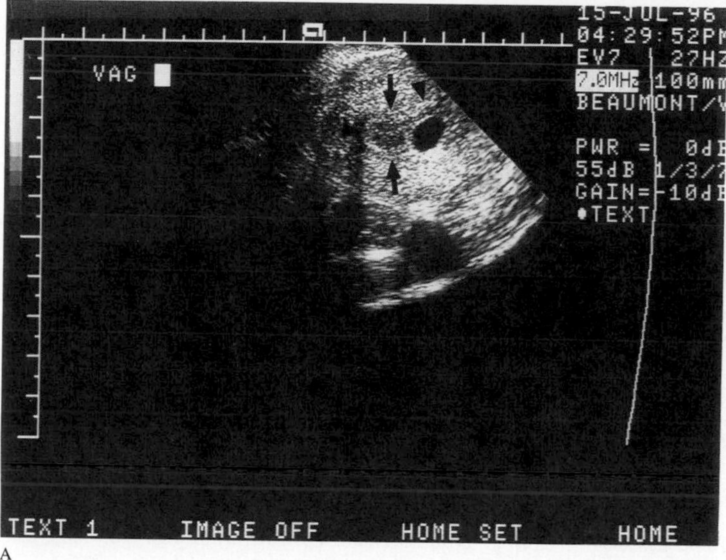

A

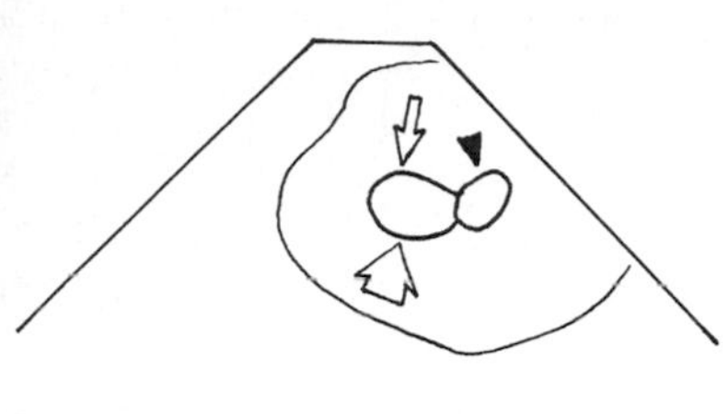

B

Fig. 4-1. *A*. On this ultrasound image, an early gestational sac appears as a black circle (*arrowhead*). Note that it is eccentrically placed in relation to the uterine cavity (*arrows*). This is an important point in differentiating a true gestational sac from a pseudosac of an ectopic pregnancy, which is centrally placed. *B*. Line drawing of same image.

with normal gestational development at various levels of β-hCG (Table 4-3). If pelvic ultrasonography confirms the presence of an intrauterine pregnancy (IUP), ectopic pregnancy is ostensibly ruled out (see Chap. 5).

The hormones of pregnancy cause an early uterine decidual reaction that may be seen soon after a missed menses by ultrasound, but this is nonspecific and occurs with both intrauterine and ectopic pregnancies.

The earliest sonographic landmark consistent with an intrauterine pregnancy is the gestational sac. With endovaginal ultrasound, this can be visualized as early as 4.5 weeks after the LMP, and reliably by 5 weeks. The gestational sac lies eccentrically within the decidua of the endometrium (Fig. 4-1), and is seen to have two sonographically distinct layers, the decidua capsularis and decidua parietalis. These two layers give a sonographic appearance of two rings, called the "double ring sign," that is diagnostic of an intrauterine gestational sac. The yolk sac seen within the gestational sac is the next sonographic landmark of the developing pregnancy, and it is seen reliably by the end of the fifth week. The embryo and cardiac activity are seen concurrently and reliably adjacent to the yolk sac by 6.5 weeks gestation by endovaginal ultrasound[17] (Fig. 4-2).

The sonographic finding that is most reassuring for a favorable prognosis is the presence of embryonic cardiac activity. For women under 35 years of age at least 8 weeks estimated gestational age (EGA), the presence of cardiac activity sonographically indicates an overall spontaneous abortion rate of 3 to 5 percent. This increases to about 8 percent for women over 35 years of age. Sonographic findings that foreshadow a poor outcome include a slow embryonic heart rate (<90 bpm), a small gestational sac for the size of the embryo, and a large yolk sac (>6 mm). Gestations with a subchorionic hematoma greater than two-thirds the circumference of the chorion have a twofold increase in their rate of spontaneous abortion (19 percent) compared to those with a small or medium sized subchorionic hematoma (9 percent).[18]

Differential Diagnosis and Emergency Department Management

Ectopic Pregnancy

Ectopic pregnancy occurs in about 3 percent of pregnancies and is discussed in detail in Chap. 5. The diagnoses to follow can only be made once ectopic pregnancy has been excluded.

Implantation Bleeding

If the bleeding is experienced around the time of or just after the expected normal menses, *implantation bleeding*

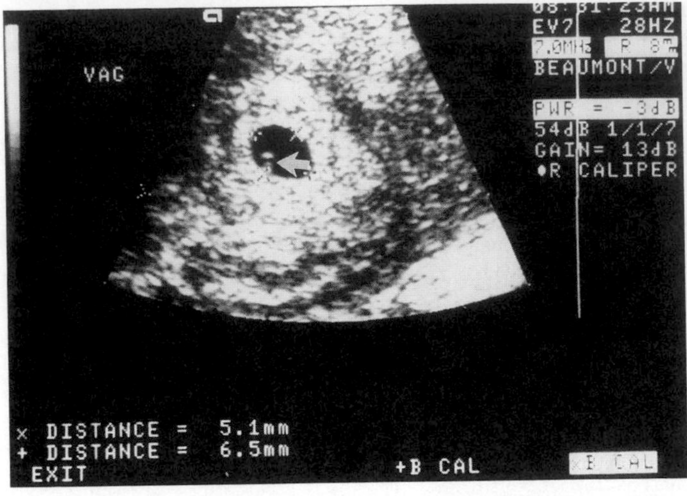

A

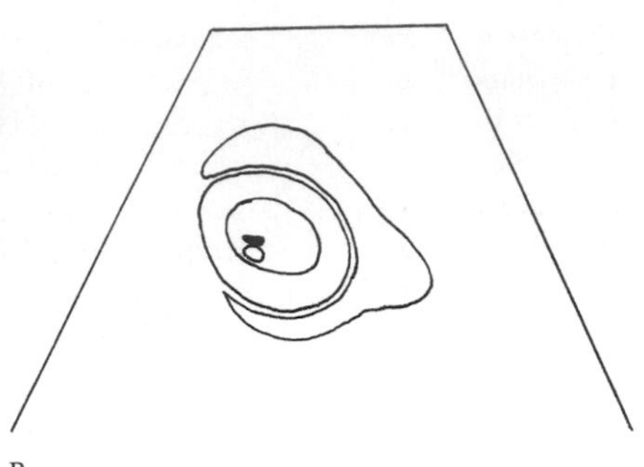

B

Fig. 4-2. *A*. Yolk sac. This can be detected by ultrasound at about 5.5 weeks (menstrual dates). It is a round, doughnut-shaped structure (*arrow*), on the surface of which the embryo will appear (*white "dash" just above tip of arrow*). *B*. Line drawing of same image.

should be considered. This is a fairly common occurrence with a benign physiologic cause. As the embryo burrows into the highly vascular decidual tissue, blood escapes into the uterine cavity and out through the cervix. It ranges from a pinkish discoloration of the vaginal discharge to bleeding equivalent to that of a menstrual period. It can last 1 or 2 days but usually not longer. Most commonly, it occurs in the fifth or sixth week after the LMP and women sometimes mistake this bleeding for normal menses; thus it is a common cause of inaccurate dating as well. The pelvic examination is normal, with a closed internal os and nontender uterus. The findings on pelvic ultrasound should correlate with the serum β-hCG level for gestational age and should demonstrate an intrauterine pregnancy. Implantation bleeding is a presumptive diagnosis of exclusion after ectopic pregnancy has been excluded. It is suggested primarily by the timing of bleeding. It is important to consider the diagnosis in order to be able to reassure patients that not all bleeding is related to abnormal pregnancies. No treatment is indicated.

Abortions

The WHO definition of abortion is "induced or spontaneous termination of pregnancy before 20 weeks gestation." Table 4-2 defines the spectrum of abortions, with their clinical, laboratory, and ultrasound findings.

Complete or Incomplete Abortion

The pelvic examination can be dramatic in the case of an abortion in progress, with products of conception in the open cervical os at the time of examination. The products may be easily removed by grasping with a ring forceps and application of gentle traction. If more than gentle traction is required, there may be incomplete separation of tissue from the endometrium. Do not simply pull harder, as mechanical separation can result in severe hemorrhage. Obtain gynecologic consultation for assistance in this instance. However, if tissue is removed manually or spontaneously, bleeding and pain quickly stop. Tissue should be sent to the laboratory for identification of chorionic villi. Routine chromosomal analysis is not necessary unless the woman has had multiple pregnancy losses. Products of conception should not be sent for genetic analysis in formalin as it destroys cells, so lactated Ringer's is a more appropriate transport medium.

Patients with an open *internal* cervical os and brisk vaginal bleeding on initial examination should have a gynecologic consultation in the ED for possible uterine evacuation of presumed incomplete abortion. If there is uncertainty as to whether a spontaneous abortion is in progress or completed, ultrasound can be helpful to determine if there is residual gestational tissue within the uterine cavity. If pain and bleeding have resolved, the internal cervical os is closed or closing, and there is no uterine tenderness, the diagnosis is completed abortion, and the patient can be discharged with gynecologic follow-up arranged in 1 week.

Blighted Ovum, Embryonic Failure, and Intrauterine Embryonic Demise

Patients with embryonic demise or blighted ovum may be managed according to the preference of the gynecologist and the patient herself. Unless she is bleeding heavily or febrile, there is no urgency to evacuate the uterus. Observation and expectant management can be continued for 2 weeks without increased complications. However, many gynecologists prefer to perform a uterine evacuation procedure sooner than 2 weeks, so management depends on the practice environment. Patients will also vary in their preferences, with some insisting on immediate evacuation, and others preferring expectant care.

Threatened Abortion

Characteristics of threatened abortion are vaginal bleeding or abdominal pain with a closed cervical os (Table 4-2). Ectopic pregnancy is always a diagnostic concern. Patients who are hemodynamically stable, with closed internal cervical os, no evidence for ectopic pregnancy, and reliable access to gynecologic follow-up may be discharged. Gynecologic follow-up should be provided in 48 hours to follow serial β-hCG levels if ectopic pregnancy has not been definitively excluded. Patients are advised to avoid strenuous activity or exertion, including sexual activity, until bleeding stops. These recommendations are primarily for patient comfort, because there is no evidence that reduction of activity or medical therapy will affect the outcome of a threatened abortion. Patients should be advised that there is no intervention that can prevent abortion at this stage of pregnancy. Any feelings of guilt expressed or exhibited by the patient or her family should be dealt with compassionately. Referral to professional counseling or support groups can be provided, and preprinted discharge instructions with appropriate referral phone numbers may be very useful. Patients should be advised to return to the ED immediately if they become dizzy or febrile, develop heavy bleeding, pass tissue, or develop severe cramping, as these symptoms suggest progression of abortion.

Septic Abortion

The estimated fatality rate from septic abortion is very low, ranging from 0.4 to 0.6 per 100,000 spontaneous abortions. Septic abortion is a polymicrobial infection and should be treated with antibiotics and evacuation of the uterus. Blood and cervical discharge should be obtained for culture. For mild endometritis, CDC recommendations[19] are ofloxacin, 400 mg PO bid plus clindamycin (450 mg PO qid) or metronidazole (500 mg PO bid) for 14 days; or ceftriaxone 250 mg IM and doxycycline 100 mg PO bid for 14 days. Patients with fever, uterine tenderness, or peritonitis require admission for IV antibiotics and evacuation of the uterus. There are several regimens: cefotetan (2 g IV) or ampicillin-sulbactam 3 g IV or imipenem 500 mg IV are common single-agent therapies. Clindamycin 900 mg IV plus gentamicin 5 mg/kg IV or ceftriaxone 2 g IV is an alternative. See Chap. 6 for additional discussion of septic abortions related to instrumentation.

GESTATIONAL TROPHOBLASTIC DISEASE

Although gestational trophoblastic disease (commonly called *molar pregnancy*) is unusual, it typically presents as bleeding in the first half of pregnancy. Also known as hydatidiform mole, it is more commonly seen in those of Asian descent, those who have had prior trophoblastic disease, and first pregnancies in the early or late years of childbearing (<15 or >35 years old). In the general population, the incidence is 1 in 1000, though it may be as high as 1 percent in the Asian population. Although usually benign, it does have malignant potential and requires long-term and careful follow-up. Abnormal proliferation of the trophoblastic cells is the underlying pathophysiology of gestational trophoblastic disease (GTD). This entity is generally divided into two categories: the complete and the partial mole. In complete molar pregnancy, fetal tissues are absent and the 46,XX karyotype is generally of duplicated paternal origin (i.e., both X chromosomes come from the sperm). In the partial mole, fetal tissues are present (there can even be a viable fetus) and, as a result of dispermy, the usual karyotype is triploidy (69,XXY). Complete moles are more likely to lead to persistent or metastatic disease. At the more serious end of the spectrum of GTD is choriocarcinoma. It usually follows a partial molar pregnancy but may follow a full-term pregnancy or can arise in the ovaries, unassociated with pregnancy. Choriocarcinoma is a malignant lesion that fortunately is usually responsive to chemotherapy. Frequently, GTD presents with abnormal bleeding mimicking an incomplete or threatened abortion. Other signs are passage of hydropic villi (that tend to have a grape-like appearance) through the vagina. Uterine size is larger (50 percent) or smaller (25 percent) than the estimated gestational age,

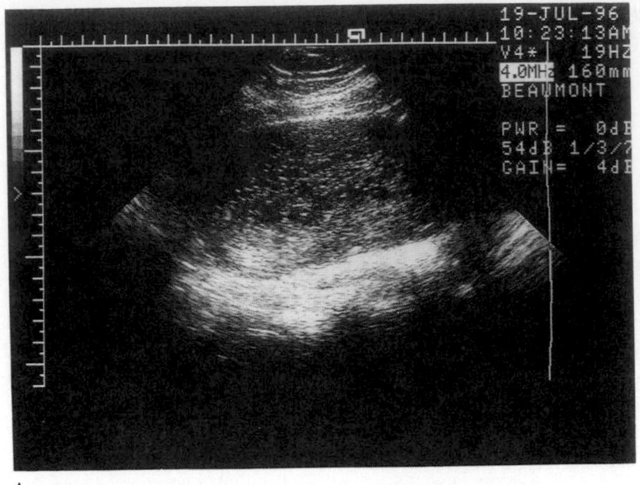

A

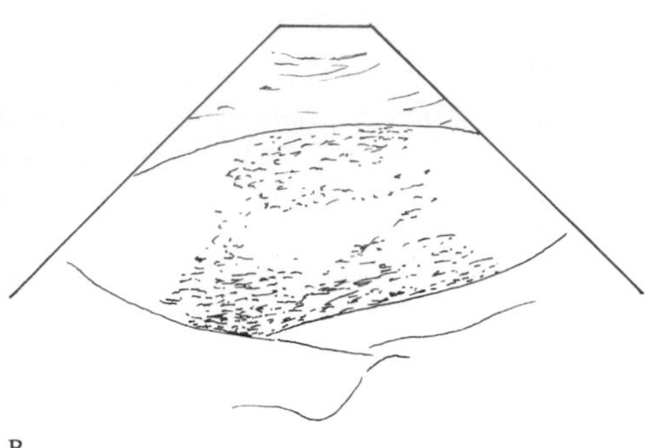

B

Fig. 4-3. *A*. Ultrasound image of hydatidiform mole (gestational trophoblastic disease). The uterus is occupied by echogenic material. *B*. Line drawing of same image.

or there may be enlarged cystic ovaries resulting from theca-lutein cysts. Additional common patient complaints include severe nausea or vomiting. Unusually, the patient may have signs of preeclampsia (see Chap. 8) or hyperthyroidism. A characteristic but unusual pattern on ultrasound ("snowstorm pattern") may accompany a molar pregnancy. The ultrasound appearance of many lucent areas interspersed with brighter areas is shown in Fig. 4-3. The β-hCG level is usually higher than expected for gestational age (generally greater than 100,000 mIU/mL). The definitive diagnosis is made by histologic evaluation of the tissue, which frequently is not done until after surgical evacuation. After removal, follow-up measurements of β-hCG should be done to ensure there is no persistent or metastatic disease. If gestational trophoblastic disease is suspected, the uterus should be evacuated as soon as possible, although this need not be done emergently unless signs of preeclampsia or hemodynamic instability are present. Nevertheless, the patient should be seen by an obstetrician-gynecologist urgently so definitive therapy can be arranged. Because some moles produce thyroid hormone, and any hyperthyroidism should be treated prior to operative intervention, thyroid studies should be obtained from the ED if there are any symptoms of hyperthyroidism.

NAUSEA AND VOMITING IN PREGNANCY

Despite the common nature of nausea and vomiting in pregnancy, most pregnant women will never become sick enough to present to the emergency department, and only 1 to 2 percent will require hospital admission.[20] The syndrome of intractable vomiting and weight loss, hypokalemia, or ketonemia is called *hyperemesis gravidarum.* The etiology is still unknown, but hormonal, neurologic, metabolic, toxic, and psychosomatic factors are all described. Most experts consider human chorionic gonadotropin (hCG) to be a causative factor,[21] though this association remains controversial.[22,23] Goodwin and associates described higher total as well as free β subunits of hCG concentrations in women with hyperemesis as compared with asymptomatic controls.[24] There is a significant difference in the incidence of nausea and vomiting in patients with spontaneous abortions (50 percent) as compared with those having induced abortions (80 percent), suggesting an inverse association with inadequate production of placental hormone.[25] Fifty to 70 percent of patients with hyperemesis gravidarum have elevated levels of free T_4 and T_3, which return to normal as soon as hyperemesis resolves.[26] Serum β-hCG levels correlate negatively with TSH and positively with free T_4 levels, though multiple studies suggest that the transient changes in free T_4 and TSH are due to the bioactivity of hCG and not secondary to primary altered thyroid function.[27–29]

Clinical Assessment

The history and physical examination should focus on assessing the severity of symptoms and findings and the need for fluid resuscitation, as well as excluding other more serious causes. The usual sequence of events of

Table 4-4. Differential Diagnosis of Nausea and Vomiting in Pregnancy

Diagnosis	Typical Key Distinguishing Clinical Diagnostic Features
Gastric mucosal irritation (NSAIDs, alcohol)	Abdominal pain decreased by food
Appendicitis	Abdominal pain, tenderness, fever
Cholelithiasis/cholecystitis	Abdominal pain increases with meals, increased LFTs
Hepatitis	Abdominal pain, increased LFTs, jaundice
Pancreatitis	Abdominal pain, increased lipase
Pyelonephritis	Dysuria, flank pain and tenderness, fever
Endocrine disorders (thyrotoxicosis, DKA, hyper-or hypoparathyroidism, adrenal insufficiency)	History, lab abnormalities
Bowel obstruction/obstipation	Abdominal pain, vomiting, constipation
Vestibular nerve stimulation/labyrinthitis	Nystagmus, vertigo
Increased intracranial pressure	Headache, papilledema
Meningeal irritation	Headache
Medications (antiseizure agents, theophylline, digitalis, salicylates)	History, drug levels
Reflux esophagitis	Retrosternal burning pain
Diaphragmatic hernia	Vomiting, abdominal pain
Achalasia	Difficulty swallowing
Psychiatric disease	History
Gastroenteritis, food poisoning	Diarrhea, fever

nausea and vomiting of pregnancy includes loss of appetite or anorexia at 5 to 6 weeks of gestation, followed by nausea and subsequently vomiting. Typically, eating or drinking quickly exacerbates these symptoms. The presence of abdominal pain suggests another etiology such as pyelonephritis, cholecystitis, appendicitis, or pancreatitis. A medication history is necessary to identify prescription, over-the-counter, or other drugs that can cause nausea and vomiting (Table 4-4).

Patients with pregnancy-induced nausea and vomiting present with few physical signs other than those of mild dehydration, or postural symptoms. Late findings such as dry mucosa or poor skin turgor may be present if symptoms are more severe or longstanding. Assessment for other diagnostic possibilities requires focused examination looking specifically for jaundice and for costovertebral tenderness. The presence of abdominal tenderness or distention must lead to assessments for gynecologic, surgical, or infectious disorders. Rectal examination may be appropriate to identify stool impaction and should include testing for occult blood. Pelvic examination is generally necessary in the presence of abdominal or pelvic pain, or vaginal bleeding or discharge, as typically ectopic pregnancy or incomplete abortion have not yet been excluded.

Laboratory testing includes a complete blood count, serum electrolytes and ketones, BUN and creatinine, and urinalysis. Elevated hematocrit and BUN may be present due to hemoconcentration. Hyper- or hyponatremia or hypokalemia may be evident. Urinalysis is important to determine the specific gravity and to identify infection. Radiographic imaging should be obtained as dictated by the clinical picture. In patients determined to have hyperemesis gravidarum, pelvic ultrasonography may be helpful to assure the presence of fetal cardiac activity, to identify multiple gestations, or to diagnose molar pregnancies. An upper abdominal ultrasound should be ordered if the clinical evaluation suggests gallbladder disease, pancreatitis, or liver disease. Obviously unnecessary radiation exposure should be avoided, but if the assessment suggests need for abdominal-pelvic CT scanning for appendicitis, diverticulitis, or other intraabdominal pathology, then the studies should be obtained. Information on relative radiation exposure is presented in Appendix 1.

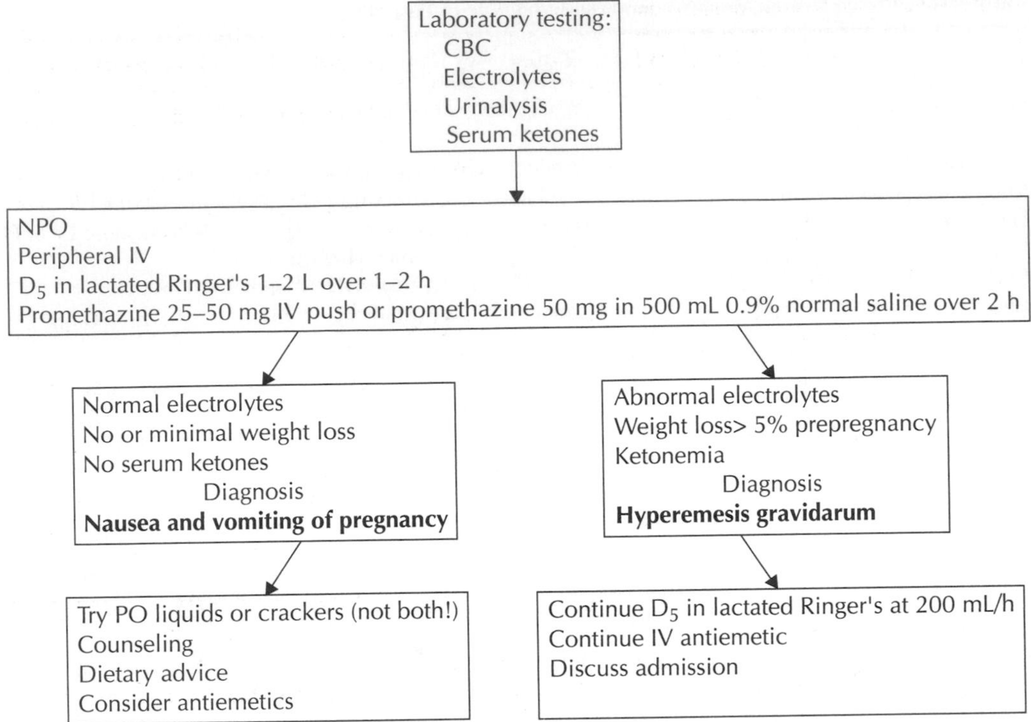

Fig. 4-4. Algorithm for the management of nausea and vomiting of pregnancy and hyperemesis gravidarum.

Emergency Department Management

This section is limited to the ED management of nausea and vomiting of pregnancy and hyperemesis gravidarum (Fig. 4-4). Management of specific intraabdominal disease states is covered elsewhere (see Chap. 14). When another etiology for the nausea and vomiting is established, management guidelines should follow a pattern similar to that followed if the patient were not pregnant. In those cases, consultation with the antenatal care provider is recommended to coordinate the care of both the patient and her fetus.

If the patient appears clinically dehydrated or when ketonuria is present, 20 mL/kg (usually 1 to 2 L) of D_5-lactated Ringer's or D_5-normal saline should be given intravenously. If laboratory studies are within normal limits, the goal is to correct the dehydration and ensure the patient is able to tolerate oral liquids prior to discharge.

When the patient has intractable vomiting and weight loss, and laboratory studies reveal hypokalemia or ketonemia, the criteria are met for the diagnosis of hyperemesis gravidarum. As solid food or liquid usually aggravates vomiting, the patient should initially take nothing by mouth. Intravenous rehydration is started with D_5LR or D_5NS. For initial rehydration, 3 to 5 L of crystalloid are commonly necessary. Because of the potential, though rare, complication of Wernicke's encephalopathy, many advocate the administration of thiamine 100 mg IV, either as part of the initial IV fluid replacement or before administration of dextrose.[30] Relief of patient symptoms is the primary end-point in initial rehydration, though correction of laboratory abnormalities is also a goal of ED management.

Antiemetics should be administered intravenously. Phenothiazines, metoclopramide, trimethobenzamide, and ondansetron are all choices with no apparent risk to the fetus[31] (Table 4-5).

Admission criteria include persistent vomiting and/or electrolyte abnormalities and/or ketosis despite fluid resuscitation, uncertainty of diagnosis, and weight loss greater than 10 percent of the prepregnancy weight. When patients have lost more than 5 to 10 percent of their prepregnancy body weight and oral feeding is not tolerated, options for inpatient management include placement of a feeding tube and total parenteral nutrition through a central line.[32–34] Some insurance plans have mandated that some of these women be discharged from the hospital for continued parenteral home care with central lines in

Table 4-5. Antiemetics for Nausea/Vomiting and Hyperemesis Gravidarum

Antiemetic	Brand Name	FDA Category	IV Dose	Oral/Rectal Dose
Promethazine	Phenergan	C	25-50 mg bolus or infused over 2 h	25 mg PO/PR q4h
Prochlorperazine	Compazine	C	10 mg bolus over 2 min, max 40 mg q24h	10 mg PO q6-8h or 25 mg PR q12h
Metoclopramide	Reglan	B	10 mg over 1-2 min q4-6h or 1 mg/kg over 30 min	Same dose IV or PO
Ondansetron[35]	Zofran	B	4-8 mg q4h	4-8 mg PO q8h
Maintenance therapy for nausea and vomiting of pregnancy				
Pyridoxine with doxylamine[36]	Vitamin B_6 Unisom	A		25 mg q8h, 25 mg qhs
Diphenhydramine	Benadryl	B		25-50 mg q6h
Maintenance therapy for hyperemesis gravidarum				
Metoclopramide	Reglan	B		As above
Trimethobenzamide	Tigan	C	200 mg IM q6-8h	250 mg PO or 200 mg PR q6-8h

place. Therefore, presentation to the emergency department with a number of complications associated with parenteral nutrition and central line problems may be seen. Catheter-induced sepsis can be an important source of morbidity in these women. Table 4-6 lists the maternal complications of hyperemesis gravidarum and its therapy with NG tube feeding and/or TPN.[37] Readmission for relapse of hyperemesis gravidarum occurs in about 27 percent of these patients.[38] Additional effective modalities for outpatient management include psychotherapy, hypnotherapy, and behavior modification.

Disposition

Teaching the usual expected events of pregnancy are important for the patient's well-being and decreases the likelihood of return visits to the ED. The average time of onset of pregnancy-associated nausea and vomiting is in weeks 4 through 6, the worst symptomatology occurs in weeks 8 through 12, and complete resolution occurs by 20 weeks.[39–42] Even though this syndrome is typically called "morning sickness," 50 percent of pregnant women with nausea and vomiting of pregnancy experience their symptoms mainly in the morning, one-third experience them throughout the day, and the remainder have symptoms mainly at night.[39] The recurrence rate in future pregnancies is 60 percent.[38] A decreased risk of miscarriage, fetal mortality, and perinatal mortality has been noted for women with nausea and vomiting during pregnancy.[38–42]

Discharge instructions should recommend follow-up for routine prenatal care. The patient should return if symptoms are severe, if she is not able to tolerate fluids, or if new symptoms such as abdominal pain or fever develop. Bed rest is not generally recommended.

Table 4-6. Maternal Complications of Hyperemesis Gravidarum and Its Therapy with TPN/Tube Feeding

Central line complications: Catheter-induced sepsis, pneumothorax, hemothorax, brachial plexus injury, catheter malposition
Medical complications: renal and hepatic insufficiency, stroke, septic emboli, retinal hemorrhage, hematemesis, gastric aspiration, Wernicke's encephalopathy
Surgical complications: esophageal rupture
Obstetric complications: persistent symptoms requiring readmission

Table 4-7. Counseling to Minimize Pregnancy-Induced Nausea and Vomiting

- Reassurance that nausea and vomiting carries minimal fetal risk
- Avoid strong odors, cigarette smoke, cooking odors, or fumes
- Decrease size and increase frequency of meals
- Stop prenatal vitamins and iron supplements until symptoms resolve
- Avoid mixing solids and liquids
- Avoid fatty foods
- Maintain oral hydration with electrolyte-rich drinks, such as Gatorade or bouillon; avoid sweet drinks
- Start oral intake with soups, followed by complex starches (pasta, rice, potatoes); add chicken or turkey for protein as tolerated

In addition to the antiemetics listed in Table 4-5, the following recommendations have been shown to be safe for treatment of mild to moderate nausea and vomiting with some efficacy: acupressure (mainly for patients with nausea and little vomiting[43]); wrist or "sea bands" (available in boating stores, automobile clubs, and some drug stores); ginger ale or capsules containing 250 mg of ginger root four times a day.[44]

Some counseling tips to minimize pregnancy-induced nausea and vomiting are given in Table 4-7.

HEADACHE AND PREGNANCY

Headaches are a leading cause of referral to primary care physicians and account for 2 to 4 percent of emergency department visits.[45] Women are affected more frequently than men, with the peak incidence in childbearing years. Headaches are classified as either primary or secondary disorders in keeping with the 1988 recommendations of the Classification Committee of the International Headache Society. In pregnant women, as in all headache sufferers, headaches are grouped into categories based on key clinical features. *Primary headaches* are those associated with absence of signs of organic disease, and *secondary headaches* are those associated with specific disease processes (Table 4-8). Headaches can be a presenting symptom of a variety of neurological or systemic disorders.[46,47] Warning signs of a potentially life-threatening disease are important to elicit during the initial evaluation, and are listed in Table 4-9.

If concerning signs or symptoms are encountered, immediate imaging studies are almost always required. CT scan of the brain can be safely performed with appropriate shielding of the fetus. CT scans are preferred for evaluation of intracranial or subarachnoid hemorrhage, while MRI is superior for evaluation of cerebral infarct, tumor, or infection. Magnetic resonance venography is a noninvasive and non-contrast-requiring tool that is excellent for diagnosing cerebral vein thrombosis. MRI is thought to be safe during pregnancy, although no systematic study has been done. Contrast agents are best avoided due to lack of available data on safety (see Appendix 1).

Primary causes of headache include migraine and tension-type headaches. ED management of these entities is no different in pregnant women than in the nonpregnant person. Secondary causes of headaches are discussed in Chapter 18.

Migraine

Clinical Assessment

Migraine headaches are usually episodic, unilateral or bilateral, and throbbing, and associated with nausea, vomiting, and photophobia, and relieved by sleep. Patients typically have a history of previous migraine headaches with a similar pattern of associated symptoms. A first-

Table 4-8. Differential Diagnosis of Headaches in Pregnancy

Primary Headaches	Secondary Headaches
Migraine	*Life-threatening*
Tension headache	Subarachnoid hemorrhage
	Intraparenchymal hemorrhage
	Central venous thrombosis
	Stroke
	CNS tumor or infection
	Preeclampsia/eclampsia
	Non-life threatening
	Sinus headache
	Benign intracranial hypertension (pseudotumor cerebri)

Table 4-9. Warning Signs in Patients with Headaches

New onset headaches in pregnancy
Headaches with different characteristics from previous headaches
Worst headache of one's life
Focal neurologic deficit
Meningismus
Fever
Altered consciousness
Papilledema or other signs of increased intracranial pressure
Retinal hemorrhages
Increased blood pressure (may herald preeclampsia or eclampsia)
Postpartum headaches (need to exclude cerebral vein thrombosis)

time migraine-type headache during pregnancy is an indication for emergent imaging, either with CT or MRI to rule out secondary life-threatening causes of headache (Table 4-8). Further testing should be guided by the clinical presentation.

Classic migraine is associated with an aura, while absence of an aura suggests the diagnosis of common migraine. The aura is usually a visual phenomenon (scintillating scotoma), but may be somatosensory or rarely motor. The aura may last for 20 to 30 minutes and may be followed by a brief period of normalcy. Typically the headache follows, lasting from a few hours to a day. Migraine may improve during pregnancy due to high levels of estrogen, but approximately 23 percent of patients worsen during this time.[48] Women with migraine *do not* have an increased incidence of fetal malformations, miscarriage, eclampsia, or spontaneous abortion relative to women without migraine.[49] New-onset headache associated with scintillating scotoma after 20 weeks' gestation may be a presentation of preeclampsia (see Chap. 8). Preeclampsia may also present in this manner prior to 20 weeks' gestation in patients with hydatidiform mole.

Emergency Department Management

Severe migraine headaches in the ED can be treated with narcotics, although propoxyphene (class D) should be avoided due to significant risk of fetal malformation. Antiemetics have become a mainstay of ED management of migraine headache, and these are appropriate in pregnancy as well. Nonsteroidal antiinflammatory agents are an option in the first and second trimester, but should be avoided in the third trimester. Acetaminophen is a safe drug, but it is frequently ineffective in standard over-the-counter doses (10 mg/kg). Better success is achieved with acetaminophen doses of 15 to 20 mg/kg (PO or PR) lean body weight. Antimigraine agents such as serotonin agonists and ergots are best avoided, even though sumatriptan is category C, because of the increased risk of thromboembolic and cerebrovascular diseases in pregnancy. The outpatient treatment of chronic migraine in pregnancy remains a challenge due to the potential toxicity of antimigraine agents. Prophylactic agents such as β-blockers and tricyclic antidepressants are classified as category C, except amitryptyline, nortriptyline, and imipramine, which are classified as category D. Obstetric and neurologic consultation is necessary to plan outpatient management for pregnant or lactating women. See Table 4-10 for medications used for chronic outpatient management of migraines.

Tension Headaches

Patients presenting with tension headaches complain of a band-like or constricting bilateral headache that may wax or wane in intensity, but is almost always persistent. Patients complain of muscular tenderness over the scalp and neck. There may be underlying psychological stress, but that may not be evident unless specifically inquired about. Pain management of tension headaches requires an approach similar to that for migraine headaches in the ED setting (Table 4-11). Nonpharmacologic treatment such as biofeedback and physical therapy are definitely preferred over chronic use of medications.[50]

Pseudotumor Cerebri

Benign intracranial hypertension, also known as pseudotumor cerebri, is primarily a disease of young, obese women. There is no increase in incidence of this disorder in pregnancy compared to the general population.[51] Classic symptoms include diffuse, unremitting headache associated with transient or progressive visual loss. Recent history of significant weight gain is common. Papilledema and marked visual field constriction are noted on examination. Usual treatment is with acetazolamide and weight loss, both of which should be avoided in pregnancy. Serial lumbar puncture or steroids are options in resistant cases.[46,47] Major morbidity is related to visual loss that can be permanent, therefore early neuro-ophthalmologic consultation should be obtained in case of rapid or progressive visual loss. Optic nerve sheath fenestration can be performed in such cases to prevent optic nerve damage.

Table 4-10. Medications for Outpatient Management of Migraine in Pregnancy and Lactation

Name	FDA Pregnancy Category	Breast-Feeding
Aspirin	C (D in third trimester)	Caution
Acetaminophen	B	Compatible
Caffeine	B	Compatible
Ibuprofen	B (D in third trimester)	Compatible
Indomethacin	B (D in third trimester)	Compatible
Naproxen	B (D in third trimester)	Compatible
Cyproheptadine	C	Concern
Promethazine	C	NA
Metoclopramide	B	Concern
Codeine	C (D if prolonged)	Compatible
Propoxyphene	D	Contraindicated
Ergotamine/dihydroergotamine	Contraindicated	Contraindicated
Sumatriptan/zolmitriptan/ naratriptan/rizatriptan	C	Caution
Propranolol	C	Compatible
Verapamil	C	Compatible
Amitriptyline/nortriptyline/imipramine	D	Concern
Fluoxetine	B	Caution
Paroxetine	C	Concern
Sertraline	B	Concern
Methysergide	D	Caution

LOW BACK PAIN

Low back pain is a common symptom during pregnancy. For the majority of women, the discomfort does not represent a harbinger of significant pathology. Prospective studies have shown that 50 to 90 percent of women develop back pain during pregnancy.[52–54] Approximately 9 percent of these women have back pain so severe that they have to discontinue work. Most back pain is worse in the evening and at night.[55] Risk factors include lack of antenatal exercise, advancing age and parity, poor posture, or improper lifting.

Several changes occur during pregnancy that make back pain more prevalent, including changes in posture and weight distribution. Enlargement of the uterus and relaxation of the abdominal muscles produce a backward displacement of the spine and increase the work of the paraspinal muscles. Additionally, the effect of increased levels of the hormone relaxin causes greater flexibility in ligaments and increases mobility of sacroiliac joints.[55–61]

Table 4-11. Medications for Emergency Department Management of Headache

Name	FDA Category	Dosage/Route
Morphine	C	0.05-0.1 mg/kg IM/IV
Meperidine	C	50-150 mg PO/IM/IV/SC
Ketorolac	C	30-60 mg IM/IV × 1
Promethazine	C	12.5-25 mg PO/PR/IM/IV
Metoclopramide	B	5-10 mg PO/IM/IV
Acetaminophen/hydrocodone	C	1-2 tabs PO q4-6h, max 8 tabs/24 h
Acetaminophen/codeine	C	1-2 tabs PO q4-6h, max 8 tabs/24 h
Ibuprofen	B	400-600 mg PO q4-6h, max 2400 mg/24 h
Acetaminophen	B	10-20 mg/kg PO/PR q4-6h

Table 4-12. Risk Factors for Serious Disorders Causing Back Pain in Pregnancy

- Motor paralysis
- Bowel or bladder incontinence
- Abdominal or pelvic pain
- Fever

Clinical Assessment

The diagnostic approach to low back pain in pregnant women should be similar to that in other patients. The history should include information regarding location and quality of pain, factors which aggravate and improve the discomfort, the diurnal pattern of the pain, and associated symptoms. Careful attention should be given to risk factors for serious disorders causing back pain, as listed in Table 4-12. Women who awaken with acute back pain may have uterine compression of the inferior vena cava, causing blood to be shunted through the vertebral venous plexus.

The physical examination should include examination of the back, with focus on the area of pain. Supporting muscles and joints (especially the sacroiliac joints) should be examined for tenderness. Maneuvers such as pressing inward, moving the pelvic brim, or the Patrick test (external rotation of the hip with knee flexed) may aid in detecting sacroiliac joint pain. Evaluation of the abdomen and pelvis should be performed, considering the possibility of pancreatic disease, renal stones, or pathology involving the reproductive tracts. The patient should have a neurologic exam focused on the motor and sensory distributions of the lower extremities. The straight leg-raising test (extension of the knee with hip flexed at 90 degrees) may elicit pain running down the back of the leg to the knee. This is commonly associated with disk disease, hamstring muscle pain, and sacroiliac disease.

The presence of fever with back pain should raise concern over possible infectious etiologies such as epidural abscess (a neurosurgical emergency) or discitis, especially in diabetic or immunocompromised patients and IV drug abusers.

Muscular pain is common, especially in the evening when muscles have been fatigued, or after a day of improper lifting or posture. This discomfort is usually paraspinal in nature and is made worse by deep palpation or use of these muscles. Bony joint pain may be demonstrated by movement of the sacroiliac joint or by putting pressure on the posterior facet joint by retroflexion of the back.[56] Neurologic deficits referable to a nerve root—such as dermatomal sensory loss, motor weakness, absent reflex, or bowel or bladder incontinence—are significant findings. Motor weakness or bowel or bladder incontinence are neurologic emergencies and warrant immediate evaluation for possible surgical intervention.

Magnetic resonance imaging of the spinal canal and neural foramen is the most appropriate means of demonstrating the disk protrusion. There is little role for plain film imaging of the spine unless the patient has been the victim of direct trauma to the spine or flexion injury with point tenderness over the vertebra.

Emergency Department Management

ED management of the pregnant woman with back pain should be first directed at relieving her discomfort, and then toward discovering the underlying pathology. Pain should be treated with analgesics and muscle spasm with benzodiazepines as necessary. Heating pads may be very useful as well. Recognition of an underlying emergency is paramount. Injection of corticosteroids into the epidural space has been proposed as a safe and effective therapy for decreasing pain in disk disease.[54] Motor paralysis or bowel or bladder incontinence are neurologic emergencies and require immediate evaluation with MRI and neurosurgical consultation. Surgical therapy for disk disease is reserved for those with motor paralysis or bowel or bladder incontinence. Patients with partial paralysis referable to a root must be followed closely.

Disposition

It is the rare pregnant patient with simple lumbar strain whose pain is unrelievable in the ED. However, if after reasonable doses of narcotic analgesics plus benzodiazepines for muscle spasm, the patient remains too uncomfortable to be discharged from the ED, further work-up to find a more serious cause of the symptoms and probable admission are necessary. For most women with back pain, nonnarcotic analgesics (acetaminophen at 10 to 20 mg/kg PO q4 to 6h) coupled with common conservative therapies provide benefit, including short-term bed rest (3 days), daily low back exercises, the practice of good posture, and avoidance of situations that may exacerbate the pain. Patients with nighttime back pain should be advised to sleep in the lateral decubitus position to relieve compression of the vena cava. If conservative measures are unsuccessful, patients may try a longer period of strict bed rest (7 to 10 days), transcutaneous electrical nerve stimulation (TENS), and physical therapy, including lumbar support while sitting, frequent changes of position, application of heat or cold, and stretching exercises.[60] Preventive measures should be encouraged in all pregnant women, especially those with a history of low back pain. Begun prior to pregnancy, exercise, good posture, and observation of the basic biomechanical principles of the back are the mainstays of prevention. Exercise—including pelvic tilts, leg lifts, modified partial sit-ups, walking, and swimming—are all aimed at strengthening the muscles and reducing the lordosis. Avoiding high heels, ensuring correct posture with minimal lordosis while walking or sitting, and proper lifting by flexing at the knees should decrease the risk of low back strain.[60,61]

Acknowledgment

The editors wish to acknowledge the contributions of Dr. Iman Ali to the content of the headache and back pain sections of this chapter.

REFERENCES

1. Everett C: Incidence and outcome of bleeding before the 20th week of pregnancy: prospective study from general practice. *BMJ* 315:32–34, 1997.
2. Ramoska EA, Sacchetti AD, Nepp M: Reliability of patient history in determining the possibility of pregnancy. *Ann Emerg Med* 18:48–50, 1989.
3. Braunstein G: False positive serum human chorionic gonadotropin results: Causes, characteristics, and recognition. *Am J Obstet Gynecol* 187:217–224, 2002.
4. Gratacos E, Torres PJ, Vila J, Alonso PL, Cararach V: Screening and treatment of asymptomatic bacteriuria in pregnancy prevent pyelonephritis. *J Infect Dis* 169:1390–1392, 1994.
5. Kuller JA, Laifer SA, Portney DL, Rulin MC: The frequency of transplacental hemorrhage in patients with threatened abortions. *Gynecol Obstet Invest* 37:229–231, 1994.
6. Grant J, Hyslop M: Underutilization of Rh prophylaxis in the emergency department: A retrospective survey. *Ann Emerg Med* 21:104–106, 1992.
7. American College of Emergency Physicians Clinical Policies Committee and the Clinical Policies Subcommittee on Early Pregnancy: Critical Issues in the Initial Management of Patients Presenting to the Emergency Department in Early Pregnancy. *Ann Emerg Med* 41; 1:123–133, 2003.
8. Cartwright PS, Victory DF, Moore, RA: Performance of a new enzyme-linked immunoassay urine pregnancy test for the detection of ectopic gestation. *Ann Emerg Med* 15:1198–1199, 1986.
9. Batemen BG, Nunley WC, Kolp LA, et al: Vaginal sonography findings and hCG dynamics of early intrauterine and tubal pregnancies. *Obstet Gynecol* 75:421–427, 1990.
10. Pittaway DE: BhCG dynamics in ectopic pregnancy. *Clin Obstet Gynecol* 30:130–135, 1987.
11. Kadar N, Romero R: Observations on the log human chorionic gonadotropin-time relationship in early pregnancy and its practical implications. *Am J Obstet Gynecol* 157:73–78, 1987.
12. Kadar N, Romero R: Further observations on serial chorionic gonadotropin patterns in ectopic pregnancies and spontaneous abortions. *Fertil Steril* 50:367–370, 1988.
13. Dart RG, Kaplan B, Cox C: Transvaginal ultrasound in patients with low B-human chorionic gonadotropin values: How often is the study diagnostic? *Ann Emerg Med* 30: 135–140, 1997.
14. Stovall T, Ling F, Carson S, et al: Serum progesterone and uterine curettage in differential diagnosis of ectopic pregnancy. *Fertil Steril* 57:456–458, 1992.
15. Gelder MS, Boots LR, Younger JB: Use of a single random serum progesterone value as a diagnostic aid for ectopic pregnancy. *Fertil Steril* 55:497–500, 1991.
16. Rulin M, Bornstein S, Cambell P, et al: The reliability of ultrasonography in the management of spontaneous abortion, clinically thought to be complete: A prospective study. *Am J Obstet Gynecol* 1993; 168:12–15.
17. Cacciatore B, Tittinen A, Stenman U, et al: Normal early pregnancy: Serum hCG levels and vaginal ultrasound findings. *Br J Obstet Gynaecol* 97:899–903, 1990.
18. Bennett GL, Bromley B, Lieberman E, Benacerraf, BR: Subchorionic hemorrhage in first trimester pregnancies: prediction of pregnancy outcome with sonography. *Radiology* 200:803–806, 1996.
19. Sexually Transmitted Diseases Treatment Guidelines—2002. May 3, 2002/mmWR 51 (RR06); 1–80.
20. Klebanoff M, Koslowe P, Kaslow R, et al: Epidemiology of vomiting in early pregnancy. *Obstet Gynecol* 66:612, 1985.
21. Kauppila A, Huhtaniemi I, Ylikorkala O: Raised serum human chorionic gonadotropin concentrations in hyperemesis gravidarum. *Br Med J* 1:1670, 1979.
22. Soules MR, Hughes CL, Garcia JA, et al: Nausea and vomiting in pregnancy: Role of human chorionic gonadotropin and 17-hydroxyprogesterone. *Obstet Gynecol* 55:696, 1980.
23. Swaminathan R, Chin RK, Lao TTH, et al: Thyroid function in hyperemesis gravidarum. *Acta Endocrinol* 120:155, 1989.
24. Goodwin TM, Hersham JM, Cole L: Increased concentration of the free beta subunit of human chorionic gonadotropin in hyperemesis gravidarum. *Acta Obstet Gynecol Scand* 73:770, 1994.
25. Jarnfelt-Samsioe A, Eriksson B, Waldenstrom J, Samsioe G: Some new aspects on hyperemesis gravidarum: Relations to clinical data, serum electrolytes, total protein and creatinine. *Gynecol Obstet Invest* 19:174, 1985.
26. Becks GP, Burrow G: Thyroid disease and pregnancy. *Med Clin North Am* 75:121, 1991.
27. Kimura M, Amino N, Tamaki H, et al: Gestational thyrotoxicosis and hyperemesis gravidarum: Possible role of hCG with higher stimulating activity. *Clin Endocrinol* 38:345, 1993.

28. Goodwin TM, Montoro M, Mestman JH, et al: The role of chorionic gonadotropin in transient hyperthyroidism of hyperemesis gravidarum. *Endocrinol Metab* 75:1333, 1992.
29. Goodwin TM, Montoro M, Mestman JH: Transient hyperthyroidism and hyperemesis gravidarum: Clinical aspects. *Am J Obstet Gynecol* 167:648, 1992.
30. Bergin PS, Harvey P: Wernicke's encephalopathy and central pontine myelinolysis associated with hyperemesis gravidarum. *BMJ* 305:517, 1992.
31. Kousen M: Treatment of nausea and vomiting in pregnancy. *Am Fam Phys* 48:1279, 1993.
32. Boyce RA: Enteral nutrition: I. Hyperemesis gravidarum—A new development. *J Am Diet Assoc* 92:733, 1992.
33. Hsu JJ, Clark-Glena R, Nelson DK, Kim CH: Nasogastric enteral feeding in the management of hyperemesis gravidarum. *Obstet Gynecol* 88:343, 1996.
34. Levine MG, Esser D: Total parenteral nutrition for the treatment of severe hyperemesis gravidarum: Marginal nutritional effects and fetal outcome. *Obstet Gynecol* 72:102, 1988.
35. Guikontes E, Spantideas A, Diakakis J: Ondansetron and hyperemesis gravidarum. *Lancet* 340:1223, 1992.
36. Vutyavanich T, Wongtra-Rjan S, Ruansri R: Pyridoxine for nausea and vomiting of pregnancy: A randomized double blind placebo controlled trial. *Am J Obstet Gynecol* 173:881, 1995.
37. Greenspoon JS, Masaki DI, Uurz CR: Cardiac tamponade in pregnancy during central hyperalimentation. *Obstet Gynecol* 73:465, 1989.
38. Godsey RK, Newman RB: Hyperemesis gravidarum: A comparison of single and multiple admissions. *J Reprod Med* 36:287, 1991.
39. Gadsby R, Barnie-Adshead AM, Jagger C: A prospective study of nausea and vomiting during pregnancy. *Br J Gen Pract* 43:245, 1993.
40. Weigel MM, Weigel RM: Nausea and vomiting of early pregnancy and pregnancy outcome: An epidemiological study. *Br J Obstet Gynecol* 96:1304, 1989.
41. Weigel MM, Weigel RM: Nausea and vomiting of early pregnancy and pregnancy outcome: A meta-analytical review. *Br J Obstet Gynecol* 96:1312, 1989.
42. Jarnfelt A, Samsioe G, Velinder GM: Nausea and vomiting in pregnancy: A contribution to its epidemiology. *Gynecol Obstet Invest* 16:221, 1983.
43. Belluomini J, Litt RC, Lee KA, Katz M: Acupressure for nausea and vomiting of pregnancy: A randomized blinded study. *Obstet Gynecol* 84:245, 1994.
44. Fischer-Rasmussen W, Kjaer SK, Dahl C, et al: Ginger treatment of hyperemesis gravidarum. *Eur J Obstet Gynecol Reprod Biol* 38:19, 1990.
45. Lipton RB, Silberstein SD, Stewart WF: An update on migraine epidemiology. *Headache* 34:319–328, 1994.
46. Hainline B: Headache. *Neurol Clin* 12:443, 1994.
47. Reik L: Headaches in pregnancy. *Semin Neurol* 8:187, 1988.
48. Sommerville BW. The role of estradiol withdrawal in the etiology of menstrual migraine. *Neurology* 1972; 22:355–365.
49. Wainscott G, Sullivan FM, Volans GN, Wilkinson M. The outcome of pregnancy in women suffering from migraine. *Postgrad Med J.* 1978; 54:98–102.
50. Marcus DA, Scharff MS, Turk DC. Nonpharmacological management of headaches during pregnancy. *Psychosom Med* 1995; 57:527 535.
51. Neurologic Disorders in Pregnancy: *American Academy of Neurology Continuum.* Vol 16; No. 1:114–127, Feb, 2000.
52. Berg G, Hammar M, Moller-Nielsen J, et al: Low back pain during pregnancy. *Obstet Gynecol* 71:71, 1988.
53. Nwuga VCB: Pregnancy and back pain among upper class Nigerian women. *Aust J Physiother* 28:8, 1982.
54. Hainline B: Low back pain in pregnancy. *Neurol Clin* 12:65, 1994.
55. Fast A, Weiss L, Parik S, Hertz G: Night backache in pregnancy: Hypothetical pathophysiological mechanisms. *Am J Phys Med Rehab* 68:227, 1989.
56. Spankus JD: The cause and treatment of low back pain during pregnancy. *Wis Med J* 64:303, 1965.
57. Sandler SE: The management of low back pain in pregnancy. *Manual Therapy* 1:178–185, 1996.
58. Wade J: Obstetrical and gynaecological back and pelvic pains especially those contracted during pregnancy. *Acta Obstet Gynecol Scand* 41(Suppl 2):11, 1962.
59. Caluneri M, Bird HA, Wright V: Changes in joint laxity occurring during pregnancy. *Ann Rheum Dis* 41:126, 1982.
60. Mantle MJ, Holmes J, Currey HLF: Backache in pregnancy: II. Prophylactic influence of back care classes. *Rheumatol Rehabil* 202:27, 1981.
61. Fitzhugh ML, Newton M: Posture in pregnancy. *Am J Obstet Gynecol* 85:1091, 1963.

5

Ectopic Pregnancy

Robert G. Dart
Pamela L. Dyne

KEY POINTS

- No combination of history or examination can reliably rule out ectopic pregnancy.
- Only 70 percent have the triad of amenorrhea, abdominal pain, and vaginal bleeding.
- Only 50 percent have risk factors for ectopic pregnancy.
- About 10 percent have a normal pelvic examination, and 20 percent have normal pelvic ultrasounds.

INTRODUCTION

An ectopic pregnancy is the implantation of a fertilized ovum outside of the endometrial cavity of the uterus. Over 100,000 ectopic pregnancies are reported annually in the U.S., and they account for 2 percent of reported pregnancies.[1] Although the mortality rate has fallen substantially over the last 30 years, it is still the number one cause of maternal death in the first trimester and is the cause of 9 percent of pregnancy-associated deaths.[1] Physicians fail to make the diagnosis of ectopic pregnancy more than 40 percent of the time on the first ED visit, and missed ectopic pregnancy is also one of the leading causes of emergency physician malpractice cases.[2,3] The principal difficulty is differentiating those with ectopic pregnancy from those with threatened abortion. The diagnostic tools available in the ED can help in differentiating the two disorders.

PATHOPHYSIOLOGY

The most common cause of ectopic pregnancy is damage to the mucosa of the fallopian tube, which prevents transport of the fertilized ovum to the endometrial cavity.[4] Mucosal damage is most often a result of tubal infection.[5–7] Tubal surgery and diethylstilbestrol exposure have been demonstrated to play a role in other cases.[5] Defects in the fertilized ovum itself may contribute to increased ectopic pregnancy risk due either to decreased tubal motility or to premature implantation prior to arrival in the endometrial cavity. Hormonal factors have also been associated with an increased risk of ectopic pregnancy. Supraphysiologic levels of estradiol or progesterone have been demonstrated to inhibit tubal migration, which may account for the increased incidence of ectopic pregnancies in patients on ovulation-inducing agents.[8] Approximately 95 percent of ectopic pregnancies implant in the fallopian tube. Of these, 80 percent implant in the ampullary portion, 12 percent in the isthmus, 5 percent in the fimbriated end of the tube, and 2 percent at the junction of the fallopian tube and uterus (Fig. 5-1). The latter site of implantation is often referred to as either an *interstitial* or a *cornual* ectopic pregnancy, though the latter term is now reserved for pregnancies that occur in the rudimentary horn of a congenital bicornuate uterus. Interstitial ectopic pregnancies deserve special consideration, because they are both rare (accounting for only 2–3 percent of ectopic pregnancies), and dangerous, with a mortality rate more than twice that of other tubal pregnancies (2.2 percent vs. <1 percent).[9] Additional sites of ectopic implantation include the abdomen, the cervix, and the ovary.

Once tubal implantation has occurred, there are four potential outcomes: (1) the ectopic pregnancy may erode through the muscularis and lamina propria of the tube, leading to tubal rupture with associated intraabdominal hemorrhage; (2) it may persist within an intact tube with or without an associated tubal hematoma and/or intraabdominal hemorrhage; (3) it may abort out the fimbriated end of the fallopian tube; or (4) it may spontaneously involute.

RISK FACTORS

Table 5-1 lists the independent risk factors for ectopic pregnancy. Evidence of chronic salpingitis secondary to pelvic inflammatory disease (PID) is the most common laparoscopic finding in patients diagnosed with ectopic pregnancy. In fact, a single episode of laparoscopically-proven PID has been demonstrated to increase the ratio of extrauterine to intrauterine pregnancies by sixfold compared to control patients who did not have evidence of salpingitis at laparoscopy.[10] A history of infertility is also a risk factor for ectopic pregnancy.[5,11] As with a history of PID, the risk of ectopic pregnancy increases further if objective evidence of tubal disease has been demonstrated

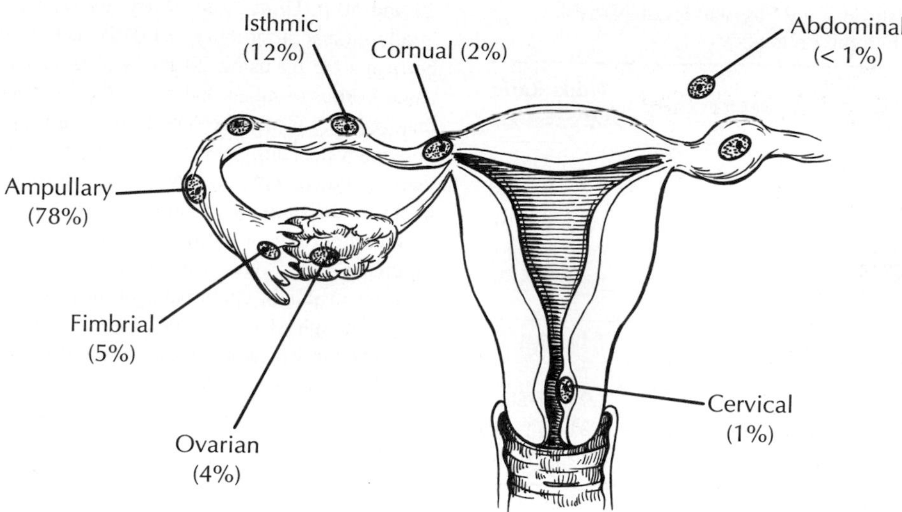

Fig. 5-1. Frequency of sites of ectopic pregnancy.

by laparoscopy. Patients who become pregnant despite a prior tubal ligation have a ninefold increased risk of ectopic pregnancy.[5] Use of an intrauterine device (IUD) increases the risk of ectopic pregnancy because of an increased susceptibility to PID, as well as by virtue of the mechanism of action of the IUD as a contraceptive (i.e., causing a fertilized ovum to be more likely to implant in the tube vs. the endometrial cavity). Increased age is also associated with ectopic pregnancy. Women aged 35 to 44 have three times the rate of ectopic pregnancy compared to those who are 15 to 24.[12] The rate of ectopic pregnancy is increased in nonwhite women,[1] with smoking and frequent douching implicated as risk factors for ectopic pregnancy in African American women.[13] Finally, The risk of ectopic pregnancy is significantly increased in individuals who undergo in vitro fertilization or use ovulation-inducing agents.[14,15] The reasons for this are likely multifactorial.

Table 5-1. Risk Factors for Ectopic Pregnancy

Prior ectopic pregnancy
History of PID/salpingitis
History of tubal ligation or tubal surgery
Current IUD
History of infertility for >2 years
Infertility treatment with IVF or ovulation induction agents
Smoking
Frequent douching
Advanced maternal age

Absence of risk factors for ectopic pregnancy should not deter the clinician from considering the diagnosis in a woman with vaginal bleeding. Only about half of women with ectopic pregnancy have one or more of the risk factors, and 25 percent of patients with threatened abortions have one or more ectopic risk factors as well.[2,15]

DIAGNOSIS

History and Physical Examination

The classic historical triad for ectopic pregnancy is that of amenorrhea, abdominal pain, and vaginal bleeding, though this combination is seen in only 65 to 70 percent of patients with ectopic pregnancy. Pain is seen in most patients with ectopic pregnancy (up to 90 percent), and vaginal bleeding occurs in 50 to 80 percent of cases.[16] Uterine size is normal on bimanual examination in 71 percent of ectopic pregnancy patients, or measures 6–8 weeks in 26 percent. Approximately 3 percent of patients with ectopic pregnancy have a uterus that measures 9 to 12 weeks.[17] Adnexal tenderness or fullness and cervical motion tenderness are each present in about 50 percent of patients.[16] Ectopic pregnancy is notoriously difficult to diagnose or exclude based on history and physical examination alone, especially given that 10 percent of patients

Table 5-2. Historical and Physical Exam Variables Predictive of Ectopic Pregnancy

Variable	Odds Ratio (95% CI)
Moderate to Severe Pain	3.4 (1.6-71.)
Pain Location Lateral	2.2 (1.2-4.0)
Pain Quality Sharp	2.0 (1.0-4.0)
Presence of CMT	3.3 (1.6-6.6)
Lateral or Bilateral Abdominal Tenderness	2.0 (1.1-3.7)
Lateral or Bilateral Pelvic Tenderness	2.4 (1.3-4.4)
Positive Peritoneal Signs	7.9 (3.1-20.0)
Pain Location Midline	0.31 (.14-.66)
Uterine Size >8 weeks	0.42 (.19-.96)

Adapted from Dart R, Kaplan B, Varakils K. Predictive value of history and physical examination in patients with suspected ectopic pregenancy. *Ann Emerg Med* 1999; 33:283–290.[11]

with ectopic pregnancy have a completely normal pelvic examination.[17] Predictive variables for ectopic pregnancy with their odds ratios are listed in Table 5-2. Ectopic pregnancy will be confirmed in only 44 percent of patients who have a combination of high-risk findings such as moderate to severe pain, cervical motion tenderness, and a closed cervical os on pelvic examination.[11] In addition, multiple studies have demonstrated that about one-half of all patients with ectopic pregnancies will have a low-risk clinical assessment.[11,18] In fact, the conclusion of one study was that the pelvic examination had little predictive value compared to US in the initial evaluation of suspected ectopic pregnancy.[19] The one exception is the obviously ruptured ectopic pregnancy, which classically presents with shock with severe abdominal pain and peritoneal signs.

DIAGNOSTIC TESTS

Beta-hCG

The beta subunit of human chorionic gonadotropin (β-hCG) is a marker for the volume of living trophoblastic tissue associated with a pregnancy. β-hCG assays are used as the initial screening test for pregnancy. Modern urine qualitative assays are highly accurate in identifying pregnancy when the quantitative serum value is >25 to 50 mIU/mL, with a sensitivity of 99.4 percent. False-negatives occur when the serum β-hCG is between 10 and 50 mIU/mL, and nearly always when the urine is dilute (specific gravity, <1.015). This limitation may be overcome by using 20 drops of urine instead of the usual 5 drops to superconcentrate the hormone on the test diaphragm.[20] Given the possibility of a ruptured ectopic pregnancy presenting with an extremely low β-hCG level, one should maintain a high suspicion of ectopic pregnancy in an appropriate clinical context (young female with peritoneal signs or syncope) despite a negative urine pregnancy test.[21] Quantitative serum β-hCG assays are useful in evaluating patients with suspected ectopic pregnancy, though a single β-hCG value alone is of limited diagnostic utility. Both ectopic and intrauterine pregnancies (IUPs) produce β-hCG. Nonviable IUPs and ectopic pregnancies tend to have lower quantitative β-hCG values compared to viable IUPs of the same gestational age.[17,22] Patients with β-hCG values <1000 mIU/mL have up to a fourfold increased risk of ectopic pregnancy compared to those with β-hCG values above this level.[15] However, this high-risk group with the lower β-hCG levels is also less likely to have a diagnostic US; about 17 percent patients with a β-hCG value <1000 mIU/mL have findings suggestive of an ectopic pregnancy or diagnostic of an IUP at initial ultrasound.[23] In addition, when ectopic pregnancy is present, one-third of patients with β-hCG values <1000 mIU/mL will have US findings suggestive of ectopic pregnancy.[23] By contrast, approximately 70 percent of ectopic pregnancy patients who have β-hCG values above 1000 mIU/mL will have US findings consistent with ectopic pregnancy.[15,22] Table 5-3 summarizes the interaction between the results of the serum β-hCG and pelvic ultrasound.

While a single value of β-hCG alone is not useful in differentiating between normal IUP, abnormal IUP, and ectopic pregnancy, a variation in the expected rate of rise of the β-hCG can be helpful.[22,24–29] The expected rate of

Table 5-3. Summary of Initial Pelvic Ultrasound and Serum β-hCG in Rule-Out Ectopic Pregnancy Patients

- If β-hCG <1000, 17 percent will have an initial US diagnostic of either an ectopic or an intrauterine pregnancy; the rest will be uncertain.
- If β-hCG <1000, 30 percent of those with an ectopic pregnancy will have US suggestive of ectopic pregnancy.
- If β-hCG >1000, 70 percent of those with an ectopic pregnancy will have US suggestive of ectopic pregnancy.

rise of β-hCG is by >66 percent in 48 hours for normal IUPs until 9 to 10 weeks gestational age, or a β-hCG of about 10,000 mIU/mL when the hormone plateaus. This is true for 85 percent of normal early IUPs, but also for about 15 percent of patients with ectopic pregnancy. Thus caution must be used in utilizing serial β-hCGs as a sole means to exclude ectopic pregnancy. The rate of rise or fall of the β-hCG value when used in concert with endometrial findings can be particularly useful when the ultrasound is indeterminate. In a study by Dart and colleagues, 22 percent of patients with a β-hCG increase of >66 percent at 48 hours and an empty uterus at US were diagnosed with ectopic pregnancy, and no patient with an increase of >66 percent but with an identified endometrial sac-like structure was diagnosed with ectopic pregnancy. When the uterus was empty and the β-hCG increased by <66 percent, ectopic pregnancy was diagnosed in 65 percent of patients.[26] The rate of fall of the β-hCG can be useful. Patients with β-hCG values that fall by >50 percent at 48 hours are at low risk for ectopic pregnancy.[25,26] This finding is most consistent with a completed abortion. β-hCG values that fall by <50 percent at 48 hours are consistent with an ectopic pregnancy or the presence of persistent trophoblastic activity within the endometrial cavity.[25,26] Evidence of an endometrial sac or debris at US suggests the later diagnosis, and these patients are at low risk for ectopic pregnancy.[26] If no endometrial contents are evident, these patients remain at risk for ectopic pregnancy.[22]

Kadar defined the term *upper discriminatory zone* as the β-hCG value above which an intrauterine sac should always be seen at US if the pregnancy is intrauterine.[30,31] Some authors have reported β-hCG values as low as 1000 mIU/mL to be an adequate cut-off when transvaginal ultrasound is employed.[32] Other authors have recommended values as high as 3000 mIU/mL before an IUP can be confidently excluded.[31,33] Even with the use of the higher value, IUPs have on rare occasion been identified in patients with an initially empty uterus at ultrasound.[34] Many institutions use a cut-off of 1500 mIU/mL as the discriminatory zone, but one should recognize that this value is based more on consensus opinion than on specific evidence, and it may be highly dependent on the sonographic skills and technology utilized by the sonologist performing the ultrasound.

Progesterone

Progesterone is produced by the corpus luteum during the first 8 weeks of pregnancy. Progesterone levels rise at the time of ovulation and are affected much less by changes in gestational age compared to β-hCG values. Numerous studies have demonstrated that both nonviable intrauterine pregnancies as well as ectopic pregnancies have significantly lower progesterone values when compared with viable intrauterine pregnancies.[28,35–38] A progesterone value >25 ng/mL is strongly associated with the diagnosis of a viable intrauterine pregnancy.[28,35,38] A progesterone <5.0 ng/mL accurately excludes the diagnosis of a viable intrauterine pregnancy, although it does not distinguish an ectopic pregnancy from a nonviable intrauterine pregnancy.[35–37]

Progesterone may be useful in two settings. The first is when pelvic ultrasound is not readily available 24 hours a day, 7 days a week. In this situation if the progesterone value is >25 ng/mL, the patient could then have an ultrasound arranged at follow-up. Emergent ultrasonography would be reserved for patients with values below this cut-off. A second role for progesterone would be in patients with an initial US that neither confirms nor excludes the diagnosis of a viable intrauterine pregnancy. As a progesterone value <5.0 ng/mL reliably excludes the diagnosis of a viable IUP, a uterine evacuation procedure may be performed without the fear of aborting a viable IUP. Identification of chorionic villi in the pathology specimen excludes the diagnosis of an ectopic pregnancy.[39] The exception to this is in the case of heterotopic pregnancy.

The major disadvantages of progesterone are twofold. First is that most hospital laboratories are unable to perform progesterone assays on a emergent basis, hence its utility as a diagnostic test in the emergency setting is limited. The other major disadvantage is that 31 percent of normal IUPs, 23 percent of abnormal IUPs, and 52 percent of ectopic pregnancies have a progesterone level between 10 and 20 ng/mL, so the diagnostic utility is also limited.[40]

Ultrasound

Transvaginal ultrasound has become the study of choice when ectopic pregnancy is suspected. Specific findings suggestive or diagnostic of ectopic pregnancy (Tables 5-4 and 5-5) will be identified in approximately 79 percent of cases.[15,41] In addition, identification of a yolk sac or fetal pole within the endometrial cavity confirms the presence of an intrauterine pregnancy, thereby excluding the diagnosis of ectopic pregnancy.[42] The one exception to this is when both an intrauterine pregnancy and an ectopic pregnancy coexist. This occurrence is termed a *heterotopic pregnancy*. Heterotopic pregnancy occurs at a rate of 1/3000 intrauterine pregnancies.[43] However, this rate

Table 5-4. Performance Characteristics of Transvaginal Ultrasound Criteria for Ectopic Pregnancy in a Referral Population when Performed in Radiology

Ultrasound finding	Sensitivity	Specificity
Adnexal embryo with cardiac activity	20.1%	100%
Adnexal mass with yolk sac or embryo	36.6%	100%
Adnexal Mass with echogenic rim ("tubal ring") or containing yolk sac or embyro	64.6%	99.5%
Adnexal mass other than simple cyst or intraovarian lesion	84.4%	98.9%

From Brown, DL and Doubilet, PM, *J Ultrasound Med* 1994; 13:256–266.[41]

may substantially increase (to as high as 1/34 intrauterine pregnancies) when in vitro fertilization or ovulation-inducing agents are used,[44,45] though this rate estimation is based on very small studies.

When the ultrasound is neither diagnostic of an intrauterine pregnancy nor suggestive or diagnostic of an ectopic pregnancy it is characterized as *indeterminate.* Categorizing the specific endometrial findings of indeterminate ultrasound studies is useful in risk stratification (Table 5-6).[46,47] Those with an empty uterus are at highest risk for ectopic pregnancy. When a well-defined sac-like structure is identified, the risk of ectopic pregnancy is low.[46]

Table 5-5. Positive Predictive Value (PPV) for Ectopic Pregnancy of Extrauterine Ultrasound Findings

Extrauterine Ultrasound Findings	PPV (%)
Extrauterine sac with yolk sac or embryo	100
Empty extrauterine sac	> 90
Complex adnexal mass discrete from ovary	70
Isolated large volume anechoic fluid or any echogenic fluid in abdomen or cul de sac	70
Isolated moderate volume anechoic fluid in cul de sac	25
Complex adenexal mass AND abnormal pelvic fluid	90

Uterine Evacuation

If the diagnosis of a viable IUP has been excluded, uterine evacuation can be performed, and the specimen evaluated for the presence or absence of chorionic villi. As chorionic villi will only be present if the pregnancy is intrauterine, their identification effectively excludes the diagnosis of ectopic pregnancy, except in the case of heterotopic pregnancy. The absence of chorionic villi is consistent with either a completed abortion or ectopic pregnancy. In most cases, obtaining a repeat β-hCG value at a 48-hour follow-up visit will clarify the diagnosis as the β-hCG should rapidly fall with a completed abortion.[39]

Laparotomy and Laparoscopy

Laparotomy and/or laparoscopy remain the gold standard for confirming the diagnosis of ectopic pregnancy. The procedure has the advantage of allowing diagnosis and surgical treatment to occur simultaneously. In addition to being invasive, the procedure also has the disadvantage of occasionally missing the ectopic pregnancy.

DIFFERENTIAL DIAGNOSIS

The differential diagnosis for ectopic pregnancy includes problems related to and unrelated to the current pregnancy. Those items in the differential list related to the current pregnancy include viable intrauterine pregnancy and nonviable intrauterine pregnancy, with or without retained products of conception. Chapter 4 covers these details in depth. Conditions not directly related to the pregnancy include ruptured corpus luteum cyst, ovarian torsion, urinary tract infection, salpingitis, gastroenteritis, and appendicitis, as well as other intraabdominal processes. See Chapter 14.

TREATMENT

Surgical

The two main surgical options for treatment of ectopic pregnancy are excision of the affected tube (salpingectomy), or performance of tube-conserving surgery. Salpingectomy is considered in three situations: when the affected tube is ruptured or severely diseased, when future fertility is not desired, or when the contralateral tube is normal. When the contralateral tube is normal, perform-

Table 5-6. Categorization of Endometrial Findings of Indeterminate Ultrasound Exams, Incidence of and Positive Predictive Value for Ectopic Pregnancy

US Category	Description	Incidence of EP (no. of EP/total no. in US category)	PPV for EP (%) (95% CI)
Empty Uterus	Empty endometrial cavity with or without a thickened endometrial stripe	36/879	13.9 (10.1-18.5)
Nonspecific Fluid	Anechoic fluid collection <10 mm in mean sac diameter without an echogenic border ("pseudogestational sac")	6/453	4.7 (1.9-9.6)
Echogenic Material	A heterogeneous collection of echogenic material within the endometerial cavity without an identifiable sac-like structure	4/323	4.5 (1.4-10.5)
Abnormal Sac	Anechoic intrauterine fluid collection >10 mm in mean sac diameter	0/349	0 (0.0-2.9)
Normal Sac	Anechoic fluid collection <10 mm in mean sac diameter with a well defined echogenic border	0/191	0 (0.0-5.5)

Adapted from Dart R et al. Subclassification of indeterminate pelvic ultrasonography: Prospective evaluation of the risk of ectopic pregnancy. *Ann Emerg Med* 2002; 39:382–388.[47]

ing a salpingectomy on the involved tube carries fertility rates similar to those seen if tube-conserving surgery is performed.[48]

The goal of tube-preserving surgery is to maximize future fertility. There are two main drawbacks to tube-preserving surgery. First, it is possible that some residual trophoblastic tissue remains in the tube, resulting in persistence of the ectopic gestation. This occurs in approximately 5 percent of patients treated in this manner.[49] Because of this potential complication, patients require postoperative β-hCG testing until their quantitative β-hCG values return to below-detectable levels. Patients with evidence of a persistent ectopic pregnancy based on rising or plateauing β-hCG values can be treated medically or surgically. The second problem with tube-conserving surgery is that the potentially abnormal tube that was the site of the initial ectopic implantation remains, and thus the patient continues to be at risk for ectopic pregnancy in the future.

Medical

Methotrexate is the primary chemotherapeutic agent used to treat ectopic pregnancy. It is a structural analogue of folic acid, which inhibits the formation of nucleotides that are necessary for DNA and RNA synthesis. Rapidly-dividing cells are particularly susceptible. Table 5-7 lists the patient-specific indications for methotrexate. Although a number of factors identified by ultrasound (absence of a fetal heart beat, mass <3.5 cm)[50] have been associated with successful treatment, the best predictor appears to be the β-hCG value at the time of treatment initiation.[51] The success rate with methotrexate is 98 percent when the β-hCG value is below 1000 mIU/mL, 92 percent when the β-hCG value ranges from 1000 to 4999 mIU/mL, and is only 81 percent when the β-hCG value is >5000 mIU/mL.[51] It should be noted that methotrexate does not prevent tubal rupture in the short term. Patients who are given methotrexate must be told to avoid vitamins containing folic acid (because it counteracts the action of methotrexate), to avoid alcohol, and to refrain from insertive vaginal or rectal intercourse (because theoretically it can precipitate rupture) until the β-hCG returns to normal.

Table 5-7. Indications for Methotrexate

Patient Hemodynamically Stable
Ectopic Mass by Transvaginal Ultrasound <4.0 cm or if fetal heart motion is present <3.5 cm
No free fluid at ultrasound outside of the pelvic cavity
Serum B-hCG value <5,000 mIU/ml
Patient does not desire surgical therapy
Patient willing and able to return weekly for follow up
No significant hepatic, renal, or hematologic disease

Methotrexate is given intramuscularly at a dose of 50 mg/m^2. β-hCG values are repeated on post-therapy days 4 and 7. If there is a <15 percent decline between days 4 and 7, a second similar dose can be given.[50]

Some additional considerations before instituting methotrexate therapy are recommended. First, patients need at least weekly follow-up with repeat β-hCG values, typically for about 4 to 6 weeks, to assure treatment success.[52] If close follow-up cannot be assured, then other treatment options should be utilized. This includes an assessment of the patient's reliability, as well as the ability to return to the hospital urgently should complications ensue. For example, access to reliable transportation, a telephone, and the living situation all must be considered in patient selection for methotrexate. Second, it is critical that the diagnosis of a viable IUP be excluded prior to initiation of methotrexate treatment. Only approximately 70 percent of patients with a complex adnexal mass actually harbor an ectopic pregnancy.[53] Abnormally rising β-hCG values (i.e., <66 percent at 48 hours) are strongly suggestive of ectopic pregnancy but are also seen with an early but viable IUP about 15 percent of the time.[24,26,27]

Emergency and primary care physicians need to be aware of the complications of methotrexate therapy, as these patients are likely to return to the ED at off-hours. The main complication is tubal rupture, which occurs in about 4 percent of cases treated.[54] Methotrexate has a variety of side effects, including abdominal pain, which occurs in up to 60 percent of patients. This is problematic, as this symptom could be indistinguishable from tubal rupture. These patients should have immediate US and gynecologic consultation to evaluate for this potentially very serious complication.[22] The other side effects of note are nausea, vomiting, and diarrhea, which occur in 5 to 20 percent of cases.[55]

Follow-Up in Patients with an Uncertain Diagnosis

Stable patients in whom the diagnosis of ectopic pregnancy has not been ruled out should be instructed to return for a follow-up β-hCG measurement in 48 hours. Clinicians should make every effort to either confirm or exclude the diagnosis of ectopic pregnancy at the first or second follow-up visit as diagnostic delays increase the risk of tubal rupture.[56] This means insisting on ready availability of ultrasound and β-hCG testing on a 24-hour basis. Patients should be informed of the warning signs that should prompt the patient to immediately return to the ED, which include increasing abdominal pain, lightheadedness or syncope, heavy vaginal bleeding, or fever.

REFERENCES

1. Current trends ectopic pregnancy—United States, 1990–1992. *MMWR* 44:46–48, 1995.
2. Abbott J, Emmans LS, Lowenstein SR: Ectopic pregnancy: Ten common pitfalls in diagnosis. *Am J Emerg Med* 8:515–522, 1990.
3. Trautlein JJ, Lambert RL, Miller J: Malpractice in the emergency department—review of 200 cases. *Ann Emerg Med* 13:709–11, 1984.
4. Joesoef M, Westrom L, Reynolds G, et al: Recurrence of ectopic pregnancy: The role of salpingitis. *Am J Obstet Gynecol* 165:46–50, 1991.
5. Ankum WM, Mol B, Van der Veen F, et al: Risk factors for ectopic pregnancy: a meta-analysis. *Fertil Steril* 65:1093–1099, 1996.
6. Kaemwendo F, Forslin L, Bodin L, et al: Epidemiology of ectopic pregnancy during a 28 year period and the role of pelvic inflammatory disease. *Sex Transm Infect* 76:28–32, 2000.
7. Weinstein L, Morris M, Dotters D, et al: Ectopic pregnancy—A new surgical epidemic. *Obstet Gynecol* 61:698–701, 1983.
8. Fernandez H, Coste J, Job-Spira N: Controlled ovarian hyperstimulation as a risk factor for ectopic pregnancy. *Obstet Gynecol* 78:656–659, 1991.
9. DeWitt C, Abbott J: "Interstitial pregnancy: A potential for misdiagnosis of ectopic pregnancy with emergency department ultrasonography." *Ann Emerg Med* 40:106–109, 2002.
10. Westrom L, Bengtssom L, Mardh P: Incidence trends and risks of ectopic pregnancy in a population of women. *Br Med J* 282:15, 1981.
11. Dart R, Kaplan B, Varaklis K: Predictive value of history and physical exam in patients with suspected ectopic pregnancy. *Ann Emerg Med* 33:283–290, 1999.
12. Dorfman S: Epidemiology of ectopic pregnancy. *Clin Obstet Gynecol* 30:173–190, 1987.
13. Kendrick JS, Atrash HK Lilo ST, et al: Vaginal douching and the risk of ectopic pregnancy among black women. *Am J Obstet Gynecol* 176:91–97, 1997.
14. American Fertility Society Assisted Reproductive Technology in the United States and Canada: 1994 results generated from the American Fertility Society Registry. *Fertil Steril* 662:697–705, 1996.
15. Kaplan B, Dart R, Moskos M, et al: Ectopic pregnancy: Prospective study with improved diagnostic accuracy. *Ann Emerg Med* 28:10–17, 1996.
16. Stovall TG, Ling FW, Carson SA, et al: Nonsurgical diagnosis and treatment of tubal pregnancy. *Fertil Steril* 54:537–538, 1990.
17. Cartwright PS: Diagnosis of ectopic pregnancy. *Obstet Gynecol Clin North Am* 18:19–37, 1991.
18. Stovall T, Kellerman A, Ling F, et al: Emergency department diagnosis of ectopic pregnancy. *Ann Emerg Med* 19:1098–1103, 1990.

19. Mol B, Hajenius P, Engelsbel S, et al: Should patients who are suspected of having ectopic pregnancy undergo physical examination? *Fertil Steril* 71:155–157, 1999.
20. Cartwright PS, Victory DF, Moore, RA: Performance of a new enzyme-linked immunoassay urine pregnancy test for the detection of ectopic gestation. *Ann Emerg Med* 15:1198–1199, 1986.
21. Kalinski, MA, Guss, DA: Hemorrhagic shock from a ruptured ectopic pregnancy in a patient with a negative urine pregnancy test result. *Ann Emerg Med* 40:102–105, 2002.
22. American College of Emergency Physicians Clinical Policies Committee and the Clinical Policies Subcommittee on Early Pregnancy: Clinical Policy: Critical Issues in the initial evaluation and management of patients presenting to the emergency department in early pregnancy. *Ann Emerg Med* 41; 1:123–133, 2003.
23. Dart R, Kaplan B, Cox C: Transvaginal ultrasonography in patients with low β-hCG values: How often is the study diagnostic? *Ann Emerg Med* 30:135–140, 1997.
24. Kadar N, Romero R: Observations on the log human chorionic gonadotropin-time relationship in early pregnancy and its practical implications. *Am J Obstet Gynecol* 157:73–78, 1987.
25. Kadar N, Romero R: Further observations on serial chorionic gonadotropin patterns in ectopic pregnancies and spontaneous abortions. *Fertil Steril* 50:367–370, 1988.
26. Dart R, Mitterando J, Dart L: Rate of change of serial B-human chorionic gonadotropin values as a predictor of ectopic pregnancy in patients with indeterminate transvaginal ultrasound findings. *Ann Emerg Med* 34:703–710, 1999.
27. Emancipator K, Bock J, Burke D: Diagnosis of ectopic pregnancy by the rate of increase of choriogonadotropin in serum: Diagnostic criteria compared. *Clin Chem* 36:2097–2101, 1990.
28. Stovall T, Ling F, Cope B, et al: Preventing ruptured ectopic pregnancy with a single serum progesterone. *Am J Obstet Gynecol* 160:1425–1431, 1989.
29. Pittaway DE: Beta-hCG dynamics in ectopic pregnancy. *Clin Obstet Gynecol* 30:130–135, 1987.
30. Kadar N, DeVore G, Romero R: The discriminatory hCG zone. Its use in the sonographic evaluation of ectopic pregnancy. *Obstet Gynecol* 50:156–161, 1980.
31. Kadar N, Bohrer M, Kemmann E, et al: The discriminatory human chorionic gonadotropin zone for endovaginal sonography: a prospective randomized study. *Fertil Steril* 61:1016–1020, 1994.
32. Cacciatore B, Stenman U, Ylostalo P: Diagnosis of ectopic pregnancy by vaginal ultrasonography in combination with a discriminatory serum hCG level of 1000 IU/L (IRP). *Brit J Obstet Gynecol* 97:904–908, 1990.
33. Dart R, Kaplan B, Ortiz L: Normal intrauterine pregnancy is unlikely in emergency department patients with either menstrual days >38 days or β-hCG >3,000, but without a gestational sac on ultrasonography. *Acad Emerg Med* 4:967–971, 1997.
34. Bateman B, Nunley W, Kolp L, et al: Vaginal sonography findings and hCG dynamics of early intrauterine and tubal pregnancies. *Obstet Gynecol* 75:421–427, 1990.
35. McCord M, Muram D, Buster J, et al: Single serum progesterone as a screen for ectopic pregnancy: Exchanging specificity and sensitivity to obtain optimal test performance. *Fertil Steril* 66:513–516, 1996.
36. Stern J, Voss F, Coulam C: Early diagnosis of ectopic pregnancy using receiver-operator characteristic curves of serum progesterone concentrations. *Hum Reprod* 8:775–779, 1993.
37. Dart R, Dart L, Segal M, et al: The ability of a single serum progesterone to identify abnormal pregnancies in patients with beta-human chorionic gonadotropin values <1,000 mIU/mL. *Acad Emerg Med* 5:304–309, 1998.
38. Buckley R, King K, Disney J, et al: Serum progesterone testing to predict ectopic pregnancy in symptomatic first trimester patients. *Ann Emerg Med* 36:95–100, 2000.
39. Stovall T, Ling F, Carson S, et al: Serum progesterone and uterine curettage in differential diagnosis of ectopic pregnancy. *Fertil Steril* 57:456–458, 1992.
40. Gelder MS, Boots LR, Younger JB: Use of a single random serum progesterone value as a diagnostic aid for ectopic pregnancy. *Fertil Steril* 55:497–500, 1991.
41. Brown DL, Doubilet PM: Transvaginal sonography for diagnosing ectopic pregnancy: Positivity criteria and performance characteristics. *J Ultrasound Med* 13:256–266, 1994.
42. Nyberg D, Mack L, Harvey D: Value of the yolk sac in evaluating early pregnancies. *J Ultrasound Med* 7:129–135, 1988.
43. Richards S, Stempel L, Carlton B: Heterotopic pregnancy: Re-appraisal of incidence. *Am J Obstet Gynecol* 142:928–930, 1982.
44. Glassner M, Aron E, Eskin B: Ovulation induction with clomiphine and the rise in heterotopic pregnancies. A report of two cases. *J Reprod Med* 35:175–178, 1990.
45. Dimitry E, Subak-Sharpe R, Mills M: Nine cases of heterotopic pregnancies in 4 years of in vitro fertilization. *Fertil Steril* 53:107–110, 1990.
46. Dart R, Howard K: Subclassification of indeterminate pelvic ultrasonograms: Stratifying the risk of ectopic pregnancy. *Acad Emerg Med* 5:313–319, 1998.
47. Dart RG, Burke G, Dart L: Subclassification of indeterminate pelvic ultrasonography: Prospective evaluation of the risk of ectopic pregnancy. *Ann Emerg Med* 39:382–388, 2002.
48. Rulin M: Is salpingostomy the surgical procedure of choice for unruptured tubal pregnancy? *Obstet Gynecol* 86:1010–1013, 1995.
49. Pouly J, Mahnes H, Mage G, et al: Conservative laparoscopic treatment of 321 ectopic pregnancies. *Fertil Steril* 46:1093–1097, 1986.
50. Stovall T, Ling F, Gray L, et al: Methotrexate treatment for unruptured ectopic pregnancy. *Obstet Gynecol* 77:749–753, 1991.
51. Lipscomb G, McCord M, Stovall T, et al: Predictors of success of methotrexate treatment in women with tubal ectopic pregnancies. *N Engl J Med* 341:1974–1978, 1999.

52. Lipscomb G, Bran D, McCord M, et al: Analysis of three hundred fifteen ectopic pregnancies treated with single-dose methotrexate. *Am J Obstet Gynecol* 178:1354–1358, 1998.
53. Huter O, Brezinka C, Solder E, et al: Diagnosis of extrauterine pregnancy with transvaginal ultrasound. *Gynecol Obstet Invest* 30:204–206, 1990.
54. Hirata AJ, Soper DE, Bump RC: Ectopic pregnancy in an urban teaching hospital: Can tubal rupture be predicted? *South Med J* 84:1467–1469, 1991.
55. Ander DS, Ward KR: Medical management of ectopic pregnancy—the role of methotrexate. *Journal of Emergency Medicine* 15:77–182, 1997.
56. Mertz H, Yalcinkaya T: Early diagnosis of ectopic pregnancy. Does use of a strict algorithm decrease the incidence of tubal rupture? *J Reprod Med* 46:29–33, 2001.

6

Complications of Induced Abortion

Phillip Stubblefield
Lynn Borgatta

KEY POINTS

- Health care providers must always maintain a professional attitude towards patients who have had elective abortions. Burdening the patient with one's personal ethical beliefs is inappropriate and impedes good patient care.
- Consider ectopic pregnancy in any patient in whom intrauterine pregnancy was not definitively demonstrated.
- Treat postabortion infection early and aggressively, as infection can progress very quickly.
- The woman with uterine tenderness, without suspected trauma and without evidence of retained intrauterine tissue, is most likely to have a postabortion infection.
- The ability to treat postabortion complications in the ED varies on the equipment available, the technical skills of the emergency physician, and the severity of the complication. Thus gynecologic or surgical consultation is frequently required.

BACKGROUND

Induced abortion as practiced in the United States is generally very safe and is therefore infrequently associated with complications.[1–4] In 1998 there were over 1,100,000 legal induced abortions performed in the United States. About 88 percent are performed before 12 weeks gestation.[5] The rate of complications increases with advancing gestational age, but serious complications are rare at any gestational age.[1–4]

The safety of abortion has improved dramatically with the legalization of abortion. Prior to its legalization, induced abortion frequently led to serious complications and death. In the 1940s, more than 1000 women died each year from abortion complications.[6] In recent years, there are fewer than 10 deaths per year from induced abortion in the U.S.[7] The risk of death from legal abortion induced prior to 16 weeks is 10 to 20 percent of the risk of death from continuing the pregnancy.[7] Because most abortions take place in the first trimester, when they are safest, the death-to-case rate for legal abortion is less than 1 per 100,000 abortions.

Abortion services are most commonly provided in freestanding specialty clinics. This pattern of care has reduced cost and made abortion services available where they would otherwise not be offered. However, when complications occur, lack of continuity of care between the clinic and the emergency department can be to the detriment of patient care.[8] Providing emergency care is more difficult if essential information from the abortion provider is not available. Management becomes simpler, and is more likely to be effective, when the abortion records can be accessed.

Emergency physicians and gynecologic consultants who do not provide abortion services may be unfamiliar with the diagnosis and management of abortion complications. Serious complications are rare, and therefore they may be easily mistaken for more common and much less severe problems. In healthy young women, serious injury may not be appreciated until secondary complications develop. On the other hand, overtreatment of normal postabortion symptoms or of minor complications is unnecessary and potentially distressing to the patient.

ATTITUDES AND BELIEFS OF HEALTH CARE PROFESSIONALS

Though induced abortion has been legal in the United States since 1973, it still arouses intense feelings. Health care professionals have a duty to put health care first when attending to the needs of such patients. The provider should assess and treat the medical issues without burdening the patient with the provider's emotional response to abortion.[9] Health care providers must maintain a professional, nonjudgmental, supportive attitude while caring for women who have sought abortion.

For some women, the abortion is a secret kept from her family and social group. The history of abortion may not be forthcoming with family present. For example, the family may have insisted on a medical evaluation for what they perceive to be prolonged or excessive bleeding. The patient may know the reason for her bleeding but may feel unable to explain the situation to others. Divulging her abortion history to her family or partner may put her at risk for disapproval or abuse. If she obtained her abortion from nonmedical providers, she may be reluctant to divulge the source of care. If the patient perceives that her caregivers are antiabortion, she may withhold information, fearing a punitive response.

If it is presumed or implied that a patient with a postabortal concern or problem had an error in management, then division and conflict between the medical providers is conveyed to the woman. This potentially increases medicolegal risk of all involved care providers.

METHODS OF INDUCED ABORTION

An explanation of common current techniques of legal abortion is necessary to anticipate possible complications and their management.

Some preabortion screening and follow-up procedures are common to all techniques. Practice with regard to screening for sexually transmitted disease (STD) varies by site, patient population, and relationships to other providers and financial institutions. If the woman has chlamydia, gonorrhea, or bacterial vaginosis, the chance of postabortal endometritis is increased. Treatment at the time of abortion decreases the risk of infection to the level seen in uninfected women.[10–12] Prophylactic antibiotics are commonly used for surgical abortion, and decrease the rates of postabortal infection.[10–15] For first-trimester medical abortion, prophylactic antibiotic use is not routine, as postabortal infection is rare.[16]

Rh-negative women are usually given Rh immune globulin at the time of abortion, or within 3 days postabortion, to prevent isoimmunization.[17]

Most abortion clinics have a 24-hour telephone number for emergencies. A treating clinician may have a list of women with unresolved problems, such as those at increased risk for ectopic pregnancy. Frequently after an abortion, the woman is given a one-page summary of her care to take to her referring physician. This summary will contain essential information such as apparent length of gestation at time of termination, how the procedure was performed, which medications are frequently administered, and any problems encountered.

Surgical Abortion in the First Trimester

First-trimester surgical abortion is usually performed by some variation of vacuum curettage.[18–22] Analgesia is usually provided by paracervical block with lidocaine or chloroprocaine. Conscious sedation with intravenous sedatives and analgesics is common. Some clinics offer general anesthesia.

In the very early first trimester, less than 6 or 7 weeks gestation, cervical dilation may not be necessary. For most women, mechanical or osmotic dilation is adequate to allow passage of an appropriate size cannula. Mechanical dilation is done with metal or plastic tapered dilators in graduated sizes. Then a hollow plastic vacuum curette 6 to 12 mm in diameter is introduced through the cervix, connected to a vacuum source, and the uterine contents evacuated. The vacuum source may be electric, using plastic tubing and a double-bottle electric pump, or a 60-mL syringe designed to fit the cannula may be used. Some operators use a sharp metal curette following the vacuum.[23] After the abortion, and before the woman leaves the facility, it is common practice to assess the aspirated tissue. The tissue is rinsed and examined with backlighting, typically by using a glass dish and light panel for sorting slides. Between 5 and 8 to 9 menstrual weeks, trophoblastic villi and membranes are visible, and are distinguishable from the uterine decidual lining. This allows immediate confirmation of products of conception, decreasing the likelihood of undiagnosed ectopic or molar pregnancy. After 8 to 9 weeks, the fetus and placenta are visible.

Medical Abortion in the First Trimester

Several agents have been used for medical abortion early in the first trimester. Medical abortion is commonly performed until 7, 8, or 9 weeks gestation according to the medication preferred by the practitioner.[24] The combination of the antiprogesterone agent mifepristone (Mifeprex®; formerly known as RU-486) and misoprostol (Cytotec®), a prostaglandin E_1 analogue, was approved by the U.S. Food and Drug Administration in 2000.[24,25] The FDA regimen is quite specific; mifepristone is approved for use up to 49 days (7 weeks) since last menstrual period, followed by oral misoprostol 2 days later with 4 hours of observation. In practice, many clinicians deviate from the FDA regimen, using a decreased dose of mifepristone and increasing the upper limit of gestational age.[24,26,27] Misoprostol may be used vaginally, administered at home, and with timing other than 2 days after mifepristone. Misoprostol is also used as a single agent.[28–30] Other techniques include using intramuscular or oral methotrexate followed in 3 to 7 days by vaginally-administered misoprostol.[16,24,31] Methotrexate has the advantage of treating ectopic pregnancy, but abortion takes longer to complete than it does with either mifepristone or misoprostol alone. The length of the abortion process is comparable for mifepristone-misoprostol and for misoprostol alone, with 75 to 80 percent of women aborting within 48 hours; abortion within 48 hours is unusual with methotrexate. The cumulative abortion rates (over 2 weeks or more) for pregnancies under 7 weeks are 92 to 98 percent for mifepristone, 90 to 96 percent for methotrexate, and 66 to 96 percent for misoprostol alone.[24–31]

All of these regimens can present problems of incomplete abortion, heavy bleeding, or prolonged bleeding after administration of the misoprostol. In several series 1 to 5 percent of women required curettage for bleeding.[16,24–31] Failed abortion, or continued growth and development of the pregnancy 2 weeks after abortion is started, occurs in a small percentage of cases (0.5 to 1.0 percent).[24,31] The need for curettage for bleeding, incomplete abortion, and failed abortion increases in frequency with increasing gestational age.[16,24,31]

Surgical Methods for Midtrimester Abortion

Dilatation and evacuation (D&E) is the most prevalent method for midtrimester abortion in the United States. More cervical dilation is necessary for second-trimester procedures than for first-trimester procedures. This is usually accomplished with osmotic dilators, made of the sea plant *Laminaria,* or a synthetic dilator, Lamicel® (Cabot, Inc.). Osmotic dilators are placed in the cervical canal where they absorb water and expand slowly over several hours or several days, producing dilation.[22,33–35] Then, under conscious sedation or general anesthesia, laminaria are removed and modified ovum forceps are inserted through the cervix to extract the fetus and placenta. Intraoperative ultrasound is commonly used to direct the forceps.[33–35] The uterus is much larger, softer, and more vascular than it is in first trimester, so the potential for both traumatic and hemorrhagic complications is greater. Blood loss increases linearly with menstrual age, from a mean of 84 mL at 13 weeks to a mean of 427 mL at 21 weeks,[36] but can be decreased with use of uterotonic agents such as vasopressin.[37] Immediate complications include uterine injury, uterine atony, and amniotic fluid embolism.

Medical Methods for Midtrimester Abortion

A variety of techniques are used to induce labor (Table 6-1).[38–41] Frequently, combinations are employed, for example, laminaria osmotic dilators to dilate the cervix and vaginal prostaglandins to produce uterine contractions. Hypertonic solutions, either saline or urea, may be instilled into the amniotic cavity in combination with

Table 6-1. Medical Regimens for Uterine Evacuation in Second Trimester

Agent	Example of Typical Use
Dinoprostone	20-mg vaginal suppositories q3h
Misoprostol	200-mcg tablets vaginally[a] q6-12h
Carboprost	250 mcg IM q4h or 250 mcg intra-amniotic initially
High-dose oxytocin[b]	• Add 50 units of oxytocin to 500 mL of 5% dextrose and normal saline. Administer over 3 hours. • Rest patient 1 h off oxytocin. • Add 100 units of oxytocin to 500 mL of dextrose/saline solution; administer over 3 hours. • Rest 1 h. • Repeat, adding another 50 units of oxytocin to each 500-mL infusion over 3 h, alternating with 1 h of rest until the patient aborts or a final solution of 300 units of oxytocin in 500 mL is reached.
Adjunctive Agents	
Mifepristone[c]	200 mg PO 12–36 hours before induction started
Hypertonic saline[d]	50–60 mL 23.4% saline intra-amniotic at start of induction
Digoxin[d]	1 mg intra-amniotic the day before induction
Potassium chloride[d]	1 mg into fetal umbilical vein or heart before procedure

[a] Oral or buccal misoprostol 200–400 mcg is less effective but may be preferred by the woman.
[b] Adapted from Winkler et al.[38]
[c] Cervical priming agent; softens and dilates cervix.
[d] Adjunctive agents cause fetal death and may accelerate the abortion process

prostaglandins. High-dose intravenous oxytocin is also used alone or in combination with other agents. The labor induction methods have complications specific to the agent used: water intoxication with concentrated oxytocin, high fever with prostaglandin E_2, and frequent vomiting and diarrhea with either prostaglandin E_2 or methyl $F_{2\alpha}$. Hemolysis, cerebral edema, and renal failure occur if hypertonic saline is inadvertently given intravascularly. Misoprostol used vaginally has fewer gastrointestinal side effects, and infrequently causes fever.[42] Some complications are common to all labor induction methods: failure of the primary method; retained placenta; and less commonly, sepsis, hemorrhage, uterine rupture, cervical laceration, and cervicovaginal fistula. Disseminated intravascular coagulation (DIC) and embolic phenomena are rare but the risk is greater with labor induction methods than with D&E.[41,43]

Selective Termination

Women carrying multifetal gestations may be offered selective termination to reduce the number of gestations usually to two, thus reducing the risk for severely premature birth for the surviving fetuses. This is done by passing a needle through the abdominal and uterine walls and into the heart of an individual fetus under ultrasound guidance. Concentrated potassium chloride is then injected into the fetal heart to produce asystole.[44] Generally the pregnancies treated in this fashion are absorbed without incident, but subsequent spontaneous loss of the remaining gestations can occur and will cause abdominal pain and vaginal bleeding.

Abortion Methods Used by Nonmedically Trained Providers

A variety of techniques are used in many cultures around the world to induce abortion.[45] Occasionally, U.S. women resort to untrained providers or attempt self-abortion. Complications from these procedures are likely to be more severe and more frequent than with legal abortion induced by a skilled provider. Insertion of a foreign body through the cervix is one such method. Rubber urinary catheters are used in this fashion. Over time, the presence of the foreign body will provide uterine contractions and expulsion of the pregnancy; however, hemorrhage and severe infection are likely. If a rigid foreign body is used, perforation of the uterus and injury to the bladder, bowel, or uterine vessels may occur. In Asia, the "massage technique" is used. The practitioner applies manual or even foot pressure to the gravid uterus through the abdominal wall. This apparently disrupts the placental attachment, leading to placental abruption and labor. Prior to legalization of abortion in the United States, transcervical instillation of chemical pastes and soap solutions into the extra-amniotic space was sometimes employed. Entry of soap solutions into the systemic circulation caused intravascular hemolysis and widespread damage to membranes, with resultant pulmonary and renal failure.[46] Sepsis is common with use of nonsterile instruments and techniques that do not immediately evacuate the uterus. Clostridial sepsis, a significant problem with illegal induced abortion, is much less frequently encountered with legal procedures. Botanical preparations may be ingested as infusions and teas in an attempt to induce abortion. In the U.S. in the nineteenth century, pennyroyal and oil of juniper were commonly taken for this purpose and are still occasionally encountered. Tablets of potassium permanganate are sometimes inserted vaginally to produce abortion. This causes sharply demarcated, deep ulcerations of the vaginal mucosa, with resultant bright red vaginal bleeding. The intent of the abortionist was to mislead medical personnel so they would perform a D& C evacuation of the uterus for a presumed incomplete spontaneous abortion.

More recently, misoprostol has been used by women to self-induce abortion.[47] Self-dosing has been reported at a variety of doses. The most common expected complications are incomplete abortion and failed abortion.

SIDE EFFECTS AND SYMPTOMS AFTER ABORTION

Bleeding and crampy lower abdominal pain are common side effects, and are experienced by most women to some degree. Increased bleeding or pain may be symptoms of either minor or major complications.

Uterine bleeding after pregnancy originates from spiral arteries in the myometrium. With myometrial contraction, the vessels are compressed and bleeding slows or stops. The type of abortion procedure used affects the bleeding amount and pattern.

After first-trimester surgical abortion, bleeding may be similar to a heavy period for 1 or 2 days; on occasion the woman may pass some clots. After the first day or two, bleeding typically diminishes to light bleeding or spotting. The total duration of bleeding is usually 3 to 10 days, and has no effect on blood indices such as hematocrit.

For early medical abortion, the situation is more variable. Before the abortion, bleeding may be absent, and if present, may vary in amount and be intermittent. The abortion itself may be accompanied by heavy bleeding with passage of clots for several hours before the abortion, usually stopping promptly after expelling the pregnancy. In contrast, some women have very little bleeding with expulsion, particularly if the pregnancy is very early (less than 6 weeks). After the abortion is complete, bleeding which seems similar to a menstrual period to the woman may continue for several days, followed by light bleeding or spotting. The mean length of bleeding is 10 to 12 days, but may vary from 2 days to 3 weeks or longer.[48] The total amount of bleeding is greater than with first-trimester surgical abortion.[32,49] This amount is not clinically significant, and is typically well tolerated by women who choose medical abortion.

After second-trimester surgical or medical abortion, bleeding in the first few days may be heavier, sometimes with passage of significant clots during the first day. However, some women have considerably less bleeding, with cessation of bleeding altogether after a few days.

Regardless of the type of abortion, many women start contraception immediately or soon afterward. All hormonal methods may induce spotting or bleeding, particularly in the first weeks of usage. Prolonged spotting or light bleeding may be due to hormonal contraceptives rather than the abortion itself.

Postabortal cramping and pain can result from uterine contraction. It can also result from pathologic uterine distention, such as hematometra, or from induration of pelvic organs. Examples of the latter would be fallopian tube distention from ectopic pregnancy, and extravasated blood or hematoma formation from injury and infection.

After first- or second-trimester surgical abortion, most women have cramping. The cramps typically subside after 10 to 30 minutes, but may recur with decreased intensity during the next several days. Acetaminophen or another nonnarcotic analgesic should be sufficient to relieve pain. Women may also have a similar pattern after completed first-trimester medical abortion. However, immediately prior to and during the medical abortion cramping can be quite severe, occasionally requiring oral narcotic medication. Women may request emergency evaluation before the medical abortion has occurred. Most women undergoing medical abortion do not have such severe cramping, requiring use of little to no nonnarcotic analgesics.

EMERGENCY FACILITIES

Many abortion providers have the capability to provide emergency care, but a woman may arrive at a different emergency facility than that arranged by the provider because of confusion about the emergency plan, ambulance directives, or family insistence. Freestanding abortion facilities may rely on a hospital emergency department as backup either by formal arrangement or referral. Even when formal arrangements are in place, women may self-refer to an emergency department without consulting the abortion provider. In any of these situations, contact with the provider may promptly provide medical history, gestational age, and details of the abortion procedure including any procedural difficulties or complications and the results of tissue examination. Although many women seeking care have a normal postabortion course, and most will have a relatively minor problem, some have illnesses that are rare but potentially life-threatening (Table 6-2).

INITIAL ASSESSMENT

Initial assessment of the woman includes the interval history since the abortion, vital signs, and evaluation of her overall appearance (Table 6-3). She should be given an opportunity to speak to staff privately. She may be unable to give an accurate history with her family or companions present.

If her medical condition appears to be unstable (i.e., with obvious heavy bleeding), or she has unstable vital signs or decreased level of consciousness, stabilization measures should start immediately. These include at least one large-bore IV line for hydration and blood replacement. If there is bleeding, high-dose intravenous oxytocin therapy should be started with 50 units of oxytocin in 500 mL of 5 percent dextrose and normal saline administered at 125 mL/h. Table 6-4 lists the other uterotonic agents. Laboratory tests include a complete blood count, blood type and screen, coagulation profiles, electrolytes. Monitoring should include pulse oximetry.

Next, the woman should receive a targeted abdominal and pelvic examination. The abdominal examination is to assess tenderness, distention, rebound, and masses; the speculum examination can reveal extruded pregnancy tissue and vaginal or cervical injury. The bimanual examination can assess uterine size, consistency, and tenderness, as well as the presence of other masses.

Ultrasound examination is frequently helpful, and is essential when the woman is critically ill. Ultrasound may demonstrate the extent of tissue remaining in the uterus and it may allow determination of gestational age if intact fetal tissue remains. It may show a large amount of fluid in the pelvis, suggesting intra-abdominal hemorrhage. The finding of large amounts of intraperitoneal fluid is an indication for immediate transfer to the operating room. Operative evaluation is almost always needed if there is known perforation, major cervical injury with continued external bleeding, or signs of peritoneal irritation such as marked tenderness and rebound.

The woman with uterine tenderness, without suspected trauma and without evidence of retained intrauterine

Table 6-2. Possible Complications after Induced Abortion

Condition	Timing	Gravity
Inability to dilate the cervix	Immediate	Not serious in itself
Inability to complete the abortion	Immediate	Generally not serious if recognized
Uterine perforation	Immediate but may not be recognized until later	Varies from asymptomatic to very serious; **potentially life-threatening**
Anaphylaxis	Immediate	**Potentially life-threatening**
Seizure	Immediate	May be serious or not serious depending on etiology and seizure type
Embolism	Immediate	**Potentially life-threatening**
Cervical laceration	Early	Usually not serious Deep lacerations or cervical fracture can be **potentially life-threatening**
Disseminated intravascular coagulation	Early	**Potentially very serious**
Uterine atony	Early	Depends on amount of blood loss
Hematometra	Early or delayed	Usually not serious
Failed abortion	Early or delayed	Not serious if pregnancy is intact
Ectopic pregnancy	Early or delayed	Serious; **potentially life-threatening**
Endometritis	Delayed	Usually not serious if treated promptly
Incomplete abortion	Delayed	Usually not serious
"Postabortal triad"	Delayed	Usually not serious
Septic incomplete abortion	Delayed	Serious; **potentially life-threatening**

tissue, is most likely to have an infection. Mild endometritis with isolated mild uterine tenderness can be treated as an outpatient; the patient should return for follow-up in 2 days to assess improvement. More extensive infection requires aggressive parenteral antibiotic treatment (see sections on endometritis, pelvic inflammatory disease, sepsis, and septic incomplete abortion, below).

Treatment of incomplete abortion depends on the amount of retained tissue and the overall status of the patient. Women with retained fetal parts in the second trimester need evacuation with analgesia in a facility equipped for second-trimester procedures, either an operating room or an abortion unit. Women with evidence of infection need IV antibiotics and admission as well as uterine evacuation by an experienced operator, because the uterus may be boggy and fragile. Fortunately, most women with incomplete abortion have undergone a first-trimester abortion, after which infection is uncommon. These patients are usually treated with repeat curettage.

Surgical Evacuation of the Uterus in the Emergency Department

An essential part of adequate treatment of most postabortal complications is prompt evacuation of any retained pregnancy tissue. Most women with incomplete abortion, and many women with postabortal pain, bleeding, or fever will require uterine evacuation. Stable patients with these complications of first-trimester abortion and no evidence of perforation can be safely treated in an emergency department or office setting.[50] Transfer to an operating room is often medically unnecessary and results in delay of care if the suction equipment is available in the ED. Many institutions now provide uterine evacuation using suction curettage with analgesia or conscious sedation in the emergency department. Vacuum curettage can be performed with conventional plastic cannulas and an electric vacuum pump or with manual vacuum systems, such as the hand-held double-valve syringe used with flexible vacuum cannula (IPAS, Chapel Hill, NC).[51] Examples of instrument sets for surgical evacuation are pictured in Figs. 6-1 and 6-2.

Paracervical block should be done; it is seldom uncomfortable provided a small gauge needle (22-gauge or smaller) is used. The anesthetic, such as 10 to 20 mL lidocaine 1 percent, is injected at multiple sites both for anesthetic efficacy and to avoid intravascular bolus. The addition of 2 units of vasopressin to the anesthetic will increase uterine contraction and decrease bleeding. Analgesia can be augmented by a nonsteroidal or a narcotic anal-

Table 6-3. General Approach to the Woman with a Postabortal Emergency Visit

Stable Condition	Acutely Ill
Assessment of history from patient and available information from abortion provider: • Preoperative examination and ultrasound findings • Procedure type • Suspected problems or complications, if any • Results of tissue examination	Assessment of history from patient and available information from abortion provider: • Preoperative examination and ultrasound findings • Procedure type • Suspected problems or complications, if any • Results of tissue examination
Vital signs	Vital signs
Focused physical examination (especially abdominal and pelvic examination)	Focused physical examination (especially abdominal and pelvic examination)
Laboratory studies: • CBC if indicated (e.g., significant bleeding) • Screen for sexually transmitted disease, as indicated (e.g., young age, pelvic pain)	Laboratory studies: • CBC • Type and screen or cross-match • Blood and endometrial cultures if febrile or septic abortion suspected
	Start intravenous line with lactated Ringer's or 0.9% saline solution
If significant bleeding present, administer uterotonics. Examples: • Methylergonovine 0.2 mg IM • Misoprostol 400 mcg orally	If significant bleeding present, administer uterotonics immediately. Examples: • Oxytocin 20–40 units in 1 L of D5NS. Run at 125 cc/hr; increasing to 100 units if hemorrhage unresponsive to lower dose • Carboprost 0.25 mg IM or into myometrium • Methylergonovine 0.2 mg IM • Misoprostol 1000 mcg rectally or misoprostol 400 mcg orally or buccally
If endometritis suspected, prescribe antibiotics. Examples: • Ceftrioxone 250 mg IM PLUS doxycycline 100 mg PO bid × 14 days • Ofloxacin 400 mg PO bid × 14 days PLUS metronidazole 500 mg PO bid for 14 days	If fever present or septic abortion suspected, begin IV antibiotics promptly. Examples: • Cefotetan 2 g IV q12h PLUS ampicillin/sulbactam 1.5 g q6h or ampicillin 1 g IV q6h • Clindamycin 900 mg IV q8h PLUS gentamicin 1.5 mg/kg q8h (2 mg/kg loading dose) or metronidazole 500 mg IV q4h PLUS other antibiotics appropriate for specific suspected organisms (e.g. β-hemolytic streptococci, *Clostridium perfringens*, enterococci, synergistic infections)
Ultrasonography, if indicated (see text) (e.g., enlarged uterus, uncertain diagnosis)	Ultrasonography
Uterine aspiration, if necessary (see text) (e.g., hematometra, incomplete abortion)	Uterine aspiration is indicated for most women
Rh immune globulin, if Rh-negative patient and Rh immune globulin not given within past 3 weeks	Rh immune globulin, if Rh-negative patient and Rh immune globulin not given within past 3 weeks
Follow-up care	Admission, if indicated, or outpatient follow-up care

Table 6-4. Uterotonic Medications

Agent	Example of Typical Use
Methylergonovine maleate	0.2 mg IM or 0.2 mg IV or 0.1–0.2 mg into cervix
Misoprostol	400 mcg orally or buccally 800–1000 mcg rectally (Note: 800 mcg vaginally can be used but may be washed out by heavy bleeding)
Carboprost	250 mcg IM
Oxytocin	10 units IV bolus or 10 units IM Continuous infusion: Initially, 20 units in 1 L IV fluid such as lactated Ringer's solution. Run at 500 mL/h (10 units per hour) until bleeding slows Increase to 40 units/L if no response May increase to 80–100 units/L for short-term use only Use medication pump for oxytocin if more than 2 liters are used; water intoxication is possible with continued infusion of oxytocin
Vasopressin	2 units vasopressin/10 mL saline or local anesthetic, injected into the cervix at several sites

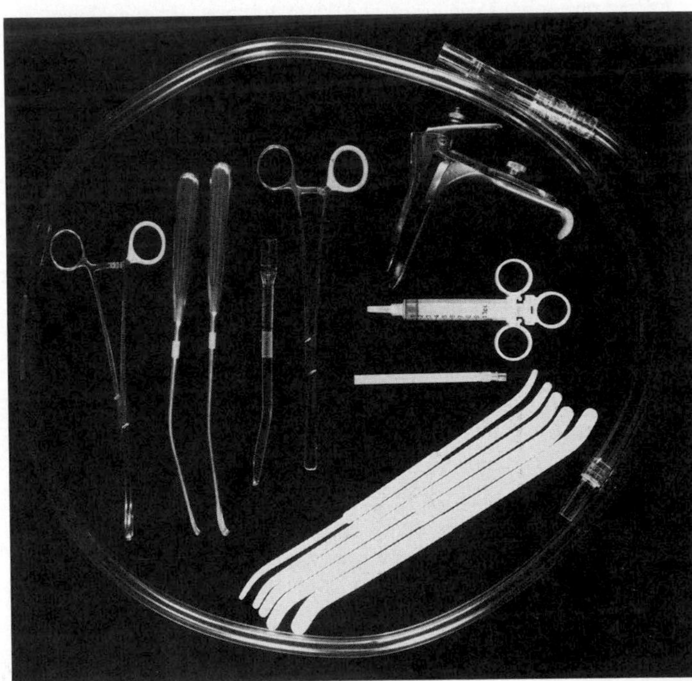

Fig. 6-1. Typical instruments for electric vacuum curettage in the emergency department. Clockwise from upper right corner: Graves vaginal speculum, 10-mL syringe, $3^1/_2$-inch 22-gauge spinal needle, Deniston uterine dilators, Forester ovum forceps, #1 curette, #3 curette, 9-mm vacuum cannula, and single-tooth tenaculum. Surrounding the instruments is disposable vacuum tubing. (Photo courtesy of P.G. Stubblefield.)

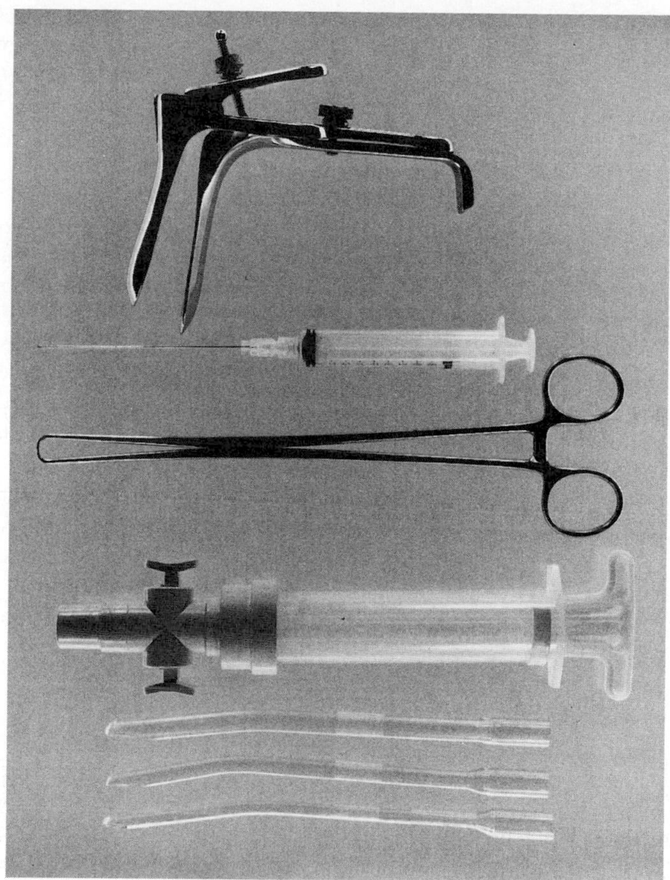

Fig. 6-2. Typical instruments for manual vacuum aspiration of incomplete abortion in the emergency department. From top to bottom: Moore-Graves speculum, 10-mL syringe, $3^1/_2$-inch 22-gauge spinal needle, single-tooth tenaculum, 60-mL vacuum syringe, semirigid vacuum curettes sizes 10, 8, and 6 mm.

gesic, administered via oral, intramuscular, or intravenous routes. Conscious sedation and analgesia can also be used; one regimen is midazolam 2 mg IV, followed with one to two doses of 50 mcg of fentanyl. When sedatives and narcotics are used in combination, monitoring of pulse, blood pressure, and pulse oximetry is needed until there is recovery from sedation following the procedure.

Once analgesia has been started, the next step is to stabilize the cervix with a tenaculum or an atraumatic grasper such as an Allis clamp, sponge forceps, or Bierer tenaculum. Gentle traction straightens the cervical canal, which facilitates safe passage of instruments. Dilatation should not be necessary. A plastic vacuum cannula is then placed through the cervix. The size of the cannula (in mm) should be equal to or slightly smaller than the number of weeks of pregnancy (e.g., a 9-week pregnancy can be evacuated by a 7-, 8-, or 9-mm cannula).

Either manual or electric suction may be used. Manual suction is inexpensive, quiet, compact, easily moved from location to location, and is usually sufficient for first-trimester procedures. Electric suction is more convenient if the amount of tissue and blood is over 100 mL. Manual suction requires more time and may require multiple insertions of the cannula because only a maximum of 50 mL can be removed with each pass. After evacuation with suction, some operators check the uterine cavity with a sharp curette. Others use sharp curettage infrequently, feeling that it is both unnecessary and that excessive curettage potentially can damage the endometrium.

At the conclusion of the procedure, bleeding should have stopped. If significant bleeding (i.e., more than a typical period) persists, either the uterus has not been evacuated completely, or there is another cause of bleeding such as atony, endometritis, or injury. Cramping from the curettage usually improves or ceases within 10 to 15 minutes.

Disposition

If not already treated at the abortion facility, Rh-negative women should be given Rh immune globulin. Plans for contraception should be reviewed, and if a pharmacologic method was selected but not obtained, it should be prescribed.[52,53] Follow-up should be arranged. Women treated on an ambulatory basis for presumed early infection should be evaluated at 48 hours to be certain of the adequacy of the clinical response to initial therapy. Women who require serial β-hCG testing typically need follow-up in 48 hours. Other women should be seen in 1 or 2 weeks. Postoperative instructions include monitoring temperature morning and evening for several days and attention to the amount of pain and vaginal bleeding. Patients should be given a 24-hour telephone contact number for questions and be instructed to call or return if body temperature exceeds 38°C, if there is persistent abdominal pain, or if there is vaginal bleeding sufficient to require changing a pad every hour.

COMPLICATIONS AND MANAGEMENT

Complications range in severity from minor to life-threatening (see Table 6-2). Complications can be divided into three groups, with considerable overlap. Early, or immediate complications are those arising during the abortion procedure or the immediate postabortion period. Some consider an immediate complication one that occurs any time during the first 24 hours postabortion. Delayed complications occur several hours to several days after abortion. Remote complications occur after the abortion period and recovery are complete (i.e., more than a month later). The distribution of complications varies by type of procedure. Advanced gestational age is related to increased complication rates for all techniques.[2–4,22,54]

Rates of complications are difficult to establish with certainty. Most estimates of complication rates are based on observational data, and tend to be reported by busy services with resources for compiling results. These centers may not be representative of abortion providers as a whole. Another barrier to assessing complication rates is fragmentation, or lack of postabortion care. In a private practice model follow-up visits may be the rule, but in many abortion clinics rates of return are low. (In the authors' institution it is under 25 percent). The abortion provider will be aware of most immediate or early complications. However the woman with a late complication may utilize another provider for a variety of reasons, such as geographic, financial, or personal reasons. If she sees another provider, the complication may not be reported back to the original facility.

Early or Immediate Complications

Inability to Complete the Abortion

The provider may begin a procedure but be unable to complete evacuation of the pregnancy. This may occur for several reasons. Anatomic abnormalities such as a septate uterus may be difficult to detect before abortion; distorted anatomy can make curettage difficult or impossible and increase the likelihood of perforation. Repeated or prolonged unsuccessful attempts to complete abortion can increase the chance of uterine injury by multiple intrauterine maneuvers. If the gestation is too advanced for the instruments available at the site, or too advanced for the amount of dilatation obtained, the procedure cannot safely be continued and the best course is patient transfer.

Cervical Laceration

Cervical lacerations are usually on the anterior lip of the cervix, and result from use of the tenaculum or clamp to provide traction during the procedure. Although lacerations are minor, lacerations worrisome enough to result in transfer should be carefully evaluated. Arterial bleeding may be intermittent. If the laceration is deep enough to cause persistent bleeding, it should be repaired using absorbable sutures. The upper extent of the laceration must be visualized prior to repair. If the laceration extends to the internal cervical os, uterine perforation or cervical rupture (a longitudinal disruption of the cervix resulting from dilation or tissue removal, also called a split or fracture) must be considered and urgent gynecologic consultation obtained. These possibilities can be evaluated by probing the laceration with a uterine sound or other small blunt instrument, preferably under ultrasound guidance (see section on uterine perforation, below). As the bladder and ureters lie adjacent to the anterior wall of the vagina, deep lacerations extending to the anterior vaginal wall require an evaluation of the integrity of these structures.

Complications Associated with Increased or Excessive Bleeding

Excessive bleeding most frequently results from inadequate uterine contraction or injury. Problems of uterine contractility are far more common. This can occur with primary uterine atony, or from inability of the uterus to contract because of retained tissue or blood clots. Severe anteflexion or retroflexion may prevent intrauterine blood from being expelled. The resultant distention prevents contraction and the uterus continues to bleed. Uterine, cervical, or other genital tract injury can also result in bleeding. Coagulopathy may result in persistent bleeding of nonclotting blood; however, mild or moderate degrees of coagulopathy usually do not cause excessive bleeding after surgical abortion when the uterus contracts well. Arteriovenous malformations may result in persistent bleeding ranging from moderate to extremely heavy; presentation may be immediate or delayed.

Uterine Atony

Increased bleeding during or immediately after the abortion procedure may indicate uterine atony, or failure of the uterus to contract normally. The occurrence of uterine atony in about 1 percent of abortions has been reported.[4,22,54,55] One of the causes of atony is incomplete abortion, therefore atony may respond to completion of the abortion. Bimanual massage is an immediate method to slow bleeding, but is usually not sufficient. Atony should respond to uterotonic agents such as methylergonovine maleate intravenously intramuscularly intrauterine oxytocin, or prostaglandin (Table 6-4). Misoprostol can be given orally, buccally, or rectally; the vaginal route is impractical if there is heavy bleeding. Carboprost can be given via intramuscular or intrauterine routes. An immediate local measure is dilute vasopressin (2 units vasopressin to 10 mL local anesthetic or saline) injected directly into the cervix. Failure to respond to these measures may indicate cervical laceration, uterine perforation, retained tissue in the uterus, or DIC.

Hematometra

Hematometra, also known as postabortal syndrome, is a type of uterine atony.[55] A hematometra consists of uterine distension with blood and an inability for the uterus to contract and expel the blood. It is characterized by increasing lower abdominal pain, absent or decreased vaginal bleeding, and at times, tachycardia and prostration. It may present immediately after the abortion, or it may be more insidious, evolving slowly over several days before reaching sufficient intensity to bring the woman to the emergency department. It appears to be more common after first-trimester abortions. Hematometra should be suspected on physical exam if there is a tense, tender midline mass arising from the cervix and absence of a tender mass lateral to the uterus. Ultrasound is not essential if the physical findings are clear-cut, but ultrasound can demonstrate the enlarged uterine cavity distended with multiechoic material (Fig. 6-3). Treatment is immediate re-evacuation of the uterine contents and administration of uterotonic agents such as intravenous oxytocin or misoprostol. The aspiration of clotted blood from the uterus with prompt uterine contraction and relief of symptoms confirm the diagnosis. Although repeat hematometra is rare, usually the should be discharged on a uterotonic agent such as methylergotamine maleate, 0.2 mg PO tid for 3 days.

Coagulopathy

Disseminated intravascular coagulation (DIC) must be considered with persistent unexplained bleeding, especially after midtrimester abortion. Passage of blood that does not clot, or persistent hemorrhage after uterine massage and uterotonic therapy are indications for evaluation of coagulopathy by measuring platelets, fibrinogen, and fibrin split products. Quick confirmation of the diagnosis is provided by a bedside clotting time, observing the length of time to formation of clot in a glass tube of blood. A firm clot should be present in 5 to 7 minutes. A longer interval or incomplete coagulation in the tube strongly suggests DIC. In most cases postabortal DIC can be treated successfully with intramuscular carboprost (250 mcg IM). This usually produces sufficient contraction of the uterus to stop the bleeding within several minutes of administration, avoiding the need for blood products and transfusion. If hemorrhage persists, treatment of the DIC with fresh frozen plasma and cryoprecipitate is indicated.

Disorders of platelet aggregation, such as von Willebrand's disease and aspirin use, present as prolonged bleeding that may continue for days after the abortion. Immediately after the abortion, the amount of bleeding may be indistinguishable from that of other women, as uterine vessels are compressed by uterine contraction. However, the bleeding may not decrease as much as expected over the first hours or days, and the cumulative blood loss may be significant.

Vascular Malformations

Vascular malformations of the uterus may present as hemorrhage or heavy bleeding immediately after the abortion, or as a more prolonged course of bleeding. Some women may have episodes of heavy bleeding that seem to stop completely. The bleeding may not be responsive

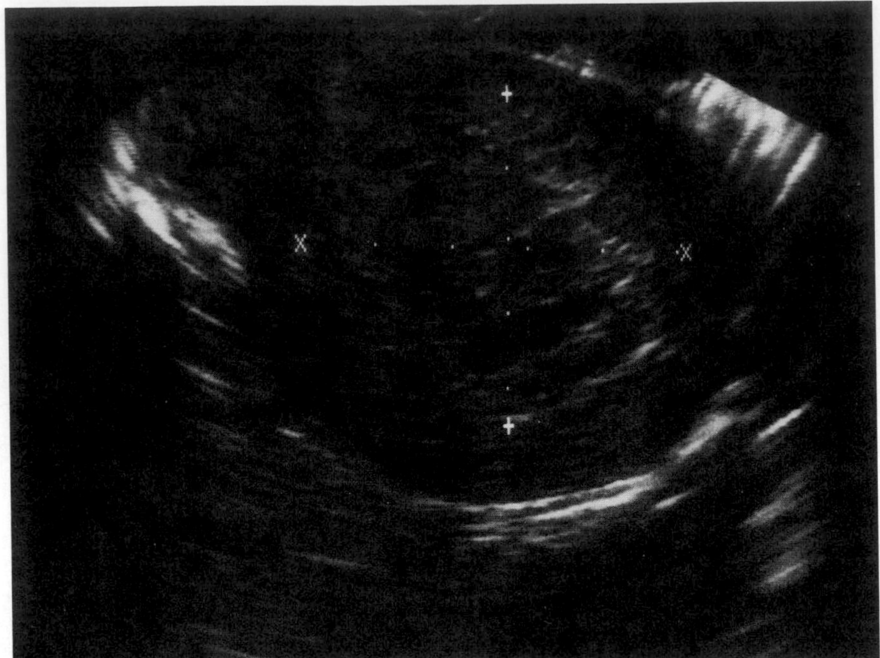

Fig. 6-3. Hematometra. The uterus is filled with a heterogeneous collection of blood several hours after a suction abortion. The cross hatches indicate the uterine cavity measures 4.6 × 5.2 cm. Collections up to 10 cm or more are not uncommon.

to uterotonic agents. Bleeding may stop as the uterus involutes and the blood supply decreases, or it may continue until it is treated with selective embolization[56] or hysterectomy.

Uterine Perforation

Uterine perforations range from a small puncture of the uterine wall without other injury to arterial laceration, or laceration of bowel, bladder, or ureters. The anatomy of uterine perforation is shown in Fig. 6-4. Fortunately most perforations in first trimester are simple punctures of the lower uterine segment or the fundus; these perforations heal without sequelae. In a study of U.S. national data on 67,175 abortions, perforation occurred at a rate of 0.9 per 1000 abortions. Perforation is more likely with procedures performed at a later gestational age, and each 2-week increase in gestational age was associated with a 1.4-fold increase in risk.[57] However, the rate of perforations may be underestimated,[58] and many simple perforations are asymptomatic.

If uterine perforation is suspected, gynecologic consultation should be obtained. The clinical challenge for the consultant is to efficiently determine the location and extent of injury and manage the injury appropriately (Fig. 6-4). When the diagnosis of perforation is unclear and physical findings are minimal, ultrasound may be of help. Suspected perforation can often be confirmed by passing a small dilator through the track with ultrasound guidance.

A midline puncture resulting from a sound or dilator, with no visceral or vascular injury, will require only evacuation of any retained pregnancy tissue under ultrasonic or laparoscopic guidance. The operator can often judge the seriousness of the puncture. If the operator did not immediately recognize uterine perforation, the vacuum cannula or forceps may injure abdominal or pelvic organs outside the uterus. Serious perforations markedly increase the risk for serious bleeding, infection, and death. Suspected perforations in which the site of perforation is not definite can be managed by immediate laparoscopy to assess the extent of injury and plan repair. The abortion can be completed at the same time under laparoscopic guidance.[59] Laparoscopy should be used to inspect the uterus, adnexa, pelvic sidewalls, and the pelvic portions of the large and small intestine. Laparotomy is indicated if the site of injury cannot be completely visualized. Perforations occurring at second trimester D&E procedures

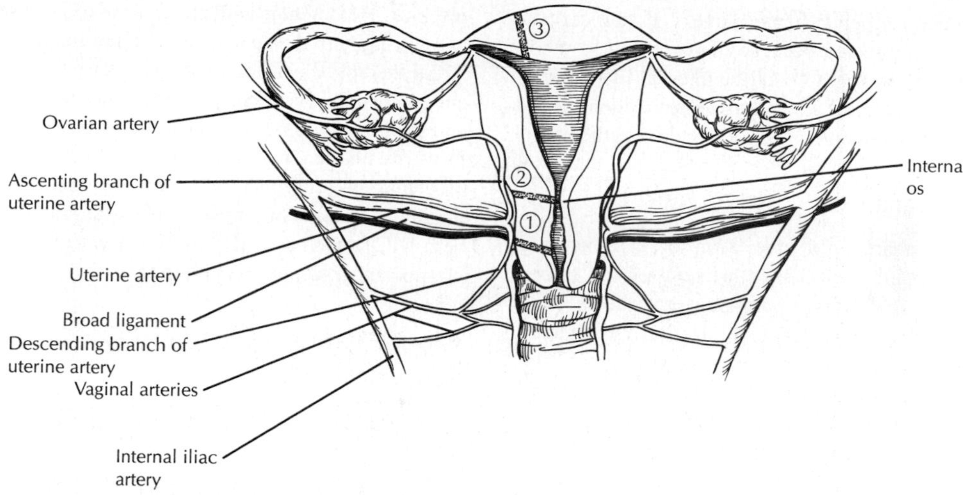

Fig. 6-4. Anatomy of uterine perforations. Possible sites of uterine perforation at abortion: 1. Lateral low cervical perforation with laceration of descending branches of the uterine artery; 2. lateral perforation at junction of cervix and lower uterine segment with laceration of ascending branch of the uterine artery; 3. fundal perforation. (After Berek and Stubblefield,[61] with permission.)

will usually require laparotomy for adequate evaluation and management.

Visceral Injury

Extrauterine instruments, including the suction cannula, may lacerate or traumatize bowel or its mesentery. If fat or bowel is recognized on tissue examination or in the vagina during the abortion, perforation has occurred. Bowel injury can also present as fever and increasing abdominal pain 24 to 48 hours after the procedure.[60] Laparotomy, and occasionally laparoscopy in expert hands, is needed for diagnosis and treatment, as there may be multiple injuries. Bladder injury during an abortion is likely to be in the region of the trigone. Suprapubic pain, anuria, bloody urine, and pain on urination are all suggestive of bladder injury. Operative consultation with an experienced surgical specialist is advised for management of these more extensive injuries. Inadequate initial management of major injury adds significant risk and may jeopardize the woman's survival.

Lateral Uterine Perforation

Lateral uterine perforations present special problems, as they may cause extensive vascular injury that may be unrecognized initially. The operator may perforate laterally with initial dilatation and note a spurt of bright blood that does not appear excessive. The operator may continue and then find the correct channel through the internal os, complete the dilatation, and successfully evacuate the pregnancy. The injured vessels constrict and bleeding stops temporarily, but it can recur minutes, hours, or days later. Lateral perforations at the junction of the cervix and lower uterine segment can lacerate an ascending branch of the uterine artery, giving rise to severe pain, a broad ligament hematoma, and intra-abdominal bleeding (Fig. 6-4).[61] They are managed by laparoscopy to confirm the nature and extent of the injury; laparotomy may be necessary to control bleeding and repair the uterine injury. Low cervical perforation can result from instrumentation during dilation or removal of tissue, causing a cervical "fracture" or rupture. This can injure the descending branch of the uterine artery, which lies within the dense collagenous tissue of the cardinal ligaments. There is no intra-abdominal bleeding seen with this injury. The bleeding is vaginal, through the cervical canal, and may subside temporarily as the artery goes into spasm. These vascular injuries produce recurrent episodes of hemorrhage that may appear to respond to repeated uterine evacuation and uterotonic agents, but recur unexpectedly. Deaths have occurred when this phenomenon was not recognized. Lateral perforations into the cervix or into the broad ligament may escape diagnosis at laparoscopy, as the injury can be retroperitoneal. Treatment by selective embolization during angiography is becoming an increasingly utilized method to control pelvic hemorrhage.[56] If low cervical perforation is suspected because of recurrent postabortal hemorrhage, angiography of the internal iliac arteries should be considered. If a bleeding vessel is identified, it can be selectively embolized via the arterial catheter.

Cervical Pregnancy

Cervical pregnancy is a rare form of ectopic pregnancy, comprising less than 1 percent of all ectopic pregnancies.[62] Treatment by potassium chloride injection, methotrexate, or uterine artery embolization may decrease vascularity enough to allow conservative therapy,[63] but cervical pregnancy may not be suspected prior to instrumentation of the cervix. An attempt at surgical abortion, without prior treatment, may result in immediate hemorrhage. Immediate hysterectomy is usually necessary.

Pulmonary Complications

Anaphylaxis

Fatal anaphylaxis has been reported in asthmatic women from allergy to the preservative sodium metabisulfite[64] and can also be provoked by preservatives found in oxytocin. These women develop severe bronchospasm immediately following an otherwise uncomplicated abortion procedure. Treatment is with oxygen, steroids, antihistamines, intubation, and agents to relieve bronchospasm. Caution must be used to avoid giving the woman more sodium metabisulfite, so epinephrine containing this preservative is absolutely contraindicated. Preservative-free compounds, such as terbutaline, a selective $beta_2$ agonist, should be used.

Embolism

Embolism of amniotic fluid (AFE) or other tissue such as the liquid fetal brain is similar to pulmonary embolism in its pathophysiology, may present as sudden cardiorespiratory collapse during the performance of a D&E, or during labor in midtrimester abortion induced with hypertonic saline or prostaglandins. Although AFE during abortion is very rare in the first trimester, it is more likely at later gestational ages.[43] Most reported cases are fatal, but reported cases probably reflect the most severe presentations. Milder forms of AFE may occur more frequently. It is not uncommon during the performance of a midtrimester D&E to have a transient, sudden drop in oxygen saturation, which spontaneously returns to normal in a few minutes with no sequelae. A woman who is awake will report sudden dyspnea and air hunger, which promptly resolves. Treatment is with oxygen and oxygen saturation monitoring until the episode is over. For major embolism, initial therapy is cardiopulmonary resuscitation, oxygen, and intubation if necessary. Differentiating between AFE and thromboembolism may be difficult, but severe respiratory difficulty leading to cardiac arrest during an abortion procedure will more likely be AFE. Women who survive the initial episode of a major embolism may develop severe DIC, which will require therapy with fresh frozen plasma and possibly cryoprecipitate.

Seizure, Reaction to Local Anesthetic, and Vasovagal Reaction

Women with epilepsy have occasionally had seizures during or after abortion procedures. This may occur if the woman discontinues her antiseizure medications because she is pregnant, and starts the abortion with inadequate levels of medication. The seizure is managed in the conventional fashion with maintenance of the airway and ventilatory support. Generalized convulsions followed by cardiorespiratory arrest may result from overdose of local anesthetic for paracervical block. Treatment is in the conventional manner, and may require intubation and cardiopulmonary support. General anesthesia or sedation may also result in respiratory arrest.[65] Despite the risks described, paracervical block is safer than general anesthesia.

Vasovagal syncope may occur during cervical dilatation under paracervical block, especially in a woman who is not sedated. The woman may have brief tonic-clonic activity and will exhibit bradycardia and marked hypotension, but quickly recovers when the painful stimulation ceases. This phenomenon is differentiated from a true seizure by its brevity, associated cardiovascular changes, and complete absence of a postictal state. Atropine (0.4 to 1 mg IV) can be administered, and the abortion procedure completed as soon as the woman feels better.

Delayed Complications

Delayed complications occur 24 hours or more from the time of abortion. Whereas many immediate complications are handled by the abortion provider, delayed complications are more likely to come to the attention of emergency care providers and may be more complex than immediate complications. There is considerable overlap between some of the conditions described as early and those described as delayed. These include, for example, hematometra, coagulopathy, vascular malformation, and genital tract injury.

Delayed Complications Associated with Increased Pain

Some cramping is normal after abortion; it is typically mild, lasts several days, and should respond to mild analgesics. Women undergoing medical abortion may have intense cramping right before and during the normal course of abortion. They may require additional analgesics, or they may simply need reassurance that the abortion process is progressing normally.

After abortion by any technique, women with a primary complaint of lower abdominal pain with little bleeding and without fever may be having normal cramping, or may have complications such as hematometra, infection, incomplete abortion, ectopic pregnancy, or genital tract injury. Another possibility is a ruptured ovarian cyst, which is most commonly a corpus luteum cyst. The rupture may occur at any point relative to the abortion, and may give unilateral or diffuse lower abdominal pain, sometimes accompanied by nausea. The pain is self-limited to 24 hours or less, and no treatment other than analgesia is required.

Another cause of pain without excessive bleeding is a degenerating leiomyoma. An enlarged uterus with point tenderness over a uterine wall mass, along with ultrasound demonstration of an enlarged empty uterus with a discrete fibroid is consistent with this diagnosis. Consideration must still be given to other possibilities such as perforation and endomyometritis, but lack of adnexal tenderness and fever, with the physical findings as described, are more suggestive of a degenerating fibroid. The treatment is a short course of nonsteroidal anti-inflammatory medication with follow-up in 48 hours.

Women with both increased cramping and increased bleeding may have uterine atony or hematometra, or extravasation or sequestration of blood. Paradoxically, women with uncontained bleeding (i.e., external or intraperitoneal) may not have severe pain.

Delayed Complications Associated with Increased Bleeding

Some of the possible causes of postprocedure excessive bleeding include uterine atony, cervical or uterine injury, hematometra, cervical pregnancy, or retained products of conception. With midtrimester abortion, DIC is a possibility. Urgent management is necessary to prevent mild to moderate bleeding, which may be alarming to the patient, from developing into severe bleeding, which is dangerous to her. As soon as a brief examination is completed, medications to control bleeding should be started. These include intramuscular or intravenous oxytocin, intramuscular carboprost (250 mcg) or oral, buccal, or rectal misoprostol (800 mcg) (Table 6-4). Another temporizing measure to control bleeding includes insertion of a Foley catheter into the uterine cavity and inflating the 30-mL balloon. However, this will only be effective if the uterus is already small and well contracted.

With the bleeding temporarily controlled, a complete history of the events should be obtained and abdominal and pelvic examination and ultrasound examination performed. An incomplete abortion or hematometra will require uterine evacuation. If perforation or ectopic pregnancy is suggested, either by the history or physical exam consistent with peritonitis, the patient should be prepared for immediate laparoscopy.

Failed Abortion

Failed abortion occurs when the procedure did not interrupt the pregnancy, and the pregnancy continues with an apparently normal growth pattern. Reasons for failed surgical abortion include removal of only one fetus of a multiple pregnancy, or inadequate tissue examination after aspiration and failure to recognize the lack of appropriate pregnancy tissue.[66] Predisposing factors for failed abortion include a distorted uterus such as a septate or fibroid uterus.[66,67] For first trimester medical abortion, the situation is more complex. A failed medical abortion is defined as normal progression and growth of the pregnancy 2 weeks after the medical agent is administered. Medical abortion patients may also have a nonviable pregnancy in which growth has stopped. This situation may persist for weeks, or even indefinitely, without detriment. In the absence of infection or bleeding, no urgent intervention is warranted. The patient should be referred to an abortion provider for follow up.

Incomplete Abortion

Incomplete abortion can occur with any abortion technique, with reported rates of 1 to 20 per 1000 women undergoing surgical abortion.[2–4,35,54] A typical presentation is increased bleeding and cramping several days after the abortion, but incomplete abortion may present weeks after the abortion was begun. The amount of bleeding and cramping is variable. Passage of recognized pregnancy tissue is less common. Examination may show some uterine enlargement or placental tissue in the cervical os, but examination is often not helpful in making the diagnosis. Ultrasound examination may not be helpful as small amounts of retained tissue are not always distinguishable from small amounts of blood and decidua normally

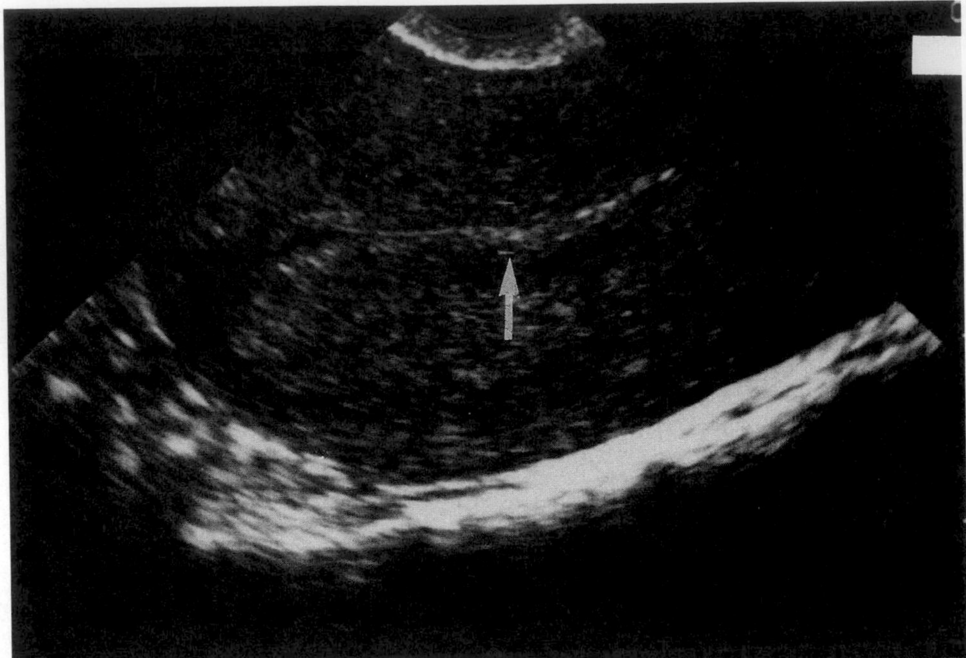

Fig. 6-5. Transvaginal ultrasound image of a uterus after suction curettage. In this example the uterine cavity is 4 mm wide between the cross hatches pointed to by the arrow. This is a normal finding soon after curettage. In the absence of hormonal contraception, the endometrium will develop and thicken during the next menstrual cycle.

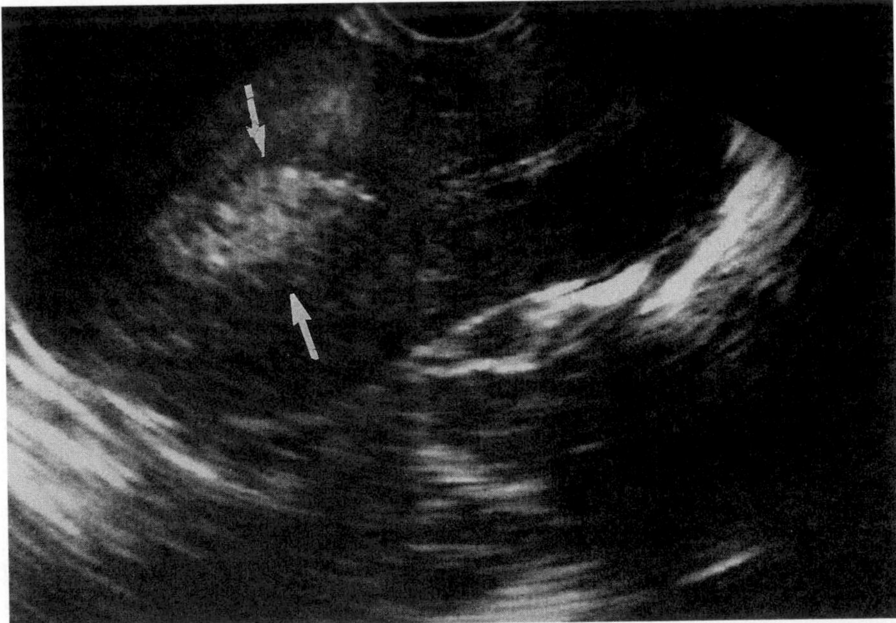

Fig. 6-6. Transvaginal ultrasound image of an incomplete abortion after suction curettage. The retained tissue is seen as a clump of tissue in the fundal part of the endometrial cavity (*arrows*).

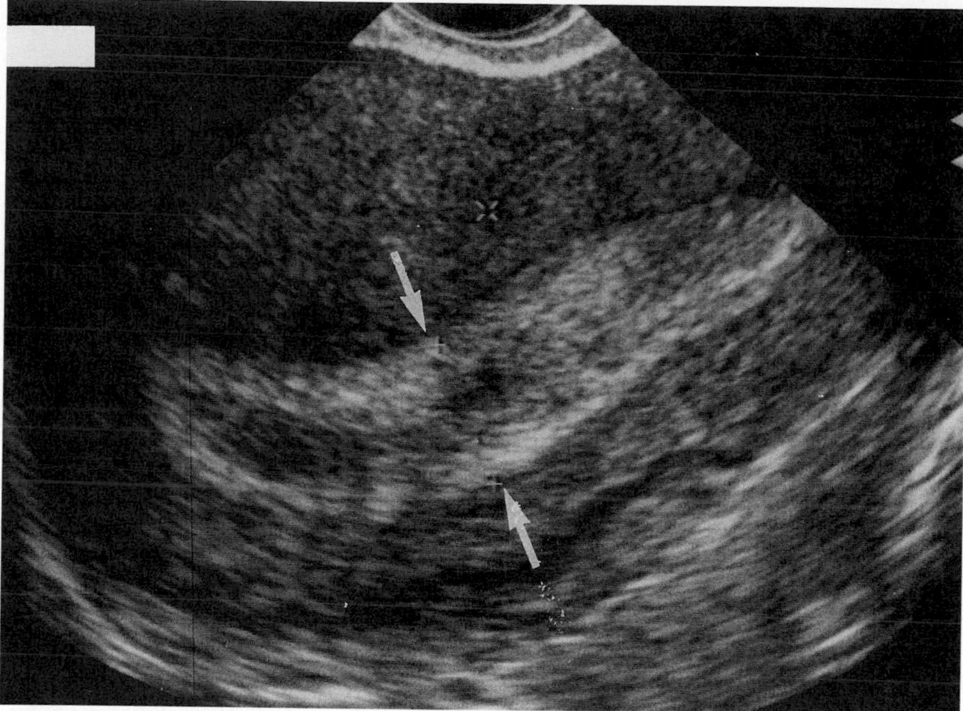

Fig. 6-7. Transvaginal ultrasound image of a uterus several days after medical abortion. In contrast to the image in Fig. 6-5, this endometrial cavity is 14 mm across (between arrows), and this is a normal finding.

present (Figs. 6-5 and 6-6). After medical abortion, the uterine cavity typically contains blood and debris, which may be confused with an incomplete abortion (Figs. 6-7 and 6-8). Hence diagnosis is usually made largely based on the history.

Treatment of incomplete abortion is usually by uterine aspiration, although uterotonic drugs may be sufficient if the amount of tissue is small and the woman wishes to avoid curettage. Curettage is generally simple as the cervix is usually already dilated, so all that is necessary is aspiration of the cavity. Electric suction can be used, but manual aspiration is suitable at most gestational ages because of the low volume of tissue. Incomplete abortion without fetal parts present is usually straightforward. If there are retained fetal parts after second-trimester abortion, an ultrasound guided D&E should be performed by a skilled provider.

Postabortal Triad

Mild to moderate lower abdominal cramping, vaginal bleeding of moderate amount (similar to a menstrual period), and low-grade temperature (38°C or less) have been described as the *postabortal triad,* and is possibly the most common complaint after an abortion. These symptoms may indicate the presence of some amount of retained tissue or blood clot within the uterus, and in some cases an associated mild endometritis (Table 6-5). If abdominal tenderness is limited to the lower abdomen and uterus, the uterus feels firm and only minimally enlarged, and transvaginal ultrasound shows no intrauterine retained tissue, the patient can be treated for possible early endometritis with appropriate antibiotics (see Table 6-3). Oral ergot (methylergonovine maleate or ergotamine, 0.2 mg PO tid for 3 days) can be prescribed to minimize bleeding.

Postabortal Infection

Endometritis and Pelvic Inflammatory Disease

Postabortal endometritis can occur after surgical abortion or second-trimester medical abortion, and appears to be rare after early first-trimester medical abortion.[68]

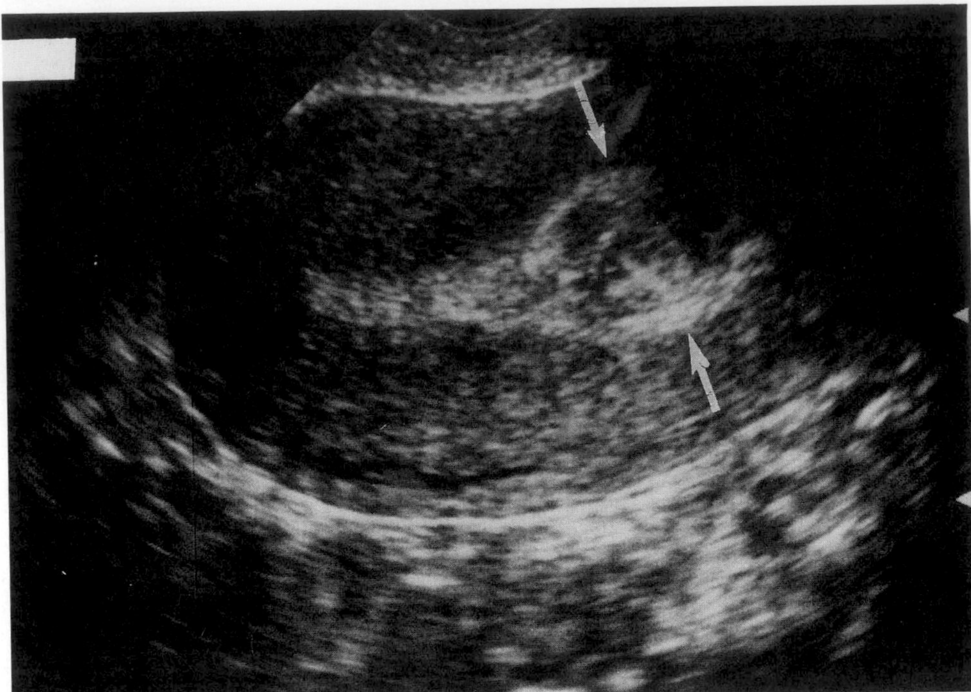

Fig. 6-8. Transvaginal ultrasound image of a uterus several days after medical abortion. In this photo there is a cluster of heterogeneous material adjacent to the internal os (*arrows*). This may represent blood clot, decidua, or an incomplete abortion. The patient was asymptomatic and the collection resolved spontaneously.

A typical presentation is increasing pelvic pain several days after the abortion. Sometimes vaginal bleeding is increased, and normal or increased bleeding obscures purulent discharge. On examination, the uterus is tender and may be slightly enlarged. The adnexa should be evaluated for tenderness or masses. Women with obvious infection 1 or 2 days after abortion may have a streptococcal or gonococcal infection. With the more usual onset of symptoms several days after abortion, the more likely organisms are enterococcal or coliform, or mixed flora.

Table 6-5. Conditions That May Present as Postabortal Triad[a]

Retained pregnancy tissue (incomplete abortion) without sepsis
Failed abortion (continued intact gestation)
Hematometra
Uterine perforation
Ectopic pregnancy
Postabortal endometritis
Early stages of septic incomplete abortion

[a]Lower abdominal pain, bleeding, and low-grade fever.

Women with endometritis should be treated immediately. Women with mild endometritis, without adnexal tenderness or high fever, can be treated as outpatients with antibiotics appropriate for the pattern of symptoms described above. An acceptable approach is to use the regimens for outpatient treatment for pelvic inflammatory disease. The current recommendations by the Centers for Disease Control and Prevention are ofloxacin (400 mg PO bid) plus either clindamycin (450 mg PO qid) or metronidazole (500 mg PO bid) for 14 days, or ceftriaxone 250 mg IM followed by 14 days of doxycycline (100 mg PO bid).[69]

Postabortal infection may progress rapidly from endometritis to endomyometritis, salpingitis, and diffuse pelvic inflammatory disease. The bacteriologic pattern of pelvic infection after abortion is similar to that of pelvic infection unrelated to pregnancy.[68] Women who have adnexal tenderness, peritonitis, high fever (e.g., over

38.5°C), or significant leukocytosis, should be hospitalized for treatment with parenteral antibiotics. Unless the infecting organism is known, broad-spectrum coverage as used for pelvic inflammatory disease should be used. Examples are gentamycin 1.5 mg/kg q8h, with either clindamycin 900 mg IV q8h or metronidazole 500 mg IV q6h.[69] Fluoroquinolones have been used for single-drug treatment.[70]

Regardless of the severity of the infection, if the woman has a coexisting incomplete abortion, it must be evacuated promptly. The infection can worsen quickly if the incomplete abortion is not treated. Antibiotic coverage for postabortal infection is unchanged with coexisting incomplete abortion.

Sepsis and Septic Incomplete Abortion

If retained pregnancy tissue is not evacuated promptly, septic incomplete abortion may develop. Septic shock and acute respiratory distress syndrome (ARDS) can ensue.[68,71] In the United States, septic incomplete abortion may be more common after spontaneous abortion than after induced abortion.[68] This condition should be suspected when a woman of childbearing age presents with sepsis, vaginal bleeding, and amenorrhea, even if there is no history of attempted abortion. Sepsis may also follow a completed abortion; the lack of retained tissue does not preclude serious infection. A variety of infecting organisms are possible, including vaginal and bowel flora, *Neisseria gonorrhoeae* and *Chlamydia,* and the more rare but extremely serious infections, such as *Clostridium perfringens* and synergistic necrotizing infections.[68,71]

To treat the infection, blood cultures and cultures from the cervix and endometrial cavity should be obtained, and high-dose broad-spectrum antibiotics begun. The Centers for Disease Control regimens for severe pelvic inflammatory disease can be used.[69] For seriously ill women triple therapy is appropriate, such as the combination of ampicillin 2 to 3 g IV q6h, gentamicin 1.5 mg/kg q8h, and either clindamycin 900 mg IV q8h or metronidazole 7.5 mg/kg IV q6h (usual adult dose, 500 mg).[68,71]

Once antibiotic coverage is started, the uterus must be emptied. In the first trimester, this can be accomplished with vacuum curettage. A retained fetus in the midtrimester creates special problems. If a physician skilled in D&E is available, D&E under ultrasound guidance may be performed; otherwise, labor can be induced with carboprost, misoprostol, or high-dose oxytocin (Table 6-1). Prostaglandin E_2 should probably be avoided in septic abortion, because it elevates body temperature.

Septic shock related to pregnancy can appear to progress rapidly, as healthy young women can maintain apparent hemodynamic stability until multisystem collapse or ARDS develop. Expert support in an intensive care unit is essential, as required with septic shock from other causes.

Clostridial sepsis should be suspected from the presence of large gram-positive rods on Gram stain from the endometrial cavity or curetted tissue. Other signs of clostridial sepsis are tachycardia that seems out of proportion to the fever, hematuria, and rapidly developing shock.[71] Severe ARDS develops rapidly in these women. Initial treatment is as described above, but with high-dose penicillin G (4 million units IV q4h) instead of ampicillin. A superficial clostridial infection will respond to these measures. If hemolysis is present, this indicates systemic release of clostridial toxins. Prompt hysterectomy and bilateral salpingo-oophorectomy are necessary. Hyperbaric oxygenation may play a role in treatment, in addition to effective surgical and medical management of clostridial sepsis.

In addition to clostridia, other severe bacterial pathogens can cause these infections. Some of these are synergistic infections with tissue necrosis and septic shock. Recognition of these rare situations, with supportive treatment and prompt surgery, can be life-saving. The woman who arrives at the emergency department in septic shock, or who deteriorates rapidly, needs immediate evaluation by both a critical care specialist and a gynecologic surgeon. Necrotic tissue from a uterus with full-thickness infection can release bacterial toxins. The woman's condition will not improve until the infected or necrotic tissue is removed surgically. This may require hysterectomy, salpingo-oophorectomy, or debridement.

Sepsis in the postabortal patient may result from infection other than in the uterus. Unrecognized bowel or urinary injury from perforation are possible, as are unrelated illnesses such as appendicitis, gallbladder disease, and pancreatitis.

Acute Respiratory Distress Syndrome

Acute respiratory distress syndrome (ARDS) occurs with septic abortion and is occasionally seen in the context of a uterine perforation with major hemorrhage. Management in an intensive care unit is required in order to have expert ventilatory support. Mortality is high even in previously healthy young women.

Ectopic Pregnancy

Women seeking abortion have rates of ectopic pregnancy ranging from 1 to 6 per 1000 women.[72] This rate is apparently lower than the overall rate for the U.S. population of 20 per 1000 women.[73] Women with ectopic pregnancy may develop symptoms and seek care elsewhere before they request abortion, contributing to this discrepancy in rates. The risk for ectopic pregnancy should have been assessed at the time of induced abortion by the woman's history, the operator's examination of the tissue, or by preabortion sonography. If an intrauterine pregnancy is not confirmed, the woman may leave the facility without appreciation of her risk of ectopic pregnancy. Later on, when pain from the ectopic pregnancy begins, the woman may initially attribute this to expected postabortal discomfort and may delay seeking help. Prior demonstration of an intrauterine pregnancy by tissue or ultrasound essentially eliminates the possibility of ectopic pregnancy,[74] with the exception of a very rare heterotopic pregnancy (a twin pregnancy in both uterus and tube at the same time).

Without prior ultrasound or tissue results, evaluating the possibility of ectopic pregnancy after an abortion can be complex. Human chorionic gonadotropin (hCG) assays will detect hCG for several weeks after an induced abortion. Most women who present with mild to moderate pain and minimal to moderate bleeding may not have an ectopic pregnancy, but rather a low-grade endometritis, some retained tissue or clot, postabortal triad, or be completely normal. Ectopic pregnancy should be suspected if ultrasound shows an empty uterus and abundant fluid in the pelvic cavity, suggestive of hemoperitoneum. Ectopic pregnancy is confirmed if ultrasound shows an adnexal mass with cardiac activity (see Chap. 5). If the woman has severe abdominal pain and peritoneal signs, then prompt evaluation by laparoscopy or laparotomy is required, as uterine or visceral injury, as well as ectopic pregnancy, are possibilities.

Until the pregnancy is confirmed as having been intrauterine, or it is demonstrated that she is no longer pregnant, the woman must be considered at risk for ectopic pregnancy. If she is clinically stable with minimal findings, she can be followed as an outpatient with serial quantitative hCG assays until it is clear that the levels are falling rapidly, consistent with a complete induced abortion. Follow-up within 48 hours is indicated as hCG levels normally fall at least 50 percent within 48 hours if the pregnancy has been removed. During this period the woman must be aware of the risk of ectopic pregnancy. If the levels plateau or start to rise, the woman should be treated as having either an ectopic pregnancy or an incomplete abortion. Uterine aspiration will remove small amounts of tissue, and demonstration of villi or an abrupt fall in hCG levels after aspiration confirms the diagnosis of incomplete abortion. Otherwise the woman has a likely ectopic pregnancy and should be treated accordingly.

Complications Remote from the Abortion Procedure

Cervical Agglutination Syndrome

Occasionally postabortal women will present several months following a surgical abortion with pelvic pain recurring monthly and no menstrual bleeding.[75] On examination, the uterus might be somewhat tender around the time of menses. Treatment is gentle passage of a small blunt cervical dilator through the cervical canal. This is followed by extrusion of mucoid old blood from the cervical canal; regular menses typically resumes. This condition is distinct from Asherman's syndrome, in which there are intrauterine adhesions and endometrial destruction. Asherman's syndrome is unlikely following uncomplicated suction abortion.

REFERENCES

1. Hakim-Elahi E, Tovell HMM, Bumhill MS: Complications of first trimester abortion: A report of 170,000 cases. *Obstet Gynecol* 76:129–135, 1990.
2. Grimes DA, Cates W: Complications from legally-induced abortion: A review. *Obstet Gynecol Surv* 34:177–191, 1979.
3. Tietze C, Lewit S: Joint Program for the Study of Abortion (JPSA): Early medical complications of legal abortion. *Stud Fam Plann* 3:97–122, 1972.
4. Lichtenberg ES, Grimes DA, Paul M. Abortion complications: Prevention and management, in Paul M, Lichtenberg ES, Borgatta L, Grimes DA, Stubblefield PG (eds): *A Clinician's Guide to Medical and Surgical Abortion*. New York: Churchill Livingstone, 1999, pp 197–216.
5. Koonin LM, Strauss LT, Chrisman CE, Parker WY: Abortion surveillance—United States, 1998. *MMWR Morb Mortal Wkly Rep* 51:1–32, 2002.
6. Cates W. Jr, Rochat RW: Illegal abortions in the United States: 1972–1974. Fam Plan Perspect 1976; 8:86–92.
7. Lawson HW, Frye A, Atrash HK, et al: Abortion mortality: United States, 1972 through 1987. *Am J Obstet Gynecol* 171:1365–1372, 1994.
8. Hodgson JE: Major complications of 20,248 consecutive induced abortions: Problems of fragmented care. *Adv Planned Parenthood* 9:52–59, 1975.
9. Susser M: Induced abortion and health as a value. *Am J Public Health* 82:1323–1324, 1992.

COLOR PLATES

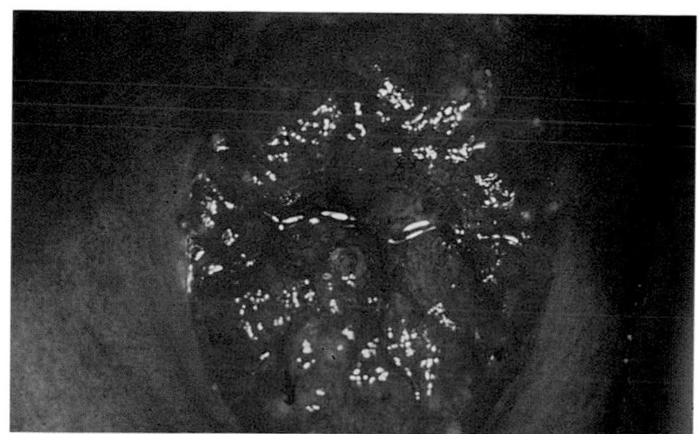

PLATE 1 Cervical ectropion. The cervical transformation zone in a woman on oral contraceptives. Note the prominent eversion of endocervical cells covering more than one half of the portio vaginalis. *(Photograph courtesy of John R.G. Gosling slide collection)*

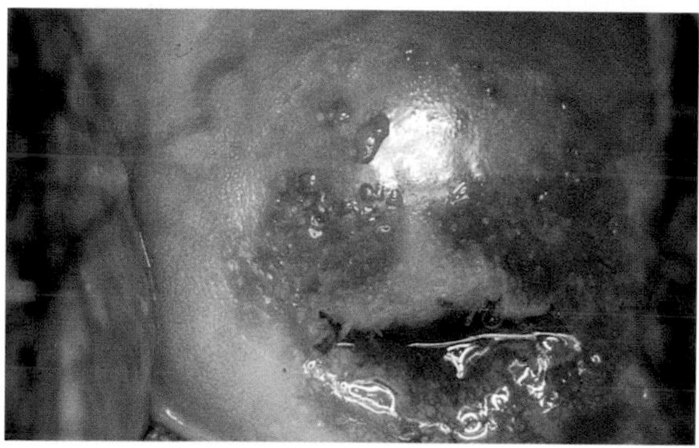

PLATE 2 Positive Chadwick sign. Note the bluish hue of the pregnant cervix. *(Photograph courtesy of John R.G. Gosling slide collection)*

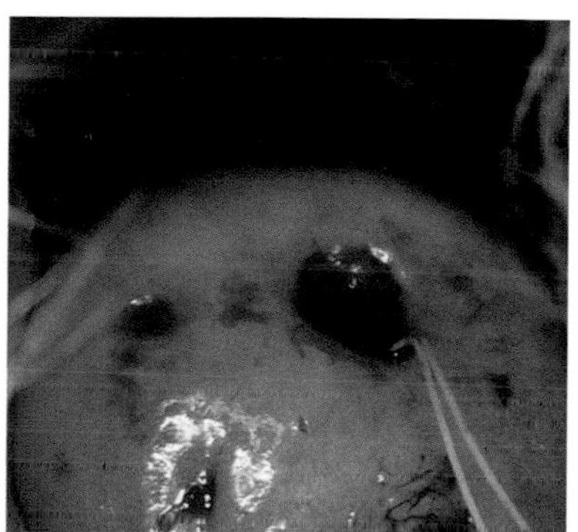

PLATE 3 Paragard IUD string protruding from the cervix.

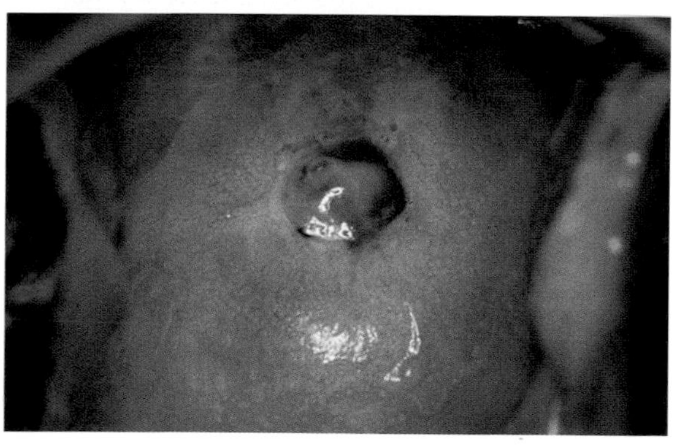

PLATE 4 Mucopurulent cervicitis. *(Photograph courtesy of Mark D. Pearlman, MD)*

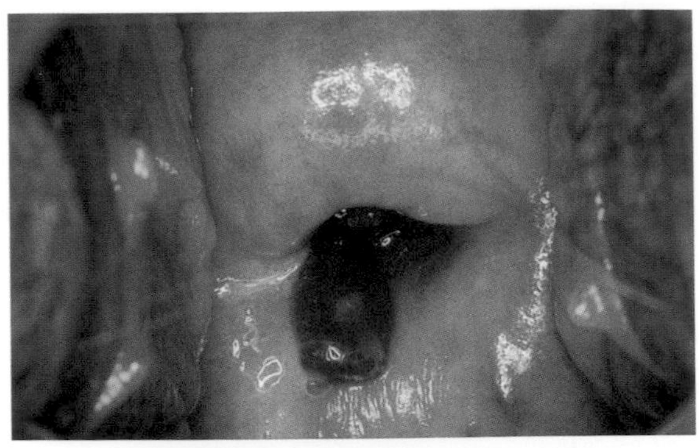

PLATE 5 Single cervical polyp.

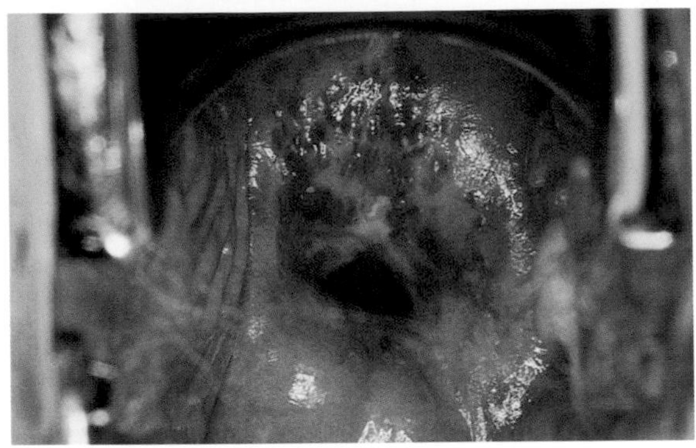

PLATE 6 Cervical endometriosis in a menstruating woman. Note the red papules on the portio vaginalis which contain blood and endometrial tissue.

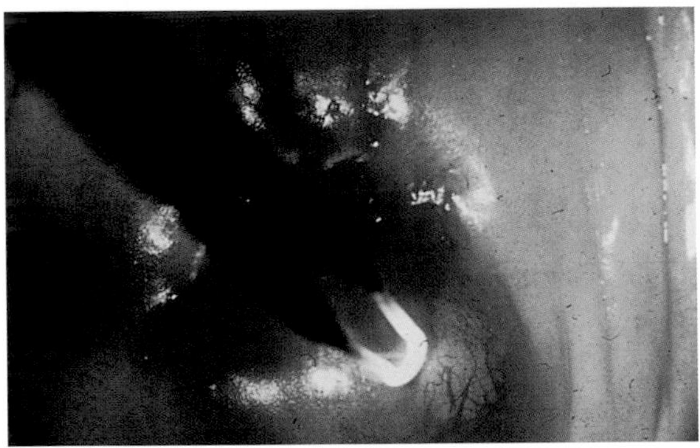

PLATE 7 Nabothian cyst. The forcep is pointed to the raised, round cyst which is yellow-white in color. Note the distinct capillaries branching over the surface of the cyst. *(Photograph courtesy of John R.G. Gosling slide collection)*

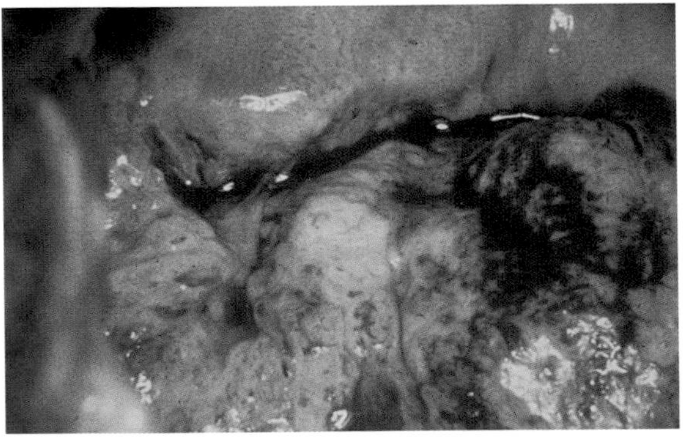

PLATE 8 Invasive squamous cell carcinoma. Note the abnormal vasculature and hemorrhage on the posterior cervical lip. *(Photograph courtesy of John R.G. Gosling slide collection)*

10. Levallois P, Rioux JE: Prophylactic antibiotics for suction curettage abortion: Results of a clinical controlled trial. *Am J Obstet Gynecol* 158:100–105, 1988.
11. Sorensen JL, Thranov I, Hoff G, Dirach J, Damsgaard M: A double-blind randomized study of the effect of erythromycin in preventing pelvic inflammatory disease after first trimester abortion. *Brit J Obstet Gynaecol* 99:434–438, 1992.
12. Larrson PG, Platz-Christensen JJ, Theijls H, Forsum U, Pahlson C: Incidence of pelvic inflammatory disease after first-trimester legal abortion in women with bacterial vaginosis after treatment with metronidazole: A double-blind, randomized trial. *Am J Obstet Gynecol* 166:100–103, 1992.
13. Darj E, Strain EB, Nilsson S: The prophylactic effect of doxycycline on postoperative infection rate after first-trimester abortion. *Obstet Gynecol* 70:755–758, 1987.
14. Brewer C: Prevention of infection after abortion with a supervised single dose of oral doxycycline. *Lancet* 281:780–781, 1980.
15. Sawaya GF, Grady DI, Kerlikowske K, Grimes DA. Antibiotics at the time of induced abortion: the case for universal prophylaxis based on meta-analysis. *Obstet Gynecol* 86: 884–889, 1996.
16. Borgatta L, Bumhill MS, Tyson J, et al: Early medical abortion with methotrexate and misoprostol. *Obstet Gynecol* 97:11–16, 2001
17. American College of Obstetricians and Gynecologists: Prevention of Rh D isoalloimmunization. ACOG Practice Bulletin No. 4, 1999.
18. Edwards JE, Damey PD, Paul M: Surgical abortion in the first trimester, in Paul M, Lichtenberg ES, Borgatta L, Grimes DA, Stubblefield PG (eds): *A Clinician's Guide to Medical and Surgical Abortion*. New York: Churchill Livingstone, 1999, pp 107–121.
19. Edwards J, Creinin MD: Surgical abortion for gestations of less than 6 weeks. *Curr Prob Obstet Gynecol* 20:11–19, 1997.
20. Damey PD, Horbach NS, Kom AP: First trimester elective abortion, in *Protocols for Office Gynecologic Surgery*. Cambridge, MA: Blackwell Science, 1996, pp 158–193.
21. Glick E: Surgical abortion. Reno, NV: West End Women's Medical Group, 1998, pp 2-43.
22. Stubblefield PG: Surgical techniques of uterine evacuation in first- and second-trimester abortion. *Clin Obstet Gynecol* 13:53–70, 1986.
23. Lichtenberg ES, Paul M, Jones H: First trimester surgical abortion practices: a survey of National Abortion Federation members. *Contraception* 64:345–352, 2001.
24. American College of Obstetricians and Gynecologists: Medical management of abortion. ACOG Practice Bulletin No. 26, 2001.
25. Christin-Maitre S, Bouchard P, Spitz IM: Drug therapy: Medical termination of pregnancy. *N Engl J Med* 342:946–956, 2000.
26. Schaff EA, Fielding SL, Eisinger SH, Stadalius LS, Fuller L: Low-dose mifepristone followed by vaginal misoprostol at 48 hours for abortion up to 63 days. *Contraception* 61:41–46, 2000.
27. Schaff EA, Fielding SL, Westhoff C, et al: Vaginal misoprostol administered 1, 2, or 3 days after mifepristone for early medical abortion: A randomized trial. *JAMA* 284:1948, 2000.
28. Blanchard K, Winikoff B, Ellertson C: Misoprostol used alone for the termination of early pregnancy: A review of the evidence. *Contraception* 59:209–217, 1999.
29. Jain JK, Harwood B, Meckstroth KR, Mishell DR: Early pregnancy termination with vaginal misoprostol combined with loperamide and acetaminophen prophylaxis. *Contraception* 63:217–223, 2001.
30. Carbonell JL, Rodriguez J, Aragon S, et al: Vaginal misoprostol 1000 μg for early abortion. *Contraception* 63:131–136, 2001.
31. Kahn JG, Becker BJ, MacIsaac L, et al: The efficacy of medical abortion: a meta-analysis. *Contraception* 61:29–40, 2000.
32. Davis A, Westhoff C, De Nonno L: Bleeding patterns after early abortion with mifepristone and misoprostol or manual vacuum aspiration. *J Am Women's Assoc* 55(Suppl):141–144, 2000.
33. Haskell MW, Easterling TR, Lichtenberg ES. Surgical abortion after the first trimester, in Paul M, Lichtenberg ES, Borgatta L, Grimes DA, Stubblefield PG (eds): *A Clinician's Guide to Medical and Surgical Abortion*. New York:, Churchill Livingstone, 1999, pp 123–138.
34. Hem WM: *Abortion Practice*. Philadelphia: JB Lippincott, 1990, pp 122–160.
35. Castadot RG: Pregnancy termination: techniques, risks, and complications and their management. *Fertil Steril* 45:5–14, 1986.
36. Schulz KF, Grimes DA, Christensen DD: Vasopressin reduces blood loss from second-trimester dilatation and evacuation abortion. *Lancet* 2(8451):353–356, 1985.
37. Woodward G: Estimation of blood loss in second-trimester dilatation and extraction. *Obstet Gynecol* 63:230–232, 1984.
38. Winkler CL, Gray SE, Hauth JC, et al: Mid second trimester labor induction: Concentrated oxytocin compared with prostaglandin E_2 vaginal suppositories. *Obstet Gynecol* 77:297–300, 1991.
39. Owen J, Hauth JC: Concentrated oxytocin plus low-dose prostaglandin E_2 compared with prostaglandin E_2 vaginal suppositories for second-trimester pregnancy termination. *Obstet Gynecol* 88:110–113, 1996.
40. Blumenthal PD, Castleman LD, Jain JK: Abortion by labor induction, in Paul M, Lichtenberg ES, Borgatta L, Grimes DA, Stubblefield PG (eds): *A Clinician's Guide to Medical and Surgical Abortion*. New York: Churchill Livingstone, 1999, pp 139–154.
41. American College of Obstetricians and Gynecologists: Methods of midtrimester abortion. ACOG Technical Bulletin No. 109, 1987.

42. Jain JK, Mishell DR: A comparison of intravaginal misoprostol with prostaglandin E_2 for termination of second trimester pregnancy. *N Engl J Med* 331:290, 1994.
43. Guidotti RJ, Grimes DA, Cates W: Fatal amniotic fluid embolism during legally induced abortion, United States, 1972–1978. *Am J Obstet Gynecol* 141:257–61, 1981.
44. Evans MI, Donunergues M, Wapner RJ, et al: Efficacy of transabdominal multifetal pregnancy reduction: Collaborative experience among the world's largest centers. *Obstet Gynecol* 82:61–66, 1993.
45. Potts M, Diggory P, Peel J: *Abortion*. New York: Cambridge University Press, 1977, p 336.
46. Bumhill MS: Treatment of women who have undergone chemically induced abortions. *J Reprod Med* 30:610–614, 1985.
47. Coelho HL, Teixeira AC, Cruz M de F, et al: Misoprostol: the experience of women in Forteleza, Brazil. *Contraception* 49:101, 1994.
48. De Nonno LJ, Westhoff C, Fielding S, Schaff EA: Timing of pain and bleeding after mifepristone-induced abortion. *Contraception* 62:305–309, 2000.
49. Elul B, Ellertson C, Winikoff B, Coyaji K: Side effects of mifepristone-misoprostol abortion versus surgical abortion. Data from a trial in China, Cuba and India. *Contraception* 59:107, 1999.
50. Farrel RG, Stonington DT, Ridgeway RA: Incomplete and inevitable abortion: treatment by suction curettage in the emergency room. *Ann Emerg Med* 11:652–8, 1982.
51. Williamson D: Resources for abortion providers, in Paul M, Lichtenberg ES, Borgatta L, Grimes D, Stubblefield P (eds): *A Clinician's Guide to Medical and Surgical Abortion*. New York: Churchill Livingstone, 1999, p 286.
52. Post-abortion family planning: a practical guide for programme managers. World Health Organization, Geneva, Switzerland, 1997.
53. Winkler J, Oliveras E, McIntosh N: *Postabortion Care: A Reference Manual for Improving Quality of Care*. Postabortion Care Consortium, c/o AVSC, New York, NY, 1995.
54. Bozorgi N: Statistical analysis of first-trimester pregnancy termination in an ambulatory surgical center. *Am J Obstet Gynecol* 127:763–768, 1977.
55. Sands RX, Bumhill MS, Hakim-Elahi E: Post-abortal uterine atony. *Obstet Gynecol* 43:595–598, 1974.
56. Borgatta L, Chen AN, Reid S, et al: Pelvic embolization for treatment of hemorrhage related to spontaneous and induced abortion. *Am J Obstet Gynecol* 185:530–536, 2001.
57. Grimes DA, Schultz KF, Cates, WJ. Prevention of uterine perforation during curettage abortion. *JAMA* 251:2108, 1984.
58. Kaali SG, Szigetvari IA, Bartfai GS: The frequency and management of uterine perforations during first-trimester abortions. *Am J Obstet Gynecol* 161:40, 1989.
59. Lindell G, Flam F: Management of uterine perforations in connection with legal abortions. *Acta Obstet Gynecol Scand* 74:373–375, 1995.
60. Leibner EC: Delayed presentation of uterine perforation. *Ann Emerg Med* 26:643, 1995.
61. Berek JS, Stubblefield PG: Anatomic and clinical correlates of uterine perforation. *Am J Obstet Gynecol* 135:181–184, 1979.
62. Cunningham FG, MacDonald PC, Gant NF, et al: Ectopic pregnancy, in *Williams Obstetrics,* 20th ed. Stamford, CT: Appleton & Lange, 1997, pp. 607–634.
63. Frates MC, Benson CB, Doubilet PM, et al: Cervical ectopic pregnancy: Results of conservative treatment. *Radiology* 191:773, 1994.
64. U.S. Food and Drug Administration: Warning for prescription drugs containing sulfite. *Drug Bull* 17:2, 1987.
65. Grimes DA, Cates W: Deaths from paracervical anesthesia used for first trimester abortion, 1972–1975. *N Engl J Med* 295:1397–1399, 1976.
66. Fielding WL, Lee SY, Borten M, Friedman EA: Continuing pregnancy after failed first-trimester abortion. *Obstet Gynecol* 63:421, 1984.
67. Kaunitz AM, Rovira EZ, Grimes DA, Schulz KF: Abortions that fail. *Obstet Gynecol* 66:533, 1985.
68. Faro S, Pearlman M: *Infections and Abortion*. New York: Elsevier, 1992.
69. Sexually Transmitted Diseases Treatment Guidelines—2002. May 3, 2002/mmWR 51 (RR06); 1–80.
70. Finch RG: Ciprofloxacin: efficacy and indications. *J Chemo Suppl* 1:5, 2000.
71. Stubblefield PG, Grimes DA: Septic abortion. *N Engl J Med* 331:310, 1994.
72. Kaall SG, Csakany GM, Szigetvari I, Barad DH: Updated screening protocol for abortion services. *Obstet Gynecol* 76:136, 1990.
73. Current Trends Ectopic Pregnancy—United States, 1990–1992. MMWR 44:46–48, 1995.
74. Edwards J, Carson SA: New technologies permit safe abortion at less than six weeks' gestation and provide timely detection of ectopic pregnancy. *Am J Obstet Gynecol* 176:1101–1106, 1997.
75. Hakim-Elahi E: Postabortal amenorrhea due to cervical stenosis. *Obstet Gynecol* 48: 723, 1976.

SECTION III
PROBLEMS AFTER 20 WEEKS OF PREGNANCY

7

Transfer and Transport of Pregnant Women

Mark J. Lowell

KEY POINTS

- EMS systems should develop protocols that identify facilities capable of caring for the pregnant woman with a medical or surgical emergency.
- Neonates cared for in a neonatal intensive care unit (NICU) beginning at birth have a greater probability of survival and a shorter length of hospitalization than those transferred after birth.
- However, if labor has progressed to the point at which delivery en route is likely, it is usually preferable to delay transport and await the arrival of the neonatal team.
- There are three interventions that should be performed on almost all pregnant patients during transport: (1) transport in the lateral tilt position, (2) administration of supplemental oxygen, and (3) administration of intravenous fluid.

TRANSPORT OF THE PREGNANT WOMAN

The need for interhospital patient transfer has grown over the past several decades. Critically ill or injured patients may require equipment and expertise that is unavailable at a smaller hospital, or deterioration in status of a previously stable patient may require advanced care that exceeds local capabilities. In the case of a sick or injured pregnant woman, the limited number of facilities equipped to care for their special needs makes the need for transfer more likely, because illness or injury frequently occurs in areas far away from tertiary care centers or centers that can provide emergency care for both the pregnant woman and her fetus. The recent development and proliferation of freestanding "birthing centers" has also contributed to the need for rapid transport. Although many birth centers are affiliated with a hospital, they may be physically separate and sometimes at great distances from the main facility. A review of care in birthing centers from 1989 reported an overall transfer rate of 15.8 percent.[1] A more recent descriptive study of a university-based center reported transfer rates of 12 percent for antepartum patients and 19 percent for intrapartum patients during a 20-month study period.[2] As the number of birthing centers increases, it is reasonable to assume that the number of transfers will rise as well. Last, the growth of health maintenance organizations (HMOs) and their practice of caring for their clients at designated institutions will assure the continued need for critical care transport.

Thus it is reasonable to assume that the need to transport pregnant women will continue to increase. This chapter focuses on some of the issues involved in the prehospital and interhospital transport of the pregnant patient.

PREHOSPITAL TRANSPORTATION

Prehospital transport refers to transport that originates at a nonmedical facility such as a residence or accident scene. The majority of transports of pregnant patients done by emergency medical technicians and paramedics are routine and uncomplicated. From a prehospital perspective, the management is based upon two principles: (1) that definitive care cannot be provided in the prehospital setting and (2) that appropriate care of the mother is the best treatment for the fetus.[3]

Most emergency medical services (EMS) systems are successful because the prehospital care providers have specific protocols that specify the care to be rendered for various medical conditions. This is known as *off-line medical control.* In the event of an unusual or unclear situation, provisions are made for direct assistance via radio or telephone from a physician or his or her designee. This is known as *on-line medical control.*

It is important for EMS systems to develop protocols that specifically identify those facilities capable of caring for the pregnant woman with a medical or surgical emergency.[3] It may be appropriate in some instances to bypass certain hospitals to get to a more comprehensive facility; for example, a woman with severe preeclampsia at 30 weeks gestation. Other patients should be transported to the closest facility for initial stabilization. For example, a pregnant patient in need of an urgent airway intervention, or a newborn in distress might best be initially cared for at the closest facility. Protocols must take into account differences in transport times and the risk that a potentially longer transport may cause adverse sequelae. Both on-line and off-line medical control should be available to assist in these situations.

Although most deliveries are uncomplicated, patients that deliver in the prehospital environment or in the emergency department do have a higher risk of complications.[4] Therefore, prehospital personnel must consider the likelihood of imminent delivery versus the ability to transport the mother to the hospital safely. If delivery appears imminent, it is usually most prudent to deliver at the scene, because delivery in the close confines of a moving ambulance, especially if there is only one caregiver, can be difficult. The prehospital caregiver should assist the delivery (see Chap. 21). Only two conditions require insertion of the sterile gloved hand into the vagina by the prehospital provider:[3] (1) in the event of a breech presentation, it may become necessary to insert a hand into the vagina to flex the fetal neck to assist in the delivery of the aftercoming head (see Chap. 21); and (2) in the event of a prolapsed umbilical cord, the provider's hand should gently displace the presenting part off the cord to restore normal umbilical cord blood flow. The mother should be placed in the knee-chest position to help decrease cord compression. In both cases, rapid transport to an obstetric facility that can perform urgent cesarean delivery is required.

INTERHOSPITAL TRANSPORTATION

The most widely recognized system of regional distribution of care designates three different levels of facility and expertise in obstetric neonatal services. The capabilities of these different levels are listed in Table 7-1.

Interhospital transports can be classified as one-way or two-way. When the patient is transferred using ambulances and personnel based at or near the referring facility, it is classified as a *one-way transport.* When a team is sent from the receiving institution to pick up and return with the patient, it is classified as a *two-way transport.*

One-way transports involve some potential disadvantages, especially for pregnant patients. When a patient is being transferred because of a complication of pregnancy, standard ambulance crews frequently lack the clinical experience to continue the level of care provided at the hospital. Furthermore, if the patient's condition should worsen en route, appropriate evaluation and intervention is dependent on the skill and expertise of the local EMS personnel. In an effort to overcome this problem, staff members from the referring institution (e.g., a nurse or physician) may accompany the patient with the ambulance crew. This, too, may not be ideal, as these personnel are usually unfamiliar with transport medicine. They are not used to working in the unstable environment of a moving ambulance, where noise, vibration, and cramped space place limitations on the ability to identify and manage changes in a patient's condition. Additionally, available equipment and resources usually do not match those available at the hospital. The nurse or physician who accompanies a patient will be absent from the institution and therefore unable to perform his or her usual hospital duties. Last, since most of these transports originate from small communities, the community will be deprived of an ambulance and its crew for several hours.[5]

Two-way transports overcome many of these problems. Two-way systems usually have dedicated transport teams that are specially trained to function in the transport environment and carry special equipment and devices to allow them to do so quickly and efficiently. Dedicated teams generally develop expertise in all types of transports. The major drawback of the two-way transport system is time: the delay in arrival of the transport team at the referring institution, followed by transport time to the receiving institution. The referring physician must consider the risks of sending an unstable (or potentially unstable) patient with an inexperienced crew using a one-way transport system versus waiting for a more experienced crew to arrive who can stabilize and prepare the patient for transport and who are better prepared to care for any problems that may arise en route.

CREW CONFIGURATION

The issue of ideal crew configuration for transport remains controversial. The most important goal is the safe and effective transfer of the patient. Regardless of the level of certification or degrees possessed, the caregiver must have general knowledge of and expertise in critical care. Furthermore, for this patient population, a working knowl-

Table 7-1. Facility Designation by Level of Obstetric Neonatal Services

	Obstetric Services	Neonatal Services	Example
Level I (Basic)	1. Ability to provide surveillance and care to all obstetric patients with a triage system to identify high-risk patients for transport to level II or III facility 2. Ability to perform cesarean section within 30 min 3. 24-h laboratory facilities including blood bank facilities	1. Care for healthy neonates 2. Resuscitation and stabilization of near-term neonates 3. Stabilization of unexpectedly small or sick neonates before transfer to a level II or III facility	1. Uncomplicated term or near-term vaginal and cesarean delivery 2. Mild preeclampsia at term
Level II (Specialty)	1. All level I services 2. Management of high-risk mothers and fetuses (generally 1500-2500 g, 32-36 weeks of gestation)	1. All level I services 2. Management of small, sick neonates with a moderate degree of illness, either admitted or transferred	1. Preterm labor at 32-36 weeks
Level III (Subspecialty)	1. All level II services 2. Comprehensive care for mothers of all risk categories 3. Evaluation of new high-risk technologies	1. All level II services 2. Management of extremely small (<1500 g) or sick neonates	1. Preterm labor <32 weeks 2. Fetal anomalies requiring correction (e.g., diaphragmatic hernia, open neural tube defects) 3. Need for maternal intensive care (e.g., severe cardiac or pulmonary disease)

Source: Modified from Gilstrap and Oh,[14] with permission.

edge of the physiology of labor and delivery, experience with drugs used during pregnancy and childbirth, familiarity with fetal heart monitors and the ability to interpret their data, and competency in newborn resuscitation are important skills to possess.

Suggested crew configuration guidelines are given in Table 7-2. Note that a low-risk patient is one in whom the risk of the development of complications or delivery en route is minimal. A moderate-risk patient is one who has been stable for several hours and in whom there is a small chance of complications developing. A high-risk patient is one who is critically ill.

The referring physician should use caution to ensure that the transporting service is as capable as it claims to be. As an example, a recent survey of air medical providers demonstrated that only half of their "standard" (i.e., nonspecialty) crews that do obstetric and neonatal transport were required to maintain certification in neonatal resuscitation.[6]

In addition to crew configuration, the mode of transport is an important consideration (Table 7-3). Options may include private automobile, ambulance, helicopter,

Table 7-2. Guidelines for Crew Configuration

Patient Category	Crew Configuration
Low-risk patient (e.g., patient with controlled diabetes mellitus)	Emergency medical technician (EMT)
Moderate-risk patient (e.g., mild preeclampsia)	Obstetrically trained provider
High-risk patient (e.g., premature labor, any patient with significantly abnormal vital signs, etc.)	Obstetrically trained critical-care transport provider

Source: Adapted from Elliott,[7] with permission.

Table 7-3. Advantages and Disadvantages of Modes of Transport

Advantages	Disadvantages
Ground ambulance	
Usually readily available Only two transfers of the patient required Adequate working environment Easily diverted and adaptable to destination changes Low maintenance costs	Lengthy travel times over long distances Limited by geographic, traffic, and weather conditions Variable capacity and capability for additional specialized equipment
Helicopter	
Rapid transport time	Adequate landing zone required Multiple patient transfers may be necessary if landing area is remote from the referring facility Prone to weather restrictions Limited working space Noise and vibration may limit evaluation and monitoring High maintenance costs
Fixed-wing aircraft	
Rapid transport time Able to fly around or over weather (assuming pressurized cabin) Cabin size usually adequate	Multiple patient transfers may be necessary if landing area is remote from the referring facility Requires airport with appropriate service availability at each end High maintenance costs May require lengthy "scramble time"

Source: Adapted from Pon and Notterman,[5] with permission.

or fixed-wing aircraft. This decision is frequently not an easy one; the type of vehicle chosen should be agreed to by both the referring and receiving physicians. Several factors must be considered in deciding the most appropriate mode of transfer. These include vehicle availability and the severity of the patient's illness, the distance between facilities, options for stopping at other facilities should problems arise during transport, total transport times, personnel availability, vehicle availability, weather limitations, traffic limitations, terrain, safety, and cost. Sometimes a combination of transport modalities may be required. One published review of air transport of pregnant patients (via helicopter and fixed-wing aircraft) demonstrated that appropriately-screened patients have an extremely low incidence of in-flight delivery.[8] A more recent review of the military experience of flying low-risk and high-risk obstetric patients demonstrated its safety at any gestational age.[9]

Another important issue is how much time should be spent at the referring facility. For patients with time-sensitive disease processes who are being transferred for specific interventions (e.g., the patient with acute trauma or a ruptured abdominal aneurysm), it is usually prudent to spend as little time as possible at the referring institution so the patient can be brought quickly to the place of definitive care. Conversely, there are transport teams whose philosophy is based on bringing the intensive care and expertise to the bedside so stabilization takes place at the referring facility prior to initiating the transfer.

A pregnant patient frequently presents an interesting dilemma. As noted above, the interhospital transport environment poses particular challenges; it is not the ideal birthing environment, especially given the restricted confines of a helicopter or airplane. If it appears that despite all interventions delivery is likely to occur during the transport, the best approach is usually to await delivery and then transfer both patients (the newborn and the postpartum woman).

LOGISTICS OF TRANSFER

In order for an interhospital transfer to proceed smoothly, adequate communication between the parties is essential. This process begins from the time of the initial request; there should be one central number answered by an appropriately-trained communications specialist (dispatcher), through whom all communications are directed. This person should provide rapid coordination of vehicles and personnel. The communications specialist should also be able to contact the receiving physician in the event that problems arise during the transport. This should include radio communications from the ambulance. It should be noted that cellular phones may cause certain medical devices to malfunction and should be avoided in this setting. Additionally, it is against federal regulations to use ordinary cellular phones aboard aircraft.

The transferring team should ensure that copies of all pertinent medical records and x-rays accompany the patient. To help the receiving facility prepare for the patient's arrival, facsimile (fax) machines may be used to send documents prior to the transport. Model step-by-step protocols for transfers have been published and can be helpful as a checklist for designing policies for interhospital transport of the pregnant woman.[10]

Table 7-4. Transport for Potential Obstetric Complications

Premature rupture of membranes
Premature labor
Severe preeclampsia, eclampsia, or hypertension
Multiple gestation
Third trimester bleeding
Medical complications
Poorly controlled diabetes or diabetic ketoacidosis
Serious infections
Heart disease or congestive heart failure
Respiratory distress[15]
Thyrotoxicosis
Renal insufficiency
Drug overdose or complications of substance abuse
Sickle cell anemia or blood dyscrasias
Liver disease
Malignancy[16]
Surgical complications
Multisystem trauma
Acute abdomen

INDICATIONS FOR TRANSPORT

Maternal transport should be considered if there is a significant chance of maternal or fetal risk that cannot be adequately addressed at the referring institution. There is overwhelming evidence that neonates cared for in a neonatal intensive care unit (NICU) beginning at birth have a greater probability of survival and a shorter length of hospitalization than those transferred after birth.[11–13] Any insult that occurs during the first 24 hours of life can have significant effects on a neonate's outcome. Even the most efficiently organized neonatal transport program is subject to logistical problems or errors that may delay care or result in adverse outcomes.

The healthy uterus is the ideal transport "incubator" and if delivery can occur at the receiving facility, immediate access to the modern care of a NICU is assured. From a logistical standpoint, it is usually easier to transport prior to delivery rather than having to assemble a neonatal team with its sophisticated but bulky and cumbersome equipment. In addition, with antepartum transfer, there is less separation of mother and infant, increasing mother-infant bonding.[12]

According to the American Academy of Pediatrics and the American College of Obstetricians and Gynecologists, the goal of interhospital transport should be "to care for high-risk perinatal patients in a facility appropriate to their needs."[14]

The decision as to who is a candidate for transfer and appropriate timing of the transfer should be agreed upon by the transferring and accepting physicians. Transport should be considered "when the resources immediately available to the maternal, fetal, or neonatal patient are not adequate to deal with the patient's actual or anticipated condition."[11] Tables 7-4 and 7-5,[14] list some of the conditions under which transport should be considered. However, the need for transport should be considered individually, based on patient condition and the capabilities of the sending physician and institution.

Transport should be arranged as soon as the decision to transfer is made. For example, patients with premature rupture of membranes should be transferred as soon as possible. Unfortunately, this is not always possible, and

Table 7-5. Transport for Potential Fetal Complications

Fetal anomalies requiring surgery or specialized care
Rh disease with or without hydrops
Fetal arrhythmia or bradycardia
Intrauterine growth restriction
Abnormal fetal stress testing
Severe oligohydramnios
Vaginal breech delivery

transport teams are frequently asked to perform rushed transports of women in active labor with advanced cervical dilatation. If labor has progressed to the point where delivery en route is likely, it is usually preferable to delay transport and await the arrival of the neonatal team. It is frequently difficult to predict whether or not the transport can be completed prior to delivery. When the transporting vehicle is a helicopter or airplane, where the space to perform delivery and/or resuscitation is severely limited, the decision becomes even more difficult. Elliott and colleagues retrospectively reviewed 1080 patients who were requested to be transported for preterm labor.[17] Of these, 54 patients were dilated 7 cm or more at the time of request for transport and 5 were delivered at the referring hospital, so 49 dilated 7 cm or more were ultimately transported. Forty were transported by helicopter (average transport time, 15 min), 8 by fixed-wing aircraft (average transport time, 90 min), and 1 by ground (transport time, 27 min). Fifteen patients had cervical dilatation of 7 cm, 9 had cervical dilatation of 8 cm, and 5 had cervical dilatation of 10 cm. The station of the presenting part was –2 in 12, –1 in 7, 0 in 10, +1 in 10, and +2 in 10. All transported patients received magnesium sulfate and terbutaline sulfate for tocolysis during transport. All patients who were completely dilated and +2 station delivered within 1 hour of arrival at the tertiary hospital. The authors concluded that when confronted with this situation, factors to consider prior to the transfer include the skill and expertise of the transport team, distance between hospitals, facilities at the transferring hospital, gestational age, and cervical examination results. The decision to transfer should be based on individual patient assessment and not on protocol. The presence of a team member with extensive labor and delivery experience (e.g., an obstetrician) is encouraged to assist in the evaluation and decision making. It is important that there be ongoing communication between the sending and receiving physicians as these issues arise. These discussions should be carefully documented in the patient's chart.[18]

Obstetric patients who are victims of trauma deserve special mention. Prehospital care providers frequently fail to recognize that pregnant multiple trauma patients with a gestational age of greater than 20 weeks should be brought to hospital with high-level trauma and obstetric capabilities even if the patient appears stable.[7] If the patient is being transferred from a hospital, information about fetal status and viability (e.g., accurate assessment of gestational age, fetal heart tones) should be obtained if possible without delaying the transfer. This information will assist the receiving hospital in determining fetal viability upon arrival there.

CARE DURING TRANSPORT

Caregivers who are called upon to transport pregnant patients must consider the physiologic changes that occur during pregnancy. These changes require alteration in the usual transport procedures. There are three interventions that should be performed on almost all pregnant patients during transport. They are (1) transport in the lateral tilt position, (2) administration of supplemental oxygen, and (3) administration of intravenous fluid.

Patient Position

Fetal compromise may result when pregnant patients are placed in the supine position. When supine, the gravid uterus (after about 20 to 24 weeks) lies directly against the vena cava and potentially the aorta, compressing both and leading to diminished venous return and decreased blood pressure.[19] Compression of the vena cava can reduce preload significantly, leading to a reduction in cardiac output of up to 25 to 30 percent.[20] Hemodynamically-compromised patients (who are usually the ones in need of transport), especially those with reduced circulating volume, will have an even lower tolerance for alterations in hemodynamics. Blood vessels in the pregnant uterus are maximally dilated at rest, and no intrinsic autoregulatory mechanism exists for increasing uterine blood flow. Therefore any decrease in cardiac output may lead to decreased uterine blood flow and possible uteroplacental insufficiency. In response to decreased cardiac output, hypotension, or hypoxia, the uterine vasculature constricts. This can cause significant fetal compromise without any detectable change in the mother's vital signs.[21] Studies in animals have demonstrated that interruption of inferior vena caval blood flow can produce placental separation.[22] Observations in humans appear to corroborated these findings.[23] It should also be noted that supine positioning of the pregnant patient may lead to respiratory compromise, as functional residual capacity is reduced by 15 to 20 percent at term.[24,25]

The problems outlined above can be avoided by transporting patients beyond 20 weeks of gestation in the left lateral tilt position (i.e., with one side of the body higher than the other). This can be accomplished by placing pillows under the mother's right or left side. If the patient requires spinal immobilization due to traumatic injuries, the backboard should be angled at approximately 15 degrees to the horizontal. This can be accomplished by placing the rolled towel, pillows, or an oxygen cylinder under one edge of the backboard. If these options are not available, the uterus can be displaced manually to one side by one of the caregivers.

Supplemental Oxygen

It seems prudent to administer supplemental oxygen to all pregnant patients being transferred. During pregnancy, increasing maternal oxygen saturation will increase fetal saturation as well.[26] Because the fetal oxygen hemoglobin dissociation curve is shifted to the left, oxygen extraction from the maternal circulation is increased.

Special consideration should be given to supplemental oxygen administration when pregnant patients are transported by air. Most commercial jet aircraft cabins are pressurized to an altitude of 8000 feet. At this altitude in a depressurized chamber, maternal Po_2 may decrease from 100 to 55 mmHg, with the fetal arterial cord Po_2 decreasing from 32 to 25.6 mmHg. Because of the differences in the fetal oxygen-hemoglobin dissociation curve, the normal fetus is able to maintain a greater degree of oxygen saturation and thus appears to be in no danger from cabin pressures used in modern jet aircraft.[27,28] Studies in animals have shown that at altitudes up to 7500 feet, there is no significant effect on oxygen exchange in a normal placenta.[29] It should also be noted that the altitudes at which most helicopter transports take place have no significant effects on maternal or fetal oxygenation. However, because women being transported or their fetuses usually have some degree of compromise, it is prudent to administer supplemental oxygen to all pregnant patients being transported, regardless of altitude.

Intravenous Fluid Therapy

All patients being transported should have at least one functioning intravenous line in place. The rate of fluid administration should be appropriate for the clinical condition of the patient and fetus. As noted above, an early maternal compensatory mechanism for hypovolemia is a decrease in uterine blood flow, resulting in potential fetal compromise with little or no change in maternal vital signs. Because maternal blood volume increases up to 45 percent during pregnancy, it is estimated that the mother can lose up to 10 to 20 percent of her circulating blood volume acutely before her vital signs become abnormal.[30] Therefore, volume replacement should be given at a rate that ensures adequate uterine perfusion. Any woman with significant hypovolemia should have at least two large-bore peripheral intravenous lines placed. Significant blood loss may require transfusion of blood in addition to crystalloid therapy.

Table 7-6. Key Factors to be Monitored During Transport[a]

Mother	Neonate
Uterine contractions and fetal heart tones	Temperature
Cardiopulmonary status	Respirations
Deep tendon reflexes	Heart rate
Infusion rates of intravenous lines	Blood pressure
Administration of medications	Color
	Activity
	Oxygen concentration

[a]Frequency of monitoring key factors will depend on patient stability, but at least every 30 min is prudent.

Special mention should be made of the use of pressor agents in pregnancy. Catecholamines cause decreased uterine blood flow[21] and thus should be used only when all other mechanisms have failed. Additionally, efforts to calm the patient in order to decrease endogenous catecholamine production may be useful.

It is important to stabilize the mother and fetus to the extent possible prior to transport. Therapeutic agents that are frequently administered safely en route include glucocorticoids, antihypertensives, anticonvulsants, antibiotics, and tocolytics.[31]

Maternal and Fetal Evaluation

While in transport, standard nursing evaluation, monitoring, and documentation should be performed, with close monitoring of the mother's cardiopulmonary status (Table 7-6). The mother should also be observed for evidence of uterine contractions. The fetal heart rate should be monitored and documented at 15- to 30-minute intervals or more often for critically ill patients. This can be done using a Doppler device or, if available, continuous electronic fetal monitoring. If a Doppler device is chosen for intermittent monitoring and the patient is contracting regularly, fetal heart tones should be documented after a uterine contraction.[32] Careful differentiation between fetal and maternal heart tones should be performed by simultaneously auscultating FHTs and palpating the pulse of the mother. These devices have been used successfully both on the ground and in the air.[28]

MEDICOLEGAL CONCERNS

The transfer of a patient from one institution to another raises many medicolegal issues. Hospitals must develop policies that comply with all applicable federal and state laws. It is best for institutions to have written letters of agreement that cover these issues.

The transfer of patients was addressed in the Consolidated Omnibus Budget Reconciliation Act of 1986, commonly referred to as the COBRA law. Under the terms of this law, the transferring physician must discuss the case with a physician at the receiving institution, who must accept the transfer. A medical screening examination must be performed prior to the transfer. Evaluation and stabilization should be performed to ensure that no harm will come to the patient (within reasonable medical probability), and that the medical benefits of transfer will outweigh the risks.[33] A patient may be transferred without being stabilized if the transfer is from a lower level to a higher level of care, and necessary interventions are beyond the capability of the sending institution.[34] Failure to comply with COBRA laws can result in fines, loss of Medicare reimbursement, and filing of a lawsuit by the patient for injuries suffered or for damages from the receiving hospital for inappropriate patient transfer.[5,35,36]

Prior to the transfer to a higher level of care, the risk and benefits of the transfer should be documented in the medical record by the sending physician. Documentation should also include the capabilities that the receiving institution has that the sending institution lacks, the options for transfer and the reasons for the mode chosen, the name of the receiving physician who accepted the transfer, and how availability of space at the receiving facility was assured.[34]

It should be noted that one-way transport systems are generally not as sophisticated as two-way systems. In general, a patient is the responsibility of the sending physician until the accepting facility assumes care of the patient. Thus the sending physician must understand and accept the risk of sending the patient with a level of care less than that provided at the sending facility, or make arrangements for transport with personnel capable of meeting the potential needs of the patient.

When members of a two-way transport service arrive at a referring hospital, questions may also arise as to when the responsibility and liability shifts to the accepting institution. Some hospitals consider a patient their responsibility when the transport team assumes care, even though they are physically outside of the home institution. Other institutions assume liability when the patient enters their ambulance. To avoid potential problems, these issues should be addressed formally and prospectively through written letters of agreement between institutions. Institutions should develop written transfer policies and procedures that are in compliance with all applicable state and federal laws.

REFERENCES

1. Rooks JP, Weatherby NL, Ernst EKM, et al: Outcomes of care in birth centers—The National Birth Center Study. *N Engl J Med* 321:1804, 1989.
2. Garite TJ, Snell BJ, Walker DL, et al: Development and experience of a university-based, freestanding birthing center. *Obstet Gynecol* 86:411, 1995.
3. Pons PT: Prehospital considerations in the pregnant patient. *Emerg Med Clin North Am* 12:1, 1994.
4. Brunette DD, Sterner SP: Prehospital and emergency department delivery: A review of eight years experience. *Ann Emerg Med* 18:1116, 1989.
5. Pon SP, Notterman DA: The organization of a pediatric critical care transport program. *Pediatr Clin North Am* 40:241, 1993.
6. Jones AE, Summers RL, Deschamp C, et al: A national survey of the air medical transport of high-risk obstetric patients. *Air Medical J* 20:17–20, 2001.
7. Elliott JP: *Maternal Air Medical Transport, Air Medical Physician's Handbook.* Salt Lake City: Air Medical Physician Association, 1996.
8. Low RB, Martin D, Brown C: Emergency air transport of pregnant patients: The national experience. *J Emerg Med* 6:41, 1988.
9. Connor SB, Lyons TJ: U.S. Air Force aeromedical evacuation of obstetric patients in Europe. Aviat Space Environ Med 66:1090–1093, 1995.
10. Bigelow LK, Anderson KC, Camp J: Maternal transport: A protocol for ambulance transfer from rural to regional facility. *J Perinatol* 17:411–415, 1997.
11. Giles HR: Maternal transport. *Clin Obstet Gynecol* 6:203, 1979.
12. Mondanlou HD, Dorchester WL, Thorosian A, et al: Antenatal versus neonatal transport to a regional perinatal center: A comparison between matched pairs. *Obstet Gynecol* 53:725, 1979.
13. Merenstein GB, Pettett G, Woodall J, et al: An analysis of air transport results in the sick newborn: II. Antenatal and neonatal referrals. *Am J Obstet Gynecol* 128:520, 1977.
14. Gilstrap LC, Oh W. (eds): Organization of Perinatal Health Care, in *Guidelines for Perinatal Care*, 5th ed. American Academy of Pediatrics and American College of Obstetricians and Gynecologists, Elk Grove Village, 2002, pp 1–16.
15. Elliott JP, Foley MR, Young L, et al: Air transport of obstetric critical care patients to tertiary centers. *J Reprod Med* 41:171–174, 1996.
16. Garmel SH, D'Alton ME: When maternal transport is necessary. *Contemp OB/GYN* 40:94, 1995.
17. Elliott JP, Sipp TL, Balazs KT: Maternal transport of patients with advanced cervical dilatation—To fly or not to fly? *Obstet Gynecol* 79:380, 1992.
18. Bowes WA, Jr: Clinical management of preterm delivery. *Clin Obstet Gynecol* 31:652, 1988.
19. Ueland K, Novy MJ, Peterson EN, et al: Maternal cardiovascular dynamics: IV. The influence of gestational age on

the maternal cardiovascular response to posture and exercise. *Am J Obstet Gynecol* 104:856, 1969.

20. Pearlman MD, Tintinalli JE, Lorenz RP: Blunt trauma during pregnancy. *N Engl J Med* 323:1609, 1990.
21. Katz VL, Hansen A: Complications in the emergency transport of pregnant women. *South Med J* 83:7, 1990.
22. Howard BK, Goodson JH: Experimental placental abruption. *Obstet Gynecol* 2:442, 1953.
23. Menger WF, Goodson JH, Campbell RG, et al: Observation on the pathogenesis of premature separation of the normally implanted placenta. *Am J Obstet Gynecol* 66:1104, 1953.
24. Novy MJ, Edwards MJ: Respiratory problems in pregnancy. *Am J Obstet Gynecol* 99:1024, 1967.
25. Cheek TG, Gutsche BB: Maternal physiologic alterations during pregnancy, in Schnider SM, Levinson G (eds): *Anesthesia for Obstetrics.* Baltimore: Williams & Wilkins, 1993, pp 3–17.
26. Shaw DB, Wheeler AS: Anesthesia for obstetric emergencies. *Clin Obstet Gynecol* 27:112, 1984.
27. Barry M, Bia F: Pregnancy and travel. *JAMA* 261:728, 1989.
28. Elliott JP, Trujillo R: Fetal monitoring during emergency obstetric transport. *Am J Obstet Gynecol* 157:245, 1987.
29. Parer JT: Effects of hypoxia on the mother and fetus with emphasis on maternal air transport. *Am J Obstet Gynecol* 142:957, 1982.
30. Baker DP: Trauma in the pregnant patient. *Surg Clin North Am* 62:275, 1992.
31. Semonin-Holleran R: *Flight Nursing: Principles and Practice,* 2d ed. St. Louis: Mosby-Year Book, 1996.
32. American College of Obstetricians and Gynecologists: *Fetal Heart Rate Patterns: Monitoring, Interpretation, and Management.* ACOG Technical Bulletin No. 207. Washington, DC: 1995.
33. American College of Emergency Physicians (ACEP) Policy Statement: Appropriate Interhospital Patient Transfer. *Ann Emerg Med* 22:766, 1993.
34. Strobos J: Tightening the screw: Statutory and legal supervision of interhospital patient transfers. *Ann Emerg Med* 20:302, 1991.
35. Frew SA, Roush WR, LaGreca K: COBRA: Implications for emergency medicine. *Ann Emerg Med* 17:835, 1988.
36. Mookini RK: Medical-legal aspects of aeromedical transport of emergency patients. *Leg Med*: 1–30, 1990.

8

Preeclampsia and Hypertensive Disorders in Pregnancy

Gary A. Dildy III

KEY POINTS

- Preeclampsia is defined by elevated blood pressure ($\geq$140 mm Hg systolic or $\geq$90 mm Hg diastolic) accompanied by proteinuria, edema, or both occurring after 20 weeks of gestation.
- Severe preeclampsia is diagnosed with severe hypertension, excess proteinuria, oliguria, cerebral or visual disturbances, pulmonary edema, impaired liver function, epigastric or right-upper–quadrant pain, thrombocytopenia or fetal growth restriction (see Table 7-5).
- Seizure prophylaxis and prompt delivery are the cornerstones of management of severe preeclampsia.
- Treatment of hypertension is usually initiated when the diastolic blood pressure exceeds 105–110 mm Hg to prevent complications of intracranial hemorrhage and abruptio placentae.
- Magnesium sulfate is usually recommended for seizure prophylaxis for patients with severe preeclampsia.
- Magnesium sulfate is also the usual first agent for treating eclamptic seizures. Other antiseizure agents (e.g., phenytoin, benzodiazepines) are reserved for second-line use.

There have been various nomenclature systems for hypertensive diseases of pregnancy. A system proposed by the National High Blood Pressure Education Program Working Group[1] is shown in Table 8-1. Hypertension is defined as a systolic blood pressure level of at least 140 mmHg or diastolic blood pressure level of at least 90 mm Hg. Preeclampsia is diagnosed when pregnancy-induced hypertension is accompanied by proteinuria. In the United States, preeclampsia complicates approximately 5 to 8 percent of pregnancies,[2,3] and is the second most common cause of maternal mortality in pregnancies beyond 20 weeks.[4] Pathophysiologic changes may adversely affect the maternal cardiovascular, renal, neurologic, hepatic, and hematologic systems.[5] Uteroplacental blood flow may also be compromised, resulting in fetal and neonatal complications including death. Eclampsia is the development of new-onset grand mal seizures in a woman with preeclampsia.[6]

PATHOPHYSIOLOGY OF PREECLAMPSIA

There are numerous known and theoretical pathophysiologic mechanisms for the development of preeclampsia: an imbalance in prostacyclin and thromboxane, immunologic abnormalities, increased vascular reactivity to vasoactive agents, hyperdynamic increase in cardiac output, abnormal placentation, genetic variations of the angiotensinogen gene, and numerous others have been proposed. However, none are proven and the exact etiology remains unknown.

The most important risk factors for preeclampsia[7] are either first pregnancy or a history of preeclampsia in a prior pregnancy. Preeclampsia rarely develops in multiparous women who did not have preeclampsia in a previous pregnancy (unless there is a different father of the baby in the current pregnancy). However, there is no accurate predictive instrument for preeclampsia. Furthermore, risk factor assessment cannot adequately distinguish those who will develop mild disease from those who will develop severe manifestations and multiorgan dysfunction.

Preeclampsia can be thought of as a process that develops because of generalized systemic vasospasm. Vasospasm leads to tissue ischemia and the various multisystem effects[8] associated with the disease (Table 8-2).

DIAGNOSIS

Preeclampsia has been classically defined based on the triad of hypertension, proteinuria, and edema. Edema is common during normal pregnancy and its presence has been eliminated as a criterion in current diagnostic schemes. Table 8-3 summarizes current criteria for the diagnosis of preeclampsia.[1,6] Recognition of the signs and varying symptoms is particularly important for health care providers not primarily involved in the management

Table 8-1. Classification of Hypertension During Pregnancy

- *Chronic hypertension*: Hypertension (BP ≥ 140/90 mmHg) that is present and observable before pregnancy or that is diagnosed before the 20th week of gestation. Hypertension diagnosed for the first time during pregnancy and persisting beyond the 42nd day postpartum.
- *Preeclampsia-eclampsia*: Increased blood pressure accompanied by proteinuria, edema, or both usually occurring after 20 weeks of gestation (or earlier with trophoblastic diseases such as hydatidiform mole or hydrops).
- *Preeclampsia superimposed on chronic hypertension*: Chronic hypertension (defined above) with increases in blood pressure (30 mmHg systolic, 15 mmHg diastolic, or 20 mmHg mean arterial pressure) together with the appearance of proteinuria or generalized edema.
- *Transient hypertension*: The development of elevated BP during pregnancy or in the first 24 h postpartum without other signs of preeclampsia or preexisting hypertension (a retrospective diagnosis).

of pregnant patients. Emergency department personnel should be aware of the pathophysiology and diagnostic criteria of preeclampsia when the pregnant woman presents for various apparently unrelated problems.

Preeclampsia is defined as either mild or severe. Mild preeclampsia is characterized by a systolic blood pressure of at least 140 mmHg or a diastolic blood pressure of at least 90 mmHg obtained on two separate occasions at least 6 hours apart. Some clinicians use a relative rise of systolic (30 mmHg) or diastolic (15 mmHg) blood pressure over prepregnancy or first-trimester levels; however, these criteria appear to be of questionable utility.[9,10]

Significant proteinuria is defined as at least 300 mg of protein in a 24-hour urine collection. While 1+ or 2+ proteinuria is frequently considered significant, the semiquantitative dipstick analysis of urine protein is poorly correlated with the actual degree of proteinuria. Classification of preeclampsia is ideally based on a 24-hour quantitative collection of urine for protein. In acute settings, urine protein dipstick ≥2+ suggests significant proteinuria, but it should be followed with a 24-hour urine collection if possible.

Preeclampsia almost always occurs after 20 weeks of gestation. An exception to this is the uncommon clinical circumstance of gestational trophoblastic disease (molar pregnancy; see Chap. 4). Severe preeclampsia is defined as existing when *any* of the manifestations listed in Table 8-4 are identified in the preeclamptic patient.[6]

HELLP SYNDROME

A diagnosis of severe preeclampsia is usually straightforward, following careful observation and monitoring of a hypertensive gravid woman who presents with complaints of severe headache, scotomata, and swelling. A variant of severe preeclampsia is HELLP (*h*emolysis, *e*levated liver enzymes, and *l*ow *p*latelets) syndrome, affecting up to 12 percent of women with preeclampsia-eclampsia. Whereas preeclampsia is usually a disease of primigravidas, HELLP syndrome has a predilection for the multigravida population. HELLP syndrome may imitate a variety of nonobstetric medical problems (Table 8-5); serious medical and surgical pathology may be misdiagnosed as preeclampsia or HELLP syndrome, or vice versa.[11,12] In addition to varying degrees of hypertension (although not always severe and sometimes not initially evident), the woman with HELLP syndrome may present with a complaint of epigastric or right upper quadrant pain. Thrombocytopenia is defined as a platelet count less than 100,000/mm^3, but a count of less than 150,000/mm^3 would be suspicious, particularly in the face of hypertension and elevated liver enzymes. Hepatic transaminase

Table 8-2. Complications of Severe Pregnancy-Induced Hypertension

Cardiovascular	Severe hypertension, pulmonary edema
Renal	Oliguria, renal failure
Hematologic	Hemolysis, thrombocytopenia, disseminated intravascular coagulation
Neurologic	Eclampsia, cerebral edema, cerebral hemorrhage, amaurosis
Hepatic	Hepatocellular dysfunction, hepatic rupture
Uteroplacental	Abruption, intrauterine growth retardation, fetal distress, fetal death

Table 8-3. Criteria for Diagnosis of Preeclampsia

- **Hypertension:** Systolic blood pressure ≥140 mmHg or diastolic blood pressure ≥90 mmHg that occurs after 20 weeks of gestation in a woman with previously normal blood pressure

and

- **Proteinuria:** urinary excretion of ≥300 mg of protein in a 24-hour specimen

or

- **Edema:** generalized edema or weight gain of at least 5 lb in 1 week

levels (AST and ALT) are not elevated during normal pregnancy and may become elevated in association with worsening preeclampsia, but not usually to the levels seen in acute viral hepatitis (i.e., in HELLP syndrome, the AST, and ALT are usually <500 IU/L). Hemolysis is due to microangiopathic hemolytic anemia, with schistocytes are frequently present on the peripheral blood smear. Hemolysis is not usually associated with anemia, since plasma volume is often decreased to a more significant degree than is loss of red cell volume in preeclamptic patients. Thus, the hematocrit may actually increase even in the face of red cell destruction.

EVALUATION AND TREATMENT OF PREECLAMPSIA

Maternal Considerations

Initial evaluation of the woman who presents with suspected preeclampsia includes several simultaneously initiated steps.[13] Maternal vital signs are monitored initially every 15 to 30 minutes. The woman is placed in the left lateral recumbent position so the gravid uterus does not produce aortocaval compression. A clean-catch specimen of urine is obtained for semiquantitative analysis of protein concentration. Initial blood laboratory evaluation is summarized in Table 8-6. If delivery is not felt to be imminent, a 24-hour urine collection should be initiated for volume, creatinine clearance, and total protein excretion.

Fetal Considerations

If the fetus is previable (e.g., less than 24 weeks of gestation), the fetal heart rate may be monitored intermittently and recorded. If the fetus is of a viable estimated gestational age, then fetal biophysical assessment (Table 8-7) should be performed via a nonstress test (NST) or biophysical profile (BPP). An evaluation of fetal condition is indicated because uteroplacental blood flow may be compromised in the preeclamptic woman, potentially producing varying degrees of fetal compromise. Initially, fetal growth may diminish as a result of chronic impairment

Table 8-4. Diagnostic Criteria for Severe Preeclampsia[a]

- Blood pressure ≥160 mmHg systolic or ≥110 mmHg diastolic on two occasions at least 6 hours apart while the patient is on bed rest
- Proteinuria ≥5000 mg in a 24-hour collection, or ≥3+ on two random urine samples collected at least 4 hours apart
- Oliguria defined as <500 mL per 24 hours
- Cerebral or visual disturbances
- Pulmonary edema or cyanosis
- Epigastric or right upper quadrant pain
- Impaired liver function
- Thrombocytopenia
- Fetal growth restriction

[a] Only one condition need be present.

Table 8-5. Differential Diagnoses of Hellp Syndrome

Autoimmune thrombocytopenic purpura
Chronic renal disease
Pyelonephritis
Cholecystitis
Gastroenteritis
Hepatitis
Pancreatitis
Thrombotic thrombocytopenic purpura
Hemolytic-uremic syndrome
Acute fatty liver of pregnancy

Table 8-6. Laboratory Evaluation for Preeclampsia

- Complete blood count with peripheral blood smear
- Platelet count
- Liver function tests (AST, ALT)
- Renal function tests (creatinine, BUN, uric acid)
- Blood type and antibody screen
- Urinalysis and microscopy
- 24-hour urine collection for protein and creatinine clearance

of placental exchange. Intrauterine growth restriction (fetal weight <10th percentile) and oligohydramnios (decreased amniotic fluid volume) may follow. Chronic severe reduction in oxygenation, uterine contractions that further decrease placental perfusion, or umbilical cord compression resulting from oligohydramnios may further compromise the fetus, leading to asphyxia or death. These fetal complications occur more frequently in pregnancies complicated by hypertension than in normotensive pregnancies.

Management of Severe Hypertension

The treatment of severe hypertension is recommended when the diastolic blood pressure exceeds 105 to 110 mmHg[6] in order to prevent complications of intracranial hemorrhage and abruptio placentae. Mild or moderate degrees of blood pressure elevation are generally not treated because of concern for obscuring worsening disease—an important determinant in management decisions such as need for delivery. In addition, treatment of mild to moderate pregnancy-induced hypertension does not necessarily improve outcome for either mother or baby.

Hypertension treatment begins when the diastolic blood pressure exceeds 105 to 110 mmHg. The treatment goal is a systolic blood pressure of 130 to 150 mmHg, diastolic 90 to 105 mmHg. Do not overtreat because hypotension can cause fetal compromise.

Although many antihypertensive agents are available, U.S. obstetricians have generally used hydralazine for primary treatment of severe hypertension during pregnancy. Recognizing that the severely hypertensive preeclamptic woman may be significantly hypovolemic, an intravenous line should be established prior to administering antihypertensive agents. Maternal volume is frequently expanded with 500 to 1000 mL of intravenous fluids before antihypertensive therapy is initiated. Hydralazine is usually administered intravenously, with an initial dose of 5 mg. The patient should be observed for 15 to 20 minutes, the usual time to onset of action of this agent. If the blood pressure is not corrected to the desired range (systolic of 130 to 150 mmHg and diastolic of 90 to 105 mmHg), then additional 5- to 10-mg boluses of hydralazine may be administered every 20 minutes up to a total dose of 40 mg. If hydralazine at this cumulative dosage is not efficacious, then a second agent such as labetalol should be considered (Table 8-8).[1,2,5,6] Care should be taken not to create hypotension or sudden drops in blood pressure, since fetal compromise may result. The use of continuous electronic fetal monitoring can help to detect adverse effects of BP treatment on the fetus. Angiotensin-converting enzyme (ACE) inhibitors should not be used during pregnancy because of potential fetal side effects (anuria or renal failure).

Seizure Prophylaxis

If severe preeclampsia is suspected during initial evaluation, most experts recommend magnesium sulfate therapy be initiated to prevent the development of eclamptic seizures. Several different regimens of magnesium sulfate ($MgSO_4$) therapy have been recommended. We generally favor an initial loading dose of 6 grams intravenously over 15 minutes, followed by a maintenance dose of 2 grams/hour IV. Maternal deep tendon reflexes, respiratory rate, and urine output should be monitored to avoid magnesium toxicity. Low urine output should result in a decrease in the infusion rate of magnesium sulfate. There is no consensus on whether to treat all mildly preeclamptic women with magnesium seizure prophylaxis;[6] however, there is substantial evidence to support the recommendation of seizure prophylaxis for women with severe preeclampsia or eclampsia.[17–22]

Normal pretreatment serum magnesium levels during pregnancy range from 1.5 to 2.0 mEq/L. The desired

Table 8-7. Tests of Fetal Condition

- *Nonstress test (NST):* The pattern of the fetal heart rate is evaluated by external electronic fetal monitoring
- *Oxytocin challenge test (OCT):* The pattern of the fetal heart rate is evaluated by external electronic fetal monitoring after uterine contractions are elicited by intravenous oxytocin infusion
- *Biophysical profile (BPP):* The fetal condition is assessed by real-time ultrasound monitoring of fetal tone, movement, breathing motions, and amniotic fluid volume
- *Ultrasound (US):* Fetal number, fetal anatomy, fetal biometric measurements, placental location, amniotic fluid volume, and other parameters are determined
- *Amniocentesis:* A sample of amniotic fluid is aspirated transabdominally under US guidance for evaluation of fetal lung maturity

therapeutic range of serum magnesium is 4 to 7 mEq/L. When serum magnesium levels exceed therapeutic ranges, toxicity may develop. Loss of deep tendon reflexes (8 to 10 mEq/L) may lead to respiratory arrest (13 mEq/L), and cardiac arrest may follow. With mild magnesium toxicity, the magnesium infusion is simply discontinued. More significant toxicity resulting in respiratory depression is treated by administration of 1 g of calcium gluconate (10 mL of a 10 percent solution) IV over 2 minutes. Respiratory support, oxygen saturation monitoring, and electrocardiographic (ECG) monitoring are indicated. Magnesium excretion may be enhanced by loop or osmotic diuretics and impaired in renal insufficiency, commonly present in preeclamptic women.

Indications for Delivery

Accurate dating of the pregnancy is of paramount importance because the ultimate management decisions for the preeclamptic woman will be based primarily on fetal maturity (gestational age), maternal well-being (mild versus severe preeclampsia), and fetal well-being (e.g., biophysical testing). Dating of the pregnancy is performed by calculating the estimated date of delivery and the estimated gestational age from the last normal menstrual period. It is important to obtain any previous data that would substantiate gestational age, such as the date of the first positive pregnancy test, first auscultation of fetal heart tones (usually at 10 weeks by Doppler or 19 weeks by fetoscope), and particularly early obstetric US biometric data. In most centers the NST remains the preferred test of fetal well-being, but it may not be reassuring (reactive) at very early gestational ages (e.g., before 28 weeks of gestation). Thus the BPP may be performed by trained personnel using real-time ultrasound to determine fetal condition. Amniocentesis for a fetal lung-maturity profile may be helpful in cases in which fetal pulmonary maturity is in question, but the disease process is not severe enough to mandate delivery.

Delivery generally benefits the preeclamptic woman but may result in serious neonatal problems in the preterm gestation. In general, mild preeclampsia remote from term may be expectantly managed. Severe preeclampsia is best managed by delivery in most cases, with the exception of very early gestational ages, in which expectant management in tertiary care centers may be appropriate, with their experienced perinatologists and the availability of appropriate neonatal services.[14–16] (See Chap. 7 for discussion of transfers.)

ECLAMPSIA

A pregnant or postpartum woman who develops new-onset seizures should be assumed to be eclamptic until proven otherwise. While most eclamptic women also demonstrate hypertension, proteinuria, and edema, up to 30 percent will not. The pathophysiology of the syndrome is poorly understood, and the occurrence of seizures does not necessarily correlate with the severity of other

Table 8-8. Antihypertensive Therapy for Preeclampsia-Eclampsia

- Hydralazine: 5- to 10-mg doses IV every 15 to 20 minutes until desired clinical response
- Labetalol: 20 mg IV bolus dose, followed by 40 mg if not effective in 10 minutes; then 80 mg every 10 minutes, until maximum total dose of 220 mg

signs. Among severe preeclamptics, approximately 3 percent will experience eclampsia if not receiving magnesium prophylaxis, versus 0.3 percent who do receive prophylaxis.[22]

Eclamptic seizures may be preceded by headache, blurred vision, or decreased visual acuity. Eclamptic seizures may be focal or generalized tonic-clonic seizures.[23] The typical pattern is a single seizure lasting <1 minute that responds to IV magnesium sulfate administration.[24]

The management of eclampsia includes treatment of seizures, hypertension, and expeditious delivery of the fetus. Emergency obstetric consultation should be obtained, and transfer to a center with resources for critical obstetric care will be necessary after maternal stabilization, if such resources are not available locally.

The initial management of eclamptic seizures is to ensure adequate maternal ventilation and oxygenation. Continuous pulse oximetry should be begun and supplemental oxygen administered to maintain the maternal oxygen saturation above 90 percent, and if undelivered above 95 percent if possible. A secure intravenous line should be established, and 6 g magnesium sulfate should be given IV over 15 minutes, with monitoring of maternal blood pressure, respirations, and pulse rate every 5 minutes during this infusion. An indwelling urinary catheter should be placed to carefully monitor urine output. This should be followed by a maintenance infusion of magnesium sulfate at 2 grams/hour. Most women should respond to this regimen, but if there is continued seizure activity, another 2 g magnesium sulfate should be given IV over 15 minutes. In Pritchard and colleagues'[17] series at Parkland Memorial Hospital, 88 percent of women had no further seizures after initial treatment with 4 grams IV magnesium sulfate, and the seizures of an additional 7 percent were controlled with another 2 g given IV. Serum magnesium levels should be monitored, but since values are unlikely to be available within minutes, the patient must be monitored closely for clinical evidence of magnesium toxicity, with frequent blood pressure readings and evaluation of respiratory rate and deep tendon reflexes. Signs and symptoms of magnesium toxicity include slurred speech, muscle weakness and areflexia, hypotension, and respiratory and cardiac depression. Endotracheal intubation and ventilation are necessary for respiratory depression that prevents adequate oxygenation that cannot be otherwise maintained with supplemental oxygen. Calcium gluconate or calcium chloride, 10 mL of 10 percent solution, should be administered IV over 5 minutes for suspected magnesium toxicity. Calcium competitively inhibits the effect of magnesium, and its effect may be transient, so measures to increase magnesium excretion and IV fluids (e.g., furosemide) may facilitate excretion. Continuous electrocardiographic monitoring is recommended in this setting.

Fetal monitoring is established as soon as possible, as fetal bradycardia is a common complication of maternal seizures. Once maternal seizures are controlled and maternal oxygenation and circulation are maintained, the fetal heart rate should return to normal. Plans for expeditious delivery should be made in consultation with an obstetrician. Vaginal delivery is generally preferred and is possible in many cases.

Reoccurrence of seizures or status epilepticus after the administration of IV magnesium sulfate is uncommon, but it poses grave risks to both mother and fetus. Hypertension must be controlled with an intravenous agent such as hydralazine or labetalol. Continued seizure activity raises the possibility of intracranial pathology, such as cerebral hemorrhage. Further treatment of acute seizures should proceed as for any adult (see Chap. 18). If seizures persist despite a therapeutic magnesium level (serum levels of 5 to 7 mEq/L), another antiepileptic agent (phenytoin or a barbiturate or benzodiazepine) should be given, with careful attention paid to maintaining adequate maternal ventilation.

Use of lorazepam and other benzodiazepines can result in neonatal respiratory depression. The use of magnesium sulfate as a standard first-line agent for treatment of eclamptic seizures is nearly universally accepted in obstetrics in the United States. Some have argued for the use of phenytoin as a first-line agent for eclamptic seizures, but recent studies evaluating the efficacy of magnesium sulfate for seizure prophylaxis or eclampsia demonstrate that it remains the agent of choice.[19,20]

Significant hemodynamic perturbations are observed in preeclamptic women (Table 8-9) who have undergone central hemodynamic monitoring.[25,26] The vast majority of severe preeclamptics do not require central monitoring. Clinical conditions that may merit central hemodynamic monitoring include severe cardiac disease, severe renal disease, pulmonary edema, refractory hypertension, or refractory oliguria.[6,8]

OBSTETRIC CONSULTATION

Any pregnant woman presenting to the emergency department with signs or symptoms consistent with preeclampsia, whether mild or severe, should have a consultation with an obstetrician or perinatologist. This is especially important for women who present with atypical signs and symptoms of medical or surgical disorders that might be confused with the HELLP syndrome (e.g., upper abdomi-

Table 8-9. Hemodynamic Profiles of Nonpregnant Women, Normal Women During the Late Third Trimester, and Severe Preeclamptics

Parameter	Normal Nonpregnant ($n = 10$),[a] Mean ± SD	Normal Late 3d Trimester ($n = 10$),[a] Mean ± SD	Severe Preeclampsia ($n = 45$),[b] Mean ± SEM
Heart rate (beats/min)	71 ± 10	83 ± 10	95 ± 10
Mean arterial BP (mmHg)	86.4 ± 7.5	90.3 ± 5.8	138 ± 3
Central venous pressure (mmHg)	3.7 ± 2.6	3.6 ± 2.5	4 ± 1
Pulmonary capillary wedge pressure (mmHg)	6.3 ± 2.1	7.5 ± 1.8	10 ± 1
Cardiac output (L/min)	4.3 ± 0.9	6.2 ± 1.0	7.5 ± 0.2
Systemic vascular resistance (dynes $\cdot$ s $\cdot$ cm^{-5})	1530 ± 520	1210 ± 266	1496 ± 64
Pulmonary vascular resistance (dynes $\cdot$ s $\cdot$ cm^{-5})	119 ± 47	78 ± 22	70 ± 5
Serum colloid osmotic pressure (mmHg)	20.8 ± 1.0	18.0 ± 1.5	19.0 ± 0.5
Left ventricular stroke work index (g $\cdot$ m $\cdot$ M^{-2})	41 ± 8	48 ± 6	81 ± 2

Sources: [a]Clark et al.,[25] [b]Cotton et al.[26]

nal pains, unexplained thrombocytopenia, or unexplained elevation of liver enzymes). Another primary reason for obstetric consultation is the ordering and interpretation of tests of fetal well-being, such as the obstetric ultrasound, NST, or BPP in the preeclamptic woman.

Three possible dispositions can be made for the woman with suspected or diagnosed preeclampsia: (1) discharge home; (2) admission to the hospital for observation; and (3) admission to the hospital for delivery.

For the preterm woman who is diagnosed with mild preeclampsia, it may be reasonable, after a period of hospital observation, to discharge her home to bed rest after ensuring continuing obstetric care and arranging for follow-up evaluation. If there is any question regarding the degree of severity of preeclampsia based on the presenting symptoms or laboratory evaluations, or any concerns regarding fetal well-being, admission to the hospital is warranted so that careful observation over a longer period of time may be performed. As previously noted, the decision for delivery will be dependent on multiple factors, including the fetal gestational age, fetal maturity, and fetal and maternal well-being.

DISCHARGE INSTRUCTIONS

When the woman with suspected mild preeclampsia is discharged from the hospital, she should be instructed to remain at bed rest and to contact her physician if symptoms arise, such as the development of headaches, scintillating scotomata or other visual changes, abdominal pain, vaginal bleeding, or decreased fetal movement. Follow-up should be arranged with the prenatal care provider within 7 days.

If the preeclamptic woman presents to a nontertiary care facility, transport to a tertiary care hospital with perinatology and neonatology services is indicated in certain clinical situations. Considering the complex clinical factors at work, consultation with a perinatologist should be attempted. In general, the patient is transferred when the fetus is viable but preterm and may need delivery (e.g., severe preeclampsia). Transport is sometimes contraindicated during acute emergencies when maternal problems (e.g., severe uncontrolled hypertension, uncontrolled eclamptic seizures, or severe hemorrhage) or fetal problems (e.g., impending delivery or significant fetal compromise) require immediate stabilization. Although maternal transport is generally preferable, in some cases delivery followed by neonatal transport may be in the patient's best interest.

REFERENCES

1. National High Blood Pressure Education Program Working Group Report on High Blood Pressure in Pregnancy. *Am J Obstet Gynecol* 163:1691–1712, 1990.
2. Hypertensive disorders in pregnancy, in Cunningham FG, Gant NF, Leveno KJ, et al (eds): *Williams Obstetrics*. New York: McGraw-Hill, 2001, pp 567–618.
3. Hauth JC, Ewell MG, Levine RJ, et al: Pregnancy outcomes in healthy nulliparas who developed hypertension. Calcium

for Preeclampsia Prevention Study Group. *Obstet Gynecol* 95:24–28, 2000.

4. Kaunitz AM, Hughes JM, Grimes DA, et al: Causes of maternal mortality in the United States. *Obstet Gynecol* 65:605–612, 1985.
5. Dildy GA, Cotton DB: Hemodynamic changes in pregnancy and pregnancy complicated by hypertension. *Acute Care* 15:26–46, 1988.
6. American College of Obstetricians and Gynecologists (ACOG) Committee on Practice Bulletins: ACOG Practice Bulletin. Diagnosis and management of preeclampsia and eclampsia. *Obstet Gynecol* 99:(suppl)159–167, 2002.
7. Committee on Technical Bulletins of the American College of Obstetricians and Gynecologists (ACOG): ACOG Technical Bulletin No. 219, Hypertension in pregnancy. January 1996.
8. Dildy GA, Cotton DB: Complications of preeclampsia, in Clark SL, Cotton DB, Hankins GDV, et al (eds): *Critical Care Obstetrics*. Boston: Blackwell Scientific Publications, 1997, pp 251–289.
9. North RA, Taylor RS, Schellenberg JC: Evaluation of a definition of pre-eclampsia. *Br J Obstet Gynaecol* 106:767–973, 1993.
10. Levine RJ, Ewell MG, Hauth JC, et al: Should the definition of preeclampsia include a rise in diastolic blood pressure of ≥15 mm Hg to a level <90 mm Hg in association with proteinuria? *Am J Obstet Gynecol* 183:787–792, 2000.
11. Goodlin RC: Preeclampsia as the great impostor. *Am J Obstet Gynecol* 164:1577–1581, 1991.
12. Sibai BM: Pitfalls in diagnosis and management of preeclampsia. *Am J Obstet Gynecol* 159:1–5, 1988.
13. Dildy GA 3d, Cotton DB: Management of severe preeclampsia and eclampsia. *Crit Care Clin* 7:829–850, 1991.
14. Sibai BM, Akl S, Fairlie F, et al: A protocol for managing severe preeclampsia in the second trimester. *Am J Obstet Gynecol* 163:733–738, 1990.
15. Sibai BM, Mercer BM, Schiff E, et al: Aggressive versus expectant management of severe preeclampsia at 28 to 32 weeks' gestation: a randomized controlled trial. *Am J Obstet Gynecol* 171:818–822, 1994.
16. Odendaal HJ, Pattinson RC, Bam R, et al: Aggressive or expectant management for patients with severe preeclampsia between 28–34 weeks' gestation: a randomized controlled trial. *Obstet Gynecol* 76:1070–1075, 1990.
17. Pritchard JA, Cunningham FG, Pritchard SA: The Parkland Memorial Hospital protocol for treatment of eclampsia: evaluation of 245 cases. *Am J Obstet Gynecol* 148:951–963, 1984.
18. Sibai BM: Magnesium sulfate is the ideal anticonvulsant in preeclampsia-eclampsia. *Am J Obstet Gynecol* 162:1141–1145, 1990.
19. Which anticonvulsant for women with eclampsia? Evidence from the Collaborative Eclampsia Trial. *Lancet* 345:1455–1463, 1995.
20. Lucas MJ, Leveno KJ, Cunningham FG: A comparison of magnesium sulfate with phenytoin for the prevention of eclampsia. *N Engl J Med* 333:201–205, 1995.
21. Witlin AG, Sibai BM: Magnesium sulfate therapy in preeclampsia and eclampsia. *Obstet Gynecol* 92:883–889, 1998.
22. Coetzee EJ, Dommisse J, Anthony J: A randomised controlled trial of intravenous magnesium sulphate versus placebo in the management of women with severe pre-eclampsia. *Br J Obstet Gynaecol* 105:300–303, 1998.
23. Kaplan PW, Repke JT: Eclampsia. *Neurol Clin* 12:565–582, 1994.
24. Usta IM, Sibai BM: Emergent management of puerperal eclampsia. *Obstet Gynecol Clin North Am* 22:315–335, 1995.
25. Clark SL, Cotton DB, Lee W, et al. Central hemodynamic assessment of normal term pregnancy. *Am J Obstet Gynecol* 161:1439–1442, 1989.
26. Cotton DB, Lee W, Huhta JC, et al: Hemodynamic profile of severe pregnancy-induced hypertension. *Am J Obstet Gynecol* 158:523–529, 1988.

9

Trauma in Pregnancy

Mark D. Pearlman

KEY POINTS

- All reproductive-age female trauma victims should have a pregnancy test because 8 percent of pregnant trauma victims have not yet had their pregnancies diagnosed.
- Pregnant women beyond 20 weeks' gestation should be placed in the lateral decubitus position or in lateral tilt to prevent supine hypotension.
- Abruptio placentae is the leading cause of fetal loss. Frequent uterine contraction, abnormal fetal heart tracing, vaginal bleeding, and uterine pain and tenderness are signs of abruption.
- All pregnant patients with a viable fetus (beyond 22 to 24 weeks' gestation) should have continuous fetal monitoring (tocodynamometry) initiated as soon as it is feasible.
- Fetal outcome is related to maternal injury severity, but even minor trauma may cause fetal loss.

Some 6 to 7 percent of pregnant women will suffer physical trauma during their pregnancy.[1] Conversely, of reproductive-age women presenting with trauma, approximately 3 percent are pregnant, 8 percent of whom were not known to be pregnant prior to presentation.[2] Because most physical trauma suffered during pregnancy is relatively minor, many of these women will not present for medical care. A critical factor to consider is that the severity of the trauma does not always accurately predict adverse fetal outcome.[3] Recognizing this, a general recommendation should be made that women who suffer any degree of truncal trauma during pregnancy should be evaluated. This is particularly true once fetal viability has been established (i.e., beyond 22 to 24 weeks of gestation). Case series of trauma during pregnancy and subsequent fetal loss bear this out, as 60 to 80 percent of all fetal losses result from relatively minor maternal trauma.[3–6]

A recent review of fetal death certificates suggest that approximately 400 to 500 fetal deaths annually in the United States resulting from trauma during pregnancy.[7] Penetrating abdominal trauma during pregnancy is particularly problematic for the fetus, because the fetus typically absorbs the brunt of penetrating energy forces, especially in the latter half of gestation. Management algorithms for penetrating trauma during pregnancy are dependent on gestational age, the penetrating object, the depth of penetration, and the maternal physical examination. Though the basic approach to the management of the gravida following trauma is largely unchanged by the pregnancy, the fetus must be considered early.

ANATOMIC AND PHYSIOLOGIC CHANGES OF PREGNANCY

While prior chapters have addressed both the anatomic and physiologic changes of pregnancy, those that affect the management of trauma in pregnancy are reviewed here.

Cardiovascular Changes

In order to compensate for the metabolic needs of the growing conceptus, fundamental changes in cardiovascular status occur during pregnancy. Changes in blood pressure, heart rate, and blood volume composition should be considered during the evaluation of the multiply-injured trauma patient. Blood pressure typically decreases 10 to 15 mm Hg systolic and 5 to 10 mm Hg diastolic during the midtrimester of pregnancy. This is largely due to a decrease in systemic vascular resistance, allowing increased blood flow to the uterus. Systolic blood pressures in the range of 80 to 90 mmHg are not uncommon in the healthy young pregnant woman and should not be mistaken for an indicator of maternal hypovolemia. This is particularly important when one considers that heart rate increases by 10 to 15 beats per minute during pregnancy. The increased heart rate is a result of the need to adequately perfuse the uterus, allowing sufficient oxygen and nutrient delivery to the fetus.

Uterine blood flow increases from 60 mL/min in the nonpregnant state to over 600 mL/min in the last third of gestation. The distribution of cardiac output to the uterus increases from 2 percent prior to pregnancy to 17 percent during pregnancy. This remarkable volume of blood flow is an important consideration if penetrating trauma transects the uterine vasculature or severe blunt abdominal trauma results in uterine rupture or uterine vascular avulsion, because rapid exsanguination may result.

The composition of blood during pregnancy changes dramatically, reaching its maximum volume change at 28 weeks of gestation. It is typical for blood volume to increase by 45 percent overall during pregnancy—even more in twins and other multiple gestations. Plasma volume increases more than does red blood cell (RBC) mass, resulting in a physiologic decrease in hematocrit during pregnancy. It is not uncommon for the normal hematocrit to vary between 33 and 36 percent during pregnancy. Taken together, the finding of a a relatively low blood pressure, increased heart rate, and low hematocrit in the multiply-injured trauma patient would understandably raise concern about potential hypovolemia. When the trauma victim is pregnant, interpretation of these findings must be made within the context of these normal physiologic changes.

Probably the most critical anatomic change during pregnancy that can affect resuscitation of the injured trauma victim is the potential for supine hypotension. Beyond 20 weeks of gestation, when the pregnant woman is lying supine the gravid uterus can compress the inferior vena cava and aorta, impeding the return of blood from the lower extremities and pelvis to the central circulation. In the healthy pregnant woman, cardiac output can decrease as much as 30 percent due to a decrease in venous return. In addition, compression of the aorta may further compromise blood flow to the uterus, potentially exacerbating fetal hypoxia. Because this is a very common position in which to evaluate and manage trauma victims (e.g., strapped to a long board), it is imperative to avoid this position. No woman beyond 20 weeks of gestation should lie supine. Either the lateral decubitus position should be used or manual displacement of the uterus should be performed (outlined below in the section about general principles of trauma management).

Gastrointestinal Changes

Gastric and intestinal motility decrease during pregnancy, presumably as a result of elevated progesterone levels (progesterone is a smooth muscle relaxant). These changes in motility cause an increase in gastric emptying time. As a result, the pregnant trauma victim with head injury and decreased sensorium is at significant risk for aspiration of gastric contents. Clinically, it is best to assume that the injured pregnant woman's stomach is full.

Progressive cephalad and lateral displacement of the small and large bowel result from the enlarging gravid uterus. Therefore penetrating trauma to the lower abdomen is less likely to result in penetrating intestinal injury during pregnancy. However, an object penetrating in the most superior or lateral aspect of the abdomen may produce complex intestinal injuries during pregnancy, with multiple entry and exit wounds to the bowel. Finally, because of the progressive distention and attenuation of the anterior abdominal wall and separation of the rectus muscles that commonly occurs during pregnancy (distasis recti), the physical response to intraperitoneal irritation may be altered. For example, rebound tenderness and involuntary guarding may be much less appreciated on physical examination, even in the presence of significant intraperitoneal injury (e.g., hemoperitoneum, ruptured viscus).

Pulmonary Changes

While tidal volume increases by 30 to 40 percent, respiratory rate does not change appreciably during pregnancy. Cephalad displacement of the diaphragm due to the enlarged gravid uterus results in a decrease in residual volume and functional residual capacity. This coupled with the increased oxygen requirements due to pregnancy can lead to a more rapid deterioration of respiratory status with significant pulmonary injury or in cases of difficult airway control. When these pulmonary changes are taken together with the risk for aspiration due to gastrointestinal changes, serious consideration should be given to early endotracheal intubation in the pregnant trauma victim with multisystem injuries.

Changes in Regional Blood Flow

The 1000 percent increase in uterine blood flow from 60 to 600 mL/min during pregnancy is an important consideration for two reasons. First, in the presence of maternal hypovolemia, the uterus is considered an expendable organ. Uterine artery vasoconstriction is an adaptive means to maintain maternal cerebral and cardiac perfusion in the presence of maternal hypovolemia, and aggressive intravascular resuscitation is mandatory to maintain adequate fetal oxygenation.

Second, uterine rupture or laceration of the uterine vessels—either through penetrating trauma to the lateral lower abdomen or severe direct abdominal impact—may result in rapid maternal exsanguination. The retroperitoneal pelvic blood vasculature is also hypertrophied during pregnancy, and maternal pelvic fracture may result in

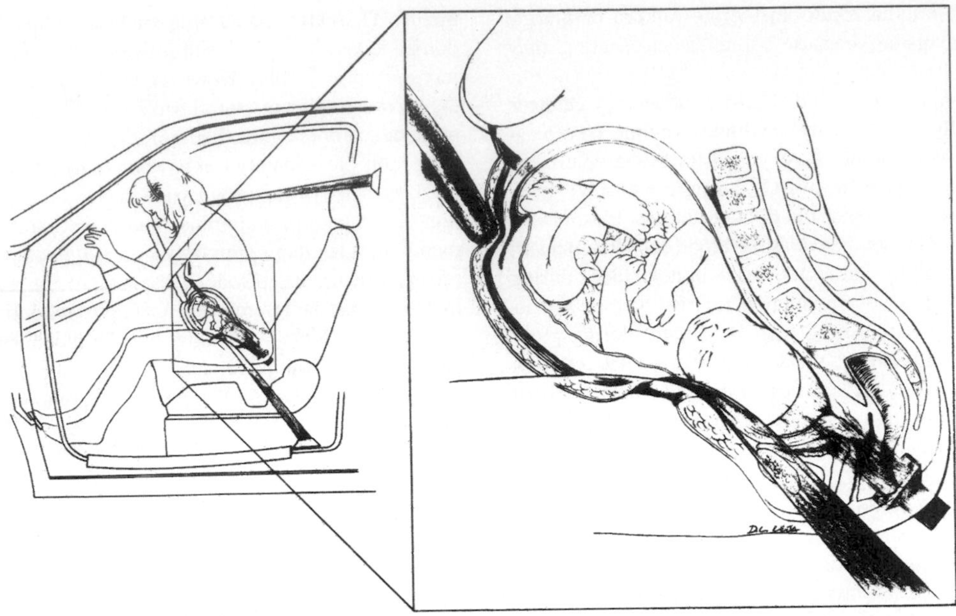

Fig. 9-1. Illustration of abruptio placentae resulting from impact with steering wheel. See text for description. (Illustration by Darryl Leja, University of Michigan. From Pearlman and Tintinalli,[14] with permission.)

impressive bleeding into the retroperitoneal space over a fairly short time.

LABORATORY CHANGES OF PREGNANCY

The most frequent and dramatic changes in maternal laboratory values are those found in the complete blood count. Both plasma volume and RBC mass increase during pregnancy, but plasma volume increases more than RBC mass. As a result, a physiologic anemia in the range of 30 to 36 percent hematocrit, or 11 to 13 g/dL hemoglobin, is normal. Furthermore, leukocytosis is common beginning in the second trimester, with white blood cell counts normally up to 15,000/mm^3. During labor, white blood cell counts in the range of 20,000 to 25,000/mm^3 are not uncommon. The platelet count is typically unchanged or minimally lower in the normal pregnancy. Likewise, prothrombin time and partial thromboplastin time are unchanged in normal pregnancy. Arterial pH is unchanged, though a slight increase in minute ventilation results in a decrease in P_{CO_2} to approximately 35 torr, To compensate for this, there is a slight increase in serum HCO_3^- due to decreased excretion of bicarbonate into the urine. Measurements Of P_{O_2} are unchanged during pregnancy (see Chap. 2 for other laboratory values in pregnancy).

INJURY PATTERNS IN PREGNANCY

Blunt Abdominal Trauma

Blunt abdominal trauma is most commonly caused by motor vehicle accidents, which account for 50 to 65 percent of all cases, followed by falls and direct blows to the abdomen.[3,5,8–11] Domestic violence is remarkably common during pregnancy; rates as high as 20 percent have been reported.[12,13] The most common adverse event resulting from blunt abdominal trauma is abruptio placentae, complicating 1 to 3 percent of non-life-threatening maternal abdominal trauma and 40 to 50 percent of life-threatening maternal trauma (Fig. 9-1). Similarly, fetal loss occurs uncommonly following trauma during pregnancy, but because most maternal trauma during pregnancy is minor (more than 90 percent), most fetal losses following trauma result from minor maternal injuries. The clinical implication of this observation is that policies should be developed to allow careful observation of the fetus following maternal trauma of any severity.[14] This specific evaluation is outlined in the management section, below.

Laboratory tests and their interpretation for a patient who has suffered blunt abdominal trauma during pregnancy is similar to that for the nonpregnant patient with two notable exceptions: (1) recognizing the differences in normal laboratory studies in the pregnant as compared with the nonpregnant patient; and (2) seeking laboratory evidence of fetomaternal hemorrhage.[3,5,15] It has been recommended that all pregnant women undergo Kleihauer-Betke testing if they suffered trauma during pregnancy.[17] This recommendation was based on the observation that evidence of fetal cells in the maternal circulation was found four times more frequently in women who suffered blunt abdominal trauma, with the presumption that identification of fetomaternal hemorrhage could impact decision making (e.g., more intensive fetal surveillance, early delivery).[3,5,15] However, subsequent experience has demonstrated that the results of a Kleihauer-Betke test rarely affect clinical decision making.[18] For example, a fetus that suffers a massive fetomaternal bleed may exsanguinate, but clinical decision making will be dictated by an abnormal fetal heart tracing rather than Kleihauer-Betke testing, as the results from the latter frequently take hours to obtain.[19] Nonetheless, in the Rh-negative woman, the possibility of isoimmunization due to fetomaternal hemorrhage is real and Rh immune globulin should be administered to Rh-negative women who have suffered blunt abdominal trauma. A 300-μg dose is sufficient to cover 30 mL of whole blood (equivalent to a 15-mL RBC bleed). Fetomaternal hemorrhage greater than that requires additional Rh immune globulin. Because the Kleihauer-Betke test can identify these occasional large bleeds, its use in the Rh-negative woman may still have utility.

Abruptio Placentae

Abruptio placentae, or separation of the placenta from the decidua basalis of the endometrium, is the most common cause of fetal loss caused by trauma, accounting for 60 to 70 percent of these losses. The pathophysiology of abruptio placentae is based on the observation that there are fundamental differences in the elastic properties of the uterus and placenta: there are substantial numbers of elastic fibers in the uterus, whereas the placenta is relatively devoid of these. When the fluid-filled uterus is struck by a deforming force (e.g., steering wheel), the noncompressible amniotic fluid transmits the force to the entire uterus, causing an outward expansion of the entire uterus except at the point of intrusion by the deforming object. An analogous situation would be attaching a piece of adhesive tape to the inside of a water balloon and squeezing the balloon. The balloon wall is stretched; however, the inelastic tape cannot. If enough stretching occurs, the tape can be sheared off of the balloon. Other mechanisms may be operative in causing placental abruption (e.g., direct placental separation of an anteriorly attached placenta from deformation of the anterior uterine wall, or a contrecoup mechanism).[16]

Table 9-1. Signs and Symptoms of Abruptio Placentae

Finding	Percent
Vaginal bleeding	78
Uterine tenderness or back pain	66
Fetal distress	60
High frequency uterine contractions	17
Uterine hypertonus	17
Fetal death	15

Source: Adapted from Hurd WW, Miodovnik M, Hertzberg V, Lavin JP: Selective management of abruptio placentae. *Obstet Gynecol* 61:467, 1983.

The signs and symptoms of abruptio placentae vary depending on the severity of separation. Vaginal bleeding is apparent in 80 percent of cases, and abdominal pain is also usually present (Table 9-1). In the most severe cases, there is fetal death associated with a tetanic uterine contraction pattern (less than 15 percent). However, the most sensitive method of diagnosing abruptio placentae following injury is by uterine contraction monitoring using a standard fetal monitor. In several studies, four or more uterine contractions in any 1 hour period in the first 4 hours of monitoring following trauma identified a group at risk for abruptio placentae.[3,5,6,8] Pregnant women beyond 22 to 24 weeks of gestation should routinely have fetal monitoring, including uterine contraction monitoring, following abdominal trauma of any severity.[17] The use of ultrasound for diagnosing abruptio placentae secondary to trauma is much less sensitive (40%) than uterine monitoring.

Uterine Rupture

Uterine rupture as a result of abdominal trauma is uncommon, complicating only about 0.6 percent of cases of severe direct abdominal trauma.[1] The clinical presentation of uterine rupture can vary considerably, from minimal abdominal tenderness in a hemodynamically stable patient to frank peritoneal signs with hypovolemic shock. If there is transmural uterine wall disruption, the fetus may be extruded from the uterus into the peritoneal cavity. Fetal death virtually always occurs in this circumstance. Uterine rupture is nearly always a second- or third-trimester event, as the first-trimester uterus is protected by the bony pelvis. Concomitant injuries to viscera such as the bladder or gastrointestinal tract can also occur.

Uterine rupture should be part of the differential diagnosis of any pregnant woman in the second or third trimester who sustains severe direct abdominal trauma. Findings of abdominal pain and tenderness, signs of hypovolemia (though not always present), and fetal distress or death are clinical clues suggestive of uterine rupture. However, these findings can also be seen in abruptio placentae. More specific findings in uterine rupture include sonographic, CT, MRI, or abdominal x-ray evidence of the fetus outside of the uterine cavity (e.g., extended fetal extremities, oblique fetal lie, or direct visualization of an extrauterine fetus) or a difficult-to-palpate uterine fundus. A history of previous uterine scarring (e.g., cesarean delivery or myomectomy) increases the risk of uterine rupture, but uterine rupture can occur in the absence of any prior uterine surgery. A positive peritoneal lavage can be suggestive of this diagnosis, but it does not differentiate between uterine rupture and other causes of intraperitoneal bleeding. Peritoneal lavage can be performed at any gestational age and has been demonstrated to be as accurate as in the nonpregnant patient.[19] However, the hemodynamically unstable patient with signs of peritoneal irritation should be taken directly for exploratory laparotomy while resuscitation efforts are ongoing.

Pelvic Fracture and Direct Fetal Injury

Pelvic fracture during pregnancy poses a significant risk of maternal mortality, because the hypertrophic vasculature can lead to significant retroperitoneal hemorrhage.[20] Aggressive hemodynamic resuscitation is paramount in the management of these women. Because of the expanded blood volume during pregnancy, blood loss can be underestimated until profound hemodynamic instability ensues. In some cases, pregnancy may result in a modification of the management of a pelvic fracture (e.g., delayed or modified operations).[21]

Pelvic fracture in late gestation also places the fetal vertex at risk for skull fracture, because the fetal head engages, or enters the bony pelvis, in late pregnancy. Direct fetal injury such as skull fracture usually results from severe maternal trauma. In addition to skull fracture, intracranial hemorrhage, fetal splenic rupture, intrathoracic injuries, and extremity fracture have been described in the fetus. Fortunately, these are rare occurrences.

Use of Ultrasound for Diagnosis of Intraabdominal Hemorrhage During Pregnancy

Ultrasound can play a valuable role in the diagnosis of intraabdominal injuries during pregnancy. However, it has a limited role in the diagnosis of abruptio placentae (sensitivity of 40 percent). Ultrasound in the nonpregnant patient has demonstrated its utility as a valuable adjunct for diagnosing intraabdominal injuries following trauma, having good sensitivity and outstanding specificity.[22] In an 8-year study at a level 1 trauma center,the utility of abdominal ultrasound (focused assessment with sonography from trauma, or FAST exam) for detecting intraabdominal hemorrhage during pregnancy appears to have comparable sensitivity and specificity to the nonpregnant setting (sensitivity 83 percent, specificity 95 percent).[23]

GENERAL PRINCIPLES OF TRAUMA MANAGEMENT

Because the fetus is wholly dependent on maternal hemodynamic stability for adequate oxygenation, all initial efforts in evaluating and managing the pregnant trauma victim should be concentrated on assessing and resuscitating maternal vital signs (Fig. 9-2). An extensive review of resuscitation of the trauma victim is not offered here because this is discussed in standard trauma texts. However, several anatomic and physiologic changes of pregnancy are discussed because they influence maternal resuscitative efforts. The supine hypotensive syndrome has been described in several chapters in this text (see Fig. 2-5). Beyond approximately 20 weeks of gestation (the uterine fundus is palpable at the umbilicus), a woman lying in the supine position can develop significant hypotension due to inferior vena caval compression by the uterus, resulting in decreased venous return from the lower extremities. This may lead to a subsequent decrease in cardiac output approaching 25 to 30 percent. In the case of a hypovolemic patient who is marginally compromised, this supine position may cause hypovolemic shock. This can be avoided by displacing the uterus to either side by placing a 4 to 6 inch roll underneath the backboard or deflecting the uterus manually. Second, the 50 percent increase in maternal blood volume by 28 weeks of gestation may allow significant blood loss before there is a change in maternal vital signs. Careful attention to the mechanism of injury and the likelihood of significant vascular injury should prompt aggressive initial efforts at maternal blood

STABILIZATION

- Maintain airway and oxygenation
- Deflect uterus to left
- Maintain circulatory volume
- Secure cervical spine if head or neck injury suspected

COMPLETE EXAMINATION

- Control external hemorrhage
- Identify/stabilize serious injuries
- Examine uterus
- Pelvic examination to identify ruptured membranes or vaginal bleeding
- Obtain initial blood work

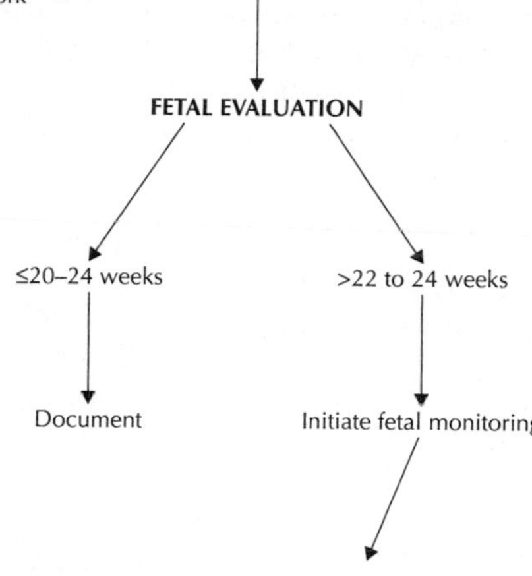

Presence of

- More than four uterine contractions in any 1 h (>22–24 weeks)
- Rupture of amniotic membranes
- Vaginal bleeding
- Serious maternal injury
- Fetal tachycardia, late decelerations, nonreactive nonstress test

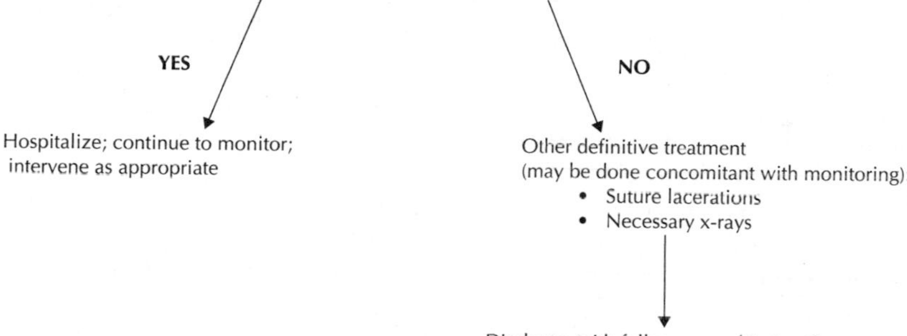

Fig. 9-2. Algorithm for management of blunt abdominal trauma during pregnancy. (From Pearlman MD: Motor vehicle crashes, pregnancy loss and preterm labor. *Int J Obstet Gynecol* 57:127, 1997. Used with permission.)

volume expansion and attention to the possible emergent need for blood products.

After assuring adequate ventilation and intravascular volume, efforts should be directed at assessing the extent of maternal injuries, followed by rapid assessment of the fetus. Particular attention should be paid to the maternal abdomen, because the finding of abdominal tenderness may indicate common injuries in accident victims (e.g., laceration of the liver or spleen) or pregnancy-specific injuries (uterine rupture or abruptio placentae) or both.

Vaginal bleeding associated with abdominal pain is highly suggestive of abruptio placentae. Beyond 20 to 24 weeks of gestation, a fetal monitor should be placed if available, because it will help to assess fetal well-being in addition to being the most sensitive test for abruptio placentae. The availability of surgical and obstetric consultation should be anticipated, particularly when the gestational age is such that the fetus is viable outside of the uterus (22 to 24 weeks).

Simultaneously with resuscitation efforts, a rapid but complete search for thoracic, intrathoracic, or intraabdominal injury, fractures, or external bleeding sites should ensue. In addition, specific efforts should be made to try to identify uterine or fetal injuries. Examination of the abdomen can be hindered by the recognized fact that findings of peritoneal irritation can be blunted in the pregnant woman because of stretching and attenuation of the abdominal musculature.

In the pregnancy that has reached viability (i.e., 22 to 24 weeks' gestation), fetal monitoring should begin as soon as maternal stabilization has occurred, because abruptio placentae is an event that usually develops early following trauma. Evidence of frequent uterine contractions (four or more in an hour), a nonreassuring fetal heart rate tracing, uterine irritability or tenderness, ruptured amniotic membranes, and vaginal bleeding are all reasons for immediate obstetric consultation. Monitoring of the fetal heart rate and uterine contractions should be interpreted by trained personnel. Monitoring is typically continued for a minimum of 4 hours. While shorter monitoring periods (e.g., 2 hours) have been utilized successfully, it is important to emphasize the critical role of fetal monitoring in diagnosing abruptio placentae following trauma during pregnancy. Patients who refuse such monitoring should understand that this refusal substantially interferes with the appropriate evaluation of the well-being of the fetus.[5]

PENETRATING TRAUMA

Knife and gunshot wounds during pregnancy are not uncommon in urban settings. Understandably, there is considerable concern for fetal well-being when gunshot or knife wounds penetrate the abdomen. Knife and gunshot wounds suffered elsewhere in the body should be managed just as they are in the nonpregnant individual except that the fetus should also be monitored if viable (beyond 22–24 weeks of gestation) once the woman has been stabilized. However, penetrating wounds to the pregnant abdomen involve different considerations, because fetal or placental injury becomes an important issue.

The proximity of the fetus and placenta to the anterior abdominal wall render them very susceptible to injury or death when there is penetrating abdominal trauma. In fact, there is disparate risk for the woman and her fetus following penetrating trauma. This is because the likelihood of fetal injury is directly related to the size of the uterus in relation to other intraabdominal organs. In this regard, the uterus is dominant in size in the second half of gestation. Furthermore, the anterior abdominal wall, uterine wall, amniotic fluid, and fetus all absorb energy of the penetrating object, protecting other maternal visceral organs. This shielding effect is manifest in the most recent series of studies of penetrating abdominal trauma during pregnancy, in which there were no maternal mortalities compared with a fetal death rate of nearly two-thirds.[24–26]

With cephalad and lateral displacement of the maternal intraabdominal viscera during pregnancy, penetrating injuries that enter superior or lateral to the uterus are likely to produce complex bowel injuries, resulting in the potential for multiple entrance and exit wounds. High-speed projectiles (e.g., bullets from high-powered rifles) can pass through the uterus, placing the organs posterior to it at risk (e.g., abdominal aorta, inferior vena cava, sigmoid colon).

Management of Penetrating Trauma

When a pregnant woman presents with penetrating abdominal trauma, three decisions must immediately be made: (1) whether to perform exploratory laparotomy; (2) whether to deliver the fetus; and (3) if delivery is planned, what the route of delivery should be.

Whether or not to perform exploratory laparotomy will depend on the patient's hemodynamic stability and the presence or absence of hemoperitoneum. It will also depend on the type of penetrating object. Most authors agree that gunshot wounds to the abdomen should be explored in all cases, since the course of the bullet cannot be predicted.[26,27] Furthermore, due to cavitation and shock waves, tissue damage well outside of the projectile's path can be significant. When extrauterine injuries do occur following penetrating abdominal trauma during pregnancy, they typically occur as a result of gunshot wounds. All gunshot wounds to the abdomen should be explored.

Knife wounds to the abdomen are much less likely to cause extrauterine injuries, and these injuries typically have a better prognosis than gunshot wounds. The individual circumstances of knife wounds should be carefully weighed prior to making a decision to perform a laparotomy. Stab wounds to the lower abdomen are much less likely to cause visceral injuries than upper abdominal wounds. However, any midline lower abdominal wound can cause bladder or ureteral injury. Grubb demonstrated that in nonpregnant patients, stab wounds to the abdomen do not penetrate the peritoneum in about one-third of cases.[28] These extraperitoneal wounds generally do not require exploration unless they have injured a large blood vessel in the abdominal wall (e.g., the inferior epigastric artery). However, because of the enlarged gravid uterus, attenuation of the abdominal wall during pregnancy makes it more susceptible to peritoneal penetration. Several invasive tests short of exploratory laparotomy can be utilized to determine if there has been significant intraperitoneal injury. Injection of radiopaque material into the entrance wound followed by a two-view radiograph may demonstrate spillage into the gastrointestinal or genitourinary tract. Such a finding would be an indication for laparotomy. Second, amniocentesis to determine whether the amniotic cavity contains blood or bacteria has been advocated. However, the presence of blood or bacteria does not necessarily mandate delivery, and careful consideration with obstetric consultation should precede this decision.

Injury to the uterine vasculature is uncommon, largely because the vessels are located quite lateral and posterior in later gestation. However, because of the tremendous volume of blood flowing through the uterine vessels, injury to these vessels is likely to result in rapid deterioration of vital signs. Unstable vital signs in the presence of a penetrating abdominal wound indicate the need for immediate laparotomy. In the absence of unstable vital signs, peritoneal lavage has been shown to accurately diagnose hemoperitoneum during pregnancy, and it can be helpful in determining whether exploratory laparotomy is necessary.

The decision to deliver depends on (1) gestational age at the time of injury, (2) penetration of the amniotic cavity by the object, (3) evidence of fetal injury or death, and (4) the extent of maternal injuries and the need to empty the uterus to explore the abdomen adequately. These decisions are best made in concert with the obstetrician and trauma surgeon. If exploratory surgery has been performed, incidental cesarean section may be indicated at term if this will improve the ability to explore the abdomen, or if there is evidence of fetal distress or injury that would likely be better dealt with in the extrauterine environment. Otherwise, it is acceptable to allow vaginal delivery. The decision to deliver in preterm gestations will depend on several considerations, mainly recognizing that if the pregnancy is allowed to continue in a gestation that is far from term, a better fetal outcome will probably result.

THERMAL AND ELECTRICAL INJURIES

There has been limited published experience with burns and electrical injuries during pregnancy. Matthews recommends that severely burned women (more than 50 percent body surface area) should be delivered immediately because maternal death is almost certain otherwise, and fetal survival is not improved by allowing the pregnancy to continue.[29] Matthews' experience was that maternal prognosis with thermal injury is worse compared with similar injuries to nonpregnant women. Other experience has suggested that pregnancy does not affect outcome in patients who have suffered burns.[30,31] More likely, the percentage of body surface area affected is a reasonably good predictor of maternal survival. In general, fetal prognosis is poor in severely burned women. Typically, spontaneous labor will develop within days to a week postburn. The approach to managing the burn victim in the first few hours after injury is similar to that in the nonpregnant woman. Several management considerations are critical in the burned pregnant patient: (1) prompt and aggressive fluid resuscitation, (2) oxygen supplementation and a low threshold for endotracheal intubation and the use of mechanical ventilation, (3) high suspicion for venous thromboembolism and appropriate preventive measures, and (4) early delivery, especially in women in the third trimester or those with extensive burns.[32]

The experience with electrical injury during pregnancy is limited. Eleven cases of lightning injury during pregnancy were summarized by Pierce and colleagues.[35] In this series, there were no maternal deaths and no long-term sequelae to the fetuses that survived. However, another series of electrical injuries suggests that there may be long-term sequelae in the fetuses who survive the initial insult.[36] In this series of six pregnancies complicated by electrical injury, there was one delayed fetal death complicated by growth retardation and oligohydramnios, and two of the three other live births were complicated by oligohydramnios. Because of this, these authors recommend serial ultrasound examinations to follow fetal growth and amniotic fluid volume.

CARBON MONOXIDE POISONING

In the United States, carbon monoxide (CO) is the leading cause of death by poisoning.[33] As many as 8.4 percent of CO poisoning victims are pregnant. CO diffuses readily across the placenta and can cause fetal tissue hypoxia. As the placental blood flow increases, so too does the diffusion of CO, such that CO diffusion capacity is directly proportional to fetal weight. Fetal hypoxia results from both accumulation of CO in the fetus and also through decreased levels of oxygen in maternal hemoglobin due to displacement by CO. Fetal carboxyhemoglobin levels are 10 to 15 percent higher than maternal levels, and elimination of CO is less rapid in the fetus. Severe acute CO poisoning can result in permanent fetal neurologic injury, or even fetal death. Chronic CO exposure (e.g., cigarette smoking) may result in intrauterine growth restriction.

Treatment of acute CO poisoning with hyperbaric oxygen works by both increasing the levels of dissolved oxygen in the blood and by increasing the rate of dissociation of CO from hemoglobin. Treatment of CO poisoning during pregnancy begins by removing the victim from the source of CO and beginning 100 percent oxygen. Strong consideration should be given to using hyperbaric oxygen for 2 hours at 2 atmospheres; this has been used successfully and safely during pregnancy.[34] Longer use of hyperbaric oxygen may be teratogenic, and abortion after first-trimester hyperbaric oxygen exposure has been reported. However, given the serious potential effects of hypoxia on the fetus, hyperbaric oxygen appears to be the treatment of choice for pregnant women suffering from CO poisoning.

REFERENCES

1. Pearlman MD, Tintinalli JE, Lorenz RP: Blunt trauma during pregnancy. *N Engl J Med* 323:1609, 1990.
2. Bochicchia GV, Napolitano LM, Haan J, Champion H, Scalea T: Incidental pregnancy in trauma patients. *J Am Coll Surg* 192:566, 2001.
3. Pearlman MD, Tintinalli JE, Lorenz RP: A prospective controlled study of outcome after trauma during pregnancy. *Am J Obstet Gynecol* 162:1502, 1990.
4. Scorpio RJ, Esposito TJ, Smith LG, Gens DR: Blunt trauma during pregnancy. Factors affecting fetal outcome. *J Trauma* 32:213, 1992.
5. GoodwinTM, Breen MT: Pregnancy outcome and fetomaternal hemorrhage after noncatastrophic trauma. *Am J Obstet Gynecol* 162:665, 1990.
6. Williams JK, McClain L, Rosemurgy AS, Colorado NM: Evaluation of blunt abdominal trauma in the third trimester of pregnancy: Maternal and fetal considerations. *Obstet Gynecol* 75:33, 1990.
7. Weiss HB, Songer TJ, Fabio A: Fetal deaths related to maternal injury. *JAMA* 286:1863, 2001.
8. Dahmus MA, Sibai BM: Blunt abdominal trauma: Are there any predictive factors for abruptio placentae or maternal-fetal distress? *Am J Obstet Gynecol* 169:1504, 1993.
9. Esposito JT, Agens DR, Smith LG, Scorpio R: Evaluation of blunt abdominal trauma occurring during pregnancy. *J Trauma* 29:1628, 1989.
10. Kissinger DP, Rozycki GS, Morris JA Jr, et al: Trauma in pregnancy: Predicting pregnancy outcome. *Arch Surg* 126:1079, 1991.
11. Rogers FB, Rozycki GS, Osler TM, et al: A multi-institutional study of factors associated with fetal death in injured pregnant patients. *Arch Surg* 134:1274, 1999.
12. Gazmararian JA, Lazorick S, Spitz AM, et al: Prevalence of violence against pregnant women. *JAMA* 275:1915, 1996.
13. Hedin LW, Janson PO: Domestic violence during pregnancy. The prevalence of physical injuries, substance use, abortions and miscarriages. *Acta Obstet Gynecol Scand* 79:625, 2000.
14. Pearlman MD, Tintinalli JE: Evaluation and treatment of the gravida and fetus following trauma during pregnancy. *Obstet Gynecol Clin North Am* 18:371, 1991.
15. Rose PG, Strohm PL, Zuspan FP: Fetomaternal hemorrhage following trauma. *Am J Obstet Gynecol* 153:844, 1985.
16. Pearlman MD, Klinich KD, Schneider LW, et al: A comprehensive program to improve safety for pregnant women and fetuses in motor vehicle crashes. *Am J Obstet Gynecol* 182:1554, 2000.
17. American College of Obstetricians and Gynecologists: Obstetric aspects of trauma management. ACOG Educational Bulletin No 251. Washington, DC ACOG, 1998.
18. Boyle J, Kim J, Walerius H, Samuels P: The clinical use of the Kleihauer-Betke test in Rh positive patients (abstract). *Am J Obstet Gynecol* 174:343, 1995.
19. Towery R, English TP, Wisner D: Evaluation of the pregnant woman after blunt injury. *J Trauma* 35:731, 1993.
20. Pearlman MD, Tintinalli JE: Trauma in pregnancy (clinical conference). *Ann Emerg Med* 17:829, 1990.
21. Pape N-C, Pohlemann T, Gansslen A, et al: Pelvic fractures in pregnant multiple trauma patients. *J Ortho Trauma* 14:238, 2000.
22. Bain IM, Kirby RM, Tiwari P, et al: Survey of abdominal ultrasound and diagnostic peritoneal lavage for suspected intra-abdominal injury following blunt trauma. *Injury* 29: 65–71, 1998.
23. Goodwin H, Holmes JF, Wisner DH: Abdominal ultrasound examination in pregnant blunt trauma paients. *J Trauma-Injury Infect Crit Care* 50:689–693, 2001.
24. Kirshon B, Young R, Gordon AN: Conservative management of abdominal gunshot wound in a pregnant woman. *Am J Perinatol* 5:232, 1988.
25. Awwad JT, Azar GB, Seoud MA, et al: High velocity penetrating wounds of the gravid uterus: Review of 16 years of civil war. *Obstet Gynecol* 83:259, 1994.
26. Buchsbaum HJ: Penetrating injury of the abdomen, in Buchsbaum HJ (ed): *Trauma in Pregnancy*. Philadelphia: Saunders, 1979, p 82.
27. Franger AL, Buchsbaum HJ, Peaceman AM: Abdominal gunshot wounds in pregnancy. *Am J Obstet Gynecol* 160:1124, 1989.
28. Grubb DK: Nonsurgical management of penetrating uterine trauma in pregnancy: A case report. *Am J Obstet Gynecol* 166:583, 1992.

29. Matthews RN: Obstetric implications of burns in pregnancy. *Br J Obstet Gynaecol* 89:603, 1982.
30. Amy BW, McManus WF, Goodwin CW, et al: Thermal injury in the pregnant patient. *Surg Gynecol Obstet* 161:209, 1985.
31. Jain ML, Gary AK: Burns with pregnancy: A review of 215 cases. *Burns* 19:166, 1993.
32. Guo SS, Greenspoon JS, Kahn AM: Management of burn injuries during pregnancy. *Burns* 27:394, 2001.
33. Cobb N, Etzel RA: Unintentional carbon monoxide related deaths in the United States, 1997 through 1998. *JAMA* 266:659, 1998.
34. Elkharrat D, Raphael JC, Korach JM, et al: Acute carbon monoxide intoxication and hyperbaric oxygen in pregnancy. *Intensive Care Med* 17:289, 1991.
35. Pierce MR, Henderson RA, Mitchell JM: Cardiopulmonary arrest secondary to lightning injury in a pregnant woman. *Ann Emerg Med* 15:597, 1986.
36. Liberman JR, Mazor M, Molcho J, et al: Electrical burns in pregnancy. *Obstet Gynecol* 67:861, 1986.

10

Bleeding After 20 Weeks' Gestation: Maternal and Fetal Assessment

Khurram S. Rehman
Timothy R.B. Johnson

Dedicated to Yasmin and Layla Rehman

KEY POINTS

- Most common causes of vaginal bleeding after 20 weeks' gestation
  - Placenta previa—painless bleeding
  - Placental abruption—bleeding with abdominal or back pain
  - Bloody show of labor
- Diagnosis of vaginal bleeding after 20 weeks' gestation
  - Never perform digital examination
  - First confirm placental location with ultrasound
  - Obtain urgent obstetric consultation
- Maternal resuscitation
  - Maternal resuscitation is the best fetal resuscitation
  - Fluid resuscitation with normal saline or Ringer's lactate
  - If class III or IV hemorrhage, administer type and cross-matched blood or O-negative blood
  - Obtain coagulation studies and correct coagulopathy
  - Administer vasopressors only if fluid and blood ineffective
  - Obtain fetal heart tones and establish cardiotocodynamometry

Vaginal bleeding after 20 weeks' gestation occurs in 3 to 5 percent of all pregnancies and is strongly associated with increased maternal and perinatal morbidity and mortality.[1] The well-being of two patients, the fetus and the mother, must be considered and managed simultaneously. Medical decisions in these cases must attempt to optimize the outcome for both patients.[2] At times, however, what is best for the mother appears not always best for the fetus. Although the mother seldom benefits from continued pregnancy when significant vaginal bleeding occurs, complications of prematurity greatly contribute to the high perinatal morbidity and mortality rates. The decision to deliver or maintain the pregnancy requires a careful assessment of the risks and benefits of all management options for both the mother and the fetus, and obstetric specialists should be involved early in decision making.

The following is a review of causes of vaginal bleeding in the second half of pregnancy, with an emphasis on the practical aspects of maternal and fetal evaluation and management in the emergency department setting.

OVERVIEW OF THE PREGNANT PATIENT WITH BLEEDING AFTER 20 WEEKS' GESTATION

The average length of human pregnancy is 40 weeks or 280 days from the first day of the last menstrual period. This is conventionally divided into three trimesters; the first trimester lasts 13 weeks, the second trimester from 14 to 26 weeks, and the third trimester after 26 weeks. The different causes of bleeding during pregnancy are gestational age-dependent. The World Health Organization (WHO) has defined abortion as termination of pregnancy (whether induced or spontaneous) before 20 weeks' gestation. Bleeding before 20 weeks gestation is thus defined as threatened abortion (see Chap. 4).

This chapter covers bleeding that occurs during the second half of pregnancy. The causes of vaginal bleeding after 20 weeks' gestation differ considerably from threatened abortion. The presence or absence of abdominal pain is helpful in the initial evaluation of the pregnant woman with bleeding (Table 10-1). The remainder of this chapter addresses the separate causes of vaginal bleeding in the second half of pregnancy and how to approach diagnosis, evaluation, and management of the pregnant woman and her fetus in the ED setting.

THE DIFFERENTIAL DIAGNOSIS

Vaginal bleeding in the second half of pregnancy can arise from either the upper or the lower genital tract. Upper genital tract bleeding may arise from the uteroplacental interface, as in placental abruption or placenta previa, or from the uterus, as with uterine rupture. Bleeding from either

Table 10-1. Causes of Vaginal Bleeding During Pregnancy

Condition	Approximate Frequency[a]	Abdominal Pain or Cramping	Associated Conditions	DIC May Occur
Placental abruption	35%	Yes, often frequent contractions	Trauma, hypertension, preeclampsia, cocaine use	Yes
Placenta previa	30%	No	Previous cesarean section, multiparity, multiple gestation	Rarely
Uterine rupture	<1%	Usually	Previous cesarean section, myomectomy, trauma	Yes
Labor "bloody show"	10%-20%	Yes		No
Lower genital tract causes (e.g., cervicitis)	5%	No	History of abnormal Pap smear	No
Blood dyscrasias	<1%	No	Usually identified before pregnancy	No
Vasa previa	<1%	No	Presents following rupture of membranes	No (fetal bleeding)

[a]Cause of bleeding is never found in up to 20 to 30 percent of cases.

the uterus or the placenta has the potential for catastrophic maternal and fetal consequences. Bleeding arising from the lower genital tract may be due to cervical changes in labor ("bloody show"), cervical erosions, cervical polyps, trauma, or cervical cancer. Vulvar varicose veins, common in pregnancy, may cause bleeding. Bleeding from the lower genital tract is usually light and is rarely immediately life-threatening. Primary systemic blood dyscrasias are a very rare cause of bleeding. Bleeding may occasionally be from fetal vessels, as in vasa previa, which are rare but life-threatening for the fetus.

Bleeding Arising from the Upper Genital Tract

Placental Abruption

Placental abruption is the premature separation of the normally implanted placenta from its uterine implantation site after 20 weeks' gestation and occurs in about 1 in 80 pregnancies. Placental separation prior to 20 weeks is considered to be part of the process of spontaneous abortion. Severe placental abruption is a leading cause of fetal death and accounts for approximately 14 percent of all stillbirths.[3] In addition, the perinatal mortality rate is up to 25 percent in these pregnancies, with problems of prematurity such as respiratory distress syndrome, intraventricular hemorrhage, and necrotizing enterocolitis accounting for a high percentage of deaths. Complications of severe hemorrhage, coagulopathy, emergent surgery, and anesthesia also render abruption a significant cause of maternal morbidity and mortality in the second and third trimester.

Risk Factors

Maternal hypertension is the greatest risk factor for placental abruption. In the abruption severe enough to cause fetal death, about 50 percent of cases are associated either with chronic or pregnancy-induced hypertension. Conditions that predispose to vascular compromise (preeclampsia, chronic hypertension, diabetes mellitus, collagen vascular disease, and chronic renal disease) are

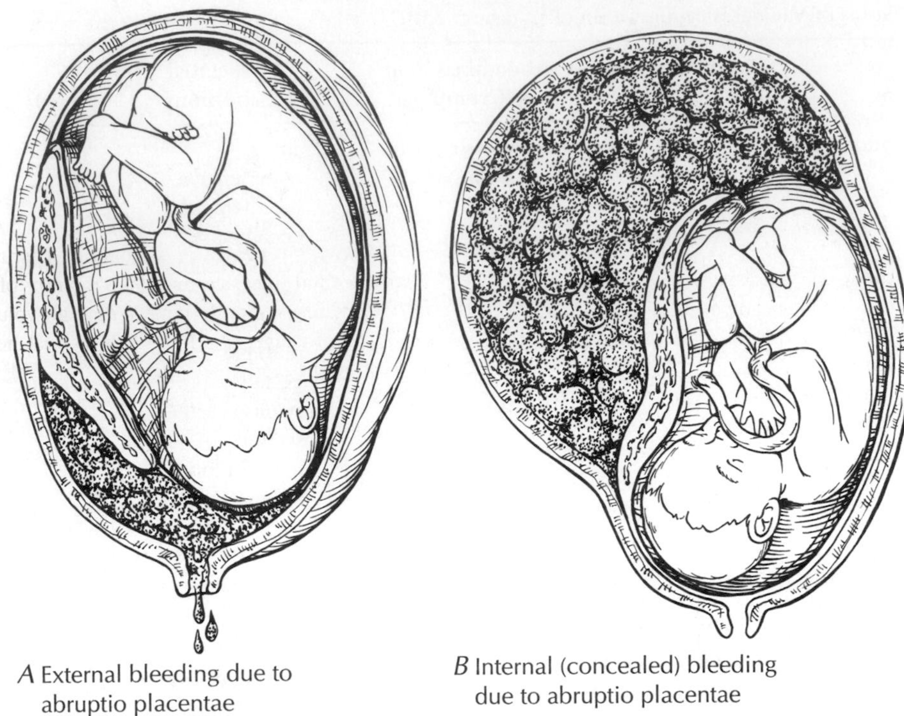

Fig. 10-1. Placental abruption. Premature separation of the normally implanted placenta after 20 weeks of gestation. *A*. External hemorrhage. *B*. Concealed hemorrhage.

associated with an increased risk for premature placental separation.

Blunt abdominal trauma from a direct blow to the abdomen or the shear force created by an acceleration-deceleration event, as in a motor vehicle accident, may also result in abruption. With severe trauma resulting in major maternal injuries, the reported incidence of abruption is as high as 35 percent, while there is a 1 to 4 percent risk of placental abruption after minor trauma.[4] Abruption may also result from partner violence or other physical abuse. Nontraumatic risk factors include placental abruption in a prior pregnancy, advanced maternal age, multiparity, cigarette smoking, and cocaine use.[5,6]

Pathophysiology

Abruption occurs after the spontaneous rupture of maternal blood vessels at the placental bed with hematoma formation. Subsequent bleeding may be external and appear vaginally (Fig. 10-1*A*), or it may be concealed (about 20 percent) (Fig. 10-1*B*). In a concealed abruption, blood does not decompress by drainage through the cervix and pressure at the placental bed increases. The adjacent myometrium is then unable to contract around the torn vessels to stop them from bleeding. Placental separation is often progressive in these cases. Under pressure, the blood may also rupture the fetal membranes and flow into the amniotic fluid (with bleeding evident only with rupture of membranes) or dissect into the myometrium (Couvelaire uterus).

Fetal hypoxia can occur as the placental disruption renders the involved placental surface inadequate for gas and metabolic exchange. Additionally, disrupted maternal and fetal vascular channels may communicate, resulting in a potentially catastrophic fetal blood loss into the maternal circulation, maternal Rh sensitization, or even a fatal amniotic fluid embolus. With significant tissue disruption or clot formation, disseminated intravascular coagulation (DIC) may occur. The inciting event is tissue thromboplastin release into the maternal circulation, with subsequent microvascular coagulation. The maternal fibrinolytic system is then activated, with critical depletion of platelets, fibrinogen, and other clotting factors. A true consumptive coagulopathy may occur at the site of a large retroplacental clot. In either case, the final result is inadequate hemostasis and an even greater maternal blood loss.

Clinical Presentation

Placental abruption is variable in its presentation, depending on the degree of the placental separation. *Severe abruption* is placental separation of such magnitude as to cause fetal death. It typically presents with a sudden onset of intense abdominal or back pain. This pain is often focal and constant, and superimposed uterine contractions are usually present. Sustained uterine tetany, described as a "woody hard" uterus on palpation, can occur. Fetal heart sounds are absent and there is no fetal cardiac activity on ultrasound. Maternal hemodynamic instability and coagulopathy are common sequelae of severe placental abruption. Clinical signs of DIC, such as mucosal bleeding, excessive bleeding at puncture sites, bruising, or hematuria may become evident. The retroplacental clot produces a true consumptive coagulopathy. In addition, sequelae of hypotension, such as acute respiratory distress syndrome and acute tubular necrosis, can occur quickly, making aggressive resuscitation, correction of coagulopathy, and prompt delivery of the fetus and placenta imperative.

Placental separations of smaller magnitude have a subtler and more variable presentation. In these cases, definitive diagnosis of abruption may be difficult. Focal abdominal or back pain and superimposed uterine contractions or irritability (high frequency, low amplitude contractions, or a uterus that contracts upon palpation) are the most common findings in these patients. Labor may progress rapidly, even in a primigravida. Pain, however, may be absent with small or marginal separations. Placental separations involving a large surface area may result in fetal compromise, and a tender, firm uterus is an important physical sign. The absence of abnormalities in fetal heart rate, however, does not exclude the diagnosis. Maternal hemodynamic instability and coagulopathy are less common with smaller degrees of placental separation.

Laboratory Studies

Although the diagnosis of placental abruption is clinical, many of the more readily apparent manifestations of this complication occur late in the disease process. The subtler presentation of minor abruption can make definitive diagnosis quite difficult therefore a high index of suspicion is required. A number of laboratory tests have been suggested to assist in the diagnosis. Although positive findings in any of these tests may predict abruption, how they should guide clinical management remains an area of controversy.

Subclinical coagulopathy seen in mild to moderate abruption may result in thrombocytopenia and prolongation of the prothrombin and partial thromboplastin times. Fibrinogen will also be consumed, with fibrin degradation products such as D-dimer appearing in the maternal circulation along with a low serum fibrinogen.[7] A fibrinogen level below 250 mg/dL is of concern. Disruption of the uteroplacental interface may lead to entry of fetal blood into the maternal circulation.[4] With high-volume fetomaternal hemorrhage, abnormalities in fetal heart rate are seen. Smaller bleeds not resulting in fetal compromise, however, are detectable only by the identification of fetal cells in the maternal circulation by using the Kleihauer-Betke test. Frequent uterine contractions with or without fetal compromise is typical.

Because of the association of cocaine use with placental abruption, a urine cocaine screen may help determine the underlying cause of bleeding.

Imaging Studies

The sensitivity of ultrasound for the diagnosis of abruption of the placenta is poor (~40%). Although ultrasound may sometimes identify a retroplacental clot, this finding is difficult to distinguish from normal placental venous lakes, and is often absent. The sensitivity is greater with severe abruption, although clinical findings should make the diagnosis straightforward in these cases. Therefore the clinical utility of ultrasound in abruption is generally limited to ruling out placenta previa as a cause of late-trimester vaginal bleeding.

Magnetic resonance imaging (MRI) has a superior ability to differentiate tissue planes and highlight blood. These properties suggest it is an attractive imaging modality for the diagnosis of abruption. However, MRI is not mobile; it is also time-consuming and expensive. These impracticalities have limited its usefulness for the evaluation of acute obstetric hemorrhage. MRI may have a limited role for patients presenting with vaginal bleeding who are clinically stable and whose diagnosis remains uncertain.[8] The use of MRI during pregnancy appears to be safe (see Appendix A-1).

Placenta Previa

Definition

Placenta previa occurs when the placenta implants in the lower uterine segment and cervix in advance of the fetal presenting part.

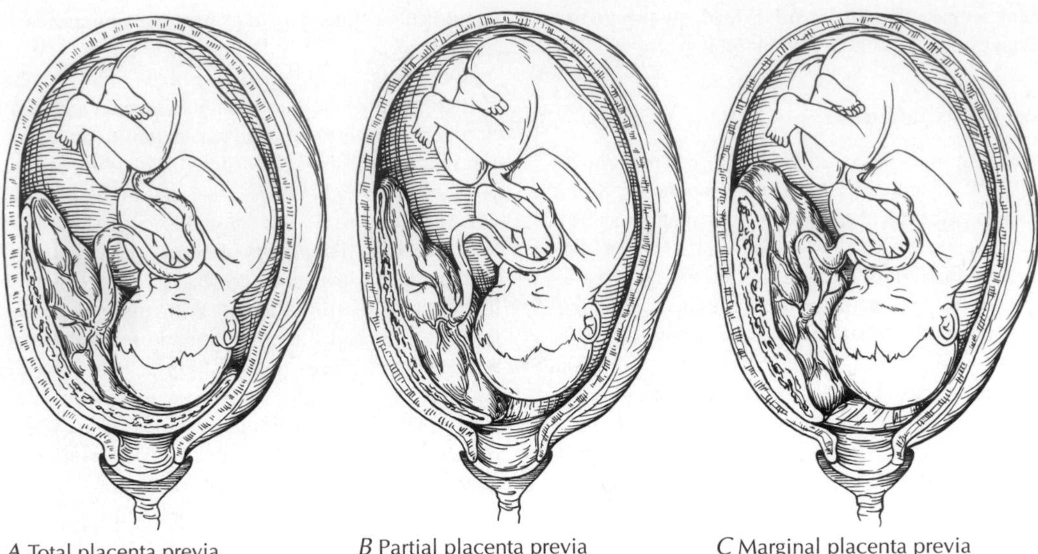

Fig. 10-2. Placenta previa. Placental separation from the lower uterine segment occurs with cervical dilation and formation of the lower uterine segment. Hemorrhage results when the lower uterine segment is unable to contract for hemostasis.

Risk Factors

Placenta previa occurs in approximately 1 in 200 term births. Previous cesarean section, a history of prior placenta previa, and multiparity all increase risk for this complication of pregnancy. Pregnancies with a large placenta, as seen in multiple gestations, erythroblastosis fetalis, and diabetics also have a higher incidence of placenta previa.

Pathophysiology

Placenta previa has been subclassified according to the relationship of the placenta to the internal cervical os:

- Total placenta previa: the placenta completely covers the internal os (Fig. 10-2*A*).
- Partial placenta previa: the placenta covers part but not all of the internal cervical os (Fig. 10-2*B*).
- Marginal placenta previa: the placenta approaches but does not cover the internal cervical os (Fig. 10-2*C*).
- Low-lying placenta: the placenta is implanted in the lower uterine segment within 2 cm of the cervical os.

Bleeding from placenta previa occurs as a result of a marginal separation of the placenta from the lower uterine segment. The relative lack of myometrial tissue in the lower uterine segment, however, renders it unable to contract effectively for hemostasis when there is separation of the placenta from its implantation site. Bleeding can occur spontaneously or be provoked by physical activity, vaginal examination, or intercourse. Uterine contractions with cervical dilation and effacement at the placental interface may also precipitate bleeding episodes.

Clinical Presentation

Placenta previa classically presents with sudden and painless vaginal bleeding in the second or third trimester of pregnancy. Pain, however, may sometimes be present. Clinically, a high fetal presenting part or fetal malpresentation, such as breech or transverse lie, supports the diagnosis. Bleeding is usually from the maternal circulation and, since the functional portion of the placenta is relatively undisturbed, fetal compromise is rare until the development of maternal hemodynamic instability.

Imaging Studies

Digital examination in a patient with placenta previa may precipitate severe hemorrhage. *Ultrasound localization of the placenta is therefore mandatory prior to any digital examination* of a patient presenting with obstetric bleeding after 20 weeks' gestation. Careful speculum examination is not contraindicated, but the speculum must *not* be inserted into the cervix. Ultrasound studies done earlier in the

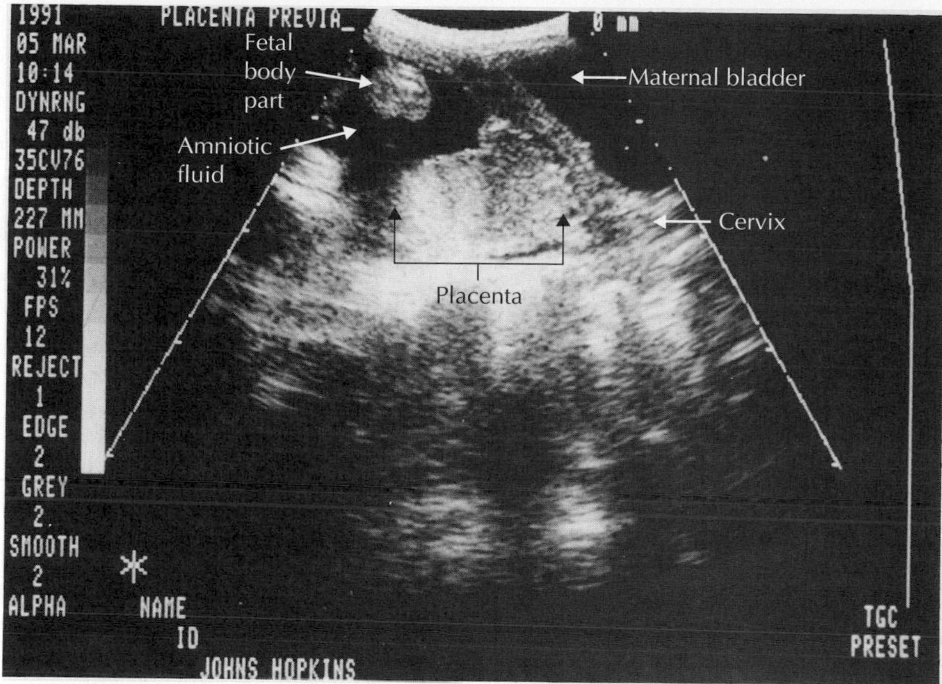

Fig. 10-3. Placenta previa. Sonographic evaluation.

pregnancy are invaluable. These may be available from the obstetric record at the time of the patient's presentation. If placenta previa was not seen on an earlier examination, then vaginal examination may safely be performed. Take note, however, that a high percentage of sonographically diagnosed cases of previa encountered early in pregnancy have resolved on repeat examination at later gestational ages.[9] This phenomenon is thought to be due to progressive thinning and stretching of the lower uterine segment with differential growth of the placenta away from the cervix. If a previa was seen at an early stage of pregnancy or reports are unavailable at presentation, ultrasound examination for placental location is indicated prior to vaginal examination. Using transabdominal sonography, a midline longitudinal scan is used to evaluate the relationship between the placental structures and the cervix (Fig. 10-3). Reported false-positive and false-negative rates of 2 to 6 percent and 2 percent, respectively, may be due to shadowing artifact from an ossified fetal presenting part, inability to distinguish a fresh blood clot located in the lower uterine segment from placenta, contractions of the lower uterine segment, maternal obesity, a posterior placenta, or an overdistended maternal bladder.[10,11] With an overdistended bladder, the anterior lower uterine segment is displaced posteriorly and may mimic a cervical os. Ultrasound examinations for the evaluation of placental location should therefore include both an initial high-resolution scan performed through a full bladder and a subsequent scan after the bladder is emptied in order to minimize distortion of the lower uterine segment.

Although digital vaginal examination of the cervix is contraindicated until placental location has been determined, translabial or transvaginal sonography may be used if the technical difficulties described above are encountered. A transvaginal probe may be safely introduced into the patient's vagina under direct sonographic visualization (stopping short of the cervix) without causing bleeding.[10] With transvaginal sonography, the shorter distance to the cervix and placenta allows for higher-resolution scans, which are helpful in differentiating the internal cervical os from placental edges. This type of examination, however, should be performed only by persons experienced with the technique and approach.

Uterine Rupture

Interruption of the integrity of the uterine cavity in pregnancy has serious consequences. Maternal mortality is

10 to 40 percent in pregnancies complicated by complete uterine rupture and fetal mortality is in excess of 50 percent.

Risk Factors

Uterine rupture occurs when there are weaknesses in the uterine wall or excessively high intrauterine pressure forces. The most common predisposing factor for rupture is previous surgery on the uterus, such as previous cesarean delivery, fibroid removal (myomectomy), resection of a uterine anomaly (metroplasty), or uterine cornual resection. Other factors that may predispose to defects in the uterine wall are placental implantation abnormalities (placenta accreta, increta, and percreta), invasive mole, or choriocarcinoma. Grand multiparity increases the risk for this complication. Uterine rupture may also occur after a dramatic increase in intrauterine pressure, as seen in severe cases of blunt abdominal trauma, such as motor vehicle crashes.

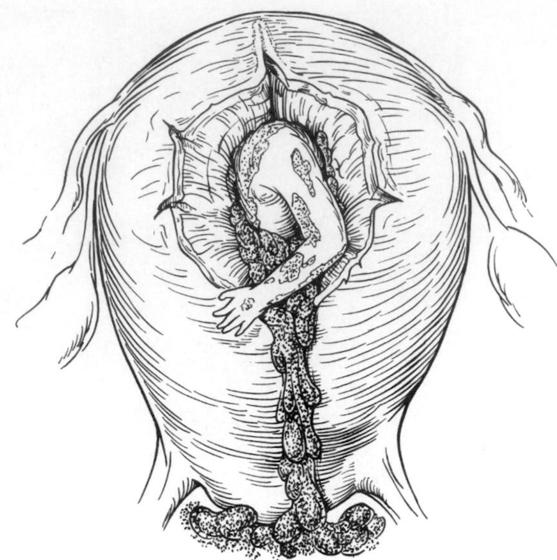

Fig. 10-4. Uterine rupture at laparotomy with partial expulsion of the fetus.

Pathophysiology

A distinction is made between uterine rupture and dehiscence. Uterine dehiscence is myometrial separation at a site of a uterine scar from previous surgery, and the uterine serosa remains intact. The vertical scar from a classic cesarean section, for example, greatly weakens the muscular active segment of the uterus. Increases in uterine pressure may result in tearing at these areas of weakness. Muscle separations may be limited to the relatively avascular scar or may extend into previously uninvolved myometrium. Uterine rupture, in contrast, involves the entire thickness of the uterine wall, resulting in communication between the uterine and peritoneal cavities (Fig. 10-4). The placenta and fetus may then be extruded into the peritoneal cavity. Bleeding usually occurs from the edges of the defect, but it may vary from minimal to massive, depending on the size and relative vascularity of the defect and whether the defect involves the placenta or extends into uterine or vaginal blood vessels. In complete uterine rupture, the defect may originate from a previous surgical scar or, less commonly, it may occur spontaneously in an unscarred uterus.

Clinical Presentation

In many cases of uterine rupture resulting in fetal or maternal death, the diagnosis is not made until laparotomy. Just as the specific anatomic defects in uterine dehiscence and rupture are variable, so is its clinical presentation. Simple uterine dehiscence at the site of a previous low transverse cesarean section may be asymptomatic and discovered incidentally at the time of repeat cesarean delivery or manual uterine exploration after vaginal delivery. Often, however, local tenderness is reported. A sudden onset of pain may be seen with an increase in uterine irritability in a previously quiescent uterus or, conversely, with cessation of an established contraction pattern in a laboring patient. Fetal heart rate abnormality is often the earliest sign of uterine rupture in the laboring patient.[12] Palpable abnormalities on abdominal examination, recession of the fetal presenting part, and loss of fetal heart tones are seen in massive rupture with extrusion of the fetus and placenta.

Vaginal bleeding is variable and rarely reflects total blood loss. Simultaneous bleeding into the abdominal cavity is common, and signs of fetal distress, maternal hypovolemia, or shock may be seen with only minor vaginal bleeding.

Imaging Studies

In cases of dramatic uterine rupture associated with abnormalities in fetal heart rate and maternal hemorrhage, ultrasound confirmation of clinical suspicions will only serve to delay treatment. Ballooning placental membranes, however, have been described by the use of ultrasound in a case of uterine dehiscence not associated with fetal or maternal compromise.[13]

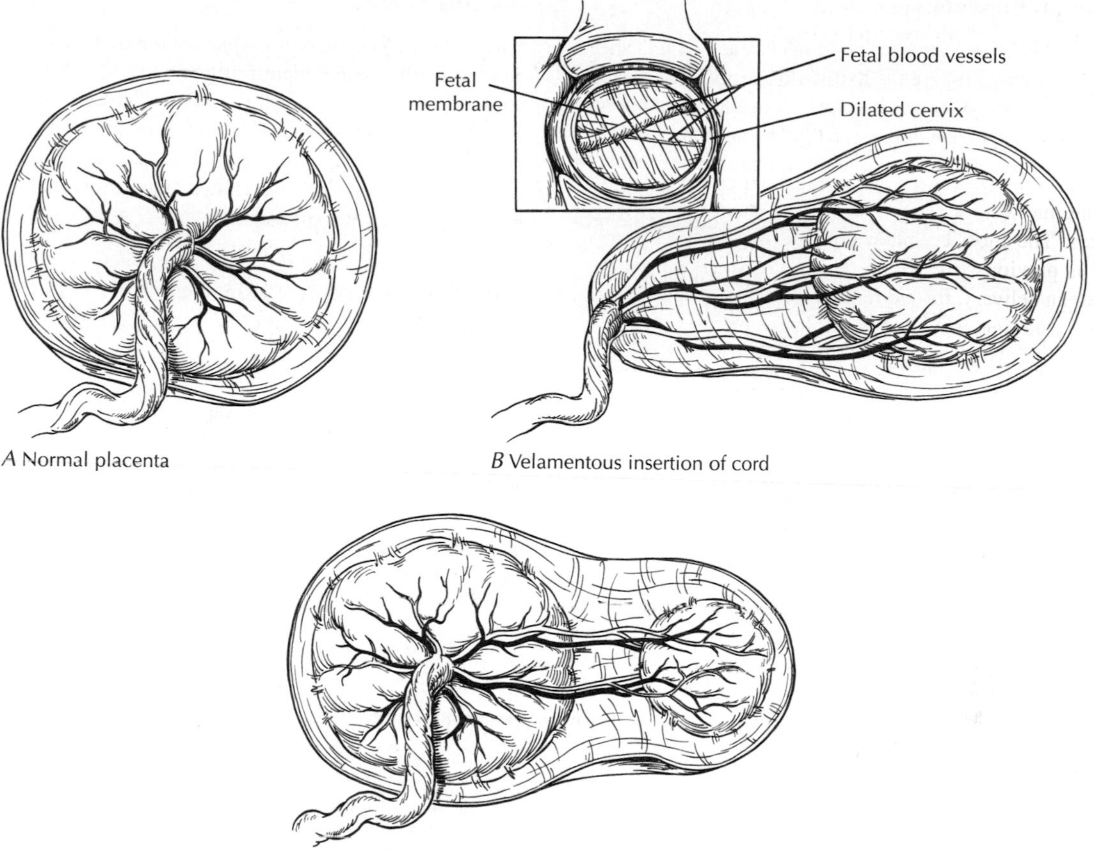

Fig. 10-5. Placental variants at risk for vasa previa. *A*. Normal placenta: central attachment of the umbilical vessels to the placenta. *B*. Velamentous insertion of the cord: fetal vessels traverse the placental membranes and divide before they reach the chorionic plate. The inset shows fetal vessels viewed during speculum examination. *C*. Succenturiate placenta: small accessory placental lobules may be joined by fetal vessels traversing the placental membranes.

Vasa Previa

Bleeding in vasa previa is from fetal vessels as they traverse the placental membranes. The bleeding is purely fetal in origin and therefore is an unusual cause of upper genital tract bleeding in that it poses almost no maternal risk, but may rapidly lead to fetal compromise and death.

Pathophysiology

Fetal umbilical vessels usually insert centrally onto the placenta (Fig. 10-5*A*). Vasa previa occurs with a lateral (velamentous) insertion of the umbilical cord onto the chorionic plate of the placenta or when there is an extra (succenturiate) lobe. With these potentially dangerous variants, fetal vessels traverse within the placental membranes prior to their insertion (Fig. 10-5*B* and *C*). If these fetal vessels cross the lower uterine segment and present in advance of the fetus, they are then vulnerable to rupture or laceration with rupture of the placental membranes. Because the circulating blood volume of a fetus is small (approximately 300 to 500 mL), relatively unimpressive amounts of vaginal bleeding may easily lead to severe fetal compromise and fetal exsanguination.

Vasa previa complicates 1 in 2000 to 5000 deliveries, and perinatal mortality due to ruptured vasa previa is reported to be as high as 50 to 75 percent.[14] This figure, however, is probably an underestimate, as deliveries complicated by vaginal bleeding and fetal compromise due to vasa previa are likely to be attributed to much more common causes, such as placental abruption.

Clinical Presentation

Vaginal bleeding and the rapid occurrence of fetal heart rate abnormalities are the hallmarks of ruptured vasa previa. A sinusoidal heart rate pattern or sudden fetal bradycardia may be seen. Occasionally, the aberrant fetal vessels are detected prior to their rupture at the time of elective cesarean section, by ultrasound as an incidental finding, or by palpation of fetal vessels overlying the presenting part during vaginal examination. Unfortunately, however, vasa previa is seldom recognized prior to vessel disruption. Spontaneous or artificial rupture of placental membranes or descent of the fetal presenting part may cause rupture of these vessels. Painless vaginal bleeding as well as the rapid occurrence of fetal compromise occur soon thereafter. However, unlike other forms of late-trimester bleeding from the upper genital tract, the potential for associated maternal hemodynamic instability is remote.

Laboratory Studies

In cases of vaginal bleeding of uncertain etiology, the Apt test may distinguish fetal from maternal red blood cells in vaginal blood. This test exploits the fact that adult oxyhemoglobin is less resistant to alkali than fetal oxyhemoglobin. It is performed by centrifugation of vaginal blood diluted with five parts water, mixing the supernatant with 0.25 M sodium hydroxide followed by a second centrifugation, and observing the color of the resulting mixture. A pink color indicates fetal origin and a yellow or brown color indicates maternal origin. This test can be time consuming, however, and is seldom practical in cases of true ruptured vasa previa associated with fetal exsanguination.

Imaging Studies

Succenturiate lobes or bilobed placentas may occasionally be seen at ultrasound, identifying patients at risk for this unusual complication. Although direct visualization of aberrant vessels using transvaginal sonography with color flow Doppler has been described,[15] ultrasound should not be considered a practical or reliable diagnostic tool for an acutely bleeding vasa previa.

Bleeding Arising from the Lower Genital Tract

Vaginal bleeding in the second half of pregnancy may originate from structures in the lower reproductive tract, rather than the uterus or placenta. A gentle bivalve speculum examination allows direct visualization of the vagina and cervix, and will typically reveal these local sources of bleeding. Unlike a digital examination, this is not contraindicated before placental localization. Care must be taken to avoid inserting the speculum into the cervix.

Obstetric Causes

Progressive cervical effacement and dilatation in term or preterm labor may result in the disruption of small blood vessels supplying the cervix. This phenomenon is known as "bloody show." The bleeding is usually relatively minor and signs of labor are often obvious.

Nonobstetric Causes

Bleeding arising from the lower genital tract may also be due to visible lesions, such as vulvar varicose veins, cervical eversion, polyps, or carcinoma (Fig. 10-6*A*, *B*, and

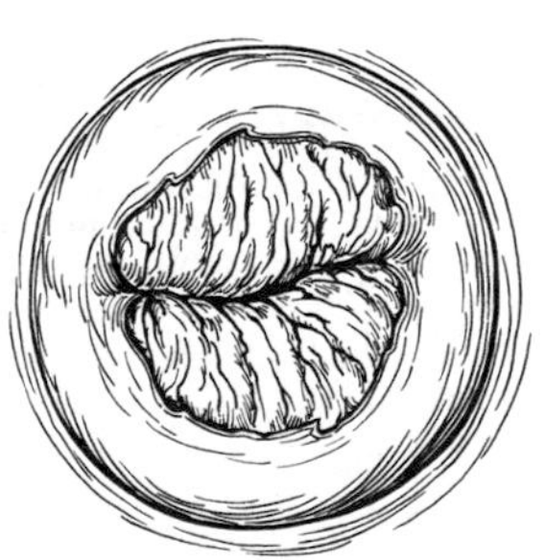

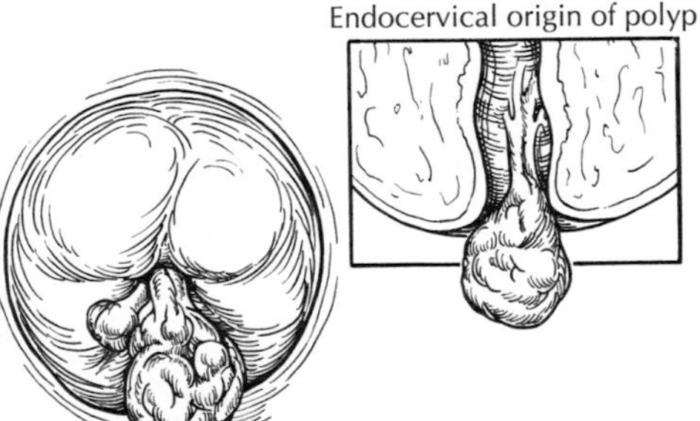

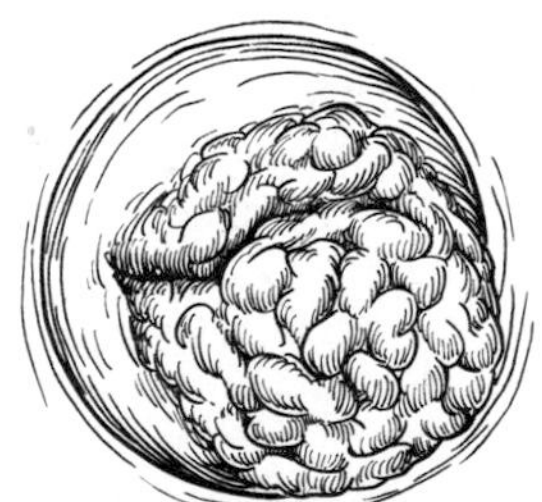

Fig. 10-6. Conditions of the cervix that may lead to bleeding in pregnancy. *A*. Erosion of a cervical ectropion. *B*. Cervical polyp. *C*. Cervical carcinoma.

C). Cervical polyps in pregnancy may present with vaginal bleeding and are easily identified on vaginal examination. Metaplastic changes due to the altered hormonal environment in pregnancy result in a cervical ectropion, or an eversion of the columnar epithelium of the cervical canal onto the ectocervix. This tissue is relatively friable and may bleed slightly, especially after intercourse or vaginal examination. Similarly, high-grade squamous intraepithelial lesions or carcinoma in situ of the cervix may be more vascular and prone to bleeding in pregnancy. Invasive cervical carcinoma of the cervix, though uncommon, may present in pregnancy with vaginal bleeding of variable amounts, vaginal discharge, or in advanced cases, pain.

Diagnosis

History may reveal recent trauma, vaginal examination, or intercourse as precipitating factors. The patient may also report a prior abnormal Pap smear or cervical lesion, possibly noted at initial obstetric evaluation earlier in the pregnancy. Direct visualization using a bivalve speculum may then reveal the source of bleeding. Of note, although cervical carcinoma is an uncommon cause of antepartum bleeding, its consideration in the differential diagnosis is essential. Stander and Lein noted a delay in diagnosis of invasive cervical cancer in 62 percent of their referrals because bleeding was attributed to other complications of pregnancy.[16]

Blood Dyscrasias

These are extremely rare causes of bleeding in pregnancy, but include Von Willebrand's disease, leukemia, Hodgkin's disease, and idiopathic thrombocytopenia. These are usually diagnosed before pregnancy, and should be managed by an obstetrician and a hematologist.

PRINCIPLES OF CARE FOR VAGINAL BLEEDING IN THE SECOND HALF OF PREGNANCY

The following is a guide for the evaluation and management of the obstetric patient who presents with vaginal bleeding in the second half of pregnancy. Management strategies are based on the etiology of the bleeding, maternal stability, fetal condition, and gestational age. Aspects of the guidelines may be modified according to the presentation and clinical severity of each individual patient. However, the basic principles that apply to the care of *all* obstetric patients who present with vaginal bleeding are listed below and in Fig. 10-11.

1. Obstetric consultation is necessary for *all* cases of bleeding in the second half of pregnancy. If the fetus is potentially viable outside the uterus ($\geq$23 to 24 weeks' gestational age), early notification of a pediatrician is also strongly encouraged.
2. Ideally, management should be done at a facility equipped to care for a compromised and possibly premature neonate.
3. Whenever an obstetric patient presents with vaginal bleeding, evaluation and resuscitation should begin *immediately*. If fetal compromise is present, maternal resuscitation is the first priority and may result in improved fetal status.
4. Remember that there are *two* patients. Evaluation and management must always take *both* patients into consideration.
5. Never perform a digital or rectal examination until placenta previa has been excluded. These examinations may provoke severe hemorrhage in a patient with placenta previa.
6. Establish gestational age as accurately as possible in all patients. Management decisions are strongly influenced by this information. Previable fetuses (less than 23 to 24 weeks' gestational age, incapable of extrauterine existence) are considered very differently from viable fetuses (24 weeks' gestation or greater). Likewise, term or near-term fetuses (37 weeks' gestation or greater) are considered differently from preterm fetuses (24 to 36 weeks' gestation).
7. The need for Rh immune globulin must also be considered.

Obstetric consultation is necessary for all cases of bleeding in the second half of pregnancy. At these advanced gestational ages, many patients will already have initiated prenatal care with an obstetrician. Clinical severity, however, may require involvement of the most readily available obstetrician. In the vast majority of cases of obstetric bleeding suspected to be from a source in the upper genital tract, obstetric admission for either delivery or observation is necessary.

Ideally, management should be done at a facility equipped to care for a compromised and possibly premature neonate. Studies have demonstrated improved outcome for premature fetuses transferred to a regional neonatal intensive care center prior to rather than after delivery.[17,18] If the initial evaluation of obstetric bleeding occurs at a facility that is not capable of the long-term management of critically ill and possibly premature neonates, then transfer to such a facility is desirable; however, this may not always be feasible if the mother is unstable. If fetal or maternal concerns require immediate delivery or render transport of the pregnant patient unsafe, then delivery, resuscitation, and postpartum neonatal transport are advised. The issues of transport are discussed elsewhere in this book (see Chap. 7).

Whenever an obstetric patient presents with hemorrhage, resuscitation should begin immediately. If fetal compromise is present, maternal resuscitation may result in improved fetal status. The position of the gravid patient greatly affects cardiac output and must always be considered. In the supine position, a large uterus may compress the inferior vena cava and reduce venous return. This is relieved by placing the patient on her left side or, if that is not possible, by displacing the uterus laterally with a pillow under one side of the maternal pelvis and lumbar spine. If hypotension is present, the Trendelenburg position may also improve venous return. As for all patients, the ABCs (*a*irway, *b*reathing, *c*irculation) of resuscitation are followed. Intravenous access is established with two large-bore intravenous catheters, and crystalloid fluid resuscitation is initiated, usually requiring 2 to 3 mL of crystalloid per milliliter of blood lost.

Maternal Hemodynamic Assessment

Visual appraisals of vaginal blood loss nearly always underestimate the actual blood loss. Additionally, maternal hemorrhage may be concealed in cases of placental abruption and uterine rupture. Clinical signs of hypovolemia must therefore be used to guide resuscitation. Pallor, cool skin, and delayed capillary refill are signs of compromised tissue perfusion. Maternal vital signs may also reflect changes in volume status. During pregnancy, however, compensatory hemodynamic mechanisms (e.g., expanded blood volume) are such that normal blood pressure and heart rate readings may be seen in the setting of dangerous hypovolemia. Normal vital signs should therefore be interpreted with caution.

Other parameters of organ perfusion, such as urine output as measured via an indwelling catheter, more accurately reflect volume status. A urine flow of at least 30 to 60 mL/h is desirable. Although maintaining a hematocrit above 30 percent is ideal, initial values may not reflect blood loss. If hemodynamic assessment remains difficult, or if urine output cannot be maintained with adequate volume replacement, invasive hemodynamic monitoring with a central venous pressure catheter is recommended.

Assessing the Severity of Hemorrhage

Blood volume in a 60-kg pregnant woman is approximately 5 liters by 30 weeks of gestation, a 40 percent expansion in blood volume compared to the nonpregnant state.

Obstetric hemorrhage can be classified into four groups.[19] In class I hemorrhage, blood loss is less than 15 percent, or about 900 mL total. The patient is usually asymptomatic. Class II hemorrhage is defined as a 20 to 25 percent blood volume loss, approximately 1200 to 1500 mL. The symptoms and signs consist of shortness of breath, dizziness, orthostatic blood pressure changes, decreased capillary refill, tachycardia, and tachypnea. Class III hemorrhage is sufficient to cause maternal hypotension, and occurs with a 30 to 35 percent acute volume loss, or 1800 to 2100 mL. Tachycardia, tachypnea, and cold skin due to peripheral vascular constriction are seen. In class IV hemorrhage, blood loss is over 40 percent, or 2400 mL. Hypovolemic shock occurs, with profound hypotension, absent peripheral pulses, and minimal urine output. Without rapid intervention, organ failure, cardiac arrest, and death may ensue.

Volume Resuscitation

Normal saline or Ringer's lactate is used for the initial resuscitation. However, when blood loss is excessive, large-volume crystalloid infusion may have deleterious effects on plasma oncotic pressure, oxygen-carrying capacity, and coagulation factor concentration. Thus when blood loss is massive, as in class III or IV hemorrhage, blood transfusion is necessary.

Whole blood is almost never available for transfusion. Packed red blood cells are prepared from whole blood by removing 200 to 250 mL of plasma, with a preservative and anticoagulant added before storage. Units of packed cells do not contain functional platelets or granulocytes, but they have the same oxygen-carrying capacity as whole blood. In the absence of ongoing blood loss, each unit will increase the hematocrit by about 3 percent.

Ideally, blood should be typed and cross-matched to avoid hemolytic transfusion reactions. However, with massive obstetric hemorrhage, urgent transfusion of O-negative, or type-specific blood may be substituted. Facilities equipped to handle obstetric emergencies should always have O-negative blood available for immediate use.

Correction of Coagulopathy

Obstetric hemorrhage, especially that due to placental abruption, can be associated with disseminated intravascular coagulopathy (DIC), where processes of coagulation and fibrinolysis become inappropriately activated. A coagulopathy should be suspected with placental abruption, uterine rupture, or when hemorrhage has been severe. The patient may demonstrate clinical evidence of an evolving coagulopathy with mucosal bleeding, excessive bleeding at puncture sites, heavy vaginal bleeding, bruising, or hematuria. Initial laboratory studies on presentation include a complete blood count and a type and cross-match. Whenever significant abruption or DIC is clinically suspected, a coagulation profile should also be sent, including PT, PTT, fibrin split products or D-dimers, and fibrinogen.

Because of increased clotting factor production, the normal fibrinogen level in pregnancy is between 400 and 450 mg/dL, and values below 300 mg/dL indicate significant defects in coagulation. However, the time needed to perform laboratory coagulation tests limits their clinical utility in the management of obstetric hemorrhage. A quick bedside assessment of clotting function may be performed with the clot observation test. Blood in a red-topped test tube (without additives) that does not clot within 6 minutes may indicate a coagulopathy with significant fibrinogen depletion.

Massive transfusion and fluid resuscitation can lead to dilutional thrombocytopenia and decreased coagulation factor concentration. Additionally, bleeding may initiate DIC or a dangerous consumptive coagulopathy. When clinical signs of inappropriate bleeding or laboratory confirmation of coagulopathy with continued obstetric hemorrhage are present, intervention is warranted. As a guideline, coagulation factors and platelets should also be replaced when transfusion of five or more units of packed red blood cells is needed in cases of severe hemorrhage.

Fresh frozen plasma (FFP), prepared by separating plasma from whole blood, is used to correct known or clinically suspected coagulation factor deficiencies. FFP is the treatment of choice in DIC, consumptive coagulopathy, and massive packed red blood cell transfusion. It contains coagulation factors II, V, VII, VIII, IX, XII, and XIII, as well as fibrinogen. Cryoprecipitate, which replaces fibrinogen, von Willebrand factor, and factors VIII and XIII, may be also be used in DIC, usually in addition to fresh frozen plasma. It allows replacement of a high dose of fibrinogen with less infusion volume than FFP.

Platelet concentrate is administered for thrombocytopenia associated with obstetric hemorrhage and coagulopathy. Each unit increases the platelet count by approximately 10,000/μL. When DIC is present, however, the half-life of each transfused unit is markedly diminished.

Clinical improvement is initially used to guide management of coagulopathy. In established DIC, repeat coagulation studies every 1 to 2 hours should include platelet count, fibrinogen, PT, and PTT, although the platelet count and fibrinogen level are more useful in assessing adequate coagulation factor replacement. Goals include a platelet count above 100,000/μL and fibrinogen above 150 mg/dL.

Transfusion Risks

Despite blood bank testing, hemolytic transfusion reactions with ABO incompatibility remain a risk of blood transfusion. Rh sensitization may also occur if an Rh-negative recipient receives Rh-positive blood. This, of course, poses a special problem for the obstetric patient with a potentially Rh-positive fetus, due to small amounts of red blood cells in platelet concentrates. Rh-negative patients should also receive only Rh-negative platelets. If this is unavailable, however, 300 μg of Rh immune globulin may be administered at the time of platelet transfusion to prevent Rh sensitization.

Transmission of viral infections, such as hepatitis, human immunodeficiency virus, and cytomegalovirus (CMV) also remains a risk with blood transfusion. In the adult, transfusion of CMV-containing blood is a concern primarily for the immunocompromised patient. In the pregnant patient who has not been previously exposed to the virus, however, there is potential for transplacental passage to the fetus and possible adverse fetal and neonatal sequelae. Transfusion of CMV-negative or frozen-thawed-deglycerolized red blood cells is ideal, but it is not practical in acute hemorrhage.

Vasopressors

With obstetric hemorrhage, hypovolemia may lead to maternal hypotension. Fluid resuscitation and blood component therapy are critical components of resuscitation. Vasopressors, if used in a hypovolemic pregnant patient, may critically compromise blood flow to vital maternal organs and to the fetus. Therefore these drugs should be used only when hypotension persists despite adequate fluid resuscitation. Invasive hemodynamic monitoring is strongly recommended to guide fluid management when these drugs are necessary.

Other Aspects of the Maternal Evaluation

History

An accurate history is invaluable to both diagnosis and clinical decision making in obstetric hemorrhage. Questions regarding the acute event are helpful in determining the cause of bleeding. Did activity, such as trauma or intercourse, precede the bleeding? If pain is present, what is its quality and character? Is the pain episodic, like uterine contractions? Did contractions precede the bleeding? Has there been fetal movement since the bleeding episode?

The prenatal history is also important. Has the patient received prenatal care? Have there been prior bleeding episodes? Is the estimated date of delivery known, and if so, how was it determined? Have there been prior ultrasounds that may have evaluated placental location? Are there any other complications, such as high blood pressure or premature contractions? Have any lower genital tract lesions been identified during the course of prenatal care?

The past obstetric history may also be useful to evaluate maternal risk for various complications. What is the patient's gravidity (how many times has she conceived) and parity (how many times has she given birth after 20 weeks' gestational age)? Have there been any cesarean sections or other surgeries on the uterus? Have prior pregnancies been complicated by placental abruption or previa?

Finally, maternal medical and social history may identify risk factors that could give clues to the etiology of the bleeding and can guide management of the mother. Are there maternal vascular disorders, such as hypertension or vasculitis? Is there any history of renal disease? Does the patient have a history of abnormal Pap smears? Does she smoke or use cocaine?

Physical Examination

In addition to the hemodynamic assessment outlined above, other aspects of the maternal physical examination are critical for both diagnosis and management of obstetric hemorrhage. Abdominal examination may identify areas of focal tenderness. A firm, tender or "woody hard" uterus suggests major abruption, and rapid assessment of fetal heart tones should ensue. Additionally, fetal movements, uterine contractions, or frank uterine tetany are identified during palpation of the gravid uterus. To identify fetal lie, Leopold's maneuvers are performed. Fetal malpresentation is diagnosed when the cephalic prominence is not presenting in the pelvis or palpation of the uterine fundus fails to identify a fetal part (transverse lie), as is often seen in placenta previa. With uterine rupture, the fetus may also be noted to be in an abnormal lie or the extruded fetus may be palpated in the maternal abdomen.

Never perform a digital vaginal or rectal examination until placenta previa has been ruled out. If placenta previa was not seen on a prior ultrasound during this pregnancy or one performed at presentation, then vaginal examination may be safely performed. Speculum examination allows for direct visualization of the site of the bleeding. Blood exiting through the uterine cervix indicates an upper genital tract source. Lesions of the vagina and cervix, on the other hand, may also be identified at this time.

After the speculum is removed, digital vaginal examination is performed to obtain information regarding cervical dilation and effacement. Confirmation of the fetal presenting part and its station in the maternal pelvis is also an important part of this examination. It is important to remember that abruption may cause rapid labor.

Tocodynamometry

Evaluation of uterine activity is an important aspect of diagnosis. Frequent uterine activity is usually present with abruption; it seldom occurs with placenta previa. Uterine contractions, however, are not always palpable. External tocodynamometry measures the change in shape of the abdominal wall with uterine contractions and is used to provide a graphic display of the frequency and duration of uterine contractions over time. If available, contraction monitoring should be used in all patients being evaluated for obstetric hemorrhage.

Initial Fetal Evaluation

Clinical decision making in obstetric hemorrhage is profoundly influenced by fetal condition and gestational age.

Assessment of Gestational Age

Establish gestational age as accurately as possible in all patients. This is critical to rational decision making in obstetrics. Term pregnancies are between 37 and 42 weeks' gestational age. Continued intrauterine existence in the setting of obstetric bleeding rarely benefits and may even harm these fetuses. The threshold of fetal viability is approximately 23 to 24 weeks (depending on the capabilities of the facility caring for the neonate). Fetuses at less than 24 weeks' gestation are incapable of extrauterine existence, and facilitation of delivery will only lead to their demise. Fetuses between 24 and 36 weeks' gestation are preterm. They may benefit from continued intrauterine existence and should be delivered only if the risk of continuation of the pregnancy to both the mother and the fetus outweighs the risk of morbidity and mortality due to complications of prematurity. It is strongly emphasized that

Table 10-2. Percent Survival by Birth Weight and Gestational Age among Neonates Born at the University of Michigan Medical Center, 1991-1994[a]

	Percent Survival	Number
Gestational age		
≤24 weeks	31	16
25 weeks	69	26
26 weeks	92	24
27 weeks	89	38
28 weeks	97	38
29 weeks	98	46
30 weeks	100	58
Birth weight		
<500 g	0	2
501-750 g	65	48
751-1000 g	92	64
1001-1250 g	96	74
1251-1500 g	100	107

[a]These data exclude neonates with congenital anomalies; those that lived to be discharged home were considered to be survivors.

Source: Data courtesy of Roger Faix, MD, University of Michigan.

within this gestational age range there is dramatic variation in potential for neonatal morbidity and mortality. This must be considered carefully when one is making management decisions in preterm pregnancies (Table 10-2).

There are several methods for estimating fetal gestational age (Table 10-3). Each method has some error associated with it; in establishing gestational age, this error must be taken into consideration. This is especially critical in patients who present at the threshold of fetal viability. For example, if a patient presents with bleeding and is found to be at 22 weeks' gestational age by a method with an error of ±2 weeks, the fetus may in fact be viable.

Last menstrual period (LMP), when known with accuracy, is a reliable clinical estimator of gestational age. *Postmenstrual weeks* is the unit of time for dating pregnancies. A known LMP will be less reliable for dating pregnancies in patients with irregular menstrual cycles or in those who conceived while using hormonal contraceptives.

When an LMP is unknown or unreliable, obstetric ultrasound may be used to establish an estimated date of confinement. Using the crown-rump length in the first trimester, ultrasound dating is accurate to approximately

Table 10-3. Assessment of Gestational Age

Test	Interpretation	Reliability/Comments
Last menstrual period	Weeks from last menstrual period	A reliable clinical estimator of gestational age if known with accuracy. *Caution*: Less reliable in patients with irregular menstrual cycles or when cycles are longer or shorter than 28 days.
Fundal height	Distance between the symphysis pubis and the uterine fundus, in centimeters. Approximates gestational age in weeks. Uterus attains the level of the umbilicus at approximately 20 weeks.	Accuracy ±3 weeks from about 18-35 weeks.
	Clinical pearl: Uterus at the umbilicus is both a proximate marker of gestational age and provides a indicator that the uterus could affect or compromise maternal hemodynamics.(e.g., for resuscitation/CPR).	*Caution*: Less reliable with maternal obesity, extremes of maternal height, transverse fetal lie, or abnormalities of fetal growth (intrauterine growth restriction, or macrosomia). Concealed bleeding from abruption may also affect this measurement.
Ultrasound	First trimester: crown-rump length (CRL).	Accuracy ±3-5 days between 6 and 10 weeks gestation
	Second trimester: biparietal diameter.	Accuracy ±2 weeks in the second trimester
	Third trimester: biparietal diameter, femur length, abdominal circumference.	Accuracy ±2-3 weeks in the third trimester.

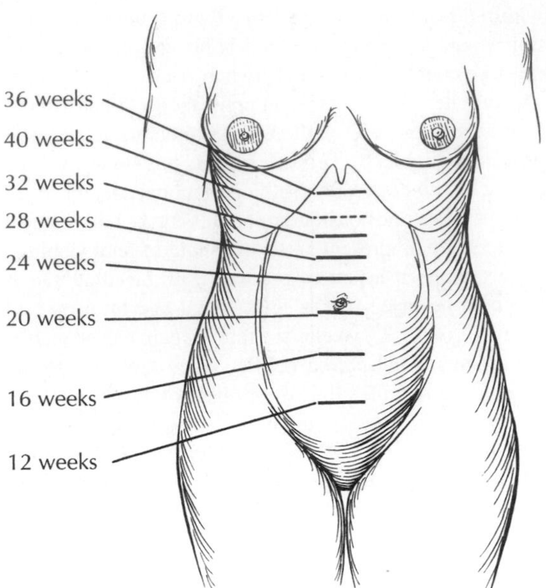

Fig. 10-7. Measurement from symphysis pubis to fundal height as a clinical estimator of gestational age.

±5 to 7 days. Assignments of gestational age using nomograms for biparietal diameter, abdominal circumference, and femur length have an accuracy of approximately ±2 weeks in the second trimester and ±2 to 3 weeks in the third. Since early ultrasound examinations are more accurate, studies performed earlier in the pregnancy are preferable.

If a patient is unable to provide a history, the prenatal record is unavailable, and the patient's clinical condition precludes a lengthy ultrasound evaluation to estimate gestational age, a fundal height measurement may be used. A simple rule is to consider gestational age in weeks to be grossly equivalent to the height in centimeters from the symphysis pubis to the uterine fundus (Fig. 10-7). However, this method is poorly reproducible, and is inaccurate with maternal obesity and multiple gestations. Additionally, with obstetric bleeding due to abruption, concealed uterine hemorrhage may increase the fundal height and render the measurement less reliable.

Evaluation of Fetal Well-Being

With obstetric bleeding, significant reductions in placental blood flow or direct fetal blood loss may result in fetal compromise or even death, so fetal well-being should be evaluated promptly. This is of great importance in any patient with a potentially viable fetus. However, maternal assessment should always be done first if simultaneous assessment cannot be performed.

During the initial evaluation, the presence of fetal heart tones must be established. A fetal Doppler device is readily available in most emergency facilities and may be used to identify fetal heart tones. Maternal pulse signals are easily obtained in the pelvis; therefore, once a signal is received, fetal and maternal pulsations should be differentiated. If Doppler is unable to locate a fetal pulse signal, ultrasound may be used to view fetal cardiac activity directly.

With continued management of the bleeding patient, more sensitive indicators of fetal well-being must be employed. Because the fetus cannot be evaluated directly, indirect methods of evaluation for potential fetal compromise have been developed. Decreased oxygen delivery to the fetus and subsequent fetal hypoxemia and/or acidemia lead to central nervous system (CNS) cellular dysfunction. The resultant decrease in fetal activity and reflex changes in cardiac activity are associated with altered fetal heart rate patterns. Therefore fetal heart rate patterns seen with continuous monitoring may reflect fetal condition and they are an important method to assess fetal well-being. When a woman carrying a potentially viable fetus presents with vaginal bleeding, continuous fetal heart rate monitoring should be employed immediately.

Fetal heart rate signals are obtained using a Doppler ultrasound probe on the maternal abdomen. The fetal cardiac wall motion detected is then electronically transformed into a continuous heart rate tracing for evaluation of temporal patterns (Fig. 10-8). Although the basic components of fetal heart rate monitoring are discussed briefly below, the interpretation of these tracings may be subtle and requires an experienced practitioner. Therefore the following discussion is intended only to familiarize the emergency physician with the basic elements of the fetal heart tracing.

The *baseline heart rate, baseline variability,* and the presence of periodic *accelerations or decelerations* are significant aspects of the fetal heart rate pattern (Table 10-4).

Fetal Heart Rate

A normal *baseline fetal heart rate* ranges from 110 to 160 beats per minute (BPM). Fetal tachycardia is a sustained elevation of the fetal heart rate above 160 BPM. Fetal activity may cause brief elevation in baseline heart rate above 160 BPM, or accelerations.These, however, are not sustained. Prolonged fetal tachycardia may be associated with maternal fever, intraamniotic infection, fetal anemia,

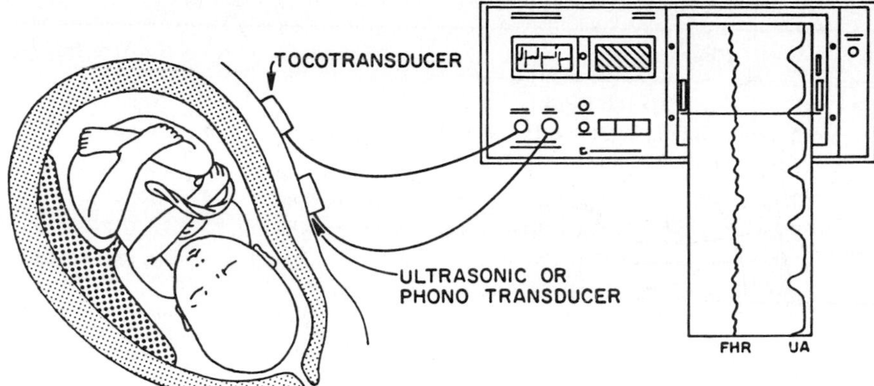

Fig. 10-8. Fetal heart rate monitoring and tocodynamometry. Ultrasound Doppler signals are obtained from the moving fetal heart valves and electronically transduced into a fetal heart rate. External uterine contraction monitoring measures uterine displacement for a graphic display of frequency and duration of contractions.

or hypoxia. Administration of certain drugs that increase maternal heart rate, such as β-sympathomimetic drugs, may also result in fetal tachycardia. Rarely, a fetal cardiac tachyarrhythmia may be present.

Fetal bradycardia is a sustained decrease in the fetal heart rate below 110 BPM. Decreased fetal heart rates may be associated with fetal hypoxia and acidemia. If bradycardia is sustained and unresponsive to in utero resuscitation measures (Table 10-4), obstetric assessment is needed without delay, as urgent delivery of the fetus is appropriate if gestational viability has been reached.

Variability

Variability in the fetal heart rate baseline represents the normal interplay between cardioinhibitory and cardiostimulatory centers in the fetal brain, and is a sensitive indicator of fetal well-being. Short-term variability is defined as a beat-to-beat variation of at least 6 BPM in fetal heart rate around an overall baseline. Minimal variability of 5 or fewer BPM may indicate fetal compromise. Other causes of decreased variability include evaluation during fetal sleep state, fetal CNS immaturity (fetuses should start to demonstrate variability in heart rate at around 28 weeks), and maternal administration of opioid analgesics.

Fetal Heart Rate Accelerations

Accelerations in fetal heart rate typically occur with movement in the healthy fetus. An acceleration is defined as an increase in fetal heart rate of at least 15 BPM over baseline and lasting at least 15 seconds. The presence of periodic accelerations is another sensitive indicator of fetal well-being. Fig. 10-9 shows a reassuring fetal heart rate pattern with accelerations.

Fetal Heart Rate Decelerations

Transient slowing of the fetal heart rate is known as a *deceleration.* Decelerations are described as early, variable, or late, depending on their relationship to uterine contractions and the morphology of the pattern (Fig. 10-10). Early decelerations are often seen in the late, active phase of labor or in the second stage of labor, reflecting fetal vagal response to head compression in the birth canal, and are generally not pathological.

Variable decelerations (Fig. 10-10*A*) and late decelerations may be associated with fetal hypoexemia acidemia, and necessitate resuscitative measures as described in Table 10-4, as well as rapid involvement of the obstetric team. Fig. 10-10*B* shows a pattern of late decelerations following uterine contractions.

The Kleihauer-Betke Test and Use of Rh Immune Globulin

The Kleihauer-Betke (K-B) test is an acid elution test that identifies the presence of fetal cells in the maternal circulation as evidence of fetomaternal hemorrhage, and can quantitate fetal blood loss if fetal cells are detected. In the Rh-negative patient, in whom fetomaternal hemorrhage of any magnitude may lead to maternal isoimmunization, the

Table 10-4. Common Patterns of the Fetal Heart Rate

FHR Pattern	Characteristic	Cause	Intervention
Normal baseline	Baseline rate 110-160 BPM	Normal	None
Acceleration	Elevation of fetal heart rate 15 BPM above baseline for 15 s	Normal, reassuring	None
Early deceleration	Shallow, symmetric slowing of the heart rate, which reaches the nadir at the peak of the uterine contraction. Appears as a "mirror image" of the uterine contraction	Fetal head compression	None
Late deceleration	U-shaped slowing of the fetal heart rate with gradual onsets and returns to baseline that are shallow (10-30 BPM). They reach their nadir after the peak of the contraction and return to baseline after uterine contraction (Fig.10-10).	Uteroplacental insufficiency; CNS hypoxia; if severe, myocardial depression	*In utero resuscitation measures*: 1. Consult obstetrician ASAP 2. Start oxygen by mask at 8-10 L/min 3. Begin intravenous lactated Ringer's solution and give 200- to 500-mL bolus of fluid 4. Change position of mother (e.g., left or right lateral decubitus) 5. Avoid supine position
Variable deceleration	Slowing of the fetal heart rate with abrupt onset and return to baseline. Varies in depth, duration, and shape, but usually occurs during a uterine contraction	Cord compression	Consult obstetrician if persistent (occurs with most uterine contractions) or if any of the "rule of 60s" are present: more than 60 s long, below 60 BPM, or more than 60 BPM drop from baseline. Begin in utero resuscitation as above.
Baseline variability	The variation of successive beats in the fetal heart rate. Usually between 6 and 25 BPM	Diminished variabilty may be asscociated with fetal hypoxia; it is normally seen in fetal sleep cycles, or in response to medications (e.g., narcotics)	Must be interpreted carefully, paying attention to baseline, accelerations, and decelerations. Prompt obstetric consultation recommended if minimal (5 BPM or less)
Tachycardia	Fetal heart rate above 160 BPM sustained for 10 minutes	Fetal hypoxemia, maternal fever, fetal arrhythmias, medications (e.g., beta-sympathomimetics)	Resuscitation measures and obstetric consultation
Bradycardia	Sustained fetal heart rate below 110 BPM for 10 minutes. Between 2 and 10 minutes is a prolonged deceleration	Fetal hypoxemia, fetal heart block, use of β-blockers	Resuscitation measures and prompt obstetric consultation, as for late decelerations

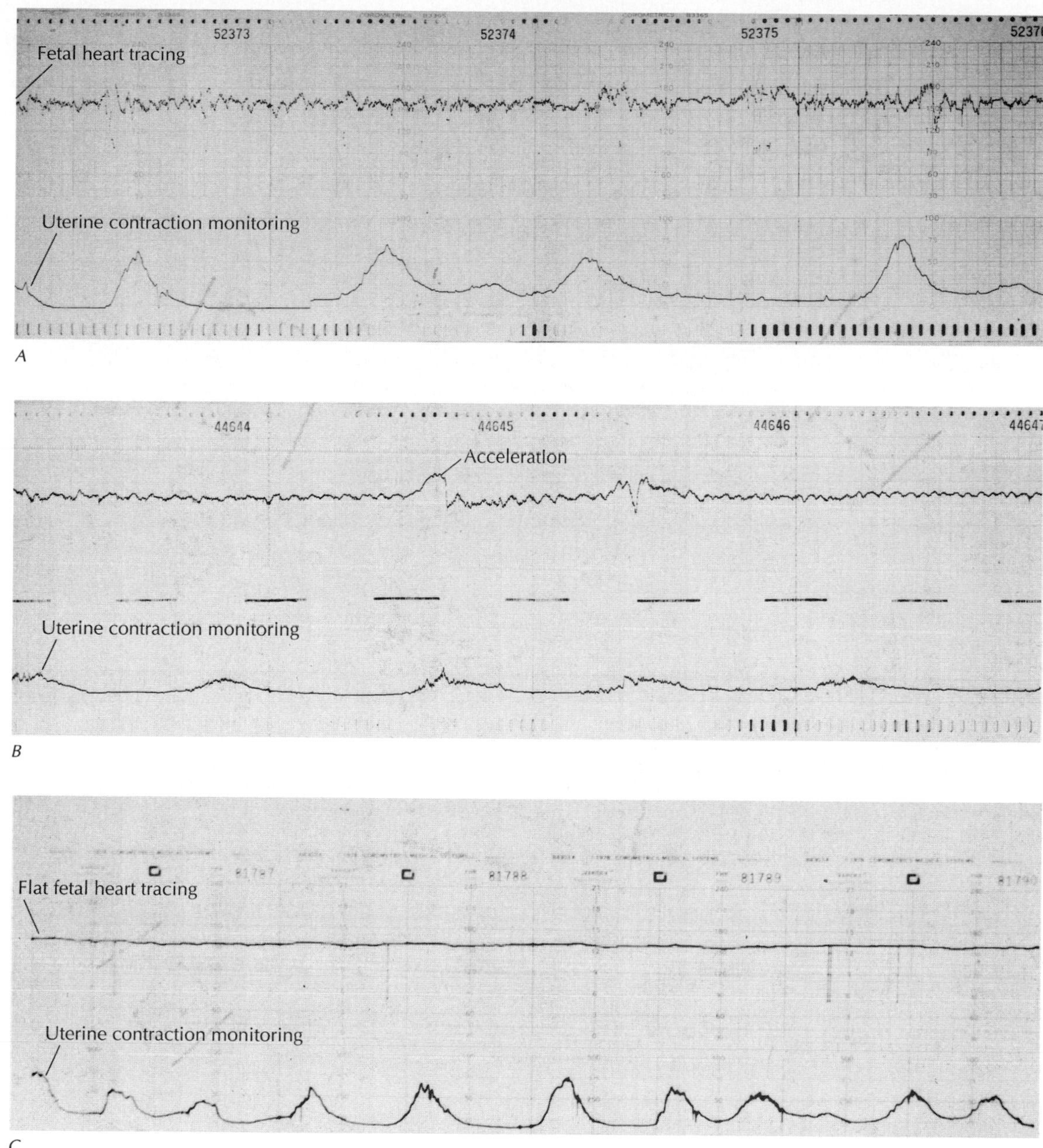

Fig. 10-9. Fetal heart rate variability patterns. *A*. Good variability. *B*. Good variability with accelerations. *C*. Poor variability.

test is employed to direct the use of Rh immune globulin. Rh immune globulin should be generally administered to all Rh-negative women with bleeding during pregnancy. A 300 μg dose of Rh immune globulin administered intramuscularly is sufficient to cover 15 mL of packed red blood cells or 30 mL of whole blood fetomaternal exchange. If the K-B test indicates a larger bleed, additional Rh immune globulin should be administered.

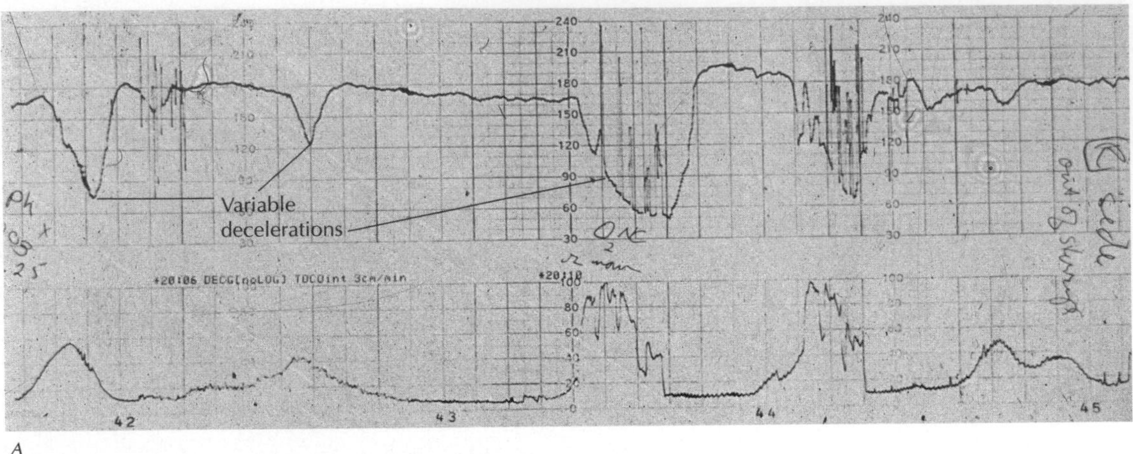

A

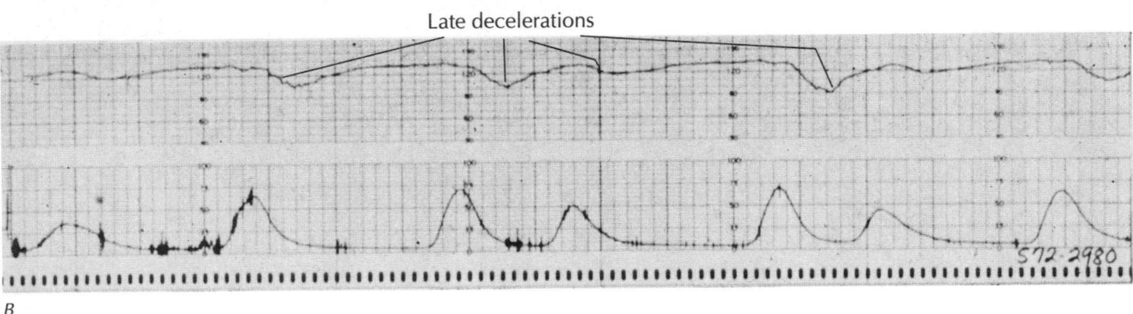

B

Fig. 10-10. Fetal heart rate deceleration patterns. Early decelerations begin with the onset of a contraction and return to baseline at the end of the contraction. *A*. Variable decelerations. There is no consistent relationship with contractions and the pattern is variable in morphology. *B*. Late decelerations. These occur after the onset of a contraction with a slow return to baseline after completion of the contraction.

Fetal blood cells last a variable amount of time in the maternal circulation, depending on the maternal-fetal ABO compatibility. When incompatibility exists, fetal cells are quickly lysed in the maternal circulation. Therefore delayed testing must be interpreted with caution. Also, because of the time needed to perform the test, it is not useful in making decisions about timing of delivery in the presence of acute vaginal bleeding, nor is it useful in known Rh D-positive mothers.

SPECIFIC MANAGEMENT PROTOCOLS

Management of Placental Abruption

The approach to managing abruption depends on three factors: (1) maternal hemodynamic status, (2) fetal condition, and (3) gestational age of the fetus. In general, the management of these cases should be directed by a physician experienced in dealing with bleeding in the second half of pregnancy, who can effect immediate operative delivery if necessary.

An algorithm for management of second- and third-trimester bleeding is presented in Fig. 10-11.

Intrauterine Fetal Demise

With severe placental abruption associated with intrauterine fetal demise (IUFD), expeditious delivery is warranted. Hemorrhage and evolution of DIC continues until the fetus and placenta are delivered. Vaginal delivery is the preferred route. Given the high incidence of DIC in severe placental abruption, surgical disruption of maternal tissues by hysterotomy may dramatically increase maternal morbidity and should be performed only if

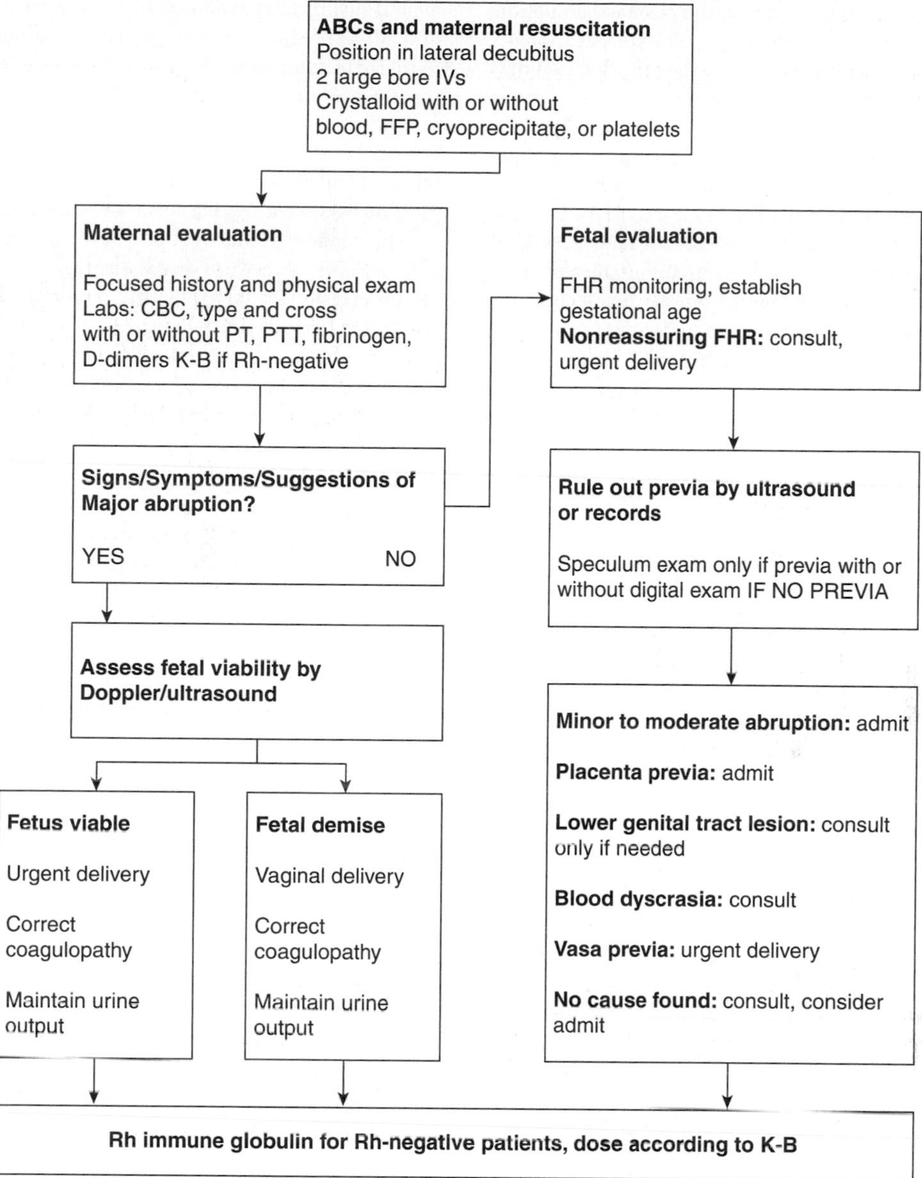

Fig. 10-11. Management algorithm for second- and third-trimester bleeding.

absolutely necessary to control hemorrhage. Ongoing blood loss may be rapid and requires aggressive replacement. Central intravenous access should be considered early, since coagulopathy can evolve, resulting in difficulties with central venous cannulation. The volume of ongoing vaginal bleeding is continuously assessed, with an understanding that occult blood loss due to concealed hemorrhage may be present. Since visual estimates of bleeding are unreliable, a disposable pad may be placed beneath the patient. Weighing these pads may provide a more objective assessment of blood loss (1 g = 1 mL). To evaluate for possible concealed hemorrhage and an enlarging uterus, serial measurements of fundal height may be helpful.

Labor is usually rapid after severe placental abruption. Contractions may be quite strong and are occasionally tetanic. Patients with uterine tetany due to abruption may also be at risk for rupture of the uterus from the high pressures generated within the cavity. Uterine decompression by artificial rupture of membranes (amniotomy) often improves this contraction pattern. Relief of the excessive intrauterine pressure may also decrease the risk of DIC and amniotic fluid embolus. The progress of labor should be monitored closely, preferably with an intrauterine pressure catheter. If uterine contractions are not adequate in strength, oxytocin should be used to expedite delivery.

In the absence of coexistent maternal medical problems or sequelae of hypovolemia and DIC, such as acute respiratory distress syndrome, acute tubular necrosis, organ infarction, or hemorrhage, recovery and correction of coagulation defects usually occur within 4 to 6 hours after delivery of the fetus and placenta.

Nonreassuring Fetal Heart Rate Patterns

Lesser degrees of placental separation may not immediately lead to fetal demise, but may compromise the fetus and be reflected in abnormal fetal heart rate patterns. In these cases, accurate knowledge of gestational age is critical. If the fetus is viable, urgent delivery by cesarean section may be warranted, although cervical dilatation should be assessed as placental abruption may cause rapid labor progress. Hypovolemia and coagulopathy should be aggressively managed in preparation for surgery.

Placental abruption in previable pregnancies is uncommon. However, if the fetus is not viable (less than 23 weeks' gestation and the gestational age is known with certainty), immediate delivery by cesarean section would not be life-saving for the fetus and management should be based on maternal considerations. If maternal hemorrhage is significant and potentially life-threatening, timely delivery is indicated. Labor is often spontaneous in these cases, but augmentation with pitocin may be necessary. If maternal bleeding is not excessive or potentially life-threatening, expectant management with close observation may be allowed. Maternal resuscitation can sometimes improve fetal condition. Prolonged fetal stress, however, may lead to compromised fetal growth or well-being.

Reassuring Fetal Heart Rate Patterns

Frequently, abruption has a less dramatic presentation, in which the fetus is not compromised and reassuring patterns of the fetal heart rate are seen. Unfortunately, the natural history and evolution of these nonacute cases is difficult to predict. Marginal sinus separations may lead to transient symptomatology that resolves without recurrence. Cases of minor abruption that may seem clinically insignificant at initial presentation, however, also have the potential to lead to progressively larger degrees of placental involvement and subsequent fetal distress. The presence of persistent uterine tenderness or uterine activity should increase suspicion of progression. Presently, there is no reliable method for distinguishing patients destined for progression of their placental abruption from those with more benign clinical courses.

If the patient is at term, facilitating a vaginal delivery is appropriate. At 34 to 37 weeks' gestation, testing of fetal lung maturity may be helpful for decision making. If the patient is remote from at term, expectant management and prolonged observation is the best strategy. Unless the fetus is previable, there must be evidence for ongoing fetal well-being, initially using continuous external fetal monitoring for expectant management to be an option. However, the risk of recurrent bleeding and premature delivery with poor perinatal outcome remains high with placental abruption managed expectantly.[20]

Maternal corticosteroid therapy has been shown to improve neonatal morbidity and mortality with premature delivery.[21,22] Antepartum administration of corticosteroids is therefore recommended in viable pregnancies prior to 34 weeks' gestational age being managed expectantly. Typically however, these are generally given once a patient is under specialist obstetric care.

Management of Placenta Previa

As with abruption, management approaches depend on maternal hemodynamic status, fetal condition, and gestational age of the fetus. If delivery is elected, cesarean section is indicated with marginal or complete placenta previa. In cases of low-lying placenta, vaginal delivery may be considered provided there is continued evidence for fetal well-being, the patient is stable, ongoing blood losses are not significant, and personnel and facilities are available should the need for operative delivery arise.

Nonreassuring Fetal Heart Rate Patterns

Fetal compromise is seen much less commonly in pregnancies complicated by placenta previa than in placental abruption. When fetal compromise is present in viable pregnancies, immediate delivery by cesarean section is indicated.

In the absence of fetal compromise, management is based on maternal hemodynamic stability and fetal maturity.

Hemorrhage with Maternal Hemodynamic Instability

Potentially life-threatening maternal hemorrhage from placenta previa is an indication for urgent cesarean delivery. Appropriate fluid and blood component replacement in preparation for surgery is essential. With severe ongoing hemorrhage from placenta previa, maternal blood loss will continue until the fetus is delivered and the placenta is removed. Surgery, therefore, should not be delayed while awaiting cross-matched blood.

Hemorrhage with Maternal Hemodynamic Stability

Historically, placenta previa complicated by vaginal bleeding was an indication for urgent delivery, without consideration for fetal maturity. In term patients, the benefits of intrauterine existence have been maximized and timely delivery is warranted. When fetal maturity status is uncertain and delivery is desired, fetal pulmonary maturity studies may be helpful. These consist of physical and biochemical testing of amniotic fluid obtained by amniocentesis, and are thus performed in relatively stable patients under specialist obstetric care.

However, complications of prematurity are the major cause of perinatal morbidity and mortality in pregnancies complicated by placenta previa. When the fetus is clearly premature by gestational age or when pulmonary maturity studies reveal an unacceptably high risk of respiratory distress syndrome if delivery were to occur, a delay in delivery may result in marked improvement in perinatal outcome.

Because significant maternal bleeding may occur in placenta previa without affecting fetal well-being, protocols for expectant management of placenta previa—using strict bed rest, volume expansion, transfusion therapy, and cautious use of tocolytic medication for selected patients—have been developed with favorable results. Since bleeding from placenta previa occurs with the development of the lower uterine segment and subsequent disruption of placental vessels, it is reasonable that tocolysis of uterine contractions would result in improved outcome. This, however, remains an area of controversy.[23–26] If expectant management is elected, fetal well-being must be assured, initially with continuous monitoring of the fetal heart rate.

Many episodes of bleeding from placenta previa are self-limited. Recurrences, however, are common and subsequent episodes tend to be more severe. Unfortunately, adverse outcomes—such as premature delivery, intrauterine fetal growth restriction, and occasional perinatal death—still occur despite aggressive expectant management. The severity of these complications tends to correlate with the number of antepartum bleeding episodes.[27] There is a high likelihood of premature delivery, and maternal corticosteroid therapy is indicated in those being managed expectantly. Delivery should be performed at a facility capable of caring for the mother and baby. In the stable patient, transfer to a facility capable of such care is appropriate.

Management of Uterine Rupture

Uterine rupture with maternal hemorrhage requires immediate laparotomy for maternal reasons, even if the fetal monitoring is reassuring. Treatment for hemorrhage, shock, and possible coagulopathy should be instituted without delay in preparation for surgery.

Management of Vasa Previa

In vasa previa diagnosed prior to vessel disruption, delivery by cesarean section is indicated. In ruptured vasa previa, if the fetus is viable, delivery should be accomplished by the most expeditious route possible, usually cesarean section. The need for intensive neonatal resuscitation, including transfusion therapy, should be anticipated.

Management of Cervical and Vulvar Lesions

Outside pregnancy, when a gross cervical lesion is present, diagnosis by removal or biopsy is encouraged. The cervix, however, is a highly vascular organ in pregnancy and removal or biopsy of a lower genital tract lesion may be complicated by profuse bleeding. Specialist consultation prior to tissue sampling is recommended when a cervical lesion is seen on speculum examination during pregnancy. Cervical erosions do not require treatment. Bleeding from vulvar varicosities can usually be controlled with pressure, and rarely requires surgical ligation.

REFERENCES

1. Lipitz S, Admon D, Menczer J, Ben-Baruch G, Oelsner G: Midtrimester bleeding—variables which affect the outcome of pregnancy. *Gynecol Obstet Invest* 32:24–27, 1991.
2. Harris LL: Rethinking maternal-fetal conflict: Gender and equality in perinatal ethics. *Obstet Gynecol* 96:786, 2000.

3. Pritchard JA, Cunningham G, Pritchard SA, Mason RA: On reducing the frequency of severe abruptio placentae. *Am J Obstet Gynecol* 165:1345, 1991.
4. Pearlman MD, Tintinalli JE, Lorenz RP: A prospective controlled study of outcome after trauma during pregnancy. *Am J Obstet Gynecol* 162:1502, 1990.
5. Kramer MS, Usher RH, Pollack R, Boyd M, Usher S: Etiologic determinants of abruptio placentae. *Obstet Gynecol* 89:221, 1997.
6. Ananth CV, Smulian JC, Vintzileos AM: Incidence of placental abruption in relation to cigarette smoking and hypertensive disorders during pregnancy: a meta-analysis of observational studies. *Obstet Gynecol* 93:622, 1999.
7. Nolan TE, Simthe RP, Devoe LD: A rapid test for abruptio placentae: Evaluation of a D-dimer latex agglutination slide test. *Am J Obstet Gynecol* 169:265, 1993.
8. Kay HH, Spritzer CE: Preliminary experience with magnetic resonance imaging in patients with third-trimester bleeding. *Obstet Gynecol* 78:424, 1991.
9. Langlois SLP, Miller AG: Placenta previa—A review with emphasis on the role of ultrasound. *Aust NZ J Obstet Gynaecol* 29:110, 1989.
10. Farine D, Fox HE, Jakobson S, Timor-Tritsch IE: Vaginal ultrasound for diagnosis of placenta previa. *Am J Obstet Gynecol* 159:566, 1988.
11. Leerentveld RA, Gilberts EC, Arnold M, Wladimiroff JW: Accuracy and safety of transvaginal monographic placental localization. *Obstet Gynecol* 76:759, 1990.
12. Ayers AW, Johnson TRBJ, Hayashi R: Characteristics of fetal heart rate tracings prior to uterine rupture. *Int J Gynecol Obstet* 74:235, 2001.
13. Shrout AB, Kopelman JN: Ultrasonographic diagnosis of uterine dehiscence during pregnancy. *J Ultrasound Med* 14:399, 1995.
14. Kouyoumkjian A: Velamentous insertion of the umbilical cord. *Obstet Gynecol* 56:737, 1980.
15. Nelson LH, Melone PJ, King M: Diagnosis of vasa previa with transvaginal and color flow Doppler ultrasound. *Obstet Gynecol* 76:506, 1990.
16. Stander RW, Lein JN: Carcinoma of the cervix and pregnancy. *Am J Obstet Gynecol* 79:164, 1960.
17. Lamont RF, Dunlop PD, Crowley P, et al: Comparative mortality and morbidity of infants transferred in utero or postnatally. *J Perinat Med* 11:200, 1983.
18. Obladen M, Luttkus A, Rey M, et al: Differences in morbidity and mortality according to type of referral of very low birthweight infants. *JPerinat Med* 22:53, 1994.
19. Baker R: Hemorrhage in obstetrics. *Obstet Gynecol Annu* 6:295, 1977.
20. Nielson EC, Vamer MW, Scott JR: The outcome of pregnancies complicated by bleeding during the second trimester. *Surg Gynecol Obstet* 173:371, 1991.
21. Collaborative Group on Antenatal Steroid Therapy: Effects of antenatal dexamethasone administration on the prevention of respiratory distress syndrome. *Am J Obstet Gynecol* 141:276, 1981.
22. Maher JE, Cliver SP, Goldenberg RL, et al: The effect of corticosteroid therapy in the very premature infant. March of Dimes Multicenter Study Group. A*m J Obstet Gynecol* 170:869, 1994.
23. Silver R, Depp R, Sabbagha RE, et al: Placenta previa: Aggressive expectant management. *Am J Obstet Gynecol* 150:15, 1984.
24. Magann EF, Johnson CA, Gookin KS, et al: Placenta previa: Does uterine activity cause bleeding? *Aust NZ J Obstet Gynaecol* 33:22, 1993.
25. Watson WJ, Cefalo RC: Magnesium sulfate tocolysis in selected patients with symptomatic placenta previa. *Am J Perinatol* 7:251, 1990.
26. Besinger R-E, Moniak CW, Paskiewicz LS, et al: The effect of tocolytic use in the management of symptomatic placenta previa. *Am J Obstet Gynecol* 172:1770, 1995.
27. Gorodeski IG, Neri A, Bahary CM: Placenta previa—The identification of low- and high-risk subgroups. *Eur J Obstet Gynecol Reprod Biol* 20:133, 1985.

11

Cardiopulmonary Resuscitation and Emergency Perimortem Cesarean Delivery

Vern L. Katz
Eric Savitsky

KEY POINTS

- Modified (pelvic-tilt) closed-chest CPR is the preferred response to maternal cardiopulmonary arrest.
- Lateral displacement of the gravid uterus during CPR minimizes aortocaval compression.
- During CPR, high-volume fluid administration must occur, as uteroplacental blood flow will not be adequate with vasoconstrictors alone.
- In an emergent setting, a uterine fundus palpated at least 2 fingerbreadths above the umbilicus is consistent with a potentially viable fetus.
- Perimortem cesarean delivery should be performed within minutes of failing to restore life-sustaining blood flow despite aggressive CPR.
- The success of the cesarean delivery demands a rapid incision, rapid delivery, and rapid closure, which are best obtained with large abdominal and uterine incisions, which are then closed with large running sutures in a single layer.

INTRODUCTION

Caring for the critically ill pregnant patient can provoke anxiety in even the most experienced emergency personnel. The anatomic and physiologic changes that occur during pregnancy as well as the psychological impact of caring for a critically ill pregnant patient makes management of these patients extremely challenging. This chapter will provide the information necessary to optimally treat a pregnant patient in cardiopulmonary arrest. This may include performance of a perimortem cesarean delivery. Indications and techniques for this procedure are also described.

Cardiopulmonary arrest is defined by the sudden loss of cardiac output and respiratory effort. It is potentially reversible with prompt restoration of oxygenated blood flow. Maternal cardiopulmonary arrest is a rare event.[1] Pregnancy-related mortality ratios in the United States range from 10 to 25 pregnancy-related deaths per 100,000 live births.[2–4] Leading causes of pregnancy-related deaths include ectopic pregnancy, pulmonary embolism, hypertensive disease (e.g., eclampsia), trauma, cerebrovascular accidents, hemorrhage and infections.[5,6]

Outcomes of cardiopulmonary resuscitation (CPR) in the general population are well described. Studies place survival to hospital discharge rates at 1 to 19 percent of patients suffering out-of-hospital cardiopulmonary arrests.[7–14] This is in contrast to studies that address the outcomes of CPR in the pregnant patient. The few case series and case reports that address this topic do not provide an accurate estimate of CPR survival rates in pregnant patients. Nonetheless, these studies have documented that appropriate and rapid resuscitative efforts may result in favorable outcomes for both the mother and fetus.[15–20]

ANATOMIC AND PHYSIOLOGIC CONSIDERATIONS

Familiarity with the pertinent anatomic and physiologic changes that occur during pregnancy will assist care providers in managing a critically ill pregnant patient. The reader is referred to Chap. 2 for a thorough discussion. Table 11-1 summarizes the cardiovascular changes during pregnancy that are pertinent to CPR, including increased blood volume, heart rate, and cardiac output.[21,22] Despite this, blood pressures during the second trimester of pregnancy are lower than in nonpregnant states. This is the result of a decrease in systemic vascular resistance (SVR) during pregnancy.[23–25] Pregnancy can be viewed as a high-flow, low systemic vascular resistance state. In addition, since the plasma volume increases to a greater extent than the red blood cell volume, a dilutional anemia of 2 to 4 percent occurs and reaches its peak (i.e., lowest ratio of RBCs to total volume) in the second trimester.[26,27] The gravid uterus lacks vascular autoregulation and is reliant on adequate perfusion pressures to maintain blood flow to

Table 11-1. Factors Affecting CPR in the Pregnant Patient

Cardiovascular	Increased blood volume
	Increased heart rate
	Increased cardiac output
	Decreased systemic vascular resistance
	Aortocaval compression by enlarging uterus
Respiratory	Primary respiratory alkalosis
	Increased respiratory rate
	Increased tidal volume
	Diminished functional residual capacity
Metabolic	Increased oxygen consumption
	Secondary compensatory metabolic acidosis
Gastrointestinal	Delayed gastric emptying
	Altered lower esophageal sphincter function

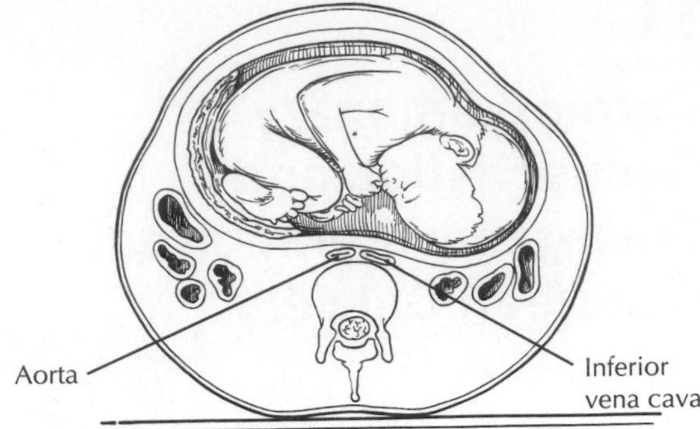

Fig. 11-1. Aortocaval compression with the mother in the supine position.

the uteroplacental unit.[23,28,29] As a result, marked reductions in circulating blood volume or elevations in SVR can have adverse effects on the fetus.[30]

Maternal oxygen consumption increases during pregnancy to meet metabolic demands.[31] Consequently, profound hypoxemia may ensue if the respiratory mechanics of a pregnant patient are compromised.[31] Maternal hypoxemia will also result in a reduction in uteroplacental perfusion.[28] Respiratory changes during pregnancy include a progesterone-mediated effect on central respiratory drive. This results in mild hyperventilation (i.e., arterial carbon dioxide tensions between 30 and 35 mmHg) and a mild compensatory metabolic acidosis (i.e., serum bicarbonate decreases by 4 mEq/L).[32–34] Intrathoracic pressure will increase secondary to displacement of the diaphragm by the enlarging gravid uterus. Tidal volumes will increase, and functional respiratory capacities will diminish. Both lower gastroesophageal sphincter function and gastric motility diminish during pregnancy.[35,36] This may predispose the critically ill pregnant patient to reflux of gastric contents. These physiologic changes underscore the importance of maintaining adequate oxygenation and airway protection in critically ill pregnant patients.

In the second half of pregnancy, the gravid patient will experience compression of her inferior vena cava (IVC), major pelvic veins, and aorta by her enlarging uterus (Fig. 11-1). As a result, pregnant patients may experience the supine hypotensive syndrome.[37] This syndrome occurs in approximately 11 percent of pregnant women.[37] It is characterized by a patient in the late stages of pregnancy assuming a supine position for several minutes, then developing hypotension and occasionally syncope. This phenomenon does not occur instantaneously as it depends on venous pooling of blood. The hypotension is the result of the IVC being compressed between the gravid uterus and the spine with a resultant decrease of preload to the heart. In most cases, an associated rise in SVR maintains a normal blood pressure.[38] Blood flow reaches the right heart via alternate routes, including the azygos vein and paraspinal venous plexus.[39] In a subset of women, these compensatory mechanisms fail, inadequate right heart filling occurs, preload is diminished, and the cardiac output decreases. Having gravid patients avoid the supine position can mitigate this effect. The left lateral decubitus position has been advocated as a treatment for the supine hypotensive syndrome (Fig. 11-2).[22,38,40,41] This position has the effect of minimizing the compressive effect of the uterus on the IVC and thus restoring adequate cardiac output.[22]

Interestingly, women during active labor tend to tolerate a supine position.[41,42] The reasons are unclear, but there are several theories. The intermittent contractions of the uterus during active labor redistribute uterine blood volume into the central circulation, restoring adequate cardiac preload.[41,42] In addition, some believe a contracted uterus minimizes its compressive effect on the IVC.[41] The deep inspiratory efforts associated with this stage of labor are also thought to augment venous return to the right heart.

Compression of the distal abdominal aorta is also a consequence of pregnancy. The aorta is compressed between

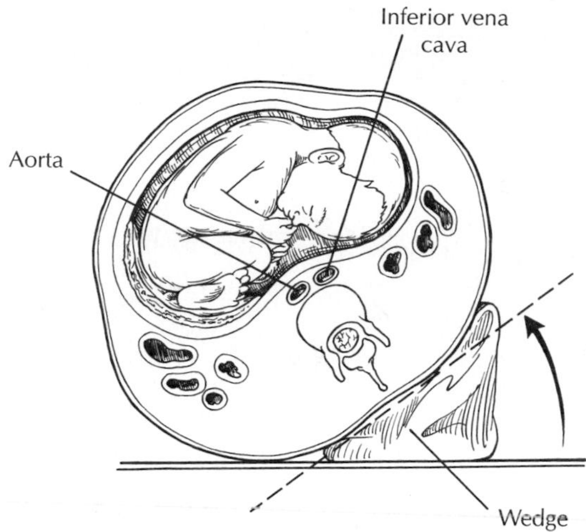

Fig. 11-2. Relief of aortocaval compression with the mother in lateral tilt.

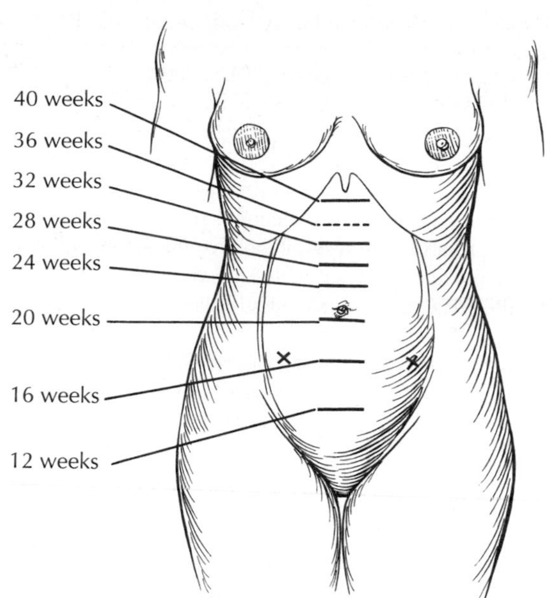

Fig. 11-3. Gestational age may be approximated by using fundal height above the umbilicus as a gauge.

the enlarging uterus and the spine.[43] This is normally of no clinical consequence; however, in cases of maternal hypotension, hypoxemia, or acidemia, it may contribute to impairment of uteroplacental blood flow.

PATIENT ASSESSMENT

Determining whether a pregnant patient is in cardiopulmonary arrest is easily assessed. Palpation of the carotid or femoral pulse in concert with visual assessment of the patient's level of responsiveness, color (e.g., cyanosis), and respiratory effort will provide a rapid answer. The absence of palpable pulses in an unresponsive patient with compromised respiratory effort warrants initiation of CPR. Cardiac telemetry, pulse oximetry, and sphygmomanometry will further assist in assessing the physiologic condition of the patient.

In the setting of maternal cardiopulmonary arrest, the first priority is maternal resuscitation; nonetheless, a rapid assessment of fetal gestational age is important (i.e., transabdominal uterine fundus palpation). The gestational age of a fetus will often dictate resuscitative interventions. Care providers should not spend time making further assessment of fetal well being until maternal resuscitative efforts are complete. The date of conception or last menstrual period is often unknown or unobtainable from critically ill pregnant patients. Assessment of uterine fundal height may be performed by directly palpating the abdomen (Fig. 11-3). In general, a uterine fundus at the level of the umbilicus it is thought to indicate a gestational age of approximately 20 weeks.[44,45] Measurement of the fundal height (i.e., the distance from the pubic symphysis to the fundus) in centimeters approximates the gestational age in weeks between 20 and 30 weeks gestation.[44] In an emergent setting, a uterine fundus palpated at least 2 fingerbreadths above the umbilicus is consistent with a potentially viable fetus. It is prudent to keep in mind that estimation of fundal height is much less reliable in obese women, and use of ultrasound or other modalities of gestational age assessment are indicated.

Methods used to document fetal well-being include assessing fetal heart tones with a stethoscope or Doppler device. Fetal heart rates between 120 and 160 beats per minute are normal. Circumstances permitting, a rapid bedside ultrasound can prove very useful as it can provide accurate information regarding fetal well-being and gestational age.[46]

CARDIOPULMONARY RESUSCITATION

While numerous articles detail CPR in children and adults, guidelines for CPR during pregnancy are scant. Traditionally, standard CPR techniques have been applied to the pregnant patient in cardiopulmonary arrest. As previously

Table 11-2. Cardiopulmonary Resuscitation (CPR) in Pregnancy

Standard CPR in Pregnancy (All stages)

- Standard closed-chest CPR is implemented
  - 100 compressions per minute
  - Sternum depressed 1.5 to 2 inches with each compression
  - 15:2 compression:ventilation ratio
- Aggressive airway protection is practiced
- Aggressive fluid resuscitation required to ensure intravascular volume repletion
- Standard cardioresuscitative pharmacotherapy is administered
- Electrical cardioversion/defibrillation is administered as necessary

CPR Modifications (implement if Gestational Age >24 weeks)

1. Ensure lateral displacement of the gravid uterus during CPR to minimize aortocaval compression
2. Consider performing perimortem cesarean section within minutes of failing to restore life-sustaining blood flow despite aggressive CPR

mentioned, while in short supply, the available literature does document that appropriate and rapid resuscitative efforts may result in survival of both the mother and fetus.

Since the initial description of closed-chest CPR, new techniques have been described. These include compression-only CPR, simultaneous ventilation and compression CPR, interposed abdominal counterpulsation CPR, and compression-decompression CPR.[14,47–49] The effects of these alternative techniques in pregnant women remain unknown.

The mechanism by which closed-chest CPR provides cardiac output is complex. Closed-chest CPR is thought to cause forward blood flow by producing phasic fluctuations in intrathoracic pressures, as well as by compression of the heart between the sternum and the spine.[50–52] Preservation of cardiac and brain function following cardiopulmonary arrest is related to the degree of coronary and cerebral perfusion attained during CPR. Myocardial perfusion during CPR is related to the coronary perfusion pressure. This is the diastolic pressure during the release phase of chest compression minus the coronary sinus pressure.[53–55] The cerebral perfusion pressure is related to the systolic pressure during the chest compression phase of CPR.

Readers are referred to standard references for a detailed discussion of Basic Life Support (BLS) and Advance Cardiac Life Support (ACLS) resuscitative algorithms.[56] The medications and dosages utilized in ACLS algorithms do not need modification in pregnancy. Recent major changes in resuscitation algorithms involve rescuers performing chest compressions at a rate of 100 per minute.[57,58] The ratio of compressions to ventilations should be 15:2 in all nonintubated patients, regardless of rescuer number. Upon intubation, compressions should be continuous and ventilations may be asynchronous. The palpation of pulses with chest compression has traditionally been used as an indicator of successful CPR technique. Capnometry has recently been described as an indicator of CPR efficacy.[59,60] End-tidal carbon dioxide levels of less than 10 mmHg following at least 20 minutes of CPR are strongly associated with death.[55,60]

There are several important modifications to CPR in pregnant patients (Table 11-2). A critical feature of the second half of pregnancy is compression of the IVC and pelvic veins by the gravid uterus. Near term, stroke volume may be decreased by up to 30 percent by this compressive effect.[22,61–63] This phenomenon may impede the efficacy of CPR performed on a supine patient.[64] The cardiac output of a near-term pregnant woman will increase by 25 percent when she is moved from a supine to left lateral decubitus position.[65] Ideally, upon determining the need for CPR, a wedge could be placed under the gravid patient's right hip and flank tilting her lower torso on an angle.[66] Alternatively, someone may be able to manually displace the uterus to the left side. This will displace the uterus off the IVC and augment return of venous blood to the heart. The upper torso remains flat on a firm surface, facilitating chest compressions. Tilting the entire body sideways or upright may minimize obstruction of venous return, but will compromise the efficacy of chest compressions. Rees and Willis demonstrated a decrease in rescuer chest compression force as the angle of a patient's body tilt increased.[67] A force equivalent to 67 percent of rescuer body weight was generated on a supine model while a force of only 36 percent of rescuer body weight was possible on a model in full lateral decubitus position. In summary, modified closed-chest CPR is the preferred response to maternal cardiopulmonary arrest. In the second half of pregnancy, lateral displacement of the gravid uterus will ensure maximal CPR efficacy.

ROLE OF PERIMORTEM CESAREAN DELIVERY

The physiologic burdens of pregnancy often preclude the successful resuscitation of pregnant patients in cardiopulmonary arrest. The performance of a perimortem cesarean delivery is a well-documented method to salvage a fetus. Several authors have described miraculously salvaging both mother and fetus from death by performing a perimortem cesarean delivery.[63,68] These authors point out that the uteroplacental unit and fetus impose tremendous physiologic limitations on the efficacy of CPR. Benefits of perimortem cesarean delivery include initiating direct resuscitative measures on the delivered fetus and restoring maternal physiology to a state that is more likely to respond to CPR.

The decision about whether to perform a perimortem cesarean delivery is partly based on the gestational age of the fetus. Newborns with a gestational age of less than 24 weeks have a less than 50 percent chance of survival and a majority of survivors will have serious neurologic sequelae.[69–71] One could argue that even if the fetus does not survive, restoration of maternal physiology to a nongravid state may improve her chances of responding to resuscitative measures. This could be used as a rationale for performing a perimortem cesarean delivery even if fetal survival is unlikely. Recommendations regarding the timing of when to perform a perimortem cesarean delivery vary from 3 minutes to 20 minutes from initiation of CPR.[68,72,73] There are numerous case reports and a strong theoretical rationale that support performing perimortem cesarean delivery within several minutes of the loss of life-sustaining blood flow.[17,61,63,68]

Based on current studies, it is recommended to perform pelvic tilt-modified CPR as a first response to a gravid patient in cardiopulmonary arrest. Standard airway interventions, cardioresuscitative medications, and resuscitative fluids should be administered. Adequate IV fluid administration must occur, as uteroplacental flow will not be adequate with use of vasoconstrictors alone.[28–30] If the patient is in the latter half of pregnancy and does not respond to resuscitative measures an emergent perimortem cesarean delivery should be considered.

Table 11-3. Equipment For A Perimortem Cesarean Delivery

Scalpel
Bandage scissors
Mayo scissors
Toothed forceps
Richardson retractors
Needle-drivers
Suture

PERFORMING A PERIMORTEM CESAREAN DELIVERY

Preparation

The materials for perimortem cesarean delivery are readily found in the trauma suite (including scalpel, clamps, Mayo scissors, large bandage scissors, suture, and needleholders; see Table 11-3). Materials for resuscitation of the baby must also be available, including a radiant warmer, neonatal laryngoscope with functioning batteries and lights, neonatal intubation tubes, cord clamp, scissors, bulb syringe, and neonatal Ambu Bag® with tubing, oxygen source, and suction source (see Chap. 21 for resuscitation of the neonate). Materials for resuscitation of the baby delivered in an emergent situation are also in the standard resuscitation pack. Notification of pediatrics, the PICU, or the NICU will aid in the resuscitation, since there will be two patients requiring attention after an emergent delivery.

Timing of the Procedure

A perimortem cesarean delivery should be initiated within 4 minutes of maternal cardiac arrest.[15–19] If a woman is brought in to the emergency department and CPR has been ongoing in the field, a cesarean delivery may be performed immediately. As discussed above, there is a double rationale for performing the perimortem delivery as part of resuscitation: First, the pregnant woman is essentially two patients, the fetus and the mother. Although fetuses can survive as long as 30 minutes after maternal cardiac arrest, the greatest likelihood of intact fetal survival requires neonatal resuscitation rapidly (4 to 5 minutes) after maternal cardiac arrest. This is because the fetus has compensatory mechanisms to prevent injury and brain damage.[5–13] Many of the situations leading to maternal cardiac arrest have already produced maternal respiratory depression and thus the fetus is already relatively hypoxic. The second reason for performing a cesarean section is that one of the greatest hindrances to effective CPR is the inability to obtain adequate cardiac output. As described above, attempts may be made to displace the uterus off the vena cava; however, these are usually only partially successful. Any alteration of a patient's supine position during chest compression leads to decreased effectiveness. Thus if the cause of the cardiac arrest is reversible—as from cerebrovascular accidents, pulmonary emboli, drug overdoses, or other forms of shock—the greatest likelihood of performing adequate resuscitation will be with the uterus emptied by cesarean section. If the cause of the cardiac arrest is irreversible—as in the case of a massive myocardial infarction or, more commonly, chest or head trauma—the sooner the baby is delivered, the better the baby's chance of survival. It will obviously not hurt the mother with irreversible cardiac arrest to perform a cesarean delivery.

Performing Cesarean Delivery

Once the decision to perform the cesarean delivery is made, the mother should not be moved to an operating suite. There is no need to scrub the abdomen. The most important aspect of the emergency delivery is speed. There is no need to administer anesthesia. The cesarean delivery will be relatively bloodless, since there is no cardiac output. Any emergency physician may perform the cesarean delivery, though if a surgeon or obstetrician is present, he or she may be most able to perform it. As stated above, chest compressions and ventilation should be continued throughout the procedure and after the delivery.

The abdominal incision should be made from approximately 4 to 5 cm below the xiphoid to 2 to 3 cm above the pubis (Fig. 11-4*A*). The incision should be stopped at the pubic hairline. The incision is made through the midline and taken down through the subcutaneous tissue and fascia. The rectus muscles are separated bluntly in the midline and the peritoneum is entered with a midline incision, usually below the umbilicus. The incision is then continued superiorly and inferiorly (Fig. 11-4*B*). Care should be taken not to injure the bladder at the most inferior aspect of the peritoneal incision (Fig. 11-4*B*). Once the peritoneal cavity is entered along the midline, the uterus will be readily visible. A vertical incision from the top of the uterine fundus to immediately above the opaque insertion of the bladder is simplest (Fig. 11-4*C*). The fetus should then be delivered from the abdomen, quickly dried, and resuscitated in the fashion of an emergency delivery (Fig. 11-4*D*). A key point is that the success of the cesarean delivery demands a rapid incision and rapid delivery. Rapid delivery is best obtained with large abdominal and uterine incisions.

After delivery of the infant, the placenta should be delivered from the uterus. The uterus should be cleaned of membranes with a sponge or towel (Fig. 11-4*E*). While CPR is continued, the uterus can be closed either by a surgical assistant or by the primary physician. The uterus should be closed in one or two layers with a large suture in a running locking stitch. The stitch may be made with either no. 0 or no. 1 semipermanent ligature, such as polyglactin or polyglycolic acid, on a large needle. It will usually take two layers to close the uterus. The most important aspect of this procedure is rapid closure. If the mother can be resuscitated and pulses return, she must be stabilized and transferred as quickly as possible. If she is not able to be resuscitated as from massive chest or head trauma, multilayered closure may not be necessary. Normally, after the uterus is closed, the fascia and peritoneum may be closed rapidly with a bulk closure and running stitch. This closure should be with a permanent or semipermanent suture. Use of no. 0 or no. 1 polyglyconate or polypropylene suture material is appropriate. The subcutaneous tissue does not need to be closed. The skin can be closed either with clips or with a running 2–0 stitch that may be revised later. Again, the rapidity of the procedure and the continuation of the code is important for the mother's survival. If necessary—prior to closure of the fascia—the liver, intestines, and other organs may be rapidly inspected to ensure that they have not been affected by trauma. If resuscitation of the mother appears to be successful, broad-spectrum antibiotics should be given. A third-generation penicillin with beta-lactamase inhibitors may be used. A third-generation cephalosporin may also be used. After the mother is resuscitated, she should be transferred to the intensive care unit and managed in the same way as any other victim of cardiac arrest or trauma.

The decision to perform a perimortem cesarean delivery is very difficult for the nonobstetrician. It is highly traumatic for the emergency physician as well as the emergency staff. We strongly recommend that a postresuscitation conference be held after any resuscitation of a pregnant trauma victim. Whether or not a perimortem cesarean delivery is performed, such a conference held within 7 to 10 days is helpful. All health providers involved, including EMTs, should be invited. This conference may function both as a quality assurance as well as an educational conference. A facilitator, chaplain, or other support staff may also be invited. The double tragedy of losing a mother and a fetus or the tragedy of losing one of them may be very difficult for the emergency staff. During the conference, a discussion of the principles of therapy and resuscitation for the emergency staff, as well as discussion of the pro-

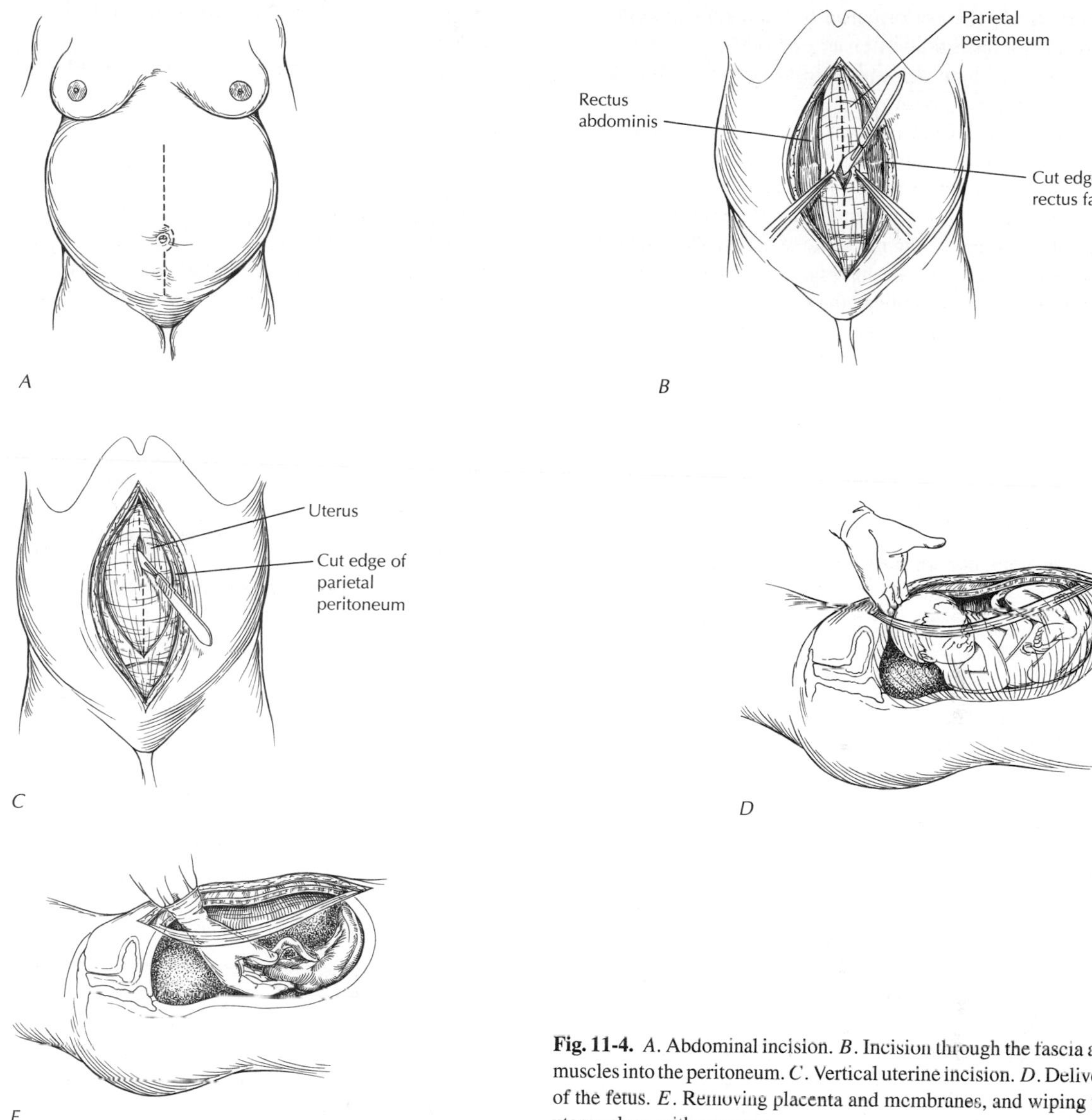

Fig. 11-4. *A*. Abdominal incision. *B*. Incision through the fascia and muscles into the peritoneum. *C*. Vertical uterine incision. *D*. Delivery of the fetus. *E*. Removing placenta and membranes, and wiping the uterus clean with a sponge.

tocols involved in the case, is helpful to both teach and relieve the emotional stress involved.

LEGAL AND ETHICAL CONSIDERATIONS FOR PERIMORTEM DELIVERY

At the time this chapter was written, there had never been litigation regarding the performance of a perimortem cesarean delivery. Legal questions have arisen when a perimortem cesarean delivery was not performed; however, to our knowledge, no litigation has arisen regarding those issues. It is inappropriate to try to obtain consent for perimortem delivery, since the life of the patient depends on prompt action. In truth, the perimortem cesarean delivery may positively influence the health of both the mother and fetus. The emergency physician would not stop or break away from resuscitation in order to obtain consent for open cardiac massage; similarly, it would be inappropriate to do this before performing a perimortem cesarean delivery. Since the performance of the cesarean section is part of the resuscitation effort and this has been documented throughout the literature, it is well within the standard of care to perform such an operation. Indeed, its timely performance (i.e., within 4 to 5 minutes of arrest) constitutes optimal care.

At least two ethical principles are involved that indicate that performance of the perimortem cesarean delivery is necessary. The first is the principle of beneficence, which involves always acting for the good of the patient. Since the pregnant mother represents two patients, the performance of a cesarean delivery in order to save the baby and potentially aid in resuscitating the mother by eliminating aortocaval compression works for the benefit of both the mother and fetus. The ethical principle of doing no harm or absence of malfeasance is also upheld by performing this operation. No major blood vessels or nerves are encountered during the cesarean delivery, given the nature of the operation. Thus performing this operation in no way potentially compromises the long-term health of the mother. Cesarean delivery does not represent a life-threatening operation, and in the setting of cardiac arrest it may be helpful in attempts at resuscitation.

SPECIAL CONSIDERATIONS

Although several cardioresuscitative medications (e.g., epinephrine) have theoretical adverse fetal consequences, use of these medications is justified in the critically ill pregnant patient. Likewise, defibrillation should be performed using the same indications as in nonpregnant patients. Reports do exist of cardioresuscitative medications and electrical cardioversion being successfully used in pregnant patients with no discernible adverse effects on mother or fetus.[20,74,75] Necessary radiographic studies should be performed as clinically indicated. Adverse fetal outcomes due to radiation are exceedingly rare with radiation doses between 5 and 10 rads.[76]

REFERENCES

1. de Swiet M: Maternal mortality: Confidential enquiries into maternal deaths in the United Kingdom. *Am J Obstet Gynecol* 182:760–766, 2000.
2. Fang J: Maternal mortality in New York City: excess mortality of black women. *J Urban Health* 77:735–744, 2000.
3. Hopkins FW: Pregnancy-related mortality in hispanic women in the United States. *Obstet Gynecol* 94:747–752, 1999.
4. Kaunitz AM, Hughes JM, Grimes DA, et al: Causes of maternal mortality in the United States. *Obstet Gynecol* 65:605–612, 1985.
5. Panchal S: Maternal mortality during hospital admission for delivery: a retrospective analysis using a state-maintained database. *Anesth Analg* 93:134–141, 2001.
6. Syverson CJ, Chavkin W, Atrash HK, et al: Pregnancy-related mortality in New York City, 1980 to 1984: Causes of death and associated risk factors. *Am J Obstet Gynecol* 164:603–608, 1991.
7. Gueugniaud PV, Mols P, Goldstein P, et al: A comparison of repeated high doses and repeated standard doses of epinephrine for cardiac arrest outside the hospital. *N Engl J Med* 339:1595–1601, 1998.
8. Thel MC, O'Connor CM: Cardiopulmonary resuscitation: Historical perspective to recent investigations. *Am Heart J* 137:39–48, 1999.
9. Barton C, Callaham M: High-dose epinephrine improves the return of spontaneous circulation rates in human victims of cardiac arrest. *Ann Emerg Med* 20:722–725, 1991.
10. Becker LB, Ostrander MP, Barrett J, et al: Outcome of CPR in a large metropolitan area—where are the survivors? *Ann Emerg Med* 20:355–361, 1991.
11. Brown CG, Martin DR, Pepe PE, et al: A comparison of standard-dose and high-dose epinephrine in cardiac arrest outside the hospital. The multicenter high-dose epinephrine study group. *N Engl J Med* 327:1051–1055, 1992.
12. Lombardi G, Gallagher J, Gennis P: Outcome of out-of hospital cardiac arrest in New York City. The Pre-Hospital Arrest Survival Evaluation (PHASE) Study. *JAMA* 271:678–683, 1994.
13. Myerburg RJ, Conde CA, Sung RJ, et al: Clinical, electrophysiologic and hemodynamic profile of patients resuscitated from prehospital cardiac arrest. *Am J Med* 68:568–576, 1980.
14. Hallstrom A, Cobb L, Johnson E, et al: Cardiopulmonary resuscitation by chest compression alone or mouth-to-mouth ventilation. *N Engl J Med* 342:1546–1553, 2000.
15. DePace NL, Betesh JS, Kotler MN: "Postmortem" cesarean section with recovery of both mother and offspring. *JAMA* 248:971–973, 1982.
16. Lindsay SL, Hanson GC: Cardiac arrest in near-term pregnancy. *Anaesthesia* 42:1074–1077, 1987.
17. Lopez-Zeno JA, Carlo WA, O'Grady JP, et al: Infant survival following delayed postmortem cesarean delivery. *Obstet Gynecol* 76:991–992, 1990.
18. O'Connor RL, Sevarino FB: Cardiopulmonary arrest in the pregnant patient: A report of a successful resuscitation. *J Clin Anesth* 6:66–68, 1994.
19. Pierce MR, Henderson RA, Mitchell JM: Cardiopulmonary arrest secondary to lightning injury in a pregnant woman. *Ann Emerg Med* 15:597–599, 1986.
20. Selden BS, Burke TJ: Complete maternal and fetal recovery after prolonged cardiac arrest. *Ann Emerg Med* 17:346–349, 1988.
21. Pritchard JA: Changes in blood volume during pregnancy and delivery. *Anesthesiology* 26:393–399, 1965.

22. Ueland K, Novy MJ, Peterson EN, et al: Maternal cardiovascular dynamics IV: The influence of gestational age on the maternal cardiovascular response to posture and exercise. *Am J Obstet Gynecol* 104:856–863, 1969.
23. Ginsburg J, Duncan SLB: Peripheral blood flow in normal pregnancy. *Cardiovasc Res* 1:132–137, 1967.
24. Duvekot JJ: Early pregnancy changes in hemodynamics and volume homeostasis are consecutive adjustments triggered by a primary fall in systemic vascular tone. *Am J Obstet Gynecol* 169:1382–1392, 1993.
25. Spaanderman ME: The effect of pregnancy on the compliance of large arteries and veins in healthy parous control subjects and women with a history of preeclampsia. *Am J Obstet Gynecol* 183:1278–1286, 2000.
26. Taylor DJ: Effect of iron supplementation on serum ferritin levels during and after pregnancy. *Br J Obstet Gynaecol* 89:1011–1017, 1982.
27. Goodman RA: Current trends—CDC criteria for anemia in children and child bearing-aged women. *MMWR Morb Mortal Wkly Rep* 38:400–405, 1989.
28. Dilts PV, Brinkman CR, Kirschbaum TH, et al: Uterine and systemic hemodynamic interrelationships and their response to hypoxia. *Am J Obstet Gynecol* 103:138–157, 1969.
29. Karlsson K: The influence of hypoxia on uterine and maternal placental blood flow, and the effect of alpha-adrenergic blockade. *J Perinat Med* 2:176–184, 1974.
30. Bernal JM, Miralles PJ: Cardiac surgery with cardiopulmonary bypass during pregnancy. *Obstet Gynecol Surv* 41: 1–6, 1986.
31. Archer GW, Marx GF: Arterial oxygen tension during apnoea in parturient women. *Br J Anaesth* 46:358–360, 1974.
32. Andersen GJ: The effect of labour on the maternal blood-gas and acid-base status. *J Obstet Gynaecol Br Commonw* 77:289–293, 1970.
33. Templeton A: Maternal blood-gases, (Pa_{O_2}-PA_{O_2}), physiological shunt and V_D/V_T in normal pregnancy. *Br J Anaesth* 48:1001–1004, 1976.
34. Weinberger SE, Weiss ST, Cohen WR, et al: Pregnancy and the lung. *Am Rev Respir Dis* 121:559–581, 1980.
35. Fisher RS, Roberts GS, Grabowski CJ, et al: Altered lower esophageal sphincter function during early pregnancy. *Gastroenterology* 74:1233–1237, 1978.
36. Chiloiro M, Darconza G, Piccioli E, et al: Gastric emptying and orocecal transit time in pregnancy. *J Gastroenterol* 36:538–543, 2001.
37. Howard BK, Goodson JH, Mengert WF: Supine hypotensive syndrome in late pregnancy. *Obstet Gynecol* 1:371–377, 1953.
38. Lees MM, Scott DB, Kerr MG, et al: The circulatory effects of recumbent postural change in late pregnancy. *Clin Sci* 32:453–465, 1967.
39. Kerr MG, Scott DB, Samuel E: Studies of the inferior vena cava in late pregnancy. *Br Med J* 1:532–533, 1964.
40. Vorys N, Ullery JC, Hanusek GE: The cardiac output changes in various positions in pregnancy. *Am J Obstet Gynecol* 82:1312–1321, 1961.
41. Ueland K, Hansen JM: Maternal cardiovascular dynamics II: Posture and uterine contractions. *Am J Obstet Gynecol* 103:1–7, 1969.
42. Hendricks CH, Quilligan EJ: Cardiac output during labor. *Am J Obstet Gynecol* 71:953–972, 1956.
43. Bieniarz J, Crottogini JJ, Curuchet E, et al: Aortocaval compression by the uterus in late human pregnancy. *Am J Obstet Gynecol* 100:203–217, 1968.
44. Jimenez JM, Tyson JE, Reisch JS: Clinical measures of gestational age in normal pregnancies. *Obstet Gynecol* 61:438–443, 1983.
45. Andersen HF, Johnson TR, Barclay ML, et al: Gestational age assessment I. Analysis of individual clinical evaluation. *Am J Obstet Gynecol* 139:173–177, 1981.
46. Campbell BA: Utilizing sonography in a general obstetric practice. *Clin Obstet Gynecol Clin* 25:598–607, 1998.
47. Chandra N, Guerci A, Weisfeldt ML, et al: Contrasts between intrathoracic pressures during chest compression and cardiac massage. *Crit Care Med* 9:789–792, 1981.
48. Babbs CF: Efficacy of interposed abdominal compression-cardiopulmonary resuscitation (CPR), active compression and decompression-CPR, and Lifestick CPR: Basic physiology in a spreadsheet model. *Crit Care Med* 28:199–202, 2000.
49. Stiell IG, Hebert PC, Wells GA, et al: The Ontario trial of active compression-decompression cardiopulmonary resuscitation for in-hospital and prehospital cardiac arrest. *JAMA* 275:1417–1423, 1996.
50. Sanders AB, Ewy GA, Taft TV: Prognostic and therapeutic importance of the aortic diastolic pressure in resuscitation from cardiac arrest. *Crit Care Med* 12:871–873, 1984.
51. Niemann JT: Artificial perfusion techniques during cardiac arrest. *Ann Emerg Med* 14:761–768, 1985.
52. Weiseldt ML, Chandra N: Physiology of cardiopulmonary resuscitation. *Ann Rev Med* 32:435–442, 1981.
53. Paradis NA, Martin GB, Rivers EP: Coronary perfusion pressure and the return of spontaneous circulation in human cardiopulmonary resuscitation. *JAMA* 263:1106–1113, 1990.
54. Eleff SM, Kim H, Shaffner DH, et al: Effect of cerebral blood flow generated during cardiopulmonary resuscitation in dogs on maintenance versus recovery of ATP and pH. *Stroke* 24:2066–2073, 1993.
55. Sanders AB, Kem KB, Otto CW, et al: End-tidal carbon dioxide monitoring during cardiopulmonary resuscitation. A prognostic indicator for survival. *JAMA* 262:1347–1351, 1989.
56. Emergency Cardiac Care Committee and Subcommittees, American Heart Association. Guidelines. Adult Advanced Cardiac Life Support. *JAMA* 268:2199–2240, 1992.
57. Kern KB, Sanders AB, Raife J, et al: A study of chest compression rates during cardiopulmonary resuscitation in humans: the importance of rate-directed chest compressions. *Arch Intern Med* 152:145–149, 1992.
58. Swenson RD, Weaver WD, Niskanen RA, et al: Hemodynamics in humans during conventional and experimen-

tal methods of cardiopulmonary resuscitation. *Circulation* 78:630–639, 1988.

59. Weil MH, Bisera J, Trevino RP, et al: Cardiac output and end-tidal carbon dioxide. *Crit Care Med* 13:907–909, 1985.
60. Levine RL, Wayne MA, Miller CC: End-tidal carbon dioxide and outcome of out-of-hospital cardiac arrest. *N Engl J Med* 337:301–306, 1997.
61. Katz VL, Dotters DJ, Droegemueller W: Perimortem cesarean delivery. *Obstet Gynecol* 68:571–576, 1986.
62. Marx GF: Cardiopulmonary resuscitation of the late pregnant woman. *Anesthesiology* 56: 1982.
63. Depace NL, Betesh JS, Kotler MN: Postmortem cesarean section with recovery of both mother and offspring. *JAMA* 248:971–973, 1982.
64. Kasten GW, Martin ST: Resuscitation from bupivacaine-induced cardiovascular toxicity during partial inferior vena cava occlusion. *Anesth Analg* 65:341–344, 1986.
65. Kerr MG: The mechanical effects of gravid uterus in late pregnancy. *J Obstet Gynaecol Br Commonw* 513–529, 1965.
66. Goodwin AP: The human wedge. A manoeuvre to relieve aortocaval compression during resuscitation in late pregnancy. *Anaesthesia* 47:433–444, 1992.
67. Rees GAD, Willis BA: Resuscitation in late pregnancy. *Anaesthesia* 43:347–349, 1988.
68. Lindsay SL, Hanson GC: Cardiac arrest in near-term pregnancy. *Anaesthesia* 42:1074–1077, 1987.
69. Berg T, Lindberg BS: Cesarean section in premature delivery. *Gynecol Obstet Invest* 11:95–101, 1980.
70. Chan K, Ohlsson A, Synnes A, et al: Survival, morbidity, and resource use of infants of 25 weeks' gestational age or less. *Am J Obstet Gynecol* 185:220–226, 2001.
71. Herschel M, Kennedy JL, Kayne HL, et al: Survival of infants born at 24 to 28 weeks' gestation. *Obstet Gynecol* 60:154–158, 1982.
72. Kam CW: Perimortem caesarean section. *J Accid Emerg Med* 11:57–58, 1994.
73. Lanoix R, Akkapeddi V, Goldfeder B: Perimortem cesarean section: Case reports and recommendations. *Acad Emerg Med* 2:1063–1067, 1995.
74. Lee RV, Rodgers BD, White LM, et al: Cardiopulmonary resuscitation of pregnant women. *Am J Med* 81:311–318, 1986.
75. Curry JJ, Quintana FJ: Myocardial infarction with ventricular fibrillation during pregnancy treated by direct current defibrillation with fetal survival. *Chest* 58:82–84, 1970.
76. Toppenberg KS, Hill DA, Miller DP: Safety of radiographic imaging during pregnancy. 59:1813–1818, 1999.

SECTION IV

MEDICAL DISORDERS IN PREGNANCY

12

Deep Venous Thrombosis and Pulmonary Embolism in Pregnancy

Marc R. Toglia

KEY POINTS

- The risk of deep venous thrombosis and pulmonary embolism is 5 times greater in pregnant than in nonpregnant women.
- D-dimer normally elevates in pregnancy and is not helpful for diagnosis.
- Compression ultrasound is currently the best screening test for deep vein thrombosis; to minimize false positives the uterus should be deflected toward the left when performing the procedure.
- In pulmonary embolism, 15 percent of patients may have normal arterial blood gases, and 40 percent may have normal P_{AO_2}-Pa_{O_2}.
- Pulmonary angiography or spiral CT is often necessary to confirm the diagnosis of pulmonary embolism.

INTRODUCTION

Deep venous thrombosis (DVT) and pulmonary embolism (PE) continue to be a leading cause of maternal morbidity.[1] Prompt recognition and treatment of DVT reduces the incidence of fatal pulmonary embolism; however, the diagnosis and management of these conditions during pregnancy remain problematic, in part due to the lack of properly performed clinical trials involving pregnant women. Fortunately, clinicians caring for pregnant women can modify the guidelines established for nonpregnant patients based on an understanding of the physiologic changes that are known to accompany pregnancy.[2] In this chapter, current diagnostic and therapeutic strategies for the evaluation of acute deep vein thrombosis and pulmonary embolism during pregnancy will be reviewed.

PATHOPHYSIOLOGY

Pregnancy is a physiologic state with a markedly elevated risk of thromboembolic events, such as DVT and PE. The risk of venous thromboembolism is five times as high among pregnant women as among nonpregnant women of similar age. Estimates of the incidence of pregnancy-associated venous thromboembolism (VTE) vary from 1 in 1000 to 1 in 3000 pregnancies.[2] Table 12-1 lists risk factors for DVT in pregnancy and the postpartum period.

Physicians have long recognized that each element of Virchow's triad for venous thrombosis—namely, stasis, endothelial damage, and hypercoagulability—is present during pregnancy. Physiologic changes associated with pregnancy result in an increase in venous distensibility and capacitance, which results in an increase in venous stasis. These changes are apparent starting in the first trimester and are thought to be hormonally mediated. As pregnancy progresses, compression of the pelvic vessels by the enlarging uterus further adds to the venous stasis in the lower extremities. Vascular wall injury may occur at the time of delivery, with placental separation, or associated with operative delivery.

Pregnancy is also associated with changes in the plasma concentrations and activities of several proteins involved in the coagulation cascade. These changes are thought to promote coagulation, decrease anticoagulation, and inhibit fibrinolysis, further contributing to a state of hypercoagulability. The levels of coagulation factors II, VII, X, and fibrin substantially increase by the middle of pregnancy. Protein S, an important coagulation inhibitor, sig-

Table 12-1. Risk Factors for Venous Thromboembolism during Pregnancy and the Puerperium

Hereditary thrombophilia
Factor V Leiden
G20210A prothrombin gene mutation
Antithrombin III deficiency
Protein C deficiency
Protein S deficiency
C677T MTHFR mutation (hyperhomocysteinemia)
Antiphospholipid antibodies, lupus anticoagulant
Personal history of VTE
Mechanical heart valve
Cesarean delivery (postpartum risk only)
Preeclampsia (postpartum risk only)

nificantly decreases throughout pregnancy, while levels of protein C and antithrombin III remain normal. Inhibition of the fibrinolytic system is also thought to occur and is greatest during the third trimester. D-dimer is formed when crosslinked fibrin is lysed by plasmin. D-dimer levels increase throughout pregnancy and remain elevated during labor and delivery and the immediate postpartum period. D-dimer levels are also elevated in abruptio placentae, preterm labor, and HELLP.[3]

Recent studies suggest that DVT and PE during pregnancy may result from the interaction of both congenital and acquired risk factors. The presence of mutations in prothrombin and factor V genes are now recognized to be independent risk factors for thromboembolism during pregnancy. Gerhardt and collegues[4] reported that the relative risk of DVT and PE was 9.3 among women with factor V Leiden mutation and 15.2 among those with G20210A prothrombin gene mutations. The authors suggested that the higher-than-expected relative risk may reflect a relationship between the presence of the mutations and pregnancy-related alterations in coagulation or fibrinolysis. In this study, antithrombin III deficiency was also identified as an independent risk factor for thromboembolism. Other studies have reported that up to half of women who have a thrombotic event during pregnancy have an underlying genetic thrombophilia.[5]

Several independent obstetric risk factors have been associated with an increased risk of DVT and PE. These include prolonged bed rest (often prescribed for preterm labor or preeclampsia), hemorrhage, sepsis, instrumental and operative delivery, and multiparity. Traditionally, it was believed that the risk for venous thromboembolism was greatest in the late third trimester and immediately postpartum. However, recent investigations using objective criteria for diagnosis have suggested that antepartum DVT occurs as commonly as postpartum thrombosis. Several studies report that deep venous thrombosis occurs with almost equal frequency in each trimester.[6–9] In contrast, the risk of pulmonary embolism is thought to be greatest postpartum, especially following cesarean delivery.

DIAGNOSIS OF DEEP VENOUS THROMBOSIS

The signs and symptoms of deep venous thrombosis are widely recognized to be nonspecific. The clinical diagnosis is further hampered because symptoms such as leg swelling and discomfort occur frequently during pregnancy. Objective testing should therefore be used liberally if DVT is suspected. Diagnostic algorithms have been well established for the nonpregnant patient.[10] Although these strategies have not been validated in pregnant patients, it is reasonable to adapt them to this population.[2,11]

During pregnancy, venous thrombosis most frequently begins in either the calf veins or the iliac and femoral veins and shows a striking predilection for the left leg.[6,8,12] The signs and symptoms that accompany DVT vary greatly and depend on the degree of vascular occlusion, the presence of collateral circulation, and the intensity of the associated inflammatory response. The most common clinical presentation of DVT in pregnancy includes the triad of pain, tenderness, and unilateral leg swelling.[6] Homan's sign may or may not be present. Severe leg and back pain associated with marked edema of the leg and thigh is concerning for iliac vein thrombosis.

The differential diagnosis of deep venous thrombosis includes many conditions of the thigh and leg that result in a painful, swollen leg, including muscular sprains and strains, superficial thrombophlebitis, impaired venous or lymphatic flow, and popliteal inflammatory cysts (Baker's cyst). Superficial thrombophlebitis may be seen in patients with varicose veins. Surprisingly, superficial phlebitis occurs uncommonly during pregnancy. It is diagnosed clinically by the presence of a warm, erythematous, tender, and indurated cord within a superficial vein. Ancillary testing should be done (see below) to determine if there is extension to the deep veins. Supportive therapy including analgesia and elastic support are all that is necessary for superficial thrombophlebitis, and the inflammatory process should resolve within a few weeks. Antibiotics and anticoagulants are not indicated. A residual cord may be palpable for several months following the resolution of the acute inflammation.

Ultrasonography

The diagnosis of deep venous thrombosis in the nonpregnant patient is typically made by the combination of a strong clinical suspicion followed by objective diagnostic testing. Currently, compressive ultrasound (CUS) is believed to be the most accurate noninvasive test to diagnose DVT in the nonpregnant patient[13]. When compared to venography, the sensitivity, specificity, and negative predictive value of ultrasonography are about 91, 99, and 95 percent, respectively.[14] Clinical models utilizing clinical suspicion and CUS have been validated in this population. However, these studies have excluded pregnant patients, and recently, concern has been expressed that these models may not be valid during pregnancy given that these patients are younger and have different risk factors for VTE and have other characteristics not considered in these models.[15] However, it is still felt that these structured models may be useful in the initial evaluation of the pregnant patient.

Currently, we recommend that CUS be performed as the initial diagnostic study in pregnant patients with suspected DVT. Starting in the late second trimester, this study should be performed with the uterus displaced toward the patient's left side, to minimize the incidence of false-positive results due to decreased flow from vena caval compression. If positive, the diagnosis is confirmed and anticoagulant therapy can be begun. Patients with a negative study should either undergo serial testing over the next 7 to 14 days or be offered a unilateral limited venography with abdominal shielding if the clinical suspicion is high. Serial studies will allow detection of calf vein thrombosis that propagate proximally and have a potential to embolize.[14] In the nonpregnant patient, only about 20 percent of isolated calf vein thrombosis have been demonstrated to propagate proximally, and the use of serial CUS without concomitant anticoagulation has been demonstrated to be safe. The safety of witholding anticoagulant therapy during serial testing is also supported by one study in pregnant patients with clinically suspected DVT.[12] This strategy has also been suggested recently by others.[15] A diagnostic algorithm for the evaluation of DVT during pregnancy is presented in Fig. 12-1.

Other Diagnostic Modalities

Compression ultrasonography is more accurate than impedance plethysmography (IPG).[13,14,16,17] Heijboer and associates prospectively compared serial IPG with serial compression ultrasonography in 985 nonpregnant patients with clinically suspected DVT. Serial ultrasonography had a positive predictive value of 94 percent compared with 83 percent for IPG.[14]

The role of venography in diagnosing DVT during pregnancy remains unresolved. Compression ultrasonography is not as reliable as venography in detecting both distal calf thrombi and proximal iliofemoral thrombi, both of which may lead to pulmonary emboli during pregnancy. Venography is also more reliable in the diagnosis of recurrent deep venous thrombosis than are noninvasive studies. However, there is a reluctance by both clinicians and pregnant women to expose the fetus to ionizing radiation, even though venography is the gold standard to which noninvasive studies have been compared. Venography is not often used because it is invasive and carries the potential risk of radiation exposure to the fetus. However, exposure data do not support this concern.[18] The estimated fetal radiation exposure with a unilateral venogram is approximately 0.314 rad (0.00314 Gy). Bilateral venography without abdominal shielding results in fetal exposure of <1.0 rad. Fetal radiation exposure of less than 5 rads has not been associated with adverse fetal outcomes.

Venography should be considered if isolated iliac vein thrombosis is suspected. Alternative methods for diagnosing this condition include CT scan and MRI. MRI has been demonstrated to have a high degree of sensitivity and specificity in the diagnosis of pelvic thrombosis in nonpregnant patients, and studies involving pregnant women appear promising.[19] The use of MRI during pregnancy has not been reported to result in any adverse effect on the fetus, but the long-term result risk of electromagnetic exposure is unknown. CT scan can also be used to diagnose iliac vein thrombosis but is associated with limited ionizing radiation to the fetus.

DIAGNOSIS OF PULMONARY EMBOLISM

The diagnosis of pulmonary embolism (PE) is complex in the nonpregnant patient and no studies have been done to validate diagnostic strategies specifically in pregnancy. The clinical diagnosis of PE has a wide spectrum of signs and symptoms that are often further confounded by the physiologic changes of pregnancy. Dyspnea, tachypnea, and pleuritic pain have high sensitivity but low specificity for PE.[20] Other common signs include pulmonary crackles or rales, tachycardia (>100 beats/min), a pleural friction rub, and an increased pulmonic second heart sound. In one study, dyspnea or tachypnea was found in 90 percent of 383 patients with PE. Dyspnea, tachypnea, or pleuritic pain was present in 97 percent.[20]

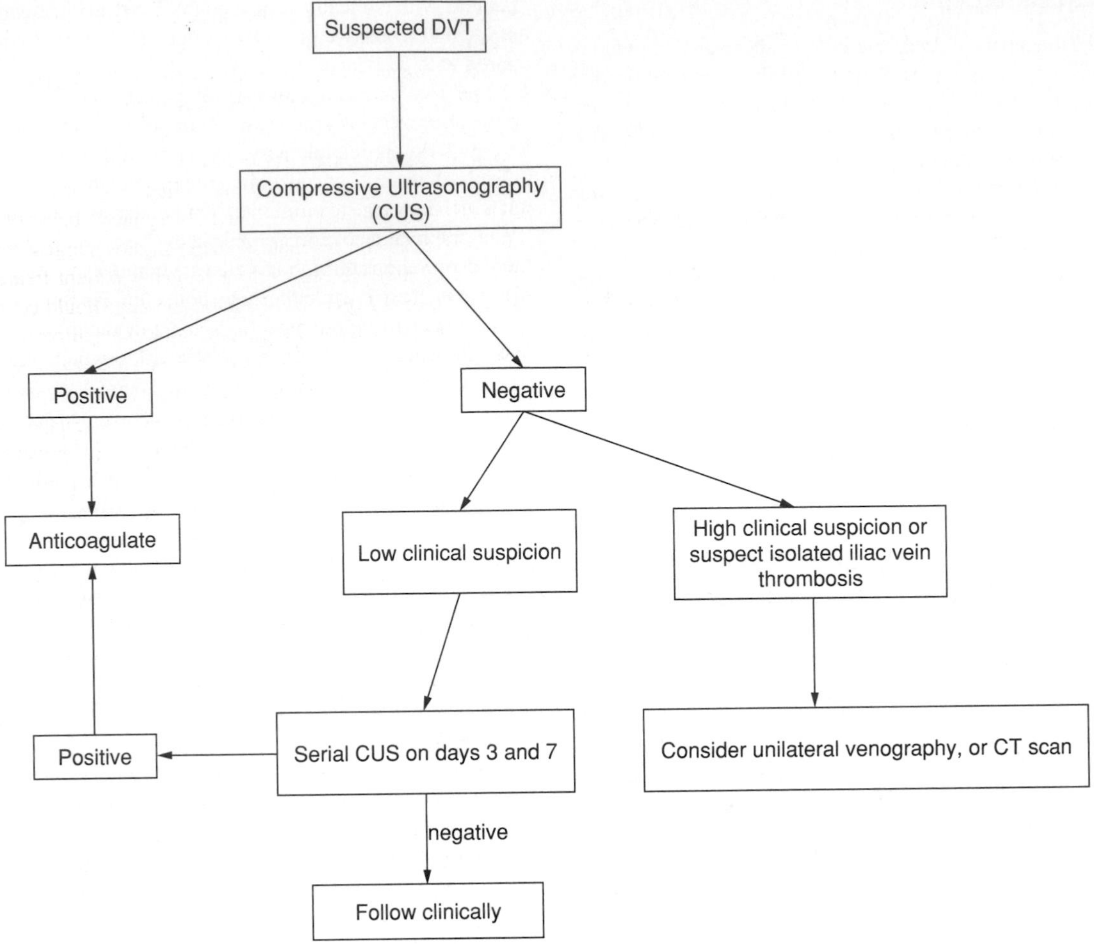

Fig. 12-1. Diagnosis of suspected DVT during pregnancy.

The signs and symptoms associated with PE can be found in a wide variety of other acute pulmonary disorders. Asthma is perhaps the most common pulmonary condition encountered in the pregnant woman, followed by pneumonia and pulmonary edema. Pneumonia and asthma can occur at any point during the pregnancy or in the postpartum period. Pulmonary edema is most frequently seen at term, in association with preeclampsia, or as a result of excess fluid administration at the time of labor and delivery. These conditions are usually excluded based on the patient's history and examination and the results of a chest radiograph.

Diagnostic tests such as electrocardiograms, chest roentgenograms, and arterial blood gases may support the diagnosis of PE or identify other etiologies for the patient's complaints. A shielded posterior-anterior chest x-ray (CXR) with lateral views should be obtained to rule out pneumonia or pulmonary edema. A CXR is also necessary for an accurate interpretation of the ventilation-perfusion (V/Q) scan. Nonspecific CXR abnormalities such as atelectasis, unilateral pleural effusions, areas of consolidation, or an elevation of the hemidiaphragm are common in patients with PE, as are nonspecific electrocardiographic changes. The characteristic $S_1Q_3T_3$ pattern is rarely present.

Most clinically significant pulmonary emboli are associated with hypoxemia (arterial Pao_2 <85 mmHg) and a widened or increased alveolar-to-arterial oxygen gradient (PAO_2-Pao_2 >20 mmHg). However, 10 to 15 percent of patients with PE can be expected to have a normal Pao_2.

During the third trimester of pregnancy, the Pa_{O_2} may be as much as 15 mmHg lower in the supine position compared to the upright condition. Therefore, during the third trimester arterial blood gases should be measured with the patient sitting upright. The alveolar-arterial oxygen gradient was reported to be <15 mmHg in 58 percent of a small series of pregnant women with documented PE, making that calculation an unreliable screening test for PE in pregnancy.[21]

Currently, the radionuclide lung imaging or ventilation-perfusion (V/Q) scan is the primary screening technique used in the evaluation for pulmonary embolism in pregnancy. If the result is normal, the diagnosis of PE can be excluded. A high-probability scan is sufficient evidence to begin anticoagulant therapy. Unfortunately, the majority of patients with PE will have a V/Q scan interpreted as either of low or intermediate (indeterminate) probability and will need to undergo pulmonary angiography or pulmonary CT scanning. Spiral CT is more sensitive and has better interobserver agreement than V/Q scanning for the diagnosis of pulmonary embolism, but it may not detect subsegmental emboli.[22,23] MR angiography is currently under investigation, but also may not be sensitive enough to detect small segmental emboli.[24]

Pregnant patients should be reassured by their physicians that the estimated radiation exposure to the fetus with the combination of chest radiograph, V/Q scanning, and pulmonary angiography is less than 0.5 rad (.005cGy).[18] The estimated radiation dose for a V/Q scan alone is about 0.1 rad. A diagnostic algorithm for the evaluation of PE during pregnancy is presented in Fig. 12-2.

MANAGEMENT

It is currently recommended that pregnant women be admitted for inpatient treatment of DVT or PE. All women who are evaluted in the ED at >12 weeks' gestation should have fetal heart tones determined as part of the initial maternal assessment. Survivable gestations (>24 weeks) should be managed closely with the obstetrics team and continuous fetal monitoring is desirable. Maternal resuscitation and stabilization is the best care for the fetus as well. Maternal oxygen saturation should be maintained at >95 percent to prevent maternal and fetal hypoxemia. Patients with hemodynamic compromise require ICU monitoring. After adequate fluid resuscitation, dopamine is the preferred agent for hypotension to maintain maternal BP >80 mmHg, although pressors may further reduce uterine blood flow. In patients with a strong suspicion of PE, anticoagulant therapy may be initiated pending confirmatory diagnostic studies. Analgesics such as morphine should be used as necessary.

Once diagnosed, venous thromboembolism requires rapid and prolonged anticoagulation to prevent extension of the thrombus, restore venous patency, and limit the risk of PE or its recurrence. Clinical experience and retrospective cohort studies have established heparin as the safest anticoagulant to use during pregnancy because it does not cross the placenta. Cohort studies suggest that the risk of major bleeding in a pregnant patient treated with heparin is 2 percent.[2] Heparin therapy should be instituted for all patients with distal deep venous thrombosis (e.g., in the calf vein), proximal venous thrombosis (e.g., in the iliofemoral or pelvic veins), and PE. One study of nonpregnant patients reported that 40 percent of distal calf vein thromboses remained isolated, 40 percent were lysed, and 20 percent propagated.[25] The risk for propagation in pregnant patients must therefore be substantial.

Since therapeutic regimens have not been well established in pregnant patients, heparin therapy should be initiated according to the current recommendations for nonpregnant patients.[2,26] However, heparin requirements appear to increase during pregnancy because of increases in heparin-binding proteins, plasma volume, and renal clearance. Heparin is a class B drug in pregnancy, and is not excreted in breast milk. The first goal of anticoagulant therapy is to provide sufficiently high starting doses to achieve therapeutic levels quickly in order to minimize the risk of recurrent thromboembolism. Therapy with unfractionated heparin should be initiated with an intravenous bolus of 5,000 U (80 U/kg) followed by a continuous infusion of at least 30,000 U per 24 hours[2,27]. Alternatively, heparin can be dosed initially according to a weight based nomogram starting at 18 U/kg/h (Table 12-2). The infusion should then be adjusted on the basis of laboratory tests, such as an activated partial thromboplastin time (aPTT), INR, or heparin level. An aPTT value 1.5 to 2.5 times the patient's baseline value, an International Normalized Ratio (INR) of 2.5, or a heparin concentration of 0.2 to 0.4 U/mL is the recommended target therapeutic range for heparin for both DVT and PE.

Heparin therapy should be monitored every 6 hours in the first 24 to 48 hours of therapy and the dose adjusted according to one of the standard nomograms for heparin therapy.[26,28] Continuous infusion heparin therapy should be continued for 5 to 7 days, followed by long-term outpatient anticoagulant therapy using subcutaneous heparin for the remainder of the pregnancy. Anticoagulation should be continued for at least 6 weeks postpartum, and the duration of treatment determined by the underlying reason for thrombosis.

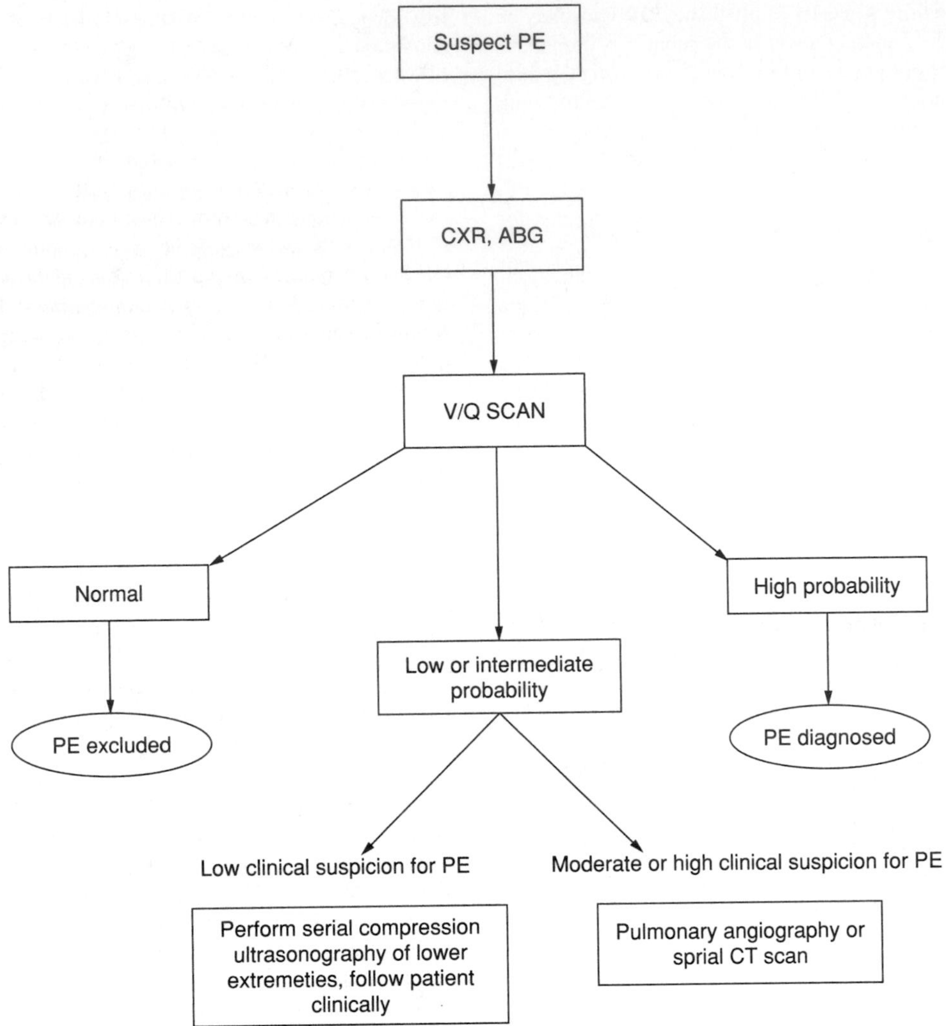

Fig. 12-2. Diagnosis of suspected PE during pregnancy.

Subcutaneous adjusted-dose heparin is typically administered either 2 or 3 three times a day to maintain a midinterval aPTT within the therapeutic range (e.g., 1.5 to 2.5 times control).

Low-molecular-weight heparin (LMWH) is an alternative treatment for acute venous thromboembolism. It has been demonstrated that LMWH does not cross the placenta, and preliminary studies involving pregnant patients have been encouraging. Although the optimal dosing is still unclear, most clinicians adjust the dosage based on maternal weight. The dose of enoxaparin is 1 mg/kg subcutaneously bid, or 1.5 mg/kg subcutaneously per day. The dose of dalteparin is 120 IU/kg subcutaneously bid or 200 IU/kg subcutaneously per day. The bioavailability of LMWH during pregnancy is improved over unfractionated heparin because of a reduction in protein binding; however, increases in renal clearance and volume of distribution of the drug may necessitate increasing the dosage throughout pregnancy.[27,29] It is suggested that peak antifactor Xa levels (drawn 3 to 4 hours after last injection) be monitored every 4 to 6 weeks and the dose be adjusted to maintain levels between 0.3 IU and 0.7 IU. Recently, it has been suggested that LMWH not be used for anticoagulation in pregnant women with prosthetic heart valves because of a lack of efficacy in these patients.[30]

Table 12-2. Doses for Anticoagulation[a]

Heparin 5,000 IU intravenous bolus, followed by 30,000 IU per 24 hours
OR
Heparin 80 U/kg actual body weight, followed by 18 U/kg/h
OR
Enoxaparin 1 mg/kg SQ bid or 1.5 mg/kg SQ qd
OR
Dalteparin 120 IU/kg SQ bid or 200 IU/kg SQ qd

[a]Warfarin is contraindicated in pregnancy.

Warfarin should not be used during pregnancy because of its adverse effects on fetal development during the first and second trimesters. In addition, warfarin readily crosses the placenta and can result in fetal and neonatal hemorrhage.

Postpartum Venous Thromboembolism

The postpartum patient is managed in the same way as the nonpregnant patient. Intravenous heparin or LMWH is initiated as described above, and warfarin may be started on the first day of heparin administration. Warfarin therapy is adjusted according to the prothrombin time (PT), expressed as the INR. In patients with venous thromboembolism, warfarin therapy should be adjusted to maintain an INR of 2.0 to 3.0. Warfarin therapy produces an early anticoagulant effect (secondary to a rapid fall in factor VII and protein C levels) before it achieves a consistent antithrombotic effect (which lags by at least 24 to 48 hours). It is therefore important to continue heparin therapy or LMWH for at least 4 days and not discontinue it until the INR has been in the therapeutic range for 2 consecutive days after the initiation of warfarin therapy.[26] Warfarin therapy is continued for at least 3 months following the acute event to minimize the risk of recurrence. Warfarin use is not a contraindication to breast-feeding. Since warfarin use during pregnancy is associated with the development of birth defects, reliable contraception should be practiced while taking this drug.

Management During Labor

Anticoagulant therapy rarely presents a problem at the time of delivery. Heparin has a short, dose-dependent half-life regardless of the route of administration. Women on a subcutaneous adjusted-dose or fixed, low-dose regimen of unfractionated heparin should be instructed to discontinue heparin use with the onset of regular uterine contractions. Upon the woman's presentation to the hospital, an aPTT or heparin level should be measured. The risk of hemorrhage at the time of vaginal delivery or cesarean section has not been reported to be significantly increased when the heparin level is less than 0.4 U/mL. Regional anesthesia is usually not contraindicated if the aPTT is normal and heparin has not been administered within 4 to 6 hours of the delivery. It has been recommended that LMWH not be used 18 to 24 hours before the administration of epidural for pain relief during labor.[30] Protamine sulfate can be administered to patients with a heparin level greater than 0.4 U/mL or an aPTT or INR greater than 2.7 times control. One milligram of protamine sulfate will neutralize 100 U of heparin with an almost immediate onset. Protamine sulfate is typically administered in small doses (less than 50 mg given intravenously over 10 minutes) and titrated against the whole-blood clotting time.

Anticoagulant therapy may be restarted within 4 to 6 hours postpartum if the patient is stable and in the absence of heavy uterine bleeding. A continuous heparin infusion should be resumed after an 80 U/kg loading dose. Warfarin therapy may be initiated on the same day or as soon as the patient can tolerate oral medications, as described above.

Thrombolytic therapy should be avoided in the pregnant patient except in life-threatening situations because of the risk of substantial maternal bleeding, especially at the time of delivery and immediately postpartum. The risk of placental abruption and fetal death due to these agents is currently unknown. Inferior vena cava filters have been used safely and effectively in pregnant women. Their use is generally restricted to those patients who have recurrent PE despite adequate anticoagulant therapy and those in whom heparin therapy is contraindicated because of a high risk of complications or a history of an adverse reaction to heparin, such as heparin-induced thrombocytopenia. Suprarenal placement has been suggested to avoid injury to the gravid uterus.

REFERENCES

1. Berg CJ, Atrash HK, Koonin LM, Tucker M: Pregnancy-related morbidity in the United States, 1987–1990. *Obstet Gynecol* 88:161, 1996.
2. Toglia MR, Weg JG: Venous thromboembolism during pregnancy. *N Engl J Med* 335:108, 1996.
3. Nolan TE, Smith RP, Devoe LD: Maternal plasma D-dimer levels in normal and uncomplicated pregnancies. *Obstet Gynecol* 81:235–238, 1993.

4. Gerhardt A, Scharf RE, Beckman MW, et al: Prothrombin and factor V mutations in women with a history of thrombosis during pregnancy and the puerperium. *N Engl J Med* 342:374, 2000.
5. Grandone E, Margaglione M, Colaizzo D, D'Andrea G, Cappucci G, Brancaccio V, et al. Genetic susceptibility to pregnancy related venous thromboembolism: roles of factor V Leiden, prothrombin G20210A, and methylenetetrahydrofolate reductase C677T mutations. *Am J Obstet Gynecol* 179:1324–1328, 1998.
6. Gherman RB, Goodwin TM, Leung B, Byrne JD, Hethumumi R, Montoro M. Incidence, clinical characteristics, and timing of objectively diagnosed venous thromboembolism during pregnancy. *Obstet Gynecol* 94:730–734, 1999.
7. Ginsberg JS, Brill-Edwards P, Burrows RF, et al: Venous thrombosis during pregnancy: Leg and trimester of presentation. *Thromb Haemost* 67:519, 1992.
8. Bergqvist A, Bergqvist D, Hallbook T: Deep vein thrombosis during pregnancy: A prospective study. *Acta Obstet Gynecol Scand* 62:443, 1983.
9. Tengborn L, Bergqvist D, Matzsch R, et al: Recurrent thromboembolism in pregnancy and the puerperium. *Am J Obstet Gynecol* 28:107, 1985.
10. Perrier A, Desmarais S, Miron MJ, et al. Non-invasive diagnosis of venous thromboembolism in outpatients. *Lancet* 353:190–95, 1999.
11. Toglia MR, Nolan TE: Venous thromboembolism during pregnancy: A current review of diagnosis and management. *Obstet Gynecol Survey* 52:1, 1997.
12. Hull RD, Raskob GE, Carter CJ: Serial impedance plethysmography in pregnant patients with clinically suspected deep-vein thrombosis: Clinical validity of negative findings. *Ann Intern Med* 112:663, 1990.
13. Lensing AWA, Prandoni P, Brandes D, et al: Detection of deep-vein thrombosis by real time B-mode ultrasonography. *N Engl J Med* 320:342, 1989.
14. Heijboer H, Buller HR, Lensing AWA, et al: A comparison of real-time compression ultrasonography with impedance plethysmography for the diagnosis of deep-vein thrombosis in symptomatic outpatients. *N Engl J Med* 329:1365, 1993.
15. Chan WS, Ginsberg JS. Diagnosis of deep vein thrombosis and pulmonary embolism in pregnancy. *Thromb Res* 107:85, 2002.
16. Polak JF, Wilkinson DL: Ultrasonographic diagnosis of symptomatic deep venous thrombosis in pregnancy. *Am J Obstet Gynecol* 165:625, 1991.
17. Kearon C, Julian JA, Newman TE, Ginsberg, JS: Noninvasive diagnosis of deep venous thrombosis. *Ann Intern Med* 128:663–677, 1998.
18. Ginsberg JS, Hirsh J, Rainbow AJ, Coates G: Risks to the fetus of radiologic procedures used in the diagnosis of maternal venous thromboembolic disease. *Thromb Haemost* 61:189, 1989.
19. Spritzer CE, Evans AC, Kay HH. Magnetic resonance imaging of deep venous thrombosis in pregnant women with lower extremity edema. *Obstet Gynecol* 85:603–607, 1995.
20. Stein PD, Terrin ML, Hales CA, et al: Clinical, laboratory, roentgenographic and electrocardiographic findings in patients with acute pulmonary embolism and no pre-existing cardiac or pulmonary disease. *Chest* 100:598, 1991.
21. Powrie R, Larson L, Rosene-Montella K, et al: Alveolar-arterial oxygen gradient in acute pulmonary embolism in pregnancy. *Am J Obstet Gynecol* 178:394–398, 1998.
22. Grenier PA, Beigelman C: Spiral computed tomographic scanning and magnetic resonance angiography for the diagnosis of pulmonary embolism. *Thorax* 53(Suppl 2):S25–S31, 1998.
23. Ferretti G, Bosson JL, Buffoz PD, et al: Acute pulmonary embolism: role of helical CT in 164 patients with intermediate probability at ventilation-perfusion scintigraphy and normal results at duplex ultrasonography of the legs. *Radiology* 205:453–458, 1997.
24. Gupta A, Frazer CK, Ferguson JM: Acute pulmonary embolism: Diagnosis with MR angiography. *Radiology* 210:353–359, 1999.
25. Lohr JM, James KV, Deshmukh RM, et al: Calf vein thrombi are not benign findings. *Am J Surg* 170:86–90, 1995.
26. Cruickshank MK, Levine MN, Hirsh J, et al: A standard heparin nomogram for the management of heparin therapy. *Arch Intern Med* 151:333, 1991.
27. American College of Obstetricians and Gynecologists. Thromboembolism in pregnancy. ACOG Practice Bulletin 19. Washington, DC. 2000.
28. Ginsberg JS: Drug therapy: Management of venous thromboembolism. *N Engl J Med* 335:1816, 1996.
29. Chan WS, Ray JG: Low molecular weight heparin use during pregnancy: Issues of safety and practicality. *Obstet Gynecol Survey* 54:649, 1999.
30. American College of Obstetricians and Gynecologists. Safety of Lovenox in pregnancy. Committee Opinion No. 276. *Obstet Gynecol* 100:845–46, 2002.

13

Pulmonary Disorders

Esam Alhamad
Fernando J. Martinez

KEY POINTS

- Symptoms of pathologic dyspnea in pregnancy
  - Acute
  - Worsen with exertion
  - Occur at rest
  - Severe
  - Associated symptoms present (e.g., chest pain, diaphoresis)
- Maternal-fetal effects of asthma
  - Preeclampsia and hypertension
  - Low birth weight
  - Preterm delivery
  - Maternal asthma status during pregnancy: one-third improve; one-third have no change; one-third worsen

PHYSIOLOGIC CHANGES DURING PREGNANCY

Structural Changes with Pregnancy

The structure of the respiratory system changes dramatically during pregnancy. This includes mucosal changes of the respiratory tract leading to hyperemia, hypersecretion, and mucosal edema, which are most prominent in the third trimester.[1] This is generally attributed to the effects of estrogen and are associated with frequent symptoms of rhinitis.[2] The progressive increase in uterine size and maternal weight result in increased circumference of the abdomen and lower chest wall (approximately 5 to 7 cm), elevation of the diaphragm (approximately 4 to 5 cm) and widening of the costal angle (approximately 50 percent).[1,2] The change in chest wall configuration peaks by 37 weeks of gestation and generally returns to normal within 24 weeks of delivery.[2] There are no changes in maximum inspiratory pressure or diaphragmatic pressure, although diaphragm fatigue has been reported to occur during labor.[3–5]

Pulmonary Function Changes During Pregnancy

By the third trimester, there is a decrease in expiratory reserve volume (ERV), residual volume (RV), and functional residual capacity (FRC) (about 17–20 percent)[6] (Fig. 13-1). At term there is no change in vital capacity (VC), but tidal volume (V_T) increases by about 500 mL. Lung compliance and diffusion capacity change little during pregnancy.[1]

The respiratory changes in ventilation are illustrated in Fig. 13-2. A dramatic increase in minute ventilation (V_E) occurs, which is predominantly caused by a rise in V_T. Respiratory rate changes little throughout pregnancy. Alveolar ventilation rises approximately 50 to 70 percent, as does metabolic rate. Alveolar hyperventilation is associated with decreases in Pa_{CO_2} from 37 to 40 mmHg to 27 to 34 mmHg, which begins by 8 to 12 weeks and plateaus by 20 weeks of gestation.[2] The fall in alveolar P_{CO_2} is associated with an increased alveolar P_{O_2} (P_{AO_2}). Moving from a sitting to supine position is associated with an increased $P(A\text{-}a)_{O_2}$ (approximately 6 mmHg) and drop in Pa_{O_2} (approximately 13 mmHg).

Dyspnea and Cough during Pregnancy

Dyspnea

Determining when dyspnea is pathologic is challenging, since it occurs frequently during normal pregnancy. Milne and colleagues assessed 62 healthy pregnant women eight times during a normal pregnancy[6] to determine the frequency of physiologic dyspnea. Before 16 weeks, the proportion of women reporting dyspnea was about 24 percent; between 16 and 19 weeks, 48 percent; and by 31 weeks, 76 percent. More than 30 percent reported moderately severe dyspnea by the thirty-sixth week of gestation. The sensation of physiologic dyspnea is presumed to be the perception of increased respiratory muscle effort.[2,5]

In contrast, pathologic dyspnea from cardiac or pulmonary disease can occur at rest, may be more severe, and interferes with the ability to exercise. Associated symptoms such as paroxysmal nocturnal dyspnea, orthopnea, and cough should be sought as they may suggest associated pulmonary or heart disease.

History and physical examination should center on the cardiovascular and pulmonary systems, with a focus on

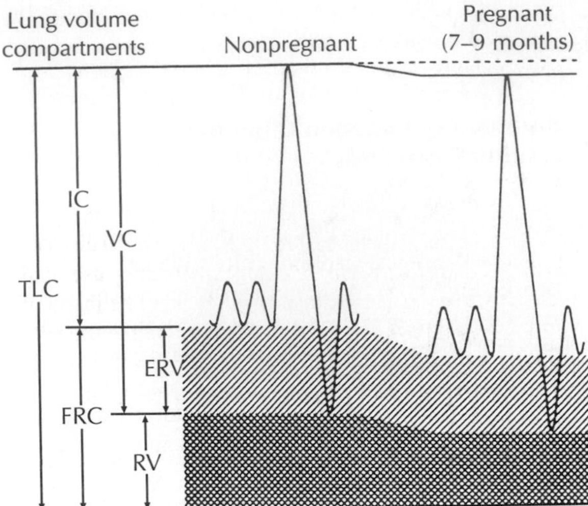

Fig. 13-1. Changes in lung volumes in women 7 to 9 months pregnant compared with nonpregnant women. TLC, total lung capacity; IC, inspiratory capacity; FRC, functional residual capacity; VC, vital capacity; RV, residual volume; ERV, expiratory reserve volume. (Adapted with permission from Elkus R, Popovich J: Respiratory physiology in pregnancy. *Clin Chest Med* 13:555–565, 1992.)[1]

differentiating normal from abnormal findings. Table 13-1 lists signs of physiologic dyspnea. Unfortunately, many of the physiologic changes of pregnancy can limit the value of physical examination. Basilar rales may be normal late in pregnancy due to basilar atelectasis. Tachypnea is abnormal. Hyperventilation is frequently seen as a normal finding but if normal, it is due to an increased V_T, not an increase in respiratory rate. If pathologic dyspnea is suspected in a previously healthy woman, pulmonary embolism, pneumonia, asthma, or pneumothorax should be considered.

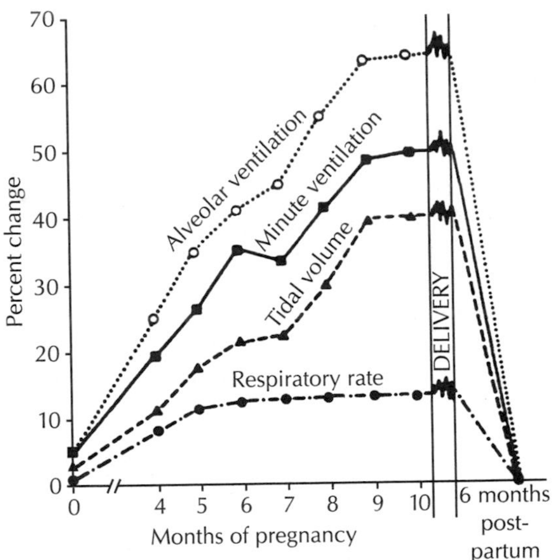

Fig. 13-2. Respiratory changes during pregnancy. (Adapted with permission from Elkus R, Popovich J: Respiratory physiology in pregnancy. *Clin Chest Med* 13:555–565, 1992.)[1]

Cough

The differential diagnosis of cough is the same in pregnant women as in nonpregnant women. Acute cough is most often due to viral infection. In women of childbearing age, atypical pathogens such as *Mycoplasma, Chlamydia,* and pertussis should be considered.[7] For severe cough with sputum production or fever, antibiotics such as amoxicillin or azithromycin can be given.

A cough lasting longer than 3 to 4 weeks in a nonsmoker suggests asthma, gastroesophageal reflux disease (GERD), or postnasal drainage. These processes account for over 90 percent of chronic cough in adults.[8]

Table 13-1. Symptoms of Physiologic Dyspnea during Normal Pregnancy

Occur frequently
Onset 1st or 2nd trimester
Greatest near term
Slowly progressive
Don't interfere with activity
Rare at rest
Not severe
No associated symptoms

Asthma is discussed subsequently and GERD is also discussed in Chap. 14. GERD is best treated during pregnancy with dietary modification, avoidance of medications that decrease lower esophageal sphincter tone, elevation of the head of the bed, and antacid therapy.[9] A recent report of 134 women exposed to omeprazole during pregnancy were compared with 1547 controls with no significant difference in the incidence of major malformations.[10] Based on current data, ranitidine remains the drug of choice.[10,11]

Antihistamines are useful for chronic cough due to postnasal drainage, but because of a high risk of adverse reactions in neonates, antihistamines should be avoided in nursing mothers because many are excreted in breast milk.[12] A recent review has determined that tripelennamine, chlorpheniramine, and clemastine are FDA Category B.[11] They can be prescribed if necessary, but should be avoided while breast-feeding. Decongestants are class C drugs. Pseudoephedrine has been reported to be associated with infant gastroschisis if used in the first trimester.[13] Nasal steroids, with the exception of triamcinolone and cromolyn, appear to be safe and effective in pregnancy.[6,14] In pregnant women with unresponsive rhinitis, asthma should be suspected. An empiric trial of bronchodilators and inhaled steroids should be considered. Bronchoprovocation testing is of unclear safety during pregnancy although methacholine likely poses little risk.

RESPIRATORY INFECTIONS DURING PREGNANCY

Bacterial Pneumonia

Bacterial pneumonia can have significant adverse effects on both the mother and fetus. Changes in cellular immunity during pregnancy include decreases in lymphocyte proliferative response, natural killer cell activity, and numbers of circulating helper T cells.[15,16] Maternal outcome from pneumonia generally depends on the presence of comorbidities such as HIV infection, cystic fibrosis, or asthma.[17] Premature labor and low birth weight are important adverse fetal outcomes.[18]

The limited data in pregnant patients with pneumonia suggests that no organism is identified in the majority of the studies. When a pathogen is recovered, the distribution appears similar to that seen in nonpregnant patients with *Streptococcus pneumoniae* the most common and *Haemophilus* species and atypical pathogens (*Mycoplasma pneumoniae* and *Legionella* species) seen less frequently.

The American Thoracic Society disease severity classification and treatment recommendations for community-acquired pneumonia are listed in Table 13-2.[19,20] The modifying factors that increase the risk of specific organisms are listed in Table 13-3.

Comorbid disorders including chronic pulmonary or cardiac disease, diabetes mellitus, hepatic or renal disease, cancer, current or recent smoking, illicit drug use, and HIV infection[17] are associated with a higher likelihood of a complicated course and should be admitted to the hospital. Multiple authors have identified an elevated respiratory rate (>20 to 30 breaths/min) as an independent predictor of complicated community-acquired pneumonia.[21] Hypotension (systolic blood pressure <90 mmHg or diastolic BP <60 mmHg) is also a useful predictor of a complicated infection.[17] Maternal hypoxia may be particularly poorly tolerated by the fetus.[22] Oxygen saturation should be measured, and patients on room air with Sa_{O_2} <92 percent should have an arterial blood gas measurement and should be admitted. A maternal P_{O_2} of >70 mmHg should be maintained to avoid maternal and fetal toxicity.[23] The need for an inspired oxygen concentration of over 60 percent to maintain adequate oxygenation, or the need to apply noninvasive positive pressure ventilation (NIPPV) are both poor prognostic indicators.[24] Other indicators of severe disease include anemia, severe leukocytosis or leukopenia, and abnormalities of electrolytes or renal or hepatic function.

Antibiotic Therapy

After disease severity is established and a decision to treat the patient is made, the physician must decide on the appropriate antibiotic therapy. The guidelines of the American Thoracic Society are useful in making this decision as illustrated in Tables 13-2 & 13-3. Antibiotic therapy in pregnant individuals is complicated by alterations in pharmacokinetics of various antibiotics due to a greater volume of distribution, reduced plasma protein concentration, more rapid clearance, increased hepatic metabolism, and erratic oral absorption of some drugs.[12,14] Additionally, antibiotics have varying effects on fetal growth and development.[11,12,14,25]

Therapeutic decisions in pneumonia have been complicated by the increasing resistance among *Streptococcus pneumoniae* isolates worldwide.[26,27] Rising *in vitro* resistance has been noted to β-lactams as well as macrolides,[28]

Table 13-2. American Thoracic Society Classification of Patients with Community-Acquired Pneumonia, Adapted for Pregnant Patients

Group	Characteristics	Likely Organisms	Appropriate Antibiotics
I	Outpatients, no cardiopulmonary disease, no modifying factors (see Table 13-3)	*Streptococcus pneumoniae* *Mycoplasma pneumoniae* *Chlamydia pneumoniae* *Haemophilus influenzae* Viruses *Legionella* spp.	PO azithromycin or erythromycin
II	Outpatient, with cardiopulmonary disease, and/or other modifying factors (see Table 13-3)	*Streptococcus pneumoniae* *Mycoplasma pneumoniae* *Chlamydia pneumoniae* Mixed infections *Haemophilus influenzae* Enteric gram-negatives Viruses *Moraxella catarrhalis* *Legionella* spp. Aspiration (anaerobes)	PO β-Lactam Cefpodoxime Cefuroxime or amoxicillin-clavulanate + Oral Erythromycin or azithromycin
IIIa	Inpatient, not in ICU; cardiopulmonary disease and/or modifying factors (see Table 13-3)	*Streptococcus pneumoniae* *Haemophilus influenzae* *Mycoplasma pneumoniae* *Chlamydia pneumoniae* Mixed infection Enteric gram-negatives Aspiration Polymicrobial Aerobic gram-negative Viruses *Legionella* spp.	IV β-lactam + IV Erythromycin or azithromycin
IIIb	Inpatient, not in ICU; no cardiopulmonary disease, no modifying factors (see Table 13-3)	*Streptococcus pneumoniae* *Haemophilus influenzae* *Mycoplasma pneumoniae* *Chlamydia pneumoniae* Mixed infection Viruses *Legionella* spp.	IV azithromycin

(*Continues*)

Table 13-2. *(Continued)* American Thoracic Society Classification of Patients with Community-Acquired Pneumonia, Adapted for Pregnant Patients

Group	Characteristics	Likely Organisms	Appropriate Antibiotics
IVa	ICU-admitted, no risks for *Pseudomonas aeruginosa* (see Table 13-3)	*Streptococcus pneumoniae* *Legionella* spp. *Haemophilus influenzae* Enteric gram-negative bacilli *Staphylococcus aureus* *Mycoplasma pneumoniae* Viruses *Chlamydia pneumoniae* *Mycobacterium tuberculosis* Endemic fungi	IV β-lactam (cefotaxime, ceftriaxone) + IV Erythromycin or azithromycin
IVb	ICU-admitted plus risk factor for *Pseudomonas aeruginosa* (see Table 13-3)	As in IVa + *Pseudomonas aeruginosa*	IV antipseudomonal β-lactam + IV aminoglycoside + IV Erythromycin or azithromycin

Source: Adapted from Niedermann et al.[19,20]

with remarkable regional difference in the prevalence of resistance.[29] Furthermore, multidrug resistance has also risen among these isolates[30] with a higher prevalence of cephalosporin and macrolide resistance in penicillin resistant pneumococcal isolates.[31] Risk factors for infection with resistant isolates have been enumerated, and include exposure to recent antibiotics or a child in day care.

Although the clinical implications of *in vitro* resistance remain controversial, there have been well-described failures (albeit limited in number) of antibiotics in the setting

Table 13-3. Modifying Factors That Increase Risk of Specific Organisms in Patients with Community-Acquired Pneumonia

Penicillin-resistant and drug-resistant pneumococci
- Age >65 years
- β-Lactam therapy within the past 3 months
- Alcoholism
- Immune-suppressive illness (including therapy with corticosteroids)
- Multiple medical comorbidities
- Exposure to a child in a day care center

Enteric gram-negatives
- Residence in a nursing home
- Underlying cardiopulmonary disease
- Multiple medical comorbidities
- Recent antibiotic therapy

Pseudomonas aeruginosa
- Structural lung disease (bronchiectasis)
- Corticosteroid therapy (>10 mg prednisone per day)
- Broad-spectrum antibiotic therapy for >7 days in the past month
- Malnutrition

Source: Adapted from Niedermann et al.[19]

of antimicrobial resistance. In addition, a recent CDC based study confirmed an increased likelihood of late hospital mortality in patients with invasive pneumococcal pneumonia with high level resistance (penicillin MIC $\geq$ 4 μg/ml).[32] Other studies, with lesser statistical power, have not confirmed an independent effect of antimicrobial resistance on mortality.[33,34] The presence of suppurative complications in patients hospitalized with CAP may be increased in the presence of pneumococcal, penicillin nonsusceptibility[34] while the likelihood of mortality in infections with resistant pneumococcus may be increased in patients infected with HIV.[35] As such, recent society recommendations have emphasized the potential clinical implications of infection with resistant isolates and targeting specific therapy to these patients. For example, in patients with a higher likelihood of β-lactam or macrolide resistance would be treated with combination, antimicrobial therapy or a fluoroquinolone.[19,36,37] The latter recommendation would be problematic for the pregnant patient.

The recommendations of the ATS can been modified for pregnancy. Group I individuals are best treated with an appropriate macrolide. A recent study examined the value of a prospective management protocol emphasizing the use of erythromycin therapy in 99/119 patients hospitalized with pneumonia.[38] This form of monotherapy was felt to be adequate in all but one of the patients. Other studies have confirmed the value of such therapy in large groups of patients with community acquired pneumonia.[39] Group II individuals are best managed with a cephalosporin and a macrolide. Group IIIa patients are best managed with a second- or third-generation cephalosporin and a macrolide. Group IIIb patients should be given intravenous macrolide. A Group IV patient is best treated with combination therapy with an antipseudomonal β-lactam antibiotic and an aminoglycoside with additional macrolide therapy to ensure coverage of atypical pathogens.

The duration of intravenous antibiotics remains controversial. Recent investigators have suggested that stability on the third hospital day, as determined by the lack of an obvious reason for continued hospitalization, high-risk pathogen or life-threatening complication, identified "low risk" individuals who could be switched to oral antibiotics. The length of stay was 4 days with no impact on survival, short and long term complications and patient satisfaction.[40] In fact, a recent meta-analysis of randomized trials confirmed a decrease in length of stay with switch therapy protocols.[39] Whether these data are applicable to the pregnant patient is unclear; clearly close outpatient follow-up is required to ensure optimal outcome after discharge.

Supportive Therapy

Supportive treatment does not differ in the pregnant patient and most include adequate hydration and antipyretics. Supplemental oxygen is crucial to maintain a maternal paO_2 greater than 70 mm Hg given the fetal intolerance of even mild decreases in maternal paO_2. Close monitoring is required and aggressive respiratory support employed if respiratory failure develops.[41] Tocolysis should be considered if preterm labor complicates pneumonia in pregnancy. There is no evidence that elective delivery will result in an overall improvement in respiratory function.[42] However if there is evidence of fetal or maternal compromise, delivery should be accomplished.

Viral Respiratory Infections

Influenza

Influenza is caused by one of the myxoviruses, types A, B, or C. Type A influenza is usually the source of epidemic infection, and as such is the most problematic. Historical data support a high mortality rate in pregnant women experiencing influenza pneumonia. In the pandemic of 1918–1919, influenza during pregnancy had a 30 percent maternal mortality, which rose to 50 percent in the presence of pneumonia. Furthermore, influenza pneumonia in the third trimester was associated with a 61 percent mortality.[43] In the 1957 Asian flu epidemic, 10 percent of all influenza deaths were in pregnant women while almost 50 percent of women of childbearing age who died were pregnant.[44] Pregnant women had twice the mortality of nonpregnant females, with a marked rise in the third trimester. More recent reports have not confirmed such high mortality rates.[45]

After an incubation period of 1 to 4 days, acute fever, malaise, coryza, headache, and cough develop. Uncomplicated cases usually resolve within 3 days without chest radiographic abnormalities. If symptoms persist longer than 5 days, particularly in a pregnant woman, complications should be suspected. Pneumonia may be a primary progression of viral infection for which pregnant women are at higher risk; or it may be a complicating secondary bacterial pneumonia. These infections are usually caused by *S. pneumoniae, S. aureus, H. influenzae,* or enteric gram-negative bacilli.[43] In the 1957–1958 epidemic, pregnant women who died generally expired of fulminant viral pneumonia, while nonpregnant patients died of secondary bacterial pneumonia.[46] Neuzil and colleagues[47] reported results of a large survey and case control study of pneumonia and/or influenza in pregnancy during epidemics. The risk of acute respiratory illness and hospitalization among women in the third trimester was 4.5 times higher, and in the second trimester it was 2.5 times higher than the risk in first-trimester pregnancies or nonpregnant women.[47]

Pneumonia complicating influenza must be managed aggressively, especially in pregnant women. Bacterial pneumonia must be treated with appropriate antibiotics using the guidelines described earlier. A picture consistent with primary viral pneumonia must be treated with aggressive oxygen therapy. Occasionally respiratory failure ensues that may require mechanical ventilation. Amantadine, an oral antiviral agent that blocks release of nucleic acids, can prevent 70 to 90 percent of infections if used prophylactically.[48] If used within 48 hours of symptom onset, the duration of symptoms can be decreased by up to 50 percent, and fever will also be lower.[48] Amantadine and the virustatic agent ribavirin have been successfully used in influenza pneumonia complicating pregnancy.[49] The safety and efficacy of the neuraminidase inhibitors zanamavir and oseltamivir in pregnancy has not been well studied (FDA category C), and these agents should be used with caution.[50]

There are no convincing data linking maternal influenzal infection with congenital malformations,[44] and the Centers for Disease Control recommends influenza vaccine for pregnant women.[51]

Varicella Zoster

Varicella zoster virus (VZV) is a herpetic DNA virus which generally infects children. It affects less than 2 percent of adults, but can be complicated by viral pneumonia in up to 50 percent of adult cases. There is an increased risk of varicella pneumonia in pregnant women with primary varicella infection.[52,53] In a review of 99 cases of varicella pneumonia, 46 were women with 28 percent pregnant.[53] A recent case control study suggested that pregnant women with varicella zoster infection were more likely to develop pneumonia if they were smokers or manifested $\geq$100 skin lesions.[54] Mortality for nonpregnant adults with varicella pneumonia ranges from 11 to 17 percent, but it has been reported to be as high as 35 to 40 percent in pregnancy.[55,56]

Varicella pneumonia usually presents 2 to 5 days after the onset of fever, rash, and malaise. Typical symptoms include cough, dyspnea, hemoptysis, and chest pain. In one series, all patients with varicella pneumonia had oral mucosal lesions in addition to the typical skin lesions. The severity of illness can range from asymptomatic to fulminant viral pneumonia with respiratory failure. The chest radiograph typically demonstrates bilateral, peribronchial, nodular infiltrates that are maximal at the height of skin eruption and usually resolve by 14 days. Diffuse pulmonary calcifications after clinical resolution is a well described syndrome.[53]

Given the potential for severe, life-threatening disease, aggressive management and observation is required in all patients. Acyclovir, a nucleoside analogue which inhibits herpesvirus DNA synthesis, decreases mortality and hospital length of stay.[54,55] Most recommend 7.5 to 10 mg/kg of intravenous acyclovir every 8 hours.[57,58] Acyclovir has been used in more than 300 pregnancies (more than 200 in the first trimester) with no increase in the number of birth defects or consistent pattern of congenital malformation.[59] Because pregnant women presenting within 96 hours of initial exposure may be more susceptible to infection, passive immunization with varicella zoster immunoglobulin (VZIG) may prevent or attenuate varicella infection.[60] As 80 to 90 percent of adult women are immune, antibody testing should be performed on exposed women and administration of VZIG limited to those who lack protective immunity.

Aggressive supportive treatment should be utilized, including appropriate hydration to minimize nephrotoxicity with acyclovir.[57] Oxygen supplementation must be optimized and mechanical ventilatory support employed in advanced respiratory failure. Extracorporeal membrane oxygenation has been successfully utilized in at least one pregnant patient with advanced acute respiratory distress syndrome complicating varicella pneumonia.[61]

Fungal Infections

The most common fungi that can cause acute pneumonia are *Blastomyces dermatitidis, Coccidioides immitis, Cryptococcus neoformans, Histoplasma capsulatum,* and *Sporothrix schenckii*.[22] In general, fungal pneumonias are characterized by cough, fever, and occasionally focal pulmonary infiltrate. Although pneumonia caused by *B. dermatitidis, C. neoformans, H. capsulatum,* and *S. schenckii* does not seem to be more common or severe in pregnant women, dissemination is more common in infections caused by *C. immitis,* which poses a significant risk for dissemination, particularly during the second and third trimesters of pregnancy.[62–64] Many infections may not require therapy because spontaneous resolution frequently occurs. Azole antibiotics should not be utilized for the treatment of histoplasmosis or blastomycosis as they are teratogenic.[65,66] For severe or disseminated fungal infection, amphotericin B is the treatment of choice. Although data are limited, amphotericin B appears to be safe for the fetus.[62]

Tuberculosis

Since the 1980s there has been a clear rise in the incidence of tuberculosis (TB). This rise is thought to be secondary to (1) the increasing incidence of HIV infection, (2) the increase in immigration from countries with a higher prevalence of TB, and (3) the decline in public health services.[67,68] The current resurgence has been particularly problematic in ethnic minorities in urban areas, the same demographic groups experiencing the highest rate of HIV infection.[68] In fact, the most populated urban areas account for 18 percent of the population and 42 percent of the TB cases.[67] Although data in pregnant women are limited, there is a potential problem with TB given CDC data confirming that the rate of reported cases increased 44 percent among patients 25 to 44 years of age.[69] All physicians caring for pregnant individuals in high risk groups must be familiar with the care of the pregnant patient with TB. Several excellent reviews of the topic have recently been published.[70,71,72]

Pregnancy per se does not appear to alter the course of acute tuberculosis, nor does it pose a risk for reactivation of TB.[67] The effect of pulmonary or extrapulmonary TB on pregnancy, however, includes prematurity, low birth weight, miscarriage, and perinatal death.[73,74] These bad outcomes were more common with late diagnosis, incomplete or irregular treatment, and advanced lesions in the mother. In fact, obstetric morbidity is increased fourfold and preterm labor ninefold with late diagnosis. Similarly, extrapulmonary involvement has been demonstrated to have a negative impact on pregnancy outcome.

In general, the clinical manifestations of TB during pregnancy are similar to those seen in nonpregnant individuals, and include cough (74 percent), weight loss (41 percent), fever (30 percent), malaise and fatigue (30 percent), and hemoptysis (19 percent).[75] Pregnant women are more likely to have asymptomatic disease.[76] Unfortunately, chest radiography is often postponed due to pregnancy, and this can impair the ability to assure an early diagnosis.[77] Therefore pregnant women should be targeted for screening if they have increased risk for tuberculous infection.[78] The tuberculin skin test (Mantoux test) is safe and reliable during pregnancy.[79] The American Thoracic Society has formulated guidelines for the evaluation of skin testing in nonpregnant individuals that should also be applicable to pregnant women.[78] These recommendations have different criteria for a positive response based on risk factors for disease. About 10 percent of individuals with TB have a negative PPD test.[68] A negative PPD and control skin test has been reported in 30 percent of women with HIV infection, so a negative PPD cannot be used to exclude TB, particularly in the setting of appropriate signs and symptoms.

Bacille Calmette-Guérin (BCG) vaccination is frequently employed in other countries, and it continues to cause confusion regarding its effect on tuberculin skin testing.[67] In general, a PPD is not contraindicated in the presence of prior BCG vaccination, and the test should be interpreted as usual if BCG vaccination occurred greater than 10 years earlier. Prior BCG vaccination should have no impact on the appropriate evaluation and treatment of suspected TB, as the PPD reaction resulting from BCG vaccination is usually less than 10 mm and wanes 3 to 5 years after vaccination.[78]

Detailed recommendations regarding management of a positive skin test have recently been published.[78] Isoniazid (INH) is 25 to 92 percent effective in prophylaxis of TB infection.[78] An increased risk of INH hepatitis has been suggested in the perinatal period.[80,81] Isoniazid is not thought to be teratogenic, even when given during the first 4 months of gestation.[78,82] Nevertheless, given the hesitancy to use unnecessary medications during pregnancy, the optimal means of TB prophylaxis remains controversial. The possible risk of hepatitis must be weighed against the risk of developing active tuberculosis.[78] Therefore INH prophylaxis is usually indicated for pregnant women at high risk for progression to active disease, such as those infected with HIV. For those women in whom the risk of active TB is lower, prophylaxis can be delayed until the postpartum period. Pregnant women taking INH should receive pyridoxine supplementation.[78]

Treatment of active TB in the pregnant woman is similar to that of nonpregnant individuals, but the potential toxicity to the fetus must be kept in mind. Nevertheless, all authorities agree that the risk of withholding therapy greatly outweighs the risks of treatment.[82] The current recommendations from the ATS are for a combination of INH, rifampin, and ethambutol.[83] INH and rifampin for 9 months are appropriate if the risk of INH resistance is small. An abbreviated regimen is also appropriate, with pyrazinamide and ethambutol in the first 2 months, in addition to INH and rifampin, which are continued for a total of 6 months of therapy[82,84] (see Table 13-4).

If INH resistance is possible, ethambutol must be added at the onset. It can be deleted from the regimen once microbiologic studies confirm pansensitivity. If multidrug resistance is possible, a regimen of at least four drugs is necessary, ideally under the supervision of a physician familiar with the management of resistant TB. The presence of HIV infection complicates treatment. A detailed discussion is beyond the scope of this chapter and interested readers should consult additional resources.

Table 13-4. Common Drugs Used to Treat Tuberculosis

Drug	Usual Dose	Possible Side Effects	FDA Category
Isoniazid	300 mg PO qd 900 mg PO 2 × weekly	GI distress, hepatotoxicity, seizures, peripheral neuritis, hypersensitivity	C
Rifampin	600 mg PO qd 600 mg PO 2 × weekly	GI distress, hepatotoxicity, headache, purpura, fever, orange secretions	C
Ethambutol	2–2.5 g PO qd 4 g PO 2 × weekly	Altered vision, red-green disturbance, optic neuritis, skin rash	B
Pyrazinamide	2–2.5 g PO qd 3 g PO 2 × weekly	Hepatotoxicity, hyperuricemia, arthralgias, gout	C
Streptomycin	1 g IM qd 1.5 g IM 2 × weekly	Ototoxicity, nephrotoxicity	D
Pyridoxine	25–50 mg PO qd		

Compiled from.[11,82,84]

ASTHMA

Asthma is one of the most common medical conditions complicating pregnancy. Management poses unique problems as both the changing thoracic mechanics of the mother and those of the developing fetus must be considered.

Asthma in pregnancy can increase maternal morbidity.[85,86] Maternal-fetal effects include preterm birth, low birth weight, increased neonatal mortality, increased neonatal hypoxia, increased hyperemesis gravidarum, vaginal hemorrhage, and increased labor complications. Some studies have confirmed increased incidence of low birth weight and an increased risk of obstetric complications. Greater prepregnancy severity of asthma is associated with greater pregnancy complications.[87,88]

In the best controlled study, Schatz and colleagues[89] reported on 486 pregnant women with asthma compared with 486 pregnant nonasthmatics with normal pulmonary function who were studied over a 12-year period at the Kaiser-Permanente Medical Center in San Diego. Asthma was managed aggressively with a stepped care approach (see below) to prevent asthma exacerbations and ensure normal sleep and activity levels. Chronic hypertension was significantly more common in the asthmatic subjects (3.7 percent) than in controls (1.0 percent). Trends towards a correlation between greater asthma severity (requiring ED therapy) and increased incidence of preeclampsia and low birth weight were found. There was no difference in perinatal mortality, overall incidence of preeclampsia or preterm births, overall low birth weight infants, intrauterine growth restriction, or congenital malformations. This suggests that aggressive management of asthma may minimize the risks from asthma during pregnancy.

Demissie and collaegues[90] found an increased incidence of adverse effect of asthma on maternal and fetal outcomes. These investigators noted an increased likelihood of preeclampsia (OR 2.18, 1.68 to 2.83), placenta previa (OR 1.71, 1.05 to 2.79), need for cesarean delivery (OR 1.62, 1.46 to 1.80), and increased maternal hospital length of stay (OR 1.86, 1.60 to 2.15).

Adverse perinatal outcomes have been linked to asthma during pregnancy. Demissie and coworkers[90] noted an increased likelihood of preterm infants (OR 1.36, 95 per cent CI 1.18 to 1.55), low birth weight (OR 1.32, 1.10 to 1.58), and small-for-gestational age infants (OR 1.26, 1.10 to 1.45) in pregnancies complicated by asthma. There does not appear to be any significant association between maternal asthma and congenital malformation.[91] Adverse fetal events appear to be predominantly seen in poorly controlled asthma,[92] so it appears that better asthma control improves pregnancy outcome.

About one-third of women with asthma experience improvement, one-third experience worsening, and one-third remain the same.[86,93]

Studies tend to agree that exacerbations are less frequent during the first trimester and the last month of pregnancy.[93] During the first 3 months postpartum the course of asthma tends to revert to the prepregnancy state.

Management of Asthma

The goals for management of asthma in pregnant individuals have been well elaborated in the NHLBI report of 1993.[94] More recent recommendations from the Working Group on Asthma and Pregnancy has enumerated the following treatment goals in pregnant asthmatics:

- Maintain normal or near normal pulmonary function
- Fully control symptoms (including nocturnal symptoms)
- Maintain near normal activity levels (including appropriate exercise)
- Prevent acute asthma episodes
- Avoid adverse effects of medication
- Give birth to a healthy infant

To achieve these goals, individuals caring for these patients need to understand the role of appropriate monitoring of airway function, the risk vs. benefit of the various medications available, and appreciate the potential role of nonpharmacologic therapy. Some have suggested that asthma during pregnancy managed by specialists results in improved outcomes.[93] Although the incidence of preeclampsia is not reduced, other complications such as perinatal mortality, preterm birth, and low birth weight do improve with such management.[93]

Monitoring of Airway Function

The role of routinely monitoring airway function has been widely accepted as standard of care in the management of patients with chronic asthma[95] due to the well known difficulty in predicting severity of airflow obstruction by both patients and physicians.[96,97]

Since pregnant women frequently experience dyspnea late in pregnancy, in pregnant asthmatics the routine measurement of peak flow is necessary to assess the status of airflow in the face of increasing symptoms.[98] In the typical physiologically-based approach, the patient measures the peak expiratory flow rate (PEFR) first thing in the morning and late in the evening over a 2-week period. In this way she establishes a personal best reading at a time of clinical stability; this period is optimally during a period of effective asthma treatment.[95] The level of subsequent PEFR readings can be used to gauge asthma severity using a zone system.[99] In the green zone, there are few asthma symptoms present and the peak flows are between 80 and 100 percent of the personal best with little variation between the morning and evening values (<20 percent). The yellow zone indicates worsening asthma and is associated with 50 to 80 percent of the personal best PEFR and a 20 to 30 percent variability between morning and evening values. The red zone is signaled by a PEFR <50 percent of personal best and a >30 percent variability between morning and evening values. This grading of asthma severity has been used to guide a "stepped care" approach to asthma therapy which will be described below.

Fetal Monitoring

Monitoring fetal function is equally as important as monitoring airflow in the mother.[100] This is particularly true in individuals with greater lability and symptoms that are more difficult to control. It is these pregnancies that are most likely to have associated fetal morbidity. Fetal monitoring should include an accurate determination of gestational age and assessment of fetal growth and activity. It should begin with careful serial measurements of fundal height, and should include sonography in poorly controlled asthma or if fetal growth restriction is suspected.[94] In the third trimester, electronic monitoring of the fetal heart rate and sonographic determinations of fetal behavior are appropriate. If an acute episode of asthma is poorly responsive to therapy, intermittent or continuous fetal monitoring should be initiated during emergency treatment.[94]

Pharmacologic Management

Table 13-5 presents data for commonly used drugs in asthma. Inhaled corticosteroids (ICS) remain the cornerstone of therapy in asthma.[101] Recent data have confirmed their important role in the management of asthma during pregnancy. In a prospective study of 504 pregnant asthmatics, those taking an ICS were four times less likely than their nontreated counterparts to experience an exacerbation.[102] A prospective study randomized 65 women hospitalized with an exacerbation of asthma during pregnancy to outpatient therapy with an oral steroid taper and inhaled albuterol (n = 31) versus an inhaled β-agonist and oral steroid taper plus inhaled beclomethasone (n = 34).[103] The latter group experienced a 55 percent reduction in subsequent exacerbations and admissions (33 percent vs. 12 percent; OR 3.63, 95 percent CI 1.01 to 13.08). Despite these data, Cydulka and colleagues[104] recently prospectively studied asthma management in 51 pregnant asthmatics and 500 nonpregnant asthmatics seen in an emergency department with an exacerbation. Only 44 percent of pregnant women were treated with cor-

Table 13-5. Risks and Benefits of Drugs Commonly Used in the Management of Asthma

Agent	Additional Data	FDA Class	Indications
Selective β_2-agonists			
Metaproterenol	May inhibit labor; fetal tachycardia, hyperglycemia, neonatal hypoglycemia	C	Short-acting reliever for symptomatic relief
Albuterol	May inhibit labor; fetal tachycardia, hyperglycemia, neonatal hypoglycemia	C	Short-acting reliever for symptomatic relief
Terbutaline	May inhibit labor; preserves placental blood flow; fetal tachycardia, hyperglycemia, neonatal hypoglycemia	B	Short-acting reliever for symptomatic relief
Pirbuterol	Fetal tachycardia, hyperglycemia, neonatal hypoglycemia	C	—
Bitolterol	Fetal tachycardia, hyperglycemia, neonatal hypoglycemia	C	—
Salmeterol	Fetal tachycardia, hyperglycemia, neonatal hypoglycemia	C	Moderate to severe asthma with good response prior to pregnancy; those inadequately controlled with medium-dose inhaled corticosteroids (ICS)
Nonselective β_2-agonists			
Epinephrine	Reduced placental blood flow in animals; may inhibit labor	C	Can be considered in anaphylaxis
Isoproterenol	Fetal tachycardia, hyperglycemia, neonatal hypoglycemia	C	—
Anticholinergic agents			
Ipratropium	—	B	Additive therapy to short acting β_2-agonists in acute asthma
Nonsteroidal antiinflammatory agents			
Cromolyn	—	B	
Nedocromil	—	—	If good response was seen prior to pregnancy
Zileuton			Not recommended
Zafirlukast		B	In recalcitrant asthma with favorable response prior to pregnancy
Montelukast		B	In recalcitrant asthma with favorable response prior to pregnancy

(*Continues*)

Table 13-5. (*Continued*) Risks and Benefits of Drugs Commonly Used in the Management of Asthma

Agent	Additional Data	FDA Class	Indications
Inhaled steroids			
Beclomethasone	Slight increase in low birth weight and premature delivery	C	Who have shown good response prior to pregnancy; starting ICS during pregnancy; require high-dose ICS for adequate control
Triamcinolone	Extensive positive animal data	D	
Flunisolide	—	C	Not recommended
Budesonide	—	B	Use in patients who have shown good response prior to pregnancy; starting ICS during pregnancy; require high-dose ICS for adequate control
Fluticasone	—	C	Use in patients who have shown good response prior to pregnancy; consider in severely symptomatic patients uncontrolled with alternative agents
Systemic steroids	Low birth weight in one series but not in another	—	
Theophylline	May inhibit labor; theophylline intoxication in newborns, particularly with blood levels $>12\ \mu g/mL$	C	

Source: Adapted from Fabre et al[11] and Dombrowski et al.[107]

ticosteroids, compared with 66 percent of nonpregnant women. Furthermore, pregnant women were more likely to be sent home without corticosteroid therapy (38 percent vs. 64 percent) and were 2.9 times more likely to report ongoing symptoms of exacerbation at a 2-week follow-up.

A recent study from Australia found a significant reduction in placental 11β-hydroxysteroid dehydrogenase type 2 (11β-HSD2) activity in a group of asthmatics not taking inhaled glucocorticoids to control their asthma.[105] 11β-HSD2 is an enzyme that converts active cortisol to inactive cortisone, thus acting as a barrier to protect the fetus from the relatively high concentrations of glucocorticoids found in the mother. This reduction in enzyme activity was associated with a 25 percent lower birth weight centile compared with a control group. There were no difference in birth weight among pregnant women who used a daily inhaled and/or periodic oral glucocorticoids compared with a control nonasthmatic group. This study delineates a biologic role for the use of inhaled glucocorticoids for asthma treatment during pregnancy.

The optimal inhaled steroids appear to be budesonide and beclomethasone.[106] This recommendation has been made based on the totality of the clinical data published to date. Six studies have been published since 1993 that examined the safety of inhaled corticosteroids in pregnancy; four of these specifically addressed safety issues.[107] In three of the studies, beclomethasone was the most frequently prescribed steroid, and the fourth study examined inhaled budesonide. In this last study, Swedish investigators reported an analysis of data from three Swedish registries comprising more than 2000 births between 1995 and 1997. No increase in the general rate of congenital malformations was noted.[106]

Oral corticosteroids may be associated with low birth weight infants and preterm delivery.[86] In a recent multivariate analysis, oral corticosteroid use was associated with preeclampsia (OR 2.0, 95 percent CI 1.11 to 3.61).[86] A systematic review of the literature suggested a 3.5 percent incidence of congenital malformations in 457 infants of mothers receiving systemic steroids.[108] In a large case control study of 20,830 infants with congenital malformations, the proportion of mothers treated with oral steroids was no different than in mothers of normal controls.[109] In contrast, a recent case control study of the Spanish Collaborative Study of Congenital Malformations noted a significant association between first-trimester use of systemic steroids and oral clefts (OR 6.55, 95 percent CI 1.44 to 29.76).[110]

Cromolyn would be an appropriate alternative antiinflammatory agent in milder disease not adequately controlled with inhaled steroids and inhaled β-agonists. Similarly, limited data have been published on nedocromil, thus it is unlikely that this agent should be chosen over cromolyn.[107] Leukotriene modifiers have assumed a prominent role in mild persistent asthma and as add-on therapy in more severe asthma.[95] Furthermore, recent comprehensive reviews have suggested that the available agents are safe in nonpregnant asthmatics.[111] Unfortunately, data in pregnancy are quite scarce. Animal studies have suggested adverse effects with zileuton, but no human data are available.[108] Similarly, limited human data are available on zafirlukast and montelukast, although animal data have been favorable. Both of these agents are currently classified as class B agents.

Theophyllines appear to be safe in pregnancy,[112] although they are no longer commonly used. Theophylline clearance may be reduced by 20 to 35 percent during the third trimester of pregnancy.[113]

Stepped-Care Approach to Asthma Management

Most experts emphasize a stepped-care approach to asthma therapy (Figs. 13-3 and 13-4) which is individualized to disease severity and symptoms.[95,114] Table 13-6 details an approach to such stepped management based on symptoms and pulmonary function.[115] In each category a short-acting β-agonist is available to all patients for use in the setting of acute symptoms. Medications are added as symptoms (including nocturnal symptoms) increase and/or as pulmonary function level decreases. Emphasis is placed on the use of appropriate antiinflammatory medications. In addition, as the patient improves, decreasing medication use is also encouraged.

Acute exacerbations must be quickly identified and managed. Monitoring remains important to assess severity of illness, with a rapid assessment of arterial hypoxemia, acid-base abnormalities, maternal dehydration, and chest pain. Patient education is paramount to facilitate appropriate management during an exacerbation. Antiinflammatory therapy including steroid therapy should be routinely used as the severity of the exacerbation increases. Aminophylline use remains controversial. Although the loading dose is no different during pregnancy, the maintenance regimen should be more conservative as clearance may be altered. If the patient does not improve with β-agonists and steroids, hospitalization should be strongly considered.[114]

Bacterial sinusitis, a well-known cause of asthma exacerbation, has been estimated to be six times more common during pregnancy than in nonpregnant patients.[116] Gastroesophageal reflux is an important comorbid factor and can be associated with exacerbation of asthma. All H_2-receptor (histamine) antagonists except nizatadine appear to be safe during pregnancy.[117]

Obstetric Management in Asthma

Most of the principles described for chronic management apply to the pregnant asthmatic during labor. The patient's regularly scheduled medications should be continued during labor and delivery. Clearly, careful fetal management is crucial to ensure a good outcome. Approximately 10 percent of asthmatics experience an asthma exacerbation during labor.

Oxytocin is the drug of choice, as both prostaglandin $F_{2\alpha}$ ($PGF_{2\alpha}$) and prostaglandin E_2 (PGE_2) have been reported to cause bronchoconstriction.[99] During an asthma exacerbation it is not unusual to experience uterine contractions, although they usually do not progress with successful treatment of the exacerbation. In preterm labor, a β-agonist, magnesium sulfate, or nifedipine can be used as tocolytic agents. In those individuals using systemic β-agonists for preterm labor, the use of two β-agonists should be avoided in preterm labor. In these individuals magnesium sulfate may be a better agent, possibly facilitating additional bronchodilation.[118]

For postpartum hemorrhage, oxytocin is the drug of choice for reasons similar to those stated above. Methylergonovine and ergonovine may cause bronchospasm and should be avoided. Prostaglandin E_2 may be used with the same caveat as discussed above; both PGE_1 and $PGF_{2\alpha}$ may precipitate bronchoconstriction.[119] For analgesia, morphine and meperidine should be avoided as they may potentially cause histamine release which could precipitate bronchospasm. Fentanyl is preferred.[120] Narcotic analgesics may be associated with respiratory depression and should be avoided if there is a concomitant

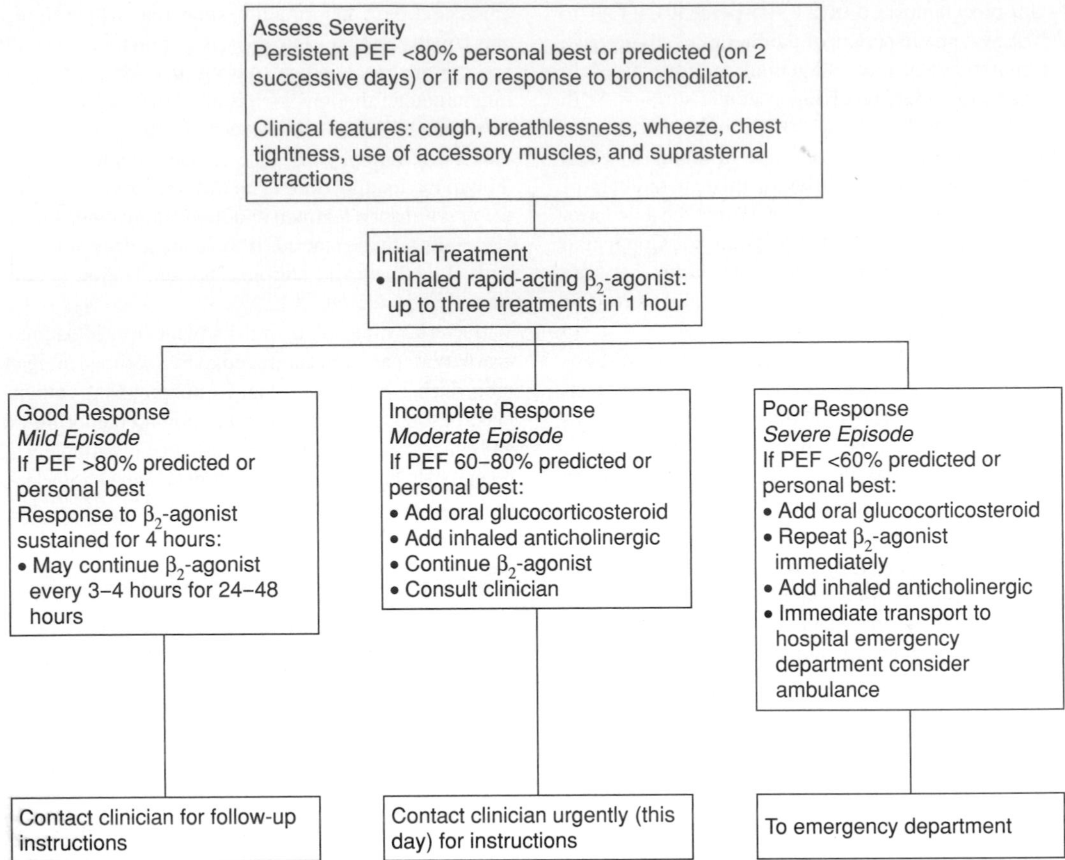

[a]Patients at high risk of asthma-related death (see text) should contact clinician promptly after initial treatment. Additional therapy may be required.

Fig. 13-3. Management of asthma exacerbations. (Adapted from National Institutes of Health.[95])

asthma exacerbation. Lumbar epidural analgesia may be the preferred technique and may enhance the response to bronchodilator therapy.[120] It should be noted, however, that bronchospasm has been reported in 2 percent of patients with asthma receiving regional anesthesia.[119] If general anesthesia is required, ketamine is the preferred agent, and low concentrations of halogenated anesthetics may provide additional bronchodilation.[121] Preanesthetic use of anticholinergic agents may provide a bronchodilatory effect.[122]

Cystic Fibrosis

Cystic fibrosis (CF) is an inherited disorder that is transmitted as an autosomal recessive trait and involves epithelial tissues of the pancreas, sweat glands, and mucous glands, as well as the exocrine glands. The lungs and pancreas are the principal organs affected, with chronic infection of the airways, bronchiectasis, airflow obstruction, and malabsoprtion, resulting in typical clinical manifestations. Progressive bronchopulmonary disease is the major cause of morbidity and mortality. Approximately 4 percent of the Caucasian population in the United States are heterozygous carriers, with disease occurring in 1 of 3000 live white births.[123]

The severity of clinical disease varies with the extent of organ involvement. Progressive bronchopulmonary involvement is characterized by recurrent infections and increasing chronic airflow obstruction. Cough and dyspnea are commonly seen. Pancreatic involvement is progressive with resulting exocrine insufficiency and malabsorption. The maldigestion of fats results in major nutritional

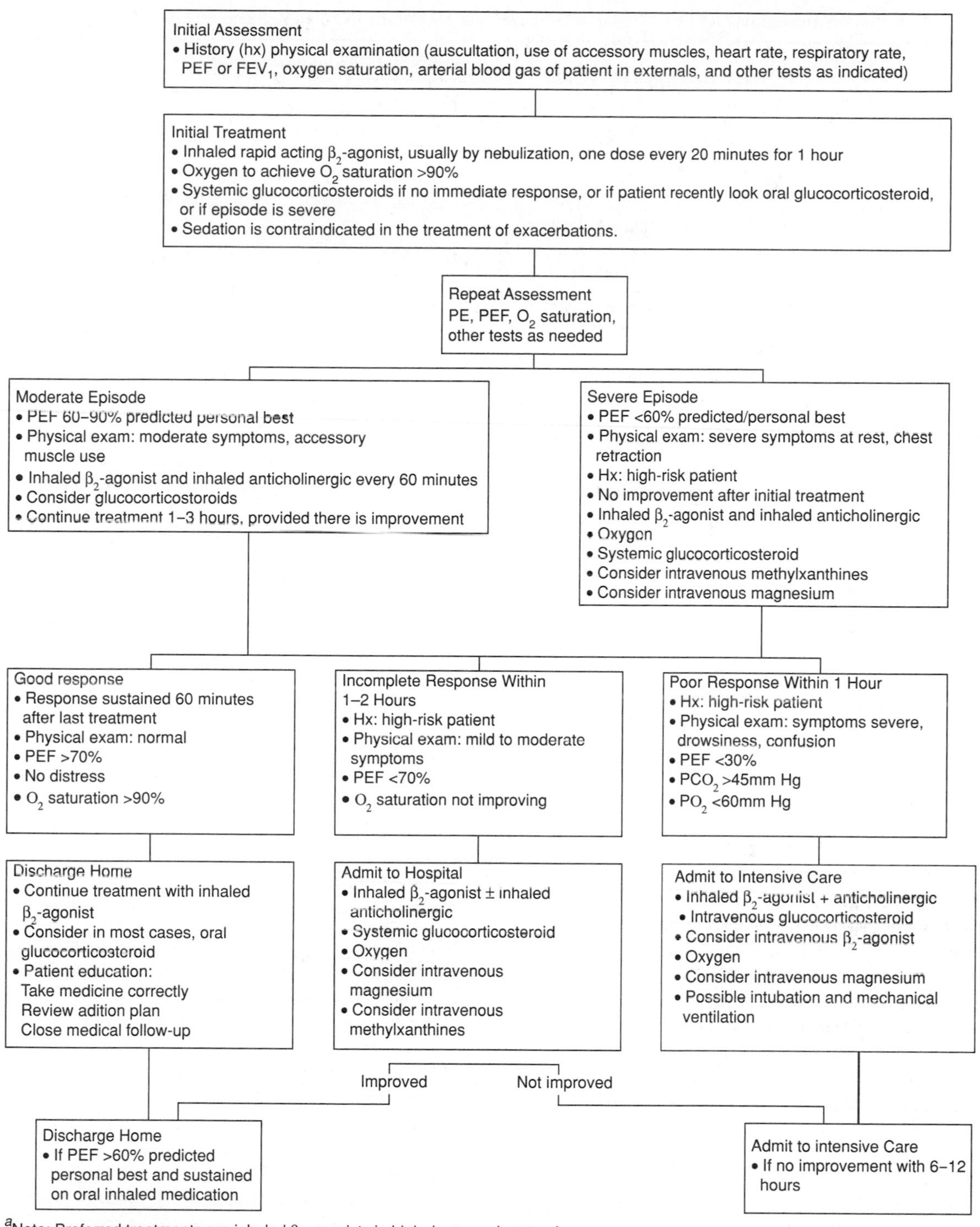

Fig. 13-4. Hospital-based management of asthma exacerbations. (Adapted from National Institutes of Health.[95])

Table 13-6. Recommendations for Pharmacologic Management of Asthma During Pregnancy

Category	Frequency/Severity of Symptoms	Pulmonary Function (FEV_1 or PEFR % of Standardized Norm or Personal Best)	Step Therapy
Mild intermittent	Symptoms ≤2/week Nocturnal symptoms ≤2/mo Brief exacerbations (few hours to days) Asymptomatic between episodes	≥80% Normal between episodes	Inhaled β_2-agonists prn (in all categories)
Mild persistent	Symptoms >2/week but not daily	≥80%	Inhaled cromolyn Substitute low-dose inhaled beclomethasone or budesonide if not adequate control
Moderate persistent	Daily symptoms Nocturnal symptoms >1/week Exacerbations affecting activity	60–80%	Inhaled beclomethasone or budesonide Add oral theophylline or inhaled salmeterol if not adequate control
Severe persistent	Continual symptoms Limited activity Frequent nocturnal symptoms Frequent acute exacerbations	<60%	Above plus oral corticosteroids (burst for active symptoms, alternate day or daily if necessary)

Source: Adapted from Luskin.[115]

deficiency. Diabetes mellitus can be seen as a late complication of cystic fibrosis.

Improved care and earlier diagnosis over the past decade has progressively improved survival such that more than one-third of patients are over the age of 16.[121] Women with CF have anatomically normal reproductive tracts. Fertility has not been systematically studied but is likely to be reduced. Despite this, multiple cases and several large series confirm that women with CF can become pregnant.[123,124]

The increased blood volume and cardiac output usually seen with pregnancy could potentially impact CF patients with advanced pulmonary disease and limited pulmonary vascular reserve. This would be particularly problematic in patients with clinical pulmonary hypertension. The increased venous return seen during and immediately after delivery would be a particularly risky time.[124,125]

Recent reports suggest a reasonable outcome of pregnancy in CF,[123–127] which may represent the higher proportion of patients with milder disease achieving successful pregnancy. Fetal outcome is strongly related to the severity of pregravid disease in the mother and the course of pulmonary function during pregnancy.

Management of the CF Patient During Pregnancy

The improving outcome of pregnancy in CF patients likely reflects, in part, the comprehensive management of these individuals. A coordinated team with knowledge of CF and the stress of pregnancy is necessary to ensure optimal outcomes. As respiratory status is closely related to pregnancy outcome, aggressive follow-up and management of respiratory disease is necessary during pregnancy. Appropriate prepregnancy evaluation is ideal and should include objective measurement of pulmonary function (spirometry and lung volumes) and gas exchange (arterial blood gas, ABG). Monitoring of pulmonary function periodically through the course of pregnancy is recommended and should include grading of subjective dyspnea and objective measurement of pulmonary function (spirometry, pulse oximetry, and ABGs, if clinically indicated). Routine respiratory management should include postural drainage and exercise to mobilize secretions. Management of bronchospasm shares many similarities to that of asthma during pregnancy (see above). Bronchodilators and anti-inflammatory medications should be utilized as clinically indicated. As in asthmatic patients, optimal airway function should take priority to the theoretical, small risk of these medications. Similarly, oxygen therapy should be utilized freely as the fetus is intolerant of even minor degrees of maternal hypoxia.

At the first sign of an exacerbation (as signaled by increased cough or dyspnea and worsened pulmonary function or weight loss) aggressive management is mandated. This should include the appropriate use of antibiotics, ideally guided by sputum microbiologic analysis. Antibiotic safety in pregnancy was described in an earlier section and these principles apply to pregnant CF patients. Several differences must be noted, however. Pharmacokinetics of multiple antibiotics are altered in patients with CF. β-lactam antibiotics are cleared more rapidly in patients with CF. The volume of distribution and the rate of clearance of aminoglycosides are also increased in CF patients. As such, higher doses of aminoglycosides and close monitoring of blood drug levels is necessary to assure optimal drug dosing.

Careful attention to nutritional status has been highlighted earlier. At each office visit, the history of caloric intake and symptoms of malabsorption should be sought. Pancreatic enzyme supplementation should be optimized. For those unable to meet nutritional goals caloric supplementation should be considered. This may include oral supplements or in more severe cases nasogastric feedings or parenteral hyperalimentation.

Given the cardiovascular stress of pregnancy, close clinical evaluation of hemodynamic status is necessary during the course of pregnancy. This is particularly important in those individuals with more severe pulmonary disease who have a greater limitation in pulmonary vascular reserve. Monitoring of blood pressure, pulse, weight, and edema is mandatory at routine office visits. During delivery and in the immediate postpartum period, additional stress and monitoring are required. The presence of ventricular dysfunction mandates aggressive diuresis and appropriate oxygen administration. A pulmonary artery catheter may aid in optimizing hemodynamics. Inhalational anesthetics, which increase pulmonary vascular tone, should be avoided in those patients requiring general anesthesia during cesarean section.

SARCOIDOSIS

Sarcoidosis is a multisystem disease of unknown etiology characterized by noncaseating granulomas in a perivascular pattern. The disease affects young adults and involves the lungs, peripheral lymph nodes, skin, eyes, and liver most commonly. The clinical manifestations are highly variable, although most commonly an asymptomatic patient presents with an abnormal chest radiograph. The most common clinical symptoms reflect lung involvement and include dyspnea, cough, and chest pain. The classic chest radiographic pattern reveals bilateral hilar adenopathy with or without parenchymal infiltration. The diagnosis is made in the appropriate clinical setting with identification of noncaseating granulomata in tissue samples.

Sarcoidosis does not appear to increase fetal or obstetric complications.[128] The management of pregnancy in patients with sarcoidosis is not generally altered. Furthermore, the course of disease is usually not altered during pregnancy,[128] with the majority of patients remaining unchanged or improving. Haynes de Regt described factors that identify high-risk individuals, including advanced maternal age, parenchymal infiltration or fibrosis on chest radiograph, low inflammatory activity, chronic (persistent) sarcoidosis with an insidious onset, and extrapulmonary disease.[129] Women should be followed closely through pregnancy and for at least 6 months after delivery, because late-onset disease progression has been reported. The indications for treatment in pregnant women are similar to the management of the nonpregnant individual, with prednisone remaining the antiinflammatory agent of choice.[130]

PNEUMOTHORAX AND PNEUMOMEDIASTINUM

Spontaneous pneumothorax should be suspected in the patient between 20 and 40 years of age with sudden, pleuritic chest pain associated with mild to moderate dyspnea.[131] The physiologic alterations of pregnancy lead to increased minute ventilation and repeated Valsalva maneuvers during labor and delivery, creating an excellent setting for pneumothorax. Given the frequency of breathlessness during pregnancy, diagnosis can be difficult. A chest radiograph is associated with minimal fetal risk and should be considered when symptoms are acute or moderate in severity.

Van Winter and colleagues recently detailed a literature survey of pneumothorax during pregnancy reported between 1957 and 1996.[132] Twenty-three cases were noted with 21 occurring in the first (18/23) or second (3/23) trimesters. Risk factors were seen in 9/23 patients, most commonly an acute respiratory infection or a history of chronic lung disease. A prior history of pneumothorax was seen in 12/23.

Treatment options are similar in pregnant women as for nonpregnant patients.[132] Given the sensitivity of the fetus to maternal hypoxia, however, initial observation is required even with a small pneumothorax (<20 percent of the hemithorax).[131,132] Supplemental oxygen during hospitalization may help accelerate pleural air resorption. If the pneumothorax is large (>20 percent of the hemithorax), aspiration is recommended with close observation over several hours.[133] If this fails or the pneumothorax recurs, treatment with tube thoracostomy is recommended. Sclerosis with tetracycline, recommended by some for nonpregnant adults, is contraindicated in pregnancy. Patients with continued air leaks, incomplete lung expansion, bilateral pneumothorax, or hemopneumothorax should be treated with surgery.[135] The optimal time for surgical intervention is the second trimester, before the increased risk of premature labor in the third trimester and after organogenesis seen during the first trimester. With careful technique, the risk of general anesthesia can be minimized during pregnancy.

Allowing spontaneous vaginal delivery with chest tubes in place or after surgery has been well described with excellent fetal and maternal outcomes.[135,136] A high rate of recurrence (30 to 50 percent) is seen after the first pneumothorax. A second pneumothorax should lead to consideration of definitive treatment, including surgery.

Pneumomediastinum, the presence of free air in the mediastinum, presents a similar spectrum of management questions in pregnancy. It is a rare phenomenon with an estimated incidence in pregnancy of 1:2000 to 1:100,000. Affected women are typically primigravidas experiencing a prolonged and difficult labor with repeated straining. Pneumomediastinum can occur any time during pregnancy but is most frequently seen during the second stage of labor.

Patients typically complain of acute substernal chest pain, frequently with a tearing sensation and radiation to the neck and arms.[137,138] Cough and dyspnea may be seen. Tachycardia and subcutaneous emphysema are common physical findings. Pneumomediastinum undergoes spontaneous resolution within 3 to 14 days without sequelae. Treatment in uncomplicated cases includes sedation, analgesics, oxygen supplementation, and elective low forceps delivery to shorten the second stage of labor. In the presence of mechanical ventilation, simultaneous pneumothorax is a distinct possibility.

POSTPARTUM PLEURAL EFFUSION

The physiologic conditions of labor and delivery appear favorable for the development of pleural effusions including an increased blood volume, decreased plasma colloid osmotic pressure, and an increased intrathoracic pressure. The techniques utilized to identify pleural fluid have ranged from simple upright radiography to thoracic ultrasonography. The true incidence is difficult to accurately determine although the frequency is likely small. In the presence of pre-eclampsia the presence of an effusion has been associated with a tenfold higher perinatal fetal mortality apparently secondary to premature labor and delivery during a shorter gestation.

KYPHOSCOLIOSIS

Kyphoscoliosis (KS) is a bony deformity of the spine that leads to excessive curvature which is usually idiopathic. Patients with untreated scoliosis are at increased risk of respiratory failure, particularly in patients with a greater degree of curvature and lower vital capacity.[139] The effects of KS on pregnancy outcome have been minimal except for a possible increase in premature birth.[140] Conflicting reports have been published addressing the risk of progression in spinal curvature during pregnancy. In general, the risk of progression appears to be increased in those with unstable scoliosis[141] or those with an initial curve greater than 25 degrees. Close observation through pregnancy is required because major respiratory complications have occurred with KS during pregnancy.[142,143] Noninvasive ventilatory support using negative pressure ventilation and nasal positive pressure ventilation have been successfully utilized during pregnancy.[143]

ACUTE RESPIRATORY FAILURE

Acute respiratory failure in pregnancy remains a major problem, accounting for 30 percent of maternal deaths.[144] Thromboembolism, amniotic fluid embolism, and venous air embolism account for the greatest proportion of maternal deaths.

The goals of management include identifying the cause and initiating therapeutic attempts to stabilize maternal physiology. Fetal oxygen delivery must also be preserved. The major determinants of oxygen delivery to fetal tissues include: oxygen content of uterine arterial blood (determined by maternal hemoglobin concentration and its saturation), uterine blood flow (determined by maternal cardiac output, blood pressure, and blood pH), placental oxygen transfer, and fetal oxygen transport. Alkalosis causes vasoconstriction of the uterine artery with decreased oxygen delivery to the placenta.[145]

Fetal oxygen content is similar to that of the mother despite a fetal umbilical vein Po_2 of 28 to 32 mmHg. Compensatory mechanisms include the high-affinity fetal hemoglobin, which is at an elevated concentration and releases oxygen to peripheral tissues more efficiently. Fetal cardiac output is also increased and is optimally distributed to fetal tissues secondary to fetal shunts.

ACUTE RESPIRATORY DISTRESS SYNDROME (ARDS)

ARDS is an acute illness characterized by the physiologic response to increased pulmonary capillary permeability and the resulting increase in lung fluid. The syndrome is defined by the presence of: (1) an appropriate risk factor, (2) radiographic infiltrates consistent with pulmonary edema, (3) impaired oxygenation with Pao_2:Fio_2 ratio $\leq$200, and (4) the absence of heart failure with a pulmonary capillary wedge pressure <18 mmHg or no clinical evidence of elevated left atrial pressure.[146]

The clinical presentation is nonspecific, with dyspnea, tachycardia, and tachypnea commonly seen.[147] Physical examination may demonstrate diffuse bibasilar rales and cyanosis. Although the chest radiograph may be normal immediately after the precipitating event, full progression to diffuse bilateral infiltrates typically occurs within 4 to 24 hours. Hypoxemia is relatively resistant to supplemental oxygen.

The overall therapeutic goals in the management of ARDS include optimizing maternal oxygen delivery while minimizing oxygen toxicity and iatrogenic complications, and preserving fetal oxygen delivery to tissues. General measures include appropriate oxygen delivery, including mechanical ventilation if necessary. The indications for intubation are similar to those of nonpregnant patients, including: (1) inability to maintain Pao_2 >70 mmHg with oxygen supplementation, (2) uncompensated respiratory acidosis, and/or (3) an inability to protect the airway and clear secretions. Intubation may be more difficult because of the hyperemia, which can narrow the upper airway of the pregnant woman. The decrease in functional residual capacity may be exacerbated during intubation. Therefore 100 percent oxygen should be administered before intubation is attempted. Hyperventilation must be avoided because alkalosis decreases uterine blood flow.

Mechanical ventilation should be initiated to maintain a relatively normal pH, which usually requires a $Paco_2$ of 30 to 32 mmHg. Ventilator settings are similar to those used in the nonpregnant patient. Small tidal volumes (6 to 10 mL/kg) are associated with lower airway pressures and potentially lower lung injury.[148] A recent ARDS Network trial showed a significant reduction in mortality from 40 percent in the traditional group (tidal volume 12 mL/kg) to about 31 percent in the lower tidal volume group (6 mL/kg).[148] The goal of low tidal volume ventilation, avoiding overdistension of the lung, is likely to be the same in the pregnant and nonpregnant patient.[148] Furthermore, it is likely that the maximum plateau pressure limit in the ARDS Network study (30 cmH_2O) should be the same in the pregnant patient.[148] It is important to maintain maternal $Paco_2$ in its usual range of 28 to 33 mmHg; thus permissive hypercapnia is not an appropriate ventilatory option in pregnant patients, as maternal hypercapnia quickly results in fetal distress.

Positive end-expiratory pressure (PEEP) can be utilized to recruit alveoli and allow the minimum Fio_2 to be used (ideally <60 percent). It should be applied in increments of 3 to 5 cmH_2O to achieve a satisfactory oxygen saturation (>90 percent) while minimizing potentially harmful peak and plateau pressures (<40 to 45 cmH_2O). Increasing PEEP can depress cardiac output, particularly in patients with intravascular depletion, and thereby decrease uterine blood flow. The minimum effective PEEP should therefore be used. When PEEP is raised above 10 cmH_2O or when hypotension and oliguria fail to respond to modest intravenous fluid challenges, placement of a pulmonary artery catheter should be considered. Although cardiac output is usually increased during pregnancy, central pressures should not be significantly different from those seen in nonpregnant women. The normal tidal volume in pregnant patients is greater than the target volume utilized in the ARDS Research Network (6 mL/kg).[148] It is likely that the optimal ventilatory strategy in pregnant patients is to increase the respiratory rate to optimize ventilation as long as severe intrinsic PEEP does not develop. If this is not adequate to maintain maternal $Paco_2$, then an increased tidal volume can be considered, as long as the plateau pressure does not exceed 30 cmH_2O.[148]

Fluid management is crucial to optimal outcome in ARDS. Recent data have suggested a better result in patients with a lower pulmonary capillary wedge pressure.[149] When fluid is required to maintain the cardiac output, blood products offer an advantage. Vasopressors may be required to optimize maternal oxygen delivery, with ephedrine providing an optimal degree of α and β stimulation to preserve uterine blood flow. Supine recumbency may cause a marked decrease in venous return during the second and third trimesters because of uterine compression of the inferior vena cava. Similarly, the Trendelenburg position may worsen hypotension. In fact, maternal position can have dramatic effects on fetal cerebral oxygenation. In one study, 14 uncomplicated term women under epidural anesthesia were moved to the supine position from the lateral position; the supine position was associated with a significantly lower fetal cerebral oxyhemoglobin concentration and saturation.[150] Ideally, the pregnant patient should be positioned with the right hip elevated 10 to 15 cm.

Specific treatment of ARDS will depend on the underlying cause. Induction of labor is not mandatory, but if the mother is critically ill and the fetus is approaching term, delivery of the fetus may facilitate management. Delivery of the fetus does not necessarily result in a therapeutic result in pregnant patients with severe respiratory distress.

ASPIRATION PNEUMONIA

The initial description of aspiration pneumonia was in obstetric patients in labor. Pregnant women are at risk of aspiration pneumonia due to several predisposing factors, including progesterone-induced relaxation of the gastroesophageal sphincter, delayed gastric emptying, raised intragastric pressure due to compression by the uterus, and as a complication of anesthesia. The use of diazepam to treat eclampsia may be associated with an increased risk of inadvertent aspiration of gastric contents.[151] The severity of aspiration depends on the volume, pH, and particulate content of the aspirate. The greater the volume, the lower the pH, and the presence of particulates will worsen the outcome. Generally, a pH <2.5 produces a chemical pneumonitis. The clinical presentation includes the development of a fever and cough during labor or the immediate postpartum period. Chest radiography confirms a radiographic infiltrate in a dependent location (basilar segments of the lower lobes, superior segments of the lower lobes, or posterior segments of the upper lobes). The clinical course generally follows one of three patterns: (1) rapid improvement in 4 to 5 days, (2) initial improvement followed by complicating bacterial pneumonia, and (3) early death from intractable hypoxemia.

Management generally emphasizes prevention of aspiration and supportive care if it occurs. The bacterial pathogens are usually oropharyngeal anaerobes that can be treated with penicillin therapy. Steroids are not indicated.

REFERENCES

1. Elkus R, Popovich J: Respiratory physiology in pregnancy. *Clin Chest Med* 13:555–565, 1992.
2. Crapo RO: Normal cardiopulmonary physiology during pregnancy. *Clin Obstet Gynecol* 39:3–16, 1996.
3. Contreras G, Guitierrez M, Beroiza T, et al: Ventilatory drive and respiratory muscle function in pregnancy. *Am Rev Respir Dis* 144:837–841, 1991.
4. Gilroy RJ, Mangura BT, Lavietes MH: Rib cage and abdominal volume displacements during breathing in pregnancy. *Am Rev Respir Dis* 137:668–672, 1988.
5. Nava S, Zanotti E, Ambrosino N, et al: Evidence of acute diaphragmatic fatigue in a "natural" condition. *Am Rev Respir Dis* 146:1226–1230, 1992.
6. Milne J, Howie A, Pack A: Dyspnea during normal pregnancy. *Br J Obstet Gynaecol* 85:260–263, 1978.
7. Granstrom G, Granstrom M, Sterner G: Whooping cough in late pregnancy. *Scand J Infect Dis* 71(Suppl):27–29, 1900.
8. Irwin RS, Curley FJ, French CL: Chronic cough. The spectrum and frequency of causes, key components of the diagnostic evaluation, and outcome of specific therapy. *Am Rev Respir Dis* 141:640–647, 1990.
9. Baron TH, Lichter JE: Gastroesophageal reflux disease in pregnancy. *Gastroenterol Clin North Am* 21:777–791, 1992.
10. Ruigomez A, Rodriguez LAG, Cattaruzzi C, et al: Use of cimetidine, omeprazole and ranitidine in pregnant women and pregnancy outcomes. *Am J Epidemiol* 150:476–481, 1999.
11. Fabre E, Tajada M, Gonzales de Aguero R: Use of drugs in pulmonary medicine in pregnant women. *Clin Pulm Med* 9:20–32, 2002.
12. Hornby PJ, Abrahams TP: Pulmonary pharmacology. *Clin Obstet Gynecol* 39:17–35, 1996.
13. Werler MM, Mitchell AA, Shapiro S: First trimester maternal medication use in relation to gastroschisis. *Teratology* 45:361–367, 1992.
14. Montella KR: Pulmonary pharmacology in pregnancy. *Clin Chest Med* 13:587–595, 1992.
15. Lederman MM: Cell-mediated immunity and pregnancy. *Chest* 86:6S–9S, 1984.
16. Lim WS, Macfarlane JT, Colthorpe CL: Pneumonia and pregnancy. *Thorax* 56:398–405, 2001.
17. Richey SD, Roberts SW, Ramin KD, et al: Pneumonia complicating pregnancy. *Obstet Gynecol* 84:525–528, 1994.
18. Munn MB, Groome LJ, Atterbury JL, et al: Pneumonia as a complication of pregnancy. *J Maternal Fetal Med* 8:151–154, 1999.
19. Niederman MS, Mandell LA, Anzueto A, et al: Guidelines for the management of adults with community-acquired pneumonia. Diagnosis, assessment of severity, antimicrobial therapy, and prevention. *Am J Respir Crit Care Med* 163:1730–1754, 2001.
20. American Thoracic Society: Guidelines for the initial management of adults with community-acquired pneumonia:

Diagnosis, assessment of severity, and initial antimicrobial therapy. *Am Rev Respir Dis* 148:1418–1426, 1993.

21. Fine MJ, Smith MA, Carson CA, et al: Prognosis and outcomes of patients with community-acquired pneumonia. A meta-analysis. *JAMA* 274:134–141, 1996.
22. Ramsey PS, Ramin KD: Pneumonia in pregnancy. *Obstet Gynecol Clin* 2001; 28:558–569.
23. Levin KP, Hanusa BH, Rotondi A, et al: Arterial blood gas and pulse oximetry in initial management of patients with community-acquired pneumonia. *J Gen Int Med* 16:590–598, 2001.
24. Neill AM, Martin IR, Weir R, et al: Community acquired pneumonia: aetiology and usefulness of severity criteria on admission. *Thorax* 51:1010–1016, 1996.
25. Chow AW, Jewesson PJ: Use and safety of antimicrobial agents during pregnancy. *West J Med* 146:761–4, 1987.
26. File Jr TM: Appropriate use of antimicrobials for drug-resistant pneumonia: focus on the significance of β-lactam-resistant *Streptococcus pneumoniae. Clin Inf Dis* 34 (Suppl 1):S17–26, 2002.
27. Doern GV, Heilman KP, Huynh HK, et al.: Antimicrobial resistance among clinical isolates of *Streptococcus pneumoniae* in the United States during 1999–2000, including a comparison of resistance rates since 1994–1995. *Antimicrob Agent Chemother* 45:1721–9, 2001.
28. Lynch III JP, Martinez FJ: Clinical relevance of macrolide-resistant *Streptococcus pneumoniae* for community-acquired pneumonia. *Clin Inf Dis* 34 (Suppl 1):S27–46, 2002.
29. Thornsberry C, Sahm DF, Kelly LJ, et al.: Regional trends in antimicrobial resistance among clinical isolates of *Streptococcus pneumoniae, Haemophilus influenzae,* and *Moraxella catarrhalis* in the United States: results from the TRUST surveillance program, 1999–2000. *Clin Inf Dis* 34 (Suppl 1):S4–16, 2002.
30. Whitney CG, Farley MM, Hadler J, et al.: Increasing prevalence of multidrug-resistant *Streptococcus pneumoniae* in the United States. *N Engl J Med* 343:1917–24, 2000.
31. Kellner JD: Drug-resistant *Streptococcus pneumoniae* infections: clinical importance, drug treatment, and prevention. *Semin Respir Infect* 16:186–95, 2001.
32. Feikin DR, Schuchat A, Kolczak M, et al.: Mortality from invasive pneumococcal pneumonia in the era of antibiotic resistance, 1995–1997. *Am J Public Health* 90:223–9, 2000.
33. Ewig S, Ruiz M, Torres A, et al.: Pneumonia acquired in the community through drug-resistant *Streptococcus pneumoniae. Am J Respir Crit Care Med* 159:1835–42, 1999.
34. Metlay JP, Hoffman J, Cetron MS, et al.: Impact of penicillin susceptibility on medical outcomes for adult patients with bacteremic pneumococcal pneumonia. *Clin Inf Dis* 30:520–8, 2000.
35. Turrett GS, Blum S, Fazal BA, et al.: Penicillin resistance and other predictors of mortality in pneumococcal bacteremia in a population with high human immunodeficiency virus seroprevalence. *Clin Inf Dis* 29:321–7, 1999.
36. Heffelfinger JD, Dowell SF, Jorgensen JH, et al.: Management of community-acquired pneumonia in the era of pneumococcal resistance. A report from the drug-resistant Streptococcus pneumoniae therapeutic working group. *Arch Int Med* 160:1399–408, 2000.
37. Bartlett JG, Dowell SF, Mandell LA, et al.: Practice guidelines for the management of community-acquired pneumonia in adults. *Clin Inf Dis* 31:347–82, 2000.
38. Yost NP, Bloom SL, Richey SD, et al: An appraisal of treatment guidelines for antepartum community-acquired pneumonia. *Am J Obstet Gynecol* 183:131–135, 2000.
39. Gleason PP, Kapoor WN, Stone RA, et al.: Medical outcomes and antimicrobial costs with the use of the American Thoracic Society guidelines for outpatients with community-acquired pneumonia. *JAMA* 278:32–9, 1997.
40. Rhew DC, Tu GS, Ofman J, et al: Early switch and early discharge strategies in patients with community-acquired pneumonia. A meta-analysis. *Arch Intern Med* 161:722–727, 2001.
41. Maccato M: Respiratory insufficiency due to pneumonia in pregnancy. *Obstet Gynecol Clinics N Amer* 18:289–99, 1991.
42. Tomlinson MW, Caruthers TJ, Whitty JE, et al.: Does delivery improve maternal condition in the respiratory-compromised gravida? *Obstet Gynecol* 91:108–11, 1998.
43. Rodrigues J, Niederman MS: Pneumonia complicating pregnancy. *Clin Chest Med* 13:679–691, 1992.
44. Rigby FB, Pastorek II JG: Pneumonia during pregnancy. *Clin Obstet Gynecol* 39:107–119, 1996.
45. McKinney P, Volkert P, Kaufman J: Fatal swine influenza pneumonia during late pregnancy. *Arch Intern Med* 150:213–215, 1990.
46. Hollingsworth HM, Pratter MR, Irwin RS: Acute respiratory failure in pregnancy. *J Intensive Care Med* 4:11–34, 1989.
47. Neuzil KM, Reed GW, Mitchell Jr EF, et al: Influenza morbidity increases in late pregnancy. Infectious Disease Society of America (IDSA) 34th Annual Meeting, 1996.
48. Mostow SR: Prevention, management, and control of influenza. Role of amantadine. *Am J Med* 82(Suppl 6A):35–41, 1987.
49. Kirshon B, Faro S, Zurawin RK, et al: Favorable outcome after treatment with amantadine and ribavirin in a pregnancy complicated by influenza pneumonia. *J Reprod Med* 33:399–401, 1988.
50. Centers for Disease Control and Prevention: Prevention and control of influenza: Recommendations of the Advisory Committee on Immunization Practices Advisory Committee (ACIP). *MMWR Morb Mortal Wkly Rep* 45:1–3, 2000.
51. Centers for Disease Control and Prevention: Prevention and control of influenza: Recommendations of the Advisory Committee on Immunization Practices (ACIP). *MMWR Morb Mortal Wkly Rep* 45(RR-5):6, 1996.
52. Cox SM, Cunningham FG, Luby J: Management of varicella pneumonia complicating pregnancy. *Am J Perinatol* 7:300–301, 1990.

53. Esmonde TF, Herdman G, Anderson G: Chickenpox pneumonia: an association with pregnancy. *Thorax* 44:812–815, 1989.
54. Harger JH, Ernest JM, Thurnau GR, et al: Risk factors and outcome of varicella-zoster virus pneumonia in pregnant women. *J Infect Dis* 185:422–427, 2002.
55. Haake DA, Zakowski PC, Haake DL, et al: Early treatment with acyclovir for varicella pneumonia in otherwise healthy adults: Retrospective controlled study and review. *Rev Infect Dis* 12:788–797, 1990.
56. Smego RA, Asperilla MO: Use of acyclovir for varicella pneumonia during pregnancy. *Obstet Gynecol* 78:1112–1116, 1991.
57. Lotshaw RR, Keegan JM, Gordon HR: Parenteral and oral acyclovir for management of varicella pneumonia in pregnancy: A case report with review of literature. *West Virginia Med J* 87:204–206, 1991.
58. Brown ZA, Baker DA: Acyclovir therapy during pregnancy. *Obstet Gynecol* 73:526–531, 1989.
59. Andrews EB, Yankaskas BC, Cordero JF, et al: Acyclovir in pregnancy registry: Six years' experience. *Obstet Gynecol* 79:7–13, 1992.
60. Centers for Disease Control and Prevention: Varicella-zoster immune globulin distribution; United States and other countries. *MMWR Morb Mortal Wkly Rep* 33:81–84, 1984.
61. Clark GPM, Dobson PM, Thickett A, et al: Chickenpox pneumonia, its complications and management. A report of three cases, including the use of extracorporeal membrane oxygenation. *Anesthesia* 46:376–380, 1991.
62. Stevens DA: Coccidioidomycosis. *N Engl J Med* 332:1077–1082, 1995.
63. Wack EE, Ampel NM, Galgiani JN, et al: Coccidioidomycosis during pregnancy. An analysis of ten cases among 47,120 pregnancies. *Chest* 94:376–379, 1988.
64. Rosenstein NE, Emery KW, Werner SB, et al: Risk factors for severe pulmonary and disseminated coccidioidomycosis: Kern County, California, 1995–1996. *Clin Infect Dis* 32:708–715, 2001.
65. Wheat J, Sarosi G, McKinsey D, et al: Practice guidelines for the management of patients with histoplasmosis. *Clin Infect Dis* 30:688–695, 2000.
66. Chapman SW, Bradsher Jr. RW, Campbell Jr. GD, et al: Practice guidelines for the management of patients with blastomycosis. *Clin Infect Dis* 30:679–683, 2000.
67. Robinson CA, Rose NC: Tuberculosis: Current implications and management in obstetrics. *Obstet Gynecol Surv* 51:115–124, 1996.
68. Vallejos JG, Starke JR: Tuberculosis and pregnancy. *Clin Chest Med* 13:693–707, 1992.
69. Jereb JA, Kelly GD, Dooley SW, et al: Tuberculosis morbidity in the United States. *MMWR Surveill Summary* 40:23, 1991.
70. Miller KS, Miller JM: Tuberculosis in pregnancy: Interactions, diagnosis, and management. *Clin Obstet Gynecol* 39:120–142, 1996.
71. Medchill MT, Gillum M: Diagnosis and management of tuberculosis during pregnancy. *Obstet Gynecol Surv* 44:81–84, 1989.
72. Ormerod P: Tuberculosis in pregnancy and the puerperium. *Thorax* 56:494–499, 2001.
73. Jana N, Vasishta K, Jindal SK, et al: Perinatal outcome in pregnancies complicated by pulmonary tuberculosis. *Int J Gynecol Obstet* 44:119–124, 1994.
74. Jana N, Vasishta K, Saha SC, et al: Obstetrical outcomes among women with extrapulmonary tuberculosis. *N Engl J Med* 341:645–649, 1999.
75. Good JT, Iseman MD, Davidson PT, et al: Tuberculosis in association with pregnancy. *Am J Obstet Gynecol* 140:492–498, 1981.
76. Carter EJ, Mates S: Tuberculosis during pregnancy. The Rhode Island experience, 1987 to 1991, *Chest* 106:1466–70, 1994.
77. Doveren RFC, Block R: Tuberculosis and pregnancy: a provincial study (1990–96). *Netherlands J Med* 52:100–106, 1998.
78. American Thoracic Society, Centers for Disease Control and Prevention: Targeted tuberculin testing and treatment of latent tuberculosis infection. *Am J Respir Crit Care Med* 161:S221–S247, 2000.
79. Present PA, Comstock GW: Tuberculin sensitivity in pregnancy. *Am Rev Respir Dis* 112:413–416, 1975.
80. Franks A, Binkin N, Snider D, et al: Isoniazid hepatitis among pregnant and postpartum Hispanic patients. *Public Health Rep* 104:151–155, 1989.
81. Snider Jr. DE, Caras GJ: Isoniazid-associated hepatitis deaths: a review of available information. *Am Rev Respir Dis* 145:494–497, 1992.
82. Bothamley G: Drug treatment for tuberculosis during pregnancy. Safety considerations. *Drug Safety* 24:553–565, 2001.
83. American Thoracic Society: Treatment of tuberculosis and tuberculosis infection in adults and children. *Am J Respir Crit Care Med* 149:1359–1374, 1994.
84. American Thoracic Society/Centers for Disease Control and Prevention/Infectious Diseases Society of America: Treatment of Tuberculosis. *Am J Respir Crit Care Med* 167:651–652, 2003.
85. Alexander S, Dodds L, Armson BA: Perinatal outcomes in women with asthma during pregnancy. *Obstet Gynecol* 92:435–440, 1998.
86. Tan KS, Thomson NC: Asthma in pregnancy. *Am J Med* 109:727–733, 2000.
87. Perlow JH, Montgomery D, Morgan MA, et al: Severity of asthma and perinatal outcome. *Am J Obstet Gynecol* 167:963–967, 1992.
88. Doucette JT, Bracken MB: Possible role of asthma in the risk of preterm labour and delivery. *Epidemiology* 4:143–150, 1993.
89. Schatz M, Zeiger RS, Hoffman CP, et al: Perinatal outcomes in the pregnancies of asthmatic women: A prospective controlled analysis. *Am J Respir Crit Care Med* 151:1170–1174, 1995.

90. Demissie K, Breckenridge MB, Rhoads GG: Infant and maternal outcomes in pregnancies of asthmatic women. *Am J Respir Crit Care Med* 158:1091–1095, 1998.
91. Liu S, Wen SW, Demissie K, et al: Maternal asthma and pregnancy outcomes: a retrospective cohort study. *Am J Obstet Gynecol* 184:90–96, 2001.
92. Fitzsimmons R, Greenberger PA, Patterson R: Outcome of pregnancy in women requiring corticosteroids for severe asthma. *J Allergy Clin Immunol* 78:349–353, 1986.
93. Schatz M: Interrelationships between asthma and pregnancy: A literature review. *J Allergy Clin Immunol* 103:S330–S336, 1999.
94. National Asthma Education Program National Heart, Lung, and Blood Institute, National Institutes of Health. Report of the Working Group on Asthma and Pregnancy. Executive summary: management of asthma during pregnancy. NIH Publications No. 93-3279A March 1993.
95. National Institutes of Health: Global Initiative for Asthma, Vol. 2002. National Heart, Blood and Lung Institute, 2002.
96. McFadden ER, Kiser R, DeGroot WJ: Acute bronchial asthma. Relations between clinical and physiologic manifestations. *N Engl J Med* 288:221–225, 1973.
97. Emerman CL, Cydulka RK: Effect of pulmonary function testing on the management of acute asthma. *Arch Intern Med* 155:2225–2228, 1995.
98. McGrath AM, Gardner DM, McCormack J: Is home peak expiratory flow monitoring effective for controlling asthma symptoms? *J Clin Pharm Therapy* 26:311–317, 2001.
99. Mabie WC: Asthma in pregnancy. *Clin Obstet Gynecol* 39:56–69, 1996.
100. Cousins L: Fetal oxygenation, assessment of fetal well-being, and obstetric management of the pregnant patient with asthma. *J Allergy Clin Immunol* 103:S343–S349, 1999.
101. Barnes PJ: Inhaled glucocorticoids for asthma. *N Engl J Med* 332:868–875, 1995.
102. Stenius-Aarniala B, Hedman J, Teramo K: Acute asthma during pregnancy. *Thorax* 51:411–414, 1996.
103. Wendel PJ, Ramin SM, Barnett-Hamm C, et al.: Asthma treatment in pregnancy. *Am J Obstet Gynecol* 175:150–154, 1996.
104. Cydulka RK, Emerman CL, Schreiber D, et al: Acute asthma among pregnant women presenting to the emergency department. *Am J Respir Crit Care Med* 160:887–892, 1999.
105. Murphy VE, Zakar T, Smith R, et al: Reduced 11beta-hydroxysteroid dehydrogenase type 2 activity is associated with decreased birth weight centile in pregnancies complicated by asthma. *J Clin Endocrinol Metab* 87:1660–1668, 2002.
106. Kallen B, Rydhstroem H, Aberg A: Congenital malformations after the use of inhaled budesonide in early pregnancy. *Obstet Gynecol* 93:392–395, 1999.
107. Dombroski MP, Huff R, Lipkowitz M, et al: The use of newer asthma and allergy medications during pregnancy. *Ann Allergy Asthma Immunol* 84:475–480, 2000.
108. Fraser FC, Sajoo A: Teratogenic potential of corticosteroids in humans. *Teratology* 51:45–46, 1995.
109. Czeizel AE, Rockenbauer M: Population-based case control study of teratogenic potential of corticosteroids. *Teratology* 56:335–340, 1997.
110. Rodriguez-Pinilla E, Martinez-Firas ML: Corticosteroids during pregnancy and oral clefts: A case-control study. *Teratology* 58:2–5, 1998.
111. Spector SL, Antileukotriene Working Group: Safety of antileukotriene agents in asthma management. *Ann Allergy Asthma Immunol* 86:18–23, 2001.
112. Schatz M, Zeiger RS, Harden K, et al: The safety of asthma and allergy medications during pregnancy. *J Allergy Clin Immunol* 100:301–306, 1997.
113. Carter BL, Driscoll CE, Smith GD: Theophylline clearance during pregnancy. *Obstet Gynecol* 68:555, 1986.
114. Greenberger PA: The management of severe asthma during pregnancy. *Immunol Allergy Clin North Am* 20:763–774, 2000.
115. Luskin AT. An overview of the recommendations of the Working Group on Asthma and Pregnancy. *J All Clin Immunol* 103:S350–3, 1999.
116. Sorri M, Bortikanen-Sorri AL, Karja J: Rhinitis during pregnancy. *Rhinology* 18:83, 1980.
117. Broussard CN, Richter JE: Treating gastro-esophageal reflux disease during pregnancy and lactation: What are the safest therapeutic options? *Drug Safety* 19:325–337, 1998.
118. Bloch H, Silverman R, Mancherje N, et al: Intravenous magnesium sulfate as an adjunct in the treatment of acute asthma. *Chest* 107:1576–1581, 1995.
119. Berg TG, Smith CV: Pharmacologic therapy for peripartum emergencies. *Clin Obstet Gynecol* 45:125–135, 2002.
120. Younker D, Clark R, Tessem J, et al: Bupivacaine-fentanyl epidural analgesia for a parturient in status asthmaticus. *Can J Anaesth* 34:609–612, 1987.
121. Fung DL: Emergency anesthesia for asthma patients. *Clin Rev Allergy* 3:127–141, 1985.
122. Gal TJ, Suratt PM: Atropine and glycopyrrolate effects on lung mechanics in normal man. *Anesth Analg* 60:85–90, 1981.
123. Kotloff RM, FitzSimmons SC, Fiel SB: Fertility and pregnancy in patients with cystic fibrosis. *Clin Chest Med* 13:623–635, 1992.
124. Hilman BC, Aitken ML, Constantinescu M: Pregnancy in patients with cystic fibrosis. *Clin Obstet Gynecol* 39:70–86, 1996.
125. Gilljam M, Antoniou M, Shin J, et al: Pregnancy in cystic fibrosis. Fetal and maternal outcome. *Chest* 118:85–91, 2000.
126. Frangolias DD, Nakielna EM, Wilcox PG: Pregnancy and cystic fibrosis. A case-controlled study. *Chest* 111:963–969, 1997.
127. Jankelson D, Robinson M, Parsons S, et al: Cystic fibrosis and pregnancy. *Aust N Z J Obstet Gynaecol* 38:180–184, 1998.

128. Selroos O: Sarcoidosis and pregnancy: A review with results of a retrospective survey. *J Intern Med* 227:221–224, 1990.
129. Haynes de Regt R: Sarcoidosis and pregnancy. *Obstet Gynecol* 70:369–372, 1987.
130. Baughman RP, Lower EE, Lynch JP III: Treatment modalities for sarcoidosis. *Clin Pulm Med* 1:223–231, 1994.
131. Terndrup TE, Bosco SF, McLean ER: Spontaneous pneumothorax complicating pregnancy. Case report and review of the literature. *J Emerg Med* 7:245–248, 1989.
132. Van Winter JT, Nichols FC, Pairolero PC, et al: Management of spontaneous pneumothorax during pregnancy: Case report and review of the literature. *Mayo Clin Proc* 71:249–252, 1996.
133. Baumann MH, Strange C, Heffner JE, et al: Management of spontaneous pneumothorax. An American College of Chest Physicians Delphi Consensus Statement. *Chest* 119:590–602, 2001.
134. Light RW: Management of spontaneous pneumothorax. *Am Rev Respir Dis* 148:245–8, 1993.
135. Dhalla SS, Teskey JM: Surgical management of recurrent spontaneous pneumothorax during pregnancy. *Chest* 89:301–302, 1985.
136. Farrell SJ: Spontaneous pneumothorax in pregnancy: A case report and review of the literature. *Obstet Gynecol* 62:43S–45S, 1983.
137. Karson EM, Saltzman D, Davis MR: Pneumomediastinum in pregnancy: Two case reports and a review of the literature, pathophysiology, and management. *Obstet Gynecol* 64:39S–43S, 1984.
138. Reeder SR: Subcutaneous emphysema, pneumomediastinum, and pneumothorax in labor and delivery. *Am J Obstet Gynecol* 154:487–489, 1986.
139. Pehrsson K, Bake B, Larsson S, et al: Lung function in adult idiopathic scoliosis: a 20 year follow up. *Thorax* 46:474–478, 1991.
140. Visscher W, Lonstein JE, Hoffman DA, et al: Reproductive outcomes in scoliosis patients. *Spine* 13:1096–1098, 1988.
141. Blount WP, Mellencamp D: The effect of pregnancy on idiopathic scoliosis. *J Bone Joint Surg [Am]* 62:1083–1087, 1980.
142. Siegler D, Zorab PA: Pregnancy in thoracic scoliosis. *Br J Dis Chest* 75:367–370, 1981.
143. Sawicka EH, Spencer GT, Branthwaite MA: Management of respiratory failure complicating pregnancy in severe kyphoscoliosis: A new use for an old technique? *Br J Dis Chest* 80:191–196, 1986.
144. Catanzarite V, Cousins L: Respiratory failure in pregnancy. *Immunol Allergy Clin North Am* 20:775–806, 2000.
145. Hollignsworth HM, Irwin RS: Acute respiratory failure in pregnancy. *Clin Chest Med* 13:723–740, 1992.
146. Kollef MH, Schuster DP: The acute respiratory distress syndrome. *N Engl J Med* 332:27–37, 1995.
147. Deblieux PM, Summer WR: Acute respiratory failure in pregnancy. *Clin Obstet Gynecol* 39:143–152, 1996.
148. Acute Respiratory Distress Syndrome Network: Ventilation with lower tidal volumes as compared with traditional tidal volumes for acute lung injury and the acute respiratory distress syndrome. *N Engl J Med* 342:1301–1308, 2000.
149. Cotton DB, Benedetti TJ: Use of the Swan-Ganz catheter in obstetrics and gynecology. *Obstet Gynecol* 56:641–5, 1980.
150. Aldrich CJ, D'Antona D, Spencer JAD, et al: The effect of maternal posture on fetal cerebral oxygenation during labor. *Br J Obstet Gynaecol* 102:14–19, 1995.
151. Crowther C: Magnesium sulfate versus diazepam in the management of eclampsia: A randomized controlled trial. *Br J Obstet Gynaecol* 97:110–115, 1990.

14

Abdominal Pain and Surgical Complications of Pregnancy

Jennifer Gunter

KEY POINTS

- Diagnostic delays are more common with surgical disorders in pregnancy, increasing both maternal and fetal morbidity and mortality.
- Physical finding of a surgical abdomen may be more difficult to elicit in pregnancy.
- Obstetric causes must always be considered in the pregnant patient with abdominal or pelvic pain, regardless of gestational age.
- Suspected appendicitis is the most common nonobstetric indication for surgery in pregnancy.
- Adnexal masses that persist beyond 18 weeks' gestation are rarely functional.
- The incidence of gallbladder disease is increased in pregnancy.
- Ultrasound (US) is the most useful imaging tool in the evaluation of abdominal pain in pregnancy.

INTRODUCTION

Abdominal pain is a common occurrence in pregnancy, with etiology ranging from benign, pregnancy-related musculoskeletal complaints to surgical emergencies with significant morbidity and mortality for both mother and fetus. The health care practitioner who first evaluates a pregnant woman with abdominal pain must be acutely aware of the anatomic and physiologic changes of pregnancy that may affect physical examination, interpretation of laboratory data, and choice of radiographic procedures. The emergency care practitioner who first evaluates a pregnant woman with abdominal pain must be able to triage patients with regard to obstetric or nonobstetric cause of pain. While the common nonobstetric causes of abdominal pain in pregnancy are generally the same medical and surgical illnesses that cause abdominal pain in all women of reproductive age and are not exacerbated by pregnancy per se, diagnostic delay is more common in the pregnant patient and may translate into increased morbidity and mortality for both mother and fetus. It is especially important that delays in diagnosis and treatment not occur in the 0.5 to 2 percent of pregnancies that are complicated by surgical illnesses, as delays in operative intervention significantly increase complications for both patients.[1,2]

PHYSICAL EVALUATION

Careful evaluation is required for all women with abdominal pain in pregnancy, especially among those patients who present to the emergency department, as this may signify a recent increase in severity of the pain. As part of the initial evaluation an estimate of gestational age should be obtained. Patients who have reached viability will generally also require an evaluation of fetal well-being, and patients who are 22 to 23 weeks and beyond may also be offered more aggressive obstetric intervention should preterm labor or fetal compromise ensue. Gestational age should also be considered when positioning a pregnant patient for physical examination. In the third trimester with increasing uterine size patients in the dorsal position may develop reduced venous return due to uterine compression of the vena cava, with resulting maternal hypotension.

Physical examination and diagnostic tools typically used for the evaluation of abdominal pain may be affected by changes in maternal anatomy and physiology. A complete review of the anatomic and physiologic alterations and adaptations of pregnancy may be found in Chaps. 1 and 2; however, some of these are of particular importance in the evaluation of patients with abdominal pain. Changes in vital signs such as physiologic dyspnea, an increase in the resting pulse rate of 10 to 15 beats per minute, and a decrease in blood pressure are all normal maternal adaptations to pregnancy and may be confused with evidence of cardiovascular dysfunction or sepsis. Conversely, the almost 50 percent increase in maternal blood volume may delay onset of symptoms and signs of hypovolemia. Pregnant women commonly experience nausea and vomiting, primarily in the first trimester, and may experience musculoskeletal abdominal pain throughout pregnancy. The enlarging uterus displaces the abdominal contents cephalad and may physically interfere with a complete examination of the abdomen and pelvis. Decreased tension of the muscles of the anterior abdominal wall and the diastasis recti may reduce abdominal findings such as rebound tenderness, rigidity, and guarding.[3–5]

Laboratory investigations may similarly be altered in pregnancy, affecting their utility in diagnosis. The white blood cell count may normally increase up to 12,000 cells/mL, limiting the usefulness of subtle increases to detect infection, and the hemodilution of pregnancy, a normal adaptation, may result in a low hematocrit in the absence of blood loss.[6] Other considerations include plasma albumin, which can be reduced to an average of 3.0 g/dL in the third trimester, and alkaline phosphatase, which may be doubled at term.

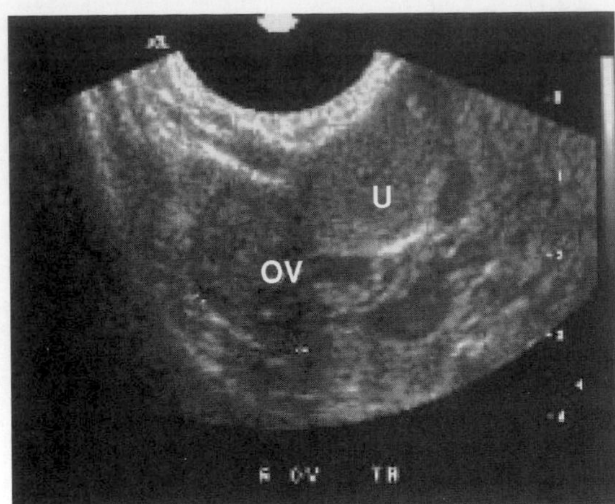

Fig. 14-1. Ultrasound image of right adnexal mass; at 8 weeks' gestation. Transverse view. OV: adnexal mass; U: uterus.

OBSTETRIC CAUSES OF ABDOMINAL PAIN

Inevitably, all pregnant women will experience abdominal pain from labor; however, other obstetric causes of abdominal pain should always be considered, especially in patients less than 37 weeks' gestational age. Conditions that produce abdominal pain in pregnancy are best divided into those that commonly occur in the first trimester and those that occur in the second and third trimesters (Table 14-1).

First Trimester Pain

Ectopic pregnancy and spontaneous abortion are common causes of abdominal pain in the first trimester and are covered in detail in Chaps. 4 and 5. The differential diagnosis for ectopic pregnancy must also include a corpus luteum, which often presents with unilateral lower quadrant pain and an adnexal mass on examination and/or ultrasound (Fig. 14-1). A ruptured corpus luteum may produce intraabdominal bleeding and even an acute abdomen. In early pregnancy before an intrauterine pregnancy can be confirmed by US, a corpus luteum may be very difficult to distinguish from an ectopic pregnancy or adnexal torsion, and frequently patients in the first trimester with pain and an adnexal mass on ultrasonography require a laparoscopy for definitive diagnosis (Fig. 14-2).

Table 14-1. Obstetric Causes of Abdominal and Pelvic Pain

First Trimester	Second and Third Trimester
Spontaneous abortion	Labor
Ectopic pregnancy	Preterm labor and contractions
Corpus luteum	Placental abruption
Musculoskeletal or ligamentous	Uterine rupture and dehiscence
	Severe preeclampsia or HELLP syndrome
	Incarcerated uterus
	Musculoskeltal or ligamentous

Second and Third Trimesters

Musculoskeletal

Musculoskeletal or ligamentous pain is very common in normal pregnancies, especially with advancing gestational age as the uterine size increases. This pain is often described as "round ligament pain"; however the exact origin of this pain many vary from patient to patient. This pain may be relieved by heat or acetaminophen, is often worse on one side, is continuous, and may be described as a stretching or pulling sensation. It is a benign and usually self-limiting occurrence that commonly causes discomfort in the second trimester.

Labor

The evaluation of all pregnant women with abdominal discomfort must always include uterine contractions as an etiology. Pain from labor is generally intermittent, occurring at decreasing intervals. However, tetanic uterine contractions, often evidence of uterine irritability, may produce sustained pain. An accurate estimation of gestational age is crucial to distinguish the normal labor antic-

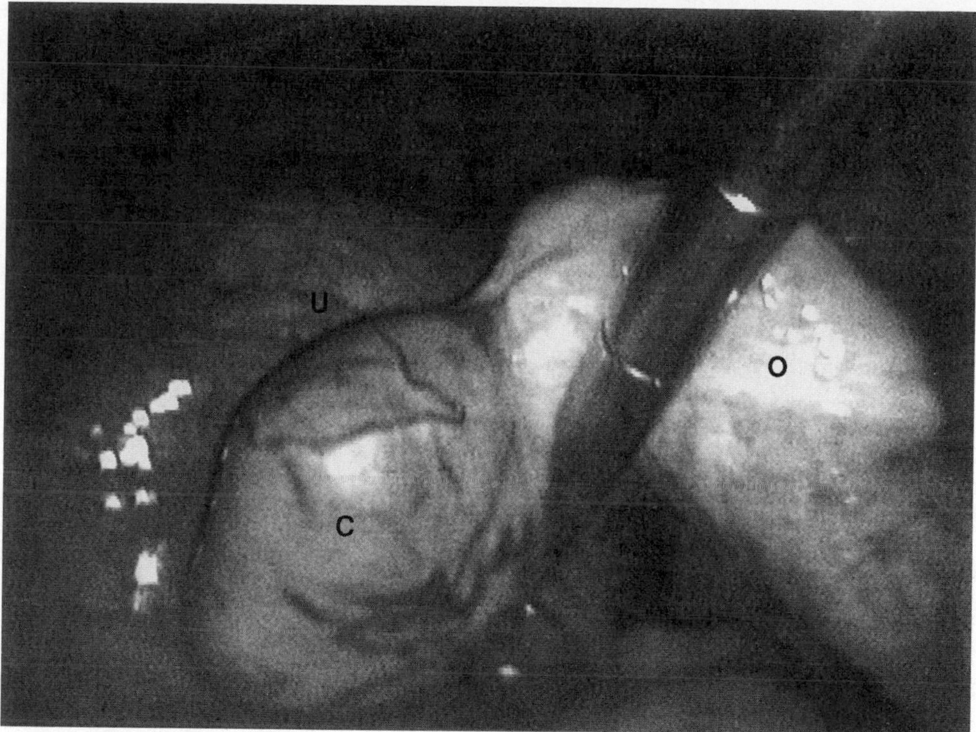

Fig. 14-2. Right ovarian mass at 8 weeks' gestational age (From Fig. 14-1) diagnosed as corpus luteum. U: pregnant uterus; O: ovary; C: corpus luteum.

ipated in a term pregnancy from preterm labor. Preterm contractions are contractions that are painful and occur by definition before 37 weeks of gestational age; preterm labor is defined as preterm contractions with associated cervical change.[7]

When contractions are suspected as a cause of abdominal pain, a cervical examination should be performed to evaluate the cervix for dilation, effacement, and if possible the station of the presenting part. A digital cervical examination should not be performed in the face of vaginal bleeding if placenta previa has not been ruled out (see Chaps. 4 and 10). Patients who are at less than 37 weeks' gestation with suspected preterm rupture of membranes should have a sterile speculum examination performed to confirm membrane rupture and to visually assess cervical dilation, because digital examinations may increase the risk of ascending infection.

While the majority of preterm labor is idiopathic, the clinician should remember that there are many conditions that may cause preterm uterine contractions and preterm labor, including placental abruption, chorioamnionitis, trauma, appendicitis, and pyelonephritis or other infection. Rapid evaluation is essential as tocolysis or other obstetric interventions may be indicated depending on gestational age.

Placental Abruption

Placental abruption is premature separation of the placenta from the uterus, resulting in bleeding from the site of placental attachment. Bleeding may be concealed if it does not occur at the edge of the placenta, and therefore some patients with significant abruptions may have no bleeding and others may bleed profusely. A significant amount of blood may be concealed in the uterus, so the degree of vaginal bleeding is not an accurate estimation of the severity of the abruption or the amount of blood lost. Patients with placental abruptions may present with severe abdominal pain, and on abdominal examination uterine tenderness is usually present. As blood is a potent uterine irritant, uterine contractions are seen. As bleeding continues, maternal hypotension and/or tachycardia may develop, fetal monitoring may indicate fetal tachycardia, and prolonged or tetanic uterine contractions may be identified on tocography. A severe abruption may produce a consumptive coagulopathy that may further potentiate bleeding from the uterus in addition to bleeding from other sites. Initial management involves ensuring adequate maternal oxygenation and hemodynamic stability. Minor abruptions with no maternal or fetal compromise may be managed conservatively, while others are true obstetric emergencies. A full discussion of management of placental abruption may be found in Chap. 10.

Uterine Rupture

Uterine rupture is fortunately an uncommon complication of pregnancy. This frequently catastrophic condition is most likely to occur in the patient laboring with a known prior cesarean section. However, uterine rupture may also happen prior to the onset of labor. The major risk factor for uterine rupture is previous uterine surgery that has affected the integrity of the myometrium, leaving the associated scar vulnerable to dehiscence with increasing uterine size. The most common surgical procedures that increase a patient's risk for uterine rupture are cesarean section and myomectomy, although spontaneous rupture of an unscarred uterus in pregnancy has also been described.[8–10] Patients who have undergone a previous pregnancy termination may also be at increased risk for uterine rupture as a delayed complication of overt or unrecognized uterine perforation.[11] The risk of uterine rupture prior to the onset of labor in a patient with a previous low-segment cesarean section is 0.16 percent, and this risk increases to 0.52 percent with spontaneous labor; classic and T-shaped uterine incisions have a spontaneous rupture rate of up to 9 percent.[8,9] While the exact rate of uterine rupture after myomectomy is unknown, spontaneous uterine rupture has been described after abdominal myomectomy, laparoscopic myomectomy, and electromyolysis.[9,12–14]

Patients with uterine rupture typically present with sudden-onset abdominal pain. There may be associated intraabdominal hemorrhage and subsequent symptoms and signs of hypovolemia; vaginal bleeding may also occur, but in no way does the absence of vaginal bleeding reduce the suspicion of uterine rupture. Fetal distress may be present if fetal heart tones can be auscultated; if fetal heart tones are inaudible, fetal demise must be suspected. Uterine rupture is a true surgical emergency for both mother and fetus, requiring prompt recognition and immediate surgical intervention.

Severe Preeclampsia

Right upper quadrant pain may be a manifestation of severe pregnancy-induced hypertension or preeclampsia, and is related to a combination of hepatic edema and ischemia.[15] In patients with advanced disease, especially with associated disseminated intravascular coagulation or thrombocytopenia, subcapsular hepatic hematomas must also be considered. Preeclampsia should always be considered in the differential diagnosis of any pregnant patient over 20 weeks' gestation with right upper quadrant or epigastric abdominal pain. Other symptoms that may raise the index of suspicion for preeclampsia include headache, visual scotomata, nausea, vomiting, worsening pedal edema, and new-onset nondependent edema (typically of the face and hands). Physical signs of preeclampsia are hypertension, a blood pressure greater than 140/90 mmHg, and hyperreflexia.[16,17] Laboratory investigations should include a complete blood count, serum electrolytes, and liver function tests including uric acid, and evaluation of urine for proteinuria. While a 24-hour urine collection with ≥300 mg of protein is diagnostic of preeclampsia, two urine dipstick tests of 2+ proteinuria (100 mg/dL) 6 hours apart are also diagonistic.[16,17]

Women with severe preeclampsia generally need to be delivered, although some exceptions may occur at the extremes of viability. When preeclampsia is suspected, early obstetric consultation is recommended so an evaluation of fetal well-being may be performed, seizure prophylaxis instituted, and preparations for delivery made as deemed appropriate.

Incarcerated Uterus

Uterine incarceration is an rare occurrence, with an incidence of 1 in 3000 pregnancies.[18,19] Classically it presents in the early second trimester, after 14 weeks' gestation in a patient with a retroflexed, retroverted uterus. While it has been postulated that uterine anomalies or pelvic pathology may increase the risk of incarceration, the exact etiology is unknown. A 1994 review of seven cases identified no causative factors.[19] An incarcerated uterus should be considered in the patient presenting in the early second trimester with complaints of severe pelvic pressure or pain. Other symptoms may include lower abdominal or back pain, symptoms of urinary retention, rectal pressure, and constipation.[19] Physical examination is usually diagnostic of incarceration; the uterus may appear small-for-dates due to the extreme retroversion and retroflexion. However, if the bladder has become obstructed from the anterior displacement of the cervix, uterine size may initially be difficult to evaluate. On vaginal examination the extreme anterior displacement of the cervix can be appreciated, often immediately behind the symphysis pubis obstructing the urethra. The fundus of the uterus will present as a bulging, soft mass in the cul-de-sac that may be tender.

While the diagnosis of uterine incarceration is largely clinical, ultrasound may be useful to rule out a prolapsed myoma or other uterine anomaly. The posterior displacement of the fundus and anterior positioning of the cervix will be visualized. Ultrasound may also be useful to document viability of the pregnancy, as fetal heart tones may be difficult to auscultate with a Doppler probe due to the extreme retroversion and retroflexion of the uterus.

Definitive management of an incarcerated uterus should be attempted as soon as the diagnosis is confirmed, as reduction is easier with a smaller uterus and complications from prolonged obstruction can occur. Initial maneuvers may be attempted in a clinic or outpatient setting. Once the bladder has been emptied, the patient should be positioned in the dorsal lithotomy position and gentle pressure applied to the fundus of the uterus with two fingers placed in the posterior fornix. If this maneuver is unsuccessful, the patient may be positioned in the knee-chest or Sims position and the attempt repeated. If initial attempts to reduce the incarceration fail, these same maneuvers may be repeated in the operating room with relaxation of the pelvic floor accomplished with a spinal or general anesthetic. Once reduction of the uterus has been successful, placement of a pessary designed to antevert a retroflexed uterus, such as a Smith-Hodge pessary, may be placed in the vagina for approximately a week to help maintain the correct abdominal position of the uterus.

NONOBSTETRIC CAUSES OF ABDOMINAL PAIN

Any condition that can produce abdominal pain in a woman of reproductive age may also cause abdominal pain in pregnancy. Many of these conditions will require surgical intervention, while others may be managed expectantly. A high index of suspicion for surgical conditions must be maintained, as delay in surgical intervention contributes significantly to both maternal and fetal complications. The main nonobstetric causes of abdominal pain to be considered in this section include gastrointestinal, gynecologic, and genitourinary causes, as these are the three organ systems most commonly involved. These are also the three organ systems most likely to be involved in nonobstetric surgery during pregnancy, with abdominal surgery accounting for 25 percent and gynecologic or urologic disorders accounting for another 19 percent.[1] Other causes of abdominal pain such as trauma and domestic violence must always be considered and are covered elsewhere in detail.

Gastrointestinal Causes of Abdominal Pain

Appendicitis

Appendicitis must be considered in the differential diagnosis of abdominal pain in pregnancy, regardless of gestational age, in any woman who has not had a previous appendectomy. Suspected appendicitis remains the most common nonobstetric indication for surgery in pregnancy, with appendectomy complicating 1 in 936 deliveries, with actual confirmed diagnosis of appendicitis in 1 in 1500 pregnancies.[20–22] The frequency of appendicitis is the same in all three trimesters; however, diagnostic delays increase with advancing gestational age.[21] A high index of suspicion and prompt surgical intervention are imperative, as delay increases both maternal and fetal risks, with perinatal mortality approaching 20 percent with appendiceal perforation.[23]

Appendicitis is often a difficult diagnosis in pregnancy as many of the symptoms such as anorexia, nausea, vomiting, and abdominal pain may be present in normal pregnancies. These symptoms are more suggestive of an underlying pathology if they are new in onset or are increasing in severity. Abdominal pain is the most common sign of appendicitis in both pregnant and nonpregnant patients. In the first trimester, pain from appendicitis is primarily localized to the right lower quadrant, or McBurney's point; however, with advancing gestational age the appendix migrates cephalad with increasing uterine size, and the point of maximal tenderness is also displaced cephalad towards the right upper quadrant by the third trimester (Fig. 2-2).[21,24] A recent retrospective review has challenged this belief, reporting an incidence of 78 to 86 percent of right lower quadrant pain in appendicitis in all three trimesters.[25] Appendicitis may also present as back or flank pain with a retrocecal appendix, and diffuse abdominal pain may be present with a ruptured appendix; thus regardless of its location, when abdominal pain is present in pregnancy, appendicitis must always be in the differential diagnosis.[21,22] Guarding and rebound tenderness may also be less frequent in the pregnant patient with appendicitis, especially later in gestation, with increasing separation of the visceral and parietal peritoneum by the gravid uterus and laxity of the muscles of the anterior abdominal wall.[21,22,26] Fever is also a very nonspecific indicator, with only 44 percent of pregnant women with histologically-confirmed appendicitis with a documented temperature greater than 37.8°C.[25]

The presence of a leukocytosis is not a sensitive indicator of appendicitis in pregnancy because the white blood cell count normally increases up to 12,000/mm^3; however, findings such as a left shift and an increase in immature forms are more specific indicators of an infectious process.[6] Similarly, a normal white blood cell count does not rule out the diagnosis of appendicitis, as patients with suppurative appendicitis may not have leukocytosis.[25,27]

Ultrasound is frequently employed in the investigation of patients with abdominal pain, and may be helpful in the diagnosis of appendicitis in the pregnant patient. Not only may ultrasound rule out other causes of abdominal pain such as an ectopic pregnancy or an adnexal mass, but it may also be used to evaluate the appendix. A noncompressible appendix greater than 6 mm in diameter with no peristalsis favors the diagnosis of appendicitis.[28–30] Unfortunately as the size of the uterus increases, visualization of the appendix becomes increasingly difficult and compression more technically challenging. Helical computed tomography (CT) of the appendix is 93 to 98 percent accurate in the diagnosis of appendicitis and is commonly used in the evaluation of a patient in the ED with right lower quadrant pain.[31] Helical CT with instillation of 3 percent contrast medium in the colon has been reported in a study of seven pregnant patients with symptoms clinically suspicious for appendicitis; two patients with appendicitis were identified and treated surgically, and the remaining five avoided surgery and recovered from their symptoms.[32] In these pregnant women select level helical scanning was employed, producing radiation exposure to the fetus of approximately 300 mrad.[32]

Once appendicitis is suspected in pregnancy, prompt surgical intervention is critical for both maternal and fetal well-being. With appendiceal rupture and peritonitis, maternal morbidity and mortality increase significantly and perforation has a 20 percent risk of fetal loss compared to a fetal loss rate of 2 to 3 percent with nonperforated appendicitis.[23,33]

Biliary Tract Disorders

Biliary tract disorders are common among women of reproductive age; however, the incidence of gallbladder disease is further increased in pregnancy due to increased production of cholesterol crystals and incomplete gallbladder emptying that produces biliary stasis.[34,35] While gallstones may be identified in 2.5 to 5 percent of pregnancies and biliary sludge seen in up to 26 percent of pregnancies, the incidence of symptomatic biliary disease is 0.16 percent in pregnancy.[36–38] Cholecystitis and choledocholithiasis are the most common gallbladder disorders in pregnancy, and the presentation may range from asymptomatic to sepsis secondary to ascending cholangitis.

Many symptoms of acute cholecystitis may be encountered in the normal pregnancy: nausea, vomiting, dyspepsia, and abdominal pain. The abdominal pain may be epigastric or in the right upper quadrant and may occur after a meal. Classically, the pain of acute cholecystitis has been described as originating in the epigastric region and radiating to the right upper quadrant, back, or scapula.[39] On examination, patients may be febrile and the presence of epigastric or right upper quadrant pain is usually confirmed; rebound tenderness is suggestive of more advanced disease with peritonitis due to abscess or perforation.[39,40] Laboratory investigation may reveal a leukocytosis; however, if a left shift is identified or an increased number of immature white cells identified, the diagnosis of cholangitis must be entertained. An elevated serum alkaline phosphatase is generally considered normal in pregnancy.

Ultrasound is the best tool for imaging the biliary tree in pregnancy and should be performed in patients with epigastric or right upper quadrant pain suggestive of gallbladder disease. While the presence of gallstones or sludge in the gallbladder are clinical findings suggestive of biliary tract disease, dilatation of the common bile duct and edema of the gallbladder are also found in patients with cholecystitis and choledocholithiasis.[3]

Initial management of uncomplicated acute cholecystitis is medical, consisting of nothing by mouth, intravenous hydration, analgesics, and nasogastric suction if required. Medical management is successful in 82 to 85 percent of cases and definitive surgical intervention can be delayed until the postpartum period.[38,40] Recurrence of symptoms is common during pregnancy, with over 50 percent of pregnant women with cholecystitis experiencing recurrences and over 25 percent hospitalized at least twice.[41] Surgical intervention is indicated in pregnancy when a hospitalized patient has failed medical management or has multiple episodes requiring hospitalization. Complications such as choledocholithiasis, ascending cholangitis, abscess, and perforation all require prompt surgical intervention. In patients with uncomplicated cholecystitis a laparoscopic approach may be possible in the first and second trimesters. Open cholecystectomy may also be safely performed in pregnancy and is generally the procedure of choice if complications are suspected or if the gestational age precludes a laparoscopic approach. Choledocholithiasis may be managed with endoscopic retrograde cholangiopancreatography (ERCP), especially because open common bile duct exploration is associated with increased maternal complications and fetal loss.

Acute Pancreatitis

The most common cause of acute pancreatitis during pregnancy is gallstones; however, other causes such as alcoholism and drug reactions should always be included in the differential diagnosis.[39,42,43] The incidence of acute pancreatitis in pregnancy is approximately 1 in 3333 pregnancies and is more commonly diagnosed with advancing gestational age.[44] Presenting complaints are similar in pregnancy and the nonpregnant state; symptoms that are suggestive of acute pancreatitis include nausea, vomiting, and epigastric abdominal pain often radiating to the back. The cornerstone of diagnosis remains a serum amylase and lipase.[42,43] Imaging the biliary tree may be helpful in identifying the etiology of acute pancreatitis as approximately two-thirds of cases in pregnancy are due to gallstones.[44]

Initial management of acute pancreatitis involves conservative therapy with nothing by mouth and intravenous hydration; some patients may require nasogastric suction for complete bowel rest. The majority of pregnant patients will respond to these initial conservative measures; however, an ERCP or surgical intervention may be required with gallstone pancreatitis or pseudocyst formation.[44,45]

Gastroesophageal Reflux and Peptic Ulcer Disease

Gastroesophageal reflux disease (GERD) is a common disorder in pregnancy. Heartburn, or pyrosis, is a sensitive and specific symptom of GERD and is present in up to 72 percent of pregnant women by the third trimester, with the incidence increasing with advancing gestational age.[46–48] The pathophysiology of increasing pyrosis with advancing gestational age appears to be primarily related to the progressive decrease in lower esophageal sphincter pressure due to the combined effect of increasing estrogen and progesterone levels; however, delays in gastric emptying and increased abdominal pressure from the enlarging uterus may have a secondary role.[46] Other risk factors for pyrosis in pregnancy include prepregnancy heartburn and parity.[48]

Heartburn is commonly described as substernal burning radiating from the xiphoid to the neck and is classically exacerbated by large meals, fatty or citrus foods, and a recumbent position or bending over.[46,49] Patients may also complain of regurgitation. While heartburn and GERD are almost synonymous, a small percentage of patients presenting with pyrosis may have biliary tract disease or peptic ulcer disease.[46] Other nonspecific symptoms that are less common but may also be due to GERD include hoarseness, cough, unexplained asthma exacerbation, and nonspecific chest pain.[46,50–52]

The diagnosis of GERD is largely based on presenting symptoms; the presence of postprandial substernal burning while recumbent or bending over is 90 percent sensitive and specific for GERD and the presence of regurgitation further increases the diagnostic accuracy.[46] Diagnostic procedures such as upper endoscopy are generally only warranted if complications are suspected.

Management of GERD in pregnancy centers on lifestyle and dietary modifications. Raising the head of the bed 6 inches, avoiding the recumbent position for 3 hours after a meal, reducing fat consumption, and avoiding foods known to aggravate GERD can bring about resolution of symptoms for 25 percent of patients.[46] When conservative measures fail, the next course of therapy is generally treatments such as antacids, alginic acid, and sulcrafate.[46] Antacids alone may improve reflux symptoms by almost 50 percent when used twice daily, and in one study of 66 pregnant women, sucralfate significantly improved heartburn symptoms in 90 percent of patients.[46,53,54] While the majority of cases of GERD will respond to conservative measures and the treatments listed above, patients who remain symptomatic are candidates for an H_2-receptor antagonist. Cimetidine, ranitidine, and famotidine are all category B drugs in pregnancy and have all been used successfully for persistent heartburn symptoms.[46,55] The proton pump inhibitor omeprazole is considered a category C drug and should therefore only be considered if H_2-receptor antagonists fail to adequately control symptoms. Omeprazole has been used as a single dose in pregnancy prior to anesthesia and several case reports describe prolonged use in pregnancy for refractory GERD without adverse fetal effects.[46,56,57]

Peptic ulcer disease should be suspected when symptoms of GERD persist despite treatment with antacids and H_2 blockers, if pyrosis is associated with abdominal pain, or if the patient develops hematemesis.[58] Rapid identification and intervention for peptic ulcer disease is essential to avoid life-threatening complications such as hemorrhage, perforation, and gastric outlet obstruction. Most peptic ulcer disease is due to infection with *Helicobacter pylori,* so identification and eradication of this bacterium is essential to the treatment of peptic ulcer disease. Though obtaining a specimen for culture via gastroscopy is the gold standard for diagnosis, several noninvasive testing methods may also be used: serology, urea breath test, and antigen detection in stool.[58] Treatment of peptic ulcer disease in pregnancy includes combination drug therapy, generally with either a H_2 receptor antagonist or a proton pump inhibitor in combination with one or more of amoxicillin, clarithromycin, and metronidazole.[58]

GYNECOLOGIC CAUSES OF ABDOMINAL PAIN

The most common gynecologic causes of abdominal pain to be considered in this chapter are adnexal masses, adnexal torsion, and complications related to leiomyomas. Though ectopic pregnancy and spontaneous abortions are considered gynecologic conditions, they are covered in detail in other chapters.

Adnexal Masses and Torsion

Adnexal disorders requiring surgical intervention occur in approximately one in 1000 pregnancies.[59] Ovarian masses may be problematic during pregnancy because of their risk for torsion, rupture, or hemorrhage. The size of the mass is an important consideration as complications increase with increasing size; large ovarian lesions may also become impacted in the pelvis and even obstruct labor. While most adnexal masses in pregnancy are functional cysts that resolve by 18 weeks' gestation, one in 328 pregnancies will be complicated by a concerning ovarian neoplasm.[60,61] The most common diagnosis in an ovarian mass large enough to warrant surgical intervention after 18 weeks' gestation is a benign cystic teratoma (Fig. 14-3), with serous cystadenoma and mucinous cystadenoma the second and third most common diagnoses respectively. Less commonly, paraovarian cysts and endometriomas may be large enough or symptomatic and thus require surgery. Malignant ovarian neoplasms are fortunately less common and are identified in 2 to 4 percent of persistent ovarian lesions removed during pregnancy.[60,62] Infertility patients who have conceived with the aid of drugs that cause ovarian hyperstimulation are at increased risk for multiple large follicular and lutein cysts, even more so if they have developed ovarian hyperstimulation syndrome (OHSS).

As most ovarian masses in pregnancy are smaller, functional cysts that are asymptomatic, they are usually identified as incidental findings on pelvic examinations in early pregnancy or on obstetric or pelvic ultrasounds ordered for other reasons. As the uterus enlarges, identification of adnexal pathology on bimanual examination becomes increasingly more difficult. Adnexal masses should be considered in the differential diagnosis of any pregnant patient with abdominal or pelvic pain. Complications of adnexal lesions, such as adnexal torsion, rupture, or hemorrhage may present with pain and also with signs of peritoneal irritation such as nausea and vomiting. Physical findings suggestive of peritoneal irritation may also be present, but as previously mentioned, these findings may be less obvious in pregnancy, especially with advancing gestational age.

Patients with pain and a suspected adnexal mass should have a complete blood count performed as bleeding from a rupture or into the mass may produce a drop in hemoglobin and hematocrit. Leukocytosis may be seen with complications that produce peritoneal irritation, such as torsion or rupture; however, this is neither a sensitive nor a specific test for either of these diagnoses. The best method for evaluating the adnexa in pregnancy is ultrasound. Simple cysts smaller than 6 cm are more likely to be functional, but extremely large functional cysts may sometimes be seen.[60] Complex masses with septations, internal echoes, and solid components may represent a hemorrhagic functional cyst or corpus luteum but may also represent a nonfunctional neoplasm such as a teratoma or cystadenoma. Findings such as surface irregularities and papillae also reduce the likelihood that an adnexal mass is a functional cyst. Ultrasound may also be useful in excluding ectopic pregnancy from the differential diagnosis of an adnexal mass in the first trimester.

Ultrasound should also be used when adnexal torsion is suspected. Adnexal torsion is more likely in the presence of an adnexal mass, and thus the identification of ovarian pathology in a pregnant patient with abdominal or pelvic pain is worrisome for torsion. Findings such as absence or a significant reduction in arterial or venous flow on color Doppler and significant ovarian enlargement are also suggestive of torsion.[63,64] Adnexal torsion should be considered a surgical emergency as delay will increase complications such as infarction and rupture, which will increase both maternal and fetal complications. It is also important not to neglect other causes of abdominal or pelvic pain when adnexal torsion is suspected as the preoperative diagnosis may be correct in as few as 27 percent of patients.[65] Treating ovarian torsion by simple unwinding of the ovary at laparotomy or laparoscopy can restore ovarian function in up to 94 percent of cases (Fig. 14-4).[66–68] Immediate surgical intervention is also warranted if rupture is suspected or in the presence of hemorrhage with hemodynamic instability.

The vast majority of adnexal masses that persist beyond 18 weeks' gestation are likely to represent benign or malignant neoplasms. Only 7 percent of those that persist beyond 18 weeks are functional.[62] Masses greater than 6 cm that persist should generally be removed in the early second trimester to reduce the risk of complications such as rupture, torsion, or hemorrhage. Large masses that are symptomatic may sometimes require earlier intervention.

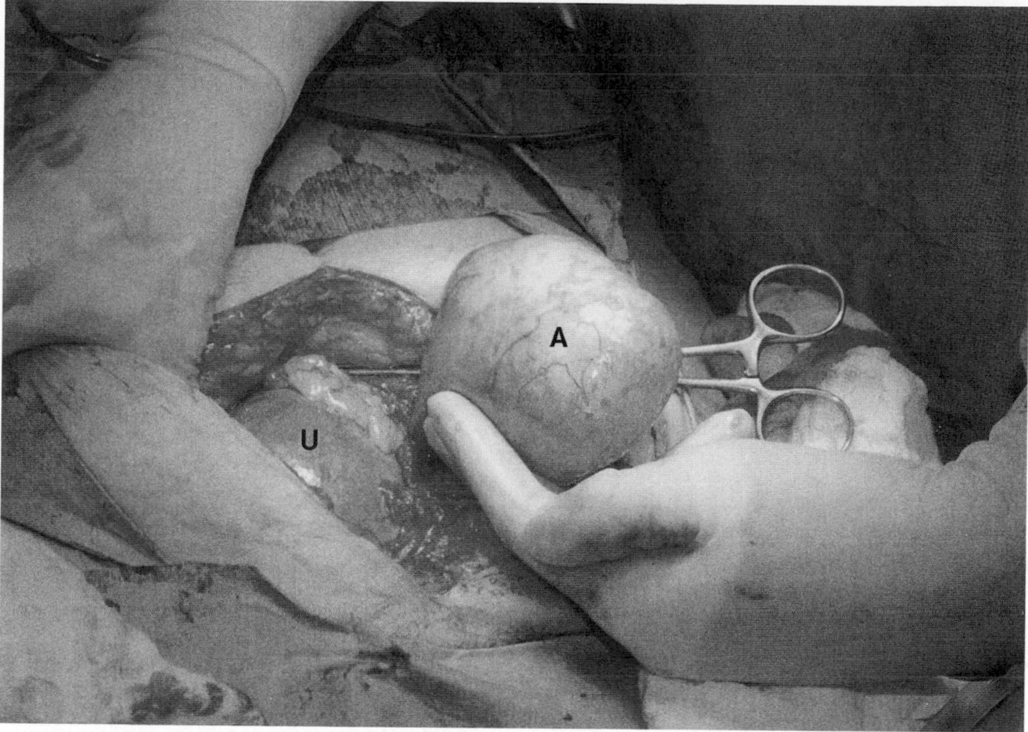

Fig. 14-3. Second trimester, 7-cm left adnexal mass diagnosed as benign cystic teratoma. U: 18 week pregnant uterus; A: adnexal mass (benign cystic teratoma).

Degenerating Leiomyomas

Uterine leiomyomas, or fibroids, may be identified in 25 to 50 percent of nonpregnant women.[69] Under the influence of the increased levels of hormones these benign neoplasms may grow significantly in pregnancy. An asymptomatic, enlarging leiomyoma may be identified on routine ultrasound, or may be suspected in a patient with a uterine size larger than anticipated for gestational age. The leiomyoma may be tender to palpation. Enlarging leiomyomas may become symptomatic, producing increasing pressure on the bladder with resulting urinary urgency and frequency. They may similarly encroach on the rectum and cause difficulties with defecation. Occasionally, as leiomyomas grow they may undergo central hemorrhagic infarction that is often very painful. Degenerating leiomyomas should be suspected in any patient with abdominal pain and uterine fibroids on ultrasound.

In patients who are not pregnant, degenerating leiomyomas are generally treated with nonsteroidal antiinflammatory drugs (NSAIDs), and while indomethacin has been used for this purpose in pregnancy, as a rule long-term use of NSAIDs should be avoided in pregnancy because of their effects on the fetus.[70] Management of the pregnant patient with a degenerating leiomyoma involves symptomatic control of pain with acetaminophen and narcotics if required. Surgical intervention is generally not recommended.

GENITOURINARY CAUSES OF ABDOMINAL PAIN

Urolithiasis

Urinary calculi or urolithiasis complicates approximately 1 in 1500 pregnancies.[71] The classic presentation is flank pain, but patients may also present with nonspecific abdominal pain. Other considerations in the differential diagnosis should include pyelonephritis, appendicitis, and ovarian cyst expansion, rupture, or torsion. Uterine contractions may also be present, further complicating the diagnosis, as the onset of preterm labor in patients with urinary calculi has been described.[72] Fever may also be

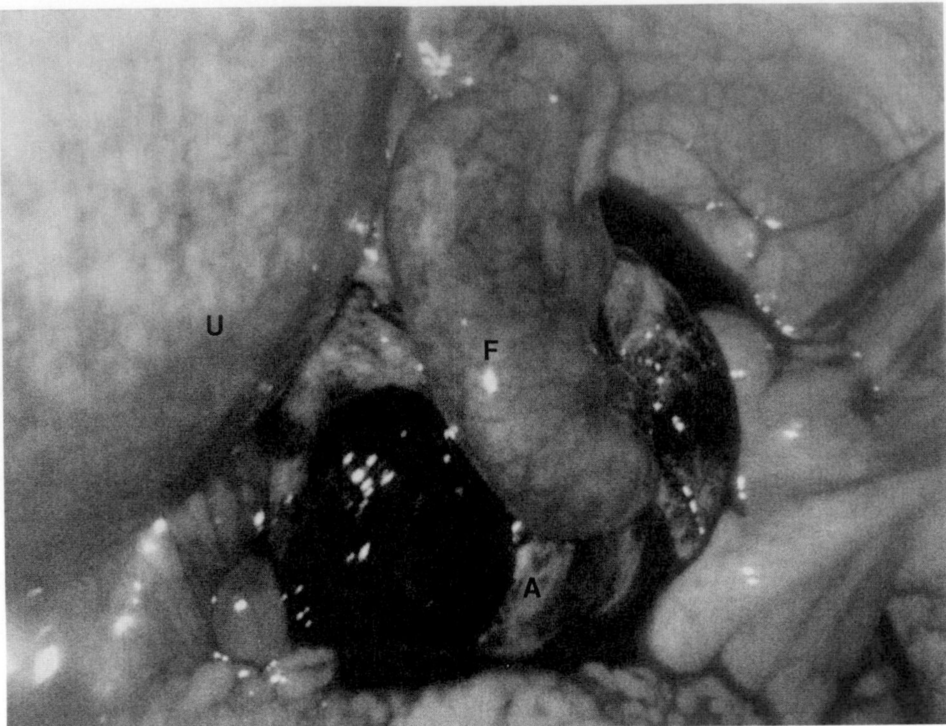

Fig. 14-4. Adnexal torsion at 14 weeks gestation. U: pregnant uterus; A: torsed adnexa; F: fallopian tube.

present and should raise the index of suspicion for a coexisting urinary tact infection. Urolithiasis should also be suspected in a patient with suspected pyelonephritis who fails to respond to antibiotic management.

Every pregnant patient with flank or abdominal pain should have urine microscopic analysis performed. The presence of blood in the absence of recent urinary tract instrumentation raises the possibility of urinary calculi and appropriate imaging studies should be used to aid in the diagnosis. Other indications for imaging the renal system include a negative urine culture with the clinical diagnosis of pyelonephritis, suspected pyelonephritis with persistent fever after 48 hours of appropriate antibiotics, increasing blood urea nitrogen (BUN) and creatinine levels, and protracted pain.[73]

Initial imaging may include a renal ultrasound. However, the finding of hydroureteronephrosis in pregnancy is often a nonspecific physiologic finding related to bolus fluid administration, mechanical obstruction from the uterus, or the smooth muscle relaxing effect of progesterone. Identification of ureteral jets with Doppler sonography may help in excluding ureteral obstruction.[74–76] If the diagnosis is still uncertain after sonographic evaluation, a noncontrast abdominal (renal protocol) CT or intravenous pyelogram (IVP) should be done. A limited IVP, a scout film and an image at 20 minutes, will result in a dose of less than 200 mrad, significantly less than the teratogenic level.[77]

Patients with urolithiasis should be hydrated and be given appropriate pain control. Antibiotics are indicated for a concomitant upper or lower urinary tract infection. The urine may also be strained to identify when the stone has passed. This conservative approach will be successful in the majority of patients.[73] Surgical intervention may be required when conservative management fails or complications of ureteral obstruction develop such as worsening renal function or a persistent infection proximal to the stone.

Acute Pyelonephritis

Acute pyelonephritis must always be considered in the differential diagnosis of abdominal or flank pain in pregnancy, and must also be considered in any patient with obstructive urinary calculi.[78] Classic symptoms include back or flank pain in association with fever, chills, nausea, vomiting, and malaise. Patients may also complain of uterine contractions. On examination the patient is often febrile, looks ill, and will have costovertebral angle tenderness on the affected side. Clinical presentation may range from mild, nonspecific discomfort to urosepsis.

Initial evaluation of the patient with suspected acute pyelonephritis should include a microscopic analysis of the unspun urine. Pyuria is almost always present and a Gram stain will often reveal bacteria, indicating $>10^5$ colony forming units per milliliter. Early identification of either gram-negative or gram-positive bacteria in this manner can also help guide initial antibiotic selection.[79,80] Leukocytosis will generally be present, often with an increase in immature forms, or bands, and urine and blood cultures should also be obtained prior to initiation of antibiotics. A serum BUN and creatinine should also be obtained for assessment of baseline renal function in any patient with suspected pyelonephritis. While urine cultures of $>10^5$ colony forming units per milliliter are generally seen with pyelonephritis, 20 percent of patients will have urine cultures with lower colony counts.[79,80]

Pregnant women with pyelonephritis generally warrant inpatient therapy. Many will require intravenous hydration, and may be too ill to tolerate oral antibiotics, and those who have reached the stage of fetal viability will require close observation for the first 24 to 48 hours for preterm labor. Initial antibiotic therapy may be guided by the Gram stain before the urine culture results are available. Second- or third-generation cephalosporins are generally effective against gram-negative bacteria, although local resistance patterns should always be considered. Demonstration of gram-positive bacteria on Gram stain is concerning for enterococci and so empiric therapy with ampicillin and gentamicin should be instituted.

REFERENCES

1. Mazze RI, Kallen B: Reproductive outcome after anesthesia and operation during pregnancy: A registry study of 5405 cases. *Am J Obstet Gynecol* 161:1178, 1989.
2. Duncan PG, Pope WDB, Cohen MM, et al: Fetal risk of anesthesia and surgery during pregnancy. *Anesthesiology* 64:790, 1996.
3. Fallon WF, Newman JS, Fallon GL, et al: The surgical management of intra-abdominal inflammatory conditions during pregnancy. *Surg Clin North Am* 75:15, 1995.
4. Babaknia A, Parsa H, Woodruff JD: Appendicitis during pregnancy. *Obstet Gynecol* 50:40, 1977.
5. Cunningham FG, McCubbin JH: Appendicitis complicating pregnancy. *Obstet Gynecol* 45:415, 1975.
6. Maternal adaptations to pregnancy, in Cunnigham FG, Gant NF, Leveno KJ, et al (eds): *Williams Obstetrics,* 21st ed. New York: McGraw-Hill, 2001, p 167.
7. American College of Obstetricians and Gynecologists: Assessment of risk factors for preterm birth. ACOG practice bulletin no. 31. *Obstet Gynecol* 98:709, 2001.
8. Lydon-Rochelle M, Holt VL, Easterling TR, Martin DP: Risk of uterine rupture during labor among women with a prior cesarean section. *N Engl J Med* 345:3, 2001.
9. American College of Obstetricians and Gynecologists: Surgical alternatives to hysterectomy in the management of leiomyomas. ACOG Practice Bulletin no. 16. Washington, DC: ACOG, 2000.
10. Singh A, Jain S: Spontaneous rupture of unscarred uterus in early pregnancy—a rare entity. *Acta Obstet Gynecol Scand* 79:431, 2000.
11. Kashyap R, Fliegner JR: Spontaneous mid-trimester uterine rupture. *Aust NZ J Surg* 69:685, 1999.
12. Hockstein S: Spontaneous uterine rupture in the early third trimester after laparoscopically assisted myomectomy. *J Reprod Med* 45:139, 2000.
13. Pelosi III MA, Pelosi MA: Spontaneous uterine rupture at thirty-three weeks subsequent to previous superficial laparoscopic myomectomy. *Am J Obstet Gynecol* 177:1547, 1997.
14. Vilos GA, Daly LJ, Tse BM: Pregnancy outcome after laparoscopic electromyolysis. *J Am Assoc Gynecol Laparosc* 5:289, 1998.
15. Rolfes DB, Ishak KG: Liver disease in toxemia of pregnancy. *Am J Gastroenterol* 81:1138, 1986.
16. American College of Obstetricians and Gynecologists: Diagnosis and management of preeclampsia and eclampsia. ACOG practice bulletin no. 33. *Obstet Gynecol* 99:159, 2002.
17. Hypertensive disorders in pregnancy, in Cunnigham FG, Gant NF, Leveno KJ, et al (eds): *Williams Obstetrics,* 21st ed. New York: McGraw-Hill, 2001, p 567.
18. Longo LD: On retroversion of the uterus by William Hunter in *Medical Observations Inquiry* 4:388, 1771. *Am J Obstet Gynecol* 113:95, 1978.
19. Lettieri L, Rodis JF, McLean DA, Campbell WA, Vintzileos AM: Incarceration of the gravid uterus. *Obstet Gynecol Survey* 49:642, 1994.
20. Mazze RI, Kallen BK: Appendectomy during pregnancy: A Swedish registry of cases. *Obstet Gynecol* 77:835, 1991.
21. Fallon WF, Newman JS, Fallon GL, et al: The surgical management of intra-abdominal inflammatory conditions during pregnancy. *Surg Clin North Am* 75:15, 1995.
22. Babaknia A, Parsa H, Woodruff JD: Appendicitis during pregnancy. *Obstet Gynecol* 50:40, 1977.
23. Mahmoodian S: Appendicitis complicating pregnancy. *South Med J* 85:19, 1992.
24. Baer JL, Reis RA, Arens RA: Appendicitis in pregnancy with changes in position and axis of the normal appendix in pregnancy. *JAMA* 98:1359, 1932.

25. Mourad J, Elliott JP, Erickson L, Lisboa L: Appendicitis in pregnancy: New information that contradicts long-held beliefs. *Am J Obstet Gynecol* 182:1027, 2000.
26. Cunningham FG, McCubbin JH: Appendicitis complicating pregnancy. *Obstet Gynecol* 45:415, 1975.
27. Wittich AC, DeSantis RA, Lockrow EG: Appendectomy during pregnancy; A survey of two army medical activities. *Military Med* 164:671, 1999.
28. Lim HK, Bae SH, Seo GS: Diagnosis of acute appendicitis in pregnant women: Value of sonography. *AJR Am J Roentgenol* 159:539, 1992.
29. Hansen GC, Toot PJ, Lynch CO: Subtle ultrasound signs of appendicitis in a pregnant patient. *J Reprod Med* 38:223, 1993.
30. Jeffrey RB Jr, Laing FC, Lewis FR: Acute appendicitis: High resolution real-time ultrasound findings. *Radiology* 163:11, 1987.
31. Rao PM, Rhea JT, Novelline RA, Mostafavi AA, McCabe CJ: Effect of computed tomography of the appendix on treatment of patients and use of hospital resources. *N Engl J Med* 338:141, 1998.
32. Castro MA, Shipp TD, Castro EE, Ouzounian J, Rao P: The use of helical computed tomography in pregnancy for the diagnosis of acute appendicitis. *Am J Obstet Gynecol* 184:954, 2001.
33. McGee TM: Acute appendicitis in pregnancy. *Aust NZ J Obstet Gynecol* 29:378, 1989.
34. Rai R, Kalloo AN: Biliary tact disease in pregnancy. *J Soc Obstet Gynaecol Can* 19:1075, 1997.
35. Braverman DZ, Johnson ML, Kern F Jr: Effects of pregnancy and contraceptive steroids on gallbladder function. *N Engl J Med* 302:362, 1980.
36. Gastrointestinal disorders, in Cunnigham FG, Gant NF, Leveno KJ, et al (eds): *Williams Obstetrics,* 21st ed. New York: McGraw-Hill, 2001, p 1273.
37. Valdivieso V, Covassubias C, Siegal F, et al: Pregnancy and cholelithiasis: pathogenesis and natural course of gallstones diagnosed in early puerperium. *Hepatology* 17:1, 1993.
38. Swisher SG, Schmit PJ, Hunt KK, et al: Biliary disease during pregnancy. *Am J Surg* 168:576, 1994.
39. DeVore GR: Acute abdominal pain in the pregnant patient due to pancreatitis, acute appendicitis, cholecystitis, or peptic ulcer disease. *Clin Perinatol* 7:349, 1980.
40. Landers D, Carmona R, Crombleholme W, Lim R: Acute cholecystitis in pregnancy. *Obstet Gynecol* 69:131, 1987.
41. Dixon NP, Faddis DM, Silberman H: Aggressive management of cholecystitis during pregnancy. *Am J Surg* 154:292, 1987.
42. Wilkinson EJ: Acute pancreatitis in pregnancy: A review of 98 cases and a report of 8 new cases. *Obstet Gynecol Surv* 28:281, 1973.
43. Scott LD: Gallstone disease and pancreatitis in pregnancy. *Gastroenterol Clin North Am* 4:803, 1992.
44. Ramin RG, Ramin SM, Richey SD, Cunningham FG: Acute pancreatitis in pregnancy. *Am J Obstet Gynecol* 173:187, 1995.
45. Fernandez-del-Castillo C, Rattner DW, Warshaw AL: Acute pancreatitis. *Lancet* 342:475, 1993.
46. Katz PO, Castell DO: Gastroesophageal reflux disease during pregnancy. *Gastroenterol Clin North Am* 27:153, 1998.
47. Klauser AG, Schindlbeck NE, Muller-Lissner SA: Symptoms in gastro-oesophageal reflux disease. *Lancet* 335:205, 1990.
48. Marrero JM, Goggin PM, de Caestecker JS, et al: Determinants of pregnancy heartburn. *Br J Obstet Gynaecol* 99:731, 1992.
49. Parkman HP, Cohen S: Heartburn, regurgitation, odynophagia, in Haubrich WS, Schattner F, Berk JE (eds): *Bockus Gastroenterolgy*, 5th ed. Philadelphia: WB Saunders, 1995, p 30.
50. Koufman JA: The otolaryngologic manifestations of gastroesophageal reflux disease: A clinical investigation of 225 patients using ambulatory 24-hour pH monitoring and an experimental investigation of the role of pepsin in the development of laryngeal injury. *Laryngoscope* 101(Suppl 53):1, 1991.
51. Peters L, Maas L, Petty D, et al: Spontaneous noncadiac pain: Evaluation by 24-hour ambulatory esophageal motility and pH monitoring. *Gastroenterology* 94:878, 1998.
52. Sontag SJ, O'Connell S, Khandewal S, et al: Most asthmatics have gastroesophageal reflux with or without bronchodilator therapy. *Gastroenterology* 99:613, 1990.
53. Lang GD, Dougall A: Comparative study of Algion suspension and magnesium trisilicate mixture in the treatment of reflux dyspepsia of pregnancy. *Br J Clin Pract Symp* 66(suppl):48, 1989.
54. Ranchet G, Gangemi O, Petronen M: Sucralfate in the treatment of gravidic pyrosis. *Giomale Italiano de Obstetrica e Ginecologia* 12:1,1990.
55. Rayburn W, Liles E, Christensen H, Robinson M: Antacids vs. antacids plus non-prescription ranitidine for heartburn during pregnancy. *Int J Obstet Gynecol* 66:35,1999.
56. Marshall JK, Thompson ABR, Armstrong D: Omeprazole for refractory gastroesophageal reflux disease during pregnancy and lactation. *Can J Gastroenterol* 12:225, 1998.
57. Harper MA, McVeigh E, Thompson W, et al: Successful pregnancy in association with Zollinger-Ellison syndrome. *Am J Obstet Gynecol* 173:863, 1995.
58. Winbery SL, Blaho KE: Dyspepsia in pregnancy. *Obstet Gynecol Clin North Am* 28:333, 2001.
59. Neoplastic diseases, in Cunnigham FG, Gant NF, Leveno KJ, et al (eds): *Williams Obstetrics,* 21st ed. New York: McGraw-Hill, 2001, p 1452.
60. Cancer in pregnancy, in Disia PJ, Creasman WT (eds): *Clinical Gynecologic Oncology*. St. Louis: Mosby Year Book, 1993, p. 544.
61. Grimes WH Jr, Bartholemew RA, Colvin ED, et al: Ovarian cysts complicating pregnancy. *Am J Obstet Gynecol* 68:594, 1954.
62. Struyk APHB, Tretters PE: Ovarian tumors in pregnancy. *Acta Obstet Gynecol Scand* 63:421, 1984.
63. Fleischer AC, Stein SM, Cullinan JA, et al: Color Doppler

sonography of adnexal torsion. *J Ultrasound Med* 14:523, 1995.

64. Tepper R, Lerner-Geva L, Zalel Y, et al: Adnexal torsion: the contribution of color Doppler sonography to diagnosis at post-operative follow-up. *Eur J Obstet Gynecol Reprod Biol* 62:121, 1995.
65. Baker TE, Copas PR: Adnexal torsion: A clinical dilemma. *J Reprod Med* 40:447, 1995.
66. Gordon JD, Hopkins KL, Jeffery RB, et al: Adnexal torsion: color Doppler diagnosis and laparoscopic treatment. *Fertil Steril* 61:383, 1994.
67. Shalev E, Bustan M, Yarom I, Peleg D. Recovery of ovarian function after laparoscopic detorsion. *Human Reprod* 10:2965, 1995.
68. Oelsner G, Bider D, Goldenberg M, et al: Long-term follow-up of the twisted adnexa managed by detorsion. *Fertil Steril* 60:976, 1993.
69. Butram VC Jr., Reiter RC: Uterine leiomyomata: etiology, symptomatology, and management. *Fertil Steril* 36:433, 1981.
70. Dildy GA III, Moise KJ, Smith LG Jr., et al: Indomethacin for the treatment of symptomatic leiomyoma uteri during pregnancy. *Am J Perinatol* 9:185, 1992.
71. Denstedt JD, Razvi H: Management of urinary calculi during pregnancy. *J Urol* 148:1072, 1992.
72. Lattanzi DR, Cook WA: Urinary calculi in pregnancy. *Obstet Gynecol* 56:462, 1980.
73. Still DK, Cumming DC: Urinary calculi in pregnancy. SOGC 13:63, 1991.
74. Weiss RM: Clinical implications of ureteral physiology. *J Urol* 121:401, 1979.
75. Asrat T, Roossin M, Miller EI: Ultrasonographic detection of ureteral jets in normal pregnancy. *Am J Obstet Gynecol* 178:1194, 1998.
76. Haddad MC, Abomelha MS, Riley PJ: Diagnosis of acute ureteral calculous obstruction in pregnant women using color and pulsed Doppler sonography. *Clin Radiol* 50:864, 1995.
77. American College of Obstetricians and Gynecologists, Committee on Obstetric Practice: Guidelines for diagnostic imaging during pregnancy. ACOG committee opinion no. 158. Washington, September 1995.
78. Lucas MJ, Cunningham FG: Urinary infection in pregnancy. *Clin Obstet Gynecol* 36:855, 1993.
79. Rubin RH, Shapiro ED, Andriole VT, Davis RJ, Stamm WE: Evaluation of new anti-infective drugs for the treatment of urinary tract infection. *Clin Infect Dis* 15(Suppl 1):S216, 1992.
80. Stamm WE, Hooton TM: Management of urinary tract infections in adults. *N Engl J Med* 329:1328, 1993.

15

Diabetes During Pregnancy

Robert P. Lorenz

KEY POINTS

- Approximately 50 percent of pregnancies in the U.S. are unplanned. All women of childbearing age should be assessed for possible pregnancy.
- Poorly controlled diabetes before and early in pregnancy increases the risk of birth defects sevenfold.
- Increasing risks of spontaneous abortion, stillbirth, and macrosomia are directly related to the severity of hyperglycemia in pregnant diabetics.
- Indications for admission in pregnant diabetics include moderate or severe hyperemesis gravidarum, persistent ketosis for any reason, diabetic ketoacidosis, and poorly controlled diabetes.

In the diabetic woman, early identification of a pregnancy is critical in providing the best possible chance for a good pregnancy outcome, because spontaneous abortion, birth defects, stillbirth, problems in labor, and illnesses in the newborn as it grows are inversely related to control of blood sugar during gestation. This is one compelling reason why women of childbearing age seen for emergency care should be evaluated for possible pregnancy.

The control of diabetes before conception can lower the risk of birth defects sevenfold.[1] The risk of birth defects was 22.4 percent for diabetic women with the highest glycosylated hemoglobin level at the first prenatal visit versus 3.5 percent for those with the lowest level.

Diabetes mellitus (DM) affects 3 to 5 percent of all pregnancies. Types 1 and 2 DM complicate approximately 0.5 percent of pregnancies; gestational DM affects 2 to 5 percent, depending on the demographics of the population. Risk factors for gestational DM include maternal age >30 years, obesity, family history of gestational or type 2 DM, previous large baby, and prior stillbirth.

PATHOPHYSIOLOGY

There is no more sensitive indicator of the metabolic stability of the pregnant diabetic than the condition of the fetus. The fetus represents a barometer, with fetal outcome directly dependent on the degree of blood sugar control from the time before conception until delivery. Table 15-1 demonstrates the potential adverse effects of maternal hyperglycemia on the fetus during various stages of gestation. In normal pregnancy, maternal glucose levels are maintained within a narrow range. Fasting levels are 8 to 10 mg/dL lower during pregnancy, while postprandial levels are slightly higher in pregnancy than otherwise. Glucose is a critical fuel for the fetus and is transported across the placenta by facilitated diffusion. The placenta is an effective barrier to insulin: maternal insulin stays in the mother's circulation for the most part, while, fetal insulin remains in the fetal compartment. In most circumstances, the fetal blood glucose level is slightly lower than the maternal level. Because of the normal stabilization of blood sugar in a nondiabetic mother, fetal insulin secretion fluctuates very little until birth.

In the diabetic pregnancy complicated by significant hyperglycemia, the fetal environment is disturbed by an excess of glucose transported from the maternal compartment to the fetal circulation. In 1954 Pederson[2] proposed a hypothesis for diabetic fetopathy that remains the basis of our understanding. It outlines the following sequence: (1) maternal hyperglycemia, which results in (2) fetal hyperglycemia, which results in (3) early stimulation of excess fetal insulin production as well as hypertrophy and hyperplasia of fetal pancreatic β cells, which results in (4) increased deposition of fetal fat and protein.

The adverse metabolic conditions involve more than glucose imbalance. There are also alterations in amino acid levels, ketone production, and fatty acid metabolism that can affect the pregnancy. The severity of these other derangements is related to the degree of hyperglycemia.

The mechanisms for pregnancy loss due to poor control of maternal glucose levels are not clearly identified. However, hyperglycemia may be more poorly tolerated by the fetus than by the mother. In the pregnant sheep model, chronic maternal hyperglycemia causes fetal acidemia before maternal acidosis develops.[3] Hyperglycemia can reduce uteroplacental blood flow acutely.[4]

Table 15-1. Effects of Hyperglycemia and/or Ketonemia on Pregnancy

Stage	Increased Risk of
Before conception	Infertility Spontaneous abortion Birth defects
First trimester	Spontaneous abortion Birth defects Neurologic sequelae Fetal growth restriction
Second trimester	Spontaneous abortion Fetal death Neurologic sequelae Excessive size Preterm birth Birth trauma
Third trimester and labor	Fetal death Neurologic sequelae Excessive size Preterm birth Birth trauma
After birth	Metabolic abnormalities in newborn Respiratory distress in newborn Childhood obesity and related diseases

Maternal diabetic vascular disease is a risk factor for fetal growth restriction due to poor perfusion and inadequate delivery of substrate. Diabetic ketoacidosis is life-threatening to the fetus. Thirty years ago, the fetal loss rate was 30 percent for maternal acidosis and 64 percent with maternal coma.[5] More recently Montoro and colleagues[6] described 20 type 1 pregnant diabetics in ketoacidosis. Of these, 7 (35 percent) had a dead fetus on admission, but all the fetuses that were alive at presentation survived the acute episode.[6] Pregnancy does predispose patients with type 1 DM to ketoacidosis.

At birth, infants of diabetic mothers exposed to hyperglycemia are susceptible to hypoglycemia in the newborn period, as their insulin production transiently remains elevated after the maternal glucose overload is removed. Related metabolic problems in infants of poorly controlled diabetics include hypocalcemia, hyperbilirubinemia, and respiratory distress.

DIAGNOSIS AND DIFFERENTIAL DIAGNOSIS

From the fetus' standpoint, the impact of DM is related to the degree of hyperglycemia, the stage of gestation, and the attendant metabolic derangements in the mother. However, from the clinician's standpoint, the type of DM present in the mother is significant for understanding the pathophysiology and proper clinical management. The three common types of DM affecting pregnancy are type 1, type 2, and gestational diabetes mellitus. They are briefly described here; readers are referred to another source for more information.[7]

Type 1 Diabetes Mellitus

Outdated synonyms that should be abandoned include insulin-dependent DM (IDDM), juvenile-onset DM, and ketosis-prone DM. The pathophysiology is a deficiency (early in the disease) or complete lack of production of insulin by the β cells in the pancreas, often due to an autoimmune process. In the absence of insulin, these patients develop ketoacidosis and die. Often the disease begins before adulthood, but not always. DM patients are at risk of developing vascular complications of all organ systems. Some patients with a long history of type 1 DM have loss of glucagon production and autonomic dysfunction, placing them at increased risk for severe hypoglycemia.

During pregnancy these patients need frequent meals and snacks, frequent blood sugar monitoring, and close observation for hypoglycemia. Any minor illness can predispose to wide fluctuations in blood sugar and increase the risk for ketoacidosis, which can result in pregnancy loss.

Type 2 Diabetes Mellitus

Outdated synonyms include non-insulin-dependent DM (NIDDM) and adult-onset DM. The pathophysiology is inappropriate utilization of insulin, usually due to insulin resistance at the cellular level.[7] Obesity is common in type 2 diabetics, and in the nonpregnant woman weight loss can cure the disease in some cases. However, weight loss is not recommended during pregnancy. Circulating insulin levels may be normal or actually above normal, but hyperglycemia occurs nevertheless. Ketoacidosis is unusual in the absence of another major illness. Treatment involves diet, exercise, and in many cases drug therapy. Oral agents are often effective but are not used during early pregnancy due to the lack of data regarding potential teratogenesis. Oral agents such as metformin hydrochloride, chlorpropamide, and glipizide cross the placenta and are associated with neonatal hypoglycemia and leukopenia. A newer agent, glyburide, does not cross the placenta and has been used effectively during the later stages of pregnancy (after organogenesis) for gestational diabetes.[8] Insulin in relatively high doses is effective and is used during pregnancy when diet and exercise are ineffective.

Gestational Diabetes Mellitus

This term should *not* be used for patients with type 1 or 2 DM who are pregnant. Gestational DM is defined as carbohydrate intolerance of variable severity with onset or first recognition during pregnancy.[9]

The pathophysiology is the same as with type 2 DM. Normal pregnancy does require increased endogenous insulin production, and this increased demand cannot be met effectively in approximately 2 to 5 percent of women, resulting in gestational DM. Many women given a diagnosis of gestational DM will continue to have carbohydrate intolerance after pregnancy and be shown to be type 2 diabetics. Within 10 to 20 years of pregnancy, up to 50 percent of women with gestational DM will be identified as type 2 diabetics. Treatment includes diet, exercise, and insulin. The specific treatment plan for gestational DM should be determined by the prenatal care provider.

Making a Diagnosis of Diabetes During Pregnancy

By definition, a pregnant woman who has DM first diagnosed during pregnancy should be identified as a gestational diabetic. She may subsequently be identified as having type 2 DM if glucose intolerance persists beyond the postpartum period. Her treatment should be based on the clinical situation rather than a simple classification. In the setting of an emergency department, there are a host of possible causes of hyperglycemia in addition to DM: infection, stress, and pharmacologic treatment (e.g., glucocorticoids, intravenously administered glucose, or parenteral nutrition). From a fetal standpoint, both the cause of the hyperglycemia (e.g., overwhelming sepsis from any source, which may cause pregnancy loss) and the elevated blood sugar are life-threatening. Thus while identifying the particular type of carbohydrate intolerance in the acute care setting is important (e.g., identifying that a patient has type 1 DM, took a large dose of insulin 6 hours ago, and has not eaten), the immediate need is to treat the underlying condition and stabilize glucose metabolism (see the management section below).

Although there is no universal agreement regarding the clinical criteria for a diagnosis of gestational DM, a widely utilized method is the 3-hour 100-g oral glucose tolerance test (GTT) administered after a 3-day carbohydrate loading diet (Table 15-2).[10–12]

Table 15-2. Gestational Diabetes Mellitus—testing Protocol[a]

I. Screening
   A. Diet: no preparation is necessary; often done as morning fasting
   B. Oral glucose (50 g) ingested quickly
   C. No smoking or vigorous activity
   D. Venous glucose drawn 1 h later
   E. Abnormal: >130 to >140 mg/dL (see text) if fasted; >130 mg/100 mL if nonfasting test[12]
   F. Abnormal values: do 3 h test with 100 g

II. Diagnosis
   A. Diet: 3-day carbohydrate loading diet
   B. Oral glucose load (100 g) ingested quickly
   C. No smoking or vigorous activity
   D. Abnormal if two or more values meet or exceed
      1. Fasting—105 mg/dL
      2. One hour—190 mg/dL
      3. Two hours—165 mg/dL
      4. Three hours—145 mg/dL

[a] All glucose measurements performed on venous plasma assayed by glucose oxidase method in a clinical laboratory.[10]

WORK-UP OF PREGNANT DIABETICS PRESENTING FOR ACUTE CARE

History

The intake history should include the last menstrual period, gestational age, any obstetric problems, past obstetric and medical history, medications, and diet. If the patient is a known diabetic, then the type of diabetes (type 1, type 2, or gestational), any diabetes-related organic disease, the type of insulin, time and route of last dose of insulin, and diet including time of last meal should be addressed. Many diabetics will carry a glucometer with them, a written record of their recent blood sugars and insulin doses, and snacks for emergency treatment of hypoglycemia. Many modern glucose reflectance meters have memory storage functions, allowing the clinician to review recent glucose levels quickly. In addition to the chief complaint on presentation for acute care, other recent minor illnesses such as a cold, flu, dental problems, or urinary tract infections may identify the cause of worsening carbohydrate intolerance.

Physical Examination

The physical examination should include temperature, pulse, respirations, blood pressure, and an estimated or measured weight. Mental status should be assessed, because severe hypoglycemia or hyperglycemia can cause confusion, lethargy, violent behavior, or coma. Examination should concentrate on possible sites of infection if clinically indicated.

A pelvic and abdominal examination should assess the fundal height, cervix, and the presence of fetal heart tones. The fetal heart rate can be auscultated by a nonamplified fetal stethoscope after 20 weeks of gestation in a nonobese patient or after 12 weeks of gestation with Doppler. If the patient is beyond 24 weeks of gestation, obstetric consultation may be appropriate to discuss the need for assessment of fetal well-being (e.g., nonstress test or biophysical profile).

Laboratory Assessment

In a pregnant diabetic presenting for emergency care for any problem, initial blood glucose measurement is advised. A bedside glucose reflectance meter, if properly calibrated, can offer a rapid estimate while the standard laboratory test is under way.

In addition to the laboratory work-up of the presenting problem, significant hyperglycemia (e.g., 200 mg/dL in a pregnant woman) in the acute setting should be further assessed for the possibility of diabetic ketoacidosis (DKA). In pregnancy, DKA can occur at glucose levels significantly lower than in the nonpregnant patient.

Diabetic ketoacidosis is defined as hyperglycemia, acidosis, and ketonemia. The laboratory assessment and principles of management of DKA in pregnancy are the same as in the nonpregnant patient.[14,15] Initial laboratory studies include a complete blood count, glucose, electrolytes, blood urea nitrogen, creatinine, venous pH, urinary and serum ketones, arterial blood gases, and urinalysis. The clinician should be aware that because of the normal physiologic changes of pregnancy, normal ranges of routine laboratory test results may change. By midpregnancy, expanded plasma volume results in a 5 to 10 percent reduction in the hemoglobin and hematocrit and a slight reduction in blood urea nitrogen and serum creatinine. The white blood cell count is often 10,000 to 15,000/mm^3 in normal pregnancy and can increase another 50 to 100 percent with labor. Maternal heart rate increases by 5 to 10 beats per minute and midtrimester blood pressures are slightly lower than normal. Increased minute ventilation causes a slight respiratory alkalosis. Small amounts of glucosuria can occur normally in the absence of DM. Once treatment of DKA is begun, 1- to 2-hour assessment of glucose, electrolytes, and pH should follow until stabilization occurs. Other laboratory studies may be repeated as frequently if they remain abnormal. In addition to metabolic therapy, a search for the cause of DKA should be undertaken. Pregnancy per se is not a cause of DKA, but it does predispose a patient to DKA (see pathophysiology section above).

If DKA is present, the patient should be placed in an obstetric intensive care area where both fetal (after about 24 weeks of gestation) and maternal evaluation and treatment can take place.

TREATMENT

Insulin

In order to understand the preexisting treatment program of a pregnant diabetic and the treatment options available in the acute care setting, the many different insulin types are reviewed. Early in pregnancy, oral hypoglycemic agents are avoided due to adverse fetal effects. If a type 2 diabetic presents early in pregnancy on an oral agent, her treatment plan should include switching to an insulin program as soon as possible. Later in pregnancy, in the third trimester, gestational diabetics have been managed successfully with the oral agent glyburide, that does not cross the placenta.[8]

Over 300 types of insulin are produced worldwide. They vary based on source, molecular structure, additives to prolong onset and duration of action, buffering agents, and recommended delivery systems. In addition, insulin can be administered intravenously, subcutaneously by single injection or infusion pump, or intramuscularly. Experimental systems include pancreatic cell transplants and other indwelling devices.

Common formulations of insulin in use include regular, insulin glargine, neutral protamine Hagedorn (NPH), Lente, and Ultralente (Table 15-3). The latter three are

Table 15-3. Insulin Types and Action

Type	Method	Time		
		Onset	Peak	Duration
Lispro	SQ	10–20 min	40 min	3 h
Regular	SQ	15–60 min	1.5 h	5 h
	IV	0–5 min	30–60 min	2–4 h
NPH	SQ	2–4 h	6–10 h	12–24 h
Lente	SQ	2–4 h	6–10 h	12–24 h
Ultralente	SQ	4–8 h	10–12 h	24–48 h
Glargine	SQ	4 h	NA[a]	24 h

[a] See text.
Note: The action of insulin given subcutaneously may vary by 25 percent in one person, and by 50 percent among individuals. The action is affected by patient activity, body location of the injection, and local injection site integrity, such as scarring due to long-term use of one site for many injections.

mixtures of regular insulin with agents that prolong onset, modulate peak action, and extend the duration of a subcutaneous injection. Lente and NPH have a nearly similar pattern of onset, peak, and duration. However, NPH has the advantage of mixing more effectively when a single injection includes a combination of a regular and a longer-acting agent. Insulin glargine is a recombinant human analogue produced by *E. coli* utilizing recombinant DNA technology. It is administered subcutaneously, should not be mixed with other insulin, and has a plateau at 4 hours with a flat profile without a peak for 24 hours. Its release is similar to a continuous infusion by subcutaneous pump of lispro (Humalog®).[13] Currently there is little published information concerning glargine in human pregnancy.

During pregnancy, when meticulous control of blood sugar has beneficial effects on pregnancy outcome, many patients are on intensive insulin therapy. Details vary based on the clinical approach in use locally, but certain aspects are uniform. Glucose measurements are frequent (often 6 to 8 times per day), and regular and intermediate insulin are used in combination or singly with scheduled administration 2 to 5 times per day. Continuous subcutaneous infusion pumps using a buffered regular insulin are occasionally utilized.

Hypoglycemia

Hypoglycemia may be present on first contact or may be iatrogenic (i.e., the result of an extended stay in the acute care setting during which ongoing glucose testing and meals are disrupted). Thus the first aspect of treatment of hypoglycemia in the pregnant diabetic is prevention. Pregnant diabetics who are well controlled by intensive insulin treatment (e.g., six feedings a day and three to five routine insulin injections per day) can quickly develop problems if the routine is disrupted. Such patients may have glucometer values of 50 to 60 mg/100 mL and be comfortable at that level, requiring only their scheduled meal or snack, as opposed to an intravenous bolus of glucose that may disrupt their diabetes for the next 24 hours. Patients with a low blood sugar who are symptomatic but are not NPO can be treated orally with crackers or milk. Candy or orange juice often causes an unnecessarily rapid rise in blood sugar, making further treatment more involved. For severe hypoglycemia associated with obtundation or coma, therapy depends on the setting. Families of type 1 diabetics (the only group at serious risk of profound hypoglycemia) are often trained and have subcutaneous glucagon available, which they may have given while waiting for the ambulance. If intravenous access can be established quickly, then intravenous glucose (e.g., 50 mL of 50 percent glucose solution) given rapidly can awaken the patient and allow further supportive treatment.

Hyperglycemia Without Ketoacidosis

Hyperglycemia without ketoacidosis may also be present on initial contact or as the result of management in the emergency department. Prevention of hyperglycemia requires knowledge of the patient's recent diet and insulin treatment and avoidance of large amounts of intravenous fluids containing glucose.

If ketoacidosis is absent, hyperglycemia can be treated on an individualized basis. Often a knowledgeable patient has an understanding of how much subcutaneously

Table 15-4. Treatment of Diabetic Ketoacidosis in Pregnancy

Simultaneously initiate all of the following:

1. Admit to obstetric intensive care area, if available.
2. Insert large-bore intravenous line.
3. Obtain initial laboratory studies (see text).
4. Place patient on her side or in left lateral tilt position to improve venous return.
5. Consider an arterial line for serial blood sampling.
6. Begin a flow sheet including vital signs, glucose, lab values (to be assessed every 1–4 h based on acuity). Glucose and potassium values should be assessed hourly initialy.
7. Oxygen by mask (3–6 L/min).
8. Foley catheter, sample to laboratory for urinalysis and culture.
9. Volume replacement (total deficit may be 5–10 L):
   a. 1000 mL normal saline over 1–2 h.
   b. If serum sodium or serum osmolality is elevated, replace with 0.45% NaCl.
   c. After 1–2 h, switch to 0.45% NaCl at 250–500 mL/h; reduce rate as glucose nears 200 mg/dL.
10. Insulin therapy:
    a. Intravenous bolus 0.4 U/kg regular insulin.
    b. Continuous intravenous infusion at 5–10 U/h regular insulin.
    c. Reduce hourly infusion rate as glucose nears 250 mg/dL.
    d. Double infusion rate if no response after first hour.
    e. Continue intravenous infusion for 12–24 h after ketoacidosis clears.
11. Potassium therapy:
    a. Give KCl 40 mEq/h if potassium is low.
    b. Give KCl 20 mEq/h if potassium is normal.
    c. Withhold KCl if potassium is elevated.
    d. ECG monitoring if KCl is given with oliguria.
12. Etiology:
    Work-up for causes of diabetic ketoacidosis.
13. Fetal assessment:
    a. Beyond 12 weeks of gestation, fetal heart rate by Doppler.
    b. Beyond 24 weeks of gestation, continuous electronic fetal monitoring and uterine monitoring.
    c. An abnormal (nonreassuring) fetal heart rate is often present in diabetic ketoacidosis and is usually best treated with intrauterine resuscitation. Maternal oxygen therapy, fluid replacement, and correction of hyperglycemia and ketoacidosis will improve fetal condition. Emergency delivery is rarely necessary and potentially hazardous to the mother.
    d. Uterine contractions are often observed and usually do not result in delivery remote from term. Tocolysis should not be undertaken unless significant cervical dilatation occurs. Avoid beta sympathomimetic agents and glucocorticoids for fetal pulmonary maturity during diabetic ketoacidosis.

administered regular insulin is necessary to normalize her blood level. In some cases, a minor modification of her usual insulin program will suffice. Intravenous insulin has a more rapid onset and shorter duration than subcutaneous insulin and can be used as a bolus or a constant infusion. If the patient is NPO and admission is likely, then an intravenous controlled infusion allows gradual and effective treatment.

Diabetic Ketoacidosis

The principles of metabolic treatment of DKA in pregnancy are the same as in the nonpregnant patient, but attention must be paid to fetal status as well.

Treatment is directed at correcting the multiple abnormalities of hyperglycemia, insulin deficiency, ketone excess, acidosis, dehydration, and electrolyte imbalance (Table 15-4).

DISCHARGE INSTRUCTIONS AND FOLLOW-UP INTERVAL

Any female diabetic of childbearing age should be encouraged to use contraception unless she is enrolled in a program to normalize her blood sugar before conception. All women of childbearing age (pregnant or not) should consume 0.4 mg of folic acid daily to reduce the incidence of neural tube defects. Diabetic women who have a normal pregnancy first identified in the emergency department need urgent follow-up to assure the best possible outcome of the pregnancy. Sometimes admission is appropriate (see below).

The goal of diet, exercise, and insulin programs is to normalize blood sugar. Consultation with a nutritionist experienced with pregnant diabetics can be very helpful. In the acute care setting, the planning of insulin therapy should be based on prior insulin doses, and ideally should be coordinated with the team who will follow the pregnancy. Insulin resistance due to hormonal changes in pregnancy does not develop until the second half of pregnancy; however, most diabetics who become pregnant find that they need more insulin than before because the goal is lower blood sugar. One or two injections a day in a type 1 or 2 diabetic who is pregnant will not be adequate to maximize control in most cases.

Home Glucose Monitoring

Any attempt at normalizing blood sugar has some risk of hypoglycemia and can only be undertaken safely with frequent self-testing. With intensive insulin therapy, measurements may be taken before and 1 or 2 hours after each of the three main meals, at bedtime, and at 3 A.M. There is little need for urinary testing at home unless the blood sugar is above 200 mg/dL, in which case urinary ketones indicate a state of increased insulin resistance.

Recordkeeping

Frequent measurements are of little benefit without an accurate record of the dates and times of insulin therapy, meals, activities, and blood glucose values.

Hypoglycemia Safeguards

Type 1 diabetics should be advised to keep a glucose meter with them at all times, along with a snack for emergencies. Family members should be instructed in the warning signs of hypoglycemia and equipped with emergency stores of oral glucose treatment and glucagon to be administered subcutaneously.

Guidelines

Diabetics under good control with a previously identified pregnancy should keep their regular appointments for follow-up care unless the acute problem dealt with in the emergency department requires other treatment.

Diabetics under less than ideal control who are pregnant and any diabetic with an early pregnancy just identified should be seen quickly, and some may be candidates for admission.

The patient should be instructed that a home-tested blood glucose value of less than 60 mg/dL, an episode of severe hypoglycemia, or blood sugar that persists above 200 mg/dL is reason to call her doctor immediately.

INDICATIONS FOR ADMISSION AND SPECIALTY CONSULTATION

Indications for admission include moderate or severe hyperemesis gravidarum, persistent ketosis for any reason, diabetic ketoacidosis, and poorly controlled diabetes mellitus (any type) in early pregnancy.

Hyperemesis gravidarum predisposes the diabetic woman to ketoacidosis because of starvation and dehydration. If a patient is unable to eat reliably and drink adequately, the risk of hypoglycemia due to mealtime nausea and vomiting after a premeal insulin dose has been taken is concerning. Hyperemesis gravidarum in a nondiabetic that can be managed on an outpatient basis often requires admission in a type 1 or 2 diabetic.

Ketosis without ketoacidosis is concerning because this may adversely affect neurodevelopmental outcome in the offspring. If ketosis can be cleared easily with hydration and the underlying cause addressed, then a trial of outpatient therapy is worthwhile. The most common cause is inadequate oral intake of fluids or calories because of vomiting or poor diet.

If an early pregnancy is first diagnosed in the emergency department and diabetic control is inadequate, admission should be considered. Organogenesis occurs in the first 6 to 8 weeks after the last menstrual period, and persistently elevated blood sugar at this time is a factor in birth defects and pregnancy loss.

If the blood sugar is elevated when the diagnosis of gestational DM is first made in the emergency department, admission is appropriate. While there are no strict guidelines, a fasting glucose of above 126 mg/dL or a random glucose of >200 mg/dL would be concerning. Urgent outpatient follow-up as soon as possible is an alternative. Diabetic ketoacidosis requires emergency admission to an obstetric intensive care area.

Specialty consultation should be used liberally for assistance in the management of DM in pregnancy for any of the above problems. In the metabolically stable patient who is already enrolled in high-risk pregnancy care, the high-risk team involved should be contacted to help plan ongoing care and address the role of admission. In many centers, there is a multidisciplinary team of obstetricians, high-risk pregnancy specialists (maternal-fetal medicine), endocrinologists, diabetes nurse educators, dieticians, and social workers who support these challenging patients. In some settings, an obstetrician along with medical consultants and others care for these patients. If the patient does not have a care team on presentation, arrangements for follow-up with experienced clinicians should ideally be made before discharge.

REFERENCES

1. Miller E, Hare JW, Cloherty JP, et al: Elevated maternal hemoglobin A1 in early pregnancy and major congenital anomalies in infants of diabetic mothers. *N Engl J Med* 304:1331, 1981.
2. Pederson J: Weight and length at birth of infants of diabetic mothers. *Acta Endocrinol* 16:30, 1954.
3. Philipps AF, Porte PJ, Stabinsky S, et al: Effects of chronic fetal hyperglycemia upon oxygen consumption in the ovine uterus and conceptus. *J Clin Invest* 74:279, 1984.
4. Nyland L, Lubell NO: Uteroplacental blood flow in diabetic pregnancy: Measurements with indium 113m and a computer-linked gamma camera. *Am J Obstet Gynecol* 144:298, 1982.
5. Kyle GC: Diabetes and pregnancy. *Ann Intern Med* 59 (Suppl 3):1, 1963.
6. Montoro MN, Myers VP, Mestmand JH, et al: Outcome of pregnancy in diabetic ketoacidosis. *Am J Perinatol* 10:17, 1993.
7. Pickup J, Williams G: *Textbook of Diabetes.* Boston: Blackwell, 1997.
8. Langer O, Conway DL, Berkus MD, et al: A comparison of glyburide and insulin in women with gestational diabetes mellitus. *N Engl J Med* 343:1134–1138, 2000.
9. National Diabetes Group: Classification and diagnosis of diabetes mellitus and other categories of glucose tolerance. *Diabetes* 28:1039, 1979.
10. American College of Obstetricians and Gynecologists: Gestational diabetes. ACOG practice bulletin no. 30. Washington: ACOG, 2001.
11. Coustan DR, Lewis SB: Insulin therapy for gestational diabetes. *Obstet Gynecol* 51:306, 1978.
12. Carpenter MW: Testing for gestational diabetes, in Reece EA Coustan DR (eds.) *Diabetes in Pregnancy* New York: Churchill Livingstone, 1995, p 267.
13. McKeage K, Goa KL: Insulin glargine: a review of its therapeutic use as a long-acting agent for the management of type 1 and 2 diabetes mellitus, *Drugs* 61:599–624, 2001.
14. Ragland G: Diabetic ketoacidosis, in Tintinalli JE, Krome RL, Ruiz E (eds): *Emergency Medicine,* 3d ed. New York: McGraw-Hill, 1992.
15. Chauhan SP, Kerry KG Jr: Management of diabetic ketoacidosis in the obstetric patient. *Obstet Gynecol Clin North Am* 21:143, 1995.

16

Common Hematologic Disorders During Pregnancy

Jeannette Wolfe
Mary E. Eberst

KEY POINTS

- A natural anemia occurs during pregnancy and a hemoglobin greater than 11 g/dL is within normal limits.
- Pregnant sickle cell disease (Hb SS) patients have an increased risk of maternal and fetal complications, including an increased risk of perinatal mortality. Sickle cell trait (HbAS) patients have an increased risk of papillary necrosis and pyelonephritis.
- Pregnancy is a hypercoagulable state that peaks in the postpartum period. All pregnancies increase the risk of thromboembolic disease with higher risks in patients with an underlying coagulation defect.
- Thrombocytopenia occurs in up to 10 percent of pregnancies and in most cases is inconsequential to both mother and fetus. Work-up focuses on the exclusion of more pathological thrombocytopenic states such as hemolysis, elevated liver enzymes and low platelets (HELLP) syndrome; thrombocytopenic thrombotic syndrome-hemolytic anemia syndrome (TTP-HUS); disseminated intravascular coagulation (DIC); and idiopathic thrombocytopenic purpura (ITP).
- Symptomatic Von Willebrand disease occurs in about one in 10,000 patients. In pregnancy, most affected patients see an improvement of their disease until after delivery, when about 20 percent develop postpartum bleeding.

REVIEW OF HEMATOLOGIC CHANGES IN NORMAL PREGNANCY

Anemia of Pregnancy

Red blood cell (RBC) mass increases 20 to 30 percent during pregnancy while plasma volume increases up to 50 percent. This causes a physiologic anemia during pregnancy that peaks during the thirtieth to thirty-fourth week of gestation with an average maternal hematocrit of about 33 to 34 percent at delivery. Anemia decreases blood viscosity, which facilitates placental perfusion, minimizes changes in perfusion with change in maternal position, decreases maternal systemic vascular resistance, and allows a buffer of blood loss during delivery (during a normal vaginal delivery average blood loss is 300 to 500 mL, which increases to 600 to 1000 mL with a cesarean section). Hemodilution and decrease in blood viscosity may also offset the increased fibrinogen levels and platelet aggregation associated with pregnancy. The expansion of RBCs results from elevated levels of erythropoietin and human placental lactogen and requires adequate levels of iron, folate, and cobalamin (B_{12}).The failure to develop this expected hemodilution may be associated with an increased risk of low birth weight and preterm delivery.[1]

Hemoglobin levels below 10.5 g/dL or hematocrit below 32 percent represent anemia beyond that expected. These levels likely represent a true anemia due to a reduction in RBC mass and should be evaluated further. Anemia is discussed more fully later in this chapter.

Leukocytosis

During normal pregnancy, leukocytosis is common. Early in pregnancy, the white blood cell (WBC) count can reach the upper limit of the normal range for nonpregnant patients. By the third trimester, the WBC may rise as high as 15,000 to 18,000/mm^3. During the last month of gestation, the WBC trends downward until the time of delivery, when it may again rise to 15,000 to 20,000/mm^3. White blood cell counts up to 25,000/mm^3 are sometimes seen during normal labor. Elevated levels of plasma cortisol are believed to be responsible for this leukocytosis. The WBC differential may reveal a rare myelocyte or metamyelocyte, and Doehle bodies may be present in the cytoplasm of the WBCs. Although elevated, the function of WBCs is often depressed, with decreased chemotaxis and adherence beginning in the second trimester and continuing throughout pregnancy. This may make pregnant women slightly more susceptible to infection and may partially explain why some autoimmune diseases improve during pregnancy.

Platelet Changes in Pregnancy

In conjunction with the increase in plasma volume during normal pregnancy, and perhaps because of compensated low-grade disseminated intravascular coagulation (DIC) within the uteroplacental unit, platelet counts decline during pregnancy as much as 20 percent from baseline values, although they usually remain within normal limits. The decline in the platelet count is most pronounced after 32 weeks of gestation. Thrombocytopenia, defined as platelet counts less than 150,000/mm^3, is present in 5 to 10 percent of pregnant patients. In about 25 percent of these women, there may be a significant cause such as preeclampsia; hemolysis, elevated liver enzymes and low platelets (HELLP) syndrome; thrombocytopenic thrombotic syndrome-hemolytic anemia syndrome (TTP-HUS); DIC; or idiopathic thrombocytopenic purpura (ITP). The vast majority of pregnant women with thrombocytopenia, however, will appear healthy and have no history of low platelet counts. If work-up reveals no identifiable cause of thrombocytopenia, these women are said to have incidental or gestational thrombocytopenia. Their platelet counts usually fall in the third trimester and return to normal soon after delivery. They have no associated fetal thrombocytopenia, and the delivery method is based solely on obstetric indications. Some patients with gestational thrombocytopenia may have a more benign form of ITP as demonstrated by the presence of maternal antiplatelet antibodies.[2] Patients with clinically significant ITP usually present earlier in pregnancy and are associated with platelet counts lower than 50,000/mm^3. This disorder is discussed later.

Hemostasis in Pregnancy

Review of Normal Coagulation

The normal hemostatic system consists of a complex process that limits blood loss by the formation of a platelet plug (primary hemostasis) and the production of cross-linked fibrin (secondary hemostasis), which strengthens the platelet plug. These reactions are counterregulated by the fibrinolytic system, which limits the size of fibrin clot that is formed, thereby preventing excessive clot formation. Congenital and acquired abnormalities occur in both of these systems and affected patients may have excessive hemorrhage, excessive thrombus formation, or both.[3]

Primary hemostasis is the platelet interaction with the vascular subendothelium that results in the formation of a platelet plug at the site of injury.[3] The components required for this to occur are normal vascular subendothelium (collagen), functional platelets (able to adhere, secrete, aggregate, and stimulate the procoagulant system), normal von Willebrand factor (connects the platelets to the endothelium via glycoprotein Ib), and normal fibrinogen (connects the platelets to each other via glycoproteins II_b through III_a). Fig. 16-1 depicts primary hemostasis.

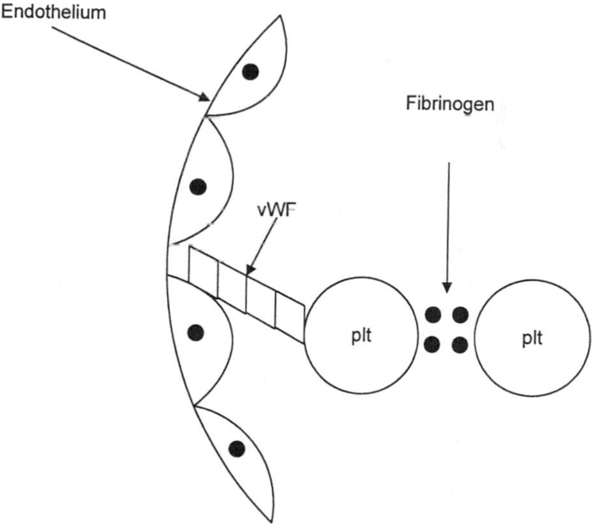

Fig. 16-1. Primary hemostasis (see text for details). vWF, von Willebrand factor; plt, platelet. (From Eberst,[30] with permission.)

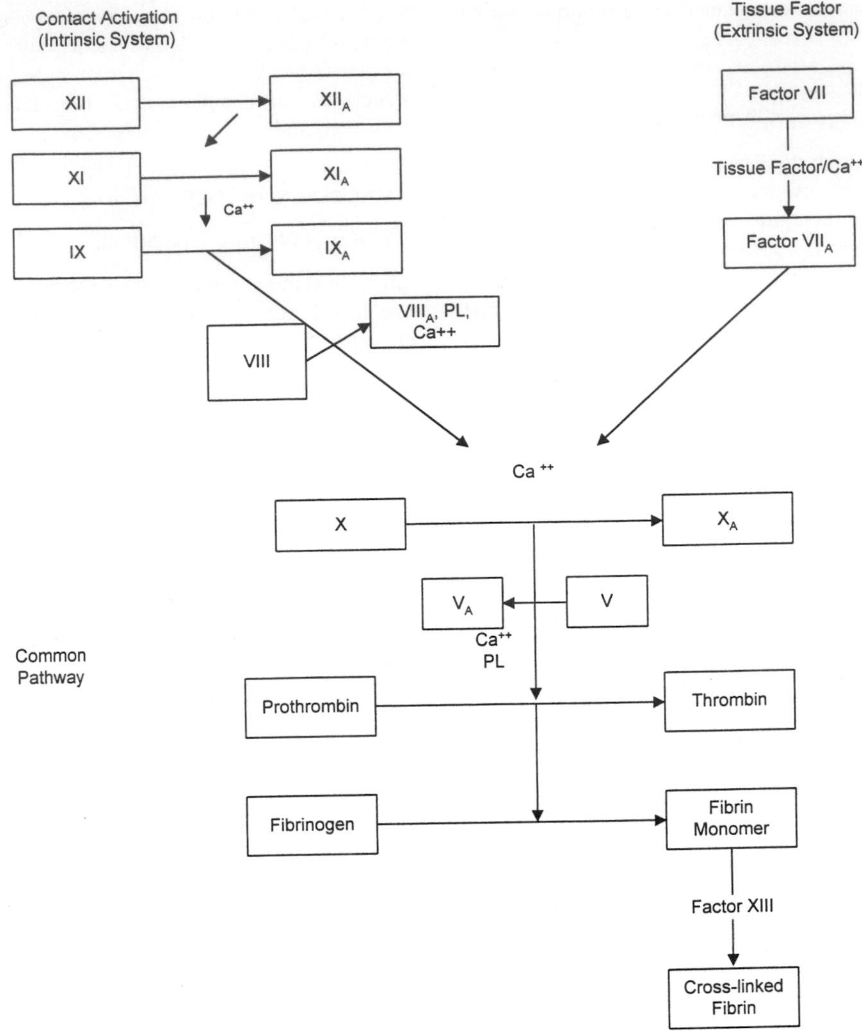

Fig. 16-2. Secondary hemostasis, also known as the *coagulation cascade.* The unactivated coagulation proteins (factors) are indicated by roman numerals; after the reaction occurs, the factor is activated and designated by subscript A. There are two independent activation pathways. The contact system is known as the *intrinsic pathway* or *augmentation stage* and the tissue factor system is known as the *extrinsic pathway* or *initiation stage.* Both pathways merge at the point of activation of factor X. This begins the common pathway, which generates the final product, cross-linked fibrin. Ca^{2++}, calcium; PL, phospholipid surface (often platelets); prothrombin is factor II; fibrinogen is factor I. (From Eberst,[30] with permission.)

Secondary hemostasis describes the reactions of the plasma coagulation proteins (factors) via a tightly regulated mechanism. This system is usually triggered by tissue factor stimulating activation of factor VII (this pathway is called the *extrinsic pathway* or the *initiation stage* of coagulation). Activated factor VII in turn stimulates both the intrinsic pathway (augmentation stage) and the common pathway before it is quickly inactivated. The final product is activated thrombin, which causes the conversion of fibrinogen to fibrin monomers and ultimately to cross-linked fibrin. The cross-linked fibrin is insoluble and strengthens the platelet plug formed in primary hemostasis. Fig. 16-2 diagrams the reactions of secondary hemostasis.

The fibrinolytic system is a complex system that regulates the hemostatic mechanism by limiting the size of

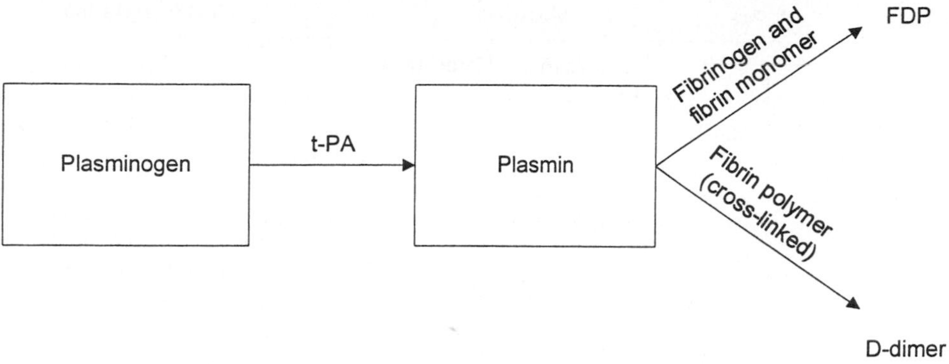

Fig. 16-3. The fibrinolytic pathway (see text for details). t-PA, tissue plasminogen activator; FDP, fibrin degradation product. (From Eberst,[30] with permission.)

fibrin clots that are formed. A simplified scheme is depicted in Fig. 16-3. The principal physiologic activator is tissue plasminogen activator (t-PA), which is released from endothelial cells. The t-PA converts plasminogen, which is synthesized in the liver and absorbed in the fibrin clot, to plasmin. Plasmin degrades fibrinogen and fibrin monomer into low-molecular-weight fragments known as *fibrin degradation products* (FDPs) and cross-linked fibrin into D-dimers.

Other physiologic inhibitors of hemostasis with relevant clinical applicability include antithrombin III and the protein C-protein S system. Antithrombin III is a protein that forms complexes with all the serine protease coagulation factors (factors XII, XI, X, IX, VII, and prothrombin) and inhibits their function. Heparin potentiates this interaction, and this is the basis for its use as an anticoagulant. Protein C, which requires the presence of protein S for activation, is capable of inactivating the two plasma cofactors, factors V and VIII, and inhibiting their participation in the coagulation cascade. Factor V Leiden, a common inherited procoagulant mutation, blocks the binding of activated protein C to factor V thereby preventing its inhibition. Patients with factor V Leiden or deficiencies of antithrombin III, protein C, or protein S may present with thromboembolic disease and often have a history of multiple pregnancy losses.[4]

The screening tests of primary and secondary hemostasis as well as other commonly used coagulation tests are outlined in Table 16-1.

Coagulation Changes in Pregnancy

Many dramatic changes in the normal hemostatic mechanism occur during pregnancy, leading to a hypercoagulable state in preparation for the hemostatic challenge that occurs at the time of delivery and placental separation. These changes lessen the amount of bleeding at the time of delivery, but increase the risk of thrombosis throughout the pregnancy and early postpartum period. As a result of these changes, the normal balance between coagulation (clot formation) and fibrinolysis (clot lysis) is tipped in favor of clot formation.[5,6] The effect of pregnancy on the coagulation factors, naturally-occurring anticoagulants, and fibrinolysis is shown in Table 16-2. In general, the factors that promote hemostasis are increased in concentration, while those that limit clot formation are unchanged or slightly reduced in concentration. The fibrinolytic system is less active overall during pregnancy, and its response to stimuli is decreased. Most of these changes in hemostasis can be detected by the third month of gestation, and return to normal levels occurs within 4 weeks after delivery. Fibrinolytic activity returns to normal levels within 1 hour after delivery of the placenta because the inhibitor of fibrinolysis, placentally-derived plasminogen activator inhibitor 2 (PAI-2), is eliminated.

D-dimer (dimerized plasmin fragment D) is a coagulation activation marker that is used to aid in the diagnosis of deep venous thrombosis and pulmonary embolism. It represents the breakdown product of cross-linked fibrin by plasmin. ELISA and latex agglutination techniques are used to measure D-dimer levels, and sensitivity and specificity for thrombosis vary with the type of assay used. In general, in the nonpregnant patient, a level less than 500 ng/mL is felt to have a high negative predictive value for thrombosis.

However, the D-dimer assay is of limited usefulness in the diagnosis of venous thromboembolism in pregnancy. Levels increase after the first trimester, and continue to rise

Table 16-1. Tests of Hemostasis

Screening Tests	Normal Value	Measures	Clinical Correlations
		Primary Hemostasis	
Platelet count	150,000 to 300,000/mm^3	Number of platelets per mm^3	*Decreased platelet count (thrombocytopenia)* Bleeding usually not a problem until platelet count <50,000; high risk of spontaneous bleeding including CNS with count <10,000 per mm^3 Causes: Decreased production—viral infections (measles); marrow infiltration; drugs (thiazides, ETOH alcohol, estrogens, alpha-interferon) Increased destruction—viral infections (mumps, varicella, EBV, HIV); ITP, TTP, DIC[a], HUS; drugs (heparin, protamine) Splenic sequestration (hypersplenism, hypothermia) Loss of platelets (hemorrhage, hemodialysis, extracorporeal circulation) Pseudothrombocytopenia—platelets are clumped but not truly decreased in number; examine blood smear to recognize this *Elevated platelet count (thrombocytosis)* Commonly reactive to inflammation or malignancy or in polycythemia vera; can be associated with hemorrhage or thrombosis
Bleeding time (BT)	2.5-10 min (template BT)	Interaction between platelets and the subendothelium	*Prolonged bleeding time caused by:* Thrombocytopenia (platelet count <50,000 per mm^3) Abnormal platelet function (vWD, ASA, NSAIDs, uremia, liver disease) Collagen abnormalities (congenital abnormality, or prolonged use of glucocorticoids)
		Secondary Hemostasis	
Prothrombin time (PT) or INR (international normalized ratio)	10-12 s, but laboratory variation INR = 1	Extrinsic system and common pathway—factors VII, X, V, prothrombin; and fibrinogen	*Prolonged PT or INR most commonly caused by:* Use of warfarin (inhibits vitamin K-dependent factors II, VII, IX and X) Advanced liver disease with decreased factor synthesis Antibiotics; some cephalosporins (moxalactam, cefamandole, cefotaxime, cefoperazone) that inhibit vitamin K-dependent factors
Activated partial thromboprastin time (aPTT)	Depends on type of thromboplastin used, "activated" with kaolin	Intrinsic system and common pathway including factors XII, XI, IX, VIII, X, V, prothrombin	*Prolongation of aPTT most commonly caused by:* Heparin therapy Factor deficiencies; factor levels have to be <30% of normal to cause prolongation "Lupus-type anticoagulant"—can occur in patients with SLE and others; can lead to recurrent pregnancy loss (see text for details)

(*Continues*)

Table 16-1. (*Continued*) Test of Hemostasis

Screening Tests	Normal Value	Measures	Clinical Correlations
			Note: High doses of heparin or warfarin can cause prolongation of both the PT and aPTT due to their activity in the common pathway
Thrombin clotting time (TCT)	10-12s	Conversion of fibrinogen to fibrin monomer	*Prolonged TCT caused by:* Low fibrinogen-level (DIC) Abnormal fibrinogen molecule (liver disease) Presence of heparin, FDPs, or a paraprotein (multiple myeloma); these interfere with the conversion Very high fibrinogen-level (acute-phase reactant)
"Mixes"	Variable	Performed when one or more of the above screening tests is prolonged; the patient's plasma ("abnormal") is mixed with "normal" plasma and the screening test is repeated	*If the "mix" corrects the screening test,* one or more factor deficiencies are present *If the "mix" does not correct the screening test,* an inhibitor is present
		Other Hemostatic Tests	
Fibrin degradation products (FDP) and D-dimer (evaluate fibrinolysis)	Variable	FDPs measure breakdown products from fibrinogen and fibrin monomer, D-dimer measures breakdown products of cross-linked fibrin	Levels of these are elevated in DIC, thrombosis, pulmonary embolus, liver disease
Factor level assays	60-130% (0.60-1.30 U/mL)	Measures the percent activity of a specified factor compared to normal	Used to identify specific factor deficiencies and in the therapeutic management of patients with deficiencies
Inhibitor screens	Variable	Verifies the presence or absence of antibodies directed against one or more of the coagulation factors	*Specific inhibitors*—directed against one coagulation factor, most commonly against factor VIII; can be found in patients with congenital or acquired deficiency *Nonspecific inhibitors*—directed against more than one of the coagulation factors, an example is the lupus-type anticoagulant

[a]There are many pregnancy-associated causes of DIC (e.g., abruptio placentae, severe preeclampsia, amniotic fluid embolism). CNS, central nervous system; ETOH, ethanol; EBV, Epstein Barr virus; HIV, human immunodeficiency virus; ITP, idiopathic thrombocytopenic purpura; TTP, thrombotic thrombocytopenic purpura; DIC, disseminated intravascular coagulation; HUS, hemolytic uremic syndrome; vWD, von Willebrand disease; ASA, aspirin; NSAIDs, nonsteroidal antiinflammatory drugs; FDPs, fibrin degradation products.

Source: Adapted from Eberst,[30] with permission.

Table 16-2. Hemostatic Changes in Normal Pregnancy

Effect on Hemostasis		Changes in Concentration (Increased Plasma Volume Taken Into Account)
	Coagulation factors	
Promote hemostasis	I (fibrinogen)	Increases (2-4 times)
	VII	Increases (up to 10 times)
	VIII	Increases (up to 2 times)
	vWF	Increases (up to 4 times)
	X	Increases
	XII	Increases
	Naturally occurring anticoagulants	
Inhibit hemostasis	Antithrombin III	Slight decrease
	Protein C	Slight increase, still in normal range
	Protein S	Slight decrease, still in normal range
	Fibrinolytic system:	
	Plasminogen activator inhibitor 2 (PAI-2) (inhibits plasminogen)	Increase (derived from placenta)

throughout the remainder of pregnancy, labor, delivery, and the immediate postpartum period.[7] D-dimer levels of 1750 ± 839 ng/mL were reported in one study of normal pregnancies.[8] Elevated D-dimer levels per se in normal pregnancies are not predictive of clinical thrombosis.[9,10] In conditions such as preterm labor, factor V Leiden, preeclampsia, abruptio placentae, and HELLP syndrome, D-dimer levels have been reported to be higher than in normal pregnant controls.[8,10,11]

RED BLOOD CELL DISORDERS

Congenital Hemolytic Anemias and Hemoglobinopathies

Sickle Cell Anemias

The sickle cell anemias include sickle cell disease (HbSS), sickle cell trait (HbAS), hemoglobin SC disease (HbSC), and sickle cell β-thalassemia. About 10 percent of African-Americans in the United States carry the sickle cell gene. The genetic abnormality that results in sickle cell disease stems from a single amino acid substitution, valine for glutamic acid, at the sixth position on the β chain of the hemoglobin molecule; the result is hemoglobin S. This genotype can be detected in fetal cells, allowing prenatal diagnosis. The inheritance of one abnormal sickle gene for sickle cell disease results in the heterozygous carrier state sickle cell trait (HbAS). When two genes are inherited, the homozygous state (HbSS) results. Homozygous sickle cell disease occurs in 0.1 to 0.2 percent of the U.S. African-American population.

Other commonly encountered heterozygous hemoglobinopathies ("major hemoglobinopathies") include hemoglobin SC disease (HbSC) and sickle cell β-thalassemia. HbSC disease is an inherited disorder of hemoglobin S (HbS) and hemoglobin C (HbC). In HbSC disease, the red blood cells contain HbC and HbS. During pregnancy, the sickle component is more clinically important and patients are managed as if they have HbSS. Patients with sickle cell β-thalassemia disease have varying degrees of anemia and clinical complications; some are as severely affected as patients with HbSS.

Most emergency department sickle cell disease patients present with pain and symptoms associated with a vaso-occlusive, infectious, or hematologic crisis. The reader is referred to standard texts on emergency medicine or hematology for an expanded discussion of the management of crises. In patients with HbSS, the sickled RBCs are rapidly removed from the circulation, resulting in a chronic hemolytic anemia. A hemoglobin of 6 to 9 g/dL is typical.

Patients with sickle cell trait (HbAS) rarely develop complications. Painful or vaso-occlusive crises can occur under conditions of extreme anoxia, dehydration, or acidosis. HbAS patients do have an increased risk of bacteriuria and cystitis, which if untreated may progress to pyelonephritis and preterm labor. They also have concentrating defects in their kidneys which lead to papillary necrosis.

The care of pregnant women with sickle cell disease or sickle cell trait begins with the identification of affected patients. Because of the profound clinical consequences, screening during early pregnancy is desirable in order to identify women who are at high risk of a difficult pregnancy and of giving birth to an affected offspring. Prenatal screening tests, including a complete blood count (CBC), will demonstrate anemia with sickled RBCs and Howell-Jolly bodies on the peripheral smear in patients with major hemoglobinopathies. Carriers of the sickle cell gene usually have a normal CBC. Hemoglobin electrophoresis is needed to identify the carrier state and is recommended as part of the prenatal screening of all African-American patients. In general, patients with higher levels of hemoglobin F demonstrated on electrophoresis will have less severe anemia. This may be due to hemoglobin F lessening intracellular polymerizations of hemoglobin S.[1] Analysis of fetal DNA can be performed as early as 7 to 13 weeks of gestation by amniocentesis or chorionic villus sampling to diagnose hemoglobinopathies in the offspring of affected patients.

Patients with hemoglobinopathies enter pregnancy with an increased risk of morbidity and mortality due to their underlying anemia and chronic organ damage. Many women with sickle cell trait (HbAS) have uncomplicated pregnancies that result in the delivery of full-term infants of normal birth weight. However, compared with hematologically normal women, pregnant women with HbSS and HbSC disease have an increased risk of both maternal and fetal complications. One recent study compared pregnant patients with HbSS or HbSC disease to a control pregnant population. Patients with HbSS or HbSC had increased risks of antepartum admission, postpartum infection, and intrauterine growth restriction.[12] In addition, HbSS patients had lower birth rates and higher rates of preterm labor and preterm delivery. About 50 percent of HbSS patients and 20 percent of HbSC patients had at least one severe painful crisis necessitating transfusion and hospital admission. There was a 15 percent combined intrauterine/perinatal mortality for HbSS patients. All of these findings are consistent with other studies in patients with significant hemoglobinopathies that suggested a maternal mortality rate of less than 1 percent, but an overall complication rate of about 30 percent with uterine and perinatal mortality of up to 30 percent.[1]

Vaso-occlusion involving the placenta is thought to be responsible for the increased incidence of low birth weight, intrauterine growth restriction, and neonatal death. Chronic hypertension and renal insufficiency may also predispose patients to preeclampsia. It is difficult to predict which women will have obstetric complications, so all require close monitoring during pregnancy.

During pregnancy, women with sickle cell disease or anemia require folic acid supplementation (1 mg/d). Levels are often marginal because of chronic accelerated erythropoiesis. Cyanocobalamin (B_{12}) deficiency may also occur but is rare. Iron supplementation may not be required. Iron deficiency should be documented with serum iron and ferritin levels prior to giving supplements in order to avoid iron overload. The management of sickle cell crises in pregnant women is the same as for nonpregnant women, with special attention paid to pregnancy-specific stressors such as an ectopic pregnancy, preeclampsia, and placental abruption, which may precipitate a crisis. An aggressive search for underlying infections should also be undertaken. The patient should be hydrated and given oxygen. Appropriate analgesia should be given. Opioids with or without antiemetics are standard. Nonsteroidal agents should not be given.

In the past, pregnant women with HbSS were given prophylactic blood transfusions in order to increase the percentage of normal circulating hemoglobin. Theoretically this was thought to lower the incidence of vaso-occlusive crises and decrease fetal wastage, but this practice has not been validated by controlled studies, and prophylactic transfusions are no longer routinely used. In addition, transfusions carry risks of alloimmunization, viral exposure, and transfusion reactions. These risks can be somewhat reduced with partial exchange transfusion using continuous flow erythrocytopheresis with buffy coat-poor blood. One study showed significantly fewer painful episodes, and decreased preterm deliveries, low birth weight infants, and perinatal death with exchange transfusion.[13] The advantage of exchange transfusions over traditional transfusion include decreased risk of hyperviscosity, hypersplenism, iron overload, and alloantibody formation. Partial exchange transfusion complications include anticoagulation effects of acid citrate buffer, rare CNS complications of unclear etiology, and risks of volume shifts and 2,3-DPG deficiency.[1] Although the role of transfusion remains unclear, most would advise transfusion or exchange transfusion for acute chest syndrome, cerebrovascular events, papillary necrosis, prolonged vaso-occlusive crises, and multiple-gestation pregnancies. Transfusion is also recommended for pregnant HbSS patients with a history of previous miscarriage and before general anesthesia or cesarean section delivery.[13] A small group of sickle cell β-thalassemia pregnant patients given erythropoietin showed an increase in hemoglobin F and a decrease of painful episodes with an improvement of pregnancy outcomes.[14]

Thalassemia

Thalassemia is an inherited hemoglobinopathy that results in reduced formation of the globin chains comprising the hemoglobin molecule. This results in both an abnormal erythropoiesis and premature red blood cell destruction resulting in a chronic hemolytic anemia. The genetic abnormality can result in decreased production of the α or β globin chains.[15]

Homozygous α-thalassemia is incompatible with life. Patients with heterozygous α-thalassemia have normal or only slightly decreased levels of hemoglobin with microcytic, hypochromic RBC indices. β-Thalassemia is more common than α-thalassemia. About 10 to 20 percent of patients with the gene for β-thalassemia have a homozygous state; no normal β chains are produced. Patients have a severe hemolytic anemia and are transfusion dependent. Survival past the teenage years is uncommon and end-organ damage from iron overload may cause decreased fertility. With transfusion and chelation therapy, however, there are now well over 60 documented cases of successful pregnancies in patients with homozygous β-thalessemia.[1] Patients with heterozygous β-thalassemia have a mild hemolytic anemia, with microcytic, hypochromic RBC indices. Some patients have a double heterozygous condition with a gene for thalassemia (usually β-thalassemia) and a gene for sickle cell hemoglobin (sickle cell β-thalassemia). Their clinical and hematologic status is variable, depending on the quantity of normal β hemoglobin chains produced.

As is the case with other hemoglobinopathies, care of the pregnant patient begins with early screening to identify carriers and offer prenatal diagnosis. The vast majority of pregnant patients encountered with thalassemia will have the heterozygous condition called thalassemia minor or trait. A screening CBC in patients with heterozygous thalassemia will show a normal to slightly decreased hemoglobin with microcytic, hypochromic indices and usually an increase in the number of absolute red blood cells (greater than 5 million). Hemoglobin electrophoresis is needed to establish the diagnosis. This anemia can easily be confused with iron-deficiency anemia. Iron studies often show elevated ferritin concentrations prepregnancy in patients with thalassemia trait. The mean cell volume (MCV) is typically lower in patients with thalassemia than in those with iron-deficiency anemia. During pregnancy, patients with thalassemia trait can become significantly more anemic than hematologically-normal women, presumably because of a larger than normal expansion of plasma volume. These patients should receive iron supplementation unless their serum ferritin level is known to be high. They also require folate supplementation; some clinicians recommend 5 mg/d. Red blood cell transfusions are sometimes needed to maintain adequate oxygen-carrying capacity. With good prenatal care, the pregnancy outcome in women with thalassemia trait is no different than that in the general population.

Nutritional Anemias

Iron-Deficiency Anemia

Anemia due to iron deficiency is the most common hematologic problem that develops during pregnancy. Among pregnant women not given iron supplementation, up to 55 percent will develop anemia (hemoglobin below 10.5 g/dL) by the end of the third trimester. This problem is greatest in women from developing countries who may have a concurrent anemia from other nutritional defects or malaria. During pregnancy, iron is used for accelerated erythropoiesis in the mother and for fetal and placental development; iron is preferentially delivered to the fetus. Iron requirements during pregnancy average 800 to 1000 mg, of which approximately one-half is used to increase maternal erythropoiesis, one-third is used for fetal erythropoiesis, and the rest is used as a buffer for anticipated blood loss during delivery and lactation. Most women of reproductive age have 300 mg in iron stores; multiparous women have less. Although iron absorption does increase during pregnancy, typically there are still not adequate supplies without supplementation. Poor appetite, poor nutrition, nausea, vomiting, multiple gestation, and chronic illness can increase the chance of iron depletion. Iron deficiency is also more common in African-Americans, Hispanics, and teenagers.

The diagnosis of iron deficiency can be difficult to establish during pregnancy. Any woman whose hemoglobin is below 10.5 g/dL should be evaluated. A low hemoglobin level is actually a late manifestation of iron deficiency. The RBC indices are not a reliable indicator of iron deficiency because microcytosis is often a late finding, and other deficiencies such as folate deficiency, which causes a macrocytosis, may mask this finding. Iron studies, such as the total iron-binding capacity (TIBC) and serum iron levels, can be artificially increased and decreased, respectively, in normal pregnancy. The serum ferritin level is the most sensitive test for diagnosing iron deficiency in pregnancy. The serum ferritin level reflects the total body iron stores. In general, patients with normal iron stores should have serum ferritin levels above 20 μg/L, but sometimes even the serum ferritin level is not reliable, with up to 20 percent of pregnant women with normal ferritin levels being iron deficient. In addition, after 34 weeks of gestation, ferritin levels as low as 15 μg/L (ferritin unit) can be seen and are not indicative of iron deficiency if the serum hemoglobin remains above 11 g/dL. In pregnancy, severe iron deficiency may be associated with an increased risk of preterm labor and delivery of a low birth weight infant.

To prevent the development of iron-deficiency anemia during pregnancy, routine prenatal care in the U.S. typically includes daily supplementation with ferrous sulfate (usually 300 mg/d), which provides 60 mg of elemental iron daily. Interestingly, it is inconclusive whether maternal or fetal outcome is improved with iron supplementation in patients with only mild to moderate iron deficiency anemia. Supplementation may theoretically decrease the absorption of other minerals and cause an increase in blood viscosity, leading some clinicians to have a more selective approach regarding supplementation.[1]

Folate Deficiency

Anemia due to folate deficiency in pregnant women is one of the most common causes of megaloblastic anemia in the world. Megaloblastic anemia in pregnancy is almost always due to folate deficiency. Deficiency of vitamin B_{12} is rare in pregnancy because it is associated with infertility, though it can occasionally be seen in patients with strict vegan diets.

Folate is a vitamin that is not naturally produced in the body. Between 10 and 60 percent of pregnant women who do not receive folate supplementation develop megaloblastic changes in their bone marrow. During pregnancy, folate requirements are at least doubled due to accelerated erythropoiesis and growth of the fetus and placenta. Even greater requirements occur in women with a history of poor nutrition; coexistent hemolytic anemias, such as sickle-cell disease; those taking anticonvulsant medications; those with twin or greater gestations; and during lactation. Total body stores of folate are small. During pregnancy, the daily folate requirement is .3 to .4 mg/d. Because the placenta has a large number of folate receptors, available folate preferentially shifts to the fetus. Nausea and vomiting during pregnancy can lead to increased loss of folate.

Folate deficiency is difficult to establish during pregnancy. Any pregnant woman with a hemoglobin below 10.5 to 11 g/dL should be considered for evaluation. Anemia purely due to folate deficiency is macrocytic and pancytopenia may be present. Many pregnant women have anemia due to a combined deficiency of folate and iron as noted above, and the resultant dimorphic population of RBCs make these indices unreliable. The presence of hypersegmented neutrophils can be a clue to the presence of folate deficiency, but these are not reliably present. Serum folate levels can be decreased in pregnancy when a true deficiency is not present. Determination of the RBC folate level is the most reliable method of diagnosing folate deficiency. In addition to anemia, low folate levels in pregnancy are associated with an increased risk of spontaneous abortion and congenital defects, particularly neural tube defects. Premature infants born with low folate stores can have feeding difficulties and infections.

Routine prenatal vitamins in the U.S. provide 0.5 to 1 mg of folic acid per day, usually in combination with iron supplementation. Women taking antiseizure medications, particularly phenytoin or phenobarbital, are at increased risk of developing anemia due to folate deficiency. They should be supplemented with 1 mg of folate daily. Women with hereditary hemolytic anemias, such as sickle cell disease or thalassemia, should receive larger doses of folate, up to 5 to 10 mg daily. Women contemplating pregnancy should begin folate supplements of 0.4 mg/d prior to pregnancy to prevent neural tube defects in the offspring they may conceive.

ACQUIRED HEMOLYTIC ANEMIAS

In this section, we explore anemias pertinent to pregnancy that result from the RBC hemolysis. Clinically, these patients all have anemia with its inherent signs and symptoms; thrombocytopenia and coagulopathy may be present, as noted below. Diagnosis of these disorders is based on the history, clinical signs and symptoms, and laboratory evaluation. The general laboratory evaluation of patients with suspected hemolytic anemia is outlined in Table 16-3. More specific tests may be required, and these are discussed below. The acquired hemolytic anemias most commonly encountered in pregnant patients are characterized in Table 16-4.

Autoimmune Hemolytic Anemia (AIHA)

This is an anemia resulting from the destruction of red blood cells by autoantibodies. It has numerous causes, and can be autoimmune, infectious, neoplastic, lymphoproliferative, inflammatory, and drug-related, but often it is idiopathic. The two types of antibody-mediated, "immune" hemolytic anemias are: (1) warm antibody hemolytic

Table 16-3. Laboratory Evaluation of Patients with Suspected Hemolytic Anemia

Study	Anticipated Result
CBC	Anemia of a variable degree; verify that WBC and platelet counts are normal
Reticulocyte count	Should be elevated, reflective of a normal bone marrow response; can be as high as 30-40%
Review of peripheral blood smear	*Spherocytes:* Most common RBC morphologic abnormality in hemolytic anemias; most abundant in warm antibody immune hemolysis and hereditary spherocytosis *Schistocytes:* Fragmented RBCs resulting from trauma within the vasculature; markers of nonimmune hemolysis
Unconjugated (indirect) bilirubin	Elevated as a result of heme catabolism
Lactic dehydrogenase (LDH)	Elevated
Haptoglobin	Low or absent in the presence of hemolysis; binds catabolized hemoglobin; is an acute-phase reactant so can be deceptively elevated
Plasma free hemoglobin	Elevated

CBC, complete blood count; WBC, white blood cells; RBC, red blood cells.

anemia–Antibodies react at body temperature and are usually IgG; and (2) cold antibody hemolytic anemia—Antibodies react with the RBCs at temperatures below normal body temperatures and are usually IgM. Hemolysis is caused by activating the complement system.

The direct Coombs test, also known as the direct antiglobulin test (DAT), is used to specifically identify immune-mediated hemolytic anemias. This test demonstrates the presence of immunoglobulin (IgG) or complement (C_3) on the surface of the RBC. The indirect Coombs test, which identifies free antibodies in the serum, is used primarily for pretransfusion screening of blood. The peripheral blood smear of patients with immune hemolysis often shows abundant spherocytes, polychromasia, erythrophagocytosis, red cell fragments, and nucleated red cells.

The treatment of AIHAs involves identification and treatment of offending factors (removal of drug, treatment of neoplasm, etc.) and immunosuppression. Initial treatment is usually with corticosteroids but plasmapheresis, immunoglobulin therapy, immunosuppressant drugs, and splenectomy may be required.

Autoimmune hemolytic anemia has rarely been reported to occur in pregnancy. Warm antibodies, since they are IgG, can cross the placenta and cause mild hemolysis in the fetus and newborn. When AIHA predates the pregnancy, the mother and fetus will require close monitoring. Ongoing therapy with glucocorticoids should continue. There is limited experience with the use of other immunosuppressives (i.e., azathioprine) in pregnancy. There are rare reports of AIHA developing only during pregnancy, remitting after delivery, and recurring during subsequent pregnancies. This has been successfully controlled with glucocorticoids, although the infant may be affected.

Table 16-4. Characteristics of Hemolytic Anemias and Idiopathic Thrombocytopenia

	HELLP	TTP-HUS	DIC	ITP	AIHA
Thrombocytopenia	+	+	+	+	*a*
Direct Coombs test	−	−	−	−	+
Antiplatelet antibodies	−	−	−	+	−
PT/PTT	Normal	Normal	Usually prolonged	Normal	Normal
Antithrombin III levels	Decreased	Normal	Decreased	Normal	Normal
Schistocytes	+	+	Usually +	−	*b*
Elevated liver transaminases	+	+/−	May be +	−	−

HELLP, hemolysis, elevated liver enzymes, low platelets; TTP-HUS, thrombotic thrombocytopenic purpura-hemolytic anemia syndrome; DIC, disseminated intravascular coagulation; ITP, idiopathic thrombocytopenic purpura; AIHA, autoimmune hemolytic anemia.

[a] Thrombocytopenia with AIHA is called Evans disease.

[b] Microspherocytes are often found on the peripheral smear.

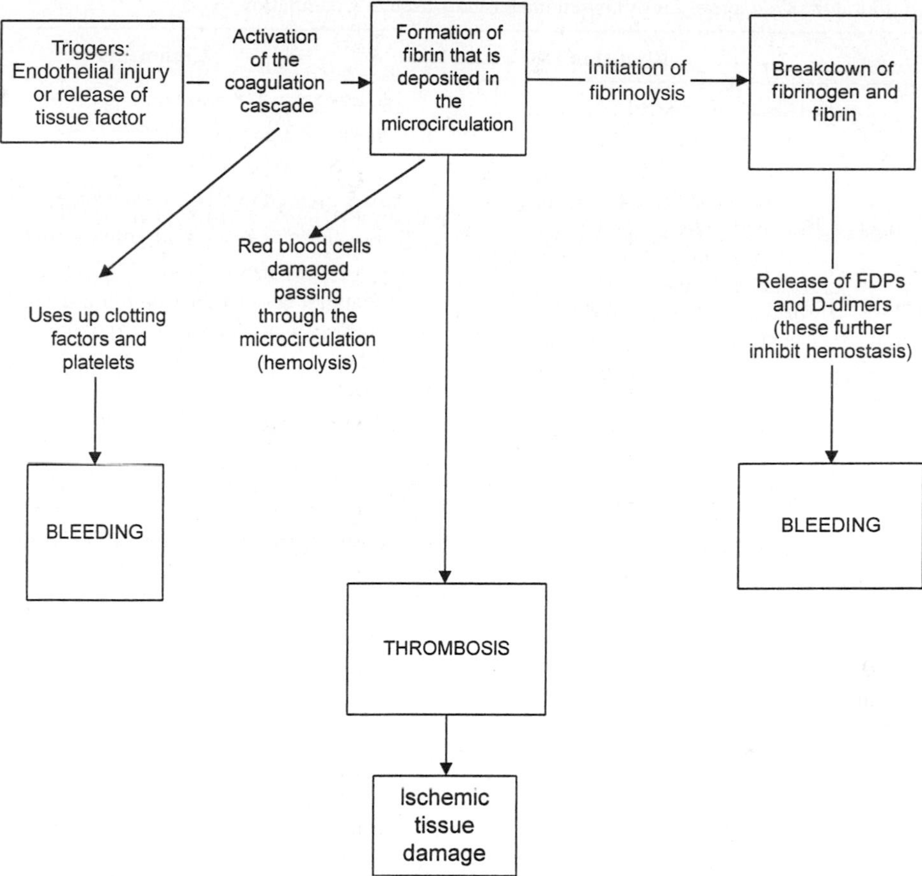

Fig. 16-4. Pathophysiology of disseminated intravascular coagulation (DIC) (see text for details). FDPs, fibrin/fibrinogen degradation products. (From Eberst,[30] with permission.)

Microangiopathic Hemolytic Anemias (MAHAs)

Although it is associated with a variety of underlying disorders, the mechanism of hemolysis in microangiopathic hemolytic anemias is consistent: vascular endothelial damage associated with platelet and fibrin clumps which cause fragmentation of RBCs (schistocytes) as they travel through the damaged vasculature. In pregnancy, MAHA is seen in the syndromes of DIC, HELLP, and TTP-HUS, which are discussed below.

Disseminated Intravascular Coagulation (DIC)

Many researchers feel that a normal pregnancy is associated with a chronic low level of well compensated disseminated intravascular coagulation. This is exemplified by an increase of fibinopeptide A (FPA), which is the first product formed by thrombin-mediated conversion of fibrinogen to fibrin and is an indirect indicator of thrombin activity.[5] Obviously, in most pregnancies this increased thrombin activity causes no problems, but it may be a contributing factor to the increased risk of pregnancy-induced thromboembolism.

DIC is not a discrete identity but rather is a systemic reaction triggered by several different etiologies. Fulminant DIC is generated when there is an excess of thrombin released into the systemic circulation, causing microvascular clot formation. It is characterized by four findings: increased coagulation leading to factor consumption, increased fibrinolysis, consumption of coagulation inhibitors (especially antithrombin III), and evidence of end-organ damage.[5,16] Resultant bleeding and thrombosis can occur simultaneously (Fig. 16-4). Although the bleeding complications may be more physically apparent,

Table 16-5. Laboratory Characteristics of Disseminated Intravascular Coagulation

Test	Results in DIC	Comments
Prothrombin fragment 1 & 2 (PF 1 & 2)	Increased	Abnormal in up to 90% of patients. PF 1 & 2 are inactivated prothrombin fragments made in the conversion of prothrombin to thrombin
Antithrombin III	Decreased in about 90%	Also decreased in HELLP syndrome
Fibrinogen	May be decreased	This is an acute phase reactant and can be normal or elevated in DIC
Fibrinogenpeptide A level FPA	Increased in about 90%	This is first product in thrombin-mediated conversion of fibrinogen to fibrin
Fibrinogen degradation products (FDPs)	Increased in 75-100%	Are only diagnostic of presence of plasmin
D-dimer	Increased in greater than 90%	Measure plasmin-mediated breakdown of cross-linked fibrin
Platelet count	Decreased	Usually also see increased size of platelets
Schistocytes	Usually present	May be absent in up to 50% of DIC patients
Protamine sulfate tests	Increased	Measures FDP binding to fibrin monomers preventing fibrin cross-linking. May also be elevated in oral contraception use and pulmonary emboli
Partial thromboplastin time (PTT)	Usually prolonged	May be normal in 25-50% of patients
Prothrombin time (PT)	Usually prolonged	May be normal in up to 50% of patients and is less sensitive than PTT

long-term morbidity is usually associated with microvascular clotting causing end-organ damage. Laboratory findings in DIC can be confusing as both the coagulation and fibrinolytic system are stimulated. This makes interpretation of individual labs difficult as many of them lack sensitivity and specificity for DIC. Lab findings commonly associated with DIC are listed in Table 16-5. Many feel that a positive D-dimer (which measures the breakdown of cross-linked fibrin by plasmin), thrombocytopenia, elevated fibrinogen peptide A levels, low levels of antithrombin III, and elevated prothrombin factors 1 and 2 (PF-1 and -2), which are inactivated prothrombin fragments produced in the conversion of prothrombin to thrombin, provide good laboratory evidence for DIC. Prolongation of prothrombin time and activated partial thromboplastin time is usually seen in DIC, but these can also be normal, as can a peripheral smear for hemolytic anemia.

Bleeding is the most common clinical presentation of DIC. Bleeding from the skin and mucous membranes is common, as well as oozing from venipuncture sites and surgical wounds, petechiae, and ecchymoses. DIC is often acute and uncompensated, because the liver and bone marrow cannot replace the rapidly consumed factors and platelets. Probably the most deadly form of DIC in pregnancy is from amniotic fluid emboli with fulminant DIC often leading to death within hours. Placental abruption can cause significant DIC in about 10 percent of cases.

Low-grade DIC is commonly seen in fetal death in utero. Fortunately, this is usually detected and the uterus evacuated before fulminant maternal DIC develops. A compensated low-grade DIC is also seen with preeclampsia due to endothelial injury. This can progress to end-stage organ damage if unrecognized (see management of HELLP syndrome below).

In general, the management of DIC in pregnancy usually involves identification of underlying cause and delivery of the fetus or evacuation of the uterus, followed by supportive care and replacement blood products.

HELLP Syndrome

This syndrome, first described in 1982, consists of *h*emolysis, *e*levated *l*iver enzymes, and *l*ow *p*latelets

(HELLP), and is usually seen with preeclampsia. However, up to 15 to 20 percent of patients diagnosed with HELLP syndrome have no evidence of antecedent hypertension or proteinuria.[17] HELLP syndrome occurs in about 0.5 to 0.9 percent of pregnancies and in about 15 to 26 percent of patients with preeclampsia. Many feel that preeclampsia, eclampsia, and HELLP syndrome represent a continuum of the same process. Although the exact etiology is unknown, it is believed to be associated with abnormal placental vascular attachment to the uterus, leading to placental ischemia and the systemic release of thromboxanes, procoagulant prostaglandins, tissue necrosis factor, endothelin-1, and angiotensin, leading to endothelial damage and thrombosis. If untreated this ultimately leads to DIC with hepatic, CNS, renal, ovarian, and placental organs at greatest risk for thrombolic involvement.[5] Most cases of HELLP occur in the third trimester, but in one study 30 percent occurred postpartum, usually within 48 hours of delivery. The maternal mortality rate is 1 to 4 percent, but the perinatal mortality may be up to 40 percent.

In general, any woman who is pregnant or newly postpartum and who presents with symptoms of upper abdominal pain, severe headache, or visual changes, especially in conjunction with hypertension and/or proteinuria, should be evaluated for HELLP syndrome. Absolute diagnostic criteria for HELLP syndrome are controversial, but commonly used diagnostic criteria developed by Sibia are displayed in Table 16-6.[18] As the name implies, HELLP syndrome is associated with microvascular hemolytic anemia with schistocytes, elevated liver enzymes (specifically transaminases) and LDH, and low platelets. Although the connection of HELLP syndrome to DIC is debatable (some claim that HELLP syndrome is an early compensated form of DIC), most patients with HELLP syndrome have normal coagulation studies. The more difficult diagnosis to exclude is thrombotic thrombocytopenic purpura (TTP) (discussed below). This distinction is important to make because therapy is different for the two disorders. Table 16-7 lists a comparison of HELLP syndrome and TTP. Of note, the antithrombin III level is decreased in most cases of HELLP syndrome and normal in most cases of TTP.

Table 16-6. Laboratory Characteristics of HELLP Syndrome

Hemolysis
Abnormal peripheral smear
Increased LDH >600 U/L
Increased bilirubin >1.2 mg/dL
Increased liver function tests
ASAT >70 U/L
LDH as above
Thrombocytopenia
$<100 \times 10^9$ cells/L

Source: From Sibia[18]

Untreated HELLP syndrome can lead to hepatic failure or rupture, coma, acute renal failure, severe hyponatremia, cortical blindness, seizures, and congestive heart failure. Patients diagnosed with HELLP syndrome should be referred to a tertiary care center that has experience with high-risk pregnancies. The optimal management of HELLP syndrome involves delivery of the fetus. Seizure prophylaxis with magnesium and close monitoring of the blood pressure are also important. In two small trials, patients with HELLP syndrome receiving dexamethasone

Table 16-7. Characteristics Differentiating HELLP Syndrome from TTP

	HELLP	TTP
Incidence	Common >1 in 200 pregnancies	Rare 1-25,000 pregnancies
Gestational age of appearance	Usually third trimester; 30% postpartum	50% less than 24 weeks
Predominant clinical symptoms	Epigastric and right upper quadrant pain Headache not infrequent	Neurological and renal symptoms
Antithrombin III	Decreased	Normal
Treatment	Magnesium, steroids, and delivery[a]	Plasmapheresis, steroids, and antiplatelet medications

[a]Delivery usually causes significant clinical improvement in the first 3 days postpartum.

(5 to 10 mg IV q12h) showed significant improvement in platelet counts and liver function in the postpartum period compared to controls. Dexamethasone has the added benefit of improving fetal lung maturation and may increase time until delivery in extreme fetal immaturity.[19–21] Patients who do not show signs of improvement within 3 to 4 days after delivery may be candidates for plasmapheresis. Experimental treatment has also been attempted with prostacyclin.

Thrombotic Thrombocytopenic Purpura (TTP) and Hemolytic Uremic Syndrome (HUS)

Thrombotic thrombocytopenic purpura (TTP) and hemolytic uremic syndrome (HUS) are diseases that reflect a similar underlying pathologic process—hyaline material composed of platelet and fibrin clumps deposited in capillaries and arterioles, causing red blood cell fragmentation, hemolytic anemia, and thrombocytopenia, but leaving the coagulation cascade intact. The initial trigger is unknown, but it may be caused by endothelial damage or platelet aggregation triggered by a direct toxin, neutrophil aggregation, or increased endothelin release. There is also growing evidence that a protease-cleaving defect is seen in many TTP patients. Normally, ultra-large von Willebrand factor (ULvWf) is released into the plasma and immediately broken down by a protease-cleaving enzyme. Many TTP patients have an antibody to this enzyme that inhibits its action. It is postulated that unchecked ULvWf then forms large multimers which trigger the above-mentioned platelet clumping and endothelial damage.[22] Unfortunately, the finding of an antibody against this protease enzyme is not specific for TTP, as it can be present in some patients with DIC, ITP, systemic lupus erythematosus, leukemia, and other disorders. Future studies are needed to determine if the presence of this antibody truly differentiates TTP from HUS.

The more important question is whether the distinction between TTP and HUS in adults needs to be made. The presence of the classic pentad of TTP, namely mental status change, fever, renal failure, hemolytic anemia, and thrombocytopenia, was initially used to help distinguish TTP from HUS, which historically was believed to involve only the renal vasculature. But because only 40 percent of patients with TTP have this pentad, and up to 30 percent of patients with HUS have neurological symptoms, this distinction has become less clear. And with the exception of childhood HUS associated with Shiga toxin-producing *E. coli* (which is often successfully treated only with dialysis), the initial treatment for TTP and HUS is the same. For these reasons the two processes are often referred to as adult TTP-HUS. As plasma exchange transfusion (PLEX) has dramatically improved mortality rates in patients with TTP-HUS (from 90 percent mortality to 70 to 85 percent complete responses), the diagnostic criteria for treatment initiation have become more liberal, with many hematologists considering PLEX in patients with thrombocytopenia and severe hemolytic anemia in the appropriate clinical context. For laboratory values that help to distinguish TTP-HUS from other forms of hemolytic anemia and thrombocytopenia, see Table 16-4.

TTP-HUS usually occurs in women aged between 10 and 60 years. In about 90 percent of cases of TTP-HUS there is no clear etiology, but in the other 10 percent there may be an association with immunologic disease, drugs (especially quinine and mitomycin), neoplasm, viral infection, diarrhea associated with Shiga toxin-producing *E. coli*, genetic predisposition, and pregnancy. Although TTP in pregnancy is rare (1 in 25,000) it is unique in that up to 60 percent will have recurrent TTP with subsequent pregnancies.

The diagnosis of TTP-HUS in a pregnant patient is a medical emergency. The foundation of therapy of TTP-HUS is daily PLEX starting at 30 to 40 mL/kg and increasing it to twice a day if there is no response. Plasma infusion alone may help some patients if PLEX is not readily available, but better outcome has been documented with PLEX. The basis for PLEX is that the exchanged fresh frozen plasma (FFP) or fresh unfrozen plasma (FUP) removes an unknown toxic substance and/or provides a substance that the patient is lacking. If the cause of TTP-HUS is an antibody to the protease-cleaving enzyme, PLEX would both remove the antibody and replace the cleaving enzyme. Daily PLEX may be required for weeks and even with a slow taper, relapses are common and PLEX needs to be restarted. Response is noted by an improvement in mental status, decreasing lactate dehydrogenase (LDH) levels, and improving platelet count, usually occurring within the first few days of therapy.

Other therapeutic measures for TTP-HUS include glucocorticoids and antiplatelet medications such as aspirin or dipyridamole. Unfortunately, most of the studies involving these medications involve the coadministration of PLEX, making it difficult to determine if and how much benefit these medications may add to therapy. Additional immunosuppressive therapy may be needed in refractory cases and may include vincristine or splenectomy. Experimental treatment includes azathioprine, cyclophosphamide, and prostacyclin.[23] Unless life-threatening bleeding is occurring, platelet transfusions should be avoided because they can aggravate the underlying platelet aggregation problem, though in reality this is less of a problem if the patient is undergoing concurrent PLEX.

TTP-HUS occurring in pregnancy is a difficult dilemma. As hyaline thrombus can affect the placental vasculature, placental insufficiency can occur, leading to intrauterine growth restriction and fetal death. Delivery of the fetus most be balanced against the risks of extreme fetal immaturity. Further complicating the picture is the fact that TTP-HUS can mimic HELLP syndrome (Table 16-7). Some obstetricians recommend delivery for gestational ages greater than 34 weeks with institution of PLEX if there is no improvement of symptoms within 2 to 3 days (delivery usually does not lead to maternal improvement in cases of TTP-HUS). If symptoms occur at less than 28 weeks and the antithrombin III is normal, they recommend steroids, antiplatelet agents, and PLEX as initial treatment. Therapy between 28 and 32 weeks is individualized, balancing the risk of maternal and fetal morbidity and mortality.[24]

OTHER RED CELL DISORDERS

Aplastic Anemia

Aplastic anemia uncommonly complicates pregnancy. Two distinct groups of patients are identified: those with a previous history of idiopathic aplastic anemia who become pregnant, and those who develop aplastic anemia during pregnancy. A recent study of pregnancy in patients with idiopathic aplastic anemia reveals that successful pregnancy can occur when these women are in remission, although relapses occurred during nearly one-third of the pregnancies. All of the infants were healthy.

Several cases of aplastic anemia that developed during pregnancy have been described. The mechanism is unknown; perhaps it is immunologic, but its occurrence is more than just random. Of these patients, approximately one-third have spontaneous remission of the aplastic anemia following abortion or delivery of the infant, but the aplasia may recur in subsequent pregnancies. When remission does not occur, bone marrow transplantation may be necessary. Maternal outcome is dependent on the severity of the aplasia and any infections that may occur. Treatment is supportive, with transfusions as necessary. The blood counts of the infant are not affected by aplastic anemia in the mother.

Polycythemia Vera in Pregnancy

Polycythemia vera (PV) is an uncommon myeloproliferative disorder that results in an elevated hematocrit and often elevated WBC and platelet counts. It is extremely rare in pregnancy, as most patients who are affected are beyond childbearing age. It is associated with hypertension and an increased risk of fetal complications including fetal demise. For further discussion refer to a perinatology text.

PRIMARY PLATELET DISORDERS

Overview of Platelet Disorders

A myriad of platelet disorders can be encountered in the pregnant patient.[2] Qualitative platelet abnormalities, characterized by abnormal platelet function, arise in many disease states that can occur in conjunction with pregnancy (Table 16-8). Quantitative disorders are more common during pregnancy, with thrombocytopenia being more common than thrombocytosis (Table 16-9). This discussion concentrates on the most common pregnancy-related causes of thrombocytopenia, specifically those due to increased platelet destruction. Table 16-4 shows characteristics of previously discussed causes of pregnancy-induced thrombocytopenia (HELLP syndrome, TTP-HUS, and DIC).

Platelet destruction is the most common mechanism causing decreased platelet count in pregnancy. The need for evaluation of thrombocytopenia in pregnant women (defined as $<150{,}000/mm^3$) is controversial. Most clin-

Table 16-8. Clinical Conditions Associated with Qualitative Platelet Abnormalities

Uremia
Liver disease
Disseminated intravascular coagulation (DIC)
Drugs (aspirin, NSAIDs, tricyclic antidepressants, phenothiazines, nitrofurantoin, prostaglandins, antihistamines)
Antiplatelet antibodies (ITP, SLE)
Cardiopulmonary bypass
Myeloproliferative disorders (PCV, CML)
Dysproteinemias (multiple myeloma, Waldenstrom's macroglobulinemia)
Preleukemias, AML, ALL
Von Willebrand disease (congenital or acquired)

ITP, idiopathic thrombocytopenic purpura; SLE, systemic lupus erythematosus; PCV, polycythemia vera; CML, chronic myelogenous leukemia; AML, acute myelogenous leukemia; ALL, acute lymphocytic leukemia.

Source: From Eberst,[31] with permission.

Table 16-9. Pathophysiologic Mechanisms of Acquired Thrombocytopenia

Mechanism	Associated Clinical Conditions
Decreased platelet production	Marrow infiltration (tumor or infections) Aplastic anemia Viral infections Drugs (thiazides, estrogens, ethanol, α-interferon, chemotherapeutic agents) Radiation Vitamin B_{12} and/or folate deficiency
Increased platelet destruction	Preeclampsia/eclampsia Idiopathic thrombocytopenic purpura (ITP) Thrombotic thrombocytopenic purpura (TTP) Hemolytic uremic syndrome (HUS) HELLP syndrome Disseminated intravascular coagulation (DIC) Viral infections (HIV, mumps, varicella, EBV) Drugs (heparin, sulfa-containing antibiotics, ethanol, aspirin, indomethacin, valproic acid, heroin, thiazides, H_2 blockers)
Splenic sequestration	Hypersplenism Hypothermia
Platelet loss	Excessive hemorrhage Hemodialysis Extracorporeal circulation
Multifactorial	Gestational or incidental thrombocytopenia in pregnancy
Pseudothrombocytopenia	Not a disease state but a laboratory phenomenon

HIV, human immunodeficiency virus; EBV, Epstein-Barr virus; HELLP, hemolysis, elevated liver enzymes, low platelets.
Note: Conditions in italic print are exclusively or commonly encountered in pregnancy.
Source: Adapted from Eberst,[30] with permission.

icians would agree that evaluation is indicated for a platelet count below 100,000/mm^3, though most women don't have significant risks of bleeding or delivery complications until their platelet counts are well below 50,000/mm^3. Patients with a stable mild thrombocytopenia (a platelet count of 100,000 to 150,000 mm^3) without any significant history or signs of significant clinical bleeding can be managed with monitoring of the platelet count. Platelet counts below 100,000/mm^3 are more likely to be due to an etiology that can potentially threaten the mother and the fetus and will lead most obstetricians to search for an underlying etiology (Table 16-10). The extent of evaluation to do in an otherwise healthy patient is debatable, but most would agree on a minimum of a CBC with a peripheral smear, liver function tests, and a urinalysis. Examination of the peripheral smear excludes pseudothrombocytopenia (due to clumping of platelets) and ensures that the WBC and RBC lines appear normal. The presence of schistocytes should lead to evaluation of a hemolytic anemia. Pregnant patients with platelet counts below 50,000/mm^3 with an identifiable pregnancy-related cause (e.g., abruptio placentae, DIC, or idiopathic thrombocytopenia) should be referred for hematologic consultation.

The management of bleeding resulting from thrombocytopenia in pregnancy is the same as for the nonpregnant patient. The risk of bleeding ascertained from an absolute platelet count may vary due to the underlying disease process (i.e., patients with aplastic anemia may actively bleed at higher counts than those with ITP), but bleeding complications are usually not seen unless the platelet count is below 50,000/mm^3. Spontaneous bleeding, including central nervous system hemorrhage, can occur with platelet levels below 10,000/mm^3. The emergency management of patients with thrombocytopenia and bleeding begins with control of the acute hemorrhage and maintenance

Table 16-10. The Evaluation of a Low Platelet Count in Pregnancy

- History
  - Rule out
    - Known thrombocytopenia
    - Hypothyroidism
    - HIV risk
    - Drug or medication exposure
- Laboratory analysis
  - Minimum
    - CBC
    - Peripheral smear
      - Rules out pseudothrombocytopenia from platelet clumping
      - Confirms normal RBC and WBC
    - If in second or third trimester, studies to rule out preeclampsia
      - Urinalysis
      - Liver function studies
  - Expanded evaluation directed by history or physical examination
    - ANA, anticardiolipin, and anti-DNA antibodies lupus anticoagulant
    - HIV serology
    - Coagulation tests
    - Coombs test
    - Antiplatelet antibodies[a]
  - Bone marrow
    - Rule out aplastic anemia, marrow infitration[b]

[a]These are positive in about 90% of patients with ITP but are not specific and their presence does not usually change treatment.
[b]In ITP a bone marrow biopsy will usually show increased megakaryocytes.

of an adequate intravascular volume to ensure hemodynamic stability. Generally, patients with active bleeding and platelet counts below 25,000 to 50,000/mm^3 should receive platelet transfusion. Each unit of platelets infused should raise the platelet count by 10,000/mm^3. Typically, platelet transfusions are given 6 units at a time. Patients with antiplatelet antibodies, such as those with idiopathic thrombocytopenic purpura (ITP), or patients with hypersplenism are unlikely to respond to platelet transfusion, and in some diseases such as DIC and TTP-HUS, thrombosis may be exacerbated by platelet transfusion. Patients with platelet counts below 10,000/mm^3 usually need platelet transfusion because of the high risk of spontaneous hemorrhage, though in TTP-HUS this should probably be discussed with a hematologist prior to administration. If surgery is necessary, patients are usually transfused until platelet counts are above 50,000/mm^3. Epidural anesthesia is also generally considered safe in patients with platelet counts greater than 50,000/mm^3.

Idiopathic Thrombocytopenic Purpura

Idiopathic thrombocytopenic purpura (ITP), also called immune thrombocytopenic purpura, is the second most common platelet abnormality encountered in pregnant patients after gestational thrombocytopenia. The true incidence is difficult to determine, especially if mild ITP is classified as a type of gestational thrombocytopenia; one estimate is from 1 in 300 to 1 in 600 pregnancies.[3] Estrogens and other hormones may play a role in this presumed immune disorder. Platelet destruction is caused by IgG antibodies directed against platelet surface antibodies, which are present in >90 percent of patients with ITP. These antibodies can cross the placenta and cause fetal thrombocytopenia (to lower than 50,000/mm^3) in about 10 percent.

The diagnosis of ITP is one of exclusion; any pregnant woman with a platelet count below 100,000/mm^3 should be evaluated. History should focus on known thrombocytopenia, potential drug or chemical exposures, connective tissue or thyroid disorders, and the possibility of HIV. Laboratory studies used to exclude other causes of thrombocytopenia are shown in Table 16-10 and are ordered as indicated by history and physical examination. Bone marrow biopsy is rarely needed, but if performed, demonstrates an increased number of megokaryocytes with the absence of infiltrative or neoplastic marrow.

As stated above, most patients with ITP have antiplatelet antibodies. The presence and quantity of maternal antiplatelet antibodies does not correlate with maternal platelet counts, is not specific for ITP (they may also be present in patients with gestational thrombocytopenia), and does not generally guide therapy. Therefore antiplatelet levels are not part of the initial evaluation of thrombocytopenia by most obstetricians.

Most pregnant patients with ITP will have a previously established diagnosis. Recurrent or new-onset ITP during pregnancy may present with easy bruising, petechiae, purpura, or bleeding from the mucous membranes. Many pregnant patients with ITP are asymptomatic; thrombocytopenia is discovered on routine prenatal screening tests.

The overall treatment of ITP in pregnancy is the same as in the nonpregnant patient, essentially with prednisone 0.5 mg/kg/d (or alternatively, dexamethasone or beclomethasone) and intravenous IgG (IV immune globulin [IVIG] 400 mg/kg for 5 days). The more controversial issue is at what point to initiate treatment. Some obstetricians will start glucocorticoid therapy when platelet counts are less than 100,000, but a 1997 recommendation by the American Society of Hematology suggests a more conservative approach, with no treatment until platelet counts fall below 30,000 or in the presence of active bleeding.[25]

Although glucocorticoids may increase maternal platelet counts, they have variable effect on fetal counts. In general, it is difficult to correlate maternal platelet counts with fetal platelet counts unless there is a maternal history of severe uncontrolled ITP, residual thrombocytopenia after splenectomy, or significant fetal thrombocytopenia in a previous birth. In these specific cases cordocentesis or fetal venous scalp sampling may be indicated. Otherwise, there is little utility in assessing fetal blood prior to delivery because most fetal platelet counts will be above 50,000/mm^3, and even in those with lower counts there appears to be minimal risk with vaginal delivery and no additional benefit with cesarean section. Fetal cord blood should be checked immediately after birth, however, to identify those neonates at risk for perinatal hemorrhage. Neonatal platelet counts fall within the first few days of life and critically low counts necessitate platelet transfusions.

For most ITP patients, delivery mode is based solely on obstetric indications and not on platelet counts. In the late third trimester, steroids and IVIG may be given to increase the maternal platelet count to 50,000/mm^3, especially if a cesarean section is planned. Patients with severe ITP may need platelet transfusions prior to delivery.

If the pregnant patient has no response with glucocorticoids or IVIG, additional treatment may be needed. Splenectomy causes remission in up to 80 percent of patients, but is rarely done in pregnancy unless all other attempts to raise the platelet count are unsuccessful. With modern surgical techniques, splenectomy can be done with minimal risk to the fetus and mother. Other medications that are used to treat ITP with some success are danazol, vincristine, and cyclophosphamide—all of which are contraindicated in pregnancy. There is some experience with the use of azathioprine in pregnancy; fetal morbidity appears to be negligible.

Thrombocytosis

Thrombocytosis is arbitrarily defined as a platelet count greater than 500,000/mm^3. Most cases (70 percent) of thrombocytosis are the result of a reactive thrombocytosis from a cytokine-driven mechanism secondary to another underlying condition such as infection or surgery.[26] Reactive thrombosis resolves with improvement of the underlying condition. Other forms of thrombocytosis are usually associated with a neoplastic or myeloproliferative disorder. Patients with consistently elevated platelet counts should be referred to a hematologist to determine if essential thrombocytosis (ET) is present. ET is a myeloproliferative variant that is associated with thromboembolism and fetal complications.

HEMATOLOGIC MALIGNANCIES

Hematologic malignancies, lymphomas or leukemias, are among the most commonly diagnosed malignancies in pregnant women. Although uncommon, these diseases represent a clinical challenge to achieve the best maternal and fetal outcome.

Lymphoma

It is estimated that lymphoma complicates 1 in 1000 to 6000 pregnancies. The vast majority of patients are diagnosed with Hodgkin's disease (HD); non-Hodgkin's lymphoma (NHL) is rare during pregnancy. There is no evidence that either type of lymphoma is directly affected by pregnancy, and there is rarely any direct effect on the fetus. Staging of the extent of disease is essential for proper treatment, although staging during pregnancy can be difficult because extensive radiographs are needed (including CT scan of the abdomen and pelvis), and staging laparotomy may be needed. Some treatment options can safely be undertaken during pregnancy, including radiotherapy above the diaphragm with abdominal shielding and some chemotherapies after the first trimester.

Women previously treated successfully for lymphoma should avoid pregnancy for 2 years after completing therapy. There is evidence that treated women have decreased fertility and may have an increased risk of spontaneous abortion and fetal abnormalities. They do not, however, have a higher rate of disease recurrence in pregnancy.

Leukemia

Leukemias are the second most common fatal malignancy of women in childbearing years and can be expected to occur in about 1 in 75,000 pregnancies. Over 300 pregnancies complicated by leukemia have been reported in the literature. The majority of new leukemias diagnosed in pregnancy, up to 88 percent, are acute leukemias; two-thirds of these are acute myelogenous leukemia (AML).

Of the chronic leukemias, chronic myelocytic leukemia (CML) accounts for almost all the cases. The prognosis for the mother and fetus depends on the type of leukemia, stage of pregnancy, clinical effects of the leukemia, and potential toxic effects of the treatment. There is no evidence that the course of leukemia is affected by pregnancy; with aggressive treatment, the prognosis should be the same as for women who are not pregnant. The earlier in pregnancy the diagnosis is made, the greater the risk to the fetus. Spontaneous abortion is common when leukemia is diagnosed during the first trimester. It is very rare for maternal leukemia cells to be transmitted to the fetus, although leukemic infiltrates are commonly found on the maternal side of the placenta. The infants of women with leukemia are commonly preterm, small for gestational age, and may be transiently cytopenic if the mother is receiving chemotherapy.

Pregnant women diagnosed with AML cannot delay treatment as the median survival of untreated patients is 2 months. Combination chemotherapy is used; it is of minimal risk to the fetus after the first trimester and of limited risk during the first trimester. The goal of aggressive chemotherapy is to attain a remission that optimizes the outcome for the mother and fetus. Some women will relapse and have a rapidly fatal course after delivery.

Chronic myelogenous leukemia typically has a more indolent course, and treatment may be delayed until later in pregnancy or the postpartum period. Alkylating agents are not without risk in the first trimester; leukopheresis may be a treatment option.

Women who have been cured of acute leukemia are usually fertile and have no increased risk of recurrent disease in pregnancy. Chronic myelogenous leukemia is typically cured only with bone marrow transplantation; successful pregnancy can subsequently occur.

HYPERCOAGULABLE STATES

Thromboembolic Disease

During a normal pregnancy the delicate balance of coagulation to fibrinolysis is tipped in favor of coagulation (Table 16-2). This may provide maternal protection against excessive hemorrhage during delivery, but unfortunately also greatly increases her risk of thromboembolic disease. This risk peaks in the postpartum period and is greater in patients with an underlying coagulation disorder or thrombophilia such as those with factor V Leiden, antithrombin III deficiency, or antiphospholipid antibodies. Such women may also have an increased risk for pregnancy loss, preeclampsia, and fetal growth restriction. For a full discussion of thromboembolic disease in pregnancy please refer to Chap. 12.

Inherited Coagulation Factor Deficiencies

Severe congenital disorders of hemostasis are nearly always diagnosed in infancy or childhood; however, milder forms may not become apparent until adulthood or when there is a significant hemostatic challenge (e.g., at menarche). Pregnant patients should be questioned about any personal or familial history of excessive bleeding with surgical procedures, menses, previous pregnancies, or dental extractions. If there has been excessive bleeding in any of these circumstances, further evaluation should be undertaken. Acquired coagulopathies due to drugs (e.g., nonsteroidal antiinflammatory drugs [NSAIDs]) or liver disease should also be considered. In this section, we discuss the most common inherited coagulopathies affecting pregnant women—von Willebrand disease (vWD), the hemophilias (factor VIII or IX deficiency), and other coagulation factor deficiencies.

The type of bleeding that occurs can give an indication of the abnormality that may be present. For example, mucosal bleeding, epistaxis, gingival bleeding, gastrointestinal bleeding, and menorrhagia occur as a result of problems with primary hemostasis, such as vWD and thrombocytopenia. Bleeding into joints (hemarthroses), fascial planes, and the retroperitoneum is associated with defects in secondary hemostasis, typically coagulation factor deficiencies. Occasionally some patients with noninherited coagulation defects will have more than one type of coagulopathy (e.g., DIC in which there is thrombocytopenia along with low coagulation factor levels).

Von Willebrand Disease (vWD)

Von Willebrand factor is a glycoprotein that is synthesized, stored, and secreted by vascular endothelial cells; it has two functions: (1) to participate in primary hemostasis, vWF allows platelets to adhere to damaged endothelium (Fig. 16-1) and (2) vWF carries factor VIII in the plasma.

Von Willebrand disease (vWD), which is caused by a deficiency or abnormality of von Willebrand factor (vWF), is the most common inherited coagulation disorder, with 1 in 100 persons having a defective gene, although only 1 in 10,000 manifests a clinically significant bleeding disorder. Usually inherited in an autosomal dominant pattern, vWD affects men and women equally. vWD is divided into three major subtypes (Table 16-11) with

Table 16-11. Von Willibrand's Disease: Types and Treatment

Type	Incidence	Deficiency	Treatment
Type I	60-80% of vWD[a]	Quantitative deficiency	Desmopressin effective in 80% of cases
Type IIA	About 2-10%	Qualitative deficiency; absence of high-molecular-weight vWF multimers (the lower-molecular-weight multimers are less hemostatically effective)	Intermediate-purity factor VIII
Type IIB	About 2-10%	Qualitative deficiency; abnormal vWF has increased affinity to bind to platelets	Intermediate-purity factor VIII; desmopressin may cause significant thrombocytopenia
Type IIM	About 1-3%	Qualitative deficiency; abnormal vWF has decreased affinity to bind to platelets	Intermediate-purity factor VIII
Type IIN	About 2-10%	Qualitiative deficiency; vWF has abnormal binding site to factor VIII	Intermediate-purity factor VIII
Type III	5-20%	Absolute quantitative deficiency with absence of VWF	Intermediate-purity factor VIII

In emergency situations if factor VIII is not available, fresh frozen plasma or cryoprecipitate can be given. The infusion of platelets may be indicated rarely.
[a] Actual occurrence percentages are difficult to estimate as methods of patient identification vary and many patients may be asymptomatic.

80 percent of patients having vWD type I. These subtypes are clinically important in that they usually dictate treatment. In general, type I is a quantitative defect of vWF, type II is a qualitative defect, and type III is characterized by a severe quantitative absence of vWF.

Clinically, the bleeding manifestations of vWD are highly variable, even among patients with the same type of vWD. Most patients have mild bleeding from mucocutaneous surfaces (such as epistaxis), easy bruising, bleeding after dental extractions, and menorrhagia. About one in a million people having type III vWD has severe, spontaneous life-threatening bleeding comparable with that of severe hemophilia. All patients with vWD should avoid NSAIDs.

A variety of laboratory tests are used to establish the diagnosis of vWD. Coagulation screening tests will usually be normal, although the PTT may be prolonged in moderate or severe vWD due to decreased circulating levels of functional vWF available to transport factor VIII. This may also cause a lower factor VIII level, as unbound factor VIII is rapidly destroyed in plasma. Bleeding time (BT) is highly variable and usually prolonged, but a normal bleeding time does not rule out vWD. Platelets are usually normal (except in vWF type IIb) and low vWF antigen and ristocetin (vWF:RCo) levels are usually noted. VWF:RCo measures the activity of vWF in the presence of the antibiotic ristocetin. Ristocetin is added to the patient's plasma along with normal donor platelets, and the amount and rate of platelet agglutination is dependent on the concentration of active vWF.[27] Multimer analysis is needed to distinguish the different types of vWD. For a definitive diagnosis, patients often have to be tested on more than one occasion as levels can be affected by estrogens, progesterone, thyroid disease, infection, and exercise.

In nonpregnant patients, the treatment of vWD depends on the type of vWD present and the severity of bleeding. Desmopressin (DDAVP) is the treatment of choice for patients with type I vWD, with 80 percent of them responding to treatment. Fortunately, many hematologists test for DDAVP responsiveness in patients when the initial diagnosis of vWD is made, and many patients will thus know if they are responsive to it. DDAVP can be given subcutaneously or intravenously at a dose of 0.3 μg/kg of body weight; a DDAVP nasal spray is also available for home use.[27] DDAVP causes the release of vWF from endothelial storage sites, and tachyphylaxis occurs when these stores become depleted. DDAVP is a synthetic product without the risks of blood products. It can cause flushing, headache, and hyponatremia due to its antidiuretic effect. It has no oxytocic activity and has been used in early pregnancy for invasive procedures. DDAVP is generally not helpful in other types of vWD and may cause severe thrombocytopenia in type IIB disease. When effective, DDAVP elevates vWF:RCo to 3 to 5 times baseline within 30 minutes and the effect lasts up to 12 hours.

Factor VIII concentrates with high levels of vWF are used to treat patients with types II or III vWD. Factor VIII replacement is usually with intermediate-purity factor VIII (which means it is virus-inactivated through heat treatment). Ultra-pure factor and recombinant factor lack the needed vWF. In an emergency, cryoprecipitate can be used to replace vWF. Each bag of cryoprecipitate contains 100 U of vWF, but its use carries a small risk of viral transmission.[3]

Fibrinolytic inhibition with ε-aminocaproic acid or tranexamic acid can be used for less severe mucosal bleeding in type I nonpregnant patients.

Von Willebrand Disease in Pregnancy

Von Willebrand disease is the most common inherited coagulation abnormality with clinical significance during pregnancy and delivery.[3] During pregnancy, most women have significant increases in their levels of vWF and factor VIII, presumably due to increased estrogen and hormonal stimulation. Although excessive bleeding can also occur after first-trimester abortions, blood levels of vWD begin to increase at about 11 weeks of gestation, with most women having normal levels of vWF and factor VIII by the time of delivery, although the bleeding time may remain prolonged. Women with type IIB disease often experience severe thrombocytopenia during pregnancy because the increased vWF produced is abnormal and leads to increased platelet binding. Pregnancy changes are not seen in type III disease, in which vWF is absent.

During pregnancy, patients with vWD should have baseline blood work done and then be followed closely in the antepartum period. Factor VIII or vWF:RCo levels can be followed. A normal vaginal delivery can be planned if factor VIII levels are >50 U/dL or vWF:RCo levels are >80 percent. If possible, episiotomy and deep injection or epidural anesthesia should be avoided. If levels fall below those stated above, DDAVP should be administered (in type I patients) and factor VIII in other vWD patients and those unresponsive to DDAVP. DDAVP may be slightly less effective in the antepartum period because many of the additional vWF stores have already been liberated through hormonal triggers. If a cesarean section is planned, DDAVP or factor VIII replacement should be given with the goal of raising of factor VIII to >50 U/dL and vWF:RCo to >100 percent. These levels should be maintained for several days after surgery.[3,27]

All patients should be watched closely for postpartum bleeding, as it occurs in about 20 percent of patients and can occur up to 1 month after birth. This delayed bleeding is correlated with the drop in vWF levels back to prepregnancy levels.

The fetus born to a mother with vWD should be assumed to have vWD until tested. This can be done prenatally or after birth. If the diagnosis is unknown, scalp electrodes and circumcision should be avoided.

Hemophilias: Deficiency of Factor VIII or Factor IX

The most common inherited coagulation factor deficiencies, hemophilia A (factor VIII deficiency) and hemophilia B (factor IX deficiency or Christmas disease), are X-linked recessive disorders and therefore are rarely of clinical significance in pregnant patients. Approximately 1 in 5000 women are carriers (85 percent with hemophilia A) of whom 10 to 20 percent will be symptomatic. Carriers of hemophilia can usually be identified based on family history. Those with low factor levels may give a history of abnormal or excessive bleeding, especially if they have been hemostatically challenged; menorrhagia is common. Coagulation screening tests, in particular PTT when screening for factor VIII or IX deficiency, will be normal unless the factor level is below 25 to 30 percent of normal. Based on history, specific factor VIII or IX levels can be obtained. Carriers of hemophilia with factor levels below 50 percent of normal should be referred to a hematologist. Patients who are hemophilia A carriers may see an increase of factor VIII levels during pregnancy and DDAVP may help them in the antenatal period. Hemophilia A and B carrier patients will often require administration of factor VIII or IX respectively, to increase their levels to >50 percent prior to delivery.

It is important to identify carriers of hemophilia early in pregnancy for testing of their factor levels and genetic counseling. Prenatal diagnosis of hemophilia is possible with fetal DNA analysis by chorionic villus sampling after 10 weeks of gestation. Of the offspring of carriers of

Table 16-12. Selected Important Hematologic Disorders and Their Maternal and Fetal Effects

Disorder	Incidence	Maternal Complications	Fetal Complications	Treatment
HbSS and HbSC	.1-.2% U.S. African-Americans	Pain crisis Chest syndrome UTI Postpartum infections Preeclampsia Folate deficiency Stroke	Preterm labor Intrauterine growth restriction ↑Perinatal mortality	Hydration Analgesics Supportive care Folate with or without iron supplementation Antibiotics Transfusion
Thalassemia minor		Anemia Folate and iron deficiency	Normal outcome	Folate and iron supplementation Transfusion
Iron deficiency anemia		Anemia	Normal outcome	Iron supplementation
Folate deficiency		Anemia exacerbated with Sickle-cell disease, poor nutrition, anticonvulsant medications, multiple gestations, lactation	Neural tube defects ↑Spontaneous abortion	Folate supplementation
HELLP syndrome (hemolysis, elevated liver enzymes, and low platelets)	.5-.9% of pregnancies, 3rd trimester or 48 hrs postpartum	Hepatic failure Coma Renal failure Hyponatremia Cortical blindness Seizures Congestive heart failure	Fetal mortality	Treat seizures Magnesium Dexamethasone Delivery
TTP-HUS	1 in 25,000 pregnancies	Altered mental status Renal failure Hemolytic anemia Thrombocytopenia	Fetal mortality	Exchange plasmapheresis Steroids Antiplatelet agents
ITP	1 in 300-600 pregnancies	Bleeding if platelets <50,000	Fetal thrombocytopenia	Steroids IVIG
Von Willebrand disease	Autosomal dominant, but 1 in 10,000 with clinical bleeding disorder	Bleeding highly variable, counteracted by increased procoagulants in pregnancy Thrombocytopenia	Anticipate bleeding until coagulopathy is ruled out	DDAVP Factor VIII

hemophilia, 50 percent of the males will have hemophilia and 50 percent of the females will be carriers.

Other Congenital Coagulation Factor Deficiencies

Although uncommon, congenital deficiency of any coagulation factor can complicate pregnancy. Best described in pregnancy are deficiencies of factors XIII, XII, and XI, and fibrinogen abnormalities. With the exception of factor XI deficiency, which may occur in up to 3 per 1000 Ashkenazi Jewish women, these are all extremely rare disorders. Deficiencies of factors XI and XII are diagnosed by a prolonged PTT and low specific factor levels. Factor XIII is essential for the cross-linking of fibrin monomer and is needed for the formation of a stable clot. It is diagnosed by clot solubility in 5 molar urea, and pregnancy in these women most be supplemented with FFP or factor XIII every several weeks.

Quantitative and qualitative fibrinogen abnormalities lead to a prolongation in PT, PTT, and thrombin clotting time (TCT), and possibly a low level of fibrinogen. Supplementation with cryoprecipitate may be necessary for a successful pregnancy. Please refer to a standard hematology text for a full discussion.

Table 16-12 is a summary of selected important hematologic disorders and their maternal-fetal effects.

Acquired Coagulation Factor Deficiencies

Inhibitors of Factor VIII

A rare cause of bleeding in previously healthy postpartum women is the development of an inhibitor to a coagulation factor. Inhibitors are circulating antibodies, usually IgG, that are directed most commonly against the factor VIII molecule, and less commonly against factor IX. These inhibitors develop in 10 to 15 percent of patients with severe hemophilia A and 10 percent of patients with severe hemophilia B. Occasionally, inhibitors develop in patients who do not have hemophilia. Interestingly, in one study 15 to 17 percent of normal adults without evidence of coagulopathy have evidence of anti-factor VIII antibodies without prolongation of PTT.[28] In patients with clinically significant disease, the presence of inhibitors is divided into types I and II. In type I patients the antibody inhibition is very potent and completely inhibits factor VIII activity. Type II disease represents weaker inhibition with some factor VIII activity.

Rarely, factor-inhibitor antibodies can occur during pregnancy, resulting in a picture clinically identical to hemophilia with massive bruising, hemarthroses, ecchymosis, or life-threatening bleeding. In most instances type II disease develops.

The diagnosis is established by laboratory findings of a normal PT, a greatly prolonged aPTT, and a normal TCT. Further studies demonstrate that the aPTT is not corrected by adding normal plasma, thereby suggesting the presence of an inhibitor. The presence of an inhibitor can be also measured by using a Bethesda assay. The factor VIII level will be very low or absent and the other factors normal or only slightly low. When an inhibitor develops during pregnancy, the IgG antibody can cross the placenta and cause a low factor VIII level in the fetus.

The etiology of inhibitor development in these patients is unknown, and in the majority of cases there is often spontaneous resolution within 30 months without recurrence in subsequent pregnancies.[29] In some patients inhibition development may herald the development of autoimmune or lymphoproliferative disease or it may represent a drug reaction. All patients suspected of having a coagulation factor inhibitor should be referred immediately to an experienced hematologist or coagulation specialist.

Treatment is based on the severity of the bleeding and whether the inhibitor has low or high titers. In type II patients, factor VIII and DDAVP are given in an attempt to overwhelm the antibody response. In type I patients treatment is usually to bypass factor VIII inhibition altogether with recombinant factor VII (which will stimulate the common pathway), or to use activated or inactivated prothrombin complexes. The use of porcine factor VIII has also been successful for both type I and II patients because it is not neutralized by anti-human factor VIII antibodies. Severe cases may require plasmapheresis followed by intravenous gamma globulin. Long-term therapy may require corticosteroids or immunosuppressive agents, but in most pregnancy-associated cases no additional treatment is needed.

REFERENCES

1. O'Reilly-Gren Christopher: Anemia, in Cherry & Merkatz's *Complications of Pregnancy*, 5th ed. Cohen, WR, ed. Philadelphia: Lippincott, Williams and Wilkins, 2000, pp 367–390.
2. George J, Rizvi M: Thrombocytopenia in pregnancy. UpToDate (www.uptodate.com), 2001, v 9.3, 1–12.
3. Kramer W, Weiner C: Disorders of hemostasis, in Cherry & Merkatz's *Complications of Pregnancy,* 5th ed. Cohen, WR, ed. Philadelphia: Lippincott, Williams and Wilkins, 2000, pp 367–390.

4. Lockwood C: Inherited thrombophilias in pregnancy. UpToDate (www.uptodate.com) 2001, v 9.3, 1–15.
5. Bick R: Syndromes of disseminated intravascular coagulation in obstetrics, pregnancy, and gynecology. Objective criteria for diagnosis and management. Hematol Oncol Clin North Am 2000;14:999–1044.
6. Lurie S, Feinstein M, Mamet Y: Disseminated intravascular coagulopathy in pregnancy: thorough comprehension of etiology and management reduces obstetricians stress. *Arch Gynecol Obstet* 2000;263:126–130.
7. Ghirardini G, Battioni M, Bertellini C, et al: D-dimer after delivery in uncomplicated pregnancies. *Clin Exp Obstet Gynecol* 1999;26:211–212.
8. Nolan TE, Smith RP, Devoe LD: Maternal plasma D-dimer levels in normal and in complicated pregnancies. *Obstet Gynecol* 1993;81:235–238.
9. Bombeli T, Raddatz-Mueller P, Fehr J: Coagulation activation markers do not correlate with the clinical risk of thrombosis in pregnant women. *Am J Obstet Gynecol* 2001;184:382–389.
10. Eichinger S, Weltermann A, Philipp K, et al: Prospective evaluation of hemostatic system activation and thrombin potential in healthy pregnant women with and without factor V Leiden. *Thromb Hemost* 1999;82:1232–1236.
11. Trofatter KF, Trofatter MO, Caudle MR, et al: Detection of fibrin D-dimer in plasma and urine of pregnant women using Dimertest latex assay. *South Med J* 1993;86:1017–1021.
12. Mou Sum P, Wilburn W, Raynor R: Sickle cell disease in pregnancy: twenty years of experience at Grady Memorial Hospital, Atlanta, Georgia. *Am J Obstet Gynecol* 2001;184:1127–1130.
13. Morrison JC, Morrison FS, Floyd RC, et al: Use of continuous flow erythrocytopheresis in pregnant patients with sickle cell diseases. *J Clin Apheresis* 1991;6:224–229.
14. Bourantas K, Markrydimas G, Georigiou J, et al: Preliminary results with administration of recombinant human erythropoietin in sickle cell/beta-thalassemia patients during pregnancy. *Eur J Haematol* 1996;56:326–328.
15. Hemphill R: Haematologic emergencies and life-threatening bleeding disorders: Differential diagnosis, evaluation, and management. Part II: Hemophilia, sickle cell anemia, and transfusion reactions. *Emerg Med Rep* 2001;22(17): 1–21.
16. Levi M, Ten Cate H: Disseminated intravascular coagulation. *N Engl J Med* 1999;341:586–592.
17. Bacq Y, Riely C: Liver in preeclampsia and HELLP. UpToDate (www.uptodate.com) 2001, v 9.3, 1–13.
18. Sibia BM: The HELLP syndrome (hemolysis, elevated liver enzymes, and low platelets): much ado about nothing? *Am J Obstet Gynecol* 1990;162:311–316.
19. Varol F, Ayden T, Gucer F; Hellp syndrome and postpartum corticosteroids. Internationaal journal of gynecology & obstetrics 2001; 73:157–159.
20. Martin JR, Perry KG, Blake PG: Better maternal outcomes are achieved with dexamethasone therapy for postpartum HELLP. *Am J Obstet Gynecol* 1997;177:1011.
21. Magann EF, Perry KG, Meydrech EF, et al: Postpartum corticosteroids: Accelerated recovery from the syndrome of HELLP. *Am J Obstet Gynecol* 1994;171:1154.
22. Rose B, George J: Causes of thrombotic thrombocytopenic purpura-hemolytic uremic syndrome. UpToDate (www.uptodate.com) 2001, v 9.3, 1–23.
23. Rock G, Porta C, Bobbio-Pallavicini E: Thrombotic thrombocytopenic purpura treatment in the year 2000. *Haematologica* 2000;85:410–419.
24. Brostrom S, Bergmann O: Thrombotic thrombocytopenic purpura: a difficult differential diagnosis in pregnancy. *Acta Obstet Gynecol Scand* 2000;79:84–85.
25. George JN, Woolf SH, Raskob GE, et al: Idiopathic thrombocytopenic purpura: a practice guideline developed by explicit methods by the American Society of Hematology. *Blood* 1996;88:3–40.
26. Tefferi A: Approach to the patient with thrombocytosis. UpToDate (www.uptodate.com) 2001, v 9.3, 1–22.
27. Sadler JE, Mannucci PM, Berbtorp E, et al: Impact, diagnosis, and treatment of von Willebrand disease' *Thromb Haemost* 2000;84:160–174.
28. Kessler C: Acquired factor VIII autoantibody inhibitors: current concepts and potential therapeutic strategies for the future. *Haematologica* 2000;85(Suppl):57–63.
29. Michiels JJ: Acquired Hemophilia A in women postpartum: Clinical manifestations diagnosis, and treatment. *Clin Appl Thromb Hemost* 2000;6:82–86.
30. Eberst ME: Evaluation of the bleeding patient in Tintinalli JE, Kelen G, Stapczynski, S (eds): *Emergency Medicine,* 5th ed. New York: McGraw-Hill, 2000, pp 1365–1370.
31. Eberst ME: Acquired bleeding disorders, in Tintinalli JE, Kelen G, Stapczynski S (eds): *Emergency Medicine*, 5th ed. New York: McGraw-Hill, 2000, pp 1370–1377.

17

Infections and Infectious Exposures in Pregnancy

David J. Weber
Mary S. Dolan
William A. Rutala

KEY POINTS

- Do not give the following attenuated live virus vaccines in pregnancy:
  - Cholera
  - Measles
  - Mumps
  - Rubella
  - Sabin polio
  - Smallpox
  - Varicella
- Immunizations or postexposure prophylaxis which are safe in pregnancy:
  - Hepatitis A and B
  - Influenza vaccine
  - Meningococcal vaccine
  - Pneumococcal polysaccharide vaccine
  - Rabies vaccine and rabies immune globulin
  - Tetanus and diphtheria toxoid (Td)

Infectious disease exposures and infections during pregnancy are common events. Infectious diseases may impact the pregnant woman in several ways, including maternal morbidity and mortality, precipitating fetal loss, and transplacental infection of the fetus. Pregnant women are at higher risk for morbidity and mortality for several infectious diseases than age-matched nonpregnant women.

The prevention and treatment of infectious diseases in pregnant women are more difficult because of limited data on the safety of therapies for mother and fetus. In general, attenuated live virus vaccines should not be administered to pregnant women. Several common antibiotic classes of drugs may adversely affect the fetus, limiting therapeutic options for clinicians.

This chapter will review pre- and postexposure prophylaxis and the use of antimicrobials in pregnant women. Infectious diseases with increased morbidity or mortality will also be reviewed. Finally, the management of the common infectious syndromes, community-acquired pneumonia, and urinary tract infections will be reviewed.

PREEXPOSURE PROPHYLAXIS

Immunization

The development and widespread use of vaccines ranks as one of the most important public health innovations of the twentieth century,[1] and has led to a dramatic decline in vaccine-preventable diseases such as mumps, measles, and rubella.[2] General guidelines for vaccine use in pregnant women are available from the Advisory Committee on Immunization Practices (ACIP),[3] the American College of Physicians,[4] and the American Academy of Pediatrics.[5] Detailed recommendations on the indications, contraindications, and administration of vaccines are available from the ACIP for diphtheria, tetanus, and pertussis;[6] hepatitis B;[7] typhoid;[8] BCG;[9] varicella;[10,11] Lyme disease; (vaccine no longer available)[12] rabies;[13] hepatitis A;[14] polio;[15] meningococcal disease;[16] and influenza.[17] Physicians prescribing vaccines should be familiar with indications, contraindications, and administration guidelines (Table 17-1).

In general, all unnecessary medications or procedures that might jeopardize the fetus should be avoided. However, the risks from immunization during pregnancy are largely theoretical.[3,4] The benefit of immunization among pregnant women usually outweighs the potential risks for adverse reactions, especially when the risk for disease exposure is high, infection would pose a special risk to the mother or fetus, and the vaccine is unlikely to cause harm. Furthermore, newer information continues to confirm the safety of vaccines given inadvertently during pregnancy.

Women of childbearing age should be immunized against measles, mumps, rubella, varicella, tetanus, diphtheria, and hepatitis B as adolescents before becoming pregnant.[3,18–20] Such women should be screened for immunity by a careful history of immunizations and childhood diseases. However, many adolescents and adults will not have reliable records or memory of childhood illnesses and immunizations. This is especially important for rubella because of the consequences of infection for the developing fetus. A history of rubella infection or undocumented immunization is often unreliable and

Table 17-1. Recommendations for Vaccine Use in Pregnant Women

Disease	Vaccines {type}	Indications	Use in Pregnancy	Adult Administration[a]
Cholera	Cholera	Travel (only if required by country to be visited)	Not recommended	Two 0.5 mL doses IM or SC, or two 0.2 mL doses ID, 1 week to 1 month apart
Diphtheria	Diphtheria {toxoid}	Universal, postexposure	If indicated[b]	Primary series, Td three 0.5 mL doses IM (0, 4–6 weeks, 6–12 months)
Hepatitis A	Hepatitis A {inactivated}	At risk[c] traveler	Data on safety in pregnancy are not available; the theoretical risk should be weighed against the risk of disease	Two 1.0 mL doses IM (0, 6–12 months)
Hepatitis B	Hepatitis B {recombinant}	Universal, at risk, traveler	If indicated	Three 1.0 mL doses IM (0, 1, 6 months)
Influenza	Influenza {inactivated whole virus or subunit}	At risk, age ≥50 years	Indicated, second and third trimester	One IM dose annually
Japanese B encephalitis	Encephalitis {inactivated}	Travel	Data on safety in pregnancy are not available; the theoretical risk should be weighed against the risk of disease	Three 1.0 mL doses SC (0, 7, 30 days)
Measles	Measles {live attenuated}	Universal	Contraindicated	—
Menigococcal meningitis	Quadrivalent meningococcal {polysaccharide, A, C, Y, W-135}	At risk, traveler	If indicated	One 0.5 mL dose SC
Mumps	Mumps {live attenuated}	Universal	Contraindicated	—
Pneumococcal infection	23 valent pneumococcal	At risk, age ≥65 years	If indicated	One 0.5 mL dose IM or SC
	7 valent pneumococcal {conjugate}	Universal (age <2 years)	Not indicated	—
Polio	Enhanced-polio (Salk) {inactivated}	Universal, traveler	If indicated	Primary series: two 0.5 mL doses SC (0, 4–8 weeks, 6–12 months)
	Polio (Sabin) {live attenuated}	No current indications	Contraindicated	—

(Continues)

Table 17-1. *(Continued)* Recommendations for Vaccine Use in Pregnant Women

Disease	Vaccines {type}	Indications	Use in Pregnancy	Adult Administration[a]
Rabies	Human diploid cell (HDCV) {human diploid cell-derived}	Pre- or postexposure, at risk	If indicated	Postexposure:[d,e] five 1.0 mL doses IM (0, 3, 7, 14, 28 days)
	Rabies absorbed (RA) {human diploid-cell-derived}	Postexposure, at risk	If indicated	Postexposure:[d,e] five 1.0 mL doses IM (0, 3, 7, 14, 28 days)
	Purified chick embryo cell culture (PCEC) {human diploid-cell derived}	Postexposure, at risk	If indicated	Postexposure:[d,e] five 1.0 mL doses IM (0, 3, 7, 14, 28 days)
Rubella	Rubella {live attenuated}	Universal	Contraindicated	—
Tuberculosis	Bacille Calmette-Guérin (BCG)	Special groups	Not recommended	—
Tetanus	Tetanus {toxoid}	Universal, postexposure	If indicated	Primary series: Td three 0.5 mL doses IM (0, 4–6 weeks, 6–12 months)
Typhoid	Ty21a {live attenuated}	Travel	Data on safety in pregnancy are not available	—
	ViCPS {polysaccharide}	Travel	If indicated (preferred typhoid vaccine)	One dose 0.5 mL IM
Smallpox	Vaccinia {live}	At risk, postexposure	Contraindicated	—
Varicella	Varicella {live attenuated}	Universal, postexposure	Contraindicated	—
Yellow fever	Yellow fever {live attenuated}	Travel	If indicated	One 0.5 mL dose SC

ID, intradermal; IM, intramuscularly; SC, subcutaneously.
[a]Booster doses may be required. See manufacturer's instructions.
[b]If indicated due to risk for exposure, occupation, lifestyle, or underlying medical disorder.
[c]At risk due to occupation, lifestyle, or underlying medical disorder.
[d]See *MMWR Morb Mortal Wkly Rep,* 1999;48(RR-1) for recommendations for pre-exposure prophylaxis.
[e]Postexposure prophylaxis in persons who have received pre-exposure prophylaxis with rabies vaccines is limited to 2 doses (0, 3 days); HRIG should be avoided. See *MMWR Morb Mortal Wkly Rep,* 1999;48(RR-1) for recommendations for postexposure prophylaxis in persons who have previously received rabies vaccine.

should not be considered evidence of immunity. In addition, hepatitis B virus (HBV) can cause asymptomatic infections, and pregnant women may be carriers of the virus without being aware of infection, thus risking perinatal infection of their newborn infants. For these reasons, all pregnant women should be screened for rubella antibody and HBV surface antigen (HBsAg). Rubella-susceptible women should be immunized immediately after delivery. Women who are HBsAg-positive should be carefully followed to ensure that the infant receives HBIG and begins the hepatitis B vaccine series ≤12 hours after birth and that the infant completes the recommended hepatitis B vaccine series.[7]

Susceptible pregnant women should receive combined tetanus and diphtheria toxoid (Td).[3,21] Previously immunized pregnant women who have not received a Td immunization in the past 10 years should receive a booster dose. Pregnant women who are unimmunized or only partially immunized against tetanus should complete the primary series. Women who are in their second or third trimester (>14 weeks pregnant) during respiratory virus season should receive influenza immunization.[17] There is no convincing evidence of risk from immunizing pregnant women with other inactivated virus or bacterial vaccines or toxoids. Susceptible pregnant women at high risk for specific infections should receive as indicated the following vaccines: hepatitis A, hepatitis B, influenza, polysaccharide pneumococcal, rabies, and polio (inactivated).[3] Thimerosol-free hepatitis B vaccine should be used. Several vaccines are recommended as part of postexposure prophylaxis including hepatitis A, hepatitis B, and rabies (Table 17-1). The same indications for use should be followed in the pregnant woman. Pregnant women should be immunized with meningococcal vaccine when there is a substantial risk of infection, such as during epidemics.[19]

Breast-feeding does not adversely affect the response to immunization and is not a contraindication for any of the currently recommended vaccines. The indications for using immune globulins, intravenous immune globulin, and specific immune globulins (e.g., tetanus immune globulin) in pregnant women are the same as those for women who are not pregnant.[22]

Because of theoretical risks to the fetus, most attenuated live virus vaccines (e.g., mumps, measles, varicella) should not be administered to pregnant women or those likely to become pregnant within 3 months. Following rubella vaccination a woman should wait 28 days before becoming pregnant. Congenital disease from maternal immunization has not been reported for any current vaccine, including rubella[20] and varicella.[23] Therefore the presence of a pregnant woman in the household no reason to avoid immunizations of household members for all vaccines including varicella.[3,24] Routine pregnancy testing of women of childbearing age before administration of a live virus vaccine is not recommended.[20] Yellow fever vaccine contains live attenuated virus, but is not known to be teratogenic. If a pregnant woman must travel to an area where yellow fever is known to be prevalent, immunization should be considered.

The administration of tetanus toxoid to the pregnant woman has been an effective method for the prevention of neonatal tetanus.[25,26] In the near future we are likely to witness the expanded use of maternal immunization to provide passive immunity of infants to agents that produce life-threatening illnesses in the neonatal period.[19,27] Vaccines under development for this purpose include *Haemophilus influenzae* type B, acellular pertussis, group B streptococcus conjugate, and respiratory syncytial virus.

Travel

Health care providers should counsel travelers to lesser-developed countries on travel-related risks and methods to prevent illness.[28–31] A risk assessment requires detailed information regarding the patient's medical condition (i.e., age, immunization history, underlying medical disorders, pregnancy status, allergies, and host defense abnormalities) and exact travel itinerary (i.e., locations to be visited, including exact length of stay, urban versus rural locales, level of accommodations, and activities such as freshwater exposure, contact with animals, and sexual activity). Special efforts should be made to identify and counsel travelers who are at high risk, such as those traveling to physically unsafe locations, persons planning a prolonged stay, those traveling off the usual tourist routes, immunocompromised persons, and the pregnant traveler. Current information regarding prevention of travel-associated diseases is available on the web site maintained by the Centers for Disease Control and Prevention (www.cdc.gov).

General risk counseling includes advice on how to avoid the following: (1) accidents, trauma, and injuries; (2) transportation-related injuries; (3) altitude illness; (4) heat, humidity, and sun-related illnesses; and (5) water-related illnesses. Counseling on avoiding infections includes the following categories of infectious diseases: (1) traveler's diarrhea; (2) respiratory tract infections; (3) arthropod-borne illnesses (especially malaria, dengue, yellow fever, and Japanese B encephalitis); (4) sexually transmitted diseases; (5) blood-borne illnesses (especially HIV); and (6) animal bites (especially

Table 17-2. Relative Contraindications to International Travel During Pregnancy

Travelers with Obstetric Risk Factors	Travelers with General Medical Risk Factors	Travelers Contemplating Travel to Potentially Hazardous Destinations
History of miscarriage	Valvular heart disease	High altitudes
Incompetent cervix	History of thromboembolic disease	Areas endemic for or with ongoing outbreaks of life-threatening food- or insect-borne infections
History of ectopic pregnancy (ectopic present pregnancy should be ruled out prior to travel)	Severe anemia	Areas where chloroquine-resistant *Plasmodium falciparum* is endemic
History of premature labor or premature rupture of membranes	Chronic organ system dysfunction that requires frequent medical interventions	Areas where live virus vaccines are required and recommended
History of placental abnormalities		
Threatened abortion or vaginal bleeding during present pregnancy		
Multiple gestation in present pregnancy		
History of toxemia, hypertension, or diabetes with any pregnancy		
Primigravida 35 years of age or older or 15 years of age or younger		

Source: Adapted from Centers for Disease Control and Prevention.[28]

rabies) and envenomations. Detailed recommendations have been published[28,30,31] including recommendations for the pregnant traveler.[28,32,33]

According to the CDC, when deciding whether to travel, a pregnant woman should be advised to consider the potential problems associated with international travel, as well as the quality of medical care available at her destination and during transit (Table 17-2).[28] According to the American College of Obstetricians and Gynecologists, the safest time for a woman to travel is during the second trimester (18 through 24 weeks) when she usually feels best and is in least danger of experiencing a spontaneous abortion or premature labor. A woman in the third trimester should be advised to stay within 300 miles of home because of concerns about access to medical care in case of problems such as hypertension, phlebitis, or false premature labor. General guidelines for the pregnant traveler include the following. First, the pregnant woman should consult with her own health care provider prior to travel; further, she should travel with at least one companion. Second, she should make sure that her health insurance is valid while abroad and during pregnancy, and that the policy covers a newborn should delivery take place while she is traveling. Third, the pregnant traveler should check medical facilities at her destination. For a woman in the last trimester, medical facilities should be able to manage complications of pregnancy, toxemia, and cesarean section. Fourth, the traveler should determine beforehand whether prenatal care will be required abroad, and if so, who will provide it. Prenatal visits requiring specific timing should not be missed. Finally, one should determine prior to traveling whether blood is screened for human immunodeficiency virus and hepatitis B at all destinations. The pregnant traveler and her companion(s) also should be advised to know their blood types. Health care providers should counsel prospective travelers regarding relative contraindications to travel (Table 17-2).

All patients should have their immunization status reviewed and if deficiencies are noted in universally recommended vaccines (e.g., diphtheria-tetanus), they should be provided. Based on a patient's individual risk assessment, they should be offered the vaccines available to prevent travel-associated illnesses (Table 17-1).[34,35] Administration of immunoglobulin can be used to protect against hepatitis A, although hepatitis vaccine is preferred provided the planned travel is sufficiently far in the future to allow the development of immunity.

Malaria in pregnancy carries significant morbidity and mortality for both mother and fetus. Pregnant women should be advised to avoid travel to malarious areas if possible. Because no antimalarial agent is completely effective, if pregnant women travel to malarious areas, they should be advised to use personal protection measures. Women traveling to areas where drug-resistant *P. falciparum* has not been reported may take chloroquine prophylaxis. Mefloquine appears to safe for use during the second and third trimesters of pregnancy and is not associated with adverse effects on fetal or pregnancy outcomes. Limited data suggest that it is also safe to use during the first trimester. Doxycycline and primaquine should not be used for prophylaxis due to fetal toxicity. There is insufficient evidence regarding the use of malarone during pregnancy to recommend this drug for prophylaxis. Small amounts of chloroquine and mefloquine are secreted in breast milk. The amount of drug transferred is not thought to be harmful to the infant, but the quantity transferred is also insufficient to provide adequate prophylaxis for the infant. Hence, breast-fed infants require additional chemoprophylaxis when traveling to a malarious area.

Breast-feeding should be advised during travel. However, nursing women should be advised that their eating and sleeping patterns, as well as stress, would inevitably affect their milk output. They need to increase their fluid intake, avoid excess alcohol and caffeine, and as much as possible avoid exposure to tobacco smoke. Nursing mothers should be advised to take the usual adult dose of the antimalarial appropriate for the country to be visited.

USE OF ANTIMICROBIAL AGENTS IN PREGNANCY

The use of all drugs, including antimicrobials, should be avoided if possible in the pregnant woman. However, infections in the pregnant woman pose a threat to both the woman and fetus and hence should be treated. Unfortunately, only limited information is available regarding the risk of adverse fetal or maternal effects for many antimicrobials. In prescribing antibiotics to the pregnant woman, the clinician should consider the following: the infectious disease or syndrome to be treated, the most effective therapy available (and if the agent is associated with potential adverse fetal or maternal effects, whether an acceptable alternative is available), the risk for adverse fetal events, the risk for adverse maternal events, and whether the dose or frequency of administration should be modified because of altered pharmacokinetics in the pregnant woman. When treating pregnant women, physicians should carefully consider the benefits and risks of individual antimicrobial agents (Table 17-3). For example, although doxycycline is listed by the Food and Drug Administration as a category D drug, it is recommended for the therapy of pregnant women with Rocky Mountain spotted fever due to its efficacy in reducing the high mortality associated with inappropriate therapy.[36]

Fetal Toxicity

Antibiotics

In the treatment of bacterial infections, penicillins (including penicillins combined with a β-lactamase inhibitor), cephalosporins, carbapenems, monobactams, and erythromycins have not been associated with fetal toxicity.[37–42] The limited data on vancomycin suggests that it does not cause fetal ototoxicity or nephrotoxicity.[38] Untreated tuberculosis in pregnancy poses a significant threat to the mother, fetus, and family. All major first-line drugs (isoniazid, rifampin, ethambutol, and pyrazinamide) have an excellent safety record in pregnancy and are not associated with human fetal abnormalities.[43,44] Women being treated for tuberculosis should be carefully monitored for drug-induced hepatitis and should receive daily pyridoxine.

Although not an antibiotic, thalidomide has been used in the therapy of leprosy and aphthous ulcerations in HIV-infected persons. Thalidomide when taken during a critical period of organogenesis (day 21 through day 40 of gestation) often results in severe limb defects and other organ dysgenesis (e.g., kidney and heart defects).[45–47] For this reason its use in pregnant women is absolutely contraindicated.

The use of tetracyclines during pregnancy may lead to teeth discoloration and retarded skeletal growth in the fetus. Oxytetracycline use has been associated with neural tube defects, cleft palate, and multiple congenital abnormalities.[48] However, use of doxycycline was not associated with any congenital abnormality.[49] Prolonged use of high-dose streptomycin has rarely been reported to result in fetal ototoxicity. The use of standard doses of gentamicin has not resulted in risk to the fetus.[50] Although tobramycin and amikacin are listed as class D drugs by their manufacturers, they more properly should be considered as class C drugs. The use of sulfa-based drugs (e.g., sulfamethoxazole) may theoretically precipitate hemolysis in G6PD-deficient fetuses. Used near term they may result in hyperbilirubinemia and neonatal kernicterus.[51] However, the weight of the scientific evidence suggests that these agents do not pose a significant teratogenic risk. Although most studies of trimethoprim have failed to demonstrate an increase in fetal abnormalities, other studies have suggested that trimethoprim use during the first trimester may result in structural defects. Maternal

Table 17-3. Use of Antimicrobials in Pregnancy

Antimicrobial Class	Antimicrobial	Pregnancy Class	Comments
Antibacterial agents			
Aminoglycosides	Streptomycin, tobramycin, amikacin	D	Rare cases of ototoxicity with high-dose streptomycin therapy (use with caution in first and second trimesters). Tobramycin and amikacin probably should be class C drugs
	Gentamicin	C	
β-Lactams	Penicillins (e.g., penicillin G, ampicillin)	B	Generally considered safe in pregnancy
	Penicillins + β-lactamase inhibitor (e.g., amoxicillin-clavulanate, piperacillin-tazobactam)	B	Generally considered safe in pregnancy
	Cephalosporins (e.g., cephalothin, cefazolin, ceftriaxone)	B	Generally considered safe in pregnancy
	Monbactam (aztreonam)	B	Generally considered safe in pregnancy
	Carbapenem (imipenem, cilastatin, ertapenem)	C	Limited data. Use if benefits exceed risks
	Carbapenem (meropenem)	B	Limited data
Quinolones	Levofloxacin, ciprofloxacin, gatifloxacin, moxifloxacin	C	Relatively contraindicated. Arthropathy in immature animals. Levofloxacin an alternative for anthrax prophylaxis
Macrolides	Erythromycin, azithromycin	B	Generally considered safe in pregnancy
	Clarithromycin	C	No reports of fetal toxicity
Tetracyclines	Tetracycline, doxycycline	D	Doxycycline preferred to tetracycline. Recommended for therapy of Rocky Mountain spotted fever and prophylaxis for anthrax
Miscellaneous	Metronidazole	B	No definitive evidence of fetal toxicity
	Linezolid	C	Limited safety data. Consider for serious VRE infections and MRSA (vancomycin intolerant)
	Quinupristin/dalfopristin	C	Limited safety data. Consider for serious VRE infections (*E faecium* only)
Folate antagonists	Trimethoprim	C	Possible antifolate effects in first trimester
	Sulfonamides	C	Risk of kernicteurs in third trimester; hemolysis in G6PD deficiency
	Trimethoprim-sulfamethoxazole	C	Possible antifolate effects in first trimester, risk of kernicterus in third trimester; hemolysis in G6PD deficiency
Glycopeptides	Vancomycin	B	No reports of fetal toxicity
Nitrofurantoin	Nitrofurantoin	B	Hemolysis in G6PD deficiency; contraindicated at term

(*Continues*)

Table 17-3. (*Continued*) Use of Antimicrobials in Pregnancy

Antimicrobial Class	Antimicrobial	Pregnancy Class	Comments
Antifungal agents			
Polyenes	Nystatin (topical vaginal agents)	A	Generally considered safe in pregnancy
	Amphotericin B preparations	B	Generally considered safe in pregnancy
Imidazoles	Miconazole, clotrimazole, butoconazole (topical agents)	B or C	Generally considered safe in pregnancy
Azoles	Fluconazole, itraconazole, ketoconazole	C	Avoid dose of fluconazole >150 mg/kg/d; use only if benefits exceed risks
Antiviral agents			
	Acyclovir, famciclovir, valacyclovir	B	Acyclovir probably safe in pregnancy; avoid other agents due to limited data
	Amantadine, rimantadine, oseltamivir, zanamivir	C	Relatively contraindicated; use only if benefits exceed risks
	Antiretrovirals[a]	—	Seek expert opinion.
Antituberculosis			
	Isoniazid, rifampin	C	Not associated with fetal toxicity (use in treatment of active tuberculosis); postpone treatment of latent tuberculous infection; follow pregnant woman for drug-induced hepatitis
	Ethambutol	C	Appears safe in pregnancy
	Pyrazinamide	C	Use with caution in treating active tuberculosis due to limited data
	Capreomycin	C	Use with extreme caution in treating active tuberculosis
	Cycloserine	C	Not recommended for use in pregnancy due to limited data
Miscellaneous			
	Thalidomide	X	Absolutely contraindicated (congenital anomalies)

FDA pregnancy categories: A, studies in pregnant women—no risk; B, animal studies—no risk, but human studies not adequate, or animal toxicity but human studies—no risk; C, animal studies show toxicity, human studies inadequate but benefit may exceed risk; D, evidence of human risk, but benefits may exceed risk; X, fetal abnormalities in human, risks outweigh benefits.
[a] See manufacturer's recommendations.

supplementation with multivitamins containing folic acid may reduce this risk.

Antifungal Agents

The imidazoles (clotrimazole, butoconazole, tioconazole, miconazole) and triazoles (terconazole, ketoconazole, itraconazole, fluconazole) are generally considered safe for topical treatment of cutaneous fungal infections in pregnancy since there is minimal systemic absorption of these compounds.[52,53] For topical vaginal therapy nystatin is considered safe in all trimesters.[52,53] The imidazoles and the triazole terconazole are widely used for topical vaginal treatment of candidiasis and are generally considered safe for use in the second and third trimesters. There is extensive experience with amphotericin B for the treatment of systemic antifungal therapy; to date there have been no reports of teratogenesis with this agent. Ketoconazole, flucytosine, and griseofulvin have been shown to be teratogenic and/or embryogenic in animals and are therefore relatively contraindicated in pregnancy.[53] Prolonged high-dose (200–400 mg/d) therapy with fluconazole has been associated with congenital limb deformities.[54] However, lower doses (<150 mg/d) have not been associated with fetal toxicity.[52,53] There are no human data on the safety of itraconazole. Iodides have been associated with congenital goiter and should not be used in pregnancy.

Antiviral Agents

Only limited data are available on the safety of most antiviral agents. Studies to date suggest that acyclovir is safe for use in pregnancy for the treatment of varicella-zoster or herpes simplex infections.[55] Because of the unknown effects of influenza antiviral drugs (amantadine, rimantadine, zanamivir, oseltamivir) on pregnant women and their fetuses, these four drugs should only be used during pregnancy if the potential benefits justify the potential risk to the embryo or fetus.[17] Antiretroviral therapy for HIV-infected pregnant women is complicated and should be administered under the care of an expert. The goal of therapy is to reduce viral replication to below detectable levels using combination therapy.[56,57] Antiretroviral therapy is associated with frequent side effects including life-threatening toxicity. The potential for fetal toxicity is unknown for many drugs.

Maternal Toxicity

Acute liver toxicity may occur in pregnant women treated with tetracycline.[58] Oral erythromycin estolate is contraindicated because of its increased risk (10 percent) of cholestatic jaundice.[59]

Antimicrobial Use in Lactating Women

Physicians should be aware of the possibility that lactating women will deliver sufficient drugs to their children to result in toxicity.[42,60,61] The American Academy of Pediatrics states that therapy with chloramphenicol and metronidazole may be of concern as these drugs have an unknown effect on the breast-feeding infant.[5] Nalidixic acid and nitrofurantoin may cause hemolysis in infants with G6PD deficiency but are usually compatible with breastfeeding. Sulfonamides should be used with caution in infants with jaundice or G6PD deficiency in ill, stressed, or premature infants.

POSTEXPOSURE PROPHYLAXIS

Postexposure prophylaxis (PEP) is available to reduce the likelihood of infection following exposure to many infectious agents (Table 17-4). Unfortunately, PEP is not available to prevent infection following exposure to cytomegalovirus, mumps, rubella, parvovirus B19, and hepatitis C.

Hepatitis A

Hepatitis A is caused by an enteric nonenveloped RNA virus (Picornaviridae, genus *Hepatovirus*) that is transmitted person to person by the fecal-oral route.[62,63] Approximately 20,000 to 30,000 cases are reported each year in the United States.[64] Infection is acquired by ingestion of contaminated food or water, close person to person contact, and uncommonly via transfusion of blood products. There are rare reports of transplacental (vertical) transmission of hepatitis A.[65–68] Persons at risk of infection include household or sexual contacts of infected people, persons living in regions of the U.S. with consistently high rates of hepatitis A, travels to countries where hepatitis A is common, men who have sex with other men, and injecting and noninjecting drug users.

After an incubation phase of 15 to 50 days (mean, 30 days), most infected persons develop nonspecific constitutional symptoms followed by gastrointestinal symptoms. Common symptoms during the icteric phase include, in addition to jaundice, fever, fatigue, abdominal pain, loss of appetite, nausea and vomiting, and diarrhea. Outbreak investigations have revealed that up to 15 percent of patients may have asymptomatic infection and in

Table 17-4. Postexposure Prophylaxis of Infectious Diseases

Disease	Indication[a]	Change in Usual Recommendations	Therapy[b]	Administration
Animal bite	Percutaneous animal bite		Tetanus immunization (if not up to date)	
Bioterrorism agents	Exposure to bioterrorism agent	Possibly (see text)	See text	See text
Hepatitis A	Household, sexual, or common-source (e.g., food) exposure	No	Immune serum globulin (time since exposure $\leq$2 weeks) and vaccine	IG 0.06 mL/kg IM and vaccine (see manufacturer's recommendations)
Hepatitis B	Sexual, mucous membrane, or percutaneous exposure to infected blood or body fluid (HBsAg-positive source); household contact of HBsAg-positive person	No	Hepatitis B immune globulin and vaccine[c]	Vaccine 1.0 mL IM at 0, 1, 6 months $\pm$ HBIG 0.06 mL/kg IM
HIV	Sexual, mucous membrane, or percutaneous exposure to infected blood or body fluid	Avoid antivirals with known teratogenicity	Antiretrovirals[d]	Orally for 4 weeks
Influenza	Close contact (droplet/airborne transmission) with infected person	Avoid antivirals	Not recommended	Not recommended
Measles	Household or close contact with infected person	Yes, avoid measles vaccine	Immune globulin (time since exposure $\leq$6 days)	IG 0.25 mL/kg IM (max 15 mL)[e]
Rabies	Mucous membrane (lick) or percutaneous (bite) exposure to a rabid animal	No	Rabies immune globulin and rabies vaccine (as soon as possible)[f]	RIG 20 IU/kg plus vaccine at 0, 3, 7, 14, and 28 days
Varicella zoster	Household or face-to-face exposure with infected person	Yes (vaccine not recommended for nonimmunocompromised adults)	VZIG (preferably with 96 hours of exposure)	125 U/10 kg IM (max 625 units)

HBIG, hepatitis B immune globulin; HIV, human immunodeciency virus; IG, immune globulin; IM, intramuscularly; RIG, rabies immune globulin; VZIG, varicella-zoster immune globulin.

[a]Postexposure prophylaxis should be provided only if source infected (or likely infected) and transmission possible. For several viral diseases the source may be infectious prior to appearing (e.g., mumps) or developing a rash (e.g., measles, varicella).

[b]Therapy is provided only to susceptible sources. May require serologic evaluation to determine susceptibility.

[c]See American Academy of Pediatrics[5] for detailed recommendations regarding postexposure prophylaxis (depends on type of exposure, immune status of exposed person).

[d]See Centers for Disease Control and Prevention (www.edc.gov).

[e]Immunocompromised persons should receive IG 0.50 mL/kg IM (max 15 mL).

[f]Persons who have receive pre-exposure prophylaxis with rabies vaccine should not be given RIG, and postexposure prophylaxis with rabies vaccine is modified (see Centers for Disease Control and Prevention[13]).

30 percent jaundice may not develop.[69] Children are much more likely than adults to have clinically inapparent infection. The fatality rate reported for hepatitis A has been <1.5 percent of all hospitalized icteric patients. Chronic infection with hepatitis A has not been reported. Hepatitis A is diagnosed via serologic testing to detect IgM antibody to the capsid proteins (anti-HAV). In most persons, IgM anti-HAV become detectable 5 to 10 days before the onset of symptoms and can persist for up to 6 months after infection.[70,71] IgG anti-HAV appears early in the course of infection, remains detectable for life, and confers lifelong protection against disease.[72] Only supportive therapy is available for the treatment of hepatitis A. The differential diagnosis of jaundice during pregnancy and an algorithm for medical evaluation has been published.[73,74]

Preexposure Prophylaxis

Preexposure prophylaxis may be provided by either immune globulin (IG) or hepatitis A vaccine, an inactivated product prepared by methods similar to those used for inactivated poliovirus vaccine. Hepatitis A vaccine is recommended for persons at high risk of hepatitis A (see above), in some outbreak settings, and for persons who have clotting factor disorders or chronic liver disease. Although hepatitis A vaccine is preferred for preexposure prophylaxis, IG may be used at a dose of 0.02 mL/kg (short-term protection, 1 to 2 months) or 0.06 mL/kg (long-term protection, 3 to 5 months) to provide preexposure prophylaxis for persons traveling to countries with a high prevalence of hepatitis A.[75]

Postexposure Prophylaxis

Persons who have been recently exposed to hepatitis A and who have not previously been administered hepatitis A vaccine should be administered a single IM dose of IG (0.02 mL/kg) as soon as possible, but no longer than 2 weeks after the last exposure.[7] Persons who have been administered one dose of hepatitis A vaccine at least 1 month before exposure do not need IG. Postexposure prophylaxis should be provided to close personal contacts (household members, sexual partners) of infected cases, staff and attendees of day care centers caring for a child with acute disease, and persons who may have ingested potentially contaminated food or water from a common-source exposure.

Hepatitis B

Hepatitis B, caused by an enveloped DNA virus (Hepadnoviridae), is a leading cause worldwide of chronic hepatitis, cirrhosis, and hepatocellular carcinoma, accounting for 1 million deaths annually.[76–78] In the United States, hepatitis B virus (HBV) infection is most commonly acquired via injection drug use, sexual activity, or occupational exposure.[79] Other routes of acquisition include household contact, hemodialysis, transfusion of blood products, organ transplantation, and mother-to-infant (vertical) transmission. In the United States, approximately 80,000 persons are infected each year and 1.25 million are estimated to be chronically infected. Chronically infected mothers give birth to 22,000 infants annually in the United States.[80] Public health interventions including increasing use of HBV vaccine, exclusion of chronically infected persons from donating blood, and the use of standard precautions in health care have resulted in a decreasing incidence of acute infections in the U.S.[81,82]

Acute hepatitis B infection is diagnosed using serologic tests. Persons with chronic HBV infection and chronic hepatitis may be candidates for therapy with interferon and lamivudine.[83]

Preexposure Prophylaxis

The currently available HBV vaccines are produced by cloning the S gene, encoding the hepatitis B surface antigen (HBsAg) through the use of a plasmid vector inserted into common baker's yeast.[84] Hepatitis B vaccine is a universally recommended vaccine for all children, with the first dose administered by 2 months of age if the mother is HBsAg negative,[24] and immunization of unvaccinated children and adolescents up to 18 years of age whenever such persons are seen for routine medical visits.[18] The vaccine may be provided by a variety of different dosage schedules including 0, 1, and 6 months; 0, 1, 2, and 12 months; and 0 and 12 months (for adolescents 11 to 15 years of age only). More than 95 percent of healthy young adults develop protective antibody levels (i.e., ≥10 mIU/mL).[84] Factors associated with reduced efficacy include older age, smoking, and increased body mass index (i.e., obesity).[81] Immunocompromised persons also have a suboptimal response. The duration of vaccine protection in healthy persons who are vaccine responders is considered lifelong and hence there is currently no recommendation for routine booster doses of vaccine.[84] The only contraindications to HBV immunization are anaphylaxis to a previous dose of vaccine or allergy to a vaccine component such as baker's yeast. In scientific evaluations, HBV vaccine was not linked with multiple sclerosis.[85,86]

All pregnant women should be tested for HBsAg. Treatment of the children of such women is highly effective in preventing acquisition of HBV infection. Currently, it is recommended that both HBV vaccine and HBIG should be administered with 12 hours of birth.

Postexposure Prophylaxis

Postexposure prophylaxis with hepatitis B immune globulin (HBIG) and/or vaccine should be considered in two situations. First, percutaneous, mucous membrane, or nonintact skin exposure to a person known or suspected to be HBsAg positive. Second, sexual exposure to a HBsAg-positive person. Needlestick or other percutaneous exposure of unvaccinated health care workers should lead to initiation of the hepatitis B vaccine series. Postexposure prophylaxis should be considered for any percutaneous, ocular, or mucous membrane exposure to blood in the workplace and is determined by the HBsAg status of the source and the vaccination and vaccine-response status of the exposed person (Table 17-5). If the source of exposure is HBsAg positive and the exposed person is unvaccinated, HBIG also should be administered as soon as possible after exposure (preferably within 24 hours) and the vaccine series started. The effectiveness of HBIG when administered >7 days after percutaneous or permucosal exposures is unknown. If the exposed person had an adequate antibody response (≥10 mIU/mL) documented after vaccination, no testing or treatment is needed, although administration of a booster dose of vaccine can be considered.

Human Immunodeficiency Virus

The care of pregnant women infected with HIV is complex and requires close collaboration among primary care physicians, high-risk obstetricians, and adult and pediatric infectious disease specialists. The medical management issues involved in the care of the pregnant woman with known or possible HIV infection include recognition and diagnosis, antiretroviral therapy, prevention and treatment of opportunistic infections, and prevention of maternal-to-child transmission.[87–92] The Public Health Service recommends universal counseling and voluntary HIV testing of all pregnant women and treatment of those infected.[93] In this section we will focus on the postexposure prophylaxis of women potentially exposed to HIV via sexually or parenteral contact.

Table 17-5. Recommended Postexposure Prophylaxis for Percutaneous or Permucosal Exposure to HBV in the United States

Vaccination and Antibody Status of Exposed Worker	Treatment when source is found to be:		
	HBsAg Positive	**HBsAg Negative**	**Not Tested or Status Unknown**
Unvaccinated	Treat with one dose of HBIG[a] and initiate HBV vaccine[b]	Initiation of HBV vaccine	Initiation of HBV vaccine
Previously vaccinated			
Known responder	No treatment	No treatment	No treatment
Known nonresponder[c]	Treat with two doses of HBIG or one dose of HBIG and initiate revaccination	No treatment	If known high-risk source, treat as if source were HBsAg positive
Antibody response unknown	Test exposed person for anti-HBsAg (if adequate, no treatment; if inadequate, treat with one dose of HBIG and vaccine booster)	No treatment	Test exposed person for anti-HBsAg (if adequate, no treatment; if inadequate, treat with vaccine booster and recheck titer in 1 to 2 months)

[a]HBIG, hepatitis B immunoglobulin (dose 0.06 mg/kg intramuscularly).
[b]Hepatitis B virus vaccine.
[c]A responder is defined as a person with adequate levels of anti-HBsAg in serum (i.e., anti-HBsAg is ≥10 mIU/mL); inadequate response is a level of anti-HBsAg in serum of <10 mIU/mL.

All primary care physicians should be aware of the signs and symptoms of primary HIV infection. They include fever, adenopathy, pharyngitis, rash, and myalgia or arthralgia. Serocoversion illness must be distinguished from acute infection with cytomegalovirus, Epstein-Barr virus, and other viral illnesses. Since laboratory findings in seroconversion disease may include a negative ELISA test with a positive RNA PCR test, physicians should obtain both a measure of antigen (i.e., HIV PCR) as well as a follow-up ELISA and Western blot.

Preexposure Prophylaxis

No vaccine has been demonstrated to effectively prevent HIV infection. Prevention depends largely on behavioral changes, including the practice of safe sex (i.e., no partners or a limited number of partners, use of condoms); for injection drug users, avoidance of sharing needles or disinfection of needles; use of standard precautions and needleless devices by health care workers; and screening and exclusion of blood and blood product donors.

All pregnant women should be screened for HIV infection.[93] Women discovered to be infected prior to labor should be referred to a high-risk obstetrician and an infectious disease expert for initiation of antiretroviral therapy and consideration of prophylaxis of opportunistic infections. In women presenting during labor without recent screening, one should consider a rapid HIV screening test and use of intrapartum antiviral therapy with agents such as nevirapine.

Postexposure Prophylaxis

The management of persons possibly exposed to HIV via sexual contact such as rape victims is controversial. Insufficient data exist on which to provide counseling regarding the risks and benefits of antiretroviral therapy.[94] Guidelines for initiating antiretroviral therapy have been published.[94]

More than 20 diseases have been transmitted by needlestick injuries. To date more than 50 health care workers have acquired HIV via occupational exposure. The risk of transmission of HIV with an HIV-infected source via percutaneous injury is ~0.3 percent (95 percent CI, 0.2 to 0.5 percent). Transmission may also occur via exposure to mucous membranes (risk ~0.09 percent) or nonintact skin. Potentially contaminated fluids include blood and blood products, cerebrospinal fluid, amniotic fluid, peritoneal fluid, synovial fluid, semen, vaginal secretions, pleural fluid, and pericardial fluid. Feces, nasal secretions, saliva, sputum, sweat, tears, urine and vomitus are not considered potentially infectious unless they contain blood. Factors increasing the risk of transmission include injury by a device visibly contaminated with blood or a needle that has been inserted directly into a vein or artery, deep injury, a source patient with terminal illness, and failure to use prophylactic therapy.

All persons with potential exposure to a possibly contaminated fluid should be evaluated. If transmission is possible, the source patient should be tested for HCV, HBsAg, and HIV. If the source is HIV-negative, PEP is not indicated. If the source is HIV-positive, PEP should be offered per CDC guidelines (Tables 17-6 and 17-7). When the source person's virus is known or suspected to be resistant to one or more of the drugs considered for the PEP regimen, the selection of drugs to which the source patient's virus is unlikely to be resistant is recommended; expert consultation is advised. If this information is not immediately available, institution of PEP, if indicated, should not be delayed. Any appropriate changes in the PEP regimen can be made after PEP has been started. The same protocol should be used if the exposed person is pregnant.[95,96] However, the decision to use any antiretroviral drug during pregnancy should involve discussion between the woman and her health care providers regarding the potential benefits and risks to her and her fetus.[97,98] Certain drugs including indinavir (taken shortly before delivery), efavirenz, and the combination of stavudine (d4T) and dideoxyinosine (ddI) should be avoided in pregnant women. In all patients with body fluid exposure, appropriate follow-up testing for viral infection should be provided. If PEP is provided, appropriate laboratory tests should be obtained to determine the risk for toxicity and repeated to assess possible adverse events.

Invasive Meningococcal Disease

Meningococcal disease is caused by *Neisseria meningitidis,* a gram-negative, aerobic diplococcus.[99] Although there are at least 13 serogroups, most cases of meningococcal disease are caused by serogroups A, B, and C. Meningococcal disease occurs worldwide as endemic infections.[100] The incidence of invasive meningococcal disease is ~1 to 3 per 100,000 population in developed countries, but may be as high as 10 to 25 per 100,000 in some developing countries. These different attack rates reflect the pathogenic properties of *N. meningitidis* strains and different socioeconomic, environmental, and climatologic conditions.[101] In the U.S. most cases occur during the winter or early spring.

Table 17-6. Recommended HIV Postexposure Prophylaxis for Percutaneous Injuries

	Infection Status of Source				
Exposure type	**HIV-Positive (Class 1[a])**	**HIV-Positive (Class 2[a])**	**Source of Unknown HIV Status[b]**	**Unknown Source[c]**	**HIV-Negative**
Less severe[d]	Basic 2-drug PEP	Expanded 3-drug PEP	Generally, no PEP warranted; however, consider basic 2 drug PEP[e] for source with HIV risk factors[f]	Generally, no PEP warranted; however, consider basic 2-drug PEP[e] in settings where exposure to HIV-infected persons is likely	No PEP warranted
More severe[g]	Expanded 3-drug PEP	Expanded 3-drug PEP	Generally, no PEP warranted; however, consider basic 2 drug PEP[e] for source with HIV risk factors[f]	Generally, no PEP warranted; however, consider basic 2-drug PEP[e] in settings where exposure to HIV-infected persons is likely	No PEP warranted

[a] HIV-positive, class 1: asymptomatic HIV infection or known viral load (e.g., <1500 RNA copies mL). HIV-positive, class 2: symptomatic HIV infection, AIDS, acute seroconversion, or known high viral-load. If drug resistance is a concern, obtain expert consultation. Initiation of postexposure prophylaxis (PEP) should not be delayed pending expert consultation, and because expert consultation alone cannot substitute for face-to-face counseling, resources should be available to provide immediate evaluation and follow-up care of all exposures.
[b] Source of unknown HIV status (e.g., deceased source person with no samples available for HIV testing).
[c] Unknown source (e.g., a needle from a sharp disposal container).
[d] Less severe (e.g., solid needle and superficial injury).
[e] The designation "consider PEP" indicates that PEP is optional and should be based on individualized decision making by the exposed persons and the treating clinician.
[f] If PEP is offered and taken and the source is later determined to be HIV-negative, PEP should be discontinued.
[g] More severe (e.g., large-bore hollow needle, deep puncture, visible blood on device, or needle used in patient's artery or vein).

Table 17-7. Recommended HIV Postexposure Prophylaxis for Mucous Membrane and Nonintact Skin[a] Exposures

	Infection Status of Source				
Exposure type	**HIV-Positive (Class 1[a])**	**HIV-Positive (Class 2[b])**	**Source of Unknown HIV Status[c]**	**Unknown Source[d]**	**HIV-Negative**
Small volume[e]	Consider basic 2-drug PEP	Basic 2-drug PEP	Generally, no PEP warranted; however, consider basic 2 drug PEP[f] for source with HIV risk factors[g]	Generally, no PEP warranted; however, consider basic 2-drug PEP[e] in settings where exposure to HIV-infected persons is likely	No PEP warranted
Large volume[h]	Basic 2-drug PEP	Expanded 3-drug PEP	Generally, no PEP warranted; however, consider basic 2-drug PEP[f] for source with HIV risk factors[g]	Generally, no PEP warranted; however, consider basic 2-drug PEP[e] in settings where exposure to HIV-infected persons is likely	No PEP warranted

[a]For skin exposures, follow-up is indicated only if there is evidence of compromised skin integrity (e.g., dermatitis, abrasion, or open wound).
[b]HIV-positive, class 1: asymptomatic HIV infection or known viral load (e.g., <1500 RNA copies/mL). HIV-positive, class: 2 symptomatic HIV infection, AIDS, acute seroconversion, or known high viral load. If drug resistance is a concern, obtain expert consultation. Initiation of postexposure prophylaxis (PEP) should not be delayed pending expert consultation, and because expert consultation alone cannot substitute for face-to-face counseling, resources should be available to provide immediate evaluation and follow-up care of all exposures.
[c]Source of unknown HIV status (e.g., deceased source person with no samples available for HIV testing).
[d]Unknown source (e.g., a needle from a sharp disposal container).
[e]Small volume (i.e., a few drops).
[f]The designation "consider PEP" indicates that PEP is optional and should be based on individualized decision making by the exposed persons and the treating clinician.
[g]If PEP is offered and taken and the source is later determined to be HIV-negative, PEP should be discontinued.
[h]Large volume (i.e., major blood splash).

The human naso-oropharyngeal mucosa is the only natural reservoir of *N. meningitidis*. During endemic periods, ~10 percent of the population harbors meningococci in the nose. However, most strains are relatively nonpathogenic. Meningococci are transferred from one person to another by direct contact or via droplet spread (up to 3 feet away). Risk of transmission of invasive strains is greatest in the first week of contact.[100] Risk factors include crowding and exposure to cigarette smoke.[100,102] For example, in households where a case of meningococcal disease has occurred, the risk of invasive disease in family members is increased by a factor of 400 to 800.[99] Risk factors for invasive disease include later terminal complement deficiencies and X-linked properdin deficiency.[100]

The highest incidence of invasive meningococcal disease occurs in children 1 to 23 months of age.[103] The incidence falls during adulthood and then increases in persons greater than 60 years of age. Over 90 percent of adult cases of meningococcal infections have meningitis, whereas in children the prevalence of meningitis is much lower, ~50 percent.[104] The mortality for meningococcal meningitis is ~3 to 10 percent, while up to 40 percent with meningococcal sepsis die.[100,105]

Acute meningococcal meningitis is characterized by the sudden onset of fever, headache, and stiffness of the neck, sometimes accompanied by nausea, vomiting, photophobia, and an altered mental status. Meningococcemia sepsis, which occurs in only 5 to 20 percent of patients with meningitis and may occur with meningeal symptoms, is characterized by an abrupt onset of fever and a petechial or purpuric rash and is often associated with the rapid onset of hypotension, acute adrenal hemorrhage (i.e., Waterhouse-Friderichsen syndrome), and multiorgan failure. Pneumonia occurs in 5 to 15 percent of patients with invasive meningococcal disease.[106] Invasive meningococcal disease is diagnosed by cultures of blood, cerebrospinal fluid, or other sites. Since the clinical presentation of meningitis due to *N. meningitidis* is similar to that of other bacteria (e.g., *Streptococcus pneumoniae*), empiric therapy must be directed at all the common pathogens. Because of the high prevalence of penicillin-resistant *S. pneumoniae,* the usual empiric coverage consists of a broad-spectrum cephalosporin (e.g., ceftriaxone, cefotaxime, or cefepime) and vancomycin.[107] If *N. meningitidis* is confirmed, high-dose penicillin may be used alone. Since invasive meningococcal disease may be rapidly fatal, starting empiric therapy should never be delayed to wait for the results of diagnostic tests (e.g., cultures, MRI, CT).

Preexposure Prophylaxis

The only meningococcal vaccine available in the U.S. contains polysaccharide to serogroups A, C, Y, and W135.[108] The vaccine does not protect against *N. meningitidis* serogroup B. The efficacy of serogroups A and C polysaccharide has been estimated at 85 to 100 percent among adults. The duration of protection is unknown; although antibodies against serogroups A and C has been detected for as long as 10 years, concentrations decline markedly in the first 3 years after immunization. Currently, meningococcal vaccine is recommended only for certain high-risk groups, including military recruits, persons with terminal complement deficiencies, persons with anatomic or functional asplenia, and laboratory personnel who are routinely exposed to *N. meningitidis*. It is also recommended for travelers to countries where disease is epidemic or hyperendemic such as sub-Saharan Africa and college students who will be living in dormitories. No fetal or maternal toxicity has been reported among pregnant women, therefore the use of meningococcal vaccine should be considered in high-risk pregnant women.

Postexposure Prophylaxis

Chemoprophylaxis should be considered for individuals intimately exposed to persons with proven invasive meningococcal disease, including household members, boyfriends and girlfriends, and health care workers with contact with secretions (e.g., those intubating the patient).[109,110] The local health department should be consulted regarding the need for prophylaxis of classmates or schoolmates of an infected person. If prophylaxis is given more than 14 days after the onset of disease, it is probably of limited or no benefit.[16] Oropharyngeal cultures or nasopharyngeal cultures are not helpful in determining the need for chemoprophylaxis and may unnecessarily delay the use of this effective preventive measure. Adult prophylactic regimens include rifampin 600 mg orally twice a day for 2 days, ceftriaxone 250 mg intramuscularly as a single dose, and ciprofloxacin 500 mg orally as a single dose. For the pregnant woman, ceftriaxone (given with lidocaine) is the preferred drug, although the risk for use of a single quinolone dose is likely minimal. In the setting of an extensive outbreak, meningococcal vaccine may be used for enhanced control.

Pertussis

In 2000, 7867 cases (2.7 per 100,000 population) of pertussis were reported to the Centers for Disease Control and Prevention.[111] High rates of pertussis, compared with other pediatric vaccine-preventable diseases, continued to occur despite the fact that since 1995 the coverage rate with at least three doses of a pertussis-containing vaccine has been greater than 95 percent among U.S. children aged 19 to 35 months.[112]

Postexposure Prophylaxis

Erythromycin is the only drug approved by the FDA for the treatment of pertussis; the estolate form is preferred by some clinicians because of superior pharmacokinetics. *Bordetella pertussis* is highly susceptible in vitro to erythromycin.[113–115] Erythromycin has been shown to decrease the duration of illness when administered early in the course of pertussis and to eliminate *B. pertussis* from the nasopharynx. For these reasons, erythromycin is considered the drug of choice for the treatment and prophylaxis of pertussis.[5,115–118] Erythromycin therapy of index cases in the community has been used successfully to reduce secondary cases of pertussis in households.[119,120] Although chemoprophylaxis of exposed household members has been recommended based on uncontrolled studies, a randomized, placebo-controlled trial of erythromycin chemoprophylaxis for household contacts of children with culture-positive *B. pertussis* failed to demonstrate a reduction in clinical pertussis.[121] Therapy of infected patients and chemoprophylaxis of exposed health care workers has been successful in terminating outbreaks in health care institutions.[122,123] The potential epidemiologic flaws in clinical trials of erythromycin prophylaxis have been reviewed.[124]

Erythromycin-resistant clinical isolates of *B. pertussis* have been reported, raising concern about the use of macrolides for therapy or prophylaxis.[125,126] However, recent surveys of *B. pertussis* strains demonstrate that macrolide resistance is uncommon.[113–115] *B. pertussis* is susceptible in vitro to trimethoprim-sulfamethoxazole,[114,115] the newer macrolides azithromycin and clarithromycin,[113,115] and the quinolones levofloxacin, ciprofloxacin, ofloxacin, and gatifloxacin.[115] Trimethoprim-sulfamethoxazole has been demonstrated to be effective in small clinical trials[127] and therefore is the recommended alternative for treatment or prophylaxis of individuals intolerant to erythromycin.[5,118] However, its efficacy as a chemoprophylactic agent has not been evaluated. Small clinical trials suggest that clarithromycin and azithromycin are also effective for the treatment of pertussis.[128] Although older studies suggested that a 14-day course of erythromycin therapy was required for eradication of *B. pertussis,* recent trials have suggested that the following shorter courses of antibiotics are as successful as the standard 14-day course of erythromycin: 7 days of erythromycin esolate (40 mg/kg/d; maximum dose 1 g),[129] 7 days of clarithromycin,[128] or 5 days of azithromycin.[128]

Rabies

Rabies is a major worldwide public health problem causing an estimated 50,000 to 60,000 deaths each year.[130] In the United States rabies is primarily a disease of animals.[131,132] The epidemiology of human rabies is a reflection of both the distribution of the disease in animals and the degree of human contact with these animals. In 1999, 49 states, the District of Columbia, and Puerto Rico reported 7067 cases of rabies in animals.[133] Wild animals accounted for 91 percent (raccoons 41 percent, skunks 29 percent, bats 14 percent, and foxes 5 percent) and domestic animals for 8.5 percent of reported cases.

Rabies is most commonly transmitted by the bite of a rabid animal. Other routes of transmission have included contamination of mucous membranes (i.e., eyes, nose, mouth), aerosol transmission during spelunking in bat-infested caves or while working in the laboratory with rabies virus, corneal transplants, and iatrogenic infection through improperly inactivated vaccine. Fomites have not been implicated in transmission. The risk of developing rabies following an animal bite or scratch by a rabid animal depends on whether a bite or scratch occurred, the number of bites, the depth of the bites, and the location of the wounds. In the absence of postexposure prophylaxis, the risk of infection has been estimated as follows: multiple severe bites around the face, 80 to 100 percent; single bites, 15 to 40 percent; superficial bites on the extremities, 5 to 10 percent; and contamination of open wounds with saliva, ~0.1 percent. Between 1981 and 1998, 37 human cases of rabies were diagnosed in the United States. Analysis of the rabies viruses revealed that all cases believed to be acquired outside of the U.S. were associated with dog strains, but 88 percent of cases acquired in the U.S. were associated with bats (1 of 22 had a known bite history).[134]

Rabies virus causes an acute encephalitis in all warm-blooded hosts, including humans, and the outcome is almost always fatal. Rabies infection is most commonly initiated by the bite of a rabid animal. Most commonly, the incubation period ranges from 20 to 90 days (range 4 days to 19 years). An initial prodromal period is characterized by fever, sore throat, chills, malaise, anorexia, headache, nausea, vomiting, dyspnea, cough, and weakness. Early in the course some patients may report symptoms suggestive of rabies, such as limb pain, limb weakness, and paresthesias at or near the presumed exposure site. The prodrome merges into the acute neurologic phase, which begins when the patient develops objective signs of central nervous system disease. Two major forms of acute neurologic disorder have been described, furious (80 percent) and paralytic (20 percent). Furious rabies is characterized by hyperactivity, disorientation, hallucinations, and bizarre behavior. Signs of autonomic dysfunction are frequently present and include hyperthermia, tachycardia, hypertension, and excessive salivation. Coma usually occurs within 10 days of the onset of symptoms. The diagnosis of rabies is frequently missed.[135]

Preexposure Prophylaxis

Preexposure prophylaxis with rabies vaccine is strongly recommended for persons whose recreational or occupational activities place them at risk for acquiring rabies, including rabies research laboratory workers, rabies biologics production workers, rabies diagnostic laboratory workers, spelunkers, veterinarians and staff members in rabies, animal-control, and wildlife work, travelers visiting foreign areas of enzootic rabies for more than 30 days, and veterinary students. Although the initial rabies preexposure vaccine regimen is similar, the need for booster doses, the timing of booster doses, and the need and timing of serologic tests to confirm immunity differs based on the degree of individual risk for exposure to rabies.[13] Preexposure vaccination does not eliminate the need for additional therapy after a rabies exposure, but simplifies PEP by eliminating the need for human rabies immune globulin (HRIG) and by decreasing the number of doses of vaccine required (see below).

Postexposure Prophylaxis

Postexposure prophylaxis is indicated for persons possibly exposed to a rabid animal. All persons presenting with an animal bite or scratch should be evaluated for the presence of a life-threatening condition such as arterial laceration, pneumothorax, or respiratory compromise. Appropriate emergency care for animal bites should be provided.[136] Key aspects include tetanus prophylaxis, wound cleansing, measures to prevent bacterial infection, and evaluation for rabies prophylaxis.

All persons bitten or scratched by an animal, whether domestic or wild, should be evaluated for the need to initiate rabies PEP. The decision to initiate rabies PEP should be based on the following: the geographic location of the incident, the type of animal that was involved, how the exposure occurred (i.e., provoked or unprovoked), the vaccination status of the animal, and whether the animal can be safely captured and tested for rabies. Excellent guidelines are often available from the local health department. For the purpose of rabies PEP, a bite exposure is defined as any penetration of the skin by the teeth of an animal. Bites to the face and hands carry the highest risk, but the site of the bite should not influence the decision to begin therapy. Scratches, abrasions, open wounds, or mucous membranes contaminated with saliva or other potentially infectious material (such as brain tissue) from a rabid animal constitute nonbite exposures. If the material containing the virus is dry, the virus can be considered noninfectious. A fully vaccinated dog or cat is unlikely to become infected with rabies, although rare cases have been reported among animals who had received only a single dose of vaccine. No documented vaccine failures have occurred among dogs or cats that had received two vaccinations. Other contact by itself, such as petting a rabid animal and contact with blood, urine, or feces (e.g., guano) of a rabid animal, does not constitute an exposure and is not an indication for prophylaxis.

Bats are increasingly implicated as an important wildlife reservoir for variants of rabies virus transmitted to humans. Minor bites by bats and awakening in a room with a bat have been associated with the development of rabies. For this reason, the CDC now recommends rabies PEP for all persons who have sustained a bite, scratch, or mucous membrane exposure to a bat unless the bat is available for testing and is negative for evidence of rabies.[13] Further, PEP is also appropriate even in the absence of a demonstrable bite, scratch, or mucous membrane exposure in situations in which there is reasonable probability that such contact occurred (e.g., a sleeping person awakens to find a bat in the room or an adult witnesses a bat in the room with a previously unattended child or mentally disabled or intoxicated person).

In the United States, PEP consists of a regimen of one dose of human rabies immune globulin (HRIG) and five doses of rabies vaccine over a 28-day period. It is critical that the CDC recommendations be followed EXACTLY. Rabies immune globulin and the first dose of rabies vaccine should be given as soon as possible after exposure, preferably within 24 hours. Rabies vaccines available in the United States include human diploid cell vaccine (HDCV; produced in human diploid cells, Imovax®, by Pasteur Merieux Connaught), rabies vaccine absorbed (RVA; produced in fetal rhesus diploid lung cells, Rabies Vaccine Absorbed®, by SmithKline

Beecham), and purified chick embryo cell culture vaccine (PCEC; produced in chick embryo cells, RabAvert,® by Chiron). All currently used vaccines are produced in cell culture and are significantly less toxic than older vaccines that were produced in neural tissue. Side effects including mild erythema and swelling and pain at the injection site and have been reported among 30 to 74 percent of vaccine recipients. Systemic reactions such as headache, nausea, abdominal pain, muscle aches, and dizziness have been reported among 5 to 40 percent of recipients. Serum sickness-like reactions (type III hypersensitivity) have been noted among approximately 6 percent of persons receiving booster doses of HDCV, 2 to 21 days after administration of the booster dose. Such reactions have not been life-threatening and have not been reported with the RVA or PCEC vaccines. Anaphylaxis and neurologic symptoms have only rarely been associated with the current rabies vaccines. Severe egg allergy is a contraindication to the use of the PCEC vaccine. Once initiated, rabies prophylaxis should not be interrupted or discontinued because of local or mild systemic adverse reactions to rabies vaccine. Usually such reactions can be successfully managed with antiinflammatory and antipyretic agents. When a person with a history of serious hypersensitivity to rabies vaccine must be revaccinated, antihistamines may be given. Epinephrine should be easily available to counteract anaphylactic reactions, and the person should be observed carefully immediately after vaccination.

Human rabies immune globulin is administered only once (at the beginning of antirabies prophylaxis) to provide immediate antibodies until the patient responds to rabies vaccine by producing antibodies. Failure to use HRIG has led to rabies, despite appropriate PEP with human diploid cell vaccine. If HRIG was not given when vaccination was begun, it can be given through the seventh day after administration of the vaccine. Beyond the seventh day, HRIG is not indicated since an antibody response is presumed to have occurred. The CDC now recommends that as much as possible of the full dose be infiltrated around the wound. HRIG should never be administered in the same syringe or into the same anatomic site as vaccine. Even if the wound has to be sutured it should be infiltrated locally with HRIG. This practice has been demonstrated to be safe and does not create an additional risk of infection. However, caution is needed when injecting into a tissue compartment such as the finger pulp because excessive HRIG can increase compartment pressure and lead to necrosis.

If exposed to rabies, persons previously vaccinated should receive two intramuscular doses (1.0 mL each) of vaccine, one immediately and one 3 days later. "Previously vaccinated" refers to persons who have received one of the recommended preexposure or PEP regimens of HDCV, RVA, or PCEC, or those who have received another vaccine and had a documented rabies antibody titer. HRIG is unnecessary and should not be given in these cases because an amnestic antibody response will follow the administration of a booster regardless of the prebooster antibody titer.

A review of the literature in 1991 reported that administering rabies vaccine to pregnant women was both safe and effective.[137] More recently rabies vaccine has been demonstrated to produce an excellent immunologic response without adverse pregnancy outcomes[138,139] and not to lead to fetal abnormalities.[140] Because of the potential consequences of inadequately treated rabies exposure, and because adverse events have not been associated with rabies PEP during pregnancy, pregnancy is not considered a contraindication to rabies PEP or HRIG.[13] If there is substantial risk of exposure to rabies, preexposure prophylaxis may also be indicated during pregnancy.

Varicella-Zoster

The incidence of varicella in the United States appears to be decreasing as coverage with the varicella vaccine increases.[141] However, varicella remains an important cause of morbidity and mortality in the United States, especially when infection occurs in neonates,[142,143] adults,[142,144] and immunocompromised persons.[145–151] Infections in otherwise healthy adults frequently result in complications including hospitalization and death. Choo and colleagues reported that approximately 1.25 percent of adults with varicella infection require hospitalization, 0.62 percent developed skin superinfection, 0.78 percent developed pneumonia, and 0.62 percent developed other complications.[142] Anecdotal evidence suggests that varicella is more severe in pregnant women than in other adults, particularly the risk of varicella pneumonia. However, there are no reliable population-based prospective studies to confirm this impression.[152] In a review of the literature, Enders and Miller concluded that the risk of varicella is approximately 2 to 3 per 1000 pregnancies, with an estimated case fatality rate of 0.5 per 1000 infections during a pregnancy (i.e., the overall mortality rate is approximately 1 per million).[153] They conclude that the risk of fatal varicella appears to be about fivefold higher in pregnant than nonpregnant immunocompetent adults.

Varicella pneumonia is the most common serious maternal complication in pregnancy,[154–158] and usually develops within 1 week of the rash. Common symptoms and signs include fever, cough, dyspnea, and tachypnea. The outcome is unpredictable and may include a rapid progression of hypoxia and respiratory failure. Case series suggest the risk to the mother may be greatest in the third trimester.[159,160] In pregnancies complicated by varicella, spontaneous abortion, stillbirth, and prematurity do not seem to be significantly increased.[161–164]

Varicella may be transmitted from mother to fetus resulting in the congenital varicella syndrome (CVS), herpes zoster in infancy or childhood, or perinatal infection.[152,153,165,166] The clinical manifestations of CVS range from severe multisystem involvement resulting in death in the neonatal period (~20 percent) to dermatomal skin scarring and/or limb hypoplasia as the only defects at birth. Major anomalies involve the skin (dermatomal lesions), skeleton (limb hypoplasia), eye (microphthalmia, chorioretinitis, cataract), and central nervous system (microcephaly, mental retardation).[167] The risk of CVS is ~1 percent for maternal varicella acquired in during the first and second trimesters, with the highest risk (~2 percent) associated with maternal infections between 13 and 20 weeks.[153] Subclinical maternal infection with varicella-zoster virus has been reported to cause congenital infection with neurologic symptoms.[168] The risk of zoster in early infancy or childhood following maternal varicella in the second or third trimester has been estimated at ~1 percent.[153] The onset of varicella in mothers from 5 days before to 2 days after delivery results in severe varicella in 17 percent[169] to 30 percent[170] of newborns. The clinical presentation of neonatal varicella varies. The interval between the onset of rash in the mother and infant is usually 12 to 13 days, but may be as brief as 2 days, suggesting transplacental infection. In the period prior to antiviral therapy, a case fatality rate of 30 percent was reported.[170] Zoster at any stage of pregnancy poses no risk for severe maternal disease, or fetal or neonatal infections.[171]

Varicella may be diagnosed by the classic rash. A positive Tzanck test supports the diagnosis, but may also be seen with infections due to herpes simplex virus. A definitive diagnosis may be provided by culture of blister fluid.

Postexposure Prophylaxis

Approximately 5 to 10 percent of the adult population in the United States is susceptible to varicella. All pregnant women exposed to varicella or zoster should be serologically screened for susceptibility. Exposed susceptible women should receive prophylaxis with varicella-zoster immune globulin (VZIG).[5,10,172] For adults, exposure is defined as residing in the same household; for playmates (friends), face-to-face indoor play (>5 minutes); and for health care workers, face-to-face contact with a person deemed contagious (i.e., with active lesions). VZIG is not known to be effective when administered more than 96 hours after exposure. Whether VZIG has any benefit in prevention of CVS is not known. Varicella vaccine may be effective as postexposure prophylaxis when administered within 72 hours of exposure, but its use in pregnant women is contraindicated.[173]

Neonates born to mothers with varicella (onset 5 days before to 2 days after birth) should be administered VZIG, 125 U/kg intramuscularly.[171] Passive immunization of the newborn may modify the clinical course of varicella, but it does not prevent the disease and although decreased, the risk of death is not eliminated. Therefore, infants with neonatal varicella should receive therapy with intravenous acyclovir 10 to 15 mg/kg every 8 hours. A small clinical trial suggested that the combination of VZIG administered after birth plus prophylactic intravenous acyclovir administered for 5 days starting 7 days after onset of maternal rash was more effective than VZIG alone in preventing neonatal varicella.[174]

Treatment

Three antivirals are available for the treatment of varicella-zoster infections: acyclovir, famciclovir, and valacyclovir. Data regarding safety during pregnancy are available only for acyclovir. In general, acyclovir is contraindicated in pregnancy. However, in varicella complicated by pneumonia or signs of disseminated disease, early treatment with acyclovir is essential and may be life-saving. To date the Acyclovir in Pregnancy Registry has not reported evidence of adverse fetal events associated with acyclovir use.[55]

Bioterrorism Agents

Recent publications have highlighted concern about the potential for biological, chemical, and nuclear terrorism.[175–178] During September through October of 2001, letters containing anthrax led to multiple cases of anthrax in the United States.[179,180] By the end of 2001, 22 cases of anthrax had been reported, including 11 cases of cutaneous anthrax and 11 cases of inhalation anthrax.[181–183] The clinical features and management (preexposure prophylaxis, postexposure prophylaxis, and treatment) have been reviewed.[184–189] The CDC has provided general recommendations for recognizing the most likely agents of bioterrorism[186] and provided detailed flow charts for the clinical evaluation of persons with possible inhalation or cutaneous anthrax. The CDC recommends that pregnant women exposed to anthrax should receive postexposure prophylaxis with ciprofloxacin 500 mg twice a day for 60 days. If the specific strain of *Bacillus anthracis* used in the attack is penicillin-susceptible, prophylactic therapy with amoxicillin 500 mg three times a day for 60 days may be used. However, the strain used in the September-October attacks in the United States demonstrated an inducible β-lactamase that might decrease the effectiveness of penicillins, hence penicillins (including amoxicillin) were not recommended. Breast-feeding mothers should be treated with ciprofloxacin or doxycycline, and in general may continue to breast-feed. However, mothers concerned about the use of ciprofloxacin or doxycycline should consider expressing and then discarding breast milk so the breast-feeding can be resumed when antimicrobial prophylaxis is completed.

The CDC has listed the following as biologic agents of highest concern for bioterrorism: *Bacillus anthracis* (anthrax), *Yersinia pestis* (plague), variola major (smallpox), *Clostridium botulinum* toxin (botulism), *Francisella tularensis* (tularemia), filoviruses (Ebola hemorrhagic fever, Marburg hemorrhagic fever), and arenaviruses (Lassa [Lassa fever], Junin [Argentine hemorrhagic fever]) and related viruses. All physicians should be knowledgeable regarding the clinical characteristics, isolation precautions, decontamination methods, diagnosis, pre- and postexposure prophylaxis for exposures, and therapy of these agents.[190] Detailed management recommendations have been published for anthrax,[191] botulism,[192] plague,[193,194] smallpox,[195] and tularemia. Current recommendations are also available on the CDC web page (www.bt.cdc.gov).

INFECTIOUS DISEASES ADVERSELY AFFECTING THE FETUS

Viral Diseases

A variety of viruses may adversely affect the fetus when they infect a pregnant woman (Table 17-8). Adverse effects may include increased maternal morbidity or mortality, fetal loss (abortion, stillbirth), congenital infections, fetal growth restriction, and prematurity. Of special importance because of their detrimental effects are human immunodeficiency virus, parvovirus B19, and rubella.

Bacterial Diseases and Parasitic Diseases

Few bacterial or parasitic diseases have a direct adverse affects on the fetus. All infections may affect the fetus when they cause serious disease in the pregnant female.

Q Fever

Q fever is caused by *Coxiella burnetii,* an obligate intracellular, small gram-negative bacterium.[196] Q fever is a zoonosis with worldwide distribution. Domestic ruminants are the most frequent source of human infection. Disease is most commonly acquired via the aerosol route (inhalation), but infection via the digestive route from eating contaminated dairy products may occur. Most infections in humans are asymptomatic. Acute symptomatic infection with *C. burnetii* usually results in acute hepatitis or pneumonia. Endocarditis is the major clinical presentation of chronic Q fever.

Several cases of Q fever during pregnancy have been described. Q fever during pregnancy frequently causes placentitis and appears to be associated with premature birth, spontaneous abortion, and death in utero.[197] Most infected pregnant women present with fever, flu-like illness,[198] severe thrombocytopenia,[199,200] and atypical pneumonia.[200] The diagnosis of Q fever relies mainly on serology.[201] Doxycycline is the treatment of choice for Q fever.[196] Fluoroquinolones are considered to be a reliable alternative. Although a macrolide compound or co-trimoxazole may be potential effective alternatives, no reliable antibiotic regimen can currently be recommended for the pregnant woman.[196]

Pregnant women should be advised to avoid contact with animals or pets, especially cats, to prevent both toxoplasmosis and Q fever.

Syphilis

Syphilis is caused by *Treponema pallidum,* a thin motile spirochete.[202] The incidence of acquired and congenital syphilis increased dramatically in the United States during the late 1980s and early 1990s, but has subsequently declined in all areas, although the rate remains disproportionately high in large urban areas and the rural South. Adult syphilis is almost always acquired through direct sexual contact with ulcerative lesions of the skin or mucous membranes of infected persons. Uncommon routes include needlestick injuries and blood transfusions. Congenital syphilis is contracted from an infected mother via transplacental transmission of *T. pallidum* at any time during pregnancy or at birth via contact of the newborn with a genital lesion. Although transmission via breast milk does not occur, babies can acquire disease via contact with maternal skin lesions while breast-feeding. Syphilis can seriously complicate pregnancy and result in spontaneous abortion, stillbirth, nonimmune hydrops, intrauterine growth restriction, and perinatal death, as well as serious sequelae in liveborn infected children.[203,204]

Table 17-8. Viral Diseases Transmitted from Mother to Child Transplacentally

Disease	Risk to Mother	Risk to Fetus	Clinical Findings	Maternal	Fetus/Neonate	Therapy
CMV	Minimal except in immunocompromised patient	Severe fetal injury with primary maternal infection transmitted antepartum	Flu-like illness with diffuse lymphadenopathy	Serology	Amniocentesis-viral culture; ultrasound	Supportive
Hepatitis B	Acute infection = hepatitis; chronic infection = cirrhosis	Perinatal transmission of infection	Acute infection = hepatitis; chronic infection = liver failure	Serology (HBsAg)	Serology (HBsAg)	
Hepatitis C	Acute infection = hepatitis; chronic infection = cirrhosis	Perinatal transmission of infection	Acute infection = hepatitis; chronic infection = liver failure	Serology (Anti-HBC)	Serology (Anti-HBC)	
Hepatitis D	Coinfection with hepatitis B increases the risk for chronic liver disease	Perinatal transmission of infection	Acute infection = hepatitis; chronic infection = liver failure	Serology (Anti-HBD)	Serology (Anti-HBD)	Supportive
Hepatitis E	Severe acute infection with 10–20% mortality	Fetal death resulting from maternal death. Perinatal transmission of infection rare	Acute infection = hepatitis	Serology (Anti-HBE)	Serology (Anti-HBE)	Supportive
Herpes simplex	Minimal except in immunocompromised patient	Severe neonatal infection when delivered to mother with primary infection	Vesicular eruption on genital mucosa	Clinical examination; culture of lesions; PCR	Clinical examination; culture of lesions; PCR	Antiviral (acyclovir, famciclovir, valacyclovir)

(Continues)

Table 17-8. (*Continued*) Viral Diseases Transmitted from Mother to Child Transplacentally

Disease	Risk to Mother	Risk to Fetus	Clinical Findings	Maternal	Fetus/Neonate	Therapy
Parvovirus B19	Aplastic crisis (hemoglobinopathy present)	Hydrops fetalis; neurologic and hematologic sequelae in neonate are rare	Rash (slapped cheeks), fever, arthralgias	Serology	Serology	Supportive
HIV	Severe disease; opportunistic infections	Prenatal, perinatal, or postnatal transmission of infection	Lymphadenopathy, wasting, opportunistic infection	Serology	Serology	Antivirals
Rubella	Minimal	Congenital rubella syndrome (greatest risk in first trimester)	Rash, fever	Clinical examination; serology	Ultrasound	Supportive
Rubeola	Rarely pneumonia or encephalitis	Minimal risk of teratogenicity	Rash, fever, pneumonia	Clinical examination; serology	—	Supportive
Variceilla	Occasionally pneumonia and encephalitis	Varicella congenital syndrome ~2%	Rash, fever	Clinical examination; Tzanck test; culture of vesicle	Ultrasound	VZIG for postexposure prophylaxis; antiviral (acyclovir, famciclovir, valacyclovir)

Infection may be divided into 3 stages. The primary stage is characterized by one or more painless ulcers (chancres) of the skin or mucous membranes at the site of inoculation, usually on the genitalia. The secondary stage that begins 1 to 2 months later is characterized by a polymorphic rash that is most commonly maculopapular and generalized, and classically involves the palms and soles. Generalized lymphadenopathy, fever, malaise, splenomegaly, sore throat, headache, and arthralgia may be present. A variable latent period follows secondary syphilis that may be divided into early latent disease (i.e., infection acquired within the preceding year) and late latent syphilis (all others). Tertiary syphilis refers to the presence of gummas and/or cardiovascular disease, but not to neurosyphilis, which may occur at any stage of disease. All pregnant women should be tested for syphilis in the first trimester with a nontreponemal test such as the rapid plasma reagin (RPR) or Venereal Disease Research Laboratory (VDRL) test, combined with confirmation of reactive persons with specific treponemal tests such as the fluorescent treponemal antibody absorption (FTA-ABS) assay. In areas with a high prevalence of syphilis, serologic testing should also be performed at the beginning of the third trimester and at delivery. In addition, any woman who delivers a stillborn infant after 20 weeks' gestation should be tested for syphilis.[205] Serologic tests may be negative if they are performed early in disease, and the VDRL may be negative in patients with late syphilis.[206] Penicillin is the drug of choice for treating infected women.[207] Patients who are allergic to penicillin should be desensitized before therapy.[204] Treatment may be complicated by the Jarisch-Herxheimer reaction, which can cause fetal distress and uterine contractions.

Pregnancy has no known effect on the clinical course of syphilis.[208] Congenital syphilis may occur when an infected woman becomes pregnant or when a pregnant woman becomes infected.[209] The risk of disease transmission to the fetus is largely dependent on the duration of disease in the mother. The rate of transmission during primary or secondary syphilis is 60 to 100 percent and decreases to ~40 percent in early latency and 10 percent in late latency. Among women with untreated early syphilis, 40 percent of pregnancies result in spontaneous abortion, stillbirth, or perinatal death. Perinatal infection with *T. pallidum* exhibits a wide range of clinical manifestations that are often divided into two clinical syndromes: early (i.e., clinical manifestations that appear within 2 years of life) and late (i.e., clinical manifestations that appear in children older than 2 years of age) congenital syphilis. Clinical findings associated with early disease include abnormal bone radiographs, hepatomegaly, splenomegaly, skin lesions, lymphadenopathy, jaundice, pseudoparalysis, and snuffles. Late clinical findings include frontal bossing, palatal deformities, dental dystrophies, interstitial keratitis, nasal deformities, eighth nerve deafness, neurosyphilitis, and joint disorders. Infants should be treated for congenital syphilis if they were born to mothers with (1) untreated syphilis at delivery, (2) serologic evidence of relapse or reinfection, (3) treatment with nonpenicillin regimens for syphilis during pregnancy, (4) treatment of syphilis within 1 month of delivery, (5) poor documentation of treatment for syphilis, or (6) insufficient serologic follow-up during pregnancy.[202] In addition, any infant with physical or laboratory findings consistent with the diagnosis of congenital syphilis should receive treatment. Despite adequate maternal treatment for syphilis, congenital infection may still occur. Risk factors for neonatal infection include high VDRL titers at treatment and delivery, earlier maternal stage of syphilis, short interval from treatment to delivery, and delivery of an infant at less than 36 weeks' gestation.[210]

Malaria

Malaria can increase the risk of adverse pregnancy outcomes including prematurity, abortion, and stillbirth (see diseases with increased maternal morbidity or mortality, below).

Toxoplasmosis

Toxoplasmosis is caused by *Toxoplasma gondii,* a ubiquitous parasite found worldwide.[211–214] The life cycle of *T. gondii* is facultatively heterogenous. Intermediate hosts probably include all warm-blooded animals (mammals and birds) including humans. Definitive hosts are members of the family Felidae, such as the domestic cat. There are three infectious stages in the life cycle of *T. gondii:*[214,215] (1) tachyzoites, the form of the parasite that invades and replicates within cells; (2) bradyzoites, the dormant form present in tissue cysts but capable of reactivation in immunocompromised persons; and (3) sporozoites, the environmentally resistant form of the parasite found within oocysts that are present in the intestinal tract of felines and shed in the stool. All three stages are infectious for both the intermediate and definitive hosts. Toxoplasmosis is acquired via one of three principal routes. First, humans can ingest bradyzoites by eating raw or inadequately cooked infected meat (especially pork, mutton, or wild game meat). Second, humans can inadvertently ingest oocysts that cats have passed in their feces, either in a cat litter box or in soil (e.g., contaminated fresh fruits or vegetables). Finally, an infected woman can transmit the infection to her fetus transplacentally.

In adults, the incubation period ranges from 10 to 23 days from ingestion of contaminated meat, and from 5 to 20 days from ingestion of oocysts from cat feces. Most infections in immunocompetent adults are asymptomatic. Symptomatic disease is characterized by nontender lymphadenopathy (typically posterior cervical), fatigue, fever, headache, malaise, and myalgia. Rarely encephalitis, myocarditis, or hepatitis may occur. In immunocompromised persons, reactivation of latent infection may lead to encephalitis or disseminated disease.

Approximately 85 percent of women of childbearing age in the United States are susceptible to *T. gondii* infection.[215] An estimated 400 to 4000 cases of congenital toxoplasmosis occur each year in the U.S. for an incidence rate of ~1 per 10,000 live births.[216] Congenital infection almost always results from primary maternal infection during pregnancy. The exception is seen in immunocompromised women (e.g., AIDS) with latent infection who may transmit *T. gondii* congenitally. The risk and manifestations of congenital infection depend on the timing of maternal infection. The average transmission rate is ~15 percent for the first trimester, 30 percent for the second trimester, and 60 percent for the third trimester. The severity of fetal disease varies inversely with the gestational age at which maternal infection occurs. Most fetuses infected early in pregnancy die in utero or in the neonatal period or have severe neurologic and ophthalmologic disease (the classic triad consists of chorioretinitis, intracranial calcifications, and hydrocephalus). Conversely, nearly all fetuses infected in the second and third trimester have mild or subclinical disease in the newborn period. In these infants the most common disease involves the eye (chorioretinitis, strabismus, blindness), the central nervous system (convulsions, neurologic deficiencies, mental retardation), or the ear (deafness).

Toxoplasmosis is most commonly diagnosed serologically, but the serologic test may be difficult to interpret.[215,217,218] Primary infection in the pregnant woman should be treated under the supervision of specialists.[5] Treatment with spiromycin should be considered (investigational drug in U.S.). If fetal infection is confirmed after 17 weeks of gestation or if the mother acquired infection in the third trimester, consideration should be given to therapy with sulfadiazine and pyrimethamine along with folinic acid.[5,217] The risks and benefits and timing of therapy must be carefully discussed with the patient.[215] The efficacy of therapy is unknown.[219] These are some measures for preventing maternal infection:[212,215] Cats should be kept indoors and the litter should be emptied every day by a nonpregnant person (pregnant persons should wear disposable gloves); children's sandboxes should be covered, and cats should only be fed dry, canned, or cooked foods. Pregnant women should avoid eating undercooked meats, thoroughly clean cutting boards and food utensils after use, and wash hands carefully after handling raw meat. Finally, pregnant women should wear gloves when gardening and wash vegetables thoroughly before eating. At present, universal screening for toxoplasmosis during pregnancy in the U.S. is not recommended.[215] The diagnosis of congenital toxoplasmosis has been reviewed.[220]

DISEASES WITH INCREASED MATERNAL MORBIDITY OR MORTALITY

Hepatitis E

Hepatitis E virus (HEV) is a small, nonenveloped RNA virus spread via the fecal-oral route usually through contaminated water.[221–227] There is no evidence of parenteral or sexual transmission. Person-to-person transmission is unusual. HEV is responsible for large epidemics (attack rates of 1 to 15 percent) of acute hepatitis in southeast and central Asia, the Middle East, parts of Africa, and Mexico. Sporadic HEV in these areas may account for 50 to 70 percent of sporadic viral hepatitis. In other parts of the world, HEV infection is infrequent and is restricted predominantly to persons who have traveled to endemic areas. Clinically, HEV generally causes an acute icteric hepatitis; chronic infection has not been observed. Overall, the mortality rate is usually low (0.07 to 0.6 percent). The disease is diagnosed serologically by finding anti-HEV IgM. Only symptomatic therapy is available for HEV infection; no vaccine is presently available. Low-dose immune serum globulin does not prevent infection.[228] Prevention therefore relies on ensuring a safe drinking water supply.

Outbreaks of HEV have been characterized by a high attack rate among pregnant women, especially among women in the second or third trimester.[229] Mortality rates for pregnant women have ranged from 10 percent to as high as 25 percent.[229–233] Mother-to-newborn (transplacental) transmission may occur.[234] Reports indicate that abortion, death of the fetus *in utero*, premature delivery, or death of the baby soon after birth are seen in women with icteric hepatitis or with fulminant hepatic failure induced by HEV.[226,229]

Listeriosis

Listeriosis is cause by *Listeria monocytogenes,* a facultative anaerobic, non-spore forming, motile, gram-positive bacteria.[235] *Listeria* spp. are ubiquitous organisms isolated from a variety of environmental sources, including soil, water, effluents, and feces of humans and animals. Human infection is acquired via ingestion of contaminated food.[236] Long-term colonization of the human gut may occur. In humans, *L. monocytogenes* may cause enteritis, meningitis, pneumonia, and sepsis. *L. monocytogenes* is the most common cause of meningitis in the immunocompromised host. Neonatal illness has early-onset and late-onset syndromes similar to those of group B streptococci. Prematurity, pneumonia, and septicemia are common in early-onset disease. Late-onset infection occurs after the first week of life and usually results in meningitis. Listeriosis may occur as both sporadic infection and outbreaks, usually due to common-source contamination of food. Incriminated foods have included coleslaw, milk, soft cheeses, paté, and jellied pork tongue. The mortality of listeriosis may be as high as 30 percent. Listeriosis may be diagnosed by culture of blood or cerebrospinal fluid. Special enrichment techniques with selective media may be needed to recover *L. monocytogenes* from sites with mixed flora (e.g., vagina, rectum). The treatment of choice for listeriosis remains either penicillin G or ampicillin.[237–240]

The incidence of listeriosis is higher in pregnant women than age-matched controls. Further, the mortality rate in pregnant women is high. Asymptomatic fecal and vaginal carriage in pregnant women can result in sporadic neonatal disease from transplacental or ascending routes of infection or from exposure during delivery. Transplacental infection of the fetus occurs which may lead to a congenitally infected infant. Maternal infection early in pregnancy poses the greatest risk to the fetus and newborn, and may lead to abortion, intrauterine death, stillbirth, and premature labor.

Recommendations for the prevention of listeriosis during pregnancy have been published and include the following:[239] (1) Pregnant women should not drink raw milk or eat dairy products made from raw milk. They should avoid soft cheeses (e.g., feta, brie, Mexican-style white cheeses). (2) Leftover foods or ready-to-eat foods such as hot dogs should be heated thoroughly until steaming before eating. (3) Foods from delicatessen counters should be avoided. Deli-style cold cuts should be heated thoroughly until steaming. (4) Precooked meals that have been subsequently stored at refrigerated temperatures should be thoroughly recooked until the product is steaming.

Malaria

Malaria is a major public health problem in tropical countries, causing 300 to 500 million infections worldwide that result in several million deaths annually. The risk of a traveler acquiring malaria depends on the intensity of transmission in the various locales visited and duration of stay. Human malaria is caused by four protozoan species belonging to the genus *Plasmodium: P. falciparum, P. vivax, P. ovale,* and *P. malariae*. *P. falciparum* is of special clinical significance because strains frequently exhibit resistance to antimalarial drugs and it is the most common species to cause death. Malaria is generally transmitted by the bite of an infected female *Anopheles* mosquito, although transmission via blood transfusion or congenitally from an infected mother to fetus may occur. Malaria is characterized clinically by fever and flu-like symptoms, including chills, headache, myalgias, and malaise. Often these symptoms occur at intervals. Malaria may be associated with anemia and jaundice; *P. falciparum* infection may result in kidney failure, coma, and death.

Worldwide, malaria in pregnancy is emerging as a major public health problem.[241,242] The prevalence of malaria parasitemia is approximately two-fold higher in the pregnant versus nonpregnant female.[243] Most malarial infections are asymptomatic. Anemia is the most common manifestation of asymptomatic infection, and this is most pronounced in primigravidas because they have a higher load of parasites.[244] The clinical manifestations of symptomatic malaria in pregnant women are similar to those seen in nonpregnant women. Hypoglycemia is a common complication of an acute malaria episode, occurring seven times more frequently in pregnant women compared to nonpregnant women.[245] In nonimmune persons or persons returning to a malarious area after an absence, disease can be symptomatic and severe.[246] Malaria increases the risk of adverse pregnancy outcomes including fetal loss (abortion and stillbirth), prematurity, intrauterine growth restriction, and congenital infection.[247]

There are relatively few data on the safety of most antimalarial agents used for therapy during pregnancy. Any pregnant traveler returning with malaria should be treated as a medical emergency. Women who have traveled to areas that have chloroquine-resistant strains of *P. falciparum* should be treated as if they have illness due to chloroquine-resistant organisms. Because of the serious nature of malaria, quinine or intravenous quinidine should be used and should be followed by Fansidar®, or even doxycycline, despite concerns regarding potential fetal problems. Frequent glucose levels and careful fluid monitoring often require admission to an intensive care unit.

MANAGEMENT OF INFECTIOUS DISEASE SYNDROMES

Pneumonia

Community-acquired pneumonia (CAP) remains an important source of morbidity and mortality in the United States.[248] Each year, 2 to 3 million cases of CAP result in approximately 10 million physician visits, 500,000 hospitalizations, and 45,000 deaths in the United States. The incidence of CAP requiring hospitalization is estimated to be 258 cases per 100,000 population, and 962 cases per 100,000 persons ≥65 years of age. The mortality of persons hospitalized is approximately 14 percent (range, 2 to 30 percent).

Pneumonia complicating pregnancy is a rare but important cause of maternal and fetal morbidity.[249–256] In the pregnant patient, pneumonia is the most frequent cause of fatal nonobstetric infection.[257] Concern has been raised that pneumonia occurring in a pregnant patient may be more frequent, exhibit atypical features, run a more severe course, or be more difficult to treat than in a nonpregnant patient.[256] An increased incidence of premature labor has been reported in pregnant women with pneumonia.[251,252,256]

Guidelines for the management of pneumonia in adults have recently been published by the American Thoracic Society[257] and the Infectious Disease Society of America.[258]

Pathophysiology

Community-acquired pneumonia may be defined as an acute infection of the pulmonary parenchyma that is associated with at least some symptoms of acute infection, and is accompanied by the presence of an acute infiltrate on a chest radiograph or auscultatory findings consistent with pneumonia (such as altered breath sounds and/or localized rales) that occurs in a patient who is not hospitalized or residing in an extended care facility for ≥14 days before the onset of symptoms.[258] The epidemiology, etiology, pathogenesis, and treatment of CAP differs from health care-associated pneumonia,[259] pneumonia in the immunocompromised host,[260] and pneumonia associated with travel outside the United States.

Epidemiology

The incidence of pneumonia complicating pregnancy has not been clearly defined. In recent reports, the incidence ranges from 1.5 to 2.5 per 1000 pregnancies.[261–263] Risk factors for pneumonia in pregnant women have been reported to include tobacco use, anemia, chronic cardiac or lung disease, substance abuse, and immunocompromised states.[251,252]

Microbiology and Clinical Presentation

Pneumonia should be suspected in patients with newly acquired lower respiratory symptoms such as cough, sputum production, and/or shortness of breath; these symptoms are frequently accompanied by fever and chills. Cough, the hallmark of pneumonia, may initially be nonproductive and become productive with disease progression. Purulent sputum most commonly occurs as a result of bacterial infection, but invasive viral illness may also result in green sputum. Signs of pneumonia may include elevated temperature, elevated respiratory and heart rates, use of accessory muscles of breathing, and generally ill appearance. Auscultatory signs of pneumonia result from alveolar infiltration and may include rales, decreased breath sounds, dullness to percussion, and egophony.

Pneumonia is traditionally divided into so called typical and atypical pneumonia. Typical pneumonia is due to extracellular bacterial pathogens, most commonly *Streptococcus pneumoniae,* but also including *Haemophilus influenzae, Klebsiella pneumoniae,* and *Staphylococcus aureus.* These infections are characterized by sudden onset, prominent pulmonary symptoms and signs, purulent sputum, and clinical and radiographic evidence of lobar consolidation. Atypical pathogens include viruses and intracellular bacteria such as *Legionella* spp., *Mycoplasma* spp., and *Chlamydia pneumoniae.* Pneumonia due to atypical pathogens is often characterized by a step-wise fever curve, prolonged prodrome, frequently extrapulmonary symptoms and signs, nonpurulent sputum (i.e., dry cough), and diffuse infiltrates on chest radiography. Often the differentiation of typical from atypical pneumonia is not clear, as some patients present with overlapping symptoms. Fungal pneumonia may rarely occur in the pregnant woman. The risk of dissemination with *Coccidioides immitis* may be two- to threefold higher in the pregnant woman.[264] There appears to be no association

Table 17-9. Diagnostic Studies for Evaluation of Community-Acquired Pneumonia

Baseline assessment:
- Chest radiograph to substantiate diagnosis of pneumonia, to detect associated lung diseases, to gain insight into the causative agent (in some cases), to assess severity, and as baseline to assess response

Outpatients:
- Sputum Gram stain and culture for conventional bacteria are optional

Inpatients:
- Determination of complete blood cell and differential counts
  - Serum creatinine blood urea nitrogen, glucose, electrolytes, bilirubin, and liver enzymes
  - HIV serologic status for persons aged 15–54 years
  - O_2 saturation and arterial blood gas values for selected patients
- Blood cultures (×2 before treatment)
- Gram stain and culture of sputum

Test for *Mycobacterium tuberculosis,* with acid-fast bacilli staining and culture for selected pathogens, especially for those with cough >1 month, other common symptoms, or suggestive radiographic changes

Test for *Legionella* in selected patients, including all seriously ill patients without an alternative diagnosis, especially if aged >40 years, immunocompromised, or nonresponsive to β-lactam antibiotics, if clinical features are suggestive of this diagnosis, or in outbreak settings

Thoracentesis with stain, culture, and determination of pH and leukocyte count differential (pleural fluid)

Alternative specimens to expectorated sputum:
- Aspirates of intubated patients, tracheostomy aspirates, and nasotracheal aspirates; manage as with expectorated sputum
- Induced sputum recommended for detection of *M. tuberculosis* or *Pneumocystis carinii*
- Bronchoscopy (see text)

Optional:

Additional cytologic or microbiologic tests may be required for diagnosis of unusual pathogens (e.g., *Chlamydia psittaci, Coxiella burnetii*) depending of epidemiologic clues (see Table 4), clinical features, available resources, and underlying conditions

Serum: To be frozen and saved for serologic analysis, if needed (useful for *Mycoplasma pneumoniae, Legionella* spp., *Chlamydia pneumoniae, Chlamydia psittaci, Coxiella burnetii,* viruses, and others)

Source: Adapted from Bartlett.[258]

between cryptococci[265] or blastomycosis[266,267] and pregnancy.

HIV-infected pregnant women are susceptible to a wide variety of opportunistic pathogens, including *Pneumocystis carinii,* CMV, and fungi such as *Cryptococcus neoformans, Histoplasma capsulatum,* and *Coccidioides immitis.*[268]

Diagnosis

The diagnosis of CAP requires a combination of clinical and laboratory assessments (including microbiologic data) (Table 17-9). Differentiation of CAP from upper respiratory tract infection is important because most upper respiratory tract infections and acute bronchitis are of viral origin and do not require antibiotic therapy. By contrast, antimicrobial therapy is usually indicated for pneumonia. A chest radiograph should be obtained in persons, including pregnant women, with symptoms and signs suggestive of lower respiratory tract infection in order to substantiate the diagnosis of pneumonia.[250,251,256] This is especially important because among adults with respiratory symptoms suggestive of pneumonitis, the likelihood of an abnormal chest radiograph ranges from 3 percent in a general outpatient setting to 28 percent in an emergency department. In addition to assisting in defining the presence of the pneumonia, a chest radiograph may occasionally be useful for determining the etiologic diagnosis, the prognosis, and for raising suspicion for an alternative diagnosis or associated conditions. Chest radiographs in patients with *Pneumocystis carinii* pneumonia (PCP) are normal (false-negative) in up to 30 percent of infected patients. PCP should be considered in the differential diagnosis of pneumonia in the severely immunocompromised host, especially persons with human immunodeficiency virus (HIV) infection, steroid use, or hematologic malignancies.

Management

The key decision concerning the treatment of patients with CAP is whether to treat such patients as outpatients or in the hospital. Prognostic scoring rules may be useful as adjunctive tools to aid in the decision regarding hospitalization, including those developed by the Pneumonia Patient Outcomes Research Team [PORT][269] and the American Thoracic Society (ATS). A modified version of the ATS guidelines for hospitalization has been evaluated in pregnant women.[263] The use of outpatient treatment requires that the patient be able to both comply with therapy as well as absorb oral antibiotics. Admission may be required for persons with cognitive impairment, history of substance abuse, nausea and vomiting, or underlying disorders that increase the risk of morbidity.

Every effort should be made to establish an etiologic diagnosis with sputum and blood cultures for the following reasons.[258] First, it permits optimal antibiotic selection specifically directed at the causative agent. Second, to allow for a rational basis for change from parenteral to oral therapy and for a change in therapy necessitated by an adverse drug reaction. Third, to permit antibiotic selection that limits the consequences of injudicious antibiotic use in terms of cost to the patient, inducible resistance, and adverse drug reactions. Finally, to identify pathogens of potential epidemiologic significance, such as *Legionella,* hantavirus, and penicillin-resistant *Streptococcus pneumoniae*. Sputum should be obtained for Gram stain (and culture) to aid in initial selection of antimicrobial therapy. Sputum should be obtained from a deep cough specimen before antibiotic therapy, rapidly transported, and properly processed in the laboratory. Sputum is considered acceptable for culture if under low-power microscopy there are >25 polymorphonuclear cells and <10 to 25 squamous epithelial cells. The Gram stain appearance of *S. pneumoniae* (lancet-shaped gram-positive diplococci), *H. influenzae* (small gram-negative coccobacilli), and *S. aureus* (clusters of gram-positive cocci) are sufficiently distinctive to allow a tentative diagnosis. Blood cultures are positive in approximately 10 percent of patients hospitalized with pneumonia. Additional diagnostic tests may be indicated, depending on the presence of epidemiologic clues, chest radiographic pattern, severity of illness, and host defense abnormalities. Diagnostic tests that are frequently useful include rapid tests for respiratory syncytial virus and/or influenza, special smears (acid-fast smears) and culture for *M. tuberculosis,* urine antigen for *Legionella,* and serologic tests for *Mycoplasma pneumoniae, Legionella,* or *Chlamydia.* Many additional tests are available to diagnose less common pathogens.[258]

Bronchoscopy is rarely indicated in immunocompetent patients with CAP. It should be considered in patients with a fulminant course without a clear etiology, who require admission to the intensive care unit, or who have complex pneumonia unresponsive to antimicrobial therapy. Bronchoscopy is particularly useful for the detection of selected pathogens, such as *P. carinii, Mycobacterium* spp., cytomegalovirus, and *Legionella* spp.

In order to help assess the physiologic status of hospitalized patients and need for intensive care, standard hematologic tests, chemistries, and oxygen saturation should be obtained. Maintaining oxygenation is crucial to protecting fetal health. The arterial oxygenation should be maintained at $\geq$70 mmHg.[249] Other supportive measures include chest physiotherapy, therapy for reactive airway disease (if present), and control of pyrexia.[251]

Therapy

Empiric antimicrobial therapy is guided by knowledge of likely pathogens and local resistance patterns. Therapy guidelines have undergone recent changes due to the increase in antimicrobial resistance of common pathogens (e.g., *S. pneumoniae*). Therapy may need to be altered or modified by host factors including age, liver or renal dysfunction, use of other medications that interact with planned antimicrobial therapy, and allergies. In general, patients who are allergic to either a penicillin or a cephalosporin should not receive a drug of either class. Other factors being equal, the least expensive therapy should be chosen. Additional factors that need to be considered for oral therapy include frequency of required dosing (for oral therapy, better compliance is achieved with once or twice per day administration), taste, and frequency of gastrointestinal irritation.

Antimicrobial therapy should be initiated promptly after the diagnosis of pneumonia is established with radiography and after Gram stain results are available to facilitate antimicrobial selection. For patients requiring hospitalization, therapy should be initiated within 8 hours (preferably after blood cultures have been drawn). Antibiotic therapy should not be withheld from acutely ill patients because of delays in obtaining appropriate specimens or the results of Gram stains and cultures. The preferred empiric therapy for an outpatient would be a macrolide (erythromycin, azithromycin); alternatives would include amoxicillin or a second-generation cephalosporin (e.g., cefuroxime).

Hospitalized patients should receive a macrolide plus an extended-spectrum cephalosporin (e.g., cefotaxime) or a β-lactam/β-lactamase inhibitor (e.g., piperacillin-tazobactam). If an etiologic agent is isolated, therapy should be altered based on the known susceptibilities of the pathogen or in vitro testing. Drug resistance is a growing problem with *S. pneumoniae* (especially resistance to ß-lactam antibiotics, macrolides, and tetracyclines) and *S. aureus* (especially resistance to ß-lactam antibiotics, macrolides, quinolones, and tetracyclines). In nonpregnant women, a fluoroquinolone with enhanced activity against pneumococci (e.g., levofloxacin) may be used alone for the therapy of CAP or when drug-resistant *S. pneumoniae* is suspected. In pregnant women, vancomycin would be preferred therapy for patients with pneumonia with known or suspected drug-resistant *S. pneumoniae*.

The duration of therapy is usually based on the pathogen, response to therapy, comorbid illness, and complications. In most cases, patients should receive therapy for ≥2 weeks. In general, hospitalized patients can be switched from intravenous therapy to oral therapy when they are clinically improved, have been afebrile (<38.3°C) for 24 hours, and have a stable or improved chest radiograph.

Tuberculosis

The clinical presentation and medical evaluation of tuberculosis is similar for the pregnant and nonpregnant woman.[252,254,270,271] Screening should include a careful history for symptoms suggestive of pulmonary tuberculosis and a Mantoux skin test. When indicated, a chest radiograph and induced sputum (x3) for smear and mycobacterial culture should be performed.

Urinary Tract Infections

Urinary tract infections are the most common medical complications of pregnancy.[272–276] While pregnant women are not predisposed to the acquisition of bacteria in the bladder (i.e., asymptomatic bacteriuria), they are predisposed to acute upper urinary tract infection (i.e., pyelonephritis) that is associated with morbidity for the woman and the fetus. Treatment of asymptomatic bacteriuria in pregnancy is effective in reducing the incidence of pyelonephritis and preterm delivery.[277]

Pathophysiology

Pregnant women are at increased risk for bacteriuria because of increased bladder volume and decreased bladder and ureteral tone that contribute to increased urinary stasis and ureterovesical reflux.[275] Asymptomatic bacteriuria (>10^5 bacteria/mL in a patient without symptoms) occurs in 5 to 10 percent of all pregnant women. Untreated asymptomatic bacteriuria leads to the development of symptomatic cystitis in ~30 percent of patients and pyelonephritis in ~25 percent. This progression from asymptomatic to symptomatic infection with pregnancy is three- to fourfold higher than the rate seen in nonpregnant women. Other adverse events reported to be associated with asymptomatic bacteriuria include prematurity or low birth weight, maternal anemia, and maternal hypertension.

Epidemiology

Risk factors for infection include low socioeconomic status,[278] sickle cell anemia, diabetes,[279] history of urinary tract infections,[288] and a neurogenic bladder.[276]

Microbiology and Clinical Manifestations

The most common pathogens involved in urinary tract infections are Enterobacteriaceae, especially *Escherichia coli* (accounts for 65 to 80 percent of cases). These enteric organisms account for ~90 percent of all urinary tract infections in pregnant women. Other pathogens include *Staphylococcus,* group B streptococci, and *Pseudomonas*.

Diagnosis

Asymptomatic bacteriuria is diagnosed by means of clean-catch urinary culture. Patients with potential pyelonephritis should have a catheterized specimen obtained for culture. Cystitis and pyelonephritis are suggested by a urinalysis that reveals hemoglobin, leukocyte esterase, or nitrate.[281] Acute pyelonephritis is suggested by bacteriuria accompanied by systemic symptoms or signs such as fever, chills, nausea, vomiting, and flank pain. Definitive therapy should be based on the results of the culture. Women with presumed pyelonephritis not responding to therapy within 48 to 72 hours should be evaluated by a noninvasive study such as renal ultrasound.

Management

Therapy should be provided to women with bacteriuria. Commonly used medications include nitrofurantoin, amoxicillin, and cephalosporins.[282] Therapy should generally be administered for 7 to 14 days.[276] All patients with asymptomatic bacteriuria should receive careful follow-up since approximately one-third will experience a recurrence. For women with frequent recurrences, continuous antibiotic suppression should be considered. Asymptomatic bacteriuria or cystitis may progress to pyelonephritis. Most patients with pyelonephritis should be hospitalized and initially receive intravenous antibiotics. Initial empiric therapy could include amoxicillin plus gentamicin, a third-generation cephalosporin (e.g., cefotaxime), or a β-lactam/β-lactamase combination (e.g., amoxicillin-clavulanate). Definitive therapy should be based on the results of the urinary culture. Most women with pyelonephritis are afebrile and asymptomatic within 48 to 72 hours. In women who do not respond to therapy within this time frame, one should consider the possibility of resistant pathogens, nephrolithiasis, perinephric abscess, obstruction, and other potential fever sources.[276]

Screening

The American College of Obstetricians and Gynecologists recommends a urine culture be obtained at the first prenatal visit.[283] A repeat culture should be obtained during the third trimester. The U.S. Preventive Services Task Force recommends a urine culture be obtained between weeks 12 and 16 of gestation.[284]

REFERENCES

1. Centers for Disease Control and Prevention: Ten great public health achievements-United States, 1900–1999. *MMWR Morb Mortal Wkly Rep* 48:241–243, 1999.
2. Centers for Disease Control and Prevention: Impact of vaccines universally recommended for children-United States, 1900–1998. *MMWR Morb Mortal Wkly Rep* 48:243–248, 1999.
3. Centers for Disease Control and Prevention: General recommendations on immunization. Recommendations of the Advisory Committee on Immunization Practices (ACIP) and the American Academy of Family Practice. *MMWR Morb Mortal Wkly Rep* 51(RR-2):1–33, 2002.
4. American College of Physicians: *Guide for Adult Immunization*. Philadelphia: American College of Physicians, 1994.
5. American Academy of Pediatrics: Pickering LK (ed): *2000 Red Book: Report of the Committee on Infectious Diseases,* 25th ed. Elk Grove Village, IL: American Academy of Pediatrics, 2000, pp 55–56.
6. Centers for Disease Control and Prevention: Diphtheria, tetanus, and pertussis: Recommendations for vaccine use and other preventive measures. Recommendations of the Immunization Practices and Advisory Committee (ACIP). *MMWR Morb Mortal Wkly Rep* 40(RR-10):1–28, 1991.
7. Centers for Disease Control and Prevention: Hepatitis B virus: A comprehensive strategy for eliminating transmission in the United States through universal childhood vaccination; recommendations of the Immunization Practices and Advisory Committee (ACIP). *MMWR Morb Mortal Wkly Rep* 40(RR-13):1–25, 1991.
8. Centers for Disease Control and Prevention: Typhoid immunization. Recommendations of the Advisory Committee on Immunization Practices (ACIP). *MMWR Morb Mortal Wkly Rep* 43l(RR-14):1–7, 1994.
9. Centers for Disease Control and Prevention: The role of BCG vaccine in the prevention and control of tuberculosis in the United States. A joint statement by the Advisory Committee for the Elimination of Tuberculosis and the Advisory Committee on Immunization Practices. *MMWR Morb Mortal Wkly Rep* 45(1–27), 1996.
10. Centers for Disease Control and Prevention: Prevention of varicella. Recommendations of the Advisory Committee on Immunization Practices (ACIP). *MMWR Morb Mortal Wkly Rep* 45(RR-11):1–27, 1996.
11. Centers for Disease Control and Prevention: Prevention of varicella. Update recommendations of the Advisory Committee on Immunization Practices (ACIP). *MMWR Morb Mortal Wkly Rep* 48(RR-6):1–5, 1999.
12. Centers for Disease Control and Prevention: Recommendations for the use of Lyme disease vaccine. Recommendations of the Advisory Committee on Immunization Practices (ACIP). *MMWR Morb Mortal Wkly Rep* 48(RR-7): 1–17, 1999.
13. Centers for Disease Control and Prevention: Human rabies prevention—United States, 1999. Recommendations of the Advisory Committee on Immunization Practices (ACIP). *MMWR Morb Mortal Wkly Rep* 48(RR-1):1–21, 1999.
14. Centers for Disease Control and Prevention: Prevention of hepatitis A through active and passive immunization: Recommendations of the Advisory Committee on Immunization Practices (ACIP). *MMWR Morb Mortal Wkly Rep* 48(RR-12):1–37, 1999.
15. Centers for Disease Control and Prevention: Poliomyelitis prevention in the United States. Updated recommendations of the Advisory Committee on Immunization Practices (ACIP). *MMWR Morb Mortal Wkly Rep* 49(RR-5): 1–22, 2000.
16. Centers for Disease Control and Prevention: Prevention and control of meningococcal disease. Recommendations of the Advisory Committee on Immunization Practices (ACIP). *MMWR Morb Mortal Wkly Rep* 49(RR-7):1–10, 2000.
17. Centers for Disease Control and Prevention: Prevention and control of influenza. Recommendations of the Advisory Committee on Immunization Practices (ACIP). *MMWR Morb Mortal Wkly Rep* 50(RR-4):1–44, 2001.
18. Centers for Disease Control and Prevention: Vaccine-preventable diseases: Improving vaccination coverage in

children, adolescents, and adults. *MMWR Morb Mortal Wkly Rep* 48(RR-8):1–15, 1999.

19. Munoz FM, Englund JA: Vaccines in pregnancy. *Infect Dis Clin North Am* 15:253–271, 2001.
20. Centers for Disease Control and Prevention: Mumps, measles, and rubella-vaccine use and strategies for elimination of measles, rubella, and congenital rubella syndrome and control of mumps: Recommendations of the Advisory Committee on Immunization Practices (ACIP). *MMWR Morb Mortal Wkly Rep* 47(RR-8):1–57, 1998.
21. Faix RG: Immunization during pregnancy. *Clin Obstet Gynecol* 45:42–58, 2002.
22. Keler M, Stiehm ER: Passive immunity in prevention and treatment of infectious diseases. *Clin Microbiol Rev* 13:602–614, 2000.
23. Shields KE, Galil K, Seward J, et al: Varicella vaccine exposure during pregnancy: data from the first 5 years of the pregnancy registry. *Obstet Gynecol* 98:14–19, 2001.
24. Centers for Disease Control and Prevention: Recommended childhood immunization schedule—United States, 2002. *MMWR Morb Mortal Wkly Rep* 51:31–33, 2002.
25. Dietz V, Galazka A, van Loon F, Cochi S: Factors affecting the immunogenicity and potency of tetanus toxoid: Implications for the elimination of neonatal and non-neonatal tetanus as public health concerns. *Bull WHO* 75:81–93, 1997.
26. Thayaparan B, Nicoll A: Prevention and control of tetanus in childhood. *Curr Opin Pediatr* 10:4–8, 1998.
27. Glezen WP, Alpers M: Maternal immunization. *Clin Infect Dis* 28:219–224, 1999.
28. Centers for Disease Control and Prevention: Health information for international travel, 2001–2002. Atlanta, GA: U.S. Department of Health and Human Services, PHS, 2001.
29. Kaplan NM, Palmer BF, Nassar NN, Keiser P, Gregg CR: Keeping travelers healthy. *Am J Med Sci* 315:327–336, 1998.
30. Ryan ET, Kain KC: Health advice and immunizations for travelers. *N Engl J Med* 342:1716–1725, 2000.
31. Virk A: Medical advice for international travelers. *Mayo Clin Proc* 76:831–840, 2001.
32. Samuel BU, Barry M: The pregnant traveler. *Infect Dis Clin North Am* 12:325–354, 1998.
33. Kozarsky PE, van Gompel A: Pregnancy, nursing, contraception, and travel, in Dupont HL, Steffen R (eds): *Textbook of Travel Medicine and Health,* 2d ed. London: BC Decker Inc, 2001, pp 444–454.
34. Jong EC: Immunizations for international travel. *Infect Dis Clin North Am* 12:249–266, 1998.
35. Wilson ME: Travel-related vaccines. *Infect Dis Clin North Am* 15:231–251, 2001.
36. Weber DJ, Walker DH: Rocky Mountain spotted fever. *Infect Dis Clin North Am* 5:19–35, 1991.
37. Lynch CM, Sinnott JT, Holt DA, Herold AH: Use of antibiotics during pregnancy. *Am Fam Pract* 43:1365–1368, 1991.
38. Korzeniowski OM: Antibacterial agents in pregnancy. *Infect Dis Clin North Am* 3:639–651, 1995.
39. Dashe JS, Gilstrap LC: Antibiotic use in pregnancy. *Obstet Gynecol Clin North Am* 24:617–629, 1997.
40. Briggs GG: Medication use during the perinatal period. *J Am Pharm Assoc* 38:717–727, 1998.
41. Roe VA: Antimicrobial agents: Pharmacology and clinical application in obstetric, gynecologic, and perinatal infections. *J Obstet Gynecol Neonatal Nurs* 28:639–648, 1999.
42. Hass DA, Pynn BR, Sands TD: Drug use for the pregnant or lactating patient. *Gen Denistry* 48:54–60, 2000.
43. Brost BC, Newman RB. The maternal and fetal effects of tuberculosis therapy. *Obstet Gynecol Clin North Am* 24:659–673, 1997.
44. Bothamley G: Drug treatment for tuberculosis during pregnancy. *Drug Safety* 24:553–565, 2001.
45. Lary JM, Daniel KL, Erickson JD, Roberts HE, Moore CA: The return of thalidomide. Can birth defects be prevented? *Drug Safety* 21:161–169, 1999.
46. Koren G, Pastuszak A, Ito A: Drugs in pregnancy. *N Engl J Med* 338:1128–1137, 1998.
47. Diggle GE: Thalidomide: 40 years on. Australasian Journal of Dermatology 55:627–631, 2001.
48. Czeizel AE, Rockenbauer M: A population-based case-control teratologic study of oxytetracycline treatment during pregnancy. *Eur J Obstet Gynecol* 88:27–33, 2000.
49. Czeizel AE, Rockenbauer M: Teratogenic study of doxycycline. *Obstet Gynecol* 89:524–528, 1997.
50. Czeizel AE, Rockenbauer M, Olsen J, Sorensen HT: A teratologic study of aminoglycoside antibiotic during pregnancy. *Scand J Infect Dis* 32:309–313, 2000.
51. Smilack JD: Trimethoprim-sulfamethoxazole. *Mayo Clin Proc* 74:730–734, 1999.
52. Sobel JD: Use of antifungal drugs in pregnancy. *Drug Safety* 23:77–85, 2000.
53. King CT, Rogers PD, Cleary JD, Chapman SW: Antifungal therapy during pregnancy. *Clin Infect Dis* 27:1151–1160, 1998.
54. Pursley TJ, Blomquist IK, Abraham J, Andersen HF, Bartley JA: Fluconazole-induced congenital anomalies in three infants. *Clin Infect Dis* 22:336–340, 1996.
55. Andrews EB, Yankaskas BC, Cordero JF, Schoeffler K, Hampp S: Acyclovir in pregnancy registry: Six years' experience. *Obstet Gynecol* 79:7–13, 1992.
56. Dattel BJ: Antiretoviral therapy during pregnancy. *Obstet Gynecol Clin North Am* 24:645–657, 1997.
57. Taylor GP, Low-Beer N: Antiretroviral therapy in pregnancy. *Drug Safety* 24:683–702, 2001.
58. Riely CA: Acute fatty liver of pregnancy. *Semin Liver Dis* 7:47–54, 1987.
59. McCormack WM, George H, Donner A, et al: Hepatotoxicity of erythromycin estolate during pregnancy. *Antimicrob Agents Chemother* 12:630–635, 1977.
60. Dillon AE, Wagner CL, Wiest D, Newman RB: Drug therapy in the nursing mother. *Obstet Gynecol Clin North Am* 24:675–696, 1997.

61. Spencer JP, Gonzalez LS, Barnhart DJ: Medications in the breast-feeding mother. *Am Fam Physician* 64:119–126, 2001.
62. Kemmer NM, Miskovisky EP: Hepatitis A. *Infect Dis Clin North Am* 14:605–615, 2000.
63. Cuthbert JA: Hepatitis A: old and new. *Clin Rev Microbiol* 14:38–58, 2001.
64. Centers for Disease Control and Prevention: Summary of notifiable diseases, United States, 1999. *MMWR Morb Mortal Wkly Rep* 48:1–101, 1999.
65. Tanaka I, Shima M, Kubota Y, et al: Vertical transmission of hepatitis A. *Lancet* 345:397, 1995.
66. Leikin E, Lysikiewicz A, Garry D, Tejani N: Intrauterine transmission of hepatitis A virus. *Obstet Gynecol* 88:690–691, 1996.
67. Erkan T, Kutlu T, Cullu F, Tumay GT: A case of vertical transmission of hepatitis A virus. *Acta Paediatrica* 87:1008–1009, 1998.
68. McDuffie RS Jr., Bader T: Fetal meconium peritonitis after maternal hepatitis A. *Am J Obstet Gynecol* 180:1031–1032, 1999.
69. Routenberg JA, Deinstag JL, Harrison WO, et al: Foodborne outbreak of hepatitis A: clinical and laboratory features of acute and protracted illness. *Am J Med Sci* 278:123–137, 1979.
70. Bower WA, Nainan OV, Han X, Margolis HS: Duration of viremia in hepatitis A virus infection. *J Infect Dis* 182:12–17, 2000.
71. Liaw YF, Yang CY, Chu CM, Huang MJ: Appearance and persistence of hepatitis A IgM antibody in acute clinical hepatitis A observed in an outbreak. *Infection* 14:156–158, 1986.
72. Stapleton JT: Host immune response to hepatitis A virus. *J Infect Dis* 171(Suppl 1):S9–S14, 1995.
73. American College of Obstetricians and Gynecologists: Viral hepatitis in pregnancy. *Int J Gynecol Obstet* 63:195–202, 1998.
74. Hunt CM, Sharara AI: Liver disease in pregnancy. *Am Fam Phys* 59:829–836, 1999.
75. Levy MJ, Herrera JL, DiPalma JA: Immune globulin and vaccine therapy to prevent hepatitis A infection. *Am J Med* 105:416–423, 1998.
76. Lee WM: Hepatitis B virus infection. *N Engl J Med* 337:1733–1745, 1997.
77. Mahoney FJ: Update on diagnosis, management, and prevention of hepatitis B virus infection. *Clin Rev Microbiol* 12:351–366, 1999.
78. Befeler AS, Bisceglie AMD: Hepatitis B. *Infect Dis Clin North Am* 14:617–632, 2000.
79. Centers for Disease Control and Prevention: Update: recommendations to prevent hepatitis B transmission—United States. *MMWR Morb Mortal Wkly Rep* 44:574–75, 1995.
80. Centers for Disease Control and Prevention: Maternal hepatitis B screening practices—California, Connecticut, Kansas, and United States, 1992–1993. *MMWR Morb Mortal Wkly Rep* 43:311, 317–20, 1994.
81. Wood RC, MacDonald KL, White KE, et al: Risk factors for lack of detectable antibody following hepatitis B vaccination of Minnesota health care workers. *JAMA* 1993;27:2935–2939.
82. Dennehy PH: Active immunization in the United States; developments over the past decade. *Clin Microbiol Rev* 14:872–908, 2001.
83. Hoofnagle JH, Bisceglie AMD: The treatment of chronic viral hepatitis. *N Engl J Med* 336:347–356, 1997.
84. Koff RS: Hepatitis vaccines. *Infect Dis Clin North Am* 15:83–95, 2001.
85. Confavreux C, Suissa S, Saddier P, Bourdes V, Vukusic S: Vaccinations and the risk of relapse in multiple sclerosis. *N Engl J Med* 344:319–326, 2001.
86. Ascherio A, Zhang SM, Hernan MA, et al. Hepatitis B vaccination and the risk of multiple sclerosis. *N Engl J Med* 344:327–332, 2001.
87. Minkoff HL: Human immunodeficiency virus infection in pregnancy. *Semin Perinatol* 22:293–308, 1998.
88. Andiman WA: Medical management of the pregnant woman infected with human immunodeficiency virus type 1 and her child. *Semin Perinatol* 22:72–86, 1998.
89. Ahdieh L: Pregnancy and infection with human immunodeficiency virus. *Clin Obstet Gynecol* 44:154–166, 2001.
90. Watts DH: Maternal therapy for HIV in pregnancy. *Clin Obstet Gynecol* 44:182–197, 2001.
91. Minkoff H: Prevention of mother-to-child transmission of HIV. *Clin Obstet Gynecol* 44:210–225, 2001.
92. Brocklehurst P: Interventions for reducing the risk of mother-to-child transmission of HIV infection, in The Cochrane Library (Cochrane Review), Issue 1. Oxford: Update Software, 2002.
93. Centers for Disease Control and Prevention: Revised guidelines for HIV counseling, testing, and referral and revised recommendations for HIV screening of pregnant women. *MMWR Morb Mortal Wkly Rep* 50(RR-19): 1–119, 2001.
94. Centers for Disease Control and Prevention: Management of possible sexual, injecting drug-use, or other nonoccupational exposure to HIV, including considerations related to antiretroviral therapy. Public Health Service Statement. *MMWR Morb Mortal Wkly Rep* 47(RR-17): 1–19, 1998.
95. Centers for Disease Control and Prevention: Updated U.S. Public Health Service guidelines for the management of occupational exposures to HBV, HCV, and HIV and recommendations for postexposure prophylaxis. *MMWR Morb Mortal Wkly Rep* 50(RR-11): 1–67, 2001.
96. Ferreiro RB, Sepkowitz KA: Management of needlestick injuries. *Clin Obstet Gynecol* 44:276–288, 2001.
97. Gerberding JL: Management of occupational exposures to blood-borne viruses. *N Engl J Med* 332:444–451, 1996.
98. Beltrami EM, Williams IT, Shapiro CN, Chamberland ME: Risk and management of blood-borne infections in health care workers. *Clin Microbiol Rev* 13:385–407, 2000.
99. Rosenstein NE, Perkins BA, Stephens DS, Popovic T, Hughes JM: Meningococcal disease. *N Engl J Med* 344:1378–1388, 2001.

100. van Deuren M, Brandtzaeg P, van der Meer JWM: Update on meningococcal disease with emphasis on pathogenesis and clinical management. *Clin Microbiol Rev* 13:144–166, 2000.
101. Hart CA: Infectious diseases: meningooccal disease. *Clin Evidence* 3:350–357, 2000.
102. Tzeng Y-L, Stephens DS: Epidemiology and pathogenesis of *Neisseria meningitidis*. *Microbes Infect* 2:687–700, 2000.
103. Schuchat A, Robinson K, Wenger JD, et al: Bacterial meningitis in the United States in 1995. *N Engl J Med* 337:970–976, 1997.
104. Ahlawat S, Kumar R, Roy P, Varma S, Sharma BK: Meningococcal meningitis outbreak control strategies. *J Commun Dis* 32:264–274, 2000.
105. Durand ML, Calderwood SB, Weber DJ, et al: Acute bacterial meningitis in adults: a review of 493 episodes. *N Engl J Med* 328:21–28, 1993.
106. Winstead JM, McKinsey DS, Tasker S, De Groote MA, Baddour LM: Meningococcal pneumonia: characterization and review of cases seen over the past 25 years. *Clin Infect Dis* 30:87–94, 2000.
107. Quaguarello VJ, Scheld WM: Treatment of bacterial meningitis. *N Engl J Med* 336:708–716, 1997.
108. Rosensetin NE, Fischer M, Tappero JW: Meningococcal vaccines. *Infect Dis Clin North Am* 15:155–69, 2001.
109. Peltola H: Prophylaxis of bacterial meningitis. *Infect Dis Clin North Am* 13:685–710, 1999.
110. Osmon DR: Antimicrobial prophylaxis in adults. *Mayo Clinic Proceedings* 75:98–109, 2000.
111. Centers for Disease Control and Prevention: Pertussis—United States, 1997–2000. *MMWR Morb Mortal Wkly Rep* 51:73–76, 2002.
112. Herrera GA, Smith P, Daniels D, et al: National, state, and urban area vaccination coverage levels among children aged 19–35 months—United States, 1998. *MMWR Morb Mortal Wkly Rep* 49(SS-9):1–23, 2000.
113. Hoppe JE, Bryskier A: In vitro susceptibilities of *Bordetella pertussis* and *Bordetella parapertussis* to two ketolides (HMR 3004 and HMR 3647), four macrolides (azithromycin, clarithromycin, erythromycin A, and roxithromycin) and two ansamycins (rifampin and rifapentine). *Antimicrob Agents Chemother* 42:965–966, 1998.
114. Brett M, Short P, Beatson S: The comparative in-vitro activity of roxithromycin and other antibiotics against *Bordetella pertussis*. *J Antimicrob Chemother* 41(suppl B):23–27, 1998.
115. Gordon KA, Fusco J, Biedenbach DJ, Pfaller MA, Jones RN: Antimicrobial susceptibility testing of clinical isolates of *Bordetella pertussis* from Northern California: Report from the SENTRY antimicrobial surveillance program. *Antimicrob Agents Chemother* 45:3599–3600, 2001.
116. Anonymous: The choice of antibacterial drugs. *Med Lett* 43:69–78, 2001.
117. Kerr JR, Preston NW: Current pharmacology of pertussis. *Exp Opin Pharmacother* 2:1275–1282, 2001.
118. Irwin RS, Madison JM: Primary care: the diagnosis and treatment of cough. *N Engl J Med* 343:1715–1721, 2000.
119. von Konig W, Postels Multani S, Bock IIL, Schmitt HJ: Pertussis in adults: frequency of transmission after household exposure. *Lancet* 346:1326–1329, 1995.
120. von Konig CHW, Postels-Multani S, Bogaerts H, et al: Factors influencing the spread of pertussis in households. *Eur J Pediatr* 157:391–394, 1998.
121. Halperin SA, Bortolussi R, Langley JM, Eastwood BJ, de Serres G: A randomized, placebo-controlled trial of erythromycin estolate chemoprophylaxis for household contacts of children with culture-positive *Bordetella pertussis* infection. *Pediatrics* 104:e42 (7 pages), 1999.
122. Linneman CC, Ramundo N, Perlstein PH, Minton SD, Englender GS: Use of pertussis vaccine in an epidemic involving hospital staff. *Lancet* 2:540–543, 1975.
123. Steketee RW, Wassilak SGF, Adkins WN, et al: Evidence for a high attack rate and efficacy of erythromycin prophylaxis in a pertussis outbreak in a facility for the developmentally disabled. *J Infect Dis* 157:434–440, 1988.
124. Dodhia H, Miller E: Review of the evidence for the use of erythromycin in the management of persons exposed to pertussis. *Epidemiol Infect* 120:143–149, 1998.
125. Lewis K, Saubolle MA, Tenover FC, et al: Pertussis caused by an erythromycin-resistant strain of *Bordetella pertussis*. *Pediatr Infect Dis J* 14:388–391, 1995.
126. Korgenski EK, Daly JA: Surveillance and detection of erythromycin resistance in *Bordetella pertussis* isolates recovered from a pediatric population in the intermountain west region of the United States. *J Clin Microbiol* 35:2989–2991, 1997.
127. Hoppe JE, Halm U, Hagedorn H-J, Kraminer-Hagedorm A: Comparison of erythromycin ethylsuccinate and co-trimoxazole for treatment of pertussis. *Infection* 7:227–231, 1989.
128. Aoyama T, Sunakawa K, Iwata S, Takeuchi Y, Fujii P: Efficacy of short-term treatment of pertussis with clarithromycin and azithromycin. *J Pediatr* 129:761–764, 1996.
129. Halperin SA, Bortolussi R, Langley JM, Miller B, Eastwood B: Seven days of erythromycin estolate is as effective as fourteen days for the treatment of *Bordetella pertussis* infections. Pediatrics 100:65–71, 1997.
130. Haupt W: Rabies—risk of exposure and current trends in prevention of human cases. *Vaccine* 17:1742–1949, 1999.
131. Fishbein DB, Robinson LE: Rabies. *N Engl J Med* 329:1632–1638, 1993.
132. Smith JS: New aspects of rabies with emphasis on epidemiology, diagnosis, and prevention of the disease in the United States. *Clin Microbiol Rev* 9:166–176, 1996.
133. Krebs JW, Rupprecht CE, Childs JE: Rabies surveillance in the United States during 1999. *J Am Vet Med Assoc* 217:1799–1811, 2000.
134. Krebs JW, Smith JS, Rupprecht CE, Childs JE: Mammalian reservoirs and epidemiology of rabies diagnosed in human

beings in the United States, 1981–1998. *Ann NY Acad Sci* 916:345–353, 2000.

135. Noah DL, Drenzek CL, Smith JS, et al: Epidemiology of human rabies in the United States, 1980 to 1996. *Ann Intern Med* 128:922–930, 1998.
136. Weber DJ, Hansen AR: Infections resulting from animal bites. *Infect Dis Clin North Am* 5:663–680, 1991.
137. Chabala S, Williams M, Amenta R, Ognjan AF: Confirmed rabies exposure during pregnancy: treatment with human rabies immune globulin and human diploid cell vaccine. *Am J Med* 91:423–424, 1991.
138. Sudarshan MK, Madhusudana SN, Mahendra BJ, Ashwathnarayana DH, Jayakumary M: Post exposure rabies prophylaxis with purified verocell rabies vaccine: a study of immunoresponse in pregnant women and their matched controls. *Ind J Public Health* 43:76–78, 1999.
139. Chutivongse S, Wilde H, Benjavongkulchai M, Chomchey P, Punthawong S: Postexposure rabies vaccination during pregnancy: effect on 202 women and their infants. *Clin Infect Dis* 20:818–820, 1995.
140. Sudarshan MK, Madhusudana SN, Mahendra BJ. Post-exposure prophylaxis with purified vero cell rabies vaccine during pregnancy-safety and immunogenicity. *J Commun Dis* 31:229–236, 1999.
141. Seward JF, Watson BM, Peterson CL, et al: Varicella disease after introduction of varicella vaccine in the United States, 1995–2000. *JAMA* 287:606–611, 2002.
142. Choo PW, Donahue JG, Manson JE, Platt R: The epidemiology of varicella and its complications. *J Infect Dis* 172:706–712, 1995
143. Wharton M: The epidemiology of varicella-zoster virus infections. *Infect Dis Clinics North Am* 10:571–581, 1996.
144. Miller E, Vardien J, Farrington P: Shift in age in chickenpox. *Lancet* 341:308–309, 1993.
145. Feldman S, Hughes WT, Daniel SB: Varicella in children with cancer: seventy-seven cases. *Pediatrics* 56:388–397, 1975.
146. Meyers JD, MacQuarrie MB, Merrigan TC, Jennison MH: Nosocomial varicella. Part I: outbreak in oncology patients at a children's hospital. *West J Med* 130:196–199, 1979.
147. Feldhoff CM, Balfour HH Jr., Simmons RL, Najarian JS, Mauer SM: Varicella in children with renal transplant. *J Pediatr* 98:25–31, 1981.
148. Whitley R, Hilty M, Haynes R, et al. Vidarabine therapy of varicella in immunosuppressed patients. *J Pediatr* 101:125–131, 1982.
149. Morgan ER, Smalley LA: Varicella in immunocompromised children: incidence of abdominal pain and organ involvement. *Am J Dis Child* 137:883–885, 1983.
150. Locksley RM, Flournoy N, Sullivan KM, Meyers JD: Infection with varicella-zoster virus after marrow transplant. *J Infect Dis* 152:1172–1181, 1985.
151. Feldman S, Lott L: Varicella in children with cancer: impact of antiviral therapy and prophylaxis. Pediatrics 80:465–472, 1987.
152. Nathwani D, Maclean A, Conway S, Carrington D: Varicella infections in pregnancy and the newborn. *J Infect* 36(Suppl 1):59–71, 1998.
153. Enders G, Miller E: Varicella and herpes zoster in pregnancy and the newborn, in Arvin AM, Gerson AA (eds): *Varicella-Zoster Virus: Virology and Clinical Management*. Cambridge: Cambridge University Press, 2000, pp 317–347.
154. Haake DA, Zakowski PC, Haake DL, Bryson YJ: Early treatment with acyclovir for varicella pneumonia in otherwise healthy adults: Retrospective controlled study and review. *Rev Infect Dis* 12:788–798, 1990.
155. Rogerson SJ, Nye FJ: Chickenpox pneumonia: An association with pregnancy. *Thorax* 45:239, 1990.
156. Haake DA, Zakowski P, Haake DL, Bryson YJ: Early treatment with acyclovir for varicella pneumonia in otherwise healthy adults: retrospective controlled study and review. *Rev Infect Dis* 12:788–798, 1990.
157. Rogerson SJ, Nye FJ, Beeching NJ: Chickenpox pneumonia: an association with pregnancy. *Thorax* 45:239, 1990.
158. Katz VL, Kuller JA, McMahon MJ, Warren MA, Wells SR: Varicella during pregnancy—maternal and fetal effects. *West J Med* 163:446–450, 1995.
159. Smego RA, Asperilla MO: Use of acyclovir for varicella pneumonia during pregnancy. *Obstet Gynecol* 78:1112–1116, 1991.
160. Esmonde TF, Herdman G, Anderson G: Chickenpox pneumonia: an association with pregnancy. *Thorax* 44:812–815, 1989.
161. Paryani SG, Arvin AM: Intrauterine infection with varicella-zoster virus after maternal varicella. *N Engl J Med* 314:1542–1546, 1986.
162. Balducci J, Rodis JF, Rosengren S, et al: Pregnancy outcome following first trimester infection. *Obstet Gynecol* 79:5–6, 1992.
163. Pastuszak AL, Levy M, Schick B, et al: Outcome of maternal varicella infection in the first 20 weeks of pregnancy. *N Engl J Med* 330:901–905, 1994.
164. Enders G, Miller E, Cradock-Watson J, Bolley I, Ridehalgh M: Consequences of varicella and herpes zoster in pregnancy: prospective study of 1739 cases. *Lancet* 343:1548–1551, 1994.
165. Sauerbrei A, Wutzler P: The congenital varicella syndrome. *J Perinatol* 20:548–554, 2000.
166. McCarter-Spaulding DE: Varicella infection in pregnancy. *J Obstet Gynecol Neonatal Nurs* 30:667–673, 2001.
167. Birthistle K, Carrington D: Fetal varicella syndrome—a reappraisal of the literature. *J Infect* 36:(Suppl 1):25–29, 1998.
168. Mustonen K, Mustakangaws P, Valanne L, Haltia M, Koskiniemi M: Congenital varicella-zoster virus infection after maternal subclinical infection: clinical and neuropathologic findings. *J Perinatol* 21:141–146, 2001.
169. Meyers JD: Congenital varicella in term infants: risk reconsidered. *J Infect Dis* 129:215–217, 1974.
170. Gershon AA: Varicella in mother and infant: problems old and new, in Krugman S, Gershon AA (eds): *Infec-*

tions of the Fetus and Newborn Infant: Progress in Clinical and Biological Research. New York: Alan R. Liss, 1975, pp 79–95.

171. Sauerbrei A, Wutzler P: Neonatal varicella. *J Perinatol* 21:545–549, 2001.
172. Ogilive MM: Antiviral prophylaxis and treatment in chickenpox. *J Infect* 36(Suppl 1):31–38, 1998.
173. American Academy of Pediatrics: Varicella vaccine update. *Pediatrics* 105:136–141, 2000.
174. Huang Y-C, Lin T-Y, Lin Y-J, Lien R-I, Chou Y-H: Prophylaxis of intravenous immunoglobulin and acyclovir in perinatal varicella. *Eur J Pediatr* 160:91–94, 2001.
175. Atlax RM: The medical threat of biological weapons. *Crit Rev Microbiol* 24:157–168, 1998.
176. Henderson DA: The looming threat of bioterrorism. *Science* 283:1279–1782, 1999.
177. Leggiadro RJ: The threat of biological terrorism: a public health and infection control reality. *Infect Control Hosp Epidemiol* 21:53–56, 2000.
178. Weber DJ, Rutala WA: Risks and prevention of nosocomial transmission of rare zoonotic diseases. *Clin Infect Dis* 32:446–456, 2001.
179. Centers for Disease Control and Prevention: Ongoing investigation of anthrax—Florida, October 2001. *MMWR Morb Mortal Wkly Rep* 50:877, 2001.
180. Centers for Disease Control and Prevention: Update: investigation of anthrax associated with intentional exposure and interim public health guidelines, October 2001. *MMWR Morb Mortal Wkly Rep* 50:889–893, 2001.
181. Centers for Disease Control and Prevention: Update: investigation of bioterrorism-related anthrax—Connecticut, 2001. *MMWR Morb Mortal Wkly Rep* 50:1077–79, 2001.
182. Centers for Disease Control and Prevention: Recognition of illness associated with the intentional release of a biologic agent. *MMWR Morb Mortal Wkly Rep* 50:893–897, 2001.
183. Centers for Disease Control and Prevention: Update: investigation of bioterrorism-related anthrax and interim guidelines for clinical evaluation of persons with possible anthrax. *MMWR Morb Mortal Wkly Rep* 50:941–948, 2001.
184. Centers for Disease Control and Prevention: Updated recommendations for antimicrobial prophylaxis among asymptomatic pregnant women and exposure to *Bacillus anthracis*. *MMWR Morb Mortal Wkly Rep* 50:960, 2001.
185. Centers for Disease Control and Prevention: Update: interim recommendations for antimicrobial prophylaxis for children and breastfeeding mothers and treatment of children with anthrax. *MMWR Morb Mortal Wkly Rep* 50:1014–1016, 2001.
186. Centers for Disease Control and Prevention: Biological and chemical terrorism: strategic plan for preparedness and response. *MMWR Morb Mortal Wkly Rep* 49(RR-4):1–26, 2000.
187. Dixon TC, Meselson M, Guilliemin J, Hanna PC: Anthrax. *N Engl J Med* 341:815–826, 1999.
188. Friedlander AM: Anthrax: clinical features, pathogenesis, and potential warfare threat. *Curr Clin Topics Infect Dis* 20:335–349, 2000.
189. Swartz MN: Recognition and management of anthrax—an update. *N Engl J Med* 345:1621–1626, 2001.
190. Franz DR, Jahrling PB, Friedlander AM, et al: Clinical recognition and management of patients exposed to biological warfare agents. *JAMA* 278:399–411, 1997.
191. Inglesby TV, Henderson DA, Bartlett JG, et al: Anthrax as a biological weapon: medical and public health consequences. *JAMA* 281:1735–1745, 1999.
192. Arnon SS, Schechter R, Inglesby TV, et al: Botulinum toxin as a biological weapon: medical and public health consequences. *JAMA* 285:1059–1070, 2001.
193. Inglesby TV, Dennis DT, Henderson DA, et al: Plague as a biological weapon: medical and public health consequences. *JAMA* 283:2281–2290, 2000.
194. Dennis DT, Inglesby TV, Henderson DA, et al: Plague as a biological weapon: medical and public health consequences. *JAMA* 285:2763–2773, 2001.
195. Henderson DA, Inglesby TV, Bartlett JG, et al: Smallpox as a biological weapon: medical and public health consequences. *JAMA* 281:2127–2137, 1999.
196. Maurin M, Raoult D: Q fever. *Clin Microbiol Rev* 12:518–553, 1999.
197. Raoult D, Tissot-Dupont H, Foucault C, et al: Q fever 1985–1998. Clinical and epidemiologic features of 1383 infections. *Medicine* 79:109–123, 2000.
198. Ludlam H, Wreghitt TG, Thornton S, et al: Q fever in pregnancy. *J Infect* 34:75–78, 1997.
199. Riechman N, Raz R, Keysary A, Goldwasser R, Flatau E: Chronic Q fever and severe thrombocytopenia in a pregnant women. *Am J Med* 85:253–254, 1988.
200. Stein A, Raoult D: Q fever during pregnancy: a public health problem in southern France. *Clin Infect Dis* 27:592–596, 1998.
201. Fournier P-E, Marrie TJ, Raoult D: Diagnosis of Q fever. *J Clin Microbiol* 36:1823–1834, 1998.
202. Singh AE, Romanowski B. Syphilis: review with emphasis on clinical, epidemiologic, and some biologic features. *Clin Microbiol Rev* 12:187–209, 1999.
203. Sheffield JS, Wendel GD: Syphilis in pregnancy. *Clin Obstet Gynecol* 1999;42:97–106.
204. Genc M, Ledger WJ: Syphilis in pregnancy. *Sex Transm Infect* 2000;76:73–79.
205. Centers for Disease Control and Prevention: Sexually transmitted disease treatment guidelines 2002 MMWR Morb Mortal Wkly Rep 51 (RR-6):1–84, 2002.
206. Birnbaum NR, Goldschmidt RH, Buffett WO: Resolving the common clinical dilemmas of syphilis. *Am Fam Physician* 59:2233–2240, 1999.
207. Walker GJA: Antibiotics for syphilis diagnosed during pregnancy, in The Cochrane Library (Cochrane Review), Issue 1. Oxford: Update Software, 2002.
208. Hollier LM, Cox SM: Syphilis. *Semin Perinatol* 22:323–331, 1998.

209. Wicher V, Wicher K: Pathogenesis of maternal-fetal syphilis revisited. *Clin Infect Dis* 33:354–363, 2001.
210. Sheffield JS, Sanchez PJ, Morris G, et al: Congenital syphilis after maternal treatment for syphilis during pregnancy. *Am J Obstet Gynecol* 186:569–573, 2002.
211. Alger LS: Toxoplasmosis and parvovirus B19. *Infect Dis Clin North Am* 11:55–75, 1997.
212. Lynfield R, Guerina NG: Toxoplasmosis. *Pediatr Rev* 18:75–83, 1997.
213. Beazley DM, Egerman RS: Toxoplasmosis. *Semin Perinatol* 22:332–338, 1998.
214. Tenter AM, Heckeroth AR, Weiss LM: *Toxoplasma gondii*: from animals to humans. *Intern J Parasitol* 30:1217–1258, 2000.
215. Jones JL, Lopez A, Wilson M, Schulkin J, Gibbs R: Congenital toxoplasmosis: a review. *Obstet Gynecol* 56:296–305. 2001.
216. Guerina NG, Hsu HW, Meissner HC, et al: Neonatal screening and early treatment for congenital *Toxoplasma gondii* infection. *N Engl J Med* 330:1856–1863, 1994.
217. Piper JM, Wen TS: Perinatal cytomegalovirus and toxoplasmosis: challenges of antepartum therapy. *Clin Obstet Gynecol* 42:81–96, 1999.
218. Boyer KM, Campbell JR: Diagnostic testing for congenital toxoplasmosis. *Pediatr Infect Dis J* 20:59–60, 2001.
219. Wallon PF, Lious C, Garner P: Treatments for toxoplasmosis in pregnancy, in The Cochrane Library, Issue 1. Oxford: Update Software, 2002.
220. Newton ER: Diagnosis of perinatal TORCH infections. *Clin Obstet Gynecol* 42:59–70, 1999
221. Duff P: Hepatitis in pregnancy. *Semin Perinatol* 22:277–283, 1998.
222. Labrique AB, Thomas DL, Stoszek SK, Nelson KE: Hepatitis E: an emerging disease. *Epidemiol Rev* 21:162–179, 1999.
223. Winn WC: Enterically transmitted hepatitis: hepatitis A and E viruses. *Clin Lab Med* 19:661–673, 1999.
224. Harrison TJ: Hepatitis E virus—an update. *Liver* 19:171–176, 1999.
225. Aggarwal R, Krawczynski K: Hepatitis E: an overview and recent advances in clinical and laboratory research. *J Gastroenterol Hepatol* 15:9–20, 2000.
226. Krawczynski K, Aggarwal R, Kamili S: Hepatitis E. *Infect Dis Clin North Am* 14:669–687, 2000.
227. Smith JL: A review of hepatitis E virus. *J Food Protection* 64:572–586, 2001.
228. Khuroo MS, Dar MY: Hepatitis E: evidence for person-to-person transmission and inability of low dose immune serum globulin from an Indian source to prevent it. *Indian J Gastroenterol* 11:109–112, 1992.
229. Naidu SS, Viswanathan R: Infectious hepatitis in pregnancy during Delhi epidemic. *Ind J Med Res* (Suppl):71–76, 1957.
230. Malkani P, Grewal AK: Observations on infectious hepatitis in pregnancy. *Ind J Med Res* (Suppl):77–84, 1957.
231. Khuroo MS: Study of an epidemic of non-A, non-B hepatitis. *Am J Med* 68:818–824, 1980.
232. Naik SR, Aggarwal R, Salunke PN, Mehrotra NM: A large waterborne viral hepatitis E epidemic in Kanpur, India. *Bull WHO* 70:597–604, 1992.
233. Rab MA, Bile MK, Mubarik M, et al: Water-borne hepatitis E virus epidemic in Islamabad, Pakistan: a common source outbreak traced to the malfunction of a modern water treatment plant. *Am J Trop Med Hyg* 57:151–157, 1997.
234. Khuroo MS, Kamili S, Jameel S: Vertical transmission of hepatitis E virus. *Lancet* 345:1025–1026, 1995.
235. Vazquez-Boland JA, Kuhn M, Berche P, et al: Listeria pathogenesis and molecular virulence determinants. *Clin Microbiol Rev* 14:584–640, 2001.
236. Hof H: *Listeria monocytogenes*: a causative agent of gastroenteritis? *Eur J Clin Microbiol Infect Dis* 20:369–373, 2001.
237. Charpentier E, Courvalin P: Antibiotic resistance in *Listeria* spp. *Antimicrob Agents Chemother* 43:2103–2108, 1999.
238. Hof H, Nichterlein T, Kretschmar M: Management of listeriosis. *Clin Microbiol Rev* 10:345–357, 1997.
239. Smith JL: Foodborne infections during pregnancy. *J Food Protect* 62.818–829, 1999.
240. Temple ME, Nahata MC: Treatment of listeriosis. *Ann Pharmacother* 34:656–661, 2000.
241. Silver HM: Malarial infections during pregnancy. *Infect Dis Clin North Am* 11:99–107, 1997.
242. Alecrim WD, Ekspinosa EM, Alecrim MGC: *Plasmodium falciparum* infection in the pregnant patient. *Infect Dis Clin North Am* 14:83–95, 2000.
243. McGregor IA: Epidemiology, malaria and pregnancy. *Am J Trop Med Hygiene* 33:517–525, 1984.
244. Guyatt HL, Snow RW: The epidemiology and burden of *Plasmodium falciparum*-related anemia among pregnant women in sub-Saharan Africa. *Am J Trop Med Hygiene* 64(1–2 Suppl):36–44, 2001.
245. Saeed BO, Atabani GS, Nawwaf A, et al: Hypoglycemia in pregnant women with malaria. *Trans Royal Soc Trop Med Hygiene* 84:349–350, 1990.
246. Looareesuwan S, Phillips RE, White NJ, et al: Quinine and severe falciparum malaria in late pregnancy. *Lancet* 2:4–8, 1985.
247. Steketee RW, Nahlen BL, Parise ME, Menendez C: The burden of malaria in pregnancy in malaria-endemic areas. *Am J Trop Med Hygiene* 64(1–2 Suppl):28–35, 2001.
248. Bartlett JG, Mundy LM: Community-acquired pneumonia. *N Engl J Med* 333:1618–1624, 1995.
249. Rigby FB, Pastorek JG: Pneumonia during pregnancy. *Clin Obstet Gynecol* 39:107–119, 1996.
250. American College of Obstetricians and Gynecologists: Pulmonary disease in pregnancy. *Int J Obstet Gynecol* 54:187–196, 1996.
251. Goodrum LA: Pneumonia in pregnancy. *Semin Perinatol* 21:276–283, 1997.
252. Riley L: Pneumonia and tuberculosis in pregnancy. *Infect Dis Clin North Am* 11:119–133, 1997.
253. Ie S, Rubino ER, Alper B, Szerlip HM: Respiratory complications of pregnancy. *Obstet Gynecol* 57:39–46, 2001.

254. Powrie RO: Respiratory disease. *Best Pract Clin Obstet Gynecol* 15:913–936, 2001.
255. Ramsey PS, Ramin KD: Pneumonia in pregnancy. *Obstet Gynecol Clin North Am* 28:553–569, 2001.
256. Lim WS, Macfarlane JT, Colthorpe CL: Pneumonia and pregnancy. *Thorax* 56:398–405, 2001.
257. American Thoracic Society: Guidelines for the management of adults with community-acquired pneumonia. *Am J Respir Crit Care Med* 163:1730–1754, 2001.
258. Bartlett JG, Dowell SF, Mandell LA, et al: Practice guidelines for the management of community-acquired pneumonia in adults. *Clin Infect Dis* 31:347–382, 2000.
259. Moreheade RS, Pinto SJ: Ventilator-associated pneumonia. *Arch Intern Med* 160:1926–1936, 2000.
260. Collin BA, Ramphal R: Pneumonia in the compromised host including cancer patients and transplant patients. *Infect Dis Clin North Am* 12:781–805, 1998.
261. Berkowitz K, LaSala A: Risk factors associated with the increasing prevalence of pneumonia during pregnancy. *Am J Obstet Gynecol* 163:981–985, 1990.
262. Richey SD, Roberts SW, Ramin KD, Cunningham FG: Pneumonia complicating pregnancy. *Obstet Gynecol* 84:525–528, 1994.
263. Yost NP, Bloom SL, Richey SD, Ramin SM, Cunningham FG: An appraisal of treatment guidelines for antepartum community-acquired pneumonia. *Am J Obstet Gynecol* 183:131–135, 2000.
264. Caldwell JW, Arsura EL, Kilgore WB, et al: Coccidioidomycosis in pregnancy during an epidemic in California. *Obstet Gynecol* 95:236–239, 2000.
265. Ely EW, Peacock JE, Haponik EF, Washburn RG: Cryptococcal pneumonia complicating pregnancy. *Medicine* 77:153–167, 1998.
266. Neiberg AD, Mavromatais F, Dyke J, Fayyad A: *Blastomyces dermatitidis* treated during pregnancy: report of a case. *Am J Obstet Gynecol* 128:911–912, 1977.
267. Daniel L, Salit IE: Blastomycosis during pregnancy. *CMAJ* 131:759–761, 1984.
268. Saade GR: Human immunodeficiency virus (HIV)-related pulmonary complications in pregnancy. *Semin Perinatol* 21:336–350, 1997.
269. Fine MJ, Auble TE, Yealy DM, et al: A prediction rule to identify low-risk patients with community-acquired pneumonia. *N Engl J Med* 336:243–250, 1997.
270. Miller KS, Miller JM: Tuberculosis in pregnancy: interactions, diagnosis, and management. *Clin Obstet Gynecol* 39:120–142, 1996.
271. Anderson GD: Tuberculosis in pregnancy. *Semin Perinatol* 21:328–335, 1997.
272. Millar LK, Cox SM: Urinary tract infections complicating pregnancy. *Infect Dis Clin North Am* 11:13–26, 1997.
273. Patterson TF, Andriole VT: Detection, significance, and therapy of bacteriuria in pregnancy. *Infect Dis Clin North Am* 11:593–608, 1997.
274. Connolly AM, Thorp JM: Urinary tract infections in pregnancy. *Urol Clin North Am* 26:779–787, 1999.
275. Delzell JE, Lefevre ML: Urinary tract infections during pregnancy. *Am Fam Physician* 61:713–721, 2000.
276. Gilstrap LC, Ramin SM: Urinary tract infections during pregnancy. *Obstet Gynecol Clin North Am* 28:581–591, 2001.
277. Smaill F: Antibiotics for asymptomatic bacteriuria in pregnancy, in The Cochrane Library, Issue 1. Oxford: Update Software, 2002.
278. Turck M, Goff BS, Petersdorf RG: Bacteriuria in pregnancy: relation to socioeconomic factors. *N Engl J Med* 266:857, 1962.
279. Whalley PJ, Martin RG, Pritchard JA: Sickle cell trait and urinary tract infection during pregnancy. *JAMA* 189:903, 1964.
280. Pastore LM, Savitz DA, Thorp JM, et al: Predictors of symptomatic urinary tract infections after 20 weeks' gestation. *J Perinatol* 19:488–493, 1999.
281. Graham JC, Galloway A: The laboratory diagnosis of urinary tract infection. *J Clin Pathol* 54:911–919, 2001.
282. Cram LF, Zapata M-I, Toy EC, Baker B: Genitourinary infections and their association with preterm labor. *Am Fam Physician* 65:241–248, 2002.
283. American College of Obstetricians and Gynecologists: Antimicrobial therapy for obstetric patients. ACOG educational bulletin no. 245. Washington, 1998, pp 8–10.
284. U.S. Preventive Services Task Force: Guide to clinical preventive services: report of the U.S. Preventive Services Task Force, 2d ed. Baltimore: Williams & Wilkins, 1996.

18

Neurologic Disorders in Pregnancy

Imran Ali
Bradley Vaughn

KEY POINTS

- Evaluation of stroke in pregnant women requires a thorough search for hematologic, cardiovascular, and neurologic causes.
- Cerebral vein thrombosis may present with headache, seizures, and focal neurologic deficits in the peri-partum or post-partum period.
- Antiepileptic drugs are associated with significant teratogenicity and require close monitoring by the neurologist and obstetrician.
- Treatment of status epilepticus in pregnancy is the same as if the patient were not pregnant. If status epilepticus develops as the first seizure, a catastrophic CNS event such as hemorrhage, tumor, or encephalitis, is likely.
- Mannitol should be avoided in the treatment of increased intracranial pressure during pregnancy because it can cause fetal dehydration and fetal bradycardia.

INTRODUCTION

There have been remarkable advances in the diagnosis and treatment of neurologic disorders in the last few years. A physician in the emergency department is likely to see most of these common neurologic disorders with increasing frequency. A firm grasp of principles of diagnosis and management of a complex group of disorders is mandatory for the practicing ED physician. Pregnancy and the postpartum period adds yet another layer of complexity, especially since there is an increasing number of drugs available to treat disorders such as migraine, epilepsy, multiple sclerosis and stroke. These drugs may be potentially harmful during pregnancy, so management of these neurologic disorders requires familiarity with the clinical presentation as well as potential treatment options.

This chapter aims to provide a brief review of common neurologic disorders in pregnancy and discuss issues that are of relevance to emergency room personnel.

NEUROLOGIC LOCALIZATION

The initial step in evaluation of neurologic problems is localization of the lesion. This localization requires a systematic approach that begins with a meticulous history and physical examination. Based on the clinical evaluation, one can usually identify the location of the lesion (Table 18-1 and Fig. 18-1). As a general rule in neurologic disorders, the location of the lesion indicates the most likely etiology and is helpful in generating a differential diagnosis.

Coma and Stupor

Stupor or coma in the pregnant patient raises concerns of possibly devastating etiologies. Begin with a detailed history, physical examination, and laboratory evaluation. A complete, but quick neurologic examination will often give clues about the diffuse or focal nature of neurologic injury.[1] Possible etiologies are listed in Table 18-2. Management includes rapid determination of possibly catastrophic reversible causes including hypoxemia, hypoglycemia, or drug intoxication, as listed in Table 18-3. Patients require supportive care until their conditions can be reversed. Once an etiology is determined, specific therapy can be undertaken. Many of these disorders are discussed further below.

Cerebrovascular Disorders in Pregnancy

Cerebral Infarction (Arterial)

The reported incidence of ischemic stroke during pregnancy varies from 5 to 200 per 100,000 deliveries[2,3] (Table 18-4). The higher estimate indicates a 10- to 13-fold increase compared to nonpregnant individuals. The incidence of stroke is likely to be higher during the third trimester and immediate postpartum period.[2–4] Most of the reviews and studies combine arterial and venous causes of ischemic strokes as well as hemorrhages, making a clear analysis of the data somewhat difficult.[5] How-

Table 18-1. Localization of Neurological Deficits

Site	Findings
Cerebral hemisphere	Contralateral hemiparesis, central facial palsy, hemianopsia and sensory findings, contralateral hyperreflexia and extensor plantar response, associated cortical function loss (aphasia, agraphia, acalculia)
Brain stem lesion	Contralateral body hemiparesis and sensory findings, contralateral hyperreflexia and extensor plantar response, ipsilateral cranial nerve findings, ataxia, hyperventilation, pinpoint pupils
Spinal cord	Paraplegia or quadriplegia, hyperreflexia below lesion, sensory level, bilateral extensor plantar responses, bladder and rectal dysfunction
Neuropathy	Distal greater than proximal weakness, loss of reflex and muscle wasting (late finding) in distribution of the nerve, polyneuropathies associated with stocking-glove distribution of functional loss usually flexor plantar or no response
Myopathy	Proximal weakness, preservation of reflexes, flexor plantar response, no sensory deficits

ever, it is well established that the incidence of ischemic stroke in pregnancy is greater than that of intracranial hemorrhage.[5,6]

The clinical presentation is variable and is dependent on the vascular territory involved. However, sudden onset of focal neurologic deficits is almost always an indication of a cerebrovascular event. Common neurologic symptoms include aphasia, focal weakness, sensory loss, diplopia, dysarthria, ataxia, vertigo, and hemifield visual loss. Rapid assessment in ischemic strokes is essential to decrease the risk of irreversible neurologic damage in a young woman. Early neurologic and obstetric consultation is necessary to confirm the diagnosis, identify the cause, and establish a treatment plan. Diagnostic evaluation requires cerebral imaging. CT scans are considered relatively safe after the first trimester as the radiation exposure is low, but appropriate shielding and informed consent are mandatory. CT scan may be normal in an acute stroke, especially in the first 24 hours. Magnetic resonance imaging (MRI) of the brain is the preferred diagnostic tool in acute stroke as it is extremely sensitive for ischemic lesions, and it is also relatively safe

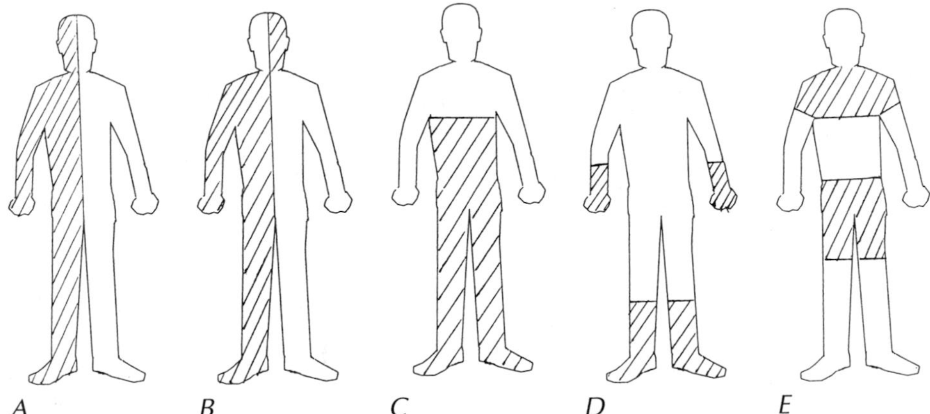

Fig. 18-1. These five figures represent the classical distribution of neurologic deficits occurring with lesions of the nervous system. *A.* Lesion of the cerebral hemisphere with body and face findings contralateral to the lesion. *B.* Brain stem lesion with body contralateral and face ipsilateral to the lesion. *C.* Spinal cord lesion with motor and sensory level. *D.* Polyneuropathy with a stocking-glove distribution of sensory and motor deficits. *E.* Myopathy showing a proximal muscle weakness (but no sensory deficits).

Table 18-2. Differential Diagnosis of Coma and Pertinent Findings

Etiology	Neurological Examination	Pertinent Findings
Anoxia	Nonlocalizing	May have posturing, seizures, and myoclonus
Carbon monoxide intoxication	Nonlocalizing	Cherry red skin, carboxyhemoglobinemia
Hypoglycemia	Nonlocalizing, can also be focal	May have seizures, posturing and signs of excessive sympathetic output, low serum glucose
Diabetic coma	Nonlocalizing	Fruity breath, Kussmal respiration, hyperglycemia, ketoacidosis, glycosuria, and ketonuria
Septic shock	Nonlocalizing	Hyperthermia, hypothermia, tachypnea, hypotension
Uremia	Nonlocalizing	Hypertension, uriniferous breath, asterixis, myoclonus, elevated BUN and creatinine
Hepatic coma	Nonlocalizing	Jaundice, ascites, elevated bilirubin and NH_3, low serum protein, hypocoagulable state
Addison's disease	Nonlocalizing	Low serum cortisol, hypotension
Hypercapnia	Nonlocalizing	Elevated CO_2 and respiratory acidosis on blood gas; may have myoclonus or asterixis; can cause papilledema
Drug intoxication	Nonlocalizing	Variable depending on the agent; seizures and encephalopathy common
Meningitis	Nonlocalizing	Meningismus, fever, headache, inflammatory pattern on CSF examination
Status epilepticus	Nonlocalizing or focal abnormalities	Electroencephalographic evidence of seizures, ongoing tonic clonic activity, or focal rhythmic twitching
Subarachnoid hemorrhage	May be focal or nonfocal	Severe headache, meningismus, subhyaloid hemorrhage, CSF shows elevated red cells or xanthochromia; CT scan shows hemorrhage
Eclampsia	May be focal or nonfocal	Headache, seizures, hypertension, proteinuria
Hypertensive encephalopathy	May be focal or nonfocal	Headache, flame hemorrhages in retina, seizures, elevated blood pressure
Intracranial mass (tumor, abscess)	Focal deficit depending on location of mass	Progressive headache, progressive neurologic deficits, papilledema or nausea and vomiting; MRI/CT scan demonstrates mass
Intraparenchymal hemorrhage	Focal depending on location of hemorrhage	Sudden onset of symptoms, seizures, hypertension, headache; CT scan demonstrates hemorrhages
Subdural hemorrhage	Focal depending on location of hemorrhage	Slow progression of symptoms, mild headache, history of trauma or anticoagulation; MRI/CT scan demonstrates subdural hemorrhage
Trauma	May be focal or nonfocal	Battle sign or other evidence of trauma
Thrombotic stroke	Focal findings depending on distribution	Abrupt onset with progression of symptoms; more likely to occur in sleep; may not be seen early on CT scan
Embolic stroke	Focal findings depending on vasculature distribution (amniotic fluid embolus may be nonfocal)	Sudden onset; maximal deficit soon after onset; may improve with time; possible risk for seizures; consider possible amniotic embolus, possible cardiac valvular or septal defect or arrhythmia; may not be seen early on CT scan
Central pontine myelinolysis	May be nonfocal or focal	Intranuclear ophthalmoplegia related to rapid correction of hyponatremia
Encephalitis	Nonfocal or focal depending on area of cerebral injury	Seizures, confusion, and fever prior to coma; CSF shows an inflammatory pattern; MRI may show abnormality

Table 18-3. Management of Acute Altered Mental Status in Pregnancy

Maternal-fetal resuscitation
- Assess and maintain adequate airway, breathing and circulation
- Obtain maternal vital signs: BP, PR, RR, core temperature, oxygen saturation
- Immobilize neck until cervical spine injury has been excluded
- Monitor cardiac rhythm and obtain ECG
- Assess fetal heart tones and determine gestational age

Initial treatment
- Administer oxygen
- Begin crystalloid infusion
- Thiamine 100 mg IV
- Glucose test strip, administer 50% dextrose if hypoglycemic
- Use naloxone 0.4 mg IV if narcotics overdose is suspected

Evaluation
- Physical examination; pelvic and rectal examination
- Neurologic examination (assess for focality)
- Reassess fetal heart tones and obtain obstetrics consultation

Diagnostics and Treatment
- CBC, type and screen, chemistries, toxicology panel, coagulation studies
- CT scan of head
- Treat seizures and infection
- Treat increased intracranial pressure
- Correct hypo- or hyperthermia
- Neurology or neurosurgery consultation

(see below). The added advantage of noninvasive imaging of both intracranial arterial (MR angiography) and venous circulation (MR venography) makes MRI an invaluable tool for evaluation of cerebrovascular disease. Diffusion-weighted imaging during MRI can be done rapidly within minutes and is able to identify acute ischemia in a majority of cases.[7]

The diagnostic approach to stroke in pregnancy is similar to that of stroke in the young. Stroke in pregnancy can be classified as embolic or thrombotic.

Embolic Stroke

Classically, embolic stroke presents with maximal deficits at onset with focal neurologic abnormalities on examination. Emboli most often are related to cardiac disease and most commonly involve the middle or posterior cerebral artery, but any vessel may be involved. Atrial fibrillation, valvular heart disease, peripartum cardiomyopathy, infectious or noninfectious endocarditis, and patent foramen ovale are some of the well-recognized causes of embolic infarction in pregnancy. A thorough general, cardiovascular, and neurologic examination is mandatory to identify the underlying cause. Transesophageal echocardiography is useful in documenting the presence of atrial or valvular thrombus as well as patent foramen ovale. Routine ECG and 24-hour telemetry are helpful in identifying arrhythmias. Definitive treatment is based on underlying etiology. Anticoagulation is recommended for embolic infarcts, but the timing and form of anticoagulation depends on the size of the infarct and underlying etiology. This will be discussed further in the section on treatment.

Thrombotic Stroke

Thrombosis in the cerebral vasculature may be related to arteriosclerosis, hypercoagulable state, vasculitis, systemic lupus erythematosus, dissection, and pregnancy-specific causes (Table 18-5). The clinical presentation is similar to embolic stroke, with sudden onset of focal neurologic deficits that may be first noted upon arousal from sleep. Premature arteriosclerosis may occur due to under-

Table 18-4. Comparison of Acute Neurologic Disorders in Pregnancy

Disorder	Incidence	Timing	Risk Factors
Embolic stroke	5-200/100,000	Third trimester or immediate postpartum	Atrial fibrillation Valvular heart disease Peripartum cardiomyopathy Endocarditis Patent foramen ovale Choriocarcinoma Amniotic fluid embolism
Thrombotic stroke	5-200/100,000	Third trimester or immediately postpartum	Arteriosclerosis Hypercoagulable state Vasculitis Carotid or aortic dissection Eclampsia Postpartum angiopathy
Cerebral venous thrombosis	10-20/100,000	Second to third week postpartum	Infection Dehydration Trauma Hypercoagulable states
Subarachnoid hemorrhage or ruptured cerebral aneurysm	10-50/100,000	Labor or immediate postpartum	Increased cardiac output Increased venous pressure Hypertension Vasodilation
Eclampsia		Second and third trimester and postpartum	Hypertension, edema, proteinuria

lying metabolic disorders such as diabetes, hypercholesterolemia, homocysteinemia, or hyperlipidemia. Hypercoagulable states may include antiphospholipid antibody syndrome, protein C or S deficiency, antithrombin III deficiency, or factor V Leiden mutation. Except for antiphospholipid antibody syndrome, all of the other causes are more commonly associated with venous infarcts. Diagnostic evaluation requires testing for all these abnormalities. Patients with systemic lupus erythematosus (SLE) or other forms of vasculitis may have systemic manifestations such as anemia, thrombocytopenia, arthropathy, rash, uremia, and elevated sedimentation rate. A postpartum angiopathy[3,8] has been described in which a young woman suddenly develops severe focal neurologic deficits a few hours to a month after delivery. Diffuse vasoconstriction is noted on angiography. This appears to be reversible, although the prognosis is poor in some cases. Precise treatment is not established, although supportive care is important to prevent worsening of neurologic symptoms. Risk factors for development of this entity include migraine and use of sympathomimetic drugs. Carotid or vertebral artery dissection may occur with mild blunt trauma to the head or neck and requires a high index of suspicion for diagnosis. Definitive diagnosis, however, requires carotid ultrasound as well as a cerebral angiogram. Patients with dissection as well as those with hypercoagulable state require anticoagulation to prevent recurrent infarction. This will be discussed further in the next section.

Table 18-5. Pregnancy-Specific Causes of Stroke

Eclampsia
Choriocarcinoma
Amniotic fluid embolism
Postpartum cerebral angiopathy
Peripartum cardiomyopathy
Hypercoagulable state

Anticoagulation with heparin is recommended for patients with underlying hypercoagulable state, carotid or vertebral artery dissections, progressing stroke, crescendo

Table 18-6. Anticoagulants in Pregnancy

Drug	Fetal Safety	Maternal Safety
Heparin	Safe	Thrombocytopenia, osteoporosis
Low-molecular-weight heparin	Probably safe	Safe
Warfarin	Avoid	Vitamin K depletion??
Aspirin	Avoid	
Nonsteroidal antiinflammatory drugs	Avoid	

transient ischemic attack (TIA), or embolic infarction (Table 18-6). Contraindications to anticoagulation are similar to those in nonpregnant individuals. Neurologists also avoid anticoagulation in the presence of a large infarct. The decision to anticoagulate in pregnancy should be based on consultations with the neurologist and obstetrician and risk-benefit analysis. Patients should be informed of these factors and consent should be obtained and documented in the chart. The risk of bleeding complications with heparin is similar in pregnant and nonpregnant individuals (2 percent).[9] Heparin is the preferred agent,[10] although long-term use may result in osteopenia. Low-molecular-weight heparin is also efficacious, although controlled studies regarding its efficacy in stroke and safety in pregnancy are not available. Warfarin should be avoided due to associated teratogenicity and long half-life.[6] The safety of aspirin or other antiplatelet agents has not been established in pregnancy and their use should be considered only after consultation with a hematologist and obstetrician.

Cerebral Venous Thrombosis

Cerebral venous thrombosis (CVT) most often occurs in the third trimester or in the immediate postpartum period. The incidence in North America and Western Europe is 10 to 20 cases per 100,000 deliveries.[3] The majority of cases (80 percent) occur in the second or third week postpartum. Clinical presentation includes headaches, seizures, encephalopathy, visual disturbances, papilledema, and focal neurologic deficits. Diagnosis requires a high index of suspicion. Risk factors for development of CVT include infection, dehydration, trauma, and hypercoagulable state. MRI is a useful noninvasive test (Fig. 18-2) that may show infarction in a venous distribution with hemorrhagic changes. MR venography can show thrombosis within the sagittal or other cerebral veins.[7] Confirmation may require conventional angiography with a venous phase. Definitive treatment for cerebral vein thrombosis is anticoagulation with heparin,[11,12] but early neurologic consultation is essential. Supportive therapy may require neurosurgical evaluation for management of elevated intracranial pressure or hematoma evacuation.

Intracranial Hemorrhage in Pregnancy

Subarachnoid Hemorrhage and Intracranial Aneurysms

The prevalence of intracranial hemorrhage in pregnancy is approximately 0.01 to 0.05 percent, but it is associated with an extremely high mortality rate (40 to 83 percent) and accounts for 5 to 12 percent of all maternal deaths during pregnancy.[13,14] This high mortality rate can be reduced with early diagnosis and timely intervention.

The most common cause of intracranial hemorrhage in pregnancy is subarachnoid hemorrhage (SAH) due a ruptured cerebral aneurysm (Fig. 18-3). The risk of rupture of an asymptomatic aneurysm is 0.4 per week during

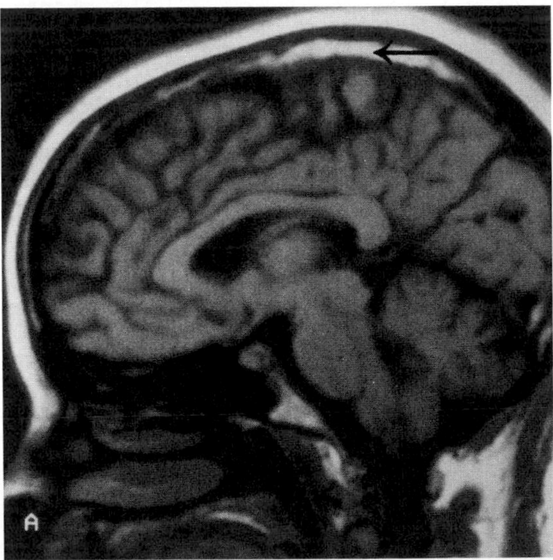

Fig. 18-2. This T1 sagittal view of the MRI demonstrates thrombosis of the sagittal sinus as seen by the bright signal noted in the sinus above the parietal region.

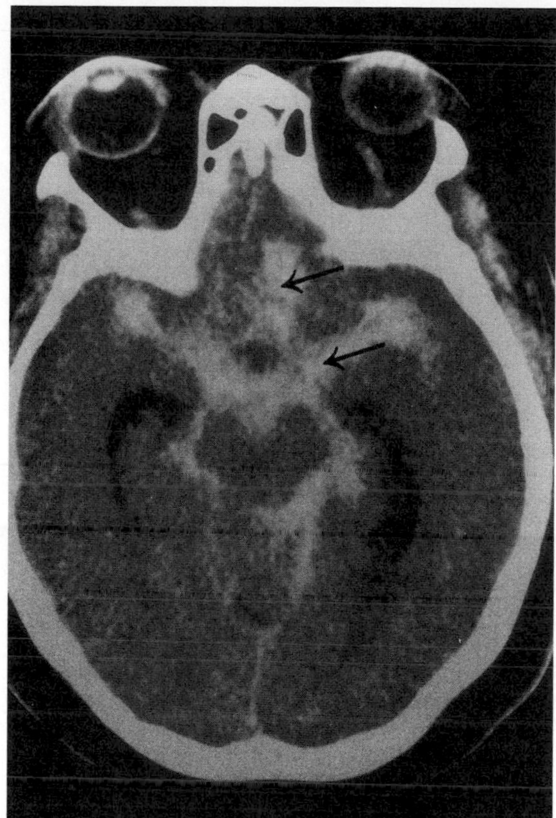

Fig. 18-3. A CT scan taken from a patient with an acute subarachnoid hemorrhage. Note the higher density in the suprasellar area and region outlining the midbrain.

pregnancy, 3.5 per week during labor and immediately postpartum, and 1.4 per week in the first 3 months after delivery. In some studies, however, the third trimester was found to be the period of greatest risk.[13–15] This may be related to hemodynamic and hormonal changes such as an increase in cardiac output, venous pressure, blood volume, and increased estrogen, resulting in vasodilatation of abnormal blood vessels. The risk of rebleeding is 33 to 50 percent with a greater than 60 percent mortality. Mortality from any SAH is also higher in gravid women compared to the nongravid population.

The clinical presentation includes severe headaches described by the patient as "the worst headache of their life." The headache is usually sudden in onset, constant in nature, and usually associated with a stiff neck (Tables 18-7 and 18-8). Nausea, vomiting, and photophobia are common. In some patients headaches may also be associated with seizures or rapid development of coma. Examination may reveal subhyaloid hemorrhages or signs of increased intracranial pressure on funduscopic examination and nuchal rigidity, as well as cranial neuropathies (most commonly third-nerve palsy due to compression of the oculomotor nerve). Focal neurologic deficits are seen in a third of the patients presenting with SAH.

The diagnosis can be made on the basis of CT scan that will reveal subarachnoid blood in 90 percent of patients with ruptured cerebral aneurysms. In those patients with suspected SAH and a negative CT, a lumbar puncture is mandatory to exclude that possibility. A cerebral angiogram is required to confirm the location of the aneurysms as well as document the presence of multiple aneurysms that are seen in 15 to 20 percent of the patients. It can be performed safely in the third trimester with appropriate precautions and informed consent.

Management of ruptured intracranial aneurysms in pregnancy requires evaluation by a neurosurgeon with expertise in neurovascular disorders. The use of nimodip-

Table 18-7. Warning Signs in Patients with Headaches

New-onset headaches in pregnancy
Headaches with different characteristics from previous headaches
"Worst headache of one's life"
Focal neurologic deficit
Meningismus
Fever
Altered consciousness
Papilledema or other signs of increased intracranial pressure
Retinal hemorrhages
Increased blood pressure (may herald preeclampsia or eclampsia)
Postpartum headaches (need to exclude cerebral venous thrombosis)

Table 18-8. Differential Diagnosis of Headaches in Pregnancy

Migraine
Tension-type headaches
Subarachnoid hemorrhage
Intraparenchymal hemorrhage
Central venous thrombosis
CNS tumor or infection
Benign intracranial hypertension
Sinus headaches
Eclampsia

ine (category C) for prevention of vasospasm is limited in pregnancy because of the concern of fetal injury, although no human data are available at present. Intracranial surgery should be performed early in women who are pregnant with ruptured aneurysms, but requires coordination with the obstetric service to avoid fetal morbidity. Surgical outcomes are good for patients with aneurysms, especially in centers with expertise in management. The role of endovascular treatment in these patients remains to be defined, but it can be considered in patients who are at a greater risk from surgical intervention. Obstetric management needs to be individualized, as there does not appear to be a significant difference in the likelihood of bleeding with vaginal or cesarean section in a patient with an untreated arteriovenous malformation (AVM) or an aneurysm.

Arteriovenous Malformations and Other Causes of Intracranial Hemorrhage

Other causes of intracranial hemorrhage include arteriovenous malformations, trauma, coagulopathy, eclampsia, and tumors such as choriocarcinoma. AVMs cause intraparenchymal hemorrhage, usually in the second trimester, the period associated with the greatest increase in cardiac output. As opposed to patients with SAH, these patients are younger, nulliparous, and more likely to bleed during labor and delivery.[14] Clinical presentation includes headaches, seizures, and focal neurologic deficits, as well as sudden onset of coma. Diagnosis requires a CT scan, which will reveal an intraparenchymal hematoma. Identification of the AVM may require a cerebral angiogram as it may be obscured on the CT by the presence of a large amount of blood. The management of a pregnant woman with AVM is similar to that in a nongravid patient. Neurosurgical consultation is required. The treatment plan should be coordinated with the obstetrician to reduce both fetal and maternal morbidity and mortality. Management of ICH from other causes in pregnancy is similar to that in nongravid women. However, mannitol should be avoided due to possible fetal toxicity (placental hypoperfusion, fetal and maternal hypernatremia, and hyperosmolarity) associated with its use in pregnancy.

Neurologic Consequences of Eclampsia

Eclampsia is a poorly understood disorder characterized by hypertension, edema, proteinuria, and convulsions or encephalopathy, most likely related to systemic vasoconstriction. This disorder usually occurs during the second or third trimester, but it can also occur days after an uneventful pregnancy and delivery.[16,17] The presence of neurologic symptoms and signs (i.e., seizure) differentiate preeclampsia from eclampsia. This disorder is considered an obstetric emergency. Immediate stabilization and expeditious delivery of the fetus are the only definitive treatment. The neurologic changes include cerebral edema, most often in the parieto-occipital region, associated with petechial hemorrhages (Fig. 18-4). Patients are clinically encephalopathic and frequently have convulsions. Either MRI with diffusion-weighted imaging or CT scan may show diffuse or focal edema, especially in the parieto-occipital region.[7,18] The scan may be completely normal in some cases.

Convulsions with eclampsia may cause fetal hypoxia and circulatory compromise. It is necessary to prevent seizure recurrence. There is considerable controversy over anticonvulsant therapy. Magnesium sulfate is the most frequently used anticonvulsant in eclampsia, but most

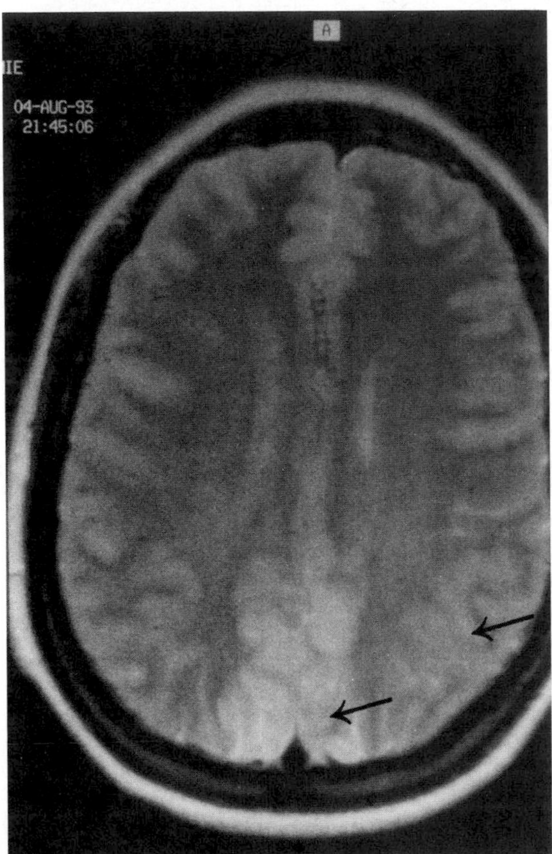

Fig. 18-4. This axial MRI taken from a patient with eclampsia demonstrates the diffuse swelling in the gray matter, indicated by the brighter T2 signal, particularly in the occipital and parietal regions.

neurologists believe that magnesium acts through neuromuscular blockade rather than as a true antiepileptogenic agent,[9] although there is some evidence to suggest that magnesium may have central inhibitory effects on glutamate receptors and may actually have some antiepileptic properties. Phenytoin is an alternative for emergency management of seizures, and most patients do not require long-term anticonvulsants.[16,17] Other issues related to eclampsia are discussed in Chap. 8.

Head Trauma

Head trauma accounts for 20 percent of nonobstetric maternal deaths.[19,20] Closed or open head injury may result in intracranial hemorrhage and CNS edema. These complications present the most acute neurologic danger to the patient. The patient's examination is a reasonable guide to the probability of good outcome. The Glasgow Coma Scale is a widely used screening tool for assessing brain function and has been correlated to outcome. The scale ranges from the normal score of 15 to a minimum of 3. Individuals who have scores of 8 or less are considered to have suffered severe head injury. Patient management should be directed toward the assessment and therapy of the most dangerous complications first.

In the pregnant patient with head trauma, the effects on the fetus should be considered in evaluation and treatment.[19–21] Fetal demise and poor outcome are correlated with the severity of maternal trauma.[21] Additionally, maternal systemic complications increase the risk of fetal complications. In every patient, the gestational age should be estimated and the mother should be checked for possible premature onset of labor. Patients who have evidence of increased intracranial pressure should be considered for intracranial pressure monitoring and CSF drainage. Hyperventilation and glucocorticoids do not appear beneficial. However, mannitol can cause fetal dehydration, contraction of blood volume, and bradycardia; its use during pregnancy should be restricted. In the event of maternal death or brain death, emergency cesarean section is indicated. This should be performed as early as possible to minimize fetal complications. Fetal demise or major morbidity has been associated with deliveries occurring 20 minutes or more after the cessation of maternal vital signs. Deliveries occurring less than 5 minutes postmortem have been associated with excellent outcome (see Chap. 11).

Seizures in Pregnancy

Seizures are defined as abnormal electrical discharges in a group of cortical neurons. By definition, epilepsy refers to recurrent and unprovoked seizures. Approximately 10 percent of the population may have a single seizure during their lifetime, but the incidence of epilepsy is about 1 percent for the entire population.[22,23] There are potentially over one million women of childbearing age in the United States. Therefore it is important for emergency department personnel to be able to diagnose and treat pregnant women with seizures (Table 18-9).

Table 18-9. Precipitants of Seizures in Pregnancy

Hypoglycemia
Hyponatremia
Hypocalcemia
Hypoxia
Drugs
Recreational
Therapeutic agents
Trauma
Brain tumor
Cerebral infarct
Intracerebral hemorrhage
Eclampsia (third trimester or postpartum)

The evaluation of new onset seizures in the emergency department requires a methodical approach.

Step 1: Is this a seizure?
The first part of the evaluation requires a focused history to evaluate whether the event being described is truly a seizure. The presence of an aura, altered awareness with automatisms, generalized tonic-clonic activity and postictal confusion or lethargy suggest a seizure. The presence of lightheadedness, dizziness, or graying of vision followed by brief loss of consciousness without postictal confusion suggests syncope rather than a seizure. This distinction is of great importance as both disorders are common, but the management in each is entirely different.

Step 2: What is the underlying cause?
Seizures may be related to numerous underlying causes (Table 18-9), some of which are rapidly reversible such as hypoglycemia, hypocalcemia, and hypoxia. The presence of a focal neurologic abnormality suggests an underlying structural abnormality such as tumor, infarct, or infection. Absence of any identifiable cause requires a neurologic consultation for planning management and follow-up.

Step 3: What is the appropriate work-up?
Evaluation of seizures in pregnancy requires a comprehensive history and physical examination as well laboratory assessment as indicated above (Table 18-10). The electroencephalogram is an important noninvasive

Table 18-10. Evaluation of New-Onset Seizures in Pregnancy

1. History and physical examination
2. Complete blood count
3. Metabolic panel (electrolytes, renal and liver function, glucose, coagulation studies)
4. Electrocardiogram (ECG)
5. CT scan or MRI
6. Neurologic and obstetric consultation
7. Electroencephalogram (EEG)

diagnostic tool as it can help in identifying the underlying cause in a certain subset of patients (e.g., focal slowing in patients with tumors or cerebral infarct or generalized spike and wave in patients with epileptic syndromes). A neurologic and obstetric consultation is important to coordinate care in the ED and after discharge. CT scan or MRI may be performed after consultation with the neurologists and obstetrician based on the risks and benefits of the procedure for that particular patient.

Step 4: What is the treatment?
Decisions regarding treatment of a single seizure are based on the underlying cause of seizure. A single seizure related to recreational drug use or hypoglycemia may not require antiepileptic therapy. However, in cases with no obvious cause for the seizure, the presence of a neurologic abnormality on examination and neuroimaging, as well as interictal epileptiform abnormalities on EEG increase the risk of recurrence. Options regarding treatment should be frankly discussed with the patient and should involve the neurologist and obstetrician as well. The teratogenic potential of some of the antiepileptic drugs in the first trimester as well as the risks of seizures in reducing placental blood flow should also be mentioned. The final decision should be based on risk and benefit analysis for that patient.

Step 5: What are the precautions recommended in the ED?
If the patient is being discharged from the ED, laws regarding driving with seizures in that locale should be discussed with the patient. Other precautions related to swimming, bathing, working around heavy machinery, heights, and dangerous equipment should also be mentioned. Close neurologic follow-up is mandatory.

Pregnancy in Women with Epilepsy

Pregnancy has a variable effect on seizure frequency. In women with epilepsy the seizure frequency is not significantly altered in 60 to 83 percent of cases. Approximately 10 to 25 percent note an increase in seizures, which is most often related to hormonal alterations, reduction in antiepileptic drug levels, stress, fatigue, and possibly sleep deprivation. Antiepileptic drug levels are reduced, possibly due to impaired absorption, increased volume of distribution, altered protein binding, and increased renal and hepatic clearance.[22–28] Compliance with the regimen may also be affected, as women often perceive antiepileptic drugs as being harmful to the baby. Tables 18-11 and 18-12 outline some of the important aspects of management of pregnant women with epilepsy.

There is a higher incidence of fetal malformations in women with epilepsy exposed to antiepileptic drugs.[24–28] These major malformations occur in 5 to 6 percent of

Table 18-11. Issues Related to Pregnancy and Epilepsy

1. Antiepileptic drug (AED) therapy should be optimized 6 months prior to pregnancy.
2. All women of childbearing age taking AEDs should be on folic acid 0.4-5 mg/d prior to pregnancy as this may reduce the incidence of fetal neural tube defects.
3. Change of AEDs should not be undertaken during pregnancy for the sole purpose of reducing teratogenic risk as these may occur with exposure in the first 4 weeks after conception.
4. Pregnant women taking valproic acid or carbamazepine as well as other AEDs should be offered prenatal testing with alpha-fetoprotein levels at 14-16 weeks' gestation, level II ultrasound at 16-20 weeks' gestation, and amniocentesis if appropriate.
5. AED levels should be monitored as levels may decrease during pregnancy and rise postpartum.
6. Increase in drug dosage should primarily be based on clinical evidence of toxicity and not on established therapeutic range alone.
7. Vitamin K should be given orally in the last month to women receiving enzyme-inducing AEDs (carbamazepine, phenytoin, primidone, and phenobarbital) to avoid neonatal coagulopathy. The neonate should also receive 1 mg vitamin K intramuscularly at birth as well.
8. Breast-feeding is not contraindicated; however, sedating effects of barbiturates may need monitoring.

Table 18-12. Potential Complications of Epilepsy in Pregnancy

Obstetric	Fetal
Vaginal bleeding	Fetal malformation
Ectopic pregnancy	Neonatal or perinatal deaths
Hyperemesis gravidarum	Low birth weight
Preeclampsia	Prematurity
Placental abruption	Neonatal coagulopathy
Anemia	Epilepsy (1-3%)
	Developmental delay and learning disorders

offspring of women with epilepsy compared to 2 to 3 percent for women without epilepsy. These include congenital heart defects, neural tube defects (spina bifida), and cleft lip and palate, as well as urogenital defects such as hypospadias. Neural tube defects are more common with valproic acid and carbamazepine compared to other drugs and can be prevented by folic acid supplementation beginning the month prior to conception and during pregnancy.[28] The risk factors associated with increased incidence of fetal malformation include use of multiple drugs, high doses, family history, folic acid deficiency, and hyperhomocystinemia (Table 18-13).

These defects are related to exposure to antiepileptic drugs (AEDs) in the first trimester, specifically with exposure in the first 4 weeks. Therefore there is no need to alter antiepileptic drug therapy after diagnosis of pregnancy as the period of greatest risk has already passed. In addition it should be stressed that more than 90 percent of pregnancies have no associated significant harmful fetal effects. Generalized tonic-clonic seizures can cause trauma to the mother as well as reduce placental blood flow, resulting in possible fetal injury. These risks should be stressed to the patient as an argument for complying with the AED regimen. The lowest effective dose of AED should be maintained. Individuals on phenytoin, carbamazepine, phenobarbital, or primidone develop vitamin K deficiency and predispose the fetus to neonatal coagulopathy. Vitamin K should be given to the mother in the last 4 weeks of the pregnancy and the baby at birth (1 mg intramuscularly) to prevent this dreaded complication.[44] There is a higher incidence of obstetric and fetal complications in women with epilepsy as well.[26] Breast-feeding is not contraindicated but should be done cautiously by patients taking barbiturates to avoid neonatal sedation and subsequent withdrawal.

Status Epilepticus

Definitions of status epilepticus vary. The classical definition of status epilepticus is seizure activity lasting for more than 30 minutes. Yet most patients with more than 5 minutes of seizure activity or two consecutive seizures

Table 18-13. Antiepileptic Drugs and Their Effects

Drug	TERATOGENIC EFFECTS
Phenytoin	Facial dysmorphism, heart and urogenital defects. Mental retardation and intrauterine growth retardation (Category D)
Phenobarbital	Cardiac defects, facial dysmorphisms, hirsutism (Category D)
Valproic acid	Dysmorphic features, craniofacial defects, neural tube defects, radial aplasia (Category D)
Carbamazepine	Neural tube defects, microcephaly and developmental delay (Category C)
Ethosuximide	Unknown (Category C)
Lamotrigine	Unknown (Category C)
Gabapentin	Unknown (Category C)
Felbamate	Unknown (Category C)
Topiramate	Unknown, limb agenesis in animals (Category C)
Levetiracetam	Unknown, growth retardation, minor skeletal abnormalities in animals (Category C)
Oxcarbazepine	Embryolethality, craniofacial, cardiovascular, and skeletal abnormalities in animals (Category C)
Zonisamide	Embryolethality, craniofacial, cardiovascular and skeletal abnormalities in animals (Category C)
Tiagabine	Unknown (Category C)

Table 18-14. Management of Status Epilepticus

	Time Frame
Resuscitation	0-5 minutes
Airway, breathing, circulation	
Oxygenate	
Initial examination	0-5 minutes
Brief history (especially anticonvulsant therapy)	
Brief physical exam (confirm seizure activity)	
Start IV (preferably 2 IV lines)	
Dextrose strip	
CBC, electrolytes, Ca, Mg, anticonvulsant levels, toxicology panel, renal and liver function	
Initial therapy	0-5 minutes
Lorazepam IV 0.05-0.1 mg/kg (may need to repeat in 20 minutes)	
Thiamine, glucose, or naloxone as indicated	10-20 minutes
Phenytoin or fosphenytoin IV if not contraindicated (15-20/mg/kg of phenytoin or 15-20 mg/kg of phenytoin equivalents [PE] over 20 minutes with ECG and blood pressure monitoring)	
Fosphenytoin is associated with reduced infusion-related adverse effects such as hypotension and arrhythmia and can be given more rapidly than phenytoin (see appropriate text for dosing rate information)	
Further assessment	10-20 minutes
Assess fetal heart tone and institute cardiotocodynamometry	
Neurology consultation	
Obstetric consultation	
Further therapy	30 minutes
Phenobarbital 20 mg/kg IV or midazolam (category D) IV infusion	
Intubate patient	

without regaining consciousness should be treated as having status epilepticus.[45] This medical emergency requires immediate attention in order to avoid complications for the mother and fetus. Table 18-14 outlines typical steps for management of status epilepticus. Intravenous loading doses of anticonvulsants should be calculated using the patient's current weight rather than basing them on absolute dose.[28]

Patients with status epilepticus generally have a history of seizures and are taking medication. If status epilepticus develops as the first seizure, a catastrophic event such as intracranial hemorrhage, tumor, or encephalitis is likely. Status epilepticus increases the risk of miscarriage and fetal demise. Greater seizure intensity and longer duration appear to affect the fetus as well as the mother adversely.

Tumors

The management of intracranial tumors during pregnancy is difficult (Table 18-15). Mass lesions of the CNS may present with a variety of neurologic deficits, systemic complaints, and seizures. Termination of the pregnancy may be indicated in patients with progressive visual loss, signs of uncontrollable rising intracranial pressure, or frequent intractable generalized seizures.[29,30] Delivery complications include decreased cerebral perfusion or herniation because of the significant increases in intracranial pressure, so cesarean section is recommended for intracranial tumors with potential mass effects.[31,32]

Movement Disorders

Movement disorders rarely occur during pregnancy.[33,34] Table 18-16 lists several movement disorders that may be seen in pregnancy. Neurologic consultation is usually not necessary in restless legs syndrome, the most common movement disorder associated with pregnancy.[33,34]

Multiple Sclerosis (MS) and Pregnancy

Multiple sclerosis is a demyelinating disease of the central nervous system that most often has a relapsing remitting

Table 18-15. Brain Tumors

Tumor Type	Symptoms	Diagnostic Evaluation	Indications for Therapy	Therapy
Meningioma	Focal neurological deficits, Seizures	MRI or enhanced CT scan show diffuse enhancing extra-axial lesion	Usually slow growing and therapy can be delayed until after delivery	Surgical excision; radiation for inoperable tumors
Gliomas	Fatigue, nausea, vomiting, headaches, seizures, and focal neurological deficits	MRI, biopsy	Mass effect (vasogenic edema), seizures (high-grade tumors)	Dexamethasone Anticonvulsants, surgical excision
Choriocarcinoma	Sudden-onset focal neurologic deficits, seizures, headache, intracranial hemorrhage, back pain, lower extremity weakness, bladder incontinence	MRI, pelvic ultrasound, serum and CSF chorionic gonadotropin levels with ratio of less than 60 to 1.	Recognition of tumor	Surgical evacuation of tumor, whole brain radiation, chemotherapy
Pituitary adenoma	Headaches, bitemporal visual field loss	MRI, CT scan of the sella, visual fields	Acute or progressive vision loss	Surgical excision, radiation for inoperable tumors

course. Two-thirds of patients are women affected mostly in the childbearing years, therefore the effect of pregnancy on MS is an important issue for all physicians involved in the care of these patients. Clinical features of MS are variable and depend on the location of the lesion. They include visual loss, focal weakness, sensory loss, diplopia, dysarthria, vertigo, ataxia, and bowel or bladder incontinence. The disease also has a variable and unpredictable clinical course. The diagnosis is based on clinical and radiologic features and exclusion of other disorders that may mimic MS (such as systemic lupus erythematosus, CNS vasculitis, neurosarcoidosis, cobalamin deficiency, Lyme disease, and neurosyphilis).

In pregnancy, the likelihood of relapse is significantly reduced. Numerous studies have shown a reduction in relapse frequency during pregnancy with an increase in relapse frequency and severity in the postpartum period.[35–38] Most of the relapses occur in the first 3 to 6 months after delivery. In a small study, postpartum relapses were dramatically reduced in patients with MS by periodic administration of intravenous immune globulin (IVIG).[38] Overall, the pregnancy does not hasten the progression of disease nor does it have a demonstrable effect on the course and outcome of pregnancy. Rates of infant mortality and congenital malformations do not differ from those seen in the general population.

Spinal Cord Injury

Chronic spinal cord injury is associated with numerous issues that require a team approach, including the neurologic specialties, obstetrics, and rehabilitative medicine. Spinal cord-injured patients may go into labor and not have any associated pain, especially if the lesion is above T10; therefore it is recommended that these patients be routinely examined after 28 weeks for cervical effacement.[39,40] Spinal cord injury in itself is not an indication for cesarean section. Important issues include respiratory support for cervical lesions, recognition of autonomic instability (autonomic hyperreflexia or autonomic stress syndrome), prevention and early treatment of urinary tract infections, and prevention of unsupervised delivery. Severe autonomic instability can occur if the lesion is above T5-T6 (i.e., above the level of the splanchnic autonomic nerves); it is characterized by uncontrolled hypertension, throbbing headaches, sweating, and flushed skin. Cardiac arrhythmias can occur during labor or as a result of infection.[39,40] Intracranial hemorrhage can

Table 18-16. Movement Disorders

Syndrome	Symptoms	Causes	Evaluation	Treatment
Restless legs	Crawling achy sensation improved with movement, associated with uncontrolled leg movement during rest and periodic limb movements during sleep	Folate deficiency, iron deficiency, uremia, peripheral vascular disease, arthritis, spinal cord lesions; stress, caffeine, and tricyclic medications can exacerbate symptoms	Serum iron, folate, BUN, creatinine levels; detailed neurologic exam to rule out central lesion	Withdraw from caffeine and tricyclic medications; stress reduction, biofeedback, folate, iron, vitamin E, gabapentin, dopaminergic agents, benzodiazepines
Chorea	Uncontrollable writhing or dance-like movements that may disappear during sleep (Chorea gravidarum is reported to clear following delivery)	Chorea gravidarum, Sydenham's chorea (rheumatic heart disease), systemic lupus erythematosus, medication-induced (neuropsychiatric medications, especially antidopaminergic agents), hyperthyroidism, Wilson's disease, vascular disease, meningovascular syphilis, Huntington's disease, neuroacanthocytosis or adult-onset Tay-Sachs disease	Detailed neurological examination and consultation, slit-lamp exam of eyes, MRI, serum thyroid function tests, ANA, anticardiolipin antibody, lupus anticoagulant, serum copper and ceruloplasmin, FTA red cell morphology for acanthocytes	Benign chorea of pregnancy (chorea gravidarum) usually clears following delivery; cases involving violent movements may cause dehydration, malnutrition, or injury and should be seen by a neurologist for consideration of haloperidol or clonazepam
Dystonia	Posturing caused by increased tone in one or more extremities or neck, focal dystonias may cause spastic dysphonia, blepharospasm, or torticollis	Dopamine-blocking agents, idiopathic torsion dystonia	Detailed neurologic exam and consultation	Levodopa/carbidopa, diphenhydramine, consideration for injection of botulinum toxin A or administration of anticholinergic agents

(*Continues*)

Table 18-16. *(Continued)* Movement Disorders

Syndrome	Symptoms	Causes	Evaluation	Treatment
Essential tremor	Oscillating movement of usually 5 to 10 Hz, accentuated with movement	Familial forms, idiopathic	Detailed neurologic exam	Withdraw of tremor-producing medication: xanthines, sympathomimetics; rarely disabling; in severe cases may wish to consider propranolol, primidone, or clonazepam
Parkinson's tremor	Resting oscillating movement of 3 to 5 Hz; improves with movement; patients also note difficulty initiating movements, hypokinesia, mask-like face, smaller handwriting	Dopamine-blocking agents, vascular disease, idiopathic	Detailed neurologic examination and consultation; MRI for new-onset symptoms	Neurologic consultation

ANA, antinuclear antibody; BUN, blood urea nitrogen; FTA, fluorescent titer antibody.

occur as a result. The use of regional anesthesia is necessary to control blood pressure.

Neuropathy

Most neuropathies in pregnancy are compressive in nature. Table 18-17 lists common compressive neuropathies associated with pregnancy or delivery.[41,42] In general, a new-onset neuropathy requires a detailed neurologic examination to fully localize the lesion and rule out the possibility of a central lesion. Underlying causes of polyneuropathies such as hypothyroidism or diabetes mellitus should also be excluded. Electromyography and nerve conduction studies may not demonstrate abnormalities until after 3 weeks of symptoms, but they are helpful in diagnosis and aid in predicting recovery.[43] Guillain-Barré syndrome (acute inflammatory polyradiculoneuropathy) is an inflammatory demyelinating neuropathy that can occur following an infection or surgery. The incidence is approximately 1.5 per 100,000 individuals and the disease course is unchanged by pregnancy.[44] It presents with subacute to acute progressive ascending paralysis associated with autonomic dysfunction, hyporeflexia, and mild distal sensory loss. Patients can decompensate within hours to ventilatory dependence. The differential diagnosis includes toxic neuropathies, porphyria, vitamin deficiencies (B_{12}, folate), or hypothyroidism. Patients should be monitored closely in the hospital, preferably in the ICU. Early plasma exchange aids in the recovery of neurologic function.[45] Intravenous immunoglobulins may be an alternative to plasma exchange.[46] Pregnant women with Guillain-Barré syndrome may require earlier ventilatory support due to loss of functional reserve capacity.[42] Patients more than 24 weeks pregnant should be positioned in the left lateral decubitus position to avoid compression of the inferior vena cava.

Lumbosacral plexopathies are most commonly associated with direct compression, although invasive tumor such as choriocarcinoma should be considered. A complete obstetric examination including pelvic ultrasound may aid in the identification of invasive tumor.

Women with preexisting peripheral neuropathies, especially diabetes, can present with several autonomic symptoms, such as orthostatic hypotension or gastroparesis.[47] Pregnancy does not appear to change the course of the diabetic neuropathy; control of glucose is the primary therapy.

Table 18-17. Compressive Neuropathies in Pregnancy

Nerve	Symptoms	Treatment
Facial (Bell's palsy)	Facial weakness, Possible hyperacusis, Loss of taste, dull ache near the ear	Protect the eye from drying and damage
Median (carpal tunnel syndrome)	Thumb, index, and long finger numbness, wrist and shoulder pain especially at night	Wrist splinting, local injection of corticosteroids, surgical release in refractory cases with significant neurologic deficits
Lateral femoral cutaneous (meralgia paresthetica)	Hyperasthesia, numbness, and pain over the lateral aspect of the thigh	Local injection of corticosteroids
Femoral	Weakness of knee extension, anterior thigh paresthesia	Physical therapy for aid with gait
Obturator	Weakness of adduction of the thigh, pain of the medial thigh and groin	Physical therapy, nerve block for severe pain
Lumbosacral plexus or sciatic (tibial or peroneal portions)	Weakness of foot dorsiflexion or plantar flexion, low back or shooting pain in posterior leg	Physical therapy, foot orthosis (if onset is during delivery, cesarean section may be considered)
Peroneal (at the fibular head)	Foot drop or weakness of dorsiflexion of the foot, numbness of anterior lateral lower leg and dorsum of the foot	Physical therapy, Foot orthosis
Pudendal	Urinary incontinence, possible pelvic pain	

Myasthenia Gravis

Myasthenia gravis is characterized by fatigable strength that causes fluctuating symptoms, especially of the extraocular, facial, bulbar, and limb muscles. A polyclonal antibody directed toward the nicotinic acetylcholine receptor and attenuating neuromuscular transmission produces this autoimmune disorder. Acetylcholinesterase inhibitors such as pyridostigmine increase synaptic acetylcholine concentrations and thus diminish the symptoms related to fewer functional acetylcholine receptors. This disorder affects approximately 1 in 10,000 individuals.[48,49] The disease is more likely to affect women in the third decade, whereas men are more likely to be affected after the fifth decade.[48,49] The diagnosis of myasthenia gravis should be suggested by the history and physical examination. Intravenous edrophonium (10 mg) will often improve the objective clinical findings for a few minutes. Repetitive nerve stimulation during nerve conduction study may provide electrophysiologic evidence of myasthenia gravis; occasionally patients will need single-fiber electromyography studies to demonstrate this neuromuscular junction abnormality.[50] Approximately 80 percent of patients will have antibodies to the acetylcholine receptor, which can be detected on serologic examination.[51]

Pregnant women with myasthenia gravis are at risk for myasthenic or cholinergic crisis during pregnancy and postpartum (Table 18-18).[52] All patients with myasthenia gravis should be closely followed by a neurologist throughout their pregnancies. Approximately one-third of patients are unchanged during pregnancy, one-third improve, and one-third become worse.[51] Mortality rates for myasthenic mothers have been estimated at between 2 and 10 percent.[50]

Myasthenic crises or exacerbations are characterized by progressive weakness and fatigability, which may become less responsive to the anticholinesterase therapy.[52] Cholinergic crisis is also characterized by progressive weakness, fasciculations, and increased salivation, as well as by gastrointestinal hypermobility (vomiting, diarrhea, and abdominal cramping). Severe exacerbations or

Table 18-18. Myasthenia in Pregnancy

	Complications Related to Myasthenia Gravis
During pregnancy	Myasthenic crisis Cholinergic crisis Medication-induced exacerbation
During delivery	Fatigability Increased weakness secondary to anesthetics Medication-induced weakness
Breast-feeding	Transfer of medication in milk Transfer of antibodies in milk (both of these are of unknown significance)
Postpartum	Neonatal myasthenia Hemorrhage Myasthenic crisis Cholinergic crisis Medication-induced exacerbation

cholinergic crises can lead to respiratory failure. If intubation is indicated, etomidate is the preferred induction agent. Depolarizing and nondepolarizing neuromuscular blocking agents can result in prolonged paralysis.

Myasthenic exacerbations require acute therapy to reduce antibody production. Emergent therapies include plasma exchange or intravenous immune globulin.[53,54] Patients also need to be educated about the possible side effects of therapies for myasthenia gravis, such as glucocorticoids, azathioprine, cyclosporine, plasma exchange, intravenous immune globulin, and thymectomy.[49,55]

Cholinergic crisis results from overmedication with anticholinesterase inhibitors. Patients will require supportive care, IV atropine for symptomatic bradycardia, and a reduction of medication. Table 18-19 lists medications that can interfere with neuromuscular transmission.[56]

Delivery also carries risks for the myasthenic patient. The uterus is composed of smooth muscle, which does not utilize nicotinic receptors. However, the use of striated muscle in the second stage of labor may cause fatigue. Addition of an acetylcholinesterase inhibitor such as pyridostigmine may be helpful. Care should be taken to avoid the possibility of cholinergic crisis from an excess of acetylcholinesterase inhibitor, which can also produce weakness. During delivery, these medications should be given either intravenously or intramuscularly. Forceps delivery or cesarean section should be considered early if the myasthenic patient starts to fatigue, but she should be given the opportunity to deliver vaginally if otherwise appropriate.[53] Anesthesia during the delivery should be used under close supervision. Medications such as benzodiazepines and narcotics may reduce the respiratory compensatory mechanism. Regional anesthesia is a safe method, and epidural anesthesia has been used successfully.[53] General anesthesia may be useful in patients undergoing cesarean section, especially patients with respiratory or bulbar symptoms who may need extra time to regain their respiratory competence and ventilatory independence following neuromuscular blockade.[57]

Neonatal myasthenia gravis has been reported in approximately 10 percent of infants born to myasthenic mothers.[52,53] Passive transmission of the antibod-

Table 18-19. Medications That Interfere with Neuromuscular Transmission

Aminoglycosides
Tetracycline
Narcotics
Lidocaine and other local anesthetics
Lithium
Phenothiazines
Magnesium sulfate
Calcium-channel blockers
Beta-blockers
Quinidine
Quinine
Depolarizing and nondepolarizing neuromuscular blocking agents

ies through the placenta accounts for development of the clinical syndrome.[58] Infants usually present with symptoms within 24 hours, but some may not show symptoms for 72 hours. These infants may demonstrate generalized weakness, poor suckling, meager cry, or respiratory distress. They require supportive care, and their condition should improve over the ensuing 3 to 4 weeks. Neonatal myasthenia gravis does not predict the subsequent development of myasthenia as an adult.[59]

Breast-feeding should be discussed with the patient. Antibodies and acetylcholinesterase inhibitors may be passed in the breast milk and thus affect the infant, but several mothers at our center have successfully breast-fed.[52] Mothers who are in an exacerbation have high antibody titers, and those who take large doses of medications may wish to avoid breast-feeding.

Myopathy

Preexisting myopathies may have a significant effect on the pregnancy and may result in a variety of clinical problems.[55,61,62] Pertinent findings on neurologic examination are proximal muscle weakness, intact deep tendon reflexes, and no sensory deficits. The most treatable myopathies in adults are inflammatory in nature. Inflammatory myopathies such as polymyositis and dermatomyositis attack striated and cardiac muscle. These disorders are associated with a variety of autoimmune, malignant, and connective tissue disorders. New-onset disease can occur at any time but is more common in the first trimester. It is usually active throughout the pregnancy and remission may occur following delivery.[55] Preexisting disease is usually unaffected by the pregnancy, but it may flare, especially in the third trimester. Little is known about pregnancy outcome, but in one report on 10 pregnancies in 7 women with polymyositis, there was a 60 percent rate of spontaneous abortion or fetal demise.[63] The benefit of treatment should be weighed against the risk. Patients with mild disease may not require therapy, whereas those with more aggressive disease should be considered for corticosteroid therapy or plasma exchange.[42,60,63] Patients should be closely co-managed by a neurologist and obstetrician during pregnancy.

Muscle Cramps

Muscle cramps are relatively common during pregnancy. They usually occur the night following exercise, fatigue, or dehydration. Rarely cramps indicate an underlying problem such as hypothyroidism, uremia, electrolyte imbalance, amyotrophic lateral sclerosis, or anterior horn cell disease such as polio, radiculopathy, or myopathy. Cramps are best treated with stretching of the affected muscle.[42] Medications are best avoided.

Connective Tissue Disorders in Pregnancy

Systemic lupus erythematosus is a disorder predominantly affecting women of childbearing age. Neurologic complications occur in 50 percent of all patients with lupus, including seizures (18 to 70 percent), occlusive infarcts (32 to 43 percent), intracerebral hemorrhage (10 to 40 percent), encephalopathy (4 to 20 percent), myelopathy (2 to 8 percent), headaches (5 to 16 percent), and cranial and peripheral nerve palsies (5 to 10 percent).[64–66] The pathogenesis of this spectrum of disorders is poorly understood.

Lupus is often associated with anticardiolipin antibodies and lupus anticoagulant.[65] These antibodies occur in about 50 percent of patients with lupus and predispose to recurrent venous or arterial thrombosis within and outside the CNS.[65,66] These antibodies are also associated with fetal heart block, stillbirth, and recurrent spontaneous abortions related to placental infarction. Frequently, these antibodies occur independently without lupus, but with the same clinical profile. Recent data indicate that these patients require aggressive anticoagulation to prevent recurrent thromboses. Intravenous immune globulin may be beneficial as well.

Data on the incidence of relapses during pregnancy are conflicting. The presence of antiphospholipid antibodies, a previous history of second-trimester abortion, and impaired renal function are poor prognostic indicators.[64] There is solid evidence now that patients with antiphospholipid antibodies require long-term anticoagulation.[65,66] Obstetric, neurologic, and rheumatologic consultation is essential for managing these very complicated patients. Other therapeutic options for CNS as well as peripheral disease include glucocorticoids, intravenous immune globulins, plasma exchange, azathioprine, and cyclophosphamide.

Acknowledgments

The authors extend their thanks to Dr. Mauricio Castillo, who supplied the MRI and CT scan images for this chapter and Jody Hamilton for preparation of this manuscript.

REFERENCES

1. Feldman E (ed): *Current Diagnosis in Neurology.* St. Louis: Mosby, 1994.
2. Donaldson JO, Lee NS: Arterial and venous stroke associated with pregnancy. *Neurol Clin* 12:583, 1994.

3. Sharshar T, Lamy C, Mas JL: Incidence and causes of strokes associated with pregnancy and puerperium. A study in public hospitals of Ile de France. *Stroke* 26:930–936, 1995.
4. Mas JL, Lamy C: Stroke in pregnancy and the puerperium. *J Neurol* 245:305–313, 1998.
5. Jaigoban C, Silver F: Stroke and pregnancy. *Stroke* 31:2948–2951, 2000.
6. Wilterdink JL, Easton JD: *Cerebral Ischemia in Neurologic Complications of Pregnancy.* New York: Raven Press, 1994, pp 1–23.
7. Kostenas A, Roth T, Hershey B, Yi JK: Imaging neurologic complications of pregnancy and puerperium. *Acad Radiol* 6:243–252, 1999.
8. Modi M, Modi G: Postpartum angiopathy in a patient with chronic migraine with aura. *Headache* 40:677–681, 2000.
9. Ginsberg J, Hirsch J: Use of antithrombotic agents during pregnancy. Anticoagulation in pregnancy and puerperium. *Chest* 102(Suppl):385–390, 1992.
10. Working Group of the Obstetric Medicine Group of Australia: Anticoagulation in pregnancy and the puerperium. *Medical Journal of Australia* 175: 258–263, 2001.
11. Einhaupl KM, Villringer A, Meister W, et al: Heparin treatment in sinus venous thrombosis. *Lancet* 338:597–600, 1991.
12. Terhaar MF, Kaut K: Perinatal superior sagittal sinus venous thrombosis. *J Perinat Neonat Nurs* 7:35, 1993.
13. Dias MS, Selchar LN: Intracranial hemorrhage from aneurysms and arteriovenous malformations during pregnancy and the puerperium. *Neurosurgery* 27:855, 1990.
14. Dias MS: Neurovascular emergencies in pregnancy. *Clin Obstet Gynecol* 37:337–354, 1994.
15. Stoodley M, Macdonald L, Weir B: Pregnancy and intracranial aneurysms. *Neurosurg Clin North Am* 9:540–556, 1998.
16. Fox MW, Harms RW, Davis D: Selected neurologic complications of pregnancy. *Mayo Clin Proc* 65:1595, 1990.
17. Kaplan PW, Repke JT: Eclampsia. *Neurol Clin* 12:565, 1994.
18. Koch S, Rabinstein A, Falcone S, Forteza A: Diffusion weighted imaging shows cytotoxic and vasogenic edema in eclampsia. *AJNR Am J Neuroradiol* 22:1068–1071, 2001.
19. Jordan BD: Maternal head trauma during pregnancy. *Adv Neurol* 64:131, 1994.
20. Kuhlmann RS, Cruikshank DP: Maternal trauma during pregnancy. *Clin Obstet Gynecol* 37:274, 1994.
21. Buschsbaum HJ, Cruikshank DP: Postmortem cesarean section, in Buschbaum HJ (ed): *Trauma in Pregnancy.* Philadelphia: Saunders, 1979, pp 236–249.
22. Yerby M, Devinsky O: Epilepsy and pregnancy, in Devinsky O, Feldman E, Hainline B (eds): *Neurologic Complications of Pregnancy.* New York: Raven Press, 1994, pp 45–63.
23. Delgado-Escueta AV, Janz D: Consensus guidelines: Preconception counseling, management and care of the pregnant woman with epilepsy. *Neurology* 42(Suppl 5):149, 1992.
24. Hiilesmaa VK: Pregnancy and birth in women with epilepsy. *Neurology* 42(Suppl 5):8, 1992.
25. Treiman DM: Current treatment strategies in selected situations in epilepsy. *Epilepsia* 34(Suppl 5):S17, 1993.
26. Zahn CA, Morrell M, Collins SJ, Labiner DM, Yerby M: Management issues for women with epilepsy. *Neurology* 51: 949–956, 1998.
27. Nulman I, Laslo D, Koren G: Treatment of epilepsy in pregnancy. *Drugs* 57:535–544, 1999.
28. Jagoda A, Riggio S: Emergency department approach to managing seizures in pregnancy. *Ann Emerg Med* 20:80, 1991.
29. DeAngelis LM: Central nervous system neoplasms in pregnancy, in Devinsky O, Feldman E, Hainline B (eds): *Neurologic Complications of Pregnancy.* New York: Raven Press, 1994, pp 139–152.
30. Weinreb HJ: Demyelinating and neoplastic diseases in pregnancy. *Neurol Clin* 12:509, 1994.
31. Finfer SR: Management of labour and delivery in patients with intracranial neoplasms. *Br J Anaesth* 67:784, 1991.
32. Prager D, Braunstein GD: Pituitary disorders in pregnancy, in Peterson LJ, Peterson CM (eds): *Endocrine Disorders in Pregnancy. Endocr Metab Clin North Am* 24:1, 1995.
33. Rogers JD, Fahn S: Movement disorders and pregnancy, in Devinsky O, Feldman E, Hainline B (eds): *Neurologic Complications of Pregnancy.* New York: Raven Press, 1994, pp 163–178.
34. Damek DM, Shuster E: Pregnancy and movement. *Mayo Clin Proc* 72: 977–989, 1997.
35. Birk K, Ford C, Smeltzer S, et al: The clinical course of multiple sclerosis during pregnancy and puerperium. *Arch Neurol* 47:738, 1990.
36. Poser S, Poser W: Multiple sclerosis and gestation. *Neurology* 33:1422, 1983.
37. Frith JA, McLeod JG: Pregnancy and multiple sclerosis. *J Neurol Neurosurg Psychiatry* 51:495, 1988.
38. Orveito R, Achiron R, Rotstein Z, et al: Pregnancy and multiple sclerosis. A 2 year experience. *Eur J Obstet Gynecol Rep Biol* 82:191–194, 1999.
39. Verduyn WH: Spinal cord injured women, pregnancy and delivery. *Paraplegia* 24:231, 1986.
40. Greenspoon JS, Paul RH: Paraplegia and quadriplegia: Special considerations during pregnancy and labor and delivery. *Am J Obstet Gynecol* 155:738, 1986.
41. Beric A: Peripheral nerve disorders in pregnancy, in Devinsky O, Feldman E, Hainline B (eds): *Neurologic Complications of Pregnancy.* New York: Raven Press, 1994, pp 179–192.
42. Rosenbaum RB, Donaldson JO: Peripheral nerve and neuromuscular disorders. *Neurol Clin* 12:461, 1994.
43. Turgut F, Cetanishan M, Turgut M, Bolukbasi O: The management of carpal tunnel syndrome in pregnancy. *J Clin Neurosci* 8:332–334, 2001.
44. Rodin A, Ferner R, Russell R: Guillain-Barré syndrome in pregnancy and the puerperium. *J Obstet Gynaecol* 9:39, 1988.
45. The Guillain-Barré Syndrome Study Group: Plasma-exchange and acute Guillain-Barré syndrome. *Neurology* 35:1096, 1985.
46. Kleyweg RP, van der Meche Meulstee J: Treatment of

Guillain-Barré syndrome with high-dose gamma globulin. *Neurology* 38:1639, 1988.

47. Steel JM: Autonomic neuropathy in pregnancy. *Diabetes Care* 12:170, 1989.
48. Kurtzke JF: Epidemiology of myasthenia gravis. *Adv Neurol* 19:545, 1978.
49. Sanders D, Howard J: Disorders of neuromuscular transmission, in Bradley WG, Daroff RB, Fenichel GM, Marsden CD (eds): *Neurologic Diseases.* Boston: Butterworth Heinemann, 1996, pp 1983–2002.
50. Sanders DB, Howard JF, Johns TR: Single fiber electromyography in myasthenia gravis. *Neurology* 29:68, 1979.
51. Lindstrom J, Shelton D, Fujii Y: Myasthenia gravis. *Adv Immunol* 42:233, 1988.
52. Plauche WC: Myasthenia gravis in mothers and their newborns. *Clin Obstet Gynaecol* 34:82, 1991.
53. Mitchell PJ, Bebbington M: Myasthenia gravis in pregnancy. *Obstet Gynecol* 80:178, 1992.
54. Esaon G, Landgraf F: Experience with intravenous immunoglobulin in myasthenia gravis: A review. *J Neurol Neurosurg Psychiatry* 57(Suppl):55, 1994.
55. Gilchrist JM: Muscle disease in the pregnant woman, in Devinsky O, Feldman E, Hainline B (eds): *Neurologic Complications of Pregnancy.* New York: Raven Press, 1994, pp 197–201.
56. Howard J: Adverse drug effects in neuromuscular transmission. *Semin Neurol* 10:89, 1990.
57. Baraka A: Anesthesia and myasthenia gravis. *Can J Anaesth* 39:476, 1992.
58. Breener T, Shahin R, Steiner I, Abramsky O: Presence of antiacetylcholine receptor antibody in human milk: Possible correlation with neonatal myasthenia gravis. *Autoimmunity* 12:315, 1992.
59. Ahlsten G, Lefvert AK, Osterman PO, et al: Follow-up study of muscle function in children of mothers with myasthenia gravis during pregnancy. *J Child Neurol* 7:264, 1992.
60. Varner M: Autoimmune disorders and pregnancy. *Semin Perinatol* 15:238, 1991.
61. Ville Y, Barbet JP, Pomidou A, et al: Limb girdle dystrophy and pregnancy: A case report. *J Gynecol Obstet Biol Reprod* 20:973, 1991.
62. Jaffe R, Mock M, Abramowitz J, Ben-Aderet N: Myotonic dystrophy and pregnancy: A review. *Obstet Gynecol Surv* 41:272, 1986.
63. Gutierrez G, Dagnino R, Mintz G: Polymyositis/dermatomyositis and pregnancy. *Arthritis Rheum* 27:291, 1984.
64. Out HJ, Bruinse HW, Christiaens GC, et al. A prospective, controlled multicenter study on the obstetric risks of pregnant women with antiphospholipid antibody. *Am J Obstet Gynecol* 167:26, 1992.
65. Futrell N, Millikan C: Neurologic disorders of pregnancy: Connective tissue disorders. *Neurol Clin* 12:520, 1994.
66. Wong KL, Chan FY, Lee CP: Outcome of pregnancy in patients with systemic lupus erythematosus. *Arch Intern Med* 151:269, 1991.

19

Mental Disorders in Pregnancy and the Postpartum Period

Diana L. Dell
Diana O. Perkins
Linda M. Nicholas

KEY POINTS

- Depressed mood and anxiety are common conditions in pregnancy and rates increase during the postpartum period.
- Medication for the treatment of moderate-to-severe anxiety or depressive symptoms should not be withheld because of pregnancy or lactation.
- Mania and psychosis pose more risk to both the fetus and neonate, and treatment for these conditions is more complex during pregnancy and lactation.
- Grief reactions accompany pregnancy loss at any stage of development and may precipitate psychiatric symptoms that require treatment.
- Substance abuse during pregnancy may have longstanding neurobehavioral implications for infants and children.

This chapter provides an overview of the psychiatric disorders that can be exacerbated by, or can affect, pregnancy. Many psychiatric medications have fetal effects. It is important to understand the scope of disorders, the treatment options in pregnancy, and the disease features that warrant psychiatric referral.

The medical literature has often characterized a woman's pregnancy year as an emotionally quiet time, emphasizing its potential joys. As a result, psychiatric complications associated with pregnancy and the postpartum period are among the most underdiagnosed pregnancy-associated complications in modern obstetrics. Recognition and treatment of psychiatric illness are essential for the proper care of pregnant and postpartum women.

MOOD DISORDERS

Description

The word *depression* can describe a wide range of conditions in pregnant as well as nonpregnant women. Depressed mood may reflect a normal reaction to loss or bereavement. It may occur in response to adverse life events over which one has no control. It may also reflect a major depressive disorder, which is a serious but treatable condition. Therefore, the differential diagnosis of depressed mood is essential to the appropriate management and protection of the patient.

Major Depressive Disorder

An episode of major depression may occur in the context of either major depressive disorder or bipolar disorder. It may develop in response to stressful life events or in the absence of a precipitating event. Symptoms reflect disturbance of biological functions, cognitive functions, and psychological well-being (Table 19-1). During an episode of major depression, behaviors governed by circadian rhythms—such as sleep, appetite, and energy level—are frequently disturbed. Depressed patients may have difficulty falling asleep; they may also experience early morning awakening or an increased need for sleep. Patients may report increased fatigue regardless of time spent sleeping. Changes related to eating include loss of appetite and weight; in severe cases, patients may stop eating and drinking altogether. A subset of depressed patients may report symptoms of increased appetite and excessive weight gain. While not considered diagnostic of a major depression, gastrointestinal pain, bloating, belching, and constipation are also common symptoms in patients with major depression.

Cognitive changes generally affect attention and concentration. Patients complain of difficulty in organizing tasks, inability to complete assigned duties, and lack of mental energy. Thought content often reflects a sustained low mood, with pessimistic ideation about oneself, the world, and the future. A patient may show cognitive and motor slowing as well.

An impaired sense of psychological well-being may be reflected in pervasive worry or guilt about present or past events. A pervasive sense of worthlessness may reach delusional intensity. Active concerns about one's physical health are common, which may reflect a misunder-

Table 19-1. Criteria for Major Depressive Episode

A. Five (or more) of the following symptoms have been present during the same 2-week period, nearly every day, and represent a change from previous functioning; at least one of the symptoms is either (1) depressed mood or (2) loss of interest or pleasure.

1. Depressed mood most of the day, by subjective report (e.g., feels sad or empty) or observation made by others (e.g., appears tearful). *Note:* In children and adolescents, can be irritable mood.
2. Markedly diminished interest or pleasure in all, or almost all, activities most of the day, by subjective report or observation.

and 3 or 4 of the following, experienced nearly every day.

3. Significant weight loss when not dieting or weight gain (e.g., a change of more than 5% of body weight in a month) or decrease or increase in appetite.
4. Insomnia or hypersomnia.
5. Psychomotor agitation or retardation (observable by others, not merely subjective feelings of restlessness or being slowed down).
6. Fatigue or loss of energy.
7. Feelings of worthlessness or excessive or inappropriate guilt (which may be delusional) (not merely self-reproach or guilt about being sick).
8. Diminished ability to think or concentrate, or indecisiveness (either by subjective account or as observed by others).
9. Recurrent thoughts of death (not just fear of dying), recurrent suicidal ideation without a specific plan, or a suicide attempt or a specific plan for committing suicide.

B. The symptoms do not meet criteria for a mixed episode.

C. The symptoms cause clinically significant distress or impairment in social, occupational, or other important areas of functioning.

D. The symptoms are not due to the direct physiologic effects of substance abuse, medication, or a general medical condition.

E. The symptoms are not better accounted for by bereavement, the symptoms persist for longer than 2 months, or are characterized by marked functional impairment, morbid preoccupation with worthlessness, suicidal ideation, psychotic symptoms, or psychomotor retardation.

Note: Do not include symptoms that are clearly due to a general medical condition or mood-incongruent delusions or hallucinations.

Source: American Psychiatric Association,[1] with permission.

standing of the biological changes that occur with major depression. Patients with major depressive disorder always complain of a dysphoric mood (e.g., feeling "low," "down," "blue"), decreased interest in their usual activities, or inability to experience pleasure. This decline in interest often includes decreased interest in sexual activity. Importantly, thoughts about death or suicide occur frequently in major depressive disorder.

Severe major depressive disorder may also be associated with psychotic symptoms such as hallucinations or paranoid ideation. Psychotic symptoms may be the presenting feature of a major depressive illness or may be symptomatic of other medical conditions, as discussed below. These symptoms usually represent a medical emergency, often requiring immediate hospitalization.

Bipolar Disorder

Bipolar disorder is evidenced by episodes of mania as well as symptoms of major depression. Mania is characterized by an expansive, elevated, elated, euphoric, or irritable mood. Cognitively, the patient experiences racing thoughts, flight of ideas, inflated self-esteem, grandiosity, distractibility, and sometimes delusions or hallucinations. His or her behavior may be marked by increased activity, excessive spending, pressured speech, intrusiveness, indiscretion, sexual promiscuity, and/or poor judgment. The patient often has decreased physical complaints, a decreased need for sleep, and increased energy. Hypomania is a milder form of these symptoms that, although less associated with impaired function, can also be quite dis-

Table 19-2. Diagnostic Criteria for Adjustment Disorder

A. The development of emotional or behavioral symptoms in response to an identifiable stressor(s) occurring within 3 months of the onset of the stressor(s).

B. These symptoms or behaviors are clinically significant as evidenced by either of the following:

1. Marked distress that is in excess of what would be expected from exposure to the stressor
2. Significant impairment in social or occupational (academic) functioning

C. The stress-related disturbance does not meet the criteria for another specific axis I disorder and is not merely an exacerbation of a preexisting axis I or axis II disorder.

D. The symptoms do not represent bereavement.

E. Once the stressor (or its consequences) has terminated, the symptoms do not persist for more than an additional 6 months.

Specify:

Acute: If the disturbance lasts less than 6 months
Chronic: If the disturbance lasts for 6 months or longer

Source: American Psychiatric Association,[1] with permission.

ruptive. Treatment options for mania are discussed under treatment of psychotic disorders.

Adjustment Disorders

In modern psychiatry, disorders are defined by the scope, severity, and longevity of symptoms. At times a patient who is overwhelmed by a stressful life event may develop some of the characteristic symptoms of a major depression (e.g., depressed mood, trouble falling asleep) without meeting the full criteria. Here, a diagnosis of adjustment disorder with depressed mood may be more appropriate.[1] The diagnostic criteria for adjustment disorder are included in Table 19-2. Major depressive disorder is distinguished from adjustment disorder by (1) the number and severity of symptoms and (2) the fact that adjustment disorder is always a reaction to stressful life events, whereas major depressive disorder often occurs without a precipitating life event.

Bereavement

In response to loss or bereavement, patients may experience symptoms similar to those of a major depressive episode. Symptoms such as loss of appetite and insomnia may become severe, interfering with function. Normal grief reactions usually improve with time. When symptoms persist longer than 2 months, a major depression may have developed, and antidepressant treatment must be considered. Cultural values often serve to interpret "normality" for the duration and intensity of these symptoms.

NORMAL ADJUSTMENT TO PREGNANCY

The physical adjustment to the hormonal and physical changes associated with pregnancy may include fluctuations of mood, including sadness, unexplained tearfulness, or irritability. The pregnant patient may express ambivalence about the changes pregnancy has made in her life. She may experience grief over the anticipated loss of her usual lifestyle and independence. These experiences are not pathologic but may be disruptive. Counseling to explore the normal change in mood is often helpful to reassure the pregnant woman.

EPIDEMIOLOGY OF MOOD DISORDERS IN PREGNANCY

Depression is the most common psychiatric disorder among reproductive-age women. Lifetime prevalence in the United States is between 9 and 20 percent.[2] Persons between the ages of 25 and 44 are at greatest risk, and rates for women are twice as high as those for men.[3]

The incidence of depression during pregnancy mirrors that in the general female population. Circumstances that may correlate with increased risk for depressive illness during pregnancy include a previous history of depressive illness, a positive family history, comorbid psychiatric diagnosis, development of a high-risk pregnancy, detection of a fetal anomaly, prior pregnancy loss, inadequate social support, inadequate finances, a changing relationship with spouse and/or mother, and multiple changes in

Table 19-3. Screening Questions for Major Depressive Disorder and Suicidality

For depressed mood:
Have you been feeling depressed or down most of the day, nearly every day?
If yes: Has that lasted for as long as 2 weeks?
Have you been a lot less interested in most things?
Are things a lot less enjoyable than they used to be? (Are things as much fun as they used to be?)
If yes: Has that lasted for as long as 2 weeks?
For suicidality:
Have things been so bad that you have been thinking you would be better off dead? Have you thought of actually killing yourself?
If yes: Have you thought of how you might kill yourself?

Source: First et al,[41] with permission.

life events.[4] The period of greatest risk for major depression is during the first 9 weeks after delivery.[5]

Risk of adjustment disorders may also be increased during pregnancy. Childbearing is a stressful life event for most women. Even when pregnancy is viewed as a positive, desired event, major life adjustments will be required throughout the pregnancy and postpartum period. Early identification and intervention in a woman experiencing an adjustment disorder may prevent the development of major depressive disorder.

ASSESSMENT OF DEPRESSIVE SYMPTOMS IN PREGNANCY

Complicating the diagnosis of major depression during pregnancy is the fact that many symptoms of major depression—such as trouble sleeping, fatigue, irritability, change in appetite, excessive nausea and vomiting, and poor concentration—are also common to the physical burden of pregnancy. The presence of any of these symptoms should prompt the clinician to inquire about other depressive symptoms. In particular, when a woman fails to meet the expected weight gain during pregnancy, major depressive disorder should be considered in the differential diagnosis. Table 19-3 gives examples of brief screening questions useful in assessing the hallmark symptoms of depressed mood. Screening is important because often, a woman may be unwilling to spontaneously discuss depressive symptoms with the physician. A positive response to any of the questions in Table 19-3 warrants a more careful evaluation. When a major depression occurs during pregnancy, the most serious emergency concern that must be assessed is suicide risk.[4]

Medical conditions associated with depressive symptoms include thyroid disease, anemia, vitamin B_{12} deficiency, folate deficiency, autoimmune disease, and substance abuse disorders. Physical examination and appropriate laboratory studies will rule out most of these causes of depressive symptoms (Table 19-4).

Women with a past history of major depressive disorder or mania are at high risk for recurrence of symptoms during the postpartum period. If this history is elicited, screening is important to identify symptoms early.

DEPRESSIVE ILLNESS IN THE POSTPARTUM PERIOD

Postpartum Blues

The postpartum period may be characterized by mild subjective depression, affective lability, irritability, anxiety, sleeplessness, and fatigue, often beginning on the third or fourth postpartum day. These symptoms usually remit within 1 to 2 days and may recur over the first few postpartum weeks. Brief supportive interventions to assess the patient's ability to cope with the demands of parenting and the adequacy of her support system usually suffice.

Table 19-4. Laboratory Evaluation of Depressive Symptoms

Thyroid-stimulating hormone
Thyroid antibodies
Complete blood count
Level of vitamin B_{12}
Level of folate
Venereal Disease Research Laboratory testing (VDRL)
Urine toxicology screen
Serum chemistry (including liver and renal function)
Human immunodeficiency virus testing

Postpartum Depression

In contrast to postpartum blues, major depressive disorder with onset during the puerperium is a much more serious illness, with major implications for both mother and infant. The exact prevalence of postpartum depression is difficult to define since recent studies have found similar rates of depression in childbearing women and nonchildbearing controls.[6] It appears that in women with biological vulnerability to major depression, however, the postpartum period is a particularly high-risk period for emergence of symptoms. The onset of depressive symptoms in childbearing women is strongly clustered within the first 9 weeks postpartum.[5] Women with a history of major depression or alcohol dependence prior to pregnancy are at particularly high risk of developing postpartum depression. In one study, 24 percent of women with a past major depression developed a postpartum major depression, compared with only 3 percent of women with no prior history.[5]

Grief Responses to Pregnancy Loss

Grieving may be intense after a spontaneous abortion or stillbirth, and is similar to the grieving process that follows the loss of a child. The normal process of bereavement may take up to 2 years to resolve. Abnormalities of bereavement may involve delayed onset of grief, symptoms that are more intense than usually encountered, prolonged symptoms, or "getting stuck" in one of the stages. The process of bereavement is more difficult when death is unexpected,[7] as typically occurs with spontaneous abortion. It is also more difficult when the pregnancy was surrounded by marked ambivalence or when there are unresolved issues related to the events surrounding the pregnancy loss. Women who have experienced pregnancy loss have higher rates of depression, anxiety, and somatization during the first 6 months, compared to women who have given birth to live infants.[8] Support groups have been widely utilized and appear to be among the most helpful modalities for patients and their partners.

When first told of the fetal death or major fetal anomaly, many parents experience shock and emotional numbing. They may express an unrealistic sense that "this is not really happening" and respond with denial and disbelief. If the obstetric condition is not an emergency, it can be very important at this stage to allow parents time to make an initial accommodation to their loss. They should be encouraged to make as many choices about the proposed obstetric intervention as feasible. This restores some sense of control in a situation in which the parents may feel out of control. Parents should be supported if they wish to see the products of conception after evacuation of the uterus. They should be encouraged to see and hold the stillborn infant after delivery; this is the only time they will ever have with their child. Seeing and holding it facilitates appropriate grieving by letting the parents claim the infant and establishing the reality of the loss. The options of pastoral care and emergency grief counseling should be offered in the emergency department. Information for continued counseling should be provided after discharge because feelings of guilt, hostility, and anger may develop and can be effectively treated with counseling.[9]

Support groups of other patients and partners who have experienced perinatal loss are especially helpful.

Psychiatric Complications of Unplanned Pregnancy and Induced Abortion

An unwanted or mistimed pregnancy may precipitate an emotional crisis for the mother. Especially for the adolescent who becomes pregnant, issues relating to the discussion of sexuality with her parents, deciding whether to abort or carry the fetus, and the limited availability of reproductive services may result in debilitating ambivalence, disturbances of sleep or appetite, and suicide.[10]

Unplanned pregnancies are often more stressful than planned ones and pose a greater risk of an adverse outcome. For example, an unwanted pregnancy may lead to economic hardships. Often, the mother may delay receiving prenatal care and may not be compliant with medical recommendations. In particular, the fetus may be more likely to be exposed to harmful substances like tobacco and alcohol. If these feelings remain unresolved, the child of an unwanted pregnancy, as distinguished from a mistimed one, is at greater risk of being born at a low birth weight, of dying within its first year of life, of being abused, and of not receiving sufficient resources for healthy development.[10]

Patients are at higher risk for depressive symptoms (usually as part of an adjustment disorder) following induced abortion if they (1) were pressured or coerced into abortion, (2) had marked ambivalence about their decision, (3) have limited social support, and (4) have had prior psychiatric illness.[11]

Treatment of Major Depression During Pregnancy and Lactation

Issues with regard to treatment of the pregnant woman with major depression are centered around a complicated risk-benefit analysis. The clinician must consider the potential risk of the therapeutic modality to the fetus versus the risks to both the mother and fetus when the psychiatric disorder goes untreated.[4]

The most significant risks of untreated major depressive disorder include suicide, nutritional impairment secondary to disturbed appetite, and neglect of self-care, including poor compliance with prenatal and postpartum medical care. During the postpartum period, a woman with a major depression is at increased risk for neglect of her infant. In addition, major depression during pregnancy may have negative behavioral effects on the newborn, especially in causing neonatal irritability.[12] These are potentially serious and life-threatening sequelae that necessitate careful evaluation and appropriate intervention.

Treatment is usually done in an outpatient setting, although admission is needed when serious suicidal ideation is present or when the patient is incapacitated. Evaluation for suicidality begins with asking the patient about suicidal ideation, since patients are often reluctant to volunteer that information. Emergency psychiatric evaluation is mandated when suicidal ideation is present or suspected. Family members may be helpful in assessing suicidal potential.

Major depressive disorder responds to pharmacologic treatment, and when symptoms are mild to moderate, to cognitive behavioral therapy. The risks and benefits of both interventions should be discussed with the patient. If symptoms of major depression become debilitating and interfere with the physical health of the mother, the risk:benefit ratio strongly favors use of antidepressant medications.

Numerous antidepressant medications are available (Table 19-5). The *selective serotonin reuptake inhibitors* (SSRIs) are commonly used because of their minimal side effects and safety in overdose. Due to their relatively recent availability, there are only preliminary data regarding their safety during pregnancy: *fluoxetine* was introduced in 1988, *sertraline* in 1992, and *paroxetine* in 1993. More information is available on fluoxetine than on the other, newer SSRIs. Available studies and a postmarketing surveillance registry maintained by the manufacturer of fluoxetine show no evidence of increased risk of congenital anomalies. Limited follow-up data are available for the SSRIs, although the evidence available is reassuring. One follow-up study of children with in utero exposure to fluoxetine did not find any associated behavioral or cognitive effects of the drug.[13] Over the last decade, the SSRIs have become the agents of choice for first-line treatment of mood and anxiety disorders in pregnancy.

Tricyclic and *heterocyclic antidepressants* are older classes of antidepressants, so more information is available about the risks they may pose during pregnancy. There is no definitive evidence for teratogenicity associated with their use. Unfortunately, the side effects (dry mouth, blurred vision, tachycardia, constipation, mental slowing, sedation) are disturbing to many patients and compliance may be poor. *Nortriptyline* and *desipramine* are generally chosen over other TCAs, because they allow monitoring of serum levels, are associated with a lower risk of orthostatic hypotension, and have fewer anticholinergic side effects. Transient urinary retention and bowel obstruction have been observed in neonates exposed to high levels of these agents. The major disadvantage to their use is the high potential lethality secondary to overdose.[14]

There are fewer data about the potential teratogenicity of the *monoamine oxidase inhibitors*. The side-effects profile includes orthostatic hypotension and potentially lethal hypertensive crisis secondary to noncompliance with strict dietary restraints. These potential adverse effects for the pregnant mother make the monoamine oxidase inhibitors a pharmacologic treatment of last resort in pregnancy.

Importantly, antidepressant medication needs to be adequately dosed. Underdosing of medication is unlikely to significantly reduce risk to the fetus and will not accomplish the goal of treatment of the major depression. Since patients who have experienced a major depression during pregnancy are at high risk of symptom exacerbation in the postpartum period, antidepressant medication should be continued for at least 6 months following delivery.

Electroconvulsive therapy (ECT) can be safely used during pregnancy and lactation. It may be administered in both inpatient and outpatient settings and offers the advantage of not exposing the fetus to long-term medications. It may be the treatment of choice for psychotic depression, especially in the first trimester.[15]

ANXIETY DISORDERS

Anxiety is an unpleasant emotional state accompanied by subjective fear and objectively measurable physical effects (e.g., tachycardia, tachypnea, sweating). Feeling anxious is a normal reaction to stressful circumstances, including pregnancy, and often may actually be adaptive. Anxiety is pathologic when it causes marked distress or interferes with an individual's relationships or ability to function. Anxiety disorders are very common, with a lifetime prevalence of 24.9 percent and a 12-month prevalence of 17.2 percent.[16] Anxiety may also be a prominent feature in adjustment disorder, major depression, and other mental disorders.

Table 19-5. Reported Teratogenicity of Antidepressant Medications

Name	Trade Name	Class[c]	Fetal Risk	Neonatal Risk	Lactation Risk
Second-generation antidepressants: Selective serotonin reuptake inhibitors (SSRIs)					
Citalopram	Celexa®	C	Not major teratogen	Transient withdrawal reported	Excreted into breast milk, infant sedation reported
Fluoxetine[a]	Prozac® Sarafem®	C	Not major teratogen	Transient irritability reported	Excreted into breast milk, slower weight gain reported
Fluvoxamine	Luvox®	C	Not major teratogen	No available data	Excreted into breast milk
Paroxetine	Paxil®	C	Not major teratogen	No available data	Excreted into breast milk
Sertraline[a]	Zoloft®	C	Not major teratogen	Transient irritability reported	Excreted into breast milk
Second-generation antidepressants: Other					
Bupropion	Wellbutrin®	B	Insufficient data	Insufficient data	Excreted into breast milk
Mirtazapine	Remeron®	C	Insufficient data	Insufficient data	Excretion into breast milk not known
Nefazadone	Serzone®	C	Insufficient data	Insufficient data	Excreted into breast milk
Trazodone	Desyrel®	C	Insufficient data	Insufficient data	Excreted into breast milk
Venlafaxine	Effexor®	C	Insufficient data	Insufficient data	Excreted into breast milk
Tricyclic antidepressants					
Amitriptyline	Elavil® Endep®	D[b]	Limb defects, causality unclear	No withdrawal reported	Excreted into breast milk
Amoxapine	Asendin®	C	Inconclusive	No data available	Excreted into breast milk
Clomipramine	Anafranil®	C	Not major teratogen	Withdrawal seizures reported	Excreted into breast milk
Desipramine[a]	Norpramin®	C[b]	Not major teratogen	Withdrawal seizures reported	Excreted into breast milk
Doxepin	Sinequan®	C[b]	Inconclusive	No withdrawal reported	Excreted into breast milk, infant respiratory depression reported
Imipramine	Tofranil®	D[b]	Reports of anomalies, causality unclear	Withdrawal seizures reported	Excreted into breast milk
Maprotiline	Ludiomil®	B	Inconclusive	No data available	Excreted into breast milk
Nortriptyline[a]	Aventyl® Pamelor®	D[b]	Reports of anomalies, causality unclear	No withdrawal reported	Excreted into breast milk
Protriptyline	Vivactil®	C[b]	No data available	No data available	No data available
Trimipramine	Surmontil®	C	No data available	No data available	No data available
Monoamine oxidase inhibitors (MAOIs)					
Phenelzine	Nardil®	C	Limited data, malformations reported	No data available	No data available
Tranylcypromine	Parnate®	C	Limited data, malformations reported	No data available	No data availble

[a]Consider for use as first-line agents.
[b]Drug not assigned to class by manufacturer; class assigned per Briggs et al.[35]
[c]Refer to Chapter 3 for definitions of categories
Source: Briggs et al,[35] with permission

Panic Attacks

A person having a panic attack experiences a discrete period of intense fear or discomfort accompanied by four of the following symptoms: (1) palpitations, pounding heart, or accelerated heart rate; (2) sweating; (3) trembling or shaking; (4) sensations of shortness of breath or smothering; (5) feeling of choking; (6) chest pain or discomfort; (7) nausea or abdominal distress; (8) feeling dizzy, unsteady, lightheaded, or faint; (9) derealization (feelings of unreality) or depersonalization (being detached from oneself); (10) fear of losing control or going crazy; (11) fear of dying; (12) paresthesias (numbness or tingling sensations); or (13) chills or hot flushes. Panic attacks develop abruptly and reach a peak within 10 minutes. They are common and may occur as isolated experiences in normal young adults or in connection with a variety of anxiety disorders. They are often easily treated, sometimes just with reassurance that the symptoms do not represent a serious physical illness. However, ongoing, untreated panic attacks can be severely debilitating.[1]

Panic Disorder

Panic disorder is a common psychiatric disorder characterized by recurrent, unexpected panic attacks. The National Comorbidity Survey[16] reported lifetime and 12-month prevalences of 3.5 and 2.3 percent, respectively, for panic disorder. Panic disorder may occur with or without agoraphobia. *Agoraphobia* is defined as anxiety about being in places or situations from which escape might be difficult (or embarrassing) or in which help may not be available in the event of a panic attack or panic-like symptoms. Such situations are either avoided or endured with marked distress and anxiety about having an attack or experiencing symptoms.

The onset of symptoms occurs in young adulthood and affects women disproportionately. Patients with panic symptoms often initially present to emergency departments or primary-care clinics with physical complaints such as chest pain, shortness of breath, increased heart rate, numbness, and/or dizziness; they often fear that they are having a heart attack or stroke. Individuals with new onset of panic symptoms must be carefully evaluated to rule out medical conditions that mimic panic attacks. Pain, hypoxia, angina, myocardial infarction, substance abuse or withdrawal, hyperthyroidism, or pheochromocytoma can cause anxiety and panic symptoms.

Obsessive Compulsive Disorder

Obsessive compulsive disorder (OCD) is characterized by recurrent obsessions or compulsions severe enough to be time-consuming, to cause marked distress, or to significantly interfere with an individual's functioning. Obsessive thoughts are usually disturbing. An example of an obsession is a recurrent thought of hurting a loved one, without anger or desire to harm that person. An example of a compulsion would be the impulse to wash the baby's bottles over and over again to make sure they were not contaminated.

ANXIETY DISORDERS IN PREGNANCY AND THE POSTPARTUM PERIOD

The effect of pregnancy on the course of panic disorder may be highly variable. A recent study examined the clinical course of 67 pregnancies occurring in 46 women with preexisting panic disorder.[17] In 43 percent of the pregnancies, women experienced improvement in their panic symptoms; in 33 percent, there was worsening; and in 23 percent there was no change. However, 63 percent of the pregnancies were associated with worsening of panic symptoms during the postpartum period, suggesting that women with panic disorder may be at risk for postpartum exacerbation. Other studies[18] have suggested that while women with mild symptoms may experience improvement, those with more severe illness may represent a subgroup at risk for persistence or worsening of symptoms.

Obsessive compulsive disorder may increase during pregnancy and the postpartum period. Some reports have suggested that obstetric complications may be relevant to the development of the disorder and that women with postpartum OCD may have significantly higher rates of aggressive obsessions about harming their infants.[19,20]

Treatment of Anxiety Disorders

Panic disorder is effectively treated by pharmacologic agents, particularly antidepressant medication and/or benzodiazepines. Cognitive-behavioral techniques have also been shown to be effective. Since cognitive-behavioral therapy may have a medication-sparing effect, this modality may be especially useful prior to and during pregnancy.

For women who are taking benzodiazepines and are contemplating pregnancy, a plan for tapering benzodiazepines prior to conception should be discussed, since use of these medications during the first trimester has been associated with fetal anomalies (Table 19-6). In particular, studies have shown approximately a 12-fold increase in the risk for cleft palate, giving an absolute risk of about 7 per 1000 births (compared with a baseline risk of 6 per 10,000 births).[13] For patients already pregnant and using benzodiazepines, recommendations must be individ-

Table 19-6. Reported Teratogenicity of Benzodiazepines and Other Anxiolytics and Hypnotics

Name	Trade Name	Class[c]	Fetal Risk	Neonatal Risk	Lactation Risk
Alprazolam	Xanax®	D	Anomalies reported, causality unlikely	Withdrawal reported	Excreted into breast milk
Buspirone	BuSpar®	B	Insufficient data	Insufficient data	Excreted into breast milk in rats, insufficient human data
Chloral hydrate	Somnote®	C	Not major teratogen	Insufficient data	Excreted into breast milk, infant drowsiness reported
Chlordiazepoxide	Librium®	D[b]	Conflicting teratogen data	Withdrawal observed occurs early and late	Presumed excretion into human breast milk
Clonazepam[a]	Klonopin®	D	No teratogen reports for this drug, positive reports in this class	Floppy infant and withdrawal reported	Excreted into breast milk
Clorazepate	Tranxene®	D[b]	Anomalies reported causality unclear	Withdrawal observed	Presumed excretion into human breast milk
Diazepam	Valium®	D[b]	Anomalies reported	Floppy infant and withdrawal reported	Excreted into breast milk, infant sedation reported
Flurazepam	Dalmane®	X	Teratogenic effect for class of drugs cited	Withdrawal predicted	Presumed excretion into human breast milk
Lorazepam[a]	Ativan®	D	No teratogen reports	Floppy infant and for this drug, positive reports in this class	Excreted into breast milk withdrawal reported
Midazolam	Versed®	D	No reports of human use before third trimester	Floppy infants reported	Excreted into breast milk
Temazepam	Restoril®	X	Teratogenic effect for class of drugs cited; ?IUFD[d] in combination with diphenhydramine	Floppy infant and withdrawal reported	Excreted into breast milk, infant sedation reported
Triazolam	Halcion®	X	Teratogenic effect for class of drugs cited	Withdrawal predicted	Excreted into breast milk
Zaleplon	Sonata®	C	Insufficient data	Insufficient data	Insufficient data
Zolpidem[a]	Ambien®	B	Limited data, no anomalies reported	Insufficient data	Excreted into breast milk

[a]Consider for use as first-line agents.
[b]Drug not assigned to class by manufacturer; class assigned per Briggs et al.[35]
[c]Refer to Chapter 3 for definitions of categories.
[d]IUFD, in utero fetal demise.
Source: Briggs et al,[35] with permission

ualized. Benzodiazepines can produce withdrawal symptoms in the infant, so gradual tapering and discontinuation of these medications prior to delivery has been recommended by some practitioners. Since the prospect of labor and delivery is anxiety-producing in its own right, this may not be possible with some patients. If a previously unmedicated patient requires pharmacotherapy, the SSRIs are reasonable choices for initial therapy. The severity of anxiety symptoms, presence of suicidality or comorbid mood disorder, concurrent medical conditions and medications, presenting stage of gestation, and other factors must be carefully considered. A retrospective study[18] has suggested that antipanic medication in the third trimester may have a protective effect in the puerperium. It has also been suggested that lactation may prevent postpartum exacerbation of anxiety disorders,[21] although clinically the opposite reaction can be seen if breast-feeding does not go well.

Like panic disorder, OCD may benefit from cognitive-behavioral strategies, and these may be used as an alternative to medications during pregnancy. Obsessive compulsive disorder is specifically responsive to drugs that inhibit serotonin reuptake. When medication is necessary, fluoxetine is an effective and reasonable treatment. Clomipramine is an effective OCD therapy in nonpregnant women, but use during pregnancy is limited by its propensity to worsen orthostatic hypotension. Furthermore, its use during labor and delivery is contraindicated, secondary to reports of seizures in neonates born to mothers who have used clomipramine during late pregnancy.[22]

EATING DISORDERS IN PREGNANCY

Anorexia nervosa is a serious and sometimes fatal disorder occurring in approximately 1 percent of reproductive-age women. Women with anorexia nervosa suffer from self-imposed starvation in pursuit of thinness and a fear of fatness. *Bulimia nervosa* occurs in 1.7 percent of reproductive-age women and is characterized by episodic binge eating followed by efforts designed to reduce calorie absorption, including self-induced vomiting, use of laxatives or diuretics, or excessive exercise. Milder versions of eating disorders occur in another 3 to 5 percent of reproductive-age women.[23] Despite the relatively high prevalence and associated morbidity of these disorders, there have been limited reports of their effects on the outcome of pregnancy.

Women with eating disorders are at increased risk for obstetric complications, including pregnancy-induced hypertension, forceps delivery, and cesarean section. Postnatally, they are at higher risk for major depression and anxiety.[24,25] The offspring of these mothers are at risk for intrauterine growth restriction, congenital malformations, failure to thrive, and low Apgar scores.[26,27]

Women with eating disorders are often reluctant to volunteer information about their condition, and those with bulimia nervosa often appear to be of normal weight. As a result, practitioners may attribute episodes of weight loss, vomiting, electrolyte imbalance, or generalized gastrointestinal disturbances to the pregnancy itself. Fluoxetine has been given an indication for the treatment of bulimia by the Food and Drug Administration. In extreme circumstances, hospitalization and feeding by nasogastric tube may become necessary.

PSYCHOSIS DURING PREGNANCY AND THE POSTPARTUM PERIOD

Psychotic symptoms include hallucinations, delusions, and severe disorganization of thought and behavior. Psychosis occurring during pregnancy and the postpartum period is most often a symptom of major depression or mania (bipolar disorder), with only a small number of cases attributable to schizophrenia or schizoaffective disorder. Psychosis is a psychiatric emergency because the patient's poor judgment and behaviors may place both her and her fetus or newborn at risk.

Psychosis and Mania During Pregnancy

Patients who have a chronic psychotic disorder or a past history of a psychotic illness continue to be at risk for psychosis during pregnancy. Patients with schizophrenia or bipolar disorder who become pregnant will often need close psychiatric and prenatal monitoring. Chronic symptoms, such as disorganization and paranoia, may interfere with the patient's ability to comply with prenatal care and to keep her medical appointments. In particular, pregnant patients with schizophrenia who develop complications of pregnancy may need more intense outpatient support in order to achieve adequate care. Psychiatric outreach services, including case management and home health nursing services, may be essential components of prenatal care.

Patients with bipolar disorder will be at risk of symptom exacerbation during pregnancy, especially if prophylactic medication (e.g., lithium carbonate, valproic acid, carbamazepine) is withheld. Manic symptoms—such as excessive energy, decreased need for sleep, sexual promiscuity, and engagement in other potentially dangerous behaviors—threaten the health and safety of both mother and fetus. Close monitoring by family and mental health professionals may be needed to reduce the risk of dangerous behaviors. Psychiatric hospitalization may be needed.

Psychosis in the Postpartum Period

As in the case of patients at risk for major depression, the postpartum period likely represents a biologically vulnerable period for patients at risk for psychosis. Women may thus present with their first episode of psychosis in the postpartum period. A population-based study in Denmark found the risk of first-episode psychosis in the month following delivery to be 1 in every 2000 deliveries (25 cases) and in the year following delivery to be 1 in every 1000 deliveries (50 cases).[28] About two-thirds of the cases met diagnostic criteria for major depression with psychotic features, with the other third split between mania and early schizophrenia.

Patients who develop first-onset psychosis in the postpartum period are at high risk for recurrent symptoms and dysfunction. While 40 percent of the women in the Danish registry had no further episodes in the 7- to 14-year follow-up period, 60 percent experienced at least one reoccurrence of a psychotic illness. Most women with recurrent illness developed nonpuerperal mania or depressive disorders; 4 percent had psychosis only in connection with subsequent deliveries. Postpartum psychotic illness led to chronic disabling illness for one-third of the affected women. Close psychiatric follow up is thus indicated for all women who experience a postpartum psychosis.[28]

Psychosis in the pregnant and postpartum woman is a psychiatric emergency. Psychosis may result in disorganization and poor judgment, with the woman at risk for engaging in behaviors that are dangerous to her and her baby. For example, of the patients reviewed in the Danish registry, 10 percent had thoughts about killing their babies and a baby was put at risk in one instance.[28]

New-onset psychotic illness requires medical evaluation. Potential causes are similar to those of major depressive disorder; laboratory screening tests are listed in Table 19-4. In particular, substance abuse (phencyclidine hydrochloride [PCP], hallucinogens, cocaine) and many prescribed medications may result in transient psychosis.

Treatment of Psychosis

Antipsychotics

Psychosis usually requires pharmacologic treatment; numerous medications are currently available in the United States for the treatment of psychosis (Table 19-7). Treatment minimizes the risk of exacerbation during pregnancy, thereby improving fetal outcomes. As discussed above, worsening of psychosis may result in poor prenatal care and dangerous psychotic behaviors that place both mother and child at risk. Thus withholding pharmacologic treatment in psychotic pregnant or postpartum patients may pose significant risk to the health of both mother and infant, since psychotic illness itself is probably a risk factor for poor fetal outcome.[13] For most women, the potential benefits of antipsychotic treatment will outweigh the potential risks.

The risks that antipsychotic medications may pose to the fetus have not been systematically studied, but a meta-analysis of small studies is available.[13] Studies of pregnant women treated for hyperemesis with low-potency antipsychotics, particularly haloperidol, suggest no increased risk for birth defects in the fetus. Phenothiazines may pose a slightly increased risk of poor outcome. Newborns exposed to antipsychotics have been reported to have transient extrapyramidal symptoms, including increased muscle tone, tremor, motor restlessness, abnormal movements, and poor feeding.[29] Functional bowel obstruction has also been reported.[30] Despite the potential risk of these effects in newborns, cessation of antipsychotic medication is usually not indicated prior to delivery. Here the risks of psychotic decompensation usually outweigh the potential for transient residual medication side effects in the newborn.

Patients with chronic psychotic illness should be maintained on their usual antipsychotic medication to minimize risk of relapse. Haloperidol should be considered first-line treatment in pregnant patients without a past pharmacologic treatment history because of more extensive experience with this drug, low risk of teratogenicity, and low risk of hypotension and other cardiovascular side effects in the pregnant woman.

Patients who develop psychosis in the postpartum period should be treated as any psychosis would be treated. The usual treatment of acute psychotic agitation includes haloperidol (dose of 2 to 5 mg orally or intramuscularly) and a benzodiazepine (e.g., lorazepam 1 to 2 mg every 2 to 4 hours until sedation occurs, up to 10 mg/d). Choice of antipsychotic agent is usually based on prior response to treatment and tolerability of side effects. The newer, atypical antipsychotic agents (risperidone, olanzapine, quetiapine, ziprasidone) may be preferable to the older agents because of their effectiveness and more favorable side-effect profiles.

Mood Stabilizers

Patients with schizophrenia, schizoaffective disorder, or mania may require a mood stabilizer, such as lithium, valproic acid, or carbamazepine, or the newer atypical antipsychotics (Table 19-8). Lithium treatment during the

Table 19-7. Reported Teratogenicity of Antipsychotic Medications

Name	Trade Name	Class[c]	Fetal Risk	Neonatal Risk	Lactation Risk
Atypical antipsychotics (second-generation)					
Clozapine	Clozaril®	B	No teratogenic effects reported	No data available	Concentrated in breast milk
Olanzapine[a]	Zyprexa®	C	Unknown	Unknown	Unknown
Quetiapine	Seroquel®	C	Unknown	Unknown	Unknown
Risperidone[a]	Risperdal®	C	Unknown	Unknown	Unknown
Ziprasidone	Geodon	C	Unknown	Unknown	Unknown
First-generation antipsychotics, high potency					
Fluphenazine[a]	Prolixin®	C[b]	Inconclusive data	EPS[d]	Excretion expected, no data available
Haloperidol[a]	Haldol®	C	Anomalies reported, causality unclear	No adverse events reported	Excreted into breast milk
Perphenazine	Trilafon®	C[b]	Conflicting teratogen data, probably safe	No data available	Excreted into breast milk
Thiothixene	Navane®	C[b]	No teratogenic reports	No data available	No data available
Trifluoperazine	Stelazine®	C[b]	Conflicting teratogen date, probably safe	? EPS[d]	No data available
First-generation antipsychotics, mid-potency					
Loxapine	Loxitane®	C[b]	No data available	No data available	Excreted into breast milk in dogs, no human data
Molindone	Moban®	C[b]	No data available	No data available	No data available
First-generation antipsychotics, low potency					
Chlorpromazine	Thorazine®	C[b]	Conflicting teratogen data; probably safe in low doses	Prolonged jaundice, EPS[d], hyper/hyporeflexia noted	Excreted into breast milk
Mesoridazine	Serentil®	C[b]	No data available	No data available	No data available
Thioridazine	Mellaril®	C[b]	Conflicting teratogen data; probably safe	? EPS[d]	No data available

[a]Consider for use as first-line agents
[b]Drug not assigned to class by manufacturer; class assigned per Briggs et al.[35]
[c]Refer to Chapter 3 for definitions of categories.
[d]EPS, extrapyramidal symptoms.
Source: Briggs et al,[35] with permission

first trimester increases the risk of Ebstein anomaly by 10- to 20-fold as compared with the risk in the general population. The absolute risk of Ebstein anomaly is very small, however, in the lithium-exposed fetus (1 in 1000 for the lithium-exposed fetus as compared with 1 in 20,000 in the unexposed fetus). Newborns exposed to lithium are at risk for "floppy infant" syndrome (cyanosis, hypertonicity).[31] A follow-up study of 60 lithium-exposed fetuses could not demonstrate long-term behavioral sequelae.[32] Treatment with valproic acid and carbamazepine has been associated with a 15-fold increased risk of spina bifida (for exposed fetuses, the risk is estimated at 5 to 10 in 1000 births) and minor malformations (e.g., rotated ears).[13] One follow-up study failed to show long-term behavioral sequelae in carbamazepine-exposed fetuses.[33]

The risk-benefit analysis for women requiring mood stabilizers should include the severity of psychiatric ill-

Table 19-8. Reported Teratogenicity of Antimania Agents (Mood Stabilizers)

Name	Trade Name	Class[c]	Fetal Risk	Neonatal Risk	Lactation Risk
Carbamazepine[a]	Tegretol® Carbatrol®	D	Major, minor malformations reported	Insufficient data	Excreted into breast milk
Gabapentin	Neurontin®	C	Limited data	Insufficient data	No data available
Lamotrigine	Lamictal®	C	Limited data, available data reassuring	Insufficient data	Excreted into breast milk
Lithium[a]	Eskalith® Lithobid® Lithonate®	D[b]	Cardiac, neural tube abnormalities	Transient lithium toxicity reported	Excreted into breast milk
Topiramate	Topamax®	C	No data available	No data available	No data available
Valproic acid	Depakote®	D	Major, minor malformations reported	Hyperbilirubinemia, hyperglycemia	Excreted into breast milk

[a]Consider for use as first-line agents
[b]Drug not assigned to class by manufacturer, multiple products listed; class assigned per Briggs et al.[35]
[c]Refer to Chapter 3 for definitions of categories.
Source: Briggs et al,[35] with permission.

ness, including past history of relapse risk if mood stabilizers have been discontinued. Women with severe, rapidly cycling mood swings may require mood-stabilizing medication throughout pregnancy. If the woman decides against this, lithium or other mood stabilizers should be slowly tapered, because this, compared with abrupt discontinuation, minimizes the risk of relapse. In addition, the dosage of lithium should be decreased by about one-third immediately prior to delivery to decease the risk of increases in the lithium level and subsequent lithium toxicity, which can occur secondary to changes in maternal blood volume after delivery.

SUBSTANCE ABUSE DISORDERS

Substance dependence or abuse occurs when a patient's pattern of use becomes maladaptive, causing impairment or distress. A patient must have at least three of the following seven symptoms to meet *substance dependence* criteria: (1) tolerance, (2) withdrawal, (3) taking more than intended, (4) a persistent desire or failure to control substance use, (5) spending a great deal of time getting the substance or recovering from its effects, (6) giving up other important activities because of substance use, and (7) continued use despite knowing that the substance use was causing persistent health problems. A patient must have at least one of following symptoms to meet *substance abuse* criteria: (1) substance use causes the patient to fail to meet obligations, (2) recurrent use when dangerous (e.g., driving when intoxicated), (3) recurrent substance-related legal problems, or (4) continued use despite social or interpersonal problems related to substance intoxication.

Alcohol

Alcohol use during pregnancy has been identified as the leading preventable cause of birth defects.[34] Alcohol crosses the placental barrier freely at all stages of gestation. Fetal effects will be reflective of the gestational timing of alcohol exposure, genetically-based differences in alcohol metabolism, the amount of alcohol consumed, and perhaps by the interaction of alcohol with other substances. Mild fetal alcohol syndrome has been induced by the consumption of as little as two drinks per day in early pregnancy. The complete syndrome is more likely when alcohol consumption exceeds four drinks per day. The complete fetal alcohol syndrome comprises a set of birth defects including craniofacial dysmorphology, prenatal and antenatal growth deficiencies, and central nervous system dysfunction. Other abnormalities include cardiac lesions, renal and genital defects, and hemangiomas, which have been reported in about 50 percent of infants. At 10-year follow up, it appeared that intellectual impairment was directly related to the degree of craniofacial abnormality. Behavioral problems are also commonly seen as long-term effects of fetal alcohol syndrome.[35] Alcohol passes freely into breast milk, and recent data indicate an untoward effect on psychomotor development

Table 19-9. "CAGE" Screen for Alcoholism

Have you ever:
C thought you should CUT back on your drinking?
A felt ANNOYED by people criticizing your drinking?
G felt GUILTY or bad about your drinking?
E had a morning EYE-OPENER to relieve hangover or nerves?

Note: A score of 2 or 3 indicates a high index of suspicion of alcohol dependence. A score of 4 is pathognomonic for dependence.
Source: From Ewing,[42] with permission.

in the neonate. Predicted short-term effects such as infant sedation are generally not noted at maternal blood alcohol levels less than 300 mg/dL.

The commonly used "CAGE" questions, shown in Table 19-9, have good reliability as a screening tool for alcohol dependence. Laboratory testing for alcohol and drugs should be done if medically indicated in the emergency department.

Positive CAGE or laboratory screening should be followed by careful diagnostic assessment. Alcohol education and warnings about fetal anomalies may not be sufficient to promote abstinence in women who are chemically dependent. Medical detoxification may be needed before entering a rehabilitation program. Alcohol withdrawal syndromes should not be treated with benzodiazepines in pregnancy. Magnesium is an alternative. Referral for treatment can be problematic, because many treatment centers will not accept pregnant women. Unemployment, lack of insurance, and lack of available care for other children may also be barriers to treatment.[36] Self-help groups like Alcoholics Anonymous and Women for Sobriety may have ongoing local programs, designed specifically for pregnancy, that can benefit these patients and their families.

Nicotine

The effects of maternal smoking on birth weight and gestational length have been clearly documented over the last 10 years.[37] More recent attention has been directed toward defining the role that chronic exposure to nicotine may have on the developing fetal brain. Nicotine freely crosses the placenta, and there is good evidence that the human fetus may actually be exposed to higher nicotine concentrations than the smoking mother. Animal studies indicate fetal tolerance to nicotine and an increase in brain nicotinic receptors.[38] Animal data also indicate a positive association between chronic intrauterine exposure to nicotine and hyperactivity in the offspring. In humans, maternal smoking has also been associated with behavioral and cognitive impairment. A recent study suggests maternal smoking may also be a risk factor for attention deficit hyperactivity disorder (ADHD), which affects 6 to 9 percent of school-age children. This association remained statistically significant even after adjusting for socioeconomic status, parental IQ, and parental ADHD status. The study also confirmed that the children of mothers who smoked during pregnancy had lower IQ scores.[38]

Marijuana

The use of marijuana by pregnant women is common, with reports stating that from 3 to 16 percent of all pregnancies are exposed to the drug. The effect of marijuana exposure on the fetus remains unclear, primarily because of the frequency of multiple substance abuse. Possible marijuana-induced complications of pregnancy are controversial, with inconsistent findings in different studies. One significant confounding variable is concurrent use of marijuana and nicotine-containing products; both can independently produce the changes in birth weight and gestational length previously attributed to marijuana alone. Animal data from the 1960s and 1970s were inconclusive with regard to teratogenicity. In humans, most researchers have concluded either that marijuana does not produce structural defects or that the available data are insufficient to reach any conclusion.[35] Early concerns about chromosomal breaks associated with marijuana use have not been confirmed.

Of great concern, however, is the 1989 report noting a tenfold increase in rates of acute nonlymphoblastic leukemia among children exposed to marijuana in utero. The exposed children had an earlier mean age of onset (37.7 months versus 96.1 months; $p = .0007$) and a disproportionate share of monocytic or myelomonocytic morphology (70 percent versus 31 percent; $p = .02$). The reasons for these findings are unclear, but the possible presence of herbicides or pesticides on the marijuana cannot be excluded.[35]

Tetrahydrocannabinol (THC), the active ingredient in marijuana, is excreted into breast milk, and metabolites are measurable in infant serum. Although no reports of adverse events secondary to exposure through breast milk have been reported, the American Academy of Pediatrics still considers breast-feeding contraindicated with ongoing marijuana use.[35]

Cocaine

Cocaine produces intense euphoria, disinhibition, an increased sense of competence as well as improved self-esteem. When used chronically, it produces less euphoria, but abstinence is associated with intense craving. Cocaine is often used in binges, which are followed by a postintoxication "crash." The crash is characterized by an intensely dysphoric mood with marked anxiety. During this phase, many cocaine users will utilize alcohol, opiates, benzodiazepines, or other sedatives to relieve the dysphoria. This is followed by a period of withdrawal, usually marked by low-grade depression, disturbed sleep, and intense cocaine craving. From a psychiatric perspective, cocaine use may precipitate mania, delirium, delusional or hallucinatory states, and organic mood and personality disorders. It can also cause exacerbation of preexisting psychiatric disorders in susceptible individuals.[39]

Cocaine is a sympathomimetic that produces hypertension and vasoconstriction directly via its cardiovascular activity. It crosses the placenta freely and can be found in numerous fetal tissues. It causes increased uterine vascular resistance, which decreases placental perfusion and may lead to fetal hypoxia. Both the hypoxia and direct effects of the cocaine have been observed to cause fetal tachycardia and hypertension. Cocaine use in pregnancy has also been associated with spontaneous abortion, preterm labor, premature delivery, abruptio placentae, premature rupture of membranes, and maternal death. It has consistently been shown to be associated with intrauterine growth restriction and low birth weight. Fetal distress during labor is not uncommon in cocaine users and the increased incidence of meconium-stained amniotic fluid has been well documented. Distinct fetal anomalies associated with cocaine use are difficult to assess, primarily because of the high incidence of multiple substance abuse in this group. The possibility of higher than expected rates of urinary tract abnormalities has been investigated, with mixed results. Numerous instances of anomalies in the brain and gastrointestinal tract that appear to be secondary to vascular accidents have been reported. Ocular and facial abnormalities have also been reported.[35]

During the neonatal period, infants of cocaine-abusing mothers tend to be irritable and tremulous, and they may experience muscular rigidity. Vomiting and diarrhea are also common. Symptoms begin on day 1 or 2 after birth, and are at maximum intensity by days 2 and 3. Increased rates of sudden infant death syndrome (SIDS) have been noted in cocaine-exposed infants during the first 6 months of life.[35]

Breast-feeding is contraindicated among cocaine users. Signs of infant cocaine toxicity secondary to ingestion of breast milk after maternal cocaine use include irritability, vomiting, diarrhea, tremulousness, increased startle reflex, hyperreflexia with clonus, and marked lability of mood. Cocaine metabolites can be found in fetal urine for a protracted period following exposure via breast milk.[35]

Opiates

Heroin crosses the placenta rapidly, but no well-defined syndrome of abnormalities has been associated with it. Acute maternal withdrawal will be associated with simultaneous fetal withdrawal, and intrauterine fetal demise can occur.

Methadone maintenance therapy is commonly used during pregnancy, and no increase in congenital anomalies has been noted among those taking methadone. The primary problems occur in the neonatal period, with withdrawal symptoms occurring in 60 to 90 percent of infants. Infants of opiate-addicted mothers are often small for gestational age. For reasons that are not yet clear, the infants of methadone-maintained mothers tend to have a higher birth weight than those of heroin-addicted mothers. This may reflect improved prenatal care in the methadone group.

Heroin crosses into breast milk in sufficient quantities to cause infant addiction. The American Academy of Pediatrics considers heroin abuse a contraindication to breast-feeding. Methadone concentrations in breast milk are sufficiently high to prevent withdrawal in breast-fed infants. But the American Academy of Pediatrics considers methadone to be compatible with breast-feeding provided that maternal doses do not exceed 20 mg/d.[35]

Treatment of Substance Abuse in Pregnancy

Women should be clearly informed about the hazards of alcohol, nicotine, and illicit drug use during pregnancy. Patients who use illegal substances or who are alcohol-dependent are also at risk for domestic violence, STD infections, and HIV.[39,40]

Patients should be encouraged to participate in regular prenatal care, since this single factor is positively related to higher birth weight and improved pregnancy outcome. Outpatient drug and alcohol rehabilitation programs designed specifically for pregnant women will often combine prenatal care and a battery of services including parenting classes, group therapy, counseling, and psychiatric management. Hospitalization may be necessary when detoxification from alcohol is needed. Methadone maintenance should be offered to heroin-addicted patients as soon as the diagnosis of opiate dependence has been made. Hospitalization may also be needed for patients with medical, obstetric, or psychiatric complications, or those with evidence of withdrawal symptoms.

REFERENCES

1. American Psychiatric Association: *Diagnostic and Statistical Manual of Mental Disorders,* 4th ed. Text Revision (DSM-IV-TR). Washington: American Psychiatric Association, 2000.
2. Kessler RC, Zhao S, Blazer DB, Swartz M: Prevalence, correlates, and course of minor depression and major depression in the national comorbidity survey. *J Affect Disord* 45: 19–30, 1997.
3. Reiger DA, Hirschfeld RMA, Goodwin FK: The NIMH depression awareness, recognition, and treatment (D/ART) program: Structure, aims, and scientific basis. *Am J Psychiatry* 145:1351, 1988.
4. Miller LJ: Psychiatric disorders during pregnancy, in Stewart DE, Stotland NL (eds): *Psychological Aspects of Women's Health Care: The Interface between Psychiatry and Obstetrics and Gynecology,* 2d ed.Washington: American Psychiatric Press, 2001, pp 51–66.
5. O'Hara MW: *Postpartum Depression: Causes and Consequences.* New York: Springer-Verlag, 1995.
6. Cox JL, Murray D, Chapman G: A controlled study of the onset, duration, and prevalence of postnatal depression. *Br J Psychiatry* 163:27, 1993.
7. Katona C, Robertson M: *Psychiatry at a Glance.* Oxford, England: Blackwell, 1995.
8. Janssen HJEM, Cuisinier MCJ, Hoogduin KAL, de Graauw KPHM: Controlled prospective study on the mental health of women following pregnancy loss. *Am J Psychiatry* 153:226, 1996.
9. American College of Obstetricians and Gynecologists: Grief related to perinatal death. ACOG technical bulletin no. 86, April 1985.
10. Brown SS, Eisenberg L (eds): *The Best Intentions: Unintended Pregnancy and the Well-Being of Children and Families.* Washington: National Academy Press, 1995.
11. Stotland NL: Induced abortion, in Stewart DE, Stotland NL (eds): *Psychological Aspects of Women's Health Care: The Interface Between Psychiatry and Obstetrics and Gynecology,* 2d ed. Washington: American Psychiatric Press, 2001, pp 219–240.
12. Zuckerman B, Bauchner H, Parker S, Cabral H: Maternal depressive symptoms during pregnancy and newborn irritability. *J Dev Behav Pediatr* 11:190, 1990.
13. Altschuler LL, Cohen LS, Szuba MP, et al: Pharmacologic management of psychiatric illness during pregnancy: Dilemmas and guidelines. *Am J Psychiatry* 153:592, 1996.
14. Rothschild AJ: Advances in the management of depression: Implications for the obstetrician/gynecologist. *Am J Obstet Gynecol* 173:659, 1995.
15. Walker R, Swartz CM: Electroconvulsive therapy during high-risk pregnancy. *Gen Hosp Psychiatry* 16:348–353, 1994.
16. Kessler RC, McGonagle KA, Zhao S, et al: Lifetime and 12-month prevalence of DSM-III-R psychiatric disorders in the United States. *Arch Gen Psychiatry* 51:8, 1994.
17. Northcott CJ, Stein MB: Panic disorder during pregnancy. *J Clin Psychiatry* 55:539, 1994.
18. Cohen LS, Sichel DA, Dimmock JA, Rosenbaum JF: Impact of pregnancy on panic disorder: A case series. *J Clin Psychiatry* 55:284, 1994.
19. Neziroglu F, Anemone R, Yaryura-Tobias JA: Onset of obsessive-compulsive disorder in pregnancy. *Am J Psychiatry* 149:947, 1992.
20. Maina G, Umberto A, Bogetto F, Vaschetto P, Ravizza L: Recent life events and obsessive-compulsive disorder (OCD): the role of pregnancy/delivery. *Psychiatry Res* 89:49–58, 1999.
21. Klein DF: Commentary: Pregnancy and panic disorder. *J Clin Psychiatry* 55:293, 1994.
22. Cowe L, Lloyd DJ, Dawling S: Neonatal convulsions caused by withdrawal from maternal clomipramine. *Br J Med* 284:1837, 1982.
23. Stewart DE, Raskin J, Garfinkel PE, et al: Anorexia nervosa, bulimia and pregnancy. *Am J Obstet Gynecol* 157:1194, 1987.
24. Abraham S, Taylor A, Conti J: Postnatal depression, eating, exercise, and vomiting before and during pregnancy. *J Eat Disord* 29:482–487, 2001.
25. Franko DL, Blais MA, Becker AE, et al: Pregnancy complications and neonatal outcomes in women with eating disorders. *Am J Psychiatry* 158:1461–1466, 2001.
26. Treasure JL, Russell GF: Intrauterine growth and neonatal weight gain in babies of women with anorexia nervosa. *Br Med J Clin Res* 296:1038, 1988.
27. Hediger ML, Scholl TO, Belsky DH, et al: Patterns of weight gain in adolescent pregnancy: Effects on birth weight and preterm delivery. *Obstet Gynecol* 74:6, 1989.
28. Videbech P, Gouliaev G: First admission with puerperal psychosis: 7–14 years of follow-up. *Acta Psychiatr Scand* 91:167, 1995.
29. Auerbach JG, Hans SL, Marcus J, Maeir S: Maternal psychotropic medication and neonatal behavior. *Neurotoxicol Teratol* 14:399, 1992.
30. Falterman LG, Richardson DJ: Small left colon syndrome associated with maternal ingestion of psychotropic drugs. *J Pediatr* 97:300, 1980.
31. Woody JN, London WL, Wilbanks GD: Lithium toxicity in a newborn. *Pediatrics* 47:94, 1971.

32. Schou M: What happened to the lithium babies? A follow-up study of children born without malformation. *Acta Psychiatr Scand* 54:193, 1976.
33. Scolnick D, Nulman I, Rover J, et al: Neurodevelopment of children exposed in utero to phenytoin and carbamazepine monotherapy. *JAMA* 271:767, 1994.
34. Centers for Disease Control and Prevention: Fetal alcohol syndrome—United States, 1979–1992. *MMWR Morb Mortal Wkly Rep* 42:339, 1993.
35. Briggs GG, Freeman RK, Yaffe SJ: *Drugs in Pregnancy and Lactation: A Reference Guide to Fetal and Neonatal Risk,* 6th ed. Philadelphia: Lippincott Williams & Wilkins, 2002.
36. Blume S, Russell M: Alcohol and substance abuse in the practice of obstetrics and gynecology, in Stewart DE, Stotland NL (eds): *Psychological Aspects of Women's Health Care: The Interface between Psychiatry and Obstetrics and Gynecology,* 2d ed. Washington: American Psychiatric Press, 2001, pp 421–440.
37. American College of Obstetricians and Gynecologists: Smoking and reproductive health. ACOG technical bulletin no. 180, May 1993.
38. Milberger SSD, Biederman J, Faraone SV, et al: Is maternal smoking during pregnancy a risk factor for attention deficit hyperactivity disorder in children? *Am J Psychiatry* 153:1138, 1996.
39. James ME, Coles CD: Cocaine abuse during pregnancy: Psychiatric considerations. *Gen Hosp Psychiatry* 13:399, 1991.
40. American College of Obstetricians and Gynecologists: Domestic violence. ACOG technical bulletin no. 209, August 1995.
41. First MB, Spitzer RL, Gibbon M, Williams JBW: *Structured Clinical Interview for DSM-IV Axis I Disorders*. Research version, patient edition (SCID-I/P). New York: Biometrics Research, New York State Psychiatric Institute, 1996.
42. Ewing JA: Detecting alcoholism: The CAGE questionnaire. *JAMA* 14:1905, 1984.

20

Cardiovascular Disorders in Pregnancy

Shannon Sovndal
Jeffrey A. Tabas

KEY POINTS

- Peripartum cardiomyopathy should be considered in any pregnant or recently postpartum patient that presents with signs and symptoms of congestive heart failure and pulmonary edema.
- The clinician should exercise extreme caution in making a *new* diagnosis of asthma during pregnancy; other more serious causes of respiratory problems should be considered.
- Pregnancy alone should not cause significant limitations of daily activities due to shortness of breath, chest pain, or dizziness, and any episode of syncope or near syncope should be thoroughly evaluated in the appropriate clinical context.

INTRODUCTION

Heart disease complicates 0.4 to 4 percent of all pregnancies in the U.S.[1] The frequency of women with heart disease becoming pregnant may be increasing due to improvements in diagnosis and treatment as well as the trend toward delayed childbearing. Pregnancy is associated with myriad physiologic alterations. Over the course of the gestation, labor, delivery, and postpartum period, there are marked changes that may have significant effects on hemodynamic function. Cardiovascular decompensation may result when previously asymptomatic pathology becomes challenged by these changes or when a cardiovascular disorder presents for the first (or only) time during pregnancy. Cardiovascular disorders in pregnancy often present a significant challenge to the clinician because many of the signs and symptoms of cardiovascular disease can be obscured or misinterpreted during pregnancy. There can also be concern over the fetal safety of standard diagnostic and therapeutic modalities.

The most common cardiovascular disorders likely to become manifest during pregnancy are hypertension, myocarditis, valvular and congenital heart disease, dysrhythmias, cardiomyopathies, arterial dissection, thromboembolic disease, and ischemic heart disease. Thromboembolic disease is discussed in detail in Chap. 12, and hypertensive disorders in pregnancy are detailed in Chap. 8. The signs and symptoms, diagnosis, treatment, and follow-up for the remainder of these disorders are addressed in this chapter.

CHANGES IN PHYSIOLOGY

The anatomy and physiology of normal pregnancy are discussed in detail in Chaps. 1 and 2. During pregnancy, intravascular volume increases by 50 percent, cardiac output increases (peaking at 20 to 26 weeks), pulse rates increase by 10 to 20 beats per minute, and systemic vascular resistance decreases (mediated by changes in endogenous hormones and uterine circulation).[2] During labor and delivery, cardiac demand may increase as much as 50 percent during uterine contractions. Rapid swings in intravascular volume occur with bleeding and with the physiologic autotransfusion of at least 500 mL of blood from the placenta after delivery. These changes are most often responsible for cardiovascular compromise from preexisting cardiac disease. However, disease that prevents any of these hemodynamic and hormonal adaptations from occurring may also compromise maternal and fetal health. Other important physiologic changes that are important to note include the potential for decreased venous return in the supine position due to uterine compression of the inferior vena cava, and the hypercoagulability of the pregnant state.[1]

PHYSICAL EXAMINATION OF THE CARDIOVASCULAR SYSTEM IN PREGNANCY

The evaluation of the pregnant patient should begin with an assessment of appearance, including any findings of distress or respiratory compromise. Abnormal skin findings such as pallor or diaphoresis should be noted.

The physical examination should continue with evaluation of the vital signs. Maternal blood pressure decreases early in pregnancy. The diastolic blood pressure and the mean arterial pressure nadir at midpregnancy (16 to 20 weeks) and return to prepregnancy levels by term.[3] Increases in the resting heart rate of 10 to 15 beats per minute occur, but physiologic rates over 100 beats per minute are unusual. The respiratory rate normally increases by 1 to 2 breaths per minute. The increase is presumably due to an increase in progesterone levels and altered pulmonary mechanics due to elevation of the diaphragm.

Examination of the pulmonary system should include pulse oximetry, respiratory rate, work of breathing, and auscultation for decreased or adventitious sounds (wheezes, rales, egophony). Systematic examination of the cardiovascular system should include inspection for elevation of the jugular venous pulse, palpation for displacement of the point of maximal impulse, right ventricular heave, delay or weakness of the carotid pulses, and auscultation for cardiac murmurs, rubs, gallops, or bruits. Cardiac flow murmurs may occur normally in pregnancy due to increased plasma volume and increased cardiac output. These are characterized as soft midsystolic murmurs without radiation to the carotids or axilla. Murmurs that are loud, radiating, or diastolic should be considered pathologic until proven otherwise.[4] The presence of an S_3 is reported to be common in pregnant patients.

Peripheral edema is common in pregnancy. Venous pressures begin to rise at 10 weeks and continue until delivery.[5] Because peripheral edema in pregnancy may be a finding of preeclampsia, the practitioner should carefully assess for other findings consistent with this diagnosis, such as an increase in blood pressure or proteinuria. However, the finding of peripheral edema is neither sensitive nor specific for preeclampsia. Peripheral edema is especially concerning when it is asymmetric (deep vein thrombosis), when it is extreme (right heart failure, left heart failure, or venous obstruction), or when it is associated with jugular venous distension or a hepatojugular reflex (right- or left-sided heart failure).

THE ELECTROCARDIOGRAM IN PREGNANCY

ECG changes that occur normally with pregnancy are largely nonspecific. These include changes in the axis and nonspecific T-wave abnormalities.[6] The presence of any ischemic-appearing changes, such as planar ST depression, inverted, symmetric T waves, tall peaked T waves (hyperacute), or ST elevation should prompt consideration of acute ischemia and an emergent evaluation for acute coronary syndrome.

PRESENTING COMPLAINTS

Shortness of Breath

Shortness of breath is a common complaint during pregnancy, especially in the third trimester, when the gravid uterus and increased intraabdominal mass impedes the mechanical function of the diaphragm. Characteristics that increase the level of concern in patients with this complaint include presentation to the emergency department, acute onset or worsening of dyspnea, or severe dyspnea. Pregnancy alone should not cause significant limitations of daily activities.

Common causes of shortness of breath are upper respiratory infection and asthma exacerbation. One should, however, exercise extreme caution in making a new diagnosis of asthma during pregnancy; other more serious causes should be considered (Table 20-1). More concerning causes of shortness of breath include pneumonia, pulmonary embolus, peripartum cardiomyopathy, pericarditis, aortic dissection, and myocarditis. The physiologic stress of pregnancy may uncover preexisting cardiopulmonary diseases such as congenital heart disease, valvular disease, pulmonary hypertension, cardiomyopathy, or pulmonary fibrosis.

Evaluation should include a careful history and physical examination. Historical factors that are common in pregnancy include fatigue and dyspnea on exertion, so historical factors must be considered in context. Extreme dyspnea or fatigue is unusual. Symptoms of cardiovascular disease that were present prior to pregnancy should also be elicited, such as dyspnea on exertion, history of rheumatic fever, and episodes of chest pain, palpitations, or lightheadedness. Complaints consistent with pulmonary or venous thromboembolism, such as unequal limb swelling, prolonged immobility, pleuritic chest pain, dyspnea, and hemoptysis should increase suspicion for this diagnosis.

In any patient with concerning cardiopulmonary signs or symptoms, it is reasonable to obtain a CBC, chemistry panel, UA, and ECG and to consider a CXR. The mean hemoglobin can be expected to fall an average of 1 g/dL based on normal physiologic changes during pregnancy. Other causes should be suspected in levels below 10 g/dL.[7] The urinalysis should be regarded closely for the presence of protein, which may prompt further evaluation for preeclampsia.

Chest Pain

The differential diagnosis for chest pain is similar to that for shortness of breath. Again, nonspecific, mild chest

Table 20-1. Cardiopulmonary Disease in Pregnancy

Serious or life-threatening cardiopulmonary diseases in pregnancy
Pneumonia
Pulmonary embolus
Peripartum cardiomyopathy
Pericarditis
Aortic dissection
Myocarditis
Acute coronary syndrome
Preexisting conditions that may be uncovered by the stress of pregnancy
Congenital heart disease
Valvular disease
Pulmonary hypertension
Cardiomyopathy

pain is not uncommon in pregnancy. Historical findings that should prompt concern include presentation to the emergency department, severe chest pain, or pain of sudden onset. See specific entities below.

Palpitations

The incidence and severity of tachyarrhythmias, both supraventricular and ventricular tachycardia, may increase during pregnancy.[8] In the pregnant patient with palpitations, determine if there is a known history of dysrhythmia, the duration of symptoms, the regularity and rate of the pulse, if known, and the presence and severity of associated symptoms, such as chest pain, shortness of breath, near syncope, or syncope. Evaluation consists of a thorough history and physical, serum electrolytes, complete blood count, ECG, and consideration of chest radiography. The presence of symptoms such as chest pain, dyspnea, syncope, near syncope, or hypertension requires admission for continuous cardiac monitoring.

Syncope or Near Syncope

Any of the disorders listed in Table 20-1 may present with syncope. Based on the physiologic changes of pregnancy, it is not uncommon for the gravid patient to experience some lightheadedness. With prolonged standing, decreased venous return due to compression by the expanding size of the uterus places patients at risk of venous pooling. This may lead to near syncopal episodes. Patients may also experience problems later in pregnancy when supine due to compression of the inferior vena cava by the gravid uterus.[3] However, any episode of syncope requires admission and thorough evaluation for serious disorders such as pulmonary embolism or cardiac arrhythmia.

RISKS OF PREGNANCY IN WOMEN WITH PREEXISTING CARDIAC DISEASE

The third trimester presents the greatest risk for the development of congestive heart failure in women with cardiac disease. In general, patients with fixed output defects, such as pulmonary hypertension, mitral stenosis, and aortic stenosis, are least tolerant to changes in circulating volume and output.[1]

One study reviewed outcomes of 562 pregnant women referred for management of heart disease and found significant maternal complications in 13 percent of pregnancies (congestive heart failure, arrhythmia, stroke, cardiac death) and neonatal complications in 20 percent of pregnancies. Four factors were found to impart significant risk for maternal cardiac events:

1. prior cardiac event or arrhythmia
2. New York Heart Association (NYHA) class >2 (Table 20-2) or cyanosis
3. left heart obstruction
4. ventricular dysfunction (ejection fraction <40 percent)

Rates of complications ranged from 5 percent with none of these risk factors, to 27 percent with one risk factor, and to 75 percent with more than one of the risk factors.

Table 20-2. New York Heart Association Clinical Classification

Class	Limitations
I	None. No anginal or symptoms of cardiac insufficiency even with vigorous activity.
II	Physical activity. Comfortable at rest, but develops symptoms with ordinary activity. Symptoms may include chest pain, dyspnea, excessive fatigue, or palpitations
III	Marked limitation of physical activity. Comfortable at rest, but develops symptoms with less than ordinary activity.
IV	Symptomatic at rest and unable to perform any physical activity without discomfort.

Factors imparting increased risk for postpartum hemorrhage included anticoagulant use and cyanosis. Finally, factors imparting risk for neonatal complications included

1. NYHA class >2
2. cyanosis
3. anticoagulant therapy
4. smoking
5. multiple gestations
6. left heart obstruction[9]

SPECIFIC DISEASE ENTITIES

Pulmonary embolism is discussed in Chap. 12.

Aortic Dissection

Although extremely rare in pregnancy, arterial dissections can be a catastrophic event. They generally occur in the third trimester and common sites of dissection include the thoracic aorta (type I), iliac artery, splenic artery, and cerebral artery. The hemodynamic stresses of pregnancy discussed previously place increased strain on weakened arteries and existing aneurysms. In late pregnancy, the gravid uterus may compress the aorta in the supine position. This combined with the increased shear stress produced by ventricular ejection into the proximal aorta predisposes to intimal tears.[10] Hormonal changes also play a role in arterial dissections. Progesterone produces structural abnormalities in vessel walls, distorting the normal vessel wall.[11] Crack cocaine use may also predispose to dissection.[12]

Aortic dissection should be suspected in a patient who presents with severe chest pain, pain that radiates to the back, or chest or upper back pain associated with a neurologic deficit.[13] Risk factors include chronic or acute hypertension, Marfan's syndrome,[9] and crack cocaine use.[14] Upon presentation, blood pressure may be elevated, normal, or low. Findings on physical examination may include an aortic insufficiency murmur, pulse deficits, or inequalities between pulses. Early diagnosis is necessary for any chance of survival. Laboratory tests should include a complete blood count, coagulation panel, chemistry panel, type and screen, and cardiac enzymes. Chest radiography may reveal a widened mediastinum suggestive of a dissection, but a normal mediastinum in the presence of suggestive symptoms does not rule out the diagnosis. ECG may show nonspecific changes and is primarily helpful to assess for findings of acute cardiac ischemia.

Angiography is the gold standard for diagnosis. However, echocardiography has gained popularity because of its high sensitivity (95 to 100 percent), specificity (85 to 95 percent), and speed of use at the bedside.[13]

Surgical repair is the only treatment for arterial rupture, which is a distinct entity from aortic dissection. The goal of medical management in aortic dissection is to reduce shear force on the dissecting vessel. This is accomplished by decreasing both cardiac inotropy and afterload. This is best accomplished with intravenous beta blockade, such as with metoprolol, esmolol, or labetalol. Labetalol has some alpha blockade effects, and some authorities prefer its use for this reason. If beta blockade is inadequate to control blood pressure, intravenous nitroprusside should be added. Continuous fetal monitoring should be initiated in the viable fetus.

Acute Coronary Syndrome

Myocardial infarction (MI) is rare in pregnancy, but when it occurs it is often devastating. *Acute coronary syndrome* (ACS) is a term used to include the spectrum of unstable angina and acute MI. The mortality rate after an MI in both the mother and fetus is relatively high, approaching 40 percent.[15] Pregnant patients may be at greater risk than their age-matched nonpregnant counterparts for a number of reasons. The increased hemodynamic strain, the stress of labor and delivery, and the rapid hemodynamic changes immediately postpartum may overly tax the heart. Etiologies include coronary atherosclerosis, coronary artery spasm, thromboembolism (pregnancy hypercoagulability), coronary artery dissection, and cocaine use. ACS may occur with increased frequency in patients who are older or diabetic, and those with a family history of premature heart disease, known atherosclerotic disease, or recent cocaine use, although ACS is possible in patients without any of these historical features. A recent review of a national database of more than 400,000 patients with myocardial infarction revealed that up to one-third presented without chest pain. Shortness of breath was found to be the most common other complaint.[16] The clinician must take into account risk factors, the history, and ECG findings in developing a level of suspicion for disease. The classic description for angina includes discomfort that is characterized as substernal, pressure-like, tight or squeezing, radiating to the jaw, neck, left arm, or both arms, improved with nitroglycerin, exacerbated by exertion or relieved with rest, and associated with shortness of breath, nausea, or diaphoresis. One should note that the "classic" descriptors for angina were determined based on male patients. There are data to suggest that the more common angina symptoms in female patients are what would otherwise be considered "atypical." There are no data on the usual presenting signs in pregnancy.

A 12-lead ECG in a patient with suspected ACS should be obtained as soon as possible. Ischemic findings such as ST elevation, ST depression, or symmetric, tall, or inverted T waves warrant immediate therapy. Chest radiography should be obtained to assess for another explanation of the symptoms and complications of ACS such as congestive heart failure.

Laboratory data should include a complete blood count, an electrolyte panel, and cardiac enzymes. These include creatine kinase MB isoenzyme (CK-MB) and cardiac troponins T or I. In the presence of acute MI, an elevation may be detected as early as a few hours after symptoms, but the diagnosis is not excluded until serial sampling is done at least 12 hours after symptom onset has occurred. Negative cardiac enzymes do not exclude a diagnosis of unstable angina. The cardiac troponins are more specific than CK-MB for myocardial injury. They remain elevated for days to weeks after MI. The most useful cardiac marker in pregnancy appears to be troponin I, based on its specificity in pregnancy.[17,18]

Pregnant patients with MI are treated similarly to nonpregnant patients with a few exceptions. Patients should be admitted to a cardiac care unit and treated with beta-blockers, nitrates, morphine, heparin, and aspirin.[19] Therapeutic trials in acute MI, as in many diseases, have specifically excluded pregnant patients, and there is controversy overtheir management. A patient with an ST elevation MI should receive urgent revascularization. Thrombolytics are relatively contraindicated in pregnancy. Therefore, cardiac catheterization for primary angioplasty should be considered in these patients, especially in the presence of hemodynamic instability, recurrent ischemia, or extensive myocardium at risk.[19] If the acute MI is associated with cocaine use, beta blockade should be avoided, and initial treatment should begin with aspirin and nitrates. Benzodiazepines can be given if maternal benefits outweigh the risks to the fetus. Glycoprotein 2b3a (GP2b3a) inhibitors should be considered by the cardiologist if percutaneous intervention is planned. There is insufficient evidence to support the use of the GP2b3a inhibitors in the absence of percutaneous intervention. The antiplatelet medication, clopidogrel has been shown to improve outcomes in patients with acute non-ST elevation MI (CURE trial).[20] However, pregnant patients were excluded from the trial, and it is unclear whether they would benefit from this intervention.

Myocarditis

Myocarditis is defined as an inflammatory process of the heart. It is most commonly caused by viral infection, although it may also be the result of hypersensitivity states such as rheumatic fever, or be caused by radiation, chemicals, or drugs. Often fulminant in pregnant women, the diagnosis is inferred from ECG changes such as ST- or T-wave changes. Sequelae include arrhythmias, heart failure, and death. It may be associated with pericarditis. Physical examination is often unremarkable unless heart failure or pericardial findings are present. Heart failure or arrhythmias should be treated as they would in the absence of myocarditis. Chagas' disease (*Trypanosoma cruzi*) is a parasite that causes myocarditis in Central and South America. It is rarely diagnosed in the acute phase, but is a common cause of cardiomyopathy in people from these regions.

Pericarditis and Pericardial Tamponade

Pericarditis should be considered in any patient with chest pain. It is classically positional in nature, described as worse when supine, and improved when sitting forward. It is often described as sharp or stabbing, may have a pleuritic component, and may last from days to weeks. It is diagnosed by characteristic ECG findings of diffuse ST-segment elevation and PR depression. An echocardiogram is necessary to rule out significant pericardial effusion. The most feared sequela is pericardial tamponade. Admission is warranted for any pregnant patient with newly diagnosed pericarditis. The presence of fever, dyspnea, signs of heart failure, or hypotension increase the level of concern.

Pericardial tamponade is defined as fluid in the pericardial space which impairs relaxation of the heart. Impaired diastolic filling occurs, leading to decreased cardiac output and increased central venous pressure. Findings suggestive of tamponade include tachycardia, hypotension, elevated jugular venous pressure, muffled heart sounds, and pulsus parodoxus (a greater than 10 mm decrease in systolic pressure during inspiration). Chest radiography reveals an enlarged cardiac silhouette, especially without other findings of heart failure. ECG may reveal low voltage and electrical alternans (alternating size and morphology of every other beat). Echocardiography is the diagnostic study of choice and demonstrates pericardial fluid with right atrial and/or ventricular collapse during diastole. Treatment includes volume resuscitation and emergent pericardiocentesis in the unstable patient.

Dysrhythmias

Although there is an increased incidence of maternal cardiac dysrhythmias during pregnancy, life-threatening dysrhythmias in the absence of preexisting heart disease are rare in the pregnant female.[21] The most common ECG findings in pregnant patients are simple ventricular and atrial ectopy, occurring in 60 percent of pregnant women. Other common findings include atrial tachycardia, paroxysmal supraventricular tachycardia (PSVT), ventricular premature contractions (VPC), and to a lesser extent ventricular tachycardia.[22] The etiology of these disturbances remains unclear. Contributing factors may be increased maternal circulatory volume resulting in increased atrial stretch and end-diastolic volume, increased plasma catecholamines, and increased adrenergic receptor sensitivity.[8] Patients with preexisting cardiomyopathy, cardiac ischemia, and valvular heart disease may present with rhythm disturbances such as atrial flutter, atrial fibrillation, and symptomatic bradycardia.

Dysrhythmia must be considered in any pregnant woman who presents with shortness of breath, syncope or near syncope, or palpitations. If the patient is experiencing the disturbance upon arrival to the emergency department, a 12-lead ECG and cardiac monitor may be all that is needed to make the diagnosis. If the patient is asymptomatic upon presentation, a 12-lead ECG as well as ambulatory cardiac monitoring is appropriate. Serum electrolytes, including sodium, potassium, chloride, magnesium, phosphorus, and calcium should be obtained. Finally, an echocardiogram should be considered to rule out structural abnormalities.

Both the type of rhythm disturbance and the patient's hemodynamic stability will guide medical management. Any disturbance resulting in hypotension is especially concerning because placental-fetal blood flow may be jeopardized. Life-threatening dysrhythmias should be treated with electrical cardioversion or defibrillation as indicated by ACLS guidelines. The fetus seems to be at little risk from the procedure and is at greatest risk from maternal hypotension.[1] Cardioversion is safe at all stages of pregnancy.[8] Because the amount of current reaching the fetus is small, the risk of causing a fetal arrhythmia is slight. Nevertheless, transient fetal arrhythmia has been reported, and fetal monitoring during the procedure is recommended.[22] Any patient with sustained dysrrhythmia that requires reversal or suppression should be hospitalized for observation.

Pharmacologic intervention is more complicated in the pregnant patient than in the nonpregnant patient. Although the mother's well being should be paramount, teratogenic risk and fetal complications must be kept in mind. The most extensively used and safest agents in pregnancy include digoxin, quinidine, and propanolol. Other relatively safe drugs include lidocaine and adenosine.[8]

For control of stable supraventricular tachycardia, adenosine is considered the drug of choice when vagal maneuvers have failed.[23] Propanolol (preferred over atenolol) and digoxin are also reasonable options. Digoxin has also been shown to be effective in controlling the maternal heart rate. Because it crosses the placenta freely, it has been used extensively to treat fetal supraventricular arrhythmias as well.[24]

For hemodynamically stable ventricular tachycardia, lidocaine is the recommended drug of choice. Occasional fetal lidocaine toxicity has been reported, but this has been primarily seen with large doses used for anesthesia.[25] Amiodarone causes fetal hypothyroidism if given chronically. The risk to the fetus with a single dose is probably small.

Bradyarrhythmias are generally the result of congenital or acquired heart block. Atropine is generally effective and the dosing regimen is similar to that for the nonpregnant patient. Both temporary and permanent transvenous pacing are safe and reasonable options in pregnancy for bradycardia and heart block.

When the patient is discharged, she should be referred to a cardiologist and a high-risk obstetrician. The risks and benefits of each medication prescribed should be discussed with the patient, and she should know how to take the drug as directed. If any recurrence of symptoms or new complaints occurs, the patient should promptly contact her doctor or return to the emergency department.

Cardiomyopathy

Peripartum cardiomyopathy is a rare form of heart failure that is unique to the pregnant woman. Reports of mortality rates in women with peripartum cardiomyopathy range from 6% to 50%.[26,27,28] Resolution of ventricular dysfunction has been reported to occur over time in 50 percent to 60 percent of patients.[26,27] There are many different types of cardiomyopathy, including hypertensive, alcoholic, viral, ischemic, hypertrophic, drug-induced, and idiopathic. The etiology of peripartum cardiomyopathy remains unclear, but it is clearly a distinct entity. Numerous hypotheses have been proposed, suggesting that peripartum cardiomyopathy may be caused by myocarditis, an abnormal immune response to pregnancy, or hemodynamic stresses of pregnancy.

The incidence of peripartum cardiomyopathy is estimated to be approximately 1 per 3000 to 4000 live births.[27] Because the disease is rare, a good history and physical examination are necessary to make the diagnosis. Obvious signs of heart failure such as pulmonary crackles, paroxysmal nocturnal dyspnea, orthopnea, chest pain, cough, new murmurs, and neck vein distention should necessitate further work-up. Multiple risk factors have been identified and include multiparity, advanced maternal age, preeclampsia, gestational hypertension, multiple gestational pregnancy, and African-American race.[27] The differential diagnosis for symptoms of heart failure in the final month of pregnancy or the first 5 months postpartum should include those mentioned above, as well as sepsis, drug toxicity, and metabolic disorders. Peripartum cardiomyopathy is diagnosed by echocardiographic evidence of new left ventricular systolic dysfunction that occurs in the peripartum period. The diagnosis is often difficult because a large percentage of healthy pregnant patients present with signs of fatigue, pedal edema, and shortness of breath in the final month of gestation. Suspicion of cardiomyopathy may be raised by the finding of increased heart size in the chest radiograph of an otherwise healthy pregnant or postpartum woman. Four criteria that have been suggested for the diagnosis of peripartum cardiomyopathy are listed in Table 20-3.[29] These criteria are important in making the correct diagnosis. Women with other types of cardiomyopathy will generally present in the second or early third trimester, when the hemodynamic stresses are the greatest. The majority of women with peripartum cardiomyopathy (75 percent) will present in the postpartum period.

Peripartum cardiomyopathy is treated similarly to other dilated cardiomyopathies. The mainstay of treatment includes sodium restriction, diuretics, vasodilators, and digoxin as needed.[27] Beta-blockers such as carvedilol have been shown to reduce mortality in dilated cardiomyopathy.[30] If thrombus is noted on echocardiography, then anticoagulation with heparin should be initiated. Warfarin can be given postpartum. Special attention must be paid to possible fetal teratogenesis and to changes in drug and drug metabolite excretion during breast-feeding. Angiotensin-converting enzyme inhibitors are contraindicated in pregnancy, but should be initiated postdelivery. Spironolactone, also recommended in patients with heart failure, is not recommended in pregnancy.

Table 20-3. Diagnostic Criteria for Peripartum Cardiomyopathy

Echocardiographic evidence of new left ventricular systolic dysfunction that occurs in the peripartum period
Onset of heart failure in the last month of pregnancy or in the first 5 months postpartum
Absence of determinable cause for cardiac failure
Absence of demonstrable heart disease before the last month of pregnancy

Aggressive treatment and follow-up are paramount for patients diagnosed with peripartum cardiomyopathy. The majority of maternal deaths occur within 3 months of the initial onset of symptoms. Consultation with specialists in obstetrics, perinatology, and cardiology are essential. If the diagnosis is made prior to delivery, hospitalization should be considered. An anesthesiologist should also be consulted for possible delivery complications. Transfer to a high-risk perinatal center is recommended.

VALVULAR DISEASE AND CONGENITAL HEART DISEASE

Pregnancy in most women with valvular and congenital heart disease has low overall fetal and maternal mortality.[31] However, there is risk for other cardiac complications such as arrhythmia, heart failure, and stroke. In the past, rheumatic heart disease led the list of cardiac diseases in pregnancy. With the reduced incidence of childhood rheumatic fever, and the advancement of medical and surgical management of congenital heart disease, the leading cardiac complication in pregnancy is now congenital heart disease.[32] Although the overall incidence of valvular and congenital heart disease in pregnancy is rare, the possible effects on maternal morbidity and mortality can be devastating. Thus in any pregnant patient that develops symptoms of dyspnea on exertion, excessive shortness of breath, palpitations, or chest discomfort, the possibility of previously undiagnosed valvular or congenital heart disease must be entertained.

A thorough history and physical examination should proceed in the patient with known or suspected valvular or congenital heart disease. This should include an assessment for sequelae of endocarditis, such as fever, Roth spots (retinal hemorrhages with central clearing), Janeway lesions (nontender plaques on palms of hands and soles of feet), and Osler nodes (tender nodules on the tips of the toes and fingers).

A transthoracic echocardiogram is an excellent tool to assess cardiac structure and function. It posses no risk to either the mother or fetus, and when coupled with Doppler ultrasound, it can provide essential information about lesions and their severity.

Valvular Heart Disease

Rheumatic fever remains the leading cause of valvular heart disease. Other causes include bacterial endocarditis and congenital lesions. Mitral stenosis is by far the most frequently discovered lesion (90 percent).[33] The next most common abnormality is mitral insufficiency, usually in combination with mitral stenosis, aortic insufficiency, and aortic stenosis. Both tricuspid and pulmonic valve disease are generally found in combination with one of the above lesions and will not be addressed separately.

Mitral stenosis may cause dyspnea, orthopnea, and paroxysmal nocturnal dyspnea. Women with severe mitral stenosis and symptoms prior to conception will predictably not tolerate the physiologic changes of pregnancy.[2] They are advised to undergo correction, such as percutaneous balloon valvotomy, prior to conception. Even in previously asymptomatic patients with mitral stenosis, complications such as left atrial enlargement with resultant atrial fibrillation and possible thrombus formation may arise. As the gradient increases across the narrowed mitral valve, the atrium grows in size.

Both aortic and mitral insufficiency are well tolerated in pregnancy when uncomplicated by another valvular lesion. Significant aortic stenosis, on the other hand, can greatly increase maternal mortality. With a pressure gradient of $\geq$70 mmHg across the aortic valve, cardiac output is greatly dependent on left ventricular end-diastolic volume. In situations in which a sudden volume loss occurs, such as maternal hemorrhage or epidural anesthesia, blood pressure may drop precipitously. In addition, ventricular arrhythmias may arise if there is left ventricle hypertrophy as a result of aortic stenosis. Because of a high complication rate, patients with symptoms prior to pregnancy are advised to delay conception until after surgical correction.[2]

Patients with bioprosthetic valves usually tolerate pregnancy well. In patients with mechanical valve prosthesis, there is an increased risk of thrombus secondary to the hypercoagulable state of pregnancy.

Congenital Heart Disease

The pathophysiology of congenital heart disease is extremely varied. Women with congenital heart disease may tolerate pregnancy well. However, in patients with pulmonary hypertension, Eisenmenger's syndrome, or Marfan's syndrome, maternal death approaches 50 percent. The most commonly seen congenital heart diseases are atrial septal defect (ASD), ventricular septal defect (VSD), and patent ductus arteriosus (PDA). All of these lesions result in left-to-right shunts, and are generally well tolerated. Other less commonly found congenital heart diseases include pulmonic stenosis, bicuspid aortic valve, coarctation of the aorta, Marfan's syndrome, and tetralogy of Fallot.

Marfan's syndrome may cause life-threatening aortic complications including dilatation, dissection, and valvular regurgitation. The pregnant patient is especially prone to complications if aortic dilatation is greater than 40 mm at baseline.[34] In tetralogy of Fallot (and other right-to-left shunts), the pregnancy-related fall in systemic vascular resistance and rise in cardiac output exacerbates the right to left shunting. The result is worsening cyanosis.

Treatment of pregnant patients with valvular or congenital heart disease will depend on the specific disorder and its severity. Prognosis is variable for any given disorder, but generally correlates with functional ability. The New York Heart Association clinical classification is a good prognostic indicator (Table 20-2). Women with New York Heart Association class I or II have a less than 1 percent mortality associated with pregnancy. In women with class III or IV symptoms, mortality approaches 5 to 15 percent.[2]

Malignant hypertension is discussed in Chap 8.

ENDOCARDITIS PROPHYLAXIS FOR LABOR AND DELIVERY

The Committee on Rheumatic Fever, Endocarditis, and Kawasaki Disease of the American Heart Association does not recommend routine antibiotic prophylaxis in patients with valvular heart disease undergoing uncomplicated vaginal delivery or cesarean section unless infection is suspected. Antibiotics are optional for high-risk patients with prosthetic heart valves, a previous history of endocarditis, complex congenital heart disease, or a surgically constructed systemic-pulmonary conduit. Antibiotic regimens include ampicillin 1 to 2 g IV and gentamicin 1.5 mg/kg (not to exceed 120 mg) before delivery and ampicillin 1 g IV 6 hours later. For penicillin-allergic patients, vancomycin 1 g q12h IV can be substituted for ampicillin.[35]

ANTICOAGULATION IN PREGNANCY

Unfractionated heparin is currently recommended for anticoagulation in pregnancy. Use of low-molecular-weight-heparin (LMWH) is also acceptable, although there is less literature support for its use. The two potential complications of anticoagulation during pregnancy are bleeding and teratogenicity. Because unfractionated heparin and LMWH do not cross the placental barrier, they are considered safe for the fetus. One study showed that the rate of major bleeding in pregnant patients treated with unfractionated heparin was 2 percent, which is consistent with the rates reported in nonpregnant patients.[36]

In women with mechanical valves, however, the management is different. The American College of Cardiology/American Heart Association guidelines for the management of mechanical valves in pregnancy recommend coumadin as first-line therapy and includes counseling the patient and her partner of the risks and benefits.[2] With heparin, there are higher rates of maternal bleeding and thrombosis, and the rates of fetal wastage are equivalent. The rate of coumadin-induced embryopathy is about 6 percent. This risk may be decreased or eliminated by switching to heparin during the sixth to twelfth week of gestation. Anticoagulation with coumadin for women with mechanical valves is used widely in Europe. In the U.S., however, the medicolegal consequences of using a medication that carries a warning of contraindication in pregnancy warrant consideration.[36]

The use of low-dose aspirin in pregnancy is considered safe, with no increase in maternal or neonatal adverse effects, but the safety of higher-dose therapy remains to be determined.

REFERENCES

1. Ramsey PS, Ramin KD, Ramin SW: Cardiac disease in pregnancy. *Am J Perinatol* 18:245–266, 2001.
2. Bonow RO, Carabello B, de Leon AC Jr, et al: Guidelines for the management of patients with valvular heart disease: executive summary. A report of the American College of Cardiology/American Heart Association Task Force on Practice Guidelines (Committee on Management of Patients with Valvular Heart Disease). *Circulation* 98:1949–1984, 1998.
3. Gabbe SG, Niebyl JR, Simpson JL: Obstetrics: *Normal and Problem Pregnancies*, 4th ed., New York: Churchill Livingstone, 2002, pp. xvii, 1429.
4. Mishra M, Chambers JB, Jackson G: Murmurs in pregnancy: an audit of echocardiography. *BMJ* 304:1413–1414, 1992.
5. Sparey C, Haddad N, Sissons G, et al: The effect of pregnancy on the lower-limb venous system of women with varicose veins. *Eur J Vasc Endovasc Surg* 18:294–299, 1999.
6. Veille JC, Kitzman DW, Bacevice AE: Effects of pregnancy on the electrocardiogram in healthy subjects during strenuous exercise. *Am J Obstet Gynecol* 175:1360–1364, 1996.
7. Recommendations to prevent and control iron deficiency in the United States. Centers for Disease Control and Prevention. *MMWR Recomm Rep* 47(RR-3):1–29, 1998.
8. Tan HL, Lie KI: Treatment of tachyarrhythmias during pregnancy and lactation. *Eur Heart J* 22:458–464, 2001.
9. Siu SC, Colman JM, Sorensen S, et al: Prospective multicenter study of pregnancy outcomes in women with heart disease. *Circulation* 104:515–521, 2001.
10. Ohlson L: Effects of the pregnant uterus on the abdominal aorta and its branches. *Acta Radiol Diagn* 19:369–376, 1978.
11. Madu EC, Kosinski DJ, Wilson WR, et al: Two-vessel coronary artery dissection in the peripartum period. Case report and literature review. *Angiology* 45:809–816, 1994.
12. Madu EC, Shala B, Baugh D: Crack-cocaine-associated aortic dissection in early pregnancy—a case report. *Angiology* 50:163–168, 1999.
13. Pretre R, Von Segesser LK: Aortic dissection. *Lancet* 349:1461–1464, 1997.
14. Hsue PY, Salinas CL, Bolger AF, et al: Acute aortic dissection related to crack cocaine. *Circulation* 105:1592–1595, 2002.
15. Soderlin MK, Purhonen S, Haring P, et al: Myocardial infarction in a parturient. A case report with emphasis on medication and management. *Anaesthesia* 49:870–872, 1994.
16. Canto JG, Shlipak MG, Rogers WJ, et al: Prevalence, clinical characteristics, and mortality among patients with myocardial infarction presenting without chest pain. JAMA 283:3223–3229, 2000.
17. Shivvers SA, Wians FH Jr, Keffer JH, et al: Maternal cardiac troponin I levels during normal labor and delivery. *Am J Obstet Gynecol* 180(1 Pt 1):122, 1999.
18. Adams JE 3rd, Abendschein DR, Jaffe AS: Biochemical markers of myocardial injury. Is MB creatine kinase the choice for the 1990s? *Circulation* 88:750–763, 1993.
19. Ryan TJ, Antman EM, Brooks NH, et al: 1999 update: ACC/AHA guidelines for the management of patients with acute myocardial infarction. A report of the American College of Cardiology/American Heart Association Task Force on Practice Guidelines (Committee on Management of Acute Myocardial Infarction). *J Am Coll Cardiol* 34: 890–911, 1999.
20. Yusuf S, Zhao F, Mehta SR, et al: Effects of clopidogrel in addition to aspirin in patients with acute coronary syndromes

without ST-segment elevation. *N Engl J Med* 345:494–502, 2001.

21. Joglar JA, Page RL: Antiarrhythmic drugs in pregnancy. *Curr Opin Cardiol* 16:40–45, 2001.
22. Page RL: Treatment of arrhythmias during pregnancy. *Am Heart J* 130:871–876, 1995.
23. Elkayam U, Goodwin TM: Adenosine therapy for supraventricular tachycardia during pregnancy. *Am J Cardiol* 75:521–523, 1995.
24. King CR, Mattioli L, Goertz KK, et al: Successful treatment of fetal supraventricular tachycardia with maternal digoxin therapy. *Chest* 85:573–575, 1984.
25. Kim WY, Pomerance JJ, Miller AA: Lidocaine intoxication in a newborn following local anesthesia for episiotomy. *Pediatrics* 64:643–645, 1979.
26. Elkayam U, Tummala PP, Rao K, et al: Maternal and fetal outcomes of subsequent pregnancies in women with peripartum cardiomyopathy. *N Engl J Med* 344:1567–1571, 2001.
27. Pearson GD, Veille JC, Rahimtoola S, et al: Peripartum cardiomyopathy: National Heart, Lung, and Blood Institute and Office of Rare Diseases (National Institutes of Health) workshop recommendations and review. *JAMA* 283:1183–1188, 2000.
28. Felker GM, Thompson RE, Hare JM, et al: Underlying causes and long-term survival in patients with initially unexplained cardiomyopathy. *N Engl J Med* 342:1077–1084, 2000.
29. Mehta NJ, Mehta RN, Khan IA: Peripartum cardiomyopathy: clinical and therapeutic aspects. *Angiology* 52:759–762, 2001.
30. Packer M, Bristow MR, Cohn JN, et al: The effect of carvedilol on morbidity and mortality in patients with chronic heart failure. U.S. Carvedilol Heart Failure Study Group. *N Engl J Med* 334:1349–1355, 1996.
31. Siu SC, Colman JM: Heart disease and pregnancy. *Heart* 85:710–715, 2001.
32. Pitkin RM, Perloff JK, Koos BJ, et al: Pregnancy and congenital heart disease. *Ann Intern Med* 112:445–454, 1990.
33. Brady K, Duff P: Rheumatic heart disease in pregnancy. *Clin Obstet Gynecol* 32:21–40, 1989.
34. Lind J, Wallenburg HC: The Marfan syndrome and pregnancy: a retrospective study in a Dutch population. *Eur J Obstet Gynecol Reprod Biol* 98:28–35, 2001.
35. Dajani AS, Taubert KA, Wilson W, et al: Prevention of bacterial endocarditis. Recommendations by the American Heart Association. *Circulation* 96:358–366, 1997.
36. Ginsberg JS, Greer I, Hirsh J: Use of antithrombotic agents during pregnancy. *Chest* 119(1 Suppl):122S–131S, 2001.

SECTION V

PROBLEMS IN LABOR, DELIVERY, AND THE POSTPARTUM PERIOD

21

Emergency Delivery, Preterm Labor, and Postpartum Hemorrhage

Keri Gardner

KEY POINTS

- A patient that may deliver before arriving at her destination should not be transferred without an attendant who is prepared to do the delivery him- or herself.
- Do not examine a woman with ruptured membranes except with a sterile speculum (preferred) and/or sterile gloves.
- A prolapsed umbilical cord is a fetal life-threatening occurrence. If a prolapsed cord is noted upon patient presentation in a viable gestation, use a sterile gloved hand to reach into the vagina and elevate the presenting part.
- Shoulder dystocia may be associated with significant fetal morbidity and mortality; thus one must have complete knowledge of the maneuvers required to reduce shoulder dystocia before it occurs.
- In the event of postpartum hemorrhage, first evaluate and treat for uterine atony. Genital lacerations and retained placenta are two other common causes of postpartum hemorrhage.

INTRODUCTION

Delivery of an infant can be one of the easiest events to occur in the emergency department or one of the most harrowing. Knowing the steps to take in case of complications during delivery will allow the emergency physician to act with a clear head and avoid potential disaster. This chapter includes discussions of routine and complicated vaginal deliveries in the ED, as well as ED management of preterm labor and postpartum hemorrhage. Most emergency physicians will not be performing most of these tasks most of the time. However, given the requirements of Emergency Medical Treatment and Active Labor Act (EMTALA) and the lack of availability of specialty back-up in all locales, it is essential that emergency physicians and physicians who practice in acute care areas be familiar with all of these concepts in the rare event they are the only provider available.

DELIVERY OF AN INFANT IN THE EMERGENCY DEPARTMENT

Normal Delivery

A full term infant is between 38 and 42 weeks gestation, and will weigh an average of 3000 to 3500 grams. Routine prenatal care provides basic screening laboratory tests, which include hemoglobin and hematocrit, blood type, Pap smear, and screening for STDs, rubella, hepatitis, group B streptococci, and in many cases HIV. Risk factors for complicated vaginal delivery such as active herpes simplex virus (HSV) lesions are identified. A screening ultrasound may or may not have been done for fetal anatomy, fetal number, or lie.

The first stage of labor is defined as the period from the moment labor begins until cervical dilation is complete (10 cm), and can last from 4 to 24 hours or more. The second stage of labor is the period from the point cervical dilation is complete until delivery is completed, and again can be highly variable in duration, from minutes to hours. The third stage of labor starts after the infant has been delivered and ends with the delivery of the placenta. This can last from 5 to 30 minutes, with ≥30 minutes defined as abnormal.

The Role of Intrapartum Monitoring

Laboring women on an obstetric service may have two types of monitoring. One is via a tocodynamometer, which is a pressure-sensitive device affixed with straps across the gravid uterus to measure the relative strength and frequency of contractions. While useful to obstetricians who are inducing or following laboring patients, this device has limited utility in the emergency department. The other fetal monitor is a Doppler device that is also placed across the abdomen and detects fetal heart motion, which is translated into the fetal heartbeat. Fetal heart tracings are followed for both the absolute number of heart beats (120 to 160 bpm being normal) and for periodic changes. A nonreassuring fetal heart may be suggested by fetal bradycardia (<120 bpm), or by patterns determined to portend poor fetal outcome (late decelerations and poor beat-to-beat variations). A full discussion of fetal heart tracing interpretations is beyond the scope of this chapter, and interpretation of fetal heart strips is best done by an obstetric provider. If a laboring patient remains in the ED for an extended period of time in the absence of a fetal monitor or one trained to interpret it, the fetal heart should be auscultated every 30 minutes and the rate recorded.

Evaluation of the Laboring Patient in the Emergency Department

The most relevant question posed to the emergency physician when presented with a patient in labor is "Is this patient able to be safely transported to labor and delivery without a physician escort and without concern for imminent delivery?" A 2-minute assessment of the laboring patient should help answer this question, and includes ascertaining gestational age, rupture of membranes, gravidity and parity, and strength and frequency of the contractions. Vaginal examination using a sterile gloved hand should be performed if the patient is >37 weeks or, in the case of preterm labor, if there is strong concern for imminent delivery (presenting part, prolapsed cord, or maternal insistence that she has to push).

Cervical dilation, effacement, and fetal descent should be estimated. *Cervical dilation* is measured with the index and middle fingers spread between the inner rim of the cervix and is expressed in centimeters. Care must be taken to accurately determine the location of the cervical rim. *Effacement* is the thinness of the cervix and is expressed as a percentage, from 0 to 100 percent. *Fetal descent* is designated by the location of the presenting bony part. At the level of the ischial spines, the station is 0, and at 1 cm below the ischial spines the station is +1, whereas if the presenting part is 1 cm above the ischial spines, it is designated −1. At 2 cm it is +2, and at 3 cm it is +3. If it is more than 3 cm below the level of the ischial spines, the infant is usually crowning.

Although it is obvious that a crowning infant (head present on the perineum) needs to remain in the emergency department for delivery, beware that the multiparous woman with 10 cm dilation and 100 percent effacement at any station can deliver very rapidly. While it is impossible to precisely predict the timing of a delivery, a fully-dilated multiparous woman probably should have a physician escort, or an obstetric consult should come to the ED if her contractions are strong and regular.

Delivery in the Emergency Department

If delivery is to occur in the emergency department, obtain the information outlined above while establishing IV access and obtaining a neonatal warmer and fetal monitor. If an OB pack is not available, obtain the equipment listed in Table 21-1.

Place the patient in the lithotomy position and assess the presenting part. Some routinely prep the perineum with povidone-iodine. Encourage the mother to breathe through her contractions while you prepare, but realize that the urge to push once the infant has crowned is almost irresistible.

Cephalic Delivery

Most infants are delivered in the cephalic, occiput anterior (OA) position. This means that the baby is delivered facing the floor, tilted slightly to one side or the other (Fig. 21-1).

Table 21-1. Required Equipment for Emergency Vaginal Delivery

Sterile gloves and gown
Povidone-iodine
Gauze pads
Two hemostats
Scissors
Bulb syringe
Blankets
Red-topped tube for cord blood

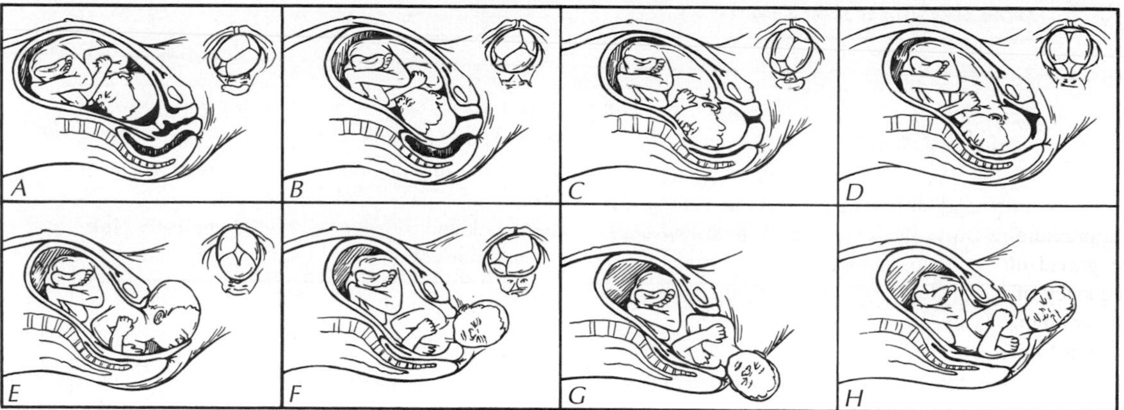

Fig. 21-1. Cardinal movements in labor. *A*. Unengaged fetal vertex in the LOA position (insct in upper-right-hand corner). *B*. Descent of the fetal vertex with flexion of the head. *C*. Further flexion and descent of the head with internal rotation of the vertex to near occiput anterior. *D*. Further internal rotation to straight occiput anterior and descent of the fetal vertex. *E*. Fetal head extension underneath the pubic symphysis. *F*. External rotation of the head (restitution). *G*. Downward gentle traction on the fetal vertex allows delivery of the anterior shoulder. *H*. Gentle upward traction on the fetal vertex allows delivery of the posterior shoulder.

Occiput posterior (OP) infants ("sunny side up") are generally slower and more difficult to deliver.

Place your dominant hand on the fetal head to provide support and control fetal descent. Your nondominant hand should grasp a gauze pad and use it to protect the perineum. This is done by placing your thumb and index finger on either side of the perineum in a pinching fashion. The best way to avoid perineal lacerations is to provide adequate pressure to control the head from crowning too quickly while protecting the perineum with the free hand.

Once the head has crossed the perineum, the head will usually rotate slightly to accommodate the shoulder. Gently continue the rotation of the fetal head so that it is facing sideways. There is usually a natural pause at this point, so use your index finger to check gently around the neck for a nuchal cord, which occurs in up to 25 percent of all deliveries. If present, it must be reduced before delivering the body. If the cord is loose around the neck, it can gently be pulled over the fetal head. Do not force this, as the cord can avulse if it is too tight. If the nuchal cord is tight, use two hemostats to clamp the cord and then cut it with scissors between the two clamps. Next, perform bulb suction of the mouth and nose if possible, but if the contractions are too close together this will not be feasible. Encourage the woman to pant through her contractions and avoid pushing. To deliver the body, place the palms of your hands on either side of the infant's, head providing support for the head and shoulders. Angle the body slightly downward to deliver the anterior shoulder and then straight upward to deliver the rest of the body. Gentle downward traction only should be applied to limit strain on the brachial plexus.

The delivered infant can comfortably rest with its head in the palm of your nondominant hand and the body on your arm, with your arm pressed against your body for stability. It is also perfectly acceptable to place the newly delivered infant on the mother's abdomen. First, use the bulb to suction the nose and mouth, and then use the free hand to clamp the umbilical cord in two places prior to cutting it between the clamps. Provide neonatal assessment and care (see below) while waiting for the placenta to deliver.

Delivery of the Placenta

After the baby is delivered, resist the urge to pull on the cord! Very gentle traction is acceptable since the placenta may be separated but not yet pushed out. Undue traction on the umbilical cord can cause uterine eversion or cord avulsion. The only time it is appropriate to hasten placental detachment is in the case of maternal hemorrhage. While it is normal to continue bleeding after delivery of the infant, any blood loss that seems to approach 500 mL is more than expected. Normal placental detachment time is usually within 15 minutes, but may normally take up to 30 minutes. If the placenta has not delivered in 30 minutes,

Table 21-2. Apgar Score Criteria[a]

Criteria	0	1	2
Heart rate	Absent	<100 bpm	>100 bpm
Respiratory effort	Absent	Slow or irregular	Normal
Muscle tone	Flaccid	Some extremity flexion	Active movement
Reflex irritability	No response	Grimace	Cry
Color	Pale or blue	Body pink and extremities blue	Completely pink

[a]The score is assessed at 1 and 5 minutes of life.

expert obstetric consultation is recommended. There are three clinical signs of placental separation:

1. A gush of blood usually occurs as the placenta separates.
2. The cord will lengthen as the placenta delivers.
3. As the placenta separates and moves from the uterus into the vagina, the uterus contracts and appears to rise up and change in shape from discoid to globular.

Once the placenta has separated and delivered, place a hand on the abdomen and massage the uterus. It should be firm. Inspect the placenta for intactness. Evaluate the perineum and rectum for lacerations. Oxytocin is routinely used to encourage uterine contraction and decrease bleeding after the placenta has delivered. It can be delivered as 10 to 20 units in 1 L of normal saline at >200 mL/h or as 10 units intramuscularly.

Immediate Postpartum Care

Immediately postpartum, maternal feeding of the infant is preferred if there are no neonatal concerns. Ensure that the infant is well bundled and wearing a hat to minimize heat loss, and is securely identified. A woman with periurethral tears or severe vaginal edema may have trouble voiding and may need a Foley catheter immediately postpartum. Ice packs applied to the perineum will help decrease labial edema. Reassess every 15 to 30 minutes for firmness of the uterus and volume of vaginal bleeding, as well as overall condition. Continue antibiotics if fever was present prior to delivery.

Neonatal Assessment and Care in the Emergency Department

Most neonates (90 percent) are vigorous at birth and only require airway clearance with a bulb syringe avoidance of heat loss with blankets and cap, and cord clamping. Apgar scores should be taken at 1 and 5 minutes of life (Table 21-2).

However, preparation is critical to allow rapid resuscitation of the 10 percent of newborns who require assistance to help with the transition from the intrauterine environment to life outside the womb. This should be a routine part of preparation for impending ED delivery. The basic equipment necessary for neonatal resuscitation is listed in Tables 21-3 and 21-4. Ideally, two persons should be assigned to care for the neonate who have no other responsibilities. Preferably a pediatrician or neonatal specialist should be in attendance, especially in the presence of preterm delivery or multiple gestations, but this is not always possible in emergent circumstances. In the absence of a pediatrician, another emergency or family physician would be helpful. Nursing support is also helpful in these situations. If there is only one physician in attendance at a delivery, then that physician will need to briefly step away from the mother to attend to the newly-delivered baby for a few minutes in order to adequately care for it.

Table 21-3. Equipment Necessary for Neonatal Resuscitation

Radiant warmer and blankets
Oxygen with tubing and flowmeter
Suction bulbs and suction source with regulator and DeLee catheters
Stethoscope
Self-inflating bag with infant masks and 100% O_2 adapter
Laryngoscope and #0 and #1 blades with functioning bulbs and batteries
Endotracheal tubes 2.5-4.0 mm internal diameter
Meds: $NaHCO_3$, epinephrine (1:10,000), naloxone, dextrose, volume expanders

Table 21-4. Endotracheal Tube Size Based on Neonatal Weight

Endotracheal Tube Size (Internal Diameter)	Infant Weight (g)
2.5 mm	<1000
3.0 mm	1000-2000
3.5 mm	2000-3000
4.0 mm	>3000

It is important to dry the infant with warm towels, then wrap the child in a clean, dry towel or sheet and place it under a radiant heat source to prevent hypothermia. Preterm infants are particularly susceptible to the effects of hypothermia. Their heads should be covered, as heat can be lost rapidly if the head is left uncovered at room temperature. Clearing the infant's oropharynx and nasal passages of mucus or fluid will provide stimulation while assisting its initial breathing efforts. The head should be placed in the sniffing position and slightly lower than the rest of the body to facilitate breathing and fluid drainage from the airway. If the amniotic fluid was meconium-stained (see below), the trachea should be intubated and suctioned directly with an appropriate-sized endotracheal tube (Table 21-4) and regulated wall suction. The endotracheal tube may be removed after suctioning, but this procedure may need to be repeated until the suctioned aspirate is no longer meconum-stained. If the infant is stable, its stomach contents should be aspirated. Breathing efforts are then promoted by the tactile stimulation of drying the amniotic fluid from the baby with towels and gently rubbing the back or flicking the soles of the baby's heels. If there is no response to two to three attempts at stimulation, further attempts are unlikely to be successful.

Evaluation of the infant's heart rate (whether it is more or less than 100 bpm) is the most reliable indicator of the need for further resuscitation. Evaluation of the newborn includes assignment of an Apgar score at 1 and 5 minutes of life. While a low 1-min Apgar score (0 to 3) indicates that the infant requires supportive care, this score does not correlate with subsequent morbidity.

A baby in need of resuscitation can be managed by following the ABCs of neonatal resuscitation, which include assessment of the infant's *a*irway, *b*reathing, and *c*irculation. In the event of delivery of a baby in need of resuscitation, renewed attempts at obtaining a neonatologist's bedside assistance is essential. A baby with spontaneous respiratory efforts and a heart rate >100 bpm should be observed for central cyanosis, which should be treated with a free flow of oxygen while continuing to monitor neonatal respiration and heart rate. If the heart rate falls below 100 bpm, begin positive pressure ventilation (PPV) as described below.

Babies making no respiratory effort should receive PPV with a well-fitting bag-valve-mask at a rate of 40 to 60 breaths per minute with 100 percent oxygen. If a pressure gauge is available, 30 to 40 cmH_2O is required for the initial breath, while subsequent breaths require only 15 to 20 cmH_2O (in normal term infants). Care should be taken not to use too much pressure with PPV, as pneumothoraces may result. Repeat assessment for spontaneous breathing should occur after 20 to 30 seconds of PPV at a rate of about one puff every 2 seconds. If the heart rate is between 60 and 100 bpm and increasing, continue PPV; if stable, check adequacy of ventilation. If the heart rate is less than 60 bpm, continue PPV and begin chest compressions. If PPV continues for more than 2 minutes and if there is a skilled provider present, place an orogastric tube to relieve abdominal distention after intubating the infant.

Chest compressions are performed by the provider placing his or her thumbs pointing toward the infant head on the chest just above the sternum. Compress the sternum (not the infant's ribs) to a depth of one-half to three-quarter's inch, at a rate of 90 compressions and 30 PPV cycles per minute. (One cycle of three compressions and one breath takes two seconds.) Check the heart rate after 30 seconds of compressions. If the heart rate is less than 60 bpm, continue compressions; if greater than 60 bpm, use PPV only, as described above, at a rate of 40 to 60 breaths per minute until the heart rate is greater than 100 bpm. If the heart rate does not improve, continue the sequence of compressions and PPV until a pediatrician arrives to continue the code. Epinephrine (0.1 to 0.3 mL/kg of 1:10,000) should be administered either intravenously or down the endotracheal tube (0.1 mL/kg of 1:1000) if there is no heart rate present.

Complications of Normal Delivery

Episiotomy

While earlier obstetric practice endorsed routine episiotomy use, current textbooks recommend that episiotomies only be used selectively for instrument delivery or complicated delivery. The notion that episiotomies resulted in smaller lacerations that healed better proved to be untrue,[1–3] so there is no reason to perform an episiotomy for a routine delivery. If an episiotomy is needed for dystocia, a midline incision is preferred to the mediolateral incision described in many American textbooks, though there are no good data to support one incision type over the other.[4,5]

Nuchal Umbilical Cord

If the umbilical cord is wrapped around the infant's neck, it must be reduced prior to delivery of the body. Have the mother breathe through contractions while attempting to slip the cord over the head. If the cord is loose this should be simple. If the cord is tight, the cord will have to be cut while the infant is on the perineum. Double clamp the cord, cut between the clamps, and deliver the infant immediately. Once the nuchal cord is reduced, check for a second loop of cord, since this is commonly present.

Retained Products or Delayed Third Stage of Labor

A delayed third stage of labor is defined as requiring >30 minutes to deliver the placenta. The first step is to place gentle traction on the umbilical cord, as close to its insertion on the placenta as possible. This is done using ring forceps or by hand. If an obstetrician is available and the patient is not bleeding heavily, it is prudent to await the arrival of the specialist, as abnormal separation may be the result of placental growth into the endo- or myometrium (placenta accreta, increta, or percreta). If the placenta has not released, the patient is bleeding heavily, and there is a delay in obtaining specialized assistance, use a long sterile glove (up to the mid-forearm) and reach into the uterus. Find the edge of the placenta and use fingers to gently separate the placenta from the endometrium. There is a cleavage plane that is juxtaposed to the endometrium and can be identified by blunt dissection with fingertips. Finding the correct plane of separation is the key to removing retained products or to encourage placental separation.

Meconium

Meconium is the infant's first stool, and it is sometimes released into the amniotic fluid either before or during the delivery. Meconium is harmless unless the infant aspirates it, so special precautions are taken if meconium staining is noted before or during birth. The emergency physician or delivery attendant should seek to obtain assistance from a neonatologist or experienced respiratory therapist at the first sign of meconium staining. In addition, the routine delivery is modified thusly: First, the infant should not be bulb suctioned on the perineum, as this may stimulate respiratory effort. Second, move the infant directly to the resuscitation area, as thick meconium contamination or meconium in the oropharynx calls for intubation or at least direct visualization of the vocal cords with suctioning of the hypopharynx. If there is only one provider, this must take priority over all else to prevent aspiration of meconium. If the baby is not vigorous (i.e., depressed respirations and depressed muscle tone and/or a heart rate of less than 100 bpm), a skilled provider should intubate the trachea and suction any meconium present (see Table 21-4 for endotracheal tube sizes). The endotracheal tube is connected to a meconium aspirator and a suction source to facilitate appropriate suctioning.

Prolapsed Umbilical Cord

A prolapsed umbilical cord is a fetal life-threatening occurrence. If a prolapsed cord is noted upon patient presentation, use a sterile gloved hand to reach into the vagina and elevate the presenting part. Replacement of the cord cannot be achieved, but alleviation of pressure on it will prevent fetal distress. While elevating the cord, make a rapid assessment of fetal heart tones and transport emergently for delivery by cesarean section.

Abnormal Presentation

Vertex or cephalic presentations account for 93 percent of births; breech presentation occurs in 2.7 percent, and face presentations account for 0.05 percent each. Compound presentations (an arm associated with a vertex presentation) occur in about 1 of 335 births.[6] Each of these presentations is associated with its own delivery management protocols. If an abnormal presentation is suspected, perform a sterile vaginal examination to make a best guess of the presenting part, and obtain ultrasonographic confirmation if available. A protocol for vaginal delivery of a breech-presentation fetus is presented in Appendix 4 for reference by emergency personnel. However, cesarean delivery for breech presentation has been shown to be safer than vaginal delivery, even by a very experienced delivery attendant (Fig. 21-2).[7] If obstetric back-up is available, perform fetal and maternal monitoring while awaiting specialty back-up. If obstetrical back-up is not available, obtain surgical consultation in case emergent cesarean delivery is needed.

Multiple Gestations

Multifetal pregnancies are at higher risk of preterm labor, cord prolapse, postpartum hemorrhage, abnormal presentations, and premature separation of the placenta. Obstetric consultation should be present for delivery of all mul-

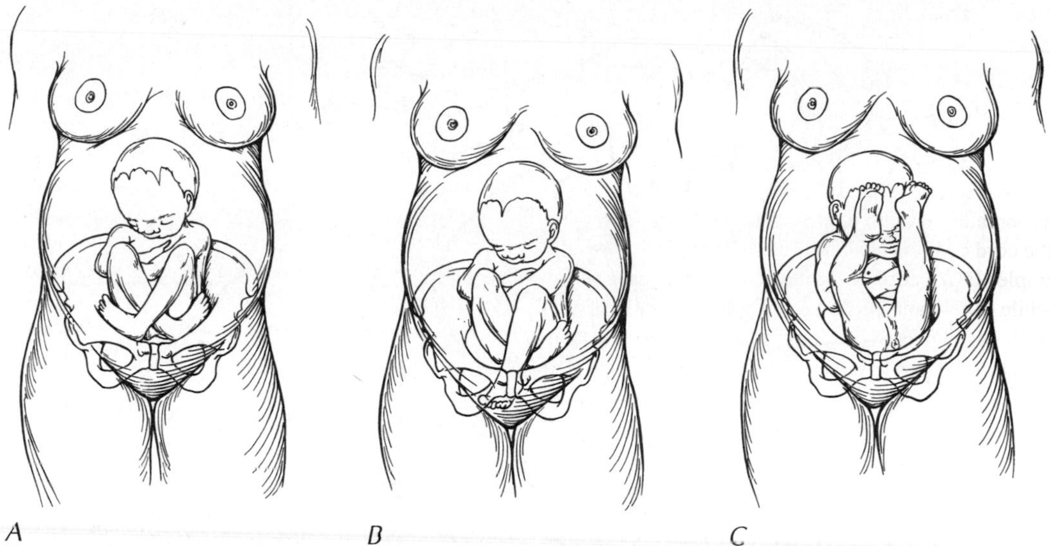

Fig. 21-2. Breech variations. *A*. A complete breech with thighs and knees flexed. *B*. An incomplete breech with one thigh partially extended and knees flexed (thighs and knees extended results in a footling breech). *C*. Frank breech with thighs flexed and knees extended.

tiple gestation pregnancies, if at all possible. The first twin presents in cephalic position in 77 percent of deliveries, but ultrasonography should be used to confirm position of the twins and their cords.[6] Delivery of the first twin is usually followed by a pause of approximately 30 minutes before the second twin delivers. Continuous fetal monitoring should be performed, as the second twin has a statistically higher incidence of fetal distress. Optimally, the descent of the second twin is guided sonographically during delivery of the first. If this isn't possible, the position of the second twin should be reconfirmed by ultrasound after delivery of the first. As the delivery of the second twin may occur at any time following the delivery of the first, the patient should not be transferred without continuous fetal monitoring until the second is delivered.

Shoulder Dystocia

Shoulder dystocia is a potentially life-threatening event in the course of a delivery, and it occurs in about 0.5 to 1 percent of births. There is no reliable method for predicting shoulder dystocia. Diagnosis is made when the fetal head retracts back into the vagina just after delivery ("turtle sign"). This occurs because the fetal shoulder becomes impacted underneath the pubic symphysis. Shoulder dystocia may be associated with significant fetal morbidity and mortality, and thus one must have complete knowledge of the maneuvers required to reduce a shoulder dystocia before it occurs. Table 21-5 lists the maneuvers described below.

Fortunately, most shoulder dystocias can be reduced with one or two simple maneuvers:

1. Call for help: a second physician if possible, and at least two persons who can assist with McRoberts maneuver; drain the bladder.
2. Perform McRoberts maneuver: Remove the maternal feet from the stirrups and sharply flex the hips so that the knees are bent and touching the abdomen (Fig. 21-3). This maneuver decreases the angle of the pelvic inclination and straightens the sacrum relative

Table 21-5. Maneuvers for Shoulder Dystocia

1. Call for assistance; drain the bladder
2. McRoberts maneuver
3. Suprapubic pressure
4. Episiotomy
5. Woods screw maneuver
6. Deliver the posterior shoulder
7. Break the clavicle
8. Zavenelli maneuver (not recommended in the ED)

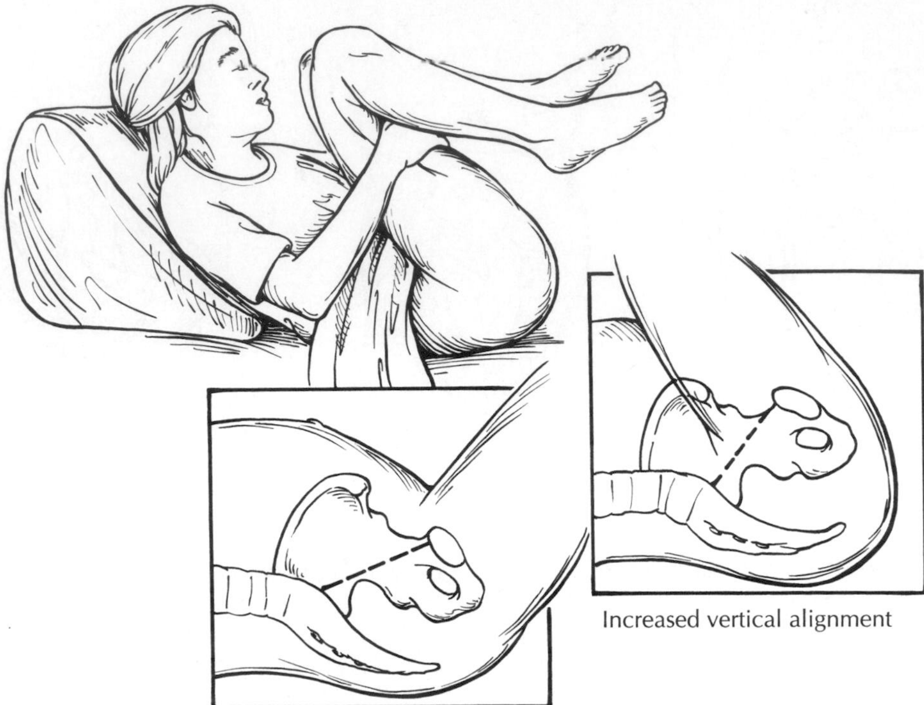

Fig. 21-3. McRoberts maneuver. Hyperflexion of the maternal thighs on the maternal abdomen changes the alignment of the pelvis relative to the anterior fetal shoulder.

to the lumbar vertebra. With an assistant holding each leg in position, the maximum angle can be achieved, and this can reduce a majority of dystocias.

3. Suprapubic pressure: An assistant places their hands just cephalad to the symphysis pubis and applies downward pressure or a rocking motion to free the impacted shoulder while the delivery attendant provides gentle downward traction on the head. Do *NOT* apply fundal pressure, as this can cause a uterine rupture. The amount of suprapubic pressure required is significant.
4. Episiotomy: A generous midline episiotomy may not itself alleviate the dystocia, but will facilitate the maneuvers that follow.
5. Woods screw maneuver: Place a finger or hand inside the uterus and behind the anterior shoulder (on the back of the baby) and rotate it in the direction of the head. It is important to place the hand posterior to the shoulder because brachial plexus injuries are more likely from anterior manipulation (Fig. 21-4).
6. Delivery of the posterior shoulder: Place a hand behind the posterior shoulder, sweep the baby's arm across the chest, grasp the baby's hand with your other hand, and deliver the arm. This alone may free the impacted shoulder or will allow rotation of the shoulder girdle to relieve pressure on the anterior shoulder (Fig. 21-5).
7. Fracture the clavicle: Deliberate fracturing of the clavicle by pressing with a finger or thumb against the mid-portion of the anterior clavicle has been described as an effective method in extreme cases of shoulder dystocia. It requires considerable force and is rarely necessary.
8. Zavenelli maneuver: This maneuver refers to replacing the head within the vagina in anticipation of a cesarean delivery. This requires rotation and flexion of the head and can be very difficult to accomplish. This is best left for the obstetrician who will be taking the patient to the operating room.

Well-known complications of shoulder dystocia are Erb's and Klumpke's paralyses. Erb's palsy is a paralysis of the shoulder and forearm muscles from lateral traction of the neck that strains the upper roots of the brachial plexus. The arm falls limply to the side of the body with

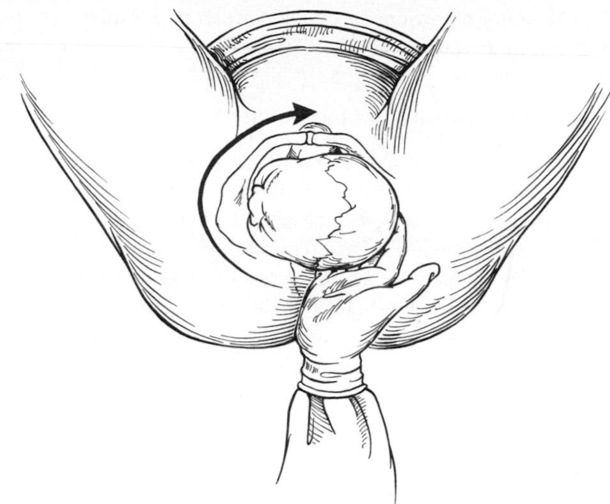

Fig. 21-4. Woods screw maneuver. A hand is placed behind the posterior shoulder and, using firm but gentle pressure, the posterior shoulder is rotated so that it becomes the anterior shoulder. This will usually allow ready delivery of either the anterior or posterior shoulder.

the forearm extended and internally rotated. Klumpke's palsy is from strain of the lower brachial plexus and results in hand and finger paralysis. The prognoses for both of these palsies depends of the severity of injury, as well as prompt identification and aggressive management of the infant's physical therapy regimen.

Group B Streptococci

Most pregnant women are routinely cultured for group B streptococci (GBS) between the thirty-fifth and thirty-seventh weeks of pregnancy. This bacterium, which commonly colonizes the vagina, is a common cause of neonatal sepsis in the United States. Women who are GBS colonized should be given chemoprophylaxis with 2 g IV ampicillin followed by 1 g every 4 hours during labor. Clindamycin 900 mg IV every 8 hours has been recommended for women with penicillin allergy. In women with unknown GBS status, treatment should be initiated in any of the following situations: preterm birth (<37 weeks' gestation), GBS bacteremia during the current pregnancy (whether treated or not), rupture of membranes for longer

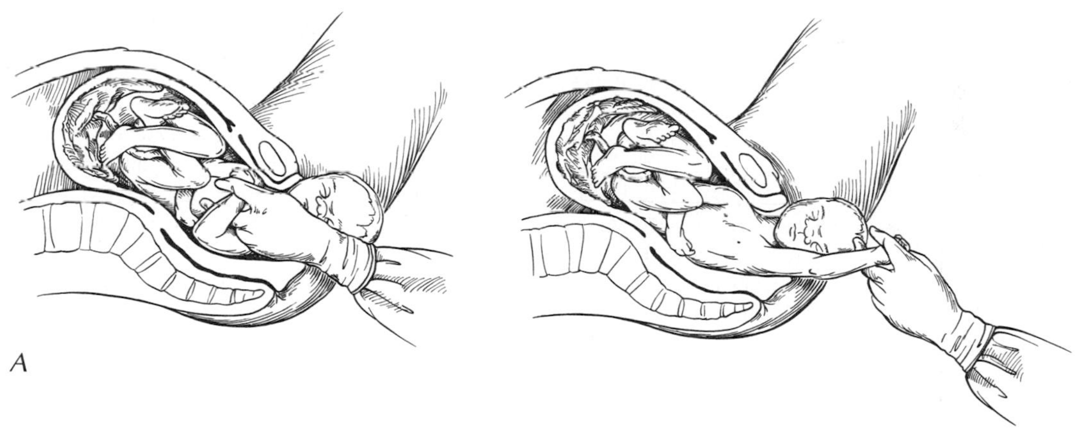

Fig. 21-5. *A* and *B*. Delivery of the posterior arm. If efforts to disimpact the anterior shoulder have failed to this point, the operator's hand is placed into the vagina, grasping the hand of the posterior arm. The arm is then swept over the fetal thorax and pulled through the maternal vagina. This will result in simultaneous delivery of the posterior shoulder.

than 18 hours, a previous infant with invasive GBS infection, or intrapartum fever ≥38°C (100.4°F).[6]

Premature Rupture of Membranes

Premature rupture of membranes (PROM) is defined as rupture of the fetal membranes resulting in leakage of amniotic fluid prior to the onset of labor. It occurs in about 10 percent of pregnancies, mostly occurring in term pregnancies. Premature labor and delivery is the most common complication of PROM, but PROM also places the infant and mother at higher risk for infection and umbilical cord prolapse or compression. The diagnosis of ruptured fetal membranes is made by an evaluation of vaginal fluid for pooling, ferning, and pH. For ED management, a woman reporting fluid leakage should be considered ruptured and at risk for early delivery. If a vaginal examination is to be performed, sterile gloves and a sterile speculum should be used to decrease the likelihood of infection. All patients with ruptured membranes require obstetric evaluation for admission and management, whether preterm or term.

Chorioamnionitis

Chorioamnionitis, or intraamniotic infection (IAI), refers to an infection of the placenta, fetal membranes, cord, or fetus. While it is most often seen after rupture of membranes and prolonged labor, it can be seen with intact membranes. Diagnosis is made by maternal temperature >38°C, maternal or fetal tachycardia, uterine tenderness, foul-smelling amniotic fluid, preterm labor or preterm PROM. Treatment is delivery and antibiotics. Ampicillin 2 g IV every 4 to 6 hours and gentamicin 1.5 mg/kg IV every 8 hours are the antibiotics of choice. Clindamycin 900 mg IV every 8 hours can be substituted for ampicillin in the penicillin-allergic patient.

Preterm Labor

A premature infant is one whose gestational age is <37 weeks or weighs <2500 grams. In 1999, 11.8 percent of births were preterm, a number that has steadily increased over the last 10 years.[6] Prematurity is second only to birth defects as the leading cause of neonatal mortality, and accounts for about 75 percent of neonatal morbidity.[8]

Diagnosis

Labor is defined by regular uterine contractions plus changes in the cervical effacement or dilation. Risk factors for preterm birth include multiple gestations, previous history of preterm labor, and PROM. Modifiable risk factors include smoking, certain vaginal infections, urinary tract infections and perhaps long periods of standing. Despite the identification of a number of risk factors, attempts to determine which patients will give birth prematurely based on a scoring system of historical factors has been unsuccessful.

A number of screening modalities have been proposed to identify patients at risk for preterm delivery. These include home uterine activity monitors (HUAM), salivary estriol levels, and screening for bacterial vaginosis, all of which have been shown not to be useful. Fetal fibronectin (fFN) is produced by the fetal membranes and is normally present in the cervical secretions until 16 to 20 weeks gestation. Subsequently, the presence of fFN in cervical secretions is associated with preterm birth, and a negative fFN test is associated with a decreased risk of preterm birth. ACOG's assessment of risk factors for preterm birth state that ultrasonography to determine cervical length may be useful in the symptomatic patient, either alone or in combination with fFN testing, for determining patients at high risk for preterm delivery.[9] Additionally, fFN testing may be useful in women with symptoms of preterm labor to identify those with negative values and a reduced risk of preterm birth. These tests may be performed in the ED if one is unable to obtain timely obstetric consultation. Utilizing the excellent negative predictive value of the fFN test may allow the nonobstetrician to transfer the patient's care to a more appropriate specialist. Fetal fibronectin levels must be collected prior to any vaginal examination and samples should not be contaminated with blood or amniotic fluid. To obtain the specimen, simply place a cotton swab in the cervical OS and collect a sample of the mucosa.

Diagnosis of preterm labor involves documenting cervical change and regular uterine contractions. Evaluation for ruptured membranes is important, and obstetric consultation may be obtained for this purpose. Once the suspicion of preterm labor is confirmed, the patient must be evaluated for imminence of delivery. If delivery is deemed likely, neonatology consultation is essential and notification of a level II or level III nursery of the impending delivery should be initiated. If delivery seems not to be impending, arrange inpatient management or transfer to a hospital with the appropriate level nursery. Level III nurseries provide the greatest technical expertise, with neonatologists available, and are recommended for early-gestational-age infants, low birth weight infants, and other high-risk pregnancies. If the facility does not have such a nursery but the preterm patient is in labor, the emergency physician should seek to obtain immediate bedside consultation by a neonatologist or pediatrician for the impending delivery of a preterm infant.

Management

Management of preterm labor is still evolving and controversial. Below is a discussion of pharmacologic agents and their relative risks and benefits. Emergency physicians in urban areas are unlikely to be initiating or managing these therapies, but those in settings in which obstetrical consultation is not readily available may need to use these agents.

Magnesium Sulfate

Magnesium sulfate remains the mainstay of treatment for preterm labor. It works as a smooth muscle relaxant at high concentrations. It is administered as 6 g/250 mL solution over 30 minutes, then as an infusion of 2 g/h. Magnesium is excreted through the urine, so magnesium sulfate should be used with caution in women with renal dysfunction. Severe toxicity of magnesium can result in apnea, cardiac arrest, neurologic depression, or pulmonary edema. Blood levels are not routinely utilized for evaluating magnesium toxicity. Instead, physical examination components should be used, specifically lung sounds, mental status, and deep tendon reflex activity. If a patient is thought to be magnesium toxic, the treatment is calcium gluconate 1 g IV push. This dose may need to be repeated, as needed, to reverse the toxic effects to a tolerable level.

Beta-Agonists

β-Agonists have been used for many years in the management of preterm labor. There have been several studies of different β-mimetics, which act via activation of the β_2-receptors to decrease muscle activity. Terbutaline is the most commonly used tocolytic, and has been shown to increase the time to delivery by 2 to 7 days, though no change in perinatal outcome has ever been demonstrated. The dosage is 0.25 to 5 mg subcutaneously or 0.01 to 0.08 mg/min IV, titrated to uterine activity and side effects. The β_1-activity of terbutaline will cause maternal and fetal tachycardia and may cause maternal pulmonary edema. Ritodrine has also been studied, but is not often used secondary to common and occasionally severe side effects.

Calcium-Channel Blockers

Calcium-channel blockers (e.g., diltiazem) have been studied for many years. In the most recent trial comparing diltiazem to terbutaline, both were found equally efficacious in delaying the onset of delivery, though no change was noted in perinatal outcome. There were, however, fewer side effects in the diltiazem group.[10]

Prostaglandin Inhibitors

Indomethacin has been used effectively to delay preterm birth. However, complications including preterm closure of the ductus arteriosus, necrotizing enterococci, and intracranial hemorrhage have been reported. Use of indomethacin as a tocolytic should be done only with consultation by an obstetrician.

Steroids

In 1995, the NIH recommended the use of corticosteroids for preterm labor between 24 and 34 weeks gestation to prevent respiratory distress syndrome (RDS). Steroids work by accelerating lung maturity and have been associated with a 50 percent reduction in RDS. However, it is not routinely recommended when there is associated premature rupture of membranes. The usual dosage is betamethasone 12 mg intramuscularly every 24 hours for two doses, or dexamethasone 6 mg intramuscularly every 12 hours for four doses. These should be administered to women at risk for preterm birth between 24 and 34 weeks gestation with intact membranes or between 24 and 32 weeks gestation with ruptured membranes.[11]

Postpartum Hemorrhage

Postpartum hemorrhage remains one of the leading causes of pregnancy-related deaths in the U.S.,[12] with 1.4 deaths per 100,000 live births. Postpartum hemorrhage is defined as >1000 mL of blood loss following a vaginal delivery or cesarean delivery.

After delivery of the placenta the uterus contracts, compressing the spiral arteries within the myometrium. Failure of the uterus to effectively contract (atony) is the most common complication resulting in hemorrhage, although retained placental tissue or placental growth into the myometrium can also occur. Bleeding may also result from lacerations, uterine rupture, or coagulopathy. Keep in mind that blood loss is notoriously underestimated, and that hypotension will be a late finding in an otherwise young healthy woman.

Table 21-6. Etiologies of Postpartum Hemorrhage

Immediate (First 24 h)	Delayed
Coagulopathy	Placental polyp
Lower genital tract laceration	Uterine subinvolution
Retained placental tissue or membranes	Von Willebrand's disease
Uterine atony	
Uterine inversion	
Uterine rupture	

Approach to the Patient with Postpartum Hemorrhage

The causes of hemorrhage are listed in Table 21-6. Because atony is by far the most common cause, first palpate the uterus for proper contraction. If the uterus feels firm, inspect the vagina and cervix for lacerations. If there are no lacerations, evaluate the placenta for completeness and obtain a bedside ultrasound to look for retained tissue. Consider coagulopathy as you call for surgical or obstetric back-up.

Atony

Atony can cause an immediate heavy blood loss or a delayed (up to 24 hours) blood loss. Risk factors for atony are multiparity, extended labor, multiple gestation, and use of oxytocin to induce labor. Diagnosis is by palpation of the uterus through the abdominal wall. The contracted uterus is globular and firm, like a softball. The first step in treatment is to massage the uterus through the abdominal wall. The uterus usually responds within 1 to 2 minutes, and if this does not happen, pharmacologic management is indicated. Bimanual massage may be used, which is done by placing one sterile gloved hand within the vagina against the cervix and one hand on the abdomen. Massage the uterus by compressing between the two hands (Fig. 21-6).

Oxytocin is routinely used postpartum to stimulate uterine contraction, and works by binding myometrial cell receptors. It is most commonly used as 10 to 20 units diluted in 1 L normal saline and run as a wide open bolus. If there is no IV access, 10 units intramuscularly may be used. Oxytocin is not usually given undiluted as an IV push, because relaxation of vascular smooth muscle can cause hypotension.

Continued hemorrhage calls for the administration of methylergonovine maleate 0.2 mg intramuscularly or directly into the uterus. There is no evidence that intrauterine administration is more effective than intramuscular, although this route should be considered if hypotension is significant enough to impair IM transport times. The usual time to onset is 7 minutes after IM administration. IV administration is not advised due to the risk of hypertension, and administration should be avoided if there is preexisting hypertension.

Further hemorrhage or the presence of hypertension requires the use of prostaglandin $F_{2\alpha}$. It is administrated as 250 mcg IM, and can be repeated in 15 to 20 minutes if atony persists. Continued bleeding after prostaglandin administration is usually due to unrecognized genital tract

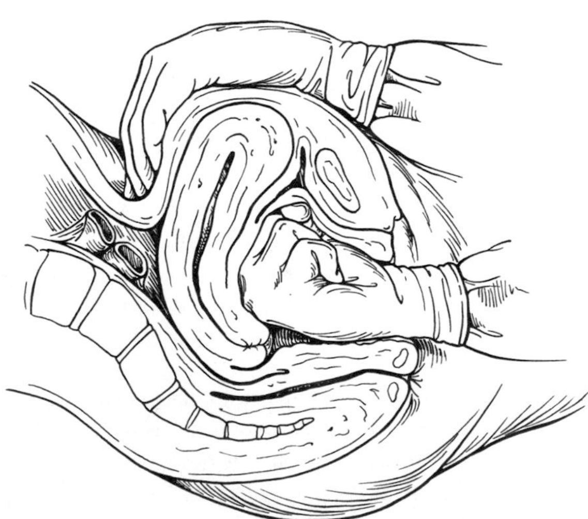

Fig. 21-6. Bimanual compression of the uterus for hemorrhage due to uterine atony.

laceration or retained placental products. Asthma is a contraindication to its use, as it is a bronchoconstrictor. Side effects are diarrhea and occasionally vomiting or pyrexia.

Lacerations

Inspection of the vagina and cervix should be routine after delivery. Lacerations of the vagina do not usually bleed as profusely as cervical lacerations. Visualization of the cervix can be difficult, but is almost always achieved with the help of an assistant and a second speculum, broken down and used to hold the vaginal sides open. This degree of inspection is essential in the ED in the setting of profuse postpartum bleeding. The lacerations found will need to be repaired immediately in order to stop the ongoing hemorrhage. If the physician who delivered the baby does not feel competent to repair the lacerations, emergent specialty consultation, either by an obstetrician-gynecologist or surgeon, is required. If the lacerations identified on routine postpartum inspection are not bleeding extensively, then it is perfectly appropriate to cover the lacerations with moist sterile gauze and transfer the patient to a facility or area where an obstetrician-gynecologist can perform the repair. If a cervical laceration is identified, absorbable suture material is used starting peripheral to the os and running towards the os (Fig. 21-7). Since bleeding can be profuse, use of an assistant is strongly advised. Ring forceps can assist in aligning the cervical tissue correctly.

Perineal lacerations are classified as first, second, third, or fourth degree. First- and second-degree lacerations involve the vaginal mucosa and muscles, respectively. Third-degree lacerations go into the anal sphincter capsule, while fourth-degree lacerations violate the rectal mucosa.

Repair of vaginal lacerations or episiotomies should be done with absorbable sutures. First- and second-degree laceration repairs should start with apposition of muscle layers first from posterior to anterior. Then the vaginal fourchette skin layers can be closed, again starting within the posterior fourchette and running forward to the edge of the vaginal opening. Next, repair the perineal layers by first opposing the deep tissue to relieve tension starting at the skin, running towards the base of the laceration. The repair is finished with a running subcutaneous stitch from base to skin (Fig. 21-8). Periurethral lacerations do not need to be repaired unless there is active bleeding from the site. If periurethral lacerations are judged to need repair, place a Foley catheter into the urethra to ensure that the meatus is not inadvertently sutured.

Third- and fourth-degree lacerations require expert closure of the sphincter and mucosal layers in order to prevent future problems with sphincter incontinence. Obstetric-gynecologic or surgical consultation is recommended.

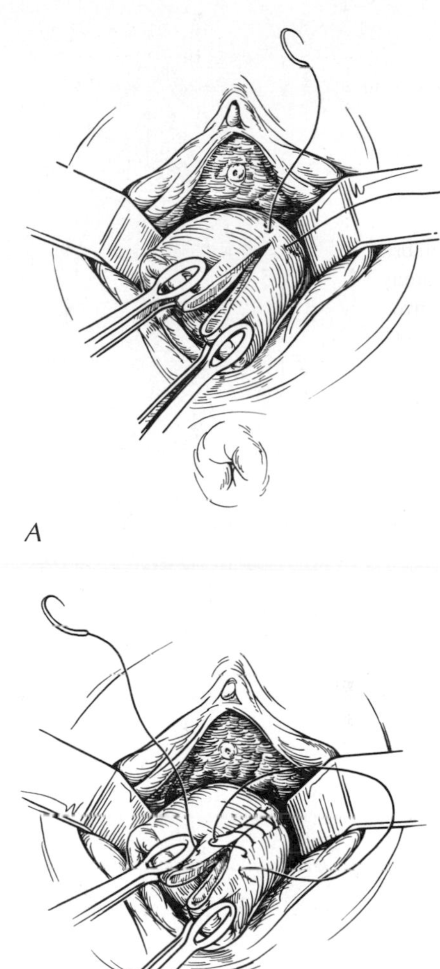

Fig. 21-7. Repair of cervical laceration.

Coagulopathy

Although a rare cause of postpartum hemorrhage, coagulopathy should be considered if no other cause of bleeding is found. In the absence of preexisting thrombocytopenia or bleeding disorder, coagulopathy may signal the onset of disseminated intravascular coagulation (DIC).

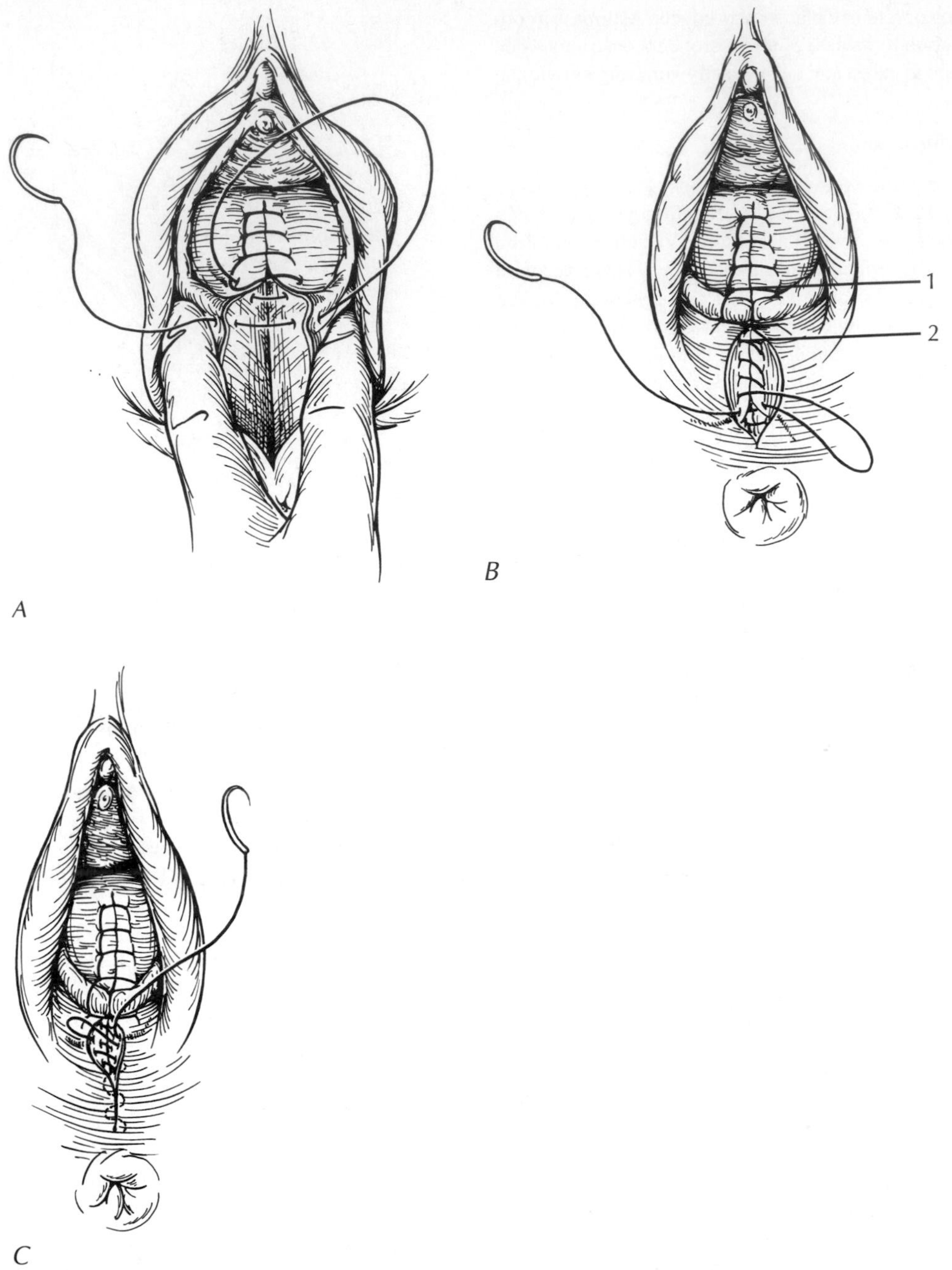

Fig. 21-8. *A*. A second-degree laceration is being repaired. Running locked absorbable suture is utilized beginning at the apex of the vaginal incision and continuing to the hymenal ring. *B*. The suture has been placed through the vaginal mucosa at point 1; it exits at point 2, allowing a continuous running suture of the perineal muscles. *C*. A continuous subcuticular closing of the perineal skin.

Though usually a complication of prolonged hemorrhage, early DIC may signal the occurrence of an amniotic fluid embolus, which is associated with respiratory distress and circulatory collapse. Amniotic fluid embolus is rare and often fatal, with no identified risk factors except rapid or tumultuous labor.

Uterine Rupture

Uterine rupture complicates about 1 in 2000 to 1 in 3000 deliveries, although the rate is higher in women who have had a previous cesarean delivery (about 1 percent). The classic description of uterine rupture is severe, tearing abdominal pain and abnormal fetal heart tones (usually bradycardia). However, many patients with uterine rupture may present without these symptoms, and may be limited to mild abdominal pain, diaphragmatic irritation, shoulder irritation, or nonreassuring fetal heart tones. The classic sign is the loss of fetal station, which is when the previously palpable fetal presenting part can no longer be palpated vaginally. Uterine rupture can range from a small tear in the uterus along a previous scar to a complete abdominal rupture with an intraabdominal fetus and massive hemorrhage. In the case of suspected uterine rupture, ultrasonography is the diagnostic modality of choice. A surgical team is needed for immediate cesarean delivery if uterine repair or hysterectomy is required.

Placenta Accreta

Placenta accreta is a result of the placenta lacking the decidua basalis, such that the placental villi are attached directly to the myometrium. This lack of a separation plane prevents a natural separation of placenta from the uterine wall. *Placenta increta* is a result of placental invasion of the myometrium, while *placenta percreta* is an invasion of the placenta completely through the uterine wall (and may involve peritoneal structures). The primary risk factor is a previous cesarean section. Diagnosis is made by finding a placenta that lacks a cleavage plane or that is incomplete upon delivery. Manual attempts to find the placental plane of separation will fail, and bleeding can be quite profuse. Treatment is replacement of blood products, and almost always hysterectomy.

Uterine Inversion

Uterine inversion complicates approximately 1 in 2500 deliveries.[13] Inversion can range in severity from simply the presence of the uterine fundus within the cervix to complete inversion of the uterus and vagina extending beyond the perineum. Most uterine inversions are believed to occur following cord traction with a fundally-implanted placenta; however, inversion can follow any delivery, even when the third stage has been managed appropriately. The hemorrhage accompanying uterine inversion can be substantial and life-threatening. The classic teaching is that uterine inversion presents with hypovolemic shock out of proportion to the visualized blood loss, although contemporary series have not substantiated this teaching.[14]

As with all forms of puerperal hemorrhage, obtaining large-bore intravenous access and initiating volume replacement are crucial. Obstetric and anesthesiologic consultation should be arranged as soon as possible. When the inversion is acute and the cervix has not contracted around the inverted uterus, it may be possible to reposition the uterus by applying manual pressure to the inverted uterine fundus (Fig. 21-9). Once the uterus has been restored to the proper anatomic location, the operator's hand should remain in the uterus to prevent reinversion while a uterotonic agent (e.g., oxytocin) is administered to obtain normal uterine tone. The blood loss is most severe in cases in which the placenta has already separated. If the placenta is still attached when the diagnosis of uterine inversion is made, it should be left in place until repositioning has been accomplished to avoid potentially catastrophic hemorrhage.

Repositioning without uterine relaxation is successful in approximately one-third of cases.[14] If the uterus cannot be replaced due to cervical contraction, a number of strategies are available to achieve uterine relaxation. Traditional methods have included either deep inhalation anesthesia or magnesium sulfate. More recently, intravenous nitroglycerine has been utilized to achieve uterine relaxation. It has the advantage of a very rapid onset of action (30 to 40 seconds) in conjunction with a short half-life of approximately 1 minute.[13] Thus, once uterine repositioning has been accomplished, uterine tone can be restored very quickly. Doses ranging from 50 to 500 mcg have been utilized, with 100 to 200 mcg appearing to be a suitable compromise between obtaining acceptable uterine relaxation while avoiding the hypotension possible with the larger doses. While hypotension does result, it is transient and can be treated with ephedrine 10 mg given intravenously.[15]

Other Methods to Control Bleeding

Persistent bleeding may be amenable to embolization of the uterine artery by interventional radiology, and has been used effectively. With severe hemorrhage, hysterectomy

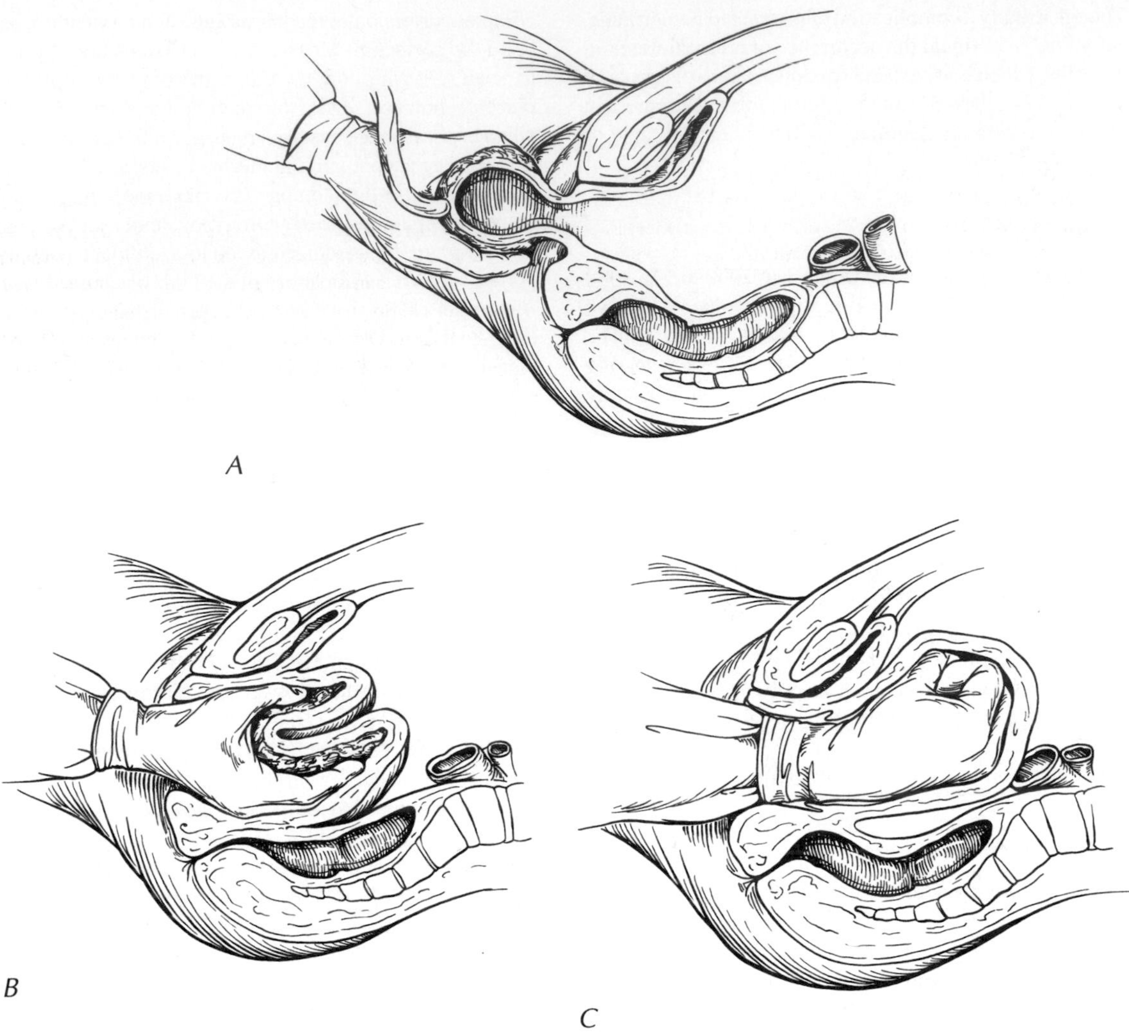

Fig. 21-9. *A*. The inverted fundus grasped in the palm of the hand with fingers directed toward the posterior fornix. The placenta is left attached, if possible. *B*. The uterus lifted out of the pelvis and directed with steady pressure toward the umbilicus after removal of the placenta. *C*. The repositioned uterus after removal of the placenta.

may provide a faster and more reliable option, especially if future fertility is not desired. Specialty consultation is essential in this scenario.

Uterine packing has occasionally been purported to be a method of providing control of postpartum hemorrhage. However, the obstetric literature does not routinely recommend this method, as it may not control bleeding and poses significant risks of infection and injury while packing is placed.

REFERENCES

1. Carroli G, Belizan J: Episiotomy for vaginal birth, in: The Cochrane Library (Cochrane Review),Issue 2, 2002.
2. Signorello LB, Harlow BL, Chekos AK, Repke JT: Midline episiotomy and anal incontinence: retrospective cohort study. *BMJ* 320:86–90, 2000.
3. Wooley RJ: Benefits and risks of episiotomy: A review of the English language literature since 1980. Parts I and II. *Obstet Gynecol Surv* 50:806–835, 1995.

4. Thacker SB: Midline vs. mediolateral episiotomy. *BMJ* 320:1615–1616, 2000.
5. Bodner-Adler B, Bodner K, Kaider A, et al: Risk factors for third-degree perineal tears in vaginal delivery, with an analysis of episiotomy types. *J Reprod Med* 46:752–755, 2001.
6. Cunningham FG, Gant NF, Leveno KJ, Gilstrap III LC, Hauth JC, Wenstrom KD: *Williams Obstetrics,* 21st ed. New York: McGraw-Hill, 2001.
7. Hannah ME, Hannah WJ, Hewson SA: Planned cesarean section versus planned vaginal birth for breech presentation at term: a randomized multicentre trial. *The Lancet* 356: 1375–1383, 2000.
8. Scott JR, Disaia PJ, Hammond CB, Spellacy WN, (eds): *Danforth's Obstetrics and Gynecology*, 8th ed. Philadelphia: Lippincott, 1999.
9. American College of Obstetricians and Gynecologists: Assessment of risk factors for preterm birth. ACOG practice bulletin no. 31. *Obstet Gynecol* 98:709–716, 2001.
10. Tsatsaris V, Papatsonis D, Goffinet F, Dekker G, Carbonne B: Tocolysis with nifedipine or beta-adrenergic agonists: A meta-analysis. *Obstet Gynecol* 97:840–847, 2001.
11. American College of Obstetricians and Gynecologists: Antenatal corticosteroid therapy for fetal maturation. ACOG committee opinion no. 273. May 2002.
12. Chichakli LO, Atrash HK, MacKay AP, Musani AS, Berg CJ: Pregnancy-related mortality in the United States due to hemorrhage: 1979–1992. *Obstet Gynecol* 94:721–725, 1999.
13. Dayan SS, Schwalbe SS: The use of small-dose intravenous nitroglycerine in a case of uterine inversion. *Anesth Analg* 82:1091, 1996.
14. Brar HS, Greenspoon JS, Platt LD, Paul RH: Acute puerperal uterine inversion: New approaches to management. *J Reprod Med* 34:173, 1989.
15. Wessen A, Elowsson P, Axemo P, Lindberg B: The use of intravenous nitroglycerine for emergency cervico-uterine relaxation. *Acta Anaesthiol Scand* 39:847, 1995.

22

Postpartum Infections

Mark D. Pearlman
Maurizio L. Maccato

KEY POINTS

- Endometritis is the most common infection in the postpartum period, complicating approximately 1 percent of vaginal deliveries and 4 to 15 percent of cesarean deliveries.
- Necrotizing fasciitis and myonecrosis are very rare but life-threatening infections which require prompt and extensive surgical debridement.
- Episiotomy infections are uncommon (<1 percent) and typically occur within the first week following delivery. Both debridement and broad-spectrum antibiotics are necessary to effect optimal outcome.
- Perineal abscesses should be surgically drained to facilitate healing.

Postpartum infections are common obstetric complications. They may involve the soft tissue of the pelvis (e.g., postpartum endometritis), the sites of surgical incisions (e.g., episiotomies or abdominal surgical incision infections), or more distant sites (e.g., urinary tract or breast infections). While absolute rates vary, the relative frequencies of these various infections is displayed in Fig. 22-1.[1] The potential seriousness of these infections demands accurate and timely diagnosis; effective antimicrobial therapy; and occasionally surgical therapy. If these infections are not adequately treated, they may spread by direct extension or through the lymphatics to cause pelvic peritonitis, septic pelvic thrombophlebitis, pelvic abscess with associated bacteremia, and sepsis. Urinary tract infections (UTI) and mastitis are covered elsewhere (Chaps. 36 and 26). With many third-party payers encouraging early discharge, women will often develop their initial signs and symptoms of postpartum endometritis after discharge, placing an increased burden on emergency departments for their initial evaluation.

POSTPARTUM ENDOMETRITIS

Postpartum endometritis (PPE) involves infection of the endometrium, myometrium, and frequently, the parametrial tissues. Its incidence varies from 0.2 to 3 percent following vaginal delivery to as high as 85 percent after high-risk cesarean deliveries.[2] More typically, PPE complicates 3 to 15 percent of cesarean deliveries. Several risk factors for PPE have been identified; the most important is cesarean delivery. Other major risk factors are chorioamnionitis, the increased duration of ruptured membranes, the presence of labor, a high number of vaginal examinations during labor, the presence of high-virulence pathogens, and the use of internal monitoring devices such as intrauterine pressure catheters.

Pathophysiology

Postpartum endometritis is an ascending polymicrobial infection caused by bacteria that have colonized the vagina and the cervix. A variety number of aerobes, facultative anaerobes, and obligate anaerobes have been recovered from the endometria of patients with PPE. The most common organisms include Group B Streptococcus, *Escherichia coli, Prevotella biva,* and *Enterococcus faecalis.* Table 22-1 lists some other common organisms that have been identified in the upper genital tract of women with PPE.

Diagnosis

The diagnosis of PPE is based primarily on the history and physical examination, with laboratory data and cultures providing supportive evidence. The physical factors contributing to a diagnosis of PPE are uterine tenderness and fever. The onset of symptoms may be slow or rapid, depending on the pathogens involved. Pertinent history includes the presence of risk factors (e.g., cesarean delivery, length of ruptured membranes in labor, chorioamnionitis) and the use of antibiotics during labor and/or delivery. Lower abdominal pain, foul-smelling purulent lochia, and rigors are frequently present. Vital signs will usually demonstrate temperature elevation, typically >38°C (100.4°F), and tachycardia. Examination of the abdomen may reveal mild to moderate distention and decreased bowel sounds may be present due to adynamic ileus.

Uterine tenderness involving the fundus of the uterus is nearly always present, though it may be limited to the lower uterine segment. Palpation of the uterine fundus abdominally will typically elicit significant tenderness. Examination of the abdomen may also identify masses

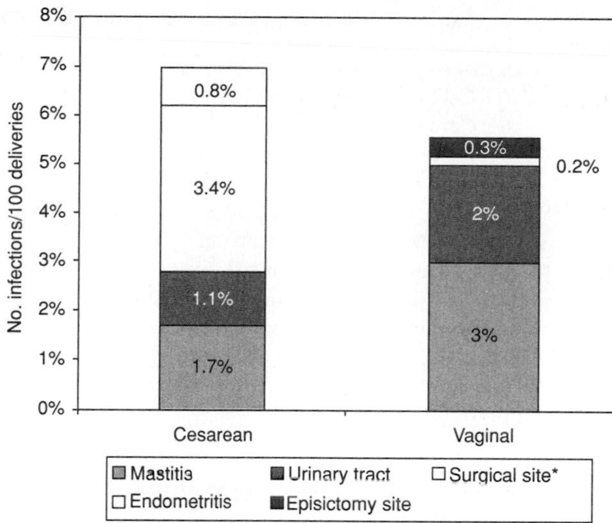

Fig. 22-1. Extrapolated site-specific infection rates following vaginal and cesarean delivery. (From the Centers for Disease Control and Prevention.)

suspicious for abscesses, though imaging (ultrasound or CT scan) is considerably more sensitive in detecting fluid collections. On pelvic examination, purulent discharge may be present in the vagina as it emanates from the cervix. The cervix is frequently softened and dilated. If the parametrial tissues are involved, tenderness and induration in the tissue lateral to the uterus will be noted.

Table 22-1. Bacteria Frequently Isolated in Postpartum Endometritis

Gram-negative rods
Escherichia coli
Klebsiella-Enterobacter species
Proteus species
Serratia species
Pseudomonas species
Haemophilus species
Anaerobes
Clostridium perfringens
Fusobacterium species
Bacteroides species
Peptococcus
Peptostreptococcus
Gram-positive cocci
Streptococci, groups A & B
Pneumococcus
Staphylococcus aureus
Enterococcus

Elevation of the white blood cell count is typical, usually in the range of 12,000 to 20,000/mm^3 or higher. Ultrasound or CT of the abdomen is usually reserved for patients who have evidence of abscess formation on physical examination and patients not responding to appropriate antibiotic therapy. The differential diagnosis of PPE includes UTI with severe cystitis, leading to lower uterine discomfort, and abdominal wound infection. A urinalysis generally provides the necessary laboratory support for the diagnosis. Infection of the abdominal wound from a cesarean delivery may also cause lower abdominal pain and fever. Evaluation of the surgical site with demonstration of erythema, purulent discharge, and induration is usually sufficient to clarify the diagnosis. Occasionally, both occur simultaneously.

Therapy

The mainstay of therapy of PPE remains the use of appropriate broad-spectrum antimicrobial agents. Because of the potential severity of the infection, outpatient treatment is usually not appropriate. Intravenous broad-spectrum antibiotics will provide the most satisfactory therapy. A number of antibiotics and antibiotic combinations have been utilized in the therapy of PPE with good success (Table 22-2). Broad-spectrum penicillin with or without a beta-lactamase inhibitor or a second-generation cephalosporin have most commonly been used. The combination of a penicillin and an aminoglycoside, typically with the addition of clindamycin or metronidazole, has

Table 22-2. Broad-Spectrum Antimicrobial Agents Commonly Used to Treat Obstetric Infections

Cefoxitin 1–2 g IV every 6 hours
Cefotetan 1–2 g IV every 12 hours
Ampicillin-sulbactam 1.5–3 g IV every 6 hours
Piperacillin-tazobactam 3.375 g IV every 6 hours
Ticarcillin-clavulanic acid 3.1 g IV every 6 hours
Clindamycin and gentamicin:
Clindamycin 900 mg IV every 8 hours + gentamicin 4.5 mg/kg IV every 24 hours[a] (assuming normal renal function)
Ampicillin 1–2 g every 6 hours + gentamicin 4.5 mg/kg every 24 hours + metronidazole 500 mg every 8 hours (assuming normal renal function)

[a] Alternative: gentamicin 2.0 mg/kg IV bolus followed by 1.5–1.7 mg/g every 8 hours.

also proved satisfactory. Favorable response to antibiotic therapy with reduction in fever and improvement in lower abdominal discomfort should be expected in 24 to 48 hours. If such a response is not present, the development of an abscess, the presence of septic pelvic venous thrombosis, or a wound complication must be considered. The therapy of abdominal abscesses requires drainage either by interventional radiology or surgically, in combination with antimicrobial therapy. In some patients, the presence of a resistant pathogen may be the cause for failure of therapy. It is important to note that enterococci are commonly isolated from the endometria of patients with PPE who have received a cephalosporin as a prophylactic agent at the time of delivery. Resistant Enterobacteriaceae have been recovered from patients given penicillin as a prophylactic agent.[3] Because PPE usually requires hospitalization and intravenous therapy, consultation with an obstetrician/gynecologist is appropriate.

An unusual but serious complication of PPE is myometrial necrosis. This infection begins with the development of microabscesses at the site of the uterine surgical incision. These abscesses will progress to a suppurative myometritis with necrosis of the tissue. The syndrome frequently involves the abdominal incision as well. Pain is minimal to mild. The physical examination will disclose both purulent vaginal discharge and a wound abscess. The cervix is generally open and bimanual palpation of the lower uterine segment will reveal necrosis of the lower uterine segment, often with fascial dehiscence. X-ray may demonstrate gas within the uterus (Fig. 22-2). CT or MRI may demonstrate disruption of the uterine wall. Therapy requires urgent surgical exploration and debridement of the uterine wound, which almost invariably leads to hysterectomy. If the abdominal wall is involved, debridement of the abdominal incision is also necessary.

POSTPARTUM ABDOMINAL WOUND INFECTIONS

Infection of the cesarean delivery abdominal incision occurs after 3 to 16 percent of operations, with an average of 7 percent. Wound infections may be caused either by bacteria present in the lower genital tract, which colonize the incision at the time of delivery, or by skin flora. Infections may or may not be associated with PPE. Risk factors for wound infection following cesarean delivery include obesity, malnutrition, diabetes mellitus, immunosuppression, and circumstances surrounding surgery (e.g., poor hemostasis, breaks in sterile techniques, improper tissue handling, etc.).

Diagnosis

Wound infection is suspected when the patient reports symptoms of incisional pain and fever. The physical examination reveals an erythematous and edematous incision. The wound may be quite indurated and usually quite tender to palpation. Frequently, purulent discharge will be noticed at the incision site.

A true wound infection must be differentiated from a seroma or hematoma. Hematomas and seromas are not typically associated with fever or cellulitis; however, the incision may be edematous. In the presence of a wound infection, the white blood cell count is typically elevated. An ultrasound of the incision site may reveal an accumulation of fluid in the subcutaneous or subfascial layers. If the accumulation of fluid is limited to the subcutaneous layer, drainage through the incision site is easily achieved and will provide a specimen for a Gram stain and culture. This will also help to diagnose uninfected seromas or hematomas. If purulent material is obtained, the incision

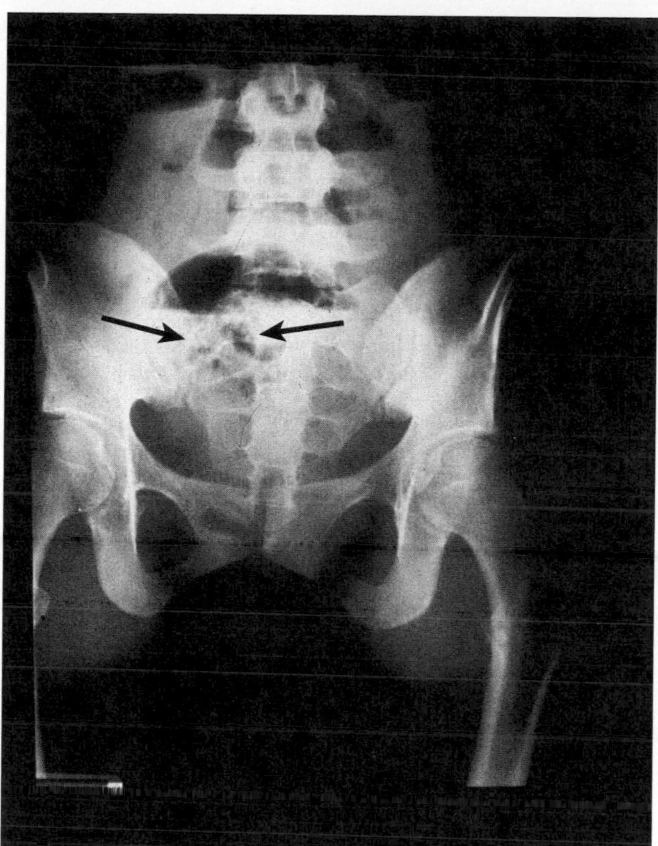

Fig. 22-2. Radiograph of abdomen with uterine gas pattern from clostridial myonecrosis. Arrows outline gas within myometrium. (Photograph courtesy of Rudi Ansbacher, M.D., University of Michigan.)

should be opened, the purulent material evacuated, and the wound debrided if necessary. Exploration of the fascia with a sterile cotton swab should be performed to ensure that it is intact. Disruption of the fascia requires repair in the operating room.

Therapy

Therapy is based on the severity of infection. If cellulitis is noted with no induration, edema, or significant fluid accumulation under the incision, antibiotic therapy alone may be satisfactory. If fluid is noted under the incision line, drainage of the fluid should be performed. Culture and Gram stain should be obtained. If the stain is positive for organisms and white blood cells or if grossly purulent material is obtained, then opening of the incision with drainage of the purulent material and packing of the incision should be initiated. If staining of the fluid reveals no white blood cells and no bacteria, then simple drainage of the pocket of fluid will frequently resolve the problem. Antimicrobial therapy is commonly used for treatment of wound infections. However, incision and drainage is usually sufficient treatment in the absence of specific indications for antibiotic treatment such as extensive cellulitis or immunosuppression (Table 22-3). If antimicrobial therapy is required (e.g., extensive cellulitis) can be empirically directed by the finding on the Gram stain. The presence of gram-positive cocci suggests staphylococci, streptococci, or enterococci as the primary responsible organisms. The finding of gram-negative bacteria suggests the presence of facultative or obligate anaerobes originating from the lower genital tract. Broad-spectrum antibiotic agents should be used pending the culture results. Hospitalization should be considered if significant temperature elevation is noted (greater than 38°C or 100.4°F orally), if local care of the incision cannot be properly performed on an outpatient basis, or if the patient is unable to tolerate oral antibiotics.

A special circumstance is the rapid development of cellulitis, usually within 24 hours of surgery. Unlike typical

Table 22-3. Indications for Antibiotics for Wound Infection

- Extensive cellulitis
- Immunosuppression (e.g., steroid use, AIDS, etc.)
- Fascial involvement (also requires surgical debridement)
- Diabetes mellitus
- Failure of incision and drainage alone (also requires evaluation for hidden fluid collection or secondary source of failure to respond)

wound infections, which present 3 to 4 days after surgery along with a fluid collection, women with cellulitis due to group A streptococci do not typically develop an abscess. Rather, they develop a rapidly-spreading cellulitis associated with high fever (38 to 40°C or 100.4 to 104°F) and tachycardia, and they appear systemically ill. Occasionally these infections will progress to develop necrotizing fasciitis, a serious life-threatening infection requiring prompt surgical intervention (see below).

Rapidly-developing cellulitis is commonly due to a single organism (e.g., Group A Streptococcus) but multiple organisms can coinfect these wounds. Therefore broad-spectrum antimicrobial therapy with good streptococcal coverage is recommended (e.g., ticarcillin-clavulanic acid, ampicillin-sulbactam, piperacillin-tazobactam, or cefotetan). In the absence of a fluid collection these wounds do not need to be opened. The use of ultrasound or other imaging (e.g., CT) can assist in determining whether a fluid accumulation is present underneath the skin. Because of the potential for significant morbidity (e.g., necrotizing fasciitis), women with rapid development of superficial cellulitis should be hospitalized for parenteral antibiotic therapy and careful observation to determine the need for surgical intervention.

If radiologic evaluation of the incision reveals a collection of fluid *below* the fascia, drainage of the fluid is necessary. This can be accomplished either by surgical exploration of the incision and subfascial tissues, or by transcutaneous drainage of the fluid under ultrasound or CT guidance. If purulent material is obtained, the patient should be taken to the operating room and the subfascial collection of pus evacuated. At that time, inspection of the uterine incision is recommended. Antimicrobial therapy will be based on culture results; however, broad-spectrum antibiotic therapy should be initiated pending culture results (see Table 22-2). Wound care of the infected postoperative incision is accomplished by a wet or dry dressing changed three to four times a day. The use of 0.25 percent acetic acid has provided good results in a high-risk population, though saline is also acceptable. If a large amount of serous fluid appears to be coming from the incision, it is important to keep in mind the potential for fascial dehiscence. The fluid volume is frequently increased by a Valsalva maneuver. If there is any question about the integrity of the fascial layer, it should be probed with a sterile cotton swab. If fascial dehiscence is suspected, the patient should be taken to the operating room for exploration of the incision. This will allow for repair of the fascial dehiscence if it is confirmed.

If there is no evidence of infection after evacuation of a seroma or a hematoma, the patient's wound can frequently be reapproximated; i.e., it does not need to be allowed to heal by secondary intention. Close follow-up is mandatory, especially during the first week to make sure that no significant infection develop. Home nurses can be particularly helpful in assisting with wound care.

EPISIOTOMY INFECTIONS

The episiotomy is one of the most common surgical procedures performed, and infection of the episiotomy site occurs in less than 1 percent of cases.[4] The severity of infection can be estimated clinically by its depth (Table 22-4 and Fig. 22-3). Most commonly, episiotomy infections are superficial and accompanied by low-grade fever and pain at the site. Physical examination will reveal edema, induration, and erythema of the perineum and vagina (Fig. 22-4). The perineal skin edges are frequently separated. Treatment of an infected episiotomy site involves debridement of the affected area and the use of a broad-spectrum antibiotic to help speed resolution of the cellulitis. Polymicrobial infection is the rule. Culture of the purulent material may identify resistant organisms and aid in the management of patients not responding to therapy. Healing by secondary intention is frequently utilized; however, some centers have used early secondary closure of an infected episiotomy site after debridement in the operating room. Satisfactory results in approximately 80

Table 22-4. Classification of Severity of Episiotomy Infection and Treatment Recommendations

Class	Anatomic Borders	Clinical Features					Treatment
		Pain	**Abscess**	**Systemic Illness**	**Fever**	**Necrosis**	
Simple	Limited to skin and superficial fascia at the incision line	Y	S	N	Y	N	Antibiotics (I) and drainage if abscess present
Superficial fascial infection	Extension to superficial fascia with spreading beyond incision line, *no* necrosis	Y	S	N	Y	N	Antibiotics (I) and drainage if abscess present; may need surgical exploration to rule out necrosis
Superficial fascial necrosis (necrotizing fasciitis)	Extension to and necrosis of the superficial fascia of the perineum (Colles' fascia), spread to the contiguous fascia of the abdominal wall (Scarpa's fascia), or the medial thighs (fascia lata) may be seen; muscle not involved	Y+/(Y−) late	N	Y	Y	Y (fascia only, not muscle)	Antibiotics (I + II) plus extensive debridement of fascia
Myonecrosis	Extension to and necrosis of fascia and underlying muscle	Y+	S	Y	Y	Y	Antibiotics (I + II) and extensive debridement of fascia and muscle; hypertonic oxygen therapy sometimes utilized.

Key: Y(−) = anesthesia; Y(+) = pain out of proportion to wound appearance; S = sometimes; Y = yes; N = no; I = broad-spectrum therapy (see Table 22-2); II = penicillin G 6–8 million units IV q4h.

to 90 percent of cases have been reported.[4,5] It is important, therefore, to obtain experienced consultation if surgical closure of the infected episiotomy site is proposed. In the absence of systemic symptoms or extensive cellulitis, outpatient therapy with close follow-up is appropriate.

Necrotizing fasciitis is a rare but frequently fatal infection most often seen in diabetics.[6,7] The hallmark of necrotizing fasciitis associated with the episiotomy site is the presence of severe pain with very mild erythema and edema of the infected area. The pain progresses from very

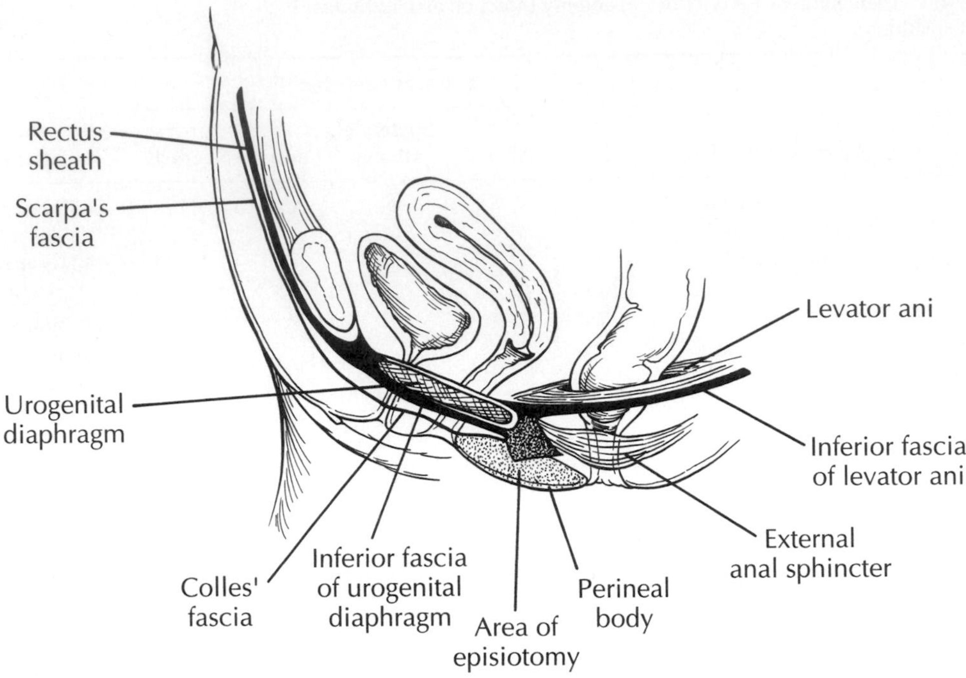

Fig. 22-3. Illustration of various fascial planes related to episiotomy infection (see Table 22-4).

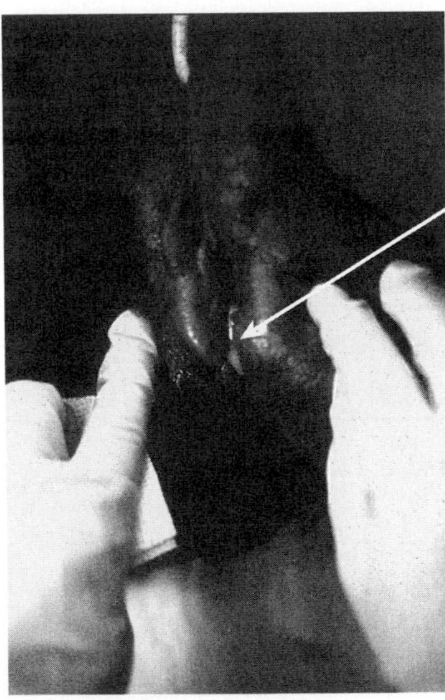

Fig. 22-4. Photo of simple episiotomy infection. Arrow points to purulent drainage at episiotomy site.

severe to very mild, frequently giving the false impression of an improvement. The skin around the area will then turn bluish and the development of necrosis is apparent toward the latter stages of the infection. Purulence is not characteristic of this condition. Serous fluid is frequently the only suspicious finding. Soft-tissue crepitance due to gas production may also be seen. Fever and tachycardia are usually present. The supportive laboratory findings include an elevation in the white blood cell count often exceeding 20,000/mm^3. The microbiology of necrotizing fasciitis involves both aerobic and anaerobic bacteria and frequently includes *Streptococcus pyogenes* or *Clostridium perfringens*. The therapy of necrotizing fasciitis demands wide debridement of the affected area and broad-spectrum antibiotic coverage. Clostridial infections should be treated with high-dose penicillin G (4 to 6 million units IV every 4 hours) in addition to surgical debridement. Immediate obstetric or surgical consultation is imperative.

Myonecrosis is a rare but life-threatening complication. It is caused by *C. perfringens* in 80 percent of cases. The hallmark of the infection is severe pain out of proportion to the wound's appearance, associated with systemic symptoms. *Clostridium perfringens* produces an exotoxin that causes not only necrosis of muscle, but also severe systemic symptoms including hypotension, tachycardia, diaphoresis, and renal tubular necrosis. Ultrasound examinations and x-rays of the pelvis will usually reveal gas at the site of infection (Fig. 22-2). Surgical debridement is mandatory, along with intravenous antibiotics (e.g., penicillin G 4 to 6 million units every 4 hours).

PERINEAL ABSCESSES

Perineal abscesses will present with development of swelling and tenderness of the perineum, frequently in association with fever and lower abdominal or leg pain. As for any other abscess, the hallmark of management is incision and drainage. If the abscess is not surgically drained, it will frequently drain spontaneously, either into the vagina or into the rectum, with the possibility of fistula formation, a significant complication of perineal abscesses. Inpatient therapy and obstetric consultation are necessary for proper care of this condition.

REFERENCES

1. Yokee DS, Christiansen RJ, Sands KE, et al: Epidemiology of and surveillance for postpartum infections. *Emerg Infect Dis* 7:837–841, 2001.
2. Casey BM, Cox SM: Chorioamnionitis and endometritis. *Infect Dis Clin North Am* 11:203, 1997.
3. Faro S, Cox SM, Phillips LE: Influence of antibiotic prophylaxis on vaginal microflora. *J Obstet Gynecol* 2(Suppl):54, 1986.
4. Arona AJ, al-Marayati L, Grimes DA, Bollard CA: Early secondary repair of third- and fourth-degree perineal lacerations after outpatient wound preparation. *Obstet Gynecol* 86:294, 1995.
5. Ramin SM, Ramus RM, Little BB, Gilstrap LC: Early repair of episiotomy dehiscence associated with infection. *Am J Obstet Gynecol* 167:1104, 1992.
6. Hauster G, Hanzal E, Dadak C, Gruber W: Necrotizing fasciitis arising from episiotomy. *Arch Gynecol Obstet* 255:153, 1994.
7. Goepfert AR, Guinn DA, Andrews WW, Hauth JC: Necrotizing fasciitis after cesarean delivery. *Obstet Gynecol* 89:409, 1997.

SECTION VI
PEDIATRIC AND ADOLESCENT GYNECOLOGY

23

Methods of Gynecologic Examination in the Young Patient

David S. Rosen

KEY POINTS

- A calm, prepared, unhurried, confident approach to the gynecologic examination of a young female will be well rewarded by a more cooperative patient.
- Although there may be reluctance on the part of the patient, family, and clinician, and despite the potential difficulties in accomplishing the examination, a gynecologic examination should not be avoided or deferred when it is clinically indicated.
- When patients do not appear able to cooperate, early consideration should be given to the use of conscious sedation or examination under anesthesia.

INTRODUCTION

The techniques used to perform gynecologic examinations of young patients in the emergency department are not substantially different from those used in the examination of older patients. Adequate preparation of the patient (and family), appropriate equipment and lighting, an unhurried approach, and sensitivity to the needs of the patient are important in either setting. Still, the clinician examining younger patients faces additional challenges not typically encountered in the care of adult women. Younger patients will likely be unaccustomed to examination of their genitalia and therefore may well be more uncomfortable or fearful than older patients. Providers, too, may be uncomfortable with the gynecologic examination of younger patients. Issues for providers include general discomfort in caring for younger patients, reluctance to broach difficult topics such as sexuality or potential abuse, lack of experience with the prepubertal or adolescent examination, and uncertainty in distinguishing between normal, variant, and abnormal findings.

In fact, the confident and prepared examiner should have little difficulty examining most younger patients. Preparation of the patient and her family are critical, and patience in this area will be well rewarded. Proper equipment—including appropriately sized vaginal specula, ample lighting, and a private, quiet, conducive environment—are essential. The clinician should be confident of his or her basic examination skills and familiar with developmental gynecologic anatomy. Finally, the clinician should anticipate and preempt difficult examinations. Care should be taken not to inadvertently traumatize younger patients in order to complete an examination. When patients do not appear able to cooperate, early consideration should be given to the use of conscious sedation or examination under anesthesia. Evaluation of alleged or suspected sexual abuse of children is best managed by a specialized team with expertise and experience in seeing these patients (see Chap. 25).

THE DECISION TO EXAMINE A YOUNGER PATIENT

It is important for the clinician to recognize that examination of the genitalia is likely to be uncomfortable for younger patients, psychologically if not physically. Many preadolescent and adolescent girls will have infrequently (or never) had their genitalia examined by their primary care provider. Understandably, discomfort arises not only from a fear of the unknown, but also from a stranger's sudden focus on the patient's "private parts." The latter will be especially true if the examination is being performed in the setting of alleged or suspected sexual abuse.

Table 23-1. Common Indications for Examination of the Genitalia in the Acute Care Setting

Vaginal discharge in the prepubescent girl
Vaginal bleeding in the prepubescent girl
Other vulvovaginal complaints
Hypermenorrhea and/or dysfunctional uterine bleeding
Suspected sexually transmitted infection
Suspected complications of pregnancy
Suspected ovarian cyst and/or torsion
Pelvic pain
Genitourinary trauma
Suspected child sexual abuse
Rape

Older children and young adolescents may be extraordinarily modest and reluctant to expose themselves for the examination. For adolescents, the complaint that brought them to the emergency department may involve disclosing behaviors that are private, potentially embarrassing to the patient, and possibly unknown to the parents. Here, assurances of confidentiality are required before the patient will reveal the actual facts of the situation. Table 23-1 lists common indications for examination of the genitalia in this age group.

Although there may be reluctance on the part of patients, families, and clinicians, and despite the potential difficulties in accomplishing the evaluation, gynecologic examinations should not be avoided or deferred when they are clinically indicated. Anecdotes abound in which significant pathology was missed and definitive diagnosis delayed because of a clinician's unwillingness to examine the genitalia. Similarly, in a recent study, 76 percent of girls seeking evaluation for blunt urogenital trauma had injuries worse than originally suspected once an adequate examination was performed.[1] If the emergency department examiner feels unprepared to perform the examination properly, or if subsequent evaluation by a specialist is expected, early consultation is appropriate so that a single satisfactory examination might be done in place of serial examinations by multiple providers.

PREPARING FOR THE EXAMINATION

Ideally, the younger patient should be evaluated in a private setting, free from distractions and interruptions. Patients should be reassured that there will be no sudden intrusions, and all efforts should be made to ensure that this is the case. Private rooms, rather than curtained examination areas, should be used if at all possible. Adequate space should be available for the patient, the examiner, a parent or other supportive person, and a chaperone or assistant.

An adequate examination table with adjustable stirrups is required. For patient comfort, it is considerate to pad the stirrups. Seating should be available for the parent and should be suitable in the event that the examination needs to be conducted with a small child in the parent's lap. Ample lighting is needed, preferably from a light source that remains cool. A fiberoptic light source is ideal, and it should be mobile to accommodate examinations that are not performed on the examination table.

A wide range of vaginal specula should be readily available (Fig. 23-1). A Pederson speculum is optimal for most adolescent examinations, while some adolescents will be more easily examined using the narrower Huffman speculum. For prepubertal children, the small Pederson speculum can sometimes be used, but more often visualization of the vagina will require the use of a smaller instrument such as a nasal speculum, a veterinary otoscope, or even a regular pediatric otoscope (without the ear speculum in place).

Supplies should be available to test for common infections such as *Neisseria gonorrhoeae, Chlamydia trachomatis,* and herpes simplex virus. In many facilities, these tests are normally done using a DNA genetic probe, immunofluorescence, or other nonculture techniques. Nevertheless, culture media should be available, since nonculture methods are not sufficiently reliable for use in the investigation of sexual abuse. See Appendix 2 for proper specimen collection and transport.

A variety of strategies have been described to facilitate the sampling of vaginal secretions from children too young to tolerate a speculum examination or even a vaginal swab. One technique employs a "catheter within a catheter" to instill and reaspirate sterile nonbacteriostatic saline from the vagina (see section below on examination of the young child).

PREPARATION OF THE FAMILY

The decision to perform a gynecologic examination on a younger patient should be based on specific clinical hypotheses that must be conclusively evaluated. Understandably, many families are anxious when the examination is suggested and will need to be reassured prior to the examination. Most families respond well to an understandable explanation of the clinical suspicions being explored

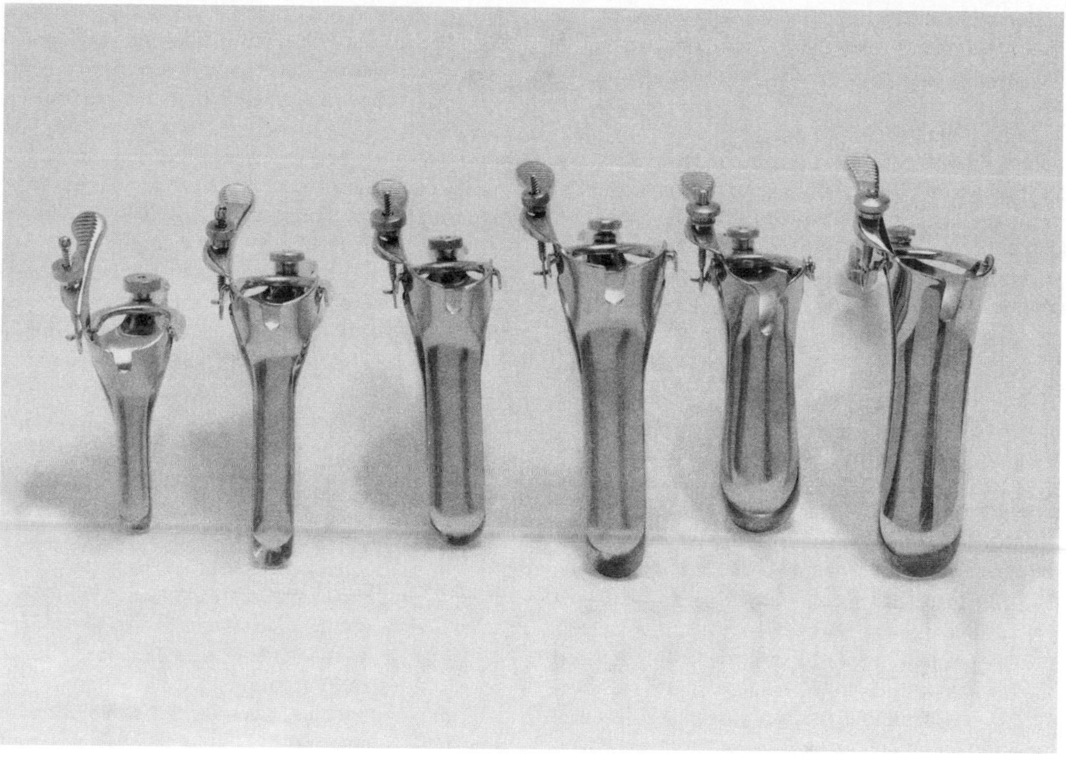

Fig. 23-1 Photo showing a variety of speculum widths and lengths.

as well as a careful description of exactly what will be done and why. Families must be helped to understand that the proposed examination is the most appropriate way to answer the clinical question. Parents are concerned that the child's examination will be identical to the complete pelvic examination with which they are most familiar, so it is important to describe the limited nature of the examination that will be done. Families are concerned that the procedure will hurt, so it is crucial to emphasize that it is unlikely to be painful. It is helpful to point out that instruments and equipment specially designed for children will be used. Finally, because some families are worried about hymenal integrity, it can be advantageous to address this issue explicitly. Important reassurance can be given by a statement such as: "We will only do those parts of the examination that are appropriate for your daughter's body; we will certainly not break or tear any tissue." Occasionally concerns regarding the patient's status as a "virgin" arise. This may be addressed by explaining the differences between the medical nature of the examination and the definition of "virgin." Frequently families with this concern need time alone to discuss this, and they should be encouraged to make contact with their clergy, as appropriate.

PREPARATION OF THE PATIENT

Adequate preparation of the patient is the single most important step in ensuring a successful gynecologic examination. A carefully conducted history offers an opportunity for the examiner to establish rapport with the patient. Talking directly to the child or adolescent is important. Clinicians who only infrequently care for pediatric patients are surprised at how well even very young children can describe their symptoms, answer questions, assent to procedures, and in general participate fully in their own care, once rapport has been established. Sitting down so that the physician is on eye level with the child, reference to age-appropriate toys or popular characters, and a friendly, engaging general style with the child are usually productive. Willingness to involve the child in the earlier parts of the visit are well rewarded later, when the child can choose to cooperate or not.

With adolescent patients, confidentiality should be discussed early in the visit and the visit should be structured so that there is some opportunity for history to be obtained from the patient alone. Often, vital information is elicited once confidentiality is assured, and the presenting complaint takes on an entirely different focus. Some adolescents will present with no parents or guardians in attendance at all. The rules related to confidentiality and consent with minor patients vary from state to state and are governed by the "mature minor" doctrine. However, every state in the United States permits clinicians to deliver reproductive health care to minors without parental consent or notification as long as the adolescents are capable of understanding and making informed decisions about their own care.[2]

When families are present, clinicians frequently worry that parents will be reluctant or unwilling to permit private discussions with their daughter. In practice, this is usually not problematic. Parents are usually quite willing to allow the clinician to speak privately with the patient; in fact, parents are usually delighted to have the clinician address the topics of sexuality and reproductive health they presume are to be discussed behind closed doors. Parents do want the opportunity to provide information they feel is relevant, they want assurances that they will be informed of any serious or life-threatening diagnoses, they want to be involved in any significant decision making, and they expect to be informed of the plans being made. Parents nearly always respond well to a statement such as "Your daughter may feel more comfortable answering some questions in private, so now I'd like to ask you to step out of the room for a few moments so that she and I can talk alone. We'll certainly bring you back when we are finished so that you can hear what we think is going on and our plans to take care of it."

The examination itself should be preceded by a complete and clear description of exactly what will be done, using simple and unambiguous language. Medical jargon should be avoided; stirrups are "foot-holders," cultures are "tests," and lesions are "sores." For very young children, it is helpful to know what words they use to denote their genitalia and to use these same words. The clinician should be alert for nonverbal cues suggesting confusion, apprehension, or discomfort and should offer additional support or explanation when necessary. For both children and adolescents, it is often helpful to demonstrate the equipment that will be used, if only to prove that there are no hidden needles.

Because of the psychosexual connotations of the genitalia and prevailing societal expectations of modesty, there is a perceived loss of control and sense of vulnerability inherent in exposure of the perineum for a gynecologic examination. To the extent possible, clinicians should endeavor to restore patients' sense of control in order to increase their comfort during the examination. Patients, for example, should be encouraged to make as many choices as possible about the conduct of their examination. Even very young patients can help to determine how they will be positioned for their examination, who will be present in the room, or even the color of their gown. Similarly, it is important for patients to retain final authority over what will or will not be done to their bodies. Patients can be told to say *"STOP"* if, during the examination, something hurts, they feel uncomfortable, or they want to interrupt the examination for any other reason.

In describing the examination, it is helpful to specifically endorse feelings of embarrassment, nervousness, and reluctance. One can say: "Nearly everyone is nervous about having this examination done, but when it's all finished, nearly everyone says it wasn't as bad as they thought it would be." One must state unequivocally that "It won't hurt" and that the examination will stop if it does. If appropriate, it is sometimes effective for the examiner to say that he or she will "just look." Of course, none of this should be promised if it is not true.

With older patients, when a more comprehensive examination is expected, it is not enough to outline what you will do; it is also important to describe how, why, and with what instruments. For patients who have never had a gynecologic examination, it is appreciated when the clinician can offer some sense of how the examination will feel as well as an account of what will be done. While a thorough explanation sometimes requires a considerable investment of time, that investment is more than repaid by a more relaxed and cooperative patient and consequently by a more efficient and productive examination.

CONDUCTING THE EXAMINATION

With proper preparation and a modicum of skill, clinicians should have little trouble in examining most children and adolescents successfully and productively. Patients are more relaxed and comfortable when the clinician is confident and unhurried. The examiner should be decisive but not forceful. Evaluation of the uncooperative patient is discussed below.

Positioning The Patient

A relevant general physical examination should be performed prior to examination of the genitalia. This information can be useful not only in making an accurate diagnosis, but also in establishing rapport and trust. The physical examination moves the clinician closer to the patient and allows the clinician to demonstrate sensitivity and gentleness prior to the gynecologic portion of the examination.

Examination of the genitalia can be successfully accomplished with patients positioned in a variety of ways. With older children and adolescents, the dorsal lithotomy position, with the feet in adjustable stirrups, is preferred. This position is usually at least somewhat familiar to patients and can be managed by most without much difficulty or distress. For younger patients, there are other options to consider. Children may be offered the choice of being examined on the table or in their parent's (usually their mother's) lap. If the examining table is chosen, children may be given the choice of putting their feet into the stirrups or use the frog leg position. Examinations done with the child arranged in the mother's lap are rarely limiting and offer some advantages. The mother may be seated in a chair (Fig. 23-2*A*) or, even better, may lie on the examining table with or without her feet in stirrups (Figs. 23-2*B* and *C*). The child lies in the mother's lap, reclining against her chest. The child's legs are abducted and draped across the mother's thighs, or they are arranged in the frog leg position. With hands resting gently on the child's legs, the mother can help to keep the legs abducted during the examination. Children are frequently more easily able to lie still when positioned with their parent.

Examining the child in the knee-chest position is sometimes very helpful. This position usually allows easy visualization of the vagina and is most useful to exclude vaginal foreign bodies, to investigate complaints of vaginal discharge, or to assess the posterior hymenal margin when sexual abuse is suspected. The knee-chest examination is more suitable for younger children than for older children or adolescents; the latter are usually reluctant to position themselves in this way. Children are draped with a sheet and are asked to lie prone on the examining table. While remaining draped, they are asked to raise the buttocks while simultaneously stretching the arms out toward the front and pulling the chest down toward the table (Fig. 23-2*D*). This position is not unlike that of a cat trying to stretch; children who have cats are usually quickly in place, while others may require more help in arranging themselves. The parent is positioned at the child's head. Once in the knee-chest position, the child should be encouraged to relax and to let her back sag down toward the table. The examiner retracts the buttocks laterally and upward. As the muscles relax, the introitus likewise relaxes, and with adequate illumination the vaginal canal (and sometimes the cervix) can be visualized. Relaxation also permits optimal visualization of the margin of the hymenal orifice and findings not seen using supine examination techniques are sometimes discovered.

Examination of the Young Child

The young child is usually examined in the mother's lap or with the mother present. A security object, favorite toy, or stuffed animal can help make the child more comfortable during her examination. The specific presenting complaint will direct the focus and extent of the examination. In general, the vulva should be examined for signs of trauma or other abnormalities. The skin should be evaluated for lesions suggestive of infection (e.g., *Candida* or human papilloma virus), infestation (e.g., scabies), or primary dermatologic conditions (e.g., eczema). The presence and configuration of pubic hair should be recorded.

The vaginal introitus is exposed by gently separating the buttocks or thighs. The clitoris, urethral meatus, fossa navicularis, posterior fourchette, and hymen should be inspected in turn for any abnormalities. Clitoromegaly (width of the clitoral glans >5 mm) should be identified. The hymenal configuration should be noted (Fig. 23-3) and unexpected anomalies of the hymenal orifice carefully described. The technique of labial traction may afford a more useful view of the hymen: the examiner gently grasps the labia majora with the thumb and forefinger of each hand and pulls outward and slightly laterally (Fig. 23-4). When done correctly, this is painless for the patient. The presence or absence of estrogen effect should be noted. The unestrogenized hymen is thin, red, and delicate, while the estrogenized hymen is dull pink, thickened, and redundant or folded. Estrogen effects may be noted well before breast budding occurs. Measurements of the hymenal orifice are controversial; at best, they are dynamic and dependent on positioning, patient relaxation, and the method of the examination. A popular rule of thumb suggests that the largest dimension of the normal hymenal orifice should be no greater than 1 mm for every year of age: thus, a normal 7-year-old girl might have a hymenal orifice of 7 mm. This guideline is generally helpful, but it should not be applied strictly; normal hymenal dimensions in a variety of examining circumstances have been published.[3] If the hymenal orifice cannot be visualized or is obscured by folds of hymenal tissue, the examiner may use a cotton or calcium alginate swab to gently probe until it is visualized. Saturating the swab with 2 percent viscous lidocaine may be helpful. The patient should be told she will feel this maneuver but that it should not hurt.

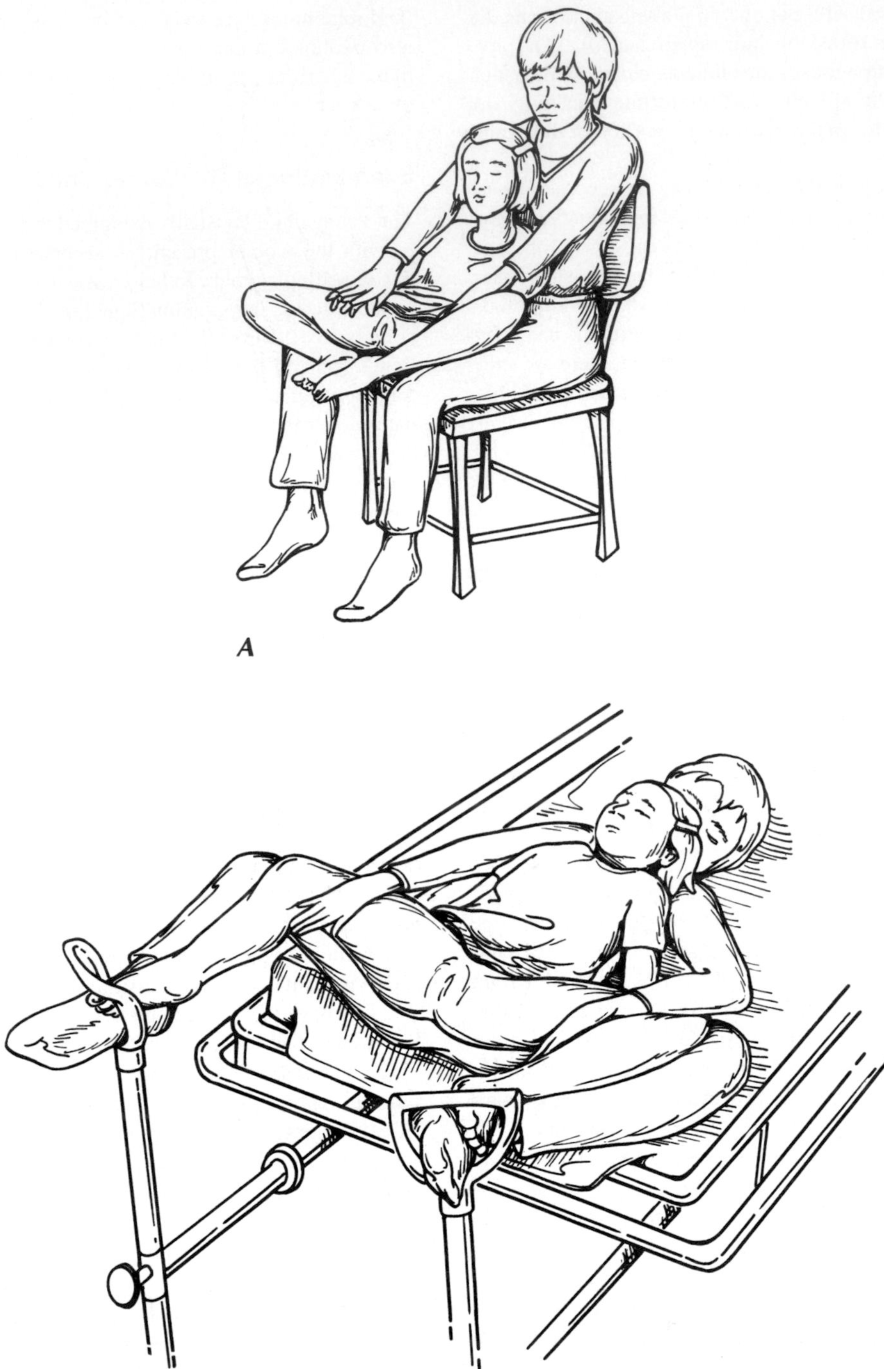

Fig. 23-2. Positioning the child for the examination. With the parent seated, the child may sit on the parent's lap with legs abducted (*A*). Alternatively, the child may lie in the parent's lap while the parent is positioned on the examining table with her feet in stirrups (*B*).

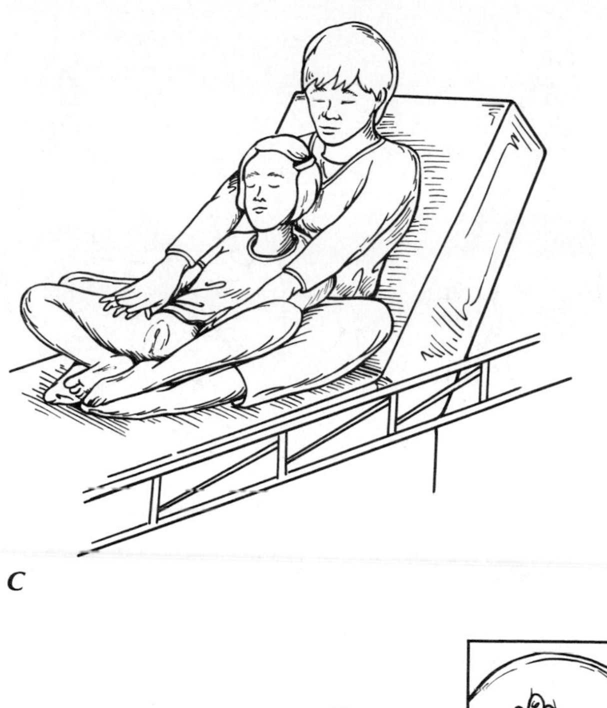

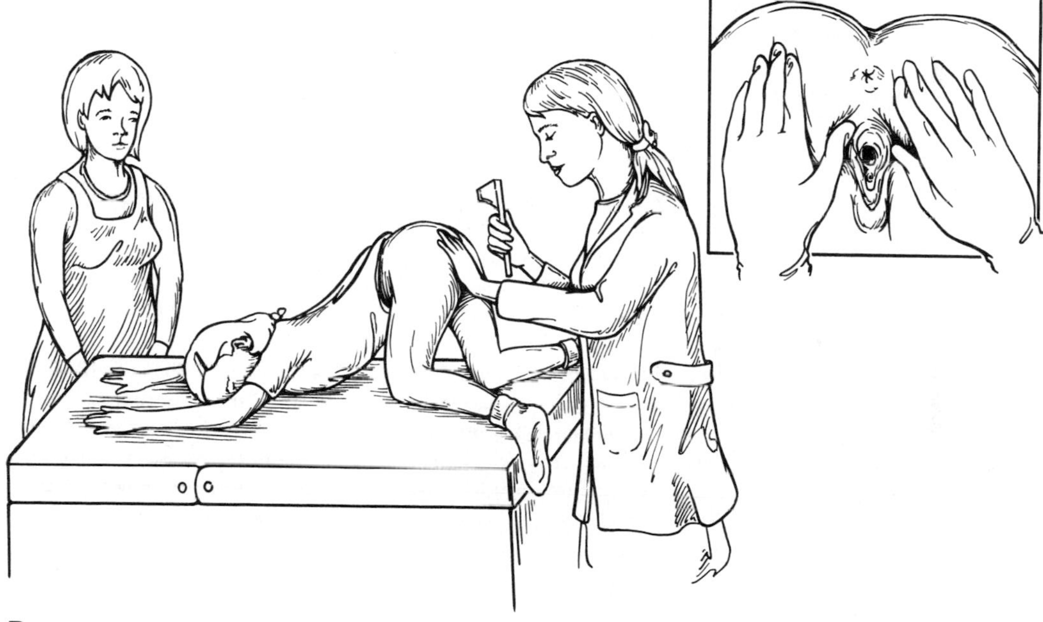

Fig. 23-2. (continued). The child may also lie in the parent's lap with legs abducted on the examining table (*C*). The knee-chest position (*D*) is sometimes useful with younger children (sheet draping is excluded for clarity; see text).

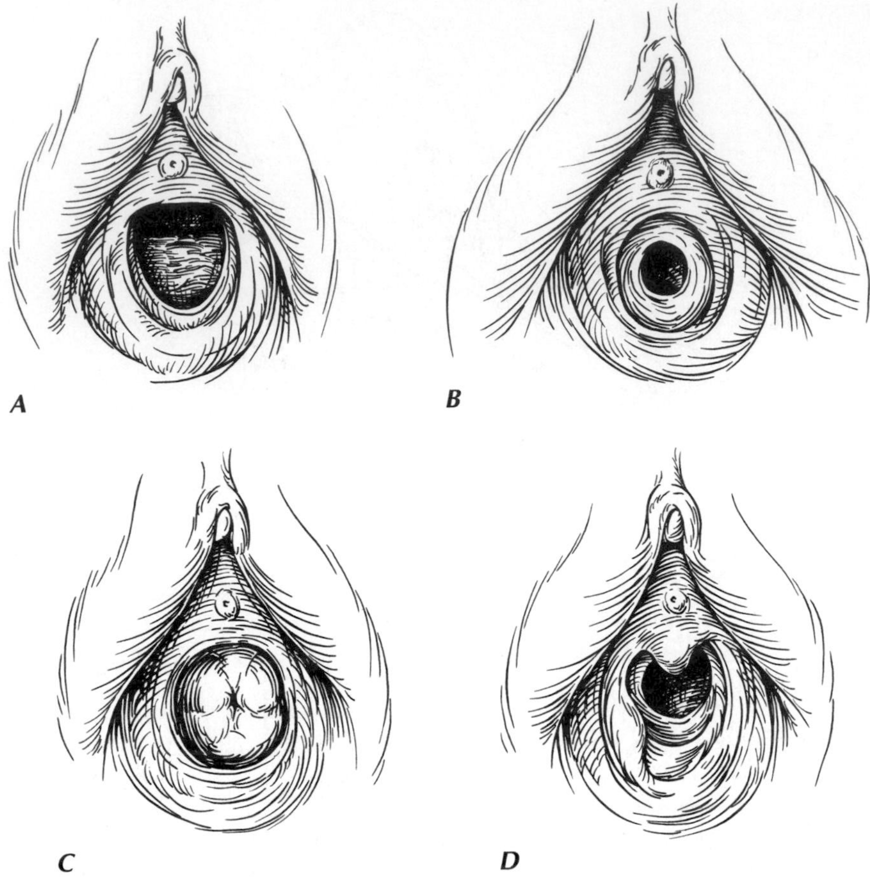

Fig. 23-3. Configuration of the hymen in young patients. Crescentic hymen (*A*); annular hymen (*B*); and redundant hymen (*C*). Sharply angulated disruptions of the hymenal contour in young children suggest hymenal trauma (*D*).

Though they may be required in some circumstances, speculum examinations of the vagina are not routinely done in prepubertal children. Likewise, digital bimanual examinations are generally not indicated. When the vagina must be visualized, examination with sedation or under anesthesia should be strongly considered, and consultation is warranted to ensure that the most experienced examiner makes the best diagnostic use of the examination. When the possibility of a pelvic mass is suspected, a rectoabdominal examination can provide nearly the same information as the vaginal bimanual examination in prepubertal patients. Not surprisingly, children have no enthusiasm for rectal examinations. Nevertheless, these can usually be managed without anesthesia or sedation in cooperative older children.

For patients whose chief complaint is vaginal discharge, various techniques have been described to collect vaginal secretions for analysis. When discharge is copious, small swabs for specimen collection can frequently be introduced through the hymenal orifice without undue difficulty or patient discomfort. In other settings, however, use of swabs can be uncomfortable or even painful when applied to the atrophic vaginal mucosa of younger children. Pokorny and Stormer[4] described a technique that can be helpful in these situations. A catheter within a catheter is constructed using the hub and tubing of a butterfly intravenous catheter and the distal 4 inches of a no. 12 red rubber urinary catheter. Using sterile technique, the needle end of the intravenous catheter is removed and slipped into the length of bladder catheter. A tuberculin syringe filled with 1 mL of sterile nonbacteriostatic saline is attached to the hub of the assembly. The procedure is carried out in the supine frog leg position after explaining to the child, in language that she can understand, that her

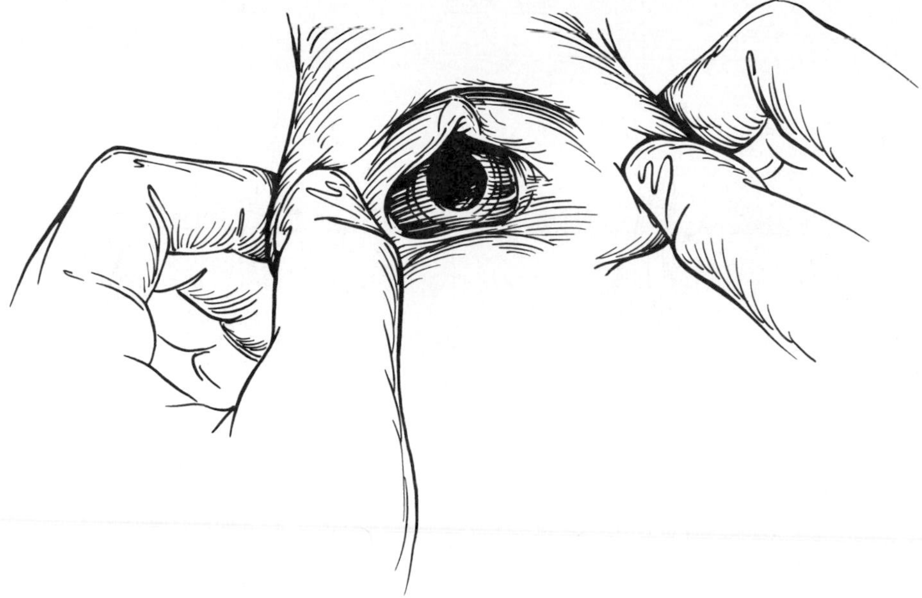

Fig. 23-4. The technique of labial traction. The examiner grasps the labia majora bilaterally between thumb and forefinger and pulls outward and slightly laterally.

vagina will be "washed with water." The vaginal introitus is exposed, and the catheter is introduced 2 to 3 cm into the vagina. Saline is injected and aspirated several times to ensure adequate mixing with vaginal secretions. The entire apparatus is then quickly removed.

Examination of the Adolescent

As discussed above, gynecologic examination of the adolescent should be undertaken only after a comprehensive confidential history has been obtained from the adolescent alone. Important components of the interview include age of menarche, menstrual history (frequency, duration, and volume of flow), sexual history and current sexual activity, history of previous sexually transmitted diseases, and previous gynecologic care (of which parents may be unaware). The examiner should be sensitive to patient concerns related to privacy, body image, and sexuality. Modesty should be respected. Some patients will ask for a female examiner, and these requests should be accommodated whenever possible. General preparation of the patient for her examination has already been discussed. For adolescents being examined for the first time, it is generally worthwhile to describe the examination in considerable detail. Emphasizing that this examination is done routinely on adolescents and that it is an examination that the patient will have done routinely throughout her life can sometimes help to normalize the experience.

Conduct of the actual examination is largely similar to the examination done in adult women. It is typical to have a chaperone present for the examination; the adolescent may or may not want her mother, sister, or friend present as well. The examination can be used as an opportunity to educate. Normal anatomy, sexual maturation, menstrual physiology, and similar topics may all be addressed as part of the visit. However, the nature of the presenting complaint, pain or discomfort, or patient receptiveness may all mitigate against the possibility of providing much in the way of education during the acute visit. It is often sufficient for the clinician to use the word "normal" frequently in describing the examination as it proceeds.

The examination is conducted in the dorsal lithotomy position with the feet in stirrups. The Tanner stage (Fig. 23-5) is recorded and careful inspection for anatomic variations or congenital anomalies is done, particularly in the girl being examined for the first time. The external genitalia are examined for evidence of trauma, infection, or other unusual findings. Clitoromegaly, inguinal lymphadenopathy, or hernias should be identified.

The hymen in adolescent girls is likely to be folded and redundant. Its orifice may not be fully visible, or it may appear smaller than it actually is. As in younger pa-

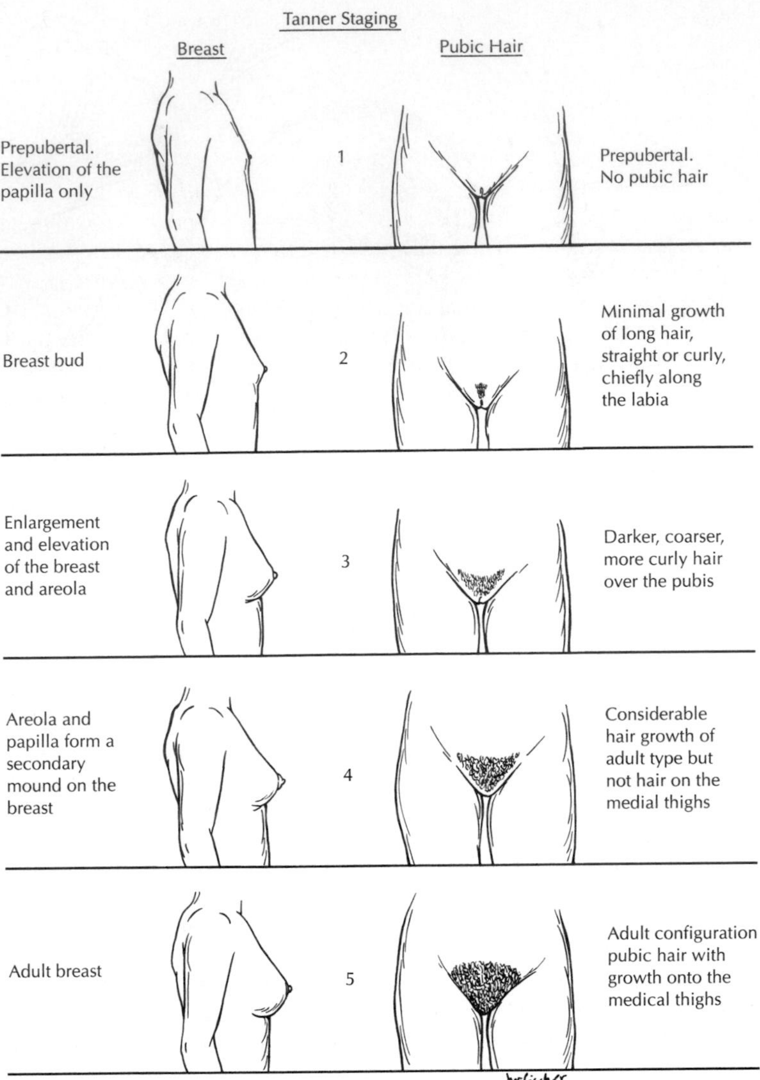

Fig. 23-5. Tanner staging.

tients, a moistened swab can be helpful in delineating the size and contour of the hymenal orifice. In adolescent patients being examined for the first time, it is frequently helpful to perform a digital vaginal examination prior to a speculum examination. One finger is used rather than two. A lubricated examining finger is less uncomfortable than a speculum and affords the examiner an opportunity to locate the cervix prior to insertion of the speculum. However, the use of lubricant precludes obtaining a satisfactory Pap smear or cultures.

For most adolescents, the straight blades of a Pederson speculum offer the best compromise between patient comfort and adequate visualization of the vagina. Some patients will tolerate the wider Graves speculum; the narrower Huffman speculum is appropriate for younger adolescents and when the hymenal orifice is smaller. The smallest pediatric specula are seldom adequate in adolescent patients, as their short length does not permit visualization of the cervix. Specula should be warmed and may be lubricated with water. Physiologic leukorrhea is a common finding in premenarchal adolescents and should not be confused with pathologic processes. Cervical ectropion, in which columnar cervical epithelium is everted onto the visible portion of the cervix, is also fairly common and should not be mistaken for cervical pathology. In young women who are sexually active, wet prep and cultures for *Chlamydia* and *N. gonorrhoeae* are usually appropriate. Pap smears may also be obtained in appropriate clinical settings or to avoid the need for a subsequent examination.

Bimanual examination is usually done with a single examining finger. The presence of cervical motion tenderness should be ascertained. The uterus and adenexa should be palpated for enlargement, discrete masses, or tenderness. Patients being examined for the first time may have difficulty distinguishing between the discomfort of the examination itself and the tenderness being sought. The examiner might say: "You will feel me press very hard on your belly. I need you to tell me whether I am pressing on something sore or whether you just feel me pressing deeply." For the most part, rectovaginal examinations are not required in adolescent patients.

SPECIAL SITUATIONS

The Uncooperative Patient or Family

When the reason for a gynecologic examination is clearly presented and the family and patient have been adequately prepared, truly uncooperative patients should be rare. In the setting of the uncooperative patient or family, the clinician should first attempt to precisely ascertain the reason for the reticence. Often, a particular concern will be at issue—one that can be resolved through additional reassurance, education, or a modification in the exam protocol. One can ask the patient (or family): "What is it about the examination that has you most worried? Maybe we can find some way to get around that for you."

Sexual abuse should also be specifically considered when concerns about the examination are unexplained or seem exaggerated. Sexual abuse may be directly or indirectly responsible for the presenting complaint, or it may have occurred far in the past and be unrelated to the current visit. Still, even remote sexual abuse can be associated with unresolved issues and may make such patients very apprehensive about the proposed examination. Patients are not always willing to disclose previous abuse to an unfamiliar provider in the emergency department; clinicians should not discount the possibility of abuse even when it is explicitly denied by patients.

If the patient's anxieties or concerns about the examination cannot be ascertained or assuaged, the help of family should be enlisted. Often, it is useful to leave the room of an uncooperative patient and allow the family some time alone. A clearer picture of the situation may emerge once the parent has had an opportunity to talk privately with the child or adolescent. For very young children, persuasion with stickers or other treats can be remarkably effective. Preadolescents and younger adolescents are often intensely modest and will be more cooperative once they are reassured that their modesty will be preserved.

Needless to say, no child or adolescent should be examined forcibly. The rights of patients to control their own bodies must be respected. Moreover, it is unlikely that an examination will be productive in the child who is resistant, tensing the muscles (including those of the perineum), and who is unwilling to relax. In such patients, an examination using sedation should be considered.

Evaluation of Alleged or Suspected Sexual Abuse

The evaluation of the sexually abused child is discussed in detail in Chap. 25. Most abused children can readily be examined using the same principles and techniques already described. Some children will be especially fearful of being examined; others, especially very young children, will be surprisingly compliant. When it is determined that the alleged or suspected abuse occurred at some time in the past, the examination may best be deferred to an established clinic or team specifically organized to evaluate these patients. Conversely, patients seen acutely (within 72 hours) after alleged or suspected abuse should be examined immediately and may require a formal forensic examination (using a rape kit). These examinations can be traumatic for patients, upsetting for families, and emotionally charged for examiners as well. Ordinarily, the forensic examination is done soon after the assault and therefore at an especially vulnerable time for the patient. Sedation for the examination may be considered, especially in the immediate aftermath of the assault, for young children or for patients who are obviously distressed.

Forensic examinations are time-consuming and require careful documentation and meticulous attention to procedures. For evidence to be admissible in court, the chain of custody must be strictly guarded and documented. The complete examination includes a full-body survey with photographs, fingernail scrapings, pubic hair combing, plucked hair, and the collection of duplicate swabs of all specimens. All bacteriologic studies should be true cultures and not genetic probes, immunofluorescent assays, or other nonculture methods. Subsequent screening for syphilis, human immunodeficiency virus, and hepatitis B is based on the history of the alleged abuse. Morning-after contraception may be offered in appropriate clinical settings (see Chap. 33).

Sedation

Examination using procedural sedation or general anesthesia should be considered when these modalities would alleviate significant discomfort and/or pain, when they would help to minimize negative psychological responses to the examination or treatment, or in other settings in which examinations could not otherwise be performed.[5] Typically, sedation is most frequently indicated in the evaluation of very young children, in the evaluation of developmentally delayed children (who may not understand the nature of the examination), or when potentially noxious procedures may be required. Only procedural sedation is discussed in detail; however, general anesthesia is a reasonable alternative when procedural sedation is not available or in situations in which extensive instrumentation is anticipated.

Safety concerns have prompted guidelines for procedural sedation from the American Academy of Pediatrics.[5] When used in children, all sedative agents are dosed by weight and care must be taken to avoid overdosing (Table 23-2). Resuscitation equipment and personnel trained in pediatric resuscitation should be immediately available. While sedated, a patient's vital signs and oxygen saturation should be continuously monitored to prevent airway and respiratory compromise. Continuous ECG monitoring is indicated for patients with a history of cardiac disease.

Choice of specific sedative agents will be determined by the nature of the examination to be conducted and its expected duration. Patient age can sometimes influence the choice of sedative but more often affects the route of administration. *Fentanyl citrate* is a narcotic that is used frequently in outpatient and emergency department settings. Its onset of action is short, its duration of action is brief, and it has potent analgesic and sedative effects, making it ideal for short, painful procedures. Its short half-life and potency make it possible to precisely titrate the drug to the desired clinical effect. Fentanyl is usually used parenterally, but it is also available in lollipop form (the Fentanyl Oralet®).[6] Respiratory depression can occur with fentanyl, is dose-dependent, and is more likely when other respiratory depressants are used concurrently. It is rapidly reversed by naloxone. Other adverse effects of fentanyl include facial pruritus, nausea and vomiting, and—rarely—anaphylaxis and profound thoracic muscular rigidity that can make ventilation difficult. Fentanyl does not cause hypotension or cardiovascular depression.

Midazolam is a short-acting benzodiazepine with sedative, anxiolytic, amnestic, and relaxant properties, but it has no analgesic effect. It has a rapid onset and a brief duration of action. Midazolam is suitable for brief, mildly noxious procedures. It can be given by nearly any route, including parenterally, intramuscularly, per rectum, and intranasally, and is frequently used orally in children. Onset of action is dependent on the route of administration, but is

Table 23-2. Useful Drugs for the Procedural Sedation of Patients in the Emergency Department

Agent	Dose	Supplement	Onset	Duration
Fentanyl				
IV	1–3 mcg/kg (over 3–5 min)	0.5 mcg/kg	3–5 min	30–40 min
PO	5–15 mcg/kg, not to exceed 15 mcg/kg (Oralet: 100, 200, 300, 400 mcg)	n/a	Variable	Variable
Midazolam				
IV	0.15 mg/kg	0.02 mg/kg	3–10 min	30–45 min
IM	0.15 mg/kg	0.1 mg/kg	5–15 min	30–45 min
PO	0.5 mg/kg, max 20 mg/does	n/a	10–30 min	Variable
Intranasal	0.2–0.3 mg/kg	n/a	5–10 min	30–45 min
PR	0.2–0.3 mg/kg	n/a	5–10 min	30–45 min
Ketamine				
IV	1–2 mg/kg	0.5–1 mg/kg	Seconds	15 min
IM	2–4 mg/kg	2–4 mg/kg	5–10 min	20 min
PO, PR, Intranasal	6–10 mg/kg		Variable	Variable

n/a, not appropriate.

usually 5 to 15 minutes. Respiratory depression is the most common adverse effect and is dose-dependent. Respiratory depression can be temporarily reversed by flumazenil, though this antagonist is not formally approved for use in children.

Ketamine is a dissociative agent with sedative, analgesic, and amnestic effects. It is useful for a wide range of diagnostic and therapeutic procedures but is short-acting. Ketamine may be given by multiple routes, but is usually used intravenously or intramuscularly. Onset is usually immediate when given intravenously, 5 to 10 minutes when given intramuscularly, and longer when administered by mouth. The dissociative state produced by ketamine may cause a trance-like effect whereby the child may appear to be wide awake and staring. The duration of action is 15 to 20 minutes. Side effects from ketamine include involuntary eye movements and motor activity as well as breath-holding during induction. Because ketamine is a secretagogue, it is recommended that glycopyrrolate or atropine be administered concurrently (in the same syringe). Emergence dysphoria and nightmares occur commonly in adults but less commonly (if at all) in children. These can be prevented and treated by the administration of benzodiazepines. Concurrent medication with midazolam is recommended, especially in older children and adolescents. Laryngospasm has been reported rarely. Ketamine does not cause respiratory or hemodynamic compromise.

Several other sedating agents can be useful in the emergency department. Short-acting barbiturates provide deep sedation but no analgesia. They usually require intravenous or intramuscular administration, though *methohexital* can be given per rectum. As with other barbiturates, respiratory and cardiac depression can occur and are dose-dependent. Use of these agents is limited by their brief duration of action and by the potential for adverse effects. When available, *nitrous oxide* can be easily administered, provides reliable analgesia, and has few adverse effects. However, nitrous oxide is not available for regular use in many emergency departments. Some older sedation protocols can no longer be recommended for routine use in children. Both chloral hydrate and "cocktails" of meperidine-promethazine-chlorpromazine were extensively used in the past to sedate children in the emergency department. These agents are seldom used today because of difficulties related to unreliable onset, prolonged sedation, and adverse effects.

REFERENCES

1. Lynch JM, Gardner MJ, Albanese CT: Blunt urogenital trauma in prepubescent female patients: More than meets the eye. *Pediatr Emerg Care* 11:372, 1995.
2. Levenberg PB, Elster AB: *Guidelines for Adolescent Preventive Services: Implementation and Resource Manual.* Chicago: American Medical Association, 1995, pp 112–118.
3. McCann J, Voris J, Simon M, Wells R: Comparison of genital examination techniques in prepubertal girls. *Pediatrics* 85:182, 1990.
4. Pokorny SF, Stormer J: Atraumatic removal of secretions from the prepubertal vagina. *Am J Obstet Gynecol* 156:581, 1987.
5. American Academy of Pediatrics Committee on Drugs: Guidelines for monitoring and management of pediatric patients during and after sedation for diagnostic and therapeutic procedures. *Pediatrics* 89:1110, 1992.
6. Schutzman SA, Burg J, Leibelt E, et al: Oral transmucosal fentanyl citrate for premedication of children undergoing laceration repair. *Ann Emerg Med* 24:1059, 1994.

24

Common Gynecologic and Urinary Problems in the Pediatric and Adolescent Female

Elisabeth H. Quint
Monica Sifuentes

KEY POINTS

- Vaginal discharge in a premenarchal girl is most commonly nonspecific if present for more than 1 month. Discharge is unlikely to be due to yeast, unless a precipitating event (like antibiotic use) occurred.
- Vaginal bleeding in a premenarchal girl is always pathologic and needs to be thoroughly evaluated to find the source.
- When interviewing an adolescent, a private discussion regarding sexuality is very important, even in an ED setting.
- About 50 percent of all adolescents that hemorrhage with their first menstrual period will have a bleeding disorder.
- Ovarian torsion does not always necessitate removal of the ovary if the diagnosis is made promptly.
- A negative urine dipstick does not exclude the diagnosis of a urinary tract infection in the pediatric patient.

Genitourinary conditions in the prepubertal girl and the adolescent are commonly encountered in the emergency department (ED). They may create diagnostic dilemmas, because the symptomatology changes with the age of the patient. As the female body changes with hormonal status and initiation of sexual activity, so do the conditions and symptomatology. Many different gynecologic and urologic disease processes have similar presentations in pediatric and adolescent girls and can be confused with one another.

Often a sensitive situation arises and it is very important to attempt to win the patient's and the family's trust. The genital examination may be a new experience for the girl and may cause physical and emotional discomfort. This chapter describes the most common gynecologic and urologic problems encountered in pediatric and adolescent patients in the ED. Some of the disease processes are similar in all women of reproductive age and are therefore only mentioned here as they relate to pediatric and adolescent patients.

PHYSIOLOGY OF THE GENITOURINARY TRACT

The genital tract of the prepubertal child is quite different from that of a woman of reproductive age. At birth, the vaginal mucosa is thick and estrogenized, due to intrauterine exposure to maternal estrogen. After several days, the estrogen level drops and the vaginal mucosa changes into smooth, atrophic, thin, and delicate tissue. The pH is between 6.5 and 7.5, and there should be no visible vaginal discharge or bleeding in a healthy prepubertal female. However, there are two points in the developmental timetable when noticeable discharge may be present. The first is in the neonatal period when white mucoid discharge may be present because of circulating maternal estrogens. As the estrogen levels fall, the discharge disappears, but there can be a small uterine estrogen withdrawal bleed which should disappear by 3 or 4 weeks of age. The typical prepubertal appearance of vulvovaginal atrophy without discharge or bleeding remains throughout childhood until ovarian stimulation occurs. At this time a noticeable whitish or slight yellow discharge may appear, which is nonodorous and nonirritating and is considered a normal physiologic discharge.

VULVOVAGINAL DISEASES IN PREMENARCHAL GIRLS

Vulvovaginitis

Prepubertal girls are at relative risk for vulvovaginitis because of the proximity of the vagina and anus, the lack of protective hair and labial fat pads, and the lack of estrogenization. Other potential contributing factors to vulvovaginitis in this age group are obesity, tight-fitting jeans or leotards, harsh soaps and bubble baths, and

Table 24-1. Etiologies of Vaginal Discharge in the Prepubertal Child

Nonspecific vulvovaginitis
Specific vulvovaginitis
- *Candida albicans*
- Respiratory pathogens
  - Group A β-streptococcis
  - *Streptococcus pneumoniae*
  - *Neisseria meningitidis*
  - *Branhamella catarrhalis*
  - *Staphylococcus aureus*
  - *Haemophilus influenzae*
- Enteric
  - *Shigella*
  - *Yersinia*
  - *Escherichia coli*
- Sexually transmitted diseases
  - *Neisseria gonorrhoeae*
  - *Chlamydia trachomatis*
  - Herpes simplex
  - *Trichomonas*
  - *Condyloma acuminatum*

Pinworms
Foreign body
Polyps, tumors
Vulvar skin disease (lichen sclerosus, contact dermatitis, psoriasis)
Systemic illness
Trauma
Prolapsed urethra
Congenital anomalies (ectopic ureter, double vagina with fistula)

poor hygiene. The normal flora of the prepubertal child has been studied and includes lactobacilli, alpha-hemolytic streptococci, and diphtheroids. Other common isolates include *Escherichia coli, Klebsiella sp.,* and other streptococci.[1,2] Etiologies for vaginal discharge are described in Table 24-1.

History and Physical Examination

The characteristics of the discharge are important: color (bloody, green, yellow), consistency (watery, creamy, flocculent), duration (more than 1 month is usually a non-specific discharge), associated pruritus (vulvar or anal), odor (fecal, urine, fishy), and staining of underwear. Has there been previous treatment and has it been effective? Is there a recent history of infection or use of antibiotics? Are there indications for suspicion of sexual abuse, including behavioral changes, abdominal pain, headaches, or enuresis? Obtain information on perineal hygiene, including wiping from front to back, use of harsh soaps and bubble baths, and urinating with the knees together, which increases urinary reflux in the vagina. The physical examination for vaginal discharge and bleeding must include special attention to Tanner staging of breasts, pubic and axillary hair, and the external genitalia (see Chap. 23, Fig. 23-5). Look for the presence of pubic hair, and note clitoral size, signs of estrogenization (lush pink vulva and vaginal tissue as opposed to premenarchal thin, red skin), discharge, bleeding, and any signs of trauma. Note the degree of perineal hygiene and perianal excoriation (suggestive of pinworm). Describe the type of hymen and look for signs of sexual abuse (described in Chap. 25). An attempt to see inside the vagina can be made by using the knee-chest position and an otoscope, as described in Chap. 23. With deep inspiration in the knee-chest position, the cervix or foreign bodies can sometimes be identified.

A rectoabdominal exam can be performed in the frog-leg position by inserting a well-lubricated index or little finger into the rectum and placing the other hand on the abdomen. In the premenarchal girl, only a small button cervix should be felt (ratio of uterus to cervix of 1:2). As the rectal finger is removed, the vagina is milked for evidence of discharge or blood.

Differential Diagnosis

The most common etiology of vaginal discharge is nonspecific vaginitis. In the case of a specific vaginitis, respiratory, enteric, and sexually transmitted pathogens are the major etiologic agents. *Shigella* and *Yersinia* can produce bloody vaginal discharge, sometimes associated with diarrhea. *Candida* in prepubertal girls is uncommon unless it is associated with risk factors such as antibiotic use or diabetes mellitus. If there is suspicion that *Neisseria gonorrhoeae* or *Chlamydia trachomatis* may be causing the discharge, a culture-proven diagnosis is crucial to pursue prosecution and positive results must be reported to local authorities according to local and state ordinance.[3–6] These infections may be acquired by colonization at birth from a mother with an active infection, but they rarely persist beyond 12 to 24 months.[6,7] Genital herpes caused by herpes simplex types 1 and 2 has been reported in children. The clinical presentation is similar to that described in adults, with painful vesicles and ulceration developing after an incubation period of 2 to 20 days. A primary infection can cause inguinal adenopathy, fever, malaise, headache, and significant discomfort with urination. Although the virus has been described as surviving in water and on plastic surfaces,[8] the majority of cases are thought to be sexually transmitted.[9,10] When a child presents with genital herpes, other sites, like the oropharynx and the hands, must be carefully inspected. When both oral and genital lesions are present, the chance of autoinoculation increases. The differential diagnosis of ulcerative lesions includes varicella, herpes zoster, dermatitis, trauma, and *Candida*. Trichomoniasis, causing a frothy yellow-green discharge, is fairly uncommon in the unestrogenized premenarchal child.[11] Approximately 5 percent of infants of mothers with vaginal trichomoniasis will become infected perinatally.[12] Onset of symptoms beyond the first few weeks of life, it is highly suspicious for sexual abuse, therefore a complete investigation must be undertaken.[13] Bacterial vaginosis (BV) generally presents as a thin grayish discharge with a fishy odor. It is caused by a mixed collection of organisms, including *Gardnerella vaginalis, Bacteroides* species, and *Mobiluncus.* It is unclear how often BV is associated with sexual abuse. Bacterial vaginosis has been described in asymptomatic girls,[2] as well as in 25 percent of abused children, compared to 4 percent of nonabused children in a case-control study.[14]

Laboratory Tests

If vaginal discharge is persistent or purulent, a Gram stain, wet preparation, and cultures should be done. In the pediatric-aged population a general genital culture is also done. If sexual abuse is suspected, cultures for *N. gonorrhoeae* (on the modified Thayer-Martin medium)[3] and *Chlamydia* need to be performed. Cultures for these and other organisms are described in Appendix 2. If there is suspicion of genital herpes, a culture must be obtained. However, this can be false-positive in a cross-reaction with varicella. False-negative results may also be seen if specimens are obtained from lesions with decreased shedding (e.g., crusted or recurrent lesions). If anal itching is an associated symptom, screening for pinworms can be done by the pediatrician.

Treatment

For nonspecific vaginitis it is important to stress the importance of hygiene measures to the parents. These include good perineal hygiene (including wiping from front to back), unscented soap products, cotton underpants, no tight-fitting clothes, and urinating with the legs spread apart. For treatment of persistent nonspecific vulvovaginitis, a broad-spectrum antibiotic (amoxicillin or cephalexin) is used for 14 days. If this is unsuccessful, an estrogen cream applied daily may help. For a specific vaginitis caused by *Shigella* or *Yersinia,* trimethoprimsulfamethoxazole, 8 mg/40 mg/kg/d orally in divided doses for 7 days is prescribed.

Candida can be treated with topical nystatin, miconazole, or clotrimazole cream. Oral fluconazole can also be used. *Neisseria gonorrhoeae* is usually treated with ceftriaxone 125 mg intramuscularly. If the child is over 8 years old, doxycycline 100 mg orally twice a day for 7 days or azithromycin 1 g orally is added. In younger children ($\leq$45 kg), *C. trachomatis* is treated with erythromycin, 50 mg/kg/d for 10 days. In children who weigh >45 kg or are $\geq$8 years old, azithromycin 1 g orally in a single dose is recommended. Treatment of genital herpes in children should be individualized. Acyclovir is unlabeled for use in children less than 2 years old. Bacterial superinfection of herpetic lesions may require antibiotics with activity against both *Streptococcus* and *Staphylococcus.* Trichomoniasis is treated with metronidazole 15 mg/kg/d in divided doses for 7 days. This same dose can also be used for the treatment of bacterial vaginosis.

Labial Agglutination

Inflammation combined with a lack of estrogen can cause labial agglutination, in which the labia minora become adherent, either in part or completely.

The diagnosis of labial agglutination or labial adhesions, has been reported in as many as 20 percent of prepubertal girls.[15] The condition is usually asymptomatic, but may present with dysuria, urinary retention, or urinary tract infections. If the agglutination is partial, it is commonly posterior; if complete, a tiny opening just below the clitoris is usually present (Fig. 24-1). Upon examination, with mild traction on the labia as described in Chapter 23, a grey line becomes easily visible where the labia are agglutinated. It can be confused with vaginal agenesis, but the presence of this midline raphe makes the diagnosis clear. Other differential diagnoses include lichen sclerosus and childhood cicatricial pemphigoid.

The treatment of labial adhesions consists of estrogen cream applied twice daily with gentle outward traction by the parent or other caregiver (Fig. 24-2). Forceful separation should be avoided. The cream makes the tissues thicker and the separation is usually complete in 7 to 14 days. After that, continued use of emollients for several months is recommended to prevent recurrence. If this is unsuccessful and there are urinary symptoms, separation

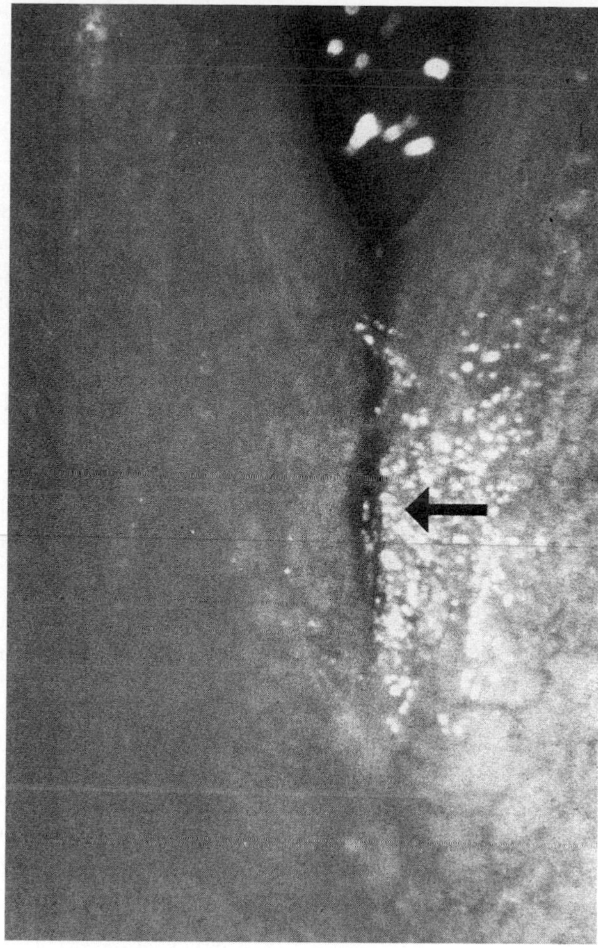

Fig. 24-1. Labial agglutination (*arrow*). With traction, the white line becomes clearly visible. Estrogen cream can be applied while traction is held on the labia. (Photograph courtesy of Pediatric and Adolescent Gynecology, Little, Brown Co. Inc., with permission).

under anesthesia is occasionally recommended, but rarely indicated.

Vaginal Bleeding

Vaginal bleeding in a prepubertal child is always abnormal after 3 or 4 weeks of age. The etiologies are listed in Table 24-2. Most bleeding in premenarchal girls occurs not because of major trauma or pathology, but result from vulvovaginitis (especially due to *Shigella* or group A β streptococci), scratching, or the introduction of a vaginal foreign body.

History and Physical Examination

The history should focus on the circumstances of bleeding, times of recurrence, and associated symptoms such as pain. Accelerated growth of weight and height or other signs of puberty suggest precocious puberty. Relevant history includes trauma, sexual abuse, history of foreign body, blood dyscrasias, and other medical problems. The physical examination should focus on all the same aspects as outlined in the section on vaginal discharge, with special attention paid to any signs of pubertal development or trauma.

Differential Diagnosis

The evaluation of a premenarchal girl with vaginal bleeding is described in the algorithm shown in Fig. 24-3. The first two circumstances that need to be ruled out are precocious puberty and genital trauma.

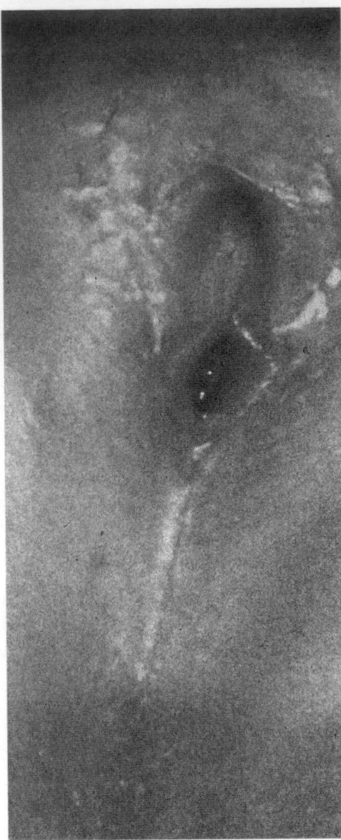

Fig. 24-2. Labial agglutination in a 9-year-old girl. (Photograph courtesy of S.F. Smith, MD and the North American Society for Pediatric and Adolescent Gynecology, with permission.)

Precocious Puberty

Traditionally, precocious puberty in girls is defined as the development of secondary sexual characteristics before the age of 8. This specific age is currently being reevaluated, however, since it has been noted that a significant number of girls from certain races (e.g., African-American) are normally starting puberty at an earlier age. The causes are numerous (Table 24-2) and referral to a pediatric endocrinologist is appropriate.

Genital Trauma

Trauma is usually evident from history and examination. Always make sure that the extent of the trauma fits with the history, otherwise abuse should be suspected. A straddle injury usually causes ecchymoses in the vulva and periclitoral folds. A hymenal tear is very uncommon without a penetrating injury (e.g., caused by a nail or a broomstick). In the absence of such a history, sexual abuse should always be suspected if a hymenal tear is present. Examination of a child with active bleeding from the vulva can be performed by wiping 2 percent lidocaine jelly on the cut and then irrigating with warm water from a syringe. If the complete extent of the wound cannot be assessed or the injury does not fit the description of the accident, an exam under sedation or anesthesia is imperative (see Chap. 23).[16] If the amount of vaginal bleeding has been significant or the patient appears unusually pale, a hematocrit and hemoglobin should be checked.

Foreign Bodies

Foreign bodies present with vaginal discharge or bleeding, occasionally associated with a foul odor. Sometimes the diagnosis can be made in the outpatient setting; often an examination under anesthesia is necessary to confirm the foreign body and for its removal.

If a foreign body is evident on physical examination, an attempt can be made to retrieve it in the emergency department. Toilet paper can be removed with a moistened cotton-tipped applicator or with irrigation. To irrigate, place a small rubber catheter in the vagina and rinse it out thoroughly with warm normal saline. Depending on the age and cooperation level of the child, this may need to be done under sedation or anesthesia (see Chap. 22).

Condyloma Acuminatum

Condyloma acuminatum (genital warts) is caused by the human papilloma virus, usually types 6 and 11 in this age group.[17] It can be transmitted perinatally (up to the age of 2 or 3 years) as well as by sexual abuse.[18] The literature is unclear about the exact age limit, but more than 50 percent of children with genital or anal warts have histories of sexual abuse.[17] Therefore every child presenting with genital warts, regardless of age, deserves a sexual abuse evaluation. The diagnosis is usually made by careful clinical inspection. The application of 3 to 5 percent acetic acid reveals the characteristic white appearance of the lesions; after it is applied, more condylomata may become apparent. The differential diagnosis includes condyloma latum due to syphilis, perineal tumors, prolapsed urethra, and molluscum contagiosum.

Genital condylomata are usually treated under general anesthesia with carbon dioxide laser. Occasionally, in a mature, cooperative girl with only a few lesions, treatment in the outpatient setting with trichloroacetic acid may be tried. The failure rate ranges from 29 to 50 percent.[17,19]

Table 24-2. Etiologies for Vaginal Bleeding in the Prepubertal Child

Associated with precocious puberty	
True	Idiopathic Cerebral disorders Tuberous sclerosis Congenital adrenal hyperplasia Primary hypothyroidism
Pseudo	Ovarian tumors Adrenal tumors McCune-Albright syndrome Gonadotropic-producing tumors Iatrogenic
Not associated with precocious puberty	
Trauma	
Accidental	
Sexual abuse	
Vulvar lesions (e.g., lichen sclerosus, condyloma)	
Vaginitis (e.g., Shigella, *Streptococcus pyogenes*)	
Foreign body	
Urethral polyps/prolapse	
Neonatal hormonal withdrawal	
Precocious menarche	
Unknown	

Podophyllin should generally be avoided in the pediatric age group.

Lichen Sclerosus

Lichen sclerosus is a skin disease of unknown etiology. It can present with itching, dysuria, irritation, and occasionally bleeding. On examination, the skin is atrophic and parchment-like, with flat ivory-colored papules that can coalesce into plaques and occasionally ulcers, inflammation, and hemorrhage is seen (Fig. 24-4). There may be an hour-glass configuration involving the anus.[20] Secondary infection and ulceration can occur, especially if itching has been present (Fig. 24-5). The differential diagnosis includes vaginitis, pinworms, sexual abuse, and vitiligo.

The treatment of lichen sclerosus consists of instituting perineal hygiene measures (see above) and the use of topical glucocorticoids. If the condition is severe, daily topical clobetasol propionate ointment 0.05 percent, may be used for short periods (2 to 4 weeks), with a taper to triamcinolone 0.1 percent ointment daily for 4 weeks.[21] The disease tends to recur unpredictably. Antibiotics may be necessary if there is secondary infection due to excoriations from scratching. Some studies have shown a spontaneous improvement with adolescence.[20]

Urethral Prolapse

Urethral prolapse is a symmetric eversion of the distal urethral mucosa through the meatus. It is seen primarily in prepubertal African-American females. A urethral prolapse usually presents with painless bleeding and complaints of dysuria, as well as pain after coughing, straining, or wiping. Occasionally it can lead to urinary retention. The urethral mucosa presents as a red-blue friable annular (doughnut-shaped) mass with a central umbilicated area representing the urethral opening. (Fig. 24-6).[22] To verify this, a small urinary catheter may be carefully introduced into this central opening. Occasionally, if the prolapse is large enough (2 to 3 cm), the vaginal introitus may be difficult to visualize. The prolapse may also appear to be fungating and neoplastic, depending on the degree of inflammation, edema, and necrosis of urethral mucosa.

The differential diagnosis includes urethral polyps, papilloma, carbuncle, prolapsed ureterocele, condyloma, sarcoma botryoides (rhabdomyosarcoma), and periurethral abscess. Urethral prolapse is usually treated by nonsurgical means including sitz-baths, 2 weeks of daily topical estrogen, and oral antibiotics for secondary infection. Manual reduction is not recommended. If there are large areas of necrosis, surgical resection is usually

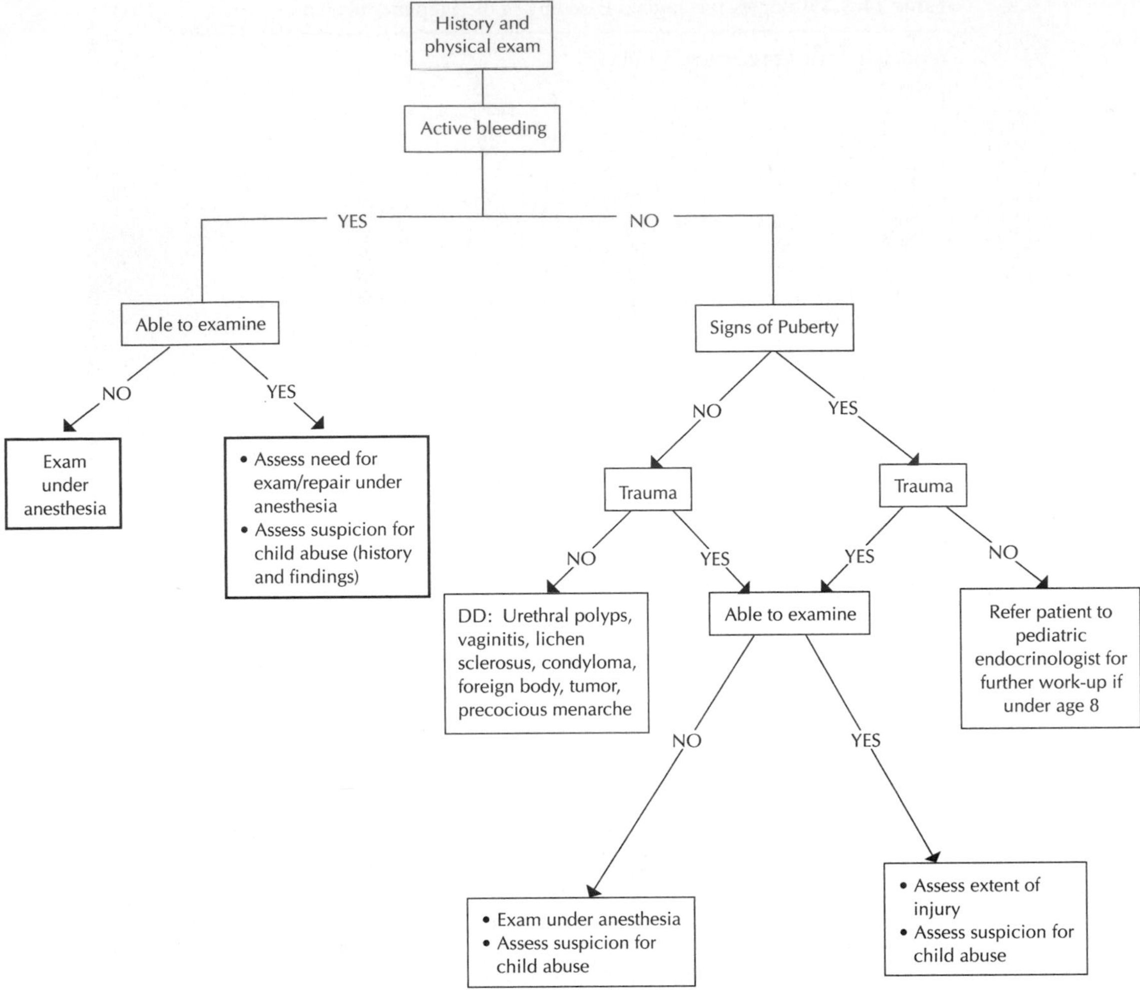

Fig. 24-3. Algorithm for the diagnosis of premenstrual vaginal bleeding. DD, differential diagnosis.

needed.[22] Follow-up with the primary care provider should occur in 1 to 2 weeks, or sooner if the patient becomes symptomatic or is not improving.

Other Disorders

Vulvar or vaginal tumors are uncommon in this age group. The most common neoplasm is sarcoma botryoides or embryonal rhabdomyosarcoma. This is a rare tumor in very young girls, involving the vagina, uterus, bladder, or urethra. The symptoms include vaginal discharge, bleeding, abdominal pain, mass, or passage of grape-like tissue. Ninety percent of these tumors occur before age 5. Sarcoma botryoides grows very rapidly and has a poor prognosis unless it is diagnosed early and aggressively treated with a combination of surgery, chemotherapy, and radiation.[23]

Blood dyscrasias are an uncommon source of vaginal bleeding, but should be considered if there are other signs of bleeding, such as epistaxis, petechiae, or hematomas.

Follow-Up

For most patients with vaginitis, follow-up is indicated only if the condition persists or returns, in which case the patient can be instructed to see her pediatrician. The patient with suspected sexually transmitted disease or

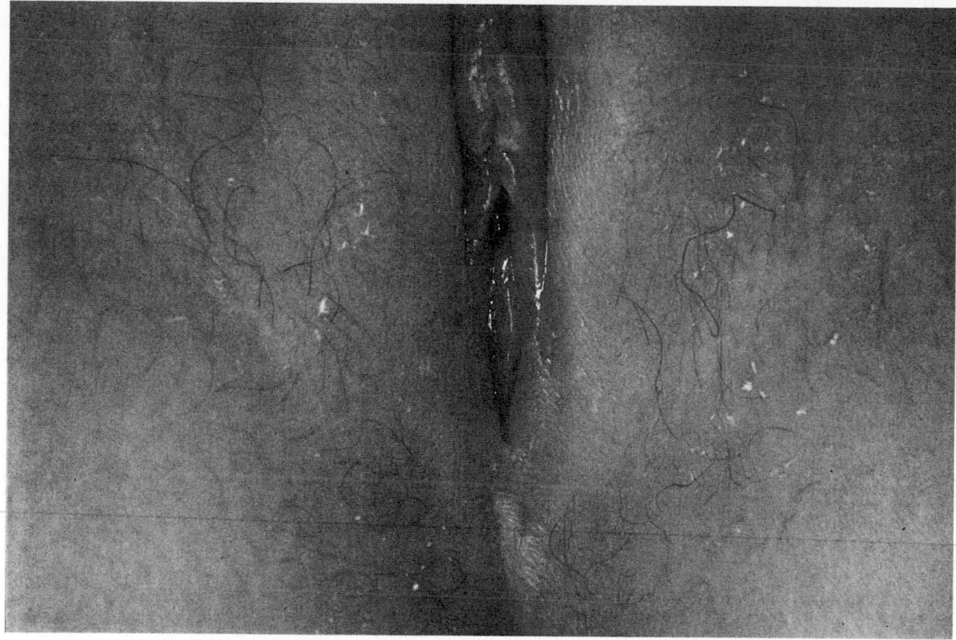

Fig. 24-4. Lichen sclerosus in an 8-year-old girl, with distribution around the labia and parchment-like skin.

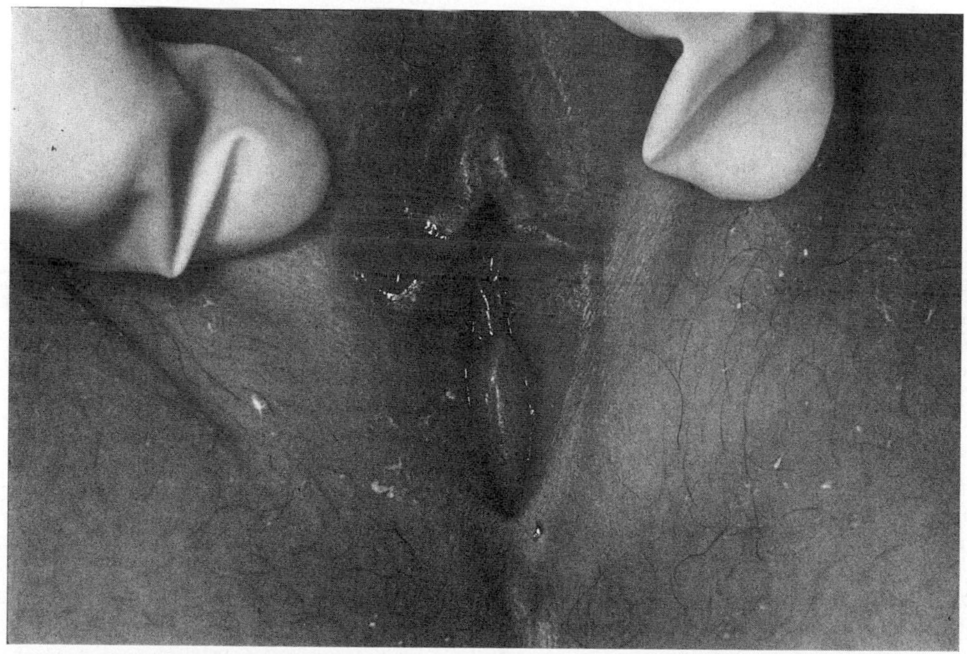

Fig. 24-5. Same patient as in Fig. 24-4. With traction, the ulcers became apparent.

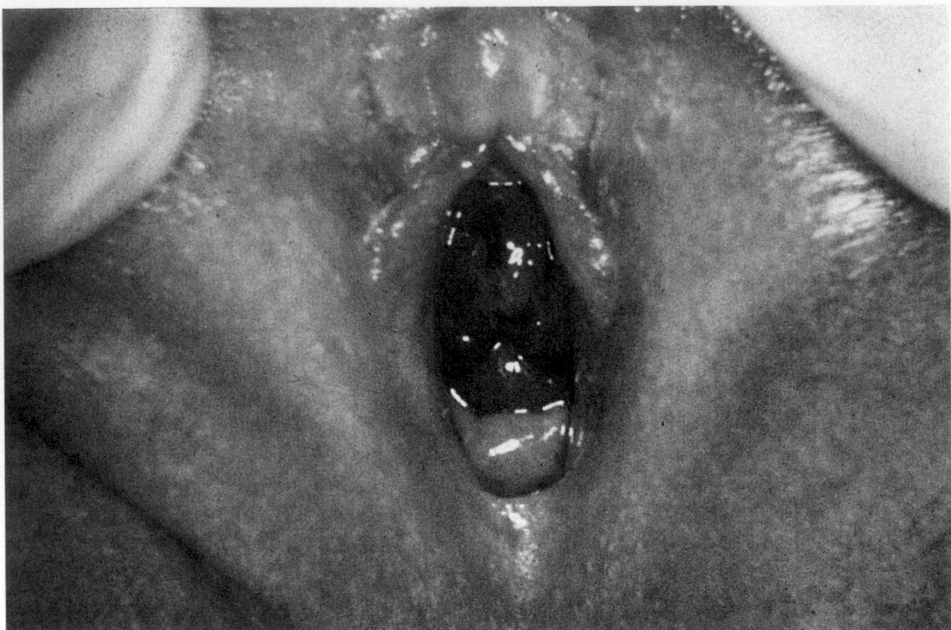

Fig. 24-6. Urethral prolapse in a prepubertal girl. A friable, red, annular mass is present around the urethra. (Photograph courtesy of M.A. Finkel, DO and the North American Society for Pediatric and Adolescent Gynecology, with permission.)

trauma due to sexual abuse will need to be reported to the local authorities—child protective services (CPS)—and follow-up of all cultures will be necessary (see Chapter 25). The patient's pediatrician will need to be involved for long-term follow-up. The patient that has experienced genital trauma needs to follow-up within 1 week with her pediatrician. Referral to a pediatrician for follow-up of chronic conditions like lichen sclerosus, labial agglutination, and urethral prolapse should be arranged in 1 to 2 weeks.

Indications for Hospitalization

Most children with vaginal discharge or bleeding will be diagnosed and treated as outpatients with follow-up as needed. If the patient is bleeding profusely and the wound or source of bleeding cannot be adequately assessed, the pediatric surgeon, gynecologist, or urologist needs to be consulted for an examination under anesthesia and possible repair. On occasion, a patient may come in with severe vulvar discomfort (e.g., severe lichen sclerosus) and cannot tolerate an examination. Depending on the patient's age, conscious sedation or an examination under anesthesia can then be performed to make a diagnosis, perform biopsies, or treat the condition.

THE ADOLESCENT

Vulvovaginitis, menstrual disorders, ovarian cyst formation, and ovarian torsion are among the most common disorders seen in female adolescents presenting to the emergency department.

Vulvovaginitis

Pathophysiology

In contrast to the nonspecific etiology of vaginitis in the prepubertal child, vaginitis and vaginal discharge in the adolescent usually have a specific etiology, most commonly related to sexual contact. Some 6 to 12 months before menarche, the physiologic vaginal secretions increase and cause a leukorrhea due to normal desquamation of epithelial cells secondary to estrogen effect. After puberty, the vaginal flora resembles that of an adult. Under normal circumstances, the pH of the vagina ranges from 3.8 to 4.5. This environment favors mainly lactobacilli.[24] Changes in pH or glycogen status affect the lactobacilli, thereby permitting other organisms to grow. Common causes for such changes include antibiotics, douches, alkaline secretions during menses, oral contraceptives, poorly controlled diabetes mellitus, and multiple sexual partners. Estrogen production during adolescence also can lead to a prominent ectropion, and these exposed columnar cervical cells are more susceptible to infection with *N. gonorrhoeae or C. trachomatis*. Thus, teenagers are at risk for vaginitis as well as sexually transmitted diseases.

Differential Diagnosis

The most common causes of vaginal discharge in a teenager are candidiasis, bacterial vaginosis, and the sexually transmitted diseases such as trichomoniasis, gonorrhea, and chlamydial infections. These infections, laboratory tests, and treatment are described in Chaps. 29 and 31. One in five cases of pelvic inflammatory disease (PID) affect sexually active adolescents.[25] The medical consequences of PID are significant for an adolescent: it is a direct cause of infertility, is associated with ectopic pregnancy, and it contributes to long-term sequelae such as chronic abdominal pain, dyspareunia, and adhesions.[26] A gynecology consult is appropriate in the adolescent, particularly in those young women whose diagnosis is uncertain, whose illness is severe, or whose symptoms are prolonged.

Follow-Up and Hospitalization

For the adolescent with gonorrhea and chlamydial infection, it is important to do a follow-up culture for a test of cure after treatment. This follow-up visit can also be used to provide education and review birth control options. Admission to the hospital has been recommended for all adolescents with PID, since compliance is often an issue and long-term sequelae of untreated or incompletely treated disease are serious, though this is controversial. Chap. 29 describes the diagnosis and management of PID in detail.

Abnormal Vaginal Bleeding

Pathophysiology

Menstrual irregularities are most commonly due to dysfunctional uterine bleeding, defined as excessive, prolonged, or unpatterned bleeding from the endometrium without an organic cause. The normal menstrual cycle usually consists of a mean interval of 28 days ($\pm$6 days) with a mean duration of 4 days ($\pm$2 to 3 days). Normal blood loss is around 30 mL per cycle with an upper limit of 80 mL. Approximately 10 to 15 percent of all gynecologic patients have dysfunctional uterine bleeding (DUB), but it is more commonly seen in adolescents. The etiology of adolescent DUB involves slow maturation of the hypothalamic-pituitary-ovarian axis. This is especially true for the first 18 months after menarche in the adolescent female, as the cycles are usually anovulatory.[27] Although menarche occurs at an average age of 12.8 years in the United States, up to 5 more years may be needed for regular ovulatory cycles to occur.[28]

Normal ovulation involves a regular cyclical production of estradiol, initiating ovarian follicular growth and endometrial proliferation, and following ovulation, causing the production of a significant increase in progesterone, which stabilizes the endometrium. Blood loss in the normal menstrual cycle is self-limited due to the action of platelets and fibrin. Without ovulation and subsequent progesterone production, a state of unopposed estrogen occurs. This leads to spontaneous superficial breakage of the thickened endometrium with random asynchronous bleeding. Eventually, increased estrogen has a negative effect on the hypothalamic-pituitary-ovarian axis, causing a decrease in follicle-stimulating hormone (FSH) and luteinizing hormone (LH) as well as estrogen. This results in a vasoconstriction and collapse of the thickened hyperplastic endometrial lining, with heavy and often prolonged bleeding.

Differential Diagnosis

Table 24-3 shows the differential diagnosis of abnormal uterine bleeding. The most common type of abnormal bleeding in teenagers is anovulatory bleeding. If a girl appears to be bleeding extremely heavily starting at the very first period and requires blood transfusions, coagulopathy (most commonly von Willebrand's disease or idiopathic thrombocytopenic purpura [ITP]) must be considered in the differential diagnosis. Nineteen percent of admissions for acute vaginal hemorrhage in this age group were the result of primary coagulation disorders.[29] Of the adolescents presenting with severe menorrhagia or hemoglobin less than 10, 25 percent were found to have a coagulation disorder; of those presenting with severe menorrhagia at the first menses, 50 percent were found to have a coagulation disorder.[29]

History

Information should be obtained regarding menstrual cycles, especially age of menarche, regularity, cycle length and duration, and heaviness of flow. Obtain information on the use of douches, tampons, and medications. The past medical history must include specific information regarding possible endocrinologic abnormalities. The subject of

Table 24-3. Differential Diagnosis of Abnormal Uterine Bleeding in the Adolescent

Pregnancy complications
Abortion
Ectopic pregnancy
Trophoblastic disease
Benign and malignant neoplasms of the genital tract
Cervical polyp
Vaginal adenosis
Vaginal carcinoma
Cervical carcinoma
Granulosa-theca cell tumors
Endometriosis
Leiomyoma
Genital tract infection
Vaginitis
Cervicitis
Vaginal foreign body
Intrauterine contraceptive device
Salpingo-oophoritis
Endocrinopathies
Polycystic ovarian disease
Hyperprolactinemia
Hypothyroidism
Hyperthyroidism
Administration of drugs or hormones
Trauma
Coagulation disorders
Idiopathic thrombocytopenic purpura
Von Willebrand disease
Thalassemia
Chronic systemic illness
Liver cirrhosis
Renal failure

sexual activity must be approached in a nonthreatening manner and confidentiality must be assured early on in the visit. It is highly preferable that the young patient be questioned about sexual activity, number of sexual partners, sexual practices, and dyspareunia without the parents present. This may be somewhat difficult in an emergency department, especially if the bleeding is heavy and the parents are very worried. However, it is of the utmost importance to obtain complete information about these sensitive matters, and therefore if possible a private interview should be made.

Physical Examination

The physical examination may be the patient's first pelvic examination and taking time to explain the procedure is essential. The initial examination includes inspection of the genitalia and noting the Tanner stage (see Chap. 23, Fig. 23-5). Any signs of inflammation, scratch effects, trauma, or discharge should be noted. After this, the labia are gently separated and the hymen and vestibule examined (the different types of hymen are described in Chap. 23). Whether or not a speculum is used depends on the size of the hymeneal opening, the use of tampons, previous sexual activity, and the amount of information that can be expected to be gained from the pelvic examination. If an adolescent is not sexually active, a moistened cotton swab can be used to obtain cultures and a specimen for wet mount. If she has used tampons in the past, it is usually possible to use a Huffman speculum (narrow but long, as opposed to a pediatric speculum, which is narrow and short) to visualize the cervix and obtain cultures. With the speculum in place it is also possible to assess the cervix and the presence and volume of active bleeding. *Chlamydia* and gonorrhea tests need to be taken from every sexually active teenager and, if possible, a Pap smear should be obtained if not performed within the last year. A rectoabdominal or vaginoabdominal bimanual exam is done to detect uterine or adnexal tenderness as well as to rule out the presence of any masses.

Laboratory Tests

The initial laboratory studies in the ED should include a CBC with platelets and a pregnancy test, regardless of the history of sexual activity. A coagulation profile is recommended if the patient is having acute hemorrhage or has a hemoglobin of less than 10 g/dL. This should include a PT, PTT, and bleeding time. If there is any evidence of an endocrinologic abnormality, a TSH, prolactin, and androgens may be considered. Screening for sexually transmitted diseases should be performed. A pelvic ultrasound can be obtained if there is a high level of suspicion for an anatomic abnormality or if it is impossible to perform a pelvic examination.

Treatment

The goals of therapy for menorrhagia once other pathology has been ruled out is to stop the bleeding, restore synchrony to the endometrium, and replenish iron stores. Most often this can be achieved with estrogen and/or progesterone therapy. The algorithm shown in Fig. 23-7 outlines the management of dysfunctional uterine bleeding in a systematic fashion.

Irregular vaginal bleeding may be controlled with oral contraceptives; usually a 35-μg ethinyl estradiol com-

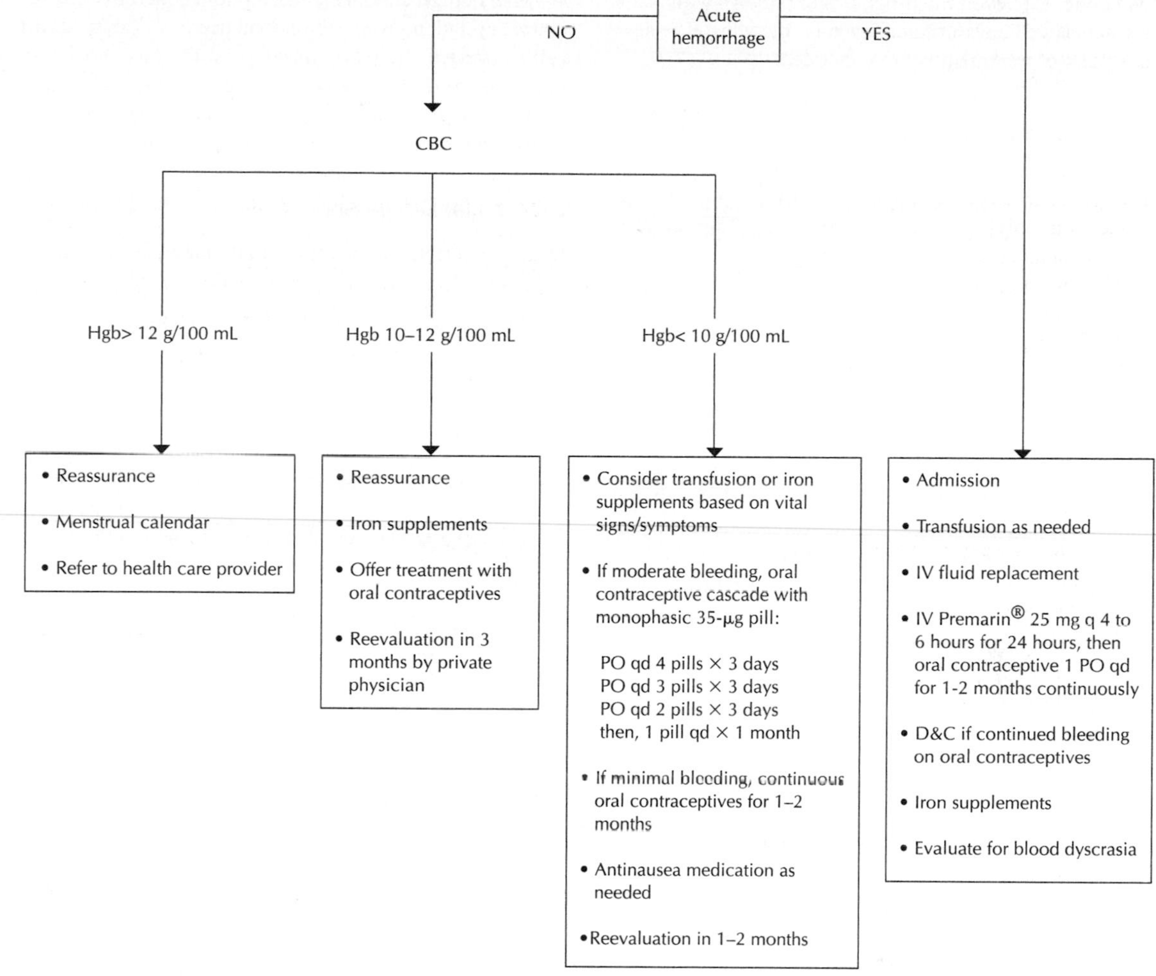

Fig. 24-7. Algorithm for the management of dysfunctional uterine bleeding in nonpregnant teenagers.

bined with a progestin preparation is adequate. If an atrophic thin uterine lining is suspected because of prolonged bleeding (several weeks, sometimes confirmed by an endometrial stripe of only several millimeters on ultrasound), the patient will require higher estrogen treatment. The estrogen can be given in the form of oral contraceptives or conjugated equine estrogen (Premarin® 2.5 mg for 7 days). An oral contraceptive taper is instituted for heavy bleeding: one pill four times a day for 3 days, then three times daily for 3 days, then twice a day for 3 days and then tapered down to one pill per day to finish off two packages of pills. An antinausea medication may be considered if high-dose estrogen is administered. Alternatively, intravenous Premarin®, 25 mg every 4 to 6 hours for 24 hours may be used if the bleeding is acute, the patient is hemodynamically unstable, and admission to the hospital is considered.

All patients with anemia also should be sent home with iron supplements. A dilatation and curettage is generally not considered in adolescents unless medical therapy is not successful.

Follow-Up

The teenager with abnormal bleeding must establish a relationship with a health care provider for long-term follow-up. This can be a gynecologist, pediatrician, internist, or adolescent specialist. The majority of patients with abnormal uterine bleeding will convert to normal menstrual cycles spontaneously within 1 to 2 years after menarche. However, the prognosis of patients with acute anemia as well as continued irregular bleeding after several years of treatment is more guarded.

Indication for Hospitalization

The adolescent patient who needs blood transfusions and intravenous estrogen will have to be admitted by the gynecology or pediatric service for treatment, close monitoring, and work-up.

Ovarian Cysts

Functional ovarian cysts are common during adolescence and include follicular as well as corpus luteum cysts. Although simple cysts are usually small (less than 5 cm) and asymptomatic, larger cysts can occur and may be complicated by torsion, rupture, or bleeding.[30] The pubertal adolescent may present with acute lower abdominal pain on the side of the involved ovary, or the pain may be described as more generalized, and have a more gradual onset.

Follicular cysts are the most common types of persistent physiologic ovarian cysts. They result either from failure of the dominant follicle to ovulate or from failure of other follicles to undergo normal atresia. Their average diameter is small (approximately 1 to 2 cm), but they may become large (6 to 8 cm). Usually follicular cysts are asymptomatic and are found incidentally on routine pelvic examination or by ultrasound performed for some other reason. If symptoms do occur, pain is usually transient, self-limited, and associated with ovulation (*mittelschmerz*). Large cysts may rupture and lead to a transient peritonitis that usually resolves in 24 hours. The patient may come in with severe abdominal pain and often appears to have an acute abdomen.[31] Ultrasonography may reveal free fluid in the pelvis, suggesting a ruptured cyst. A pelvic examination is not always indicated.

Corpus luteum cysts are less common than follicular cysts, but may be seen more frequently on an acute basis because they are larger than follicular cysts and their propensity for rupture can cause intraperitoneal hemorrhage. They result from abnormally long persistent corpora lutea.[31] Corpus luteum cysts are usually large (5 to 10 cm in diameter) and are often associated with hemorrhage into the cyst or rupture into the peritoneal cavity. Large cysts may cause acute lower abdominal pain from rupture complicated by ovarian hemorrhage and may require surgical intervention. Peritoneal signs may be present as a signal of intraperitoneal fluid or hemorrhages.[30]

Other benign tumors include teratomas, serous and mucinous cystadenomas, and endometriomas. Rarely, germ cell tumors of the ovary develop in adolescents. These malignant tumors are typically large (>5 cm) and solid or complex on ultrasound. They are usually asymptomatic unless they produce torsion or grow very rapidly.

Differential Diagnosis

Other conditions in the differential diagnosis of abdominal pain with peritoneal signs include appendicitis, ovarian torsion, PID, and ectopic pregnancy.

Follow-Up

Both parents and patient should be told that all young women of reproductive age have ovarian cysts and their presence does not necessarily indicate pathology. Since most functional cysts will resolve spontaneously over 4 to 8 weeks, the adolescent should be reexamined during a subsequent menstrual cycle by her primary care physician. Treatment with oral contraceptives can be offered if a physiologic cyst is suspected. If the mass is large or appears consistent with more serious pathology (e.g., solid on ultrasound), the patient should be urgently referred to a gynecologic or pediatric surgeon.

Consultation and Hospitalization

A gynecologic consult should be obtained for the adolescent with acute lower abdominal pain and a tender adnexal mass or evidence of peritonitis on physical examination. An ultrasound can be extremely helpful in identifying the nature of the cyst. Large masses may warrant surgery. Laparoscopy may be necessary if the diagnosis is uncertain.

Ovarian Torsion

Torsion of the uterine adnexa is a well-described surgical emergency that can involve the fallopian tube and ovary either separately or together. This disease process is described in Chap. 28 with the differential diagnosis on abdominal pain. This section discusses the issues as they pertain to children and adolescents. Although reported as occurring rarely in prepubescent girls, torsion should be a consideration in the differential diagnosis of acute abdominal pain in female children and adolescents.[32] Approximately 15 percent of adnexal torsion occurs during infancy or childhood, with the majority of cases seen in the 7- to 10-year-old group, and some of these cases do not involve a tumor or cyst.[32]

In young women the most common tumors include the benign cystic teratoma, a large functional ovarian cyst, or a germ cell neoplasm.[33] The surgical management of twisted adnexa is somewhat controversial, especially if there has been a delay in diagnosis. Laparoscopy and sometimes laparotomy are always necessary to assess the adnexa.[34] Although in the past, most women were treated by salpingo-oophorectomy because of concern that untwisting adnexa might precipitate thromboembolic events such as a pulmonary embolus,[35] a more conservative approach has now been advocated. Thromboembolic phenomena rarely occur, and most torsions do not involve a malignant neoplasm.[32] At least an initial attempt to untwist the adnexum is now used to allow preservation of the ovary and/or tube and is finding increased acceptance in all but necrotic adnexal torsions. If torsion occurs in a normal ovary and oviduct in a young patient, the physician should be aware of the possibility of its recurrence and consider fixation of the other mesosalpinx. Plication may anchor a mobile oviduct and prevent further torsion and infarction. The disadvantage of plication is that in some cases it may lead to tubal compromise, and theoretically might cause future problems with fertility.[36] In a patient with a benign neoplasm associated with ovarian torsion, cystectomy is preferred if the ovary is viable.

Indications for Admission and Specialty Consultation

The presence of a palpable abdominal mass should not delay surgical consultation and operation in the patient with symptoms consistent with adnexal torsion. The challenge remains to distinguish ovarian torsion from other more common causes of acute abdominal pain in children and adolescents, such as appendicitis. Ultrasonography may be helpful,[37] but abdominopelvic CT scanning or direct visualization remains often the only means of definitive diagnosis; therefore a gynecologist or pediatric surgeon should be notified early in the course of the work-up.

URINARY TRACT INFECTION IN PEDIATRIC AND ADOLESCENT GIRLS

Urinary tract infection is a common condition seen in children and adolescents. It is the most common serious bacterial illness among febrile infants and young children who present without an obvious source of infection.[38,39] The ongoing challenge for the clinician remains to differentiate between lower urinary tract disease (cystitis) and involvement of the upper urinary tract (pyelonephritis). Timely diagnosis and the proper management of both of these conditions will prevent morbidity and decrease the need for more expensive medical care in the future, such as dialysis or renal transplantation.[40]

Epidemiology

An estimated 40 percent of urinary tract infections are asymptomatic. The prevalence of symptomatic UTIs in pediatric patients varies with age and gender.[41] During the neonatal period, there is a male predominance, with UTIs seen primarily in uncircumcised boys. Urinary tract infections become more common in females later in infancy and childhood, with approximately 1 percent of school-aged girls developing symptomatic infections each year.[42]

The incidence of UTI increases during adolescence, when females become sexually active. Ten to 20 percent of females have at least one episode of cystitis during adolescence or young adulthood.[45]

Among febrile infants and young children, the prevalence of UTI has been reported to be between 4 and 7.5 percent.

Risk Factors

Anatomic abnormalities of the urinary tract are an important risk factor in the development of UTIs in children and adolescents. They include vesicoureteral reflux (VUR) and obstructive lesions such as obstruction of the ureterovesical or ureteropelvic junction. Posterior urethral valves also lead to obstruction, but rarely occur in females.

Nonstructural risk factors for the development of UTI in females include constipation, stool incontinence, poor hygiene, use of chemical irritants such as bubble baths, pinworms, dysfunctional voiding (infrequent or incomplete voiding), sexual abuse, sexual intercourse, and the use of diaphragms.[46]

A familial risk factor for UTI is the presence of VUR in a parent or sibling. Up to 45 percent of siblings of children with persistent VUR will have reflux themselves, compared with less than 1 percent of the general population.[47] UTI recurs in approximately 30 percent of children after an acute infection. This is especially important if the child has had three or more previous UTIs, as the risk then increases to 75 percent.[41]

Pathophysiology

A combination of both bacterial and individual host factors contributes to the development of UTIs in children and adolescents. In neonates, infections are usually blood-borne and bacteria are hematogenously spread to the kidneys. In older female children and adolescents, the usual route is by ascension of bacteria via the short urethra directly into the bladder. These bacteria are augmented by the abundance of vaginal and rectal microorganisms in the periurethral area. Any condition that leads to urinary stasis may predispose to the development of cystitis in certain hosts.[40,43]

Although viruses such as adenovirus have been known to cause hemorrhagic cystitis, bacterial enteric pathogens cause most urinary infections. By far the most common bacterial organism is *Escherichia coli,* which is responsible for 80 to 90 percent of acute UTIs in children and adolescents. Specific cell wall properties of pathogenic *E. coli* prevent it from being cleared from the bladder during voiding.[48]

Other gram-negative organisms that can cause UTIs in healthy children and adolescents are *Klebsiella, Proteus,* and *Enterobacter* species. Gram-positive cocci include enterococci and *Staphylococcus epidermidis,* which are seen primarily in adolescents. In addition, *Staphylococcus saprophyticus,* a coagulase-negative organism, has also been recognized as a common cause of UTI in sexually active adolescents and young women.[42,45]

Chronic infections or infections in patients receiving antimicrobial suppression are frequently caused by *Proteus, Pseudomonas,* or *Candida* species or enterococci.[41]

Differential Diagnosis

Several conditions may mimic UTI in females, but the differential diagnosis can be tailored depending on the age of the patient. Emergent conditions leading to an acute abdomen, such as appendicitis, ectopic pregnancy, or ovarian torsion can usually be sorted out in the adolescent by taking a careful history. Less emergent conditions like pinworm infestations may lead to local excoriation from scratching and dysuria as the urine touches the raw perineal surface during voiding.

History and Physical Examination

Symptomatic urinary tract infections are associated with a number of complaints such as low-grade fever and abdominal pain as well as nausea and vomiting. Other gastrointestinal complaints may include persistent diarrhea. The classic urinary symptoms of dysuria, increased hesitancy, frequency, or urgency, and the sudden onset of enuresis are seen only in older children and adolescents. Particularly in young children and infants, the presentation is much more subtle (Table 24-4) and it is difficult to differentiate upper from lower tract disease. In older children, however, upper tract disease is usually accompanied by more serious constitutional symptoms such as high fever, chills, costovertebral or lower abdominal tenderness, and dehydration.

A past history of UTI increases the likelihood of recurrent disease. A voiding history is important to obtain since poor habits such as infrequent or incomplete voiding or poor hygiene can predispose to UTI. Dysfunctional voiding may be manifest by urinary dribbling, daytime enuresis, or a weak urine stream at the time of micturition.[42] In all patients overall growth should be noted, since renal insufficiency can lead to poor growth. The blood pressure also should be checked for hypertension.

The physical examination should include an assessment of the patient's hydration status and general clinical appearance. Any evidence of costovertebral tenderness, lower abdominal or suprapubic pain, abdominal masses (congenital anomaly of the kidney), and edema should be noted. The external genitalia should be examined as previously described. Labial adhesions or local irritation should be documented as they may be etiologic (e.g., labial ad-

Table 24-4. Common Signs and Symptoms of Urinary Tract Infection

Neonates	Infants/Children	School-Age Children/Adolescents
Poor feeding	Fever	Abdominal pain
Lethargy	Vomiting	Enuresis
Irritability	Diarrhea	Fever and/or chills
Jaundice	Abdominal pain	Dysuria
Vomiting	Failure to thrive	Urgency
Persistent diarrhea	Foul or strong-smelling urine	Frequency
Fever or hypothermia		Hematuria
Poor weight gain		Flank pain

Source: Adapted from Todd[42] and Batisky[40]

hesions resulting in poor urinary outflow) or may provide clues about the etiology (e.g., periurethral excoriations associated with pinworms).

Laboratory Data

Controversy exists regarding whether an acute infection can be readily diagnosed or excluded by urine dipstick or microscopic analysis alone.

Urine Dipstick

It is well established that a positive dipstick for nitrites, leukocyte esterase, or blood may be indicative of UTI. The leukocyte esterase test detects esterase released from leukocytes, an indirect test for the presence of white blood cells.[50] The nitrite test is more specific and is positive when nitrate is converted to nitrite in the bladder by certain bacteria. Since most gram-negative organisms are capable of reducing nitrates to nitrites, the dipstick will be positive in most UTIs. Most gram-positive organisms, however, are not capable of reducing nitrates and nitrites will not be detected.[50]

In children below the age of 2 years, the false-negative rate is too high to use the urine dipstick as a primary screen for deciding when to get a culture or when to make a diagnosis of UTI without a culture.[38,51] The differences between adult women and young children and the usefulness of the dipstick may be related to the degree of pyuria in the two age groups, the enzyme content of immature leukocytes, or both.[39] In addition, bacteria must be present in the bladder for a period sufficient to reduce nitrates to nitrites. The low sensitivity of dipstick nitrite testing in young children may be the result of random urine sampling usually obtained by catheter rather than the first-morning voids frequently recommended for adult women.[39]

Microscopic urinalysis is important for the detection of significant numbers of WBCs, RBCs, casts, and bacteria. The presence of pyuria or hematuria is more indirect evidence of UTI and is neither sensitive nor specific.[42] More than 100 bacteria per high-powered field corresponds to $>10^5$ colony-forming units per milliliter on culture. This demonstration of bacteria microscopically is the most reliable and fastest means of establishing the diagnosis of UTI before the urine culture is available.[41]

Urine Culture

In the young, non-toilet-trained female, urethral catheterization is often necessary to make an accurate diagnosis. In toilet-trained school-age and adolescent females, carefully collected midstream urine specimens are acceptable.

As in adults, a positive urine culture is the gold standard for making a diagnosis of UTI in female children and adolescents. Any growth from a suprapubic tap aspiration is evidence of an infection; $\geq 10^4$ colonies from an "in-and-out" catheterization should be considered positive; and $\geq 10^5$ colonies from a midstream clean-catch urine specimen is diagnostic of UTI. The presence of multiple organisms or skin flora usually indicates contamination of the urine specimen except in adolescent females, in whom *S. saprophyticus* and *S. epidermidis* can cause symptomatic UTIs. In addition, some patients with structural urologic abnormalities may in fact have polymicrobial infections. Culture sensitivities are important to assure appropriate antibiotic coverage and should be obtained on all urine specimens.

Blood Tests

Routine blood tests such as a serum blood urea nitrogen (BUN) and creatinine are not necessary in an uncomplicated first episode of UTI. If the patient is being hospitalized, however, or if there is a previous history of urinary infections, these studies may be obtained to evaluate renal function. In addition, a complete blood count (CBC) and blood culture should be obtained if the child is febrile ($\geq$39.5°C, $\geq$103.1°F) or requires hospitalization.

Procedures

Suprapubic Bladder Aspiration

A suprapubic bladder aspiration may be performed in children less than 2 years of age.

Bladder Catheterization

Bladder catheterization in the infant or younger child should be attempted atraumatically with the child in the parent's lap or on the examination table. It is imperative to indicate on the laboratory slip that it is a catheterized specimen. This procedure is not usually associated with an increased risk of nosocomial infection.

Radiographic Studies

Emergent radiographic studies are not necessary to make a diagnosis of UTI or to treat it adequately. Studies such as ultrasounds, cystoureterograms, and nuclear renal cortical scans are useful during the subsequent radiographic workup of the child with UTI, but are rarely helpful in the acute

Table 24-5. Outpatient Treatment of Urinary Tract Infection

Antibiotic	Dose/Interval
Preadolescents	
Trimethoprim-sulfamethoxazole	8-10 mg/kg (based on TMP) PO BID for 10 days
Cefixime	8 mg/kg PO once-twice daily for 10 days
Cephalexin	20-50 mg/kg PO QID for 10 days
Nitrofurantoin	5-7 mg/kg PO QID for 10 days
Sulfisoxazole	120-150 mg/kg PO q 4-6 hours for 10 days
Adolescents	
Ciprofloxacin	250 mg BID for 3-7 days
Ofloxacin	200 mg BID for 3-7 days

presentation. Functional and structural abnormalities of the urinary tract are often diagnosed at that time.[40,43]

Treatment

Acute Infections

The outpatient management of uncomplicated UTI is the use of a single broad-spectrum oral agent. This agent should adequately cover what is likely to be the causative organism. If the infection is recurrent, the antibiotic coverage should take into account sensitivity studies on the organism that caused infection in the past. Antibiotic duration for young and school-age children is 10 days. Since it is often difficult to localize the infection in this age group and short-course therapy has been associated with treatment failures in prepubertal girls with acute cystitis, single-dose or short-course therapy is currently not recommended.[52]

Single-dose oral therapy may be used in the adolescent female with an uncomplicated UTI. It consists of either amoxicillin 3 g or trimethoprim-sulfamethoxazole (TMP-SMX) 320 mg/1600 mg (two double-strength tablets). A 3-day oral regimen with TMP-SMX or nitrofurantoin has also been suggested. The advantages of single-dose treatment include increased compliance with medication and follow-up, decreased cost and side effects, as well as a more rapid resolution of symptoms. Side effects such as vaginitis will almost certainly contribute to poor compliance in the adolescent population. Development of resistance to TMP-SMX has diminished the usefulness of this drug in many practice settings. Alternative agents include cephalosporin (e.g., cephalexin 20 to 50 mg/kg daily, divided into four doses for 3 days), or in adolescents, ciprofloxacin 250 mg twice a day for 5 days or ofloxacin 200 mg twice a day for 3 days.

The preferred drug for conventional oral administration is TMP-SMX because of its excellent absorption and tissue penetration. In addition, most urinary pathogens causing uncomplicated UTIs are highly susceptible to TMP-SMX.[41] Other oral antibiotics that can be used are sulfisoxazole, nitrofurantoin, cephalexin, and cefixime (Table 24-5). In most communities, amoxicillin is no longer used because of strains of *E. coli* that are resistant. Initial treatment with one dose of intramuscular ceftriaxone or gentamicin has also been proposed by some authors. This is followed by the initiation of an oral agent within the next 12 to 18 hours.[49]

Symptomatic treatments are important for patient comfort and compliance. Phenazopyridine hydrochloride may be used for 2 days in older children and adolescents as a urinary analgesic. The dose is 12 mg/kg/d over 24 hours divided tid for children 6 to 12 years of age and 200 mg tid for adolescent women. Patients should be warned about the change in urine color that accompanies use of this agent. It should not be used for longer than 48 hours because of the risk of methemoglobinemia, hemolytic anemia, and other toxic reactions.[49] Although there are conflicting reports on the mechanism by which cranberry juice produces a bacteriostatic effect, drinking large amounts of it has been shown to be beneficial in the reduction of bacteriuria.[53] Antipyretics (acetaminophen or ibuprofen) can be used to control fever, which may persist for the first 24 to 48 hours after beginning antimicrobial therapy. Finally, sitz-baths in warm water for 20 to 30 minutes three to four times a day may offer relief of dysuria.[49]

Recurrent Infections

Treatment for recurrent infections or in children at risk for recurrent infections should include consideration of the organisms responsible for previous infections as well as the antibiotics to which the child has recently been exposed.

Radiographic Follow-Up

Should all UTIs be evaluated radiographically? Guidelines for pursuing radiographic studies in patients with UTI have been developed and include: (1) the first febrile UTI in girls younger than 3 to 5 years; (2) older girls of any age with recurrent UTIs; and (3) the child with suspected pyelonephritis.[40,41,54,55] Girls older than 10 should have at least a second UTI before any studies are initiated. In most cases, sexually active adolescents do not warrant a radiologic work-up. An exception is if the adolescent has two to three episodes of cystitis in a 12- to 18-month period.[49]

Indications for Admission and Specialty Consultation

In considering the possibility of inpatient treatment, several factors must be taken into account: (1) the patient's clinical appearance; (2) the age of the patient (the risk of permanent renal damage as a consequence of infection is inversely related to the child's age); and (3) compliance and the reliability of follow up.[48] Parenteral antibiotics may be required in infants less than 2 to 3 months of age; suspected pyelonephritis at any age (complicated UTI); patients who are moderately or severely dehydrated, appear toxic, or are in shock; in patients with a history of recurrent infection or known renal disease; and in those with an infection involving an organism that is resistant to oral antibiotics. Hospitalization should also be considered when there is no improvement on oral therapy or symptoms are worsening.

Hospitalized patients should initially be treated with two antibiotics that provide broad-spectrum coverage for both gram-negative and gram-positive organisms, such as ampicillin and gentamicin. A third-generation cephalosporin, such as cefotaxime or ceftriaxone, may also be used. Specialty consultation should be considered for patients with evidence of urinary tract obstruction, renal scarring, significant voiding problems, or anatomic abnormalities. In addition, children at any age with a solitary, small, or atrophic kidney or who have hypertension should be referred to the specialist for consultation.

Follow-Up

All pediatric patients should follow-up with their primary care provider within 48 to 72 hours after the initiation of antibiotic treatment. This is especially important for the patient with recurrent infection. Adolescent patients should see the pediatrician in 2 to 3 weeks.

REFERENCES

1. Paradik JE, Campa JM, Friedman HM, Grishmuth G: Vulvovaginitis in premenarchal girls: Clinical features and diagnostic evaluation. *Pediatrics* 70:193, 1982.
2. Hammerschlag MR, Albert S, Rosner I, et al: Microbiology of vagina in children: Normal and potentially pathogenic organisms. *Pediatrics* 68:57, 1978.
3. Whittington WL, Rice RJ, Biddle JW, et al: Incorrect identification of *Neisseria gonorrhoeae* from infants and children. *Pediatr Infect Dis* 7:3, 1988.
4. Alexander ER: Misidentification of sexually transmitted organisms in children: Medicolegal implications. *Pediatr Infect Dis* 7:1, 1988.
5. Ingram DL, White ST, Occhiuti AC, et al: Childhood vaginal infections: Association of *Chlamydia trachomatis* with sexual contact. *Pediatr Infect Dis* 5:226, 1986.
6. Fuster CD, Neinstein LS: Vaginal *Chlamydia trachomatis* prevalence in sexually abused prepubertal girls. *Pediatrics* 79:235, 1987.
7. Bell TA, Stamm WE, Kuo CC, et al: Delayed appearance of *Chlamydia trachomatis* infection acquired at birth. *Pediatr Infect Dis J* 6:928, 1987.
8. Nerurkar LS, West F, May M, et al: Survival of herpes simplex virus in water specimens collected from hot tubs in spa facilities and on plastic surfaces. *JAMA* 250:3081, 1983.
9. Gushurst CA: The problem of genital herpes in prepubertal children. *Am J Dis Child* 139:542, 1985.
10. Hibbard RA: Herpetic vulvovaginitis and child abuse. *Am J Dis Child* 139:542, 1985.
11. Jones JG, Yamauchi T, Lambert B: *Trichomonas vaginalis* infestation in sexually abused girls. *Am J Dis Child* 139:846, 1985.
12. Al-Salihi FL, Curran JP, Wang J: Neonatal *Trichomonas vaginalis*: Report of three cases and review of the literature. *Pediatrics* 53:196, 1974.
13. Ross JD, Scott GR, Busuttil A: *Trichomonas vaginalis* infection in prepubertal girls. *Med Sci Law* 33:82, 1993.
14. Hammerschlag MR, Cummings M, Doraiswamy B, et al: Nonspecific vaginitis following sexual abuse in children. *Pediatrics* 75:1028, 1985.
15. Berensen AB, Hegar AH, Hayes TM et al: Appearance of the hymen in prepubertal girls. *Pediatrics* 89:387, 1993.
16. Merritt D: Evaluating and managing genital trauma in premenarchal girls. T. *Pediatr Adolesc* 12:237, 1999.
17. Armstrong DK, Handley JM: Anogenital warts in prepubertal children: pathogen, HPV typing and management. *Int J STD AIDS* 8:78, 1997.
18. Gutman LT, Herman-Giddens ME, Phelps WC: Transmission of human genital papillomavirus disease: Comparison of data from adults and children. *Pediatrics* 91:31, 1993.

19. Gale C, Muram D: The surgical treatment of condyloma acuminata in children. *Adolesc Pediatr Gynecol* 3:189, 1990.
20. Berth-Jones J, Graham-Brown RAC, Burns DA: Lichen sclerosus et atrophicus—A review of 15 cases in young girls. *Clin Exp Dermatol* 16:14, 1991.
21. Smith YR, Quint EH: Clobetasol propionate in the treatment of premenarchal vulvar lichen sclerosus. *Obstet Gynecol* 98:588, 2001.
22. Anveden-Hertzberg L, Gauderer MW, Elder JS: Urethral prolapse: an often misdiagnosed cause of urogenital bleeding in girls. *Pediatr Emergency Care* 11:212, 1995.
23. Martelli H, Oberlin O, Rey A, et al: Conservative treatment for girls with non-metastatic rhabdomyosarcoma of the genital tract: A report from the study committee of the international society of pediatric oncology. *J Clin Oncol* 17:2117, 1999.
24. Fredrich EG: Vaginitis. *Am J Obstet Gynecol* 152:247, 1985.
25. Igra V: Pelvic inflammatory disease in adolescents. *AIDS Patient Care and STDs* 12:109, 1998.
26. Rome ES: Sexually transmitted diseases: Testing and Treating. *Adolesc Med* 10:231, 1999.
27. Venturoli S, Porcu E, Fabbri R, et al: Menstrual irregularities in adolescents: Hormonal patterns and ovarian morphology. *Horm Res* 24:269, 1986.
28. Minjarez DA, Bradshaw KD: Abnormal bleeding in adolescents. *Obstet Gynecol Clin North Am* 27:63, 2000.
29. Claessens EA, Cowell CA: Acute adolescent menorrhagia. *Am J Obstet Gynecol* 139:277, 1981.
30. Ludwig S, Selbst SM, Lavelle J: Adolescent emergency conditions, in McAnarney ER, Kreipe RE, Orr D. et al: (eds): *Textbook of Adolescent Medicine.* Philadelphia: Saunders, 1992, pp 932–954.
31. Horowitz IR, Sainz de la Cuesta R: Benign and malignant tumors of the ovary, in Carpenter SEK, Rock JA (eds): *Pediatric and Adolescent Gynecology.* New York: Raven Press, 1992, pp 397–416.
32. Templeman C, Fallat ME, Blinchevsky A, Hertweck SP: Noninflammatory ovarian masses in girls and young women. *Obstet Gynecol* 96:229, 2000.
33. Cass DL, Hawkins E, Brandt ML, Chintagumpala M, et al: Surgery for ovarian masses in infants, children, and adolescents: 102 consecutive patients treated in a 15-year period. *J Pediatr Surg* 36:593, 2001.
34. Cohen Z, Shidhar D, Kopernik G, et al: The laparoscopic approach to uterine adnexal torsion in childhood. J *Pediatr Surg* 13:1557, 1996.
35. Zweizig J: Conservative management of adnexal torsion. *Am J Obstet Gynecol* 168:1791, 1993.
36. Wakamatsu M, Wolf P, Benirschke K: Bilateral torsion of the normal ovary and oviduct in a young girl. *J Fam Pract* 28:101, 1989.
37. Stark JE, Siegel MJ: Ovarian torsion in prepubertal and pubertal girls: monographic findings. *Amer J Roentgenol* 163:1479–1482, 1994.
38. Hoberman A, Chao HP, Keller DM, et al: Prevalence of urinary tract infections in febrile infants. *J Pediatr* 123:17, 1993.
39. Hoberman A, Wald ER, Reynolds EA, et al: Pyuria and bacteriuria in urine specimens obtained by catheter from young children with fever. *J Pediatr* 124:513, 1994.
40. Batisky D: Pediatric urinary tract infections. *Pediatr Ann* 25:266, 1996.
41. McCracken GH: Diagnosis and management of acute urinary tract infections in infants and children. *Pediatr Infect Dis J* 6:107, 1987.
42. Todd JK: Management of urinary tract infections: Children are different. *Pediatr Rev* 16:190, 1995.
43. Lerner GR: Urinary tract infections in children. *Pediatr Ann* 23:463, 1994.
44. D'Angelo LJ, Neinstein LS: Genitourinary tract infections, in Neinstein LS (ed): *Adolescent Health Care.* Baltimore: Williams & Wilkins, 2002, pp 551–559.
45. Hooton TM, Scholes D, Hughes JP, et al: A prospective study of risk factors for symptomatic urinary tract infection in young women. *N Engl J Med* 335:468, 1996.
46. Van den Abbeele AD, Treves ST, Lebowitz RL, et al: Vesicoureteral reflux in asymptomatic siblings of patients with known reflux: Radionuclide cystography. *Pediatrics* 79:147, 1987.
47. Shapiro ED: Infections of the urinary tract. *Pediatr Infect Dis J* 11:165, 1992.
48. Hellerstein S: Urinary tract infections. *Pediatr Clin North Am* 42:1433, 1995.
49. Lohr JA: Use of routine urinalysis in making a presumptive diagnosis of urinary tract infection in children. *Pediatr Infect Dis J* 10:646, 1991.
50. Shaw KN, Hexter D, McGowan KL, et al: Clinical evaluation of a rapid screening test for urinary infections in children. *J Pediatr* 118:733, 1991.
51. Keren R, Chan E: A meta-analysis of randomized, controlled trials comparing short- and long-course antibiotic therapy for urinary tract infections in children. *Pediatrics* 109:E70, 2002.
52. Avorn J, Monane M, Gurwitz JH, et al: Reduction of bacteriuria and pyuria after ingestion of cranberry juice. *JAMA* 271:751, 1994.
53. Hellerstein S: Evolving concepts in the evaluation of the child with a urinary tract infection. *J Pediatr* 124:589, 1994.
54. Altemeier WA: A backward look at urinary tract infections. *Pediatr Ann* 24:255, 1996.

25

Sexual Abuse and Assault In the Pediatric Patient

Rona Molodow
Daphne Wong

KEY POINTS

- First and foremost, the emotional and physical well-being of a child who has been the victim of abuse or assault must take precedence, and if possible the assessment should be delayed if a team is not familiar with the pediatric gynecologic examination and no acute injuries are suspected.
- The practitioner may face civil or criminal liability for failure to report suspected abuse. Most states protect the provider against false reporting suits as long as the report is made in good faith.
- When evidence is collected, it is important that the examiner follow the protocol of the appropriate jurisdiction, with close attention to maintaining the chain of evidence.
- Fastidious documentation, including photographs, preserves a record for future legal action while minimizing the child's exposure to repeated questions and examinations.

"There's a pediatric sexual abuse case in triage."

Few pronouncements can produce such trepidation in the emergency department, portending a time consuming, emotionally charged encounter with which few providers are comfortable. Rarely do psychosocial, medical, and legal concerns so blatantly intersect in the ED.

The pediatric victim of alleged sexual abuse can present to the emergency department in a variety of ways. Sometimes the child comes to the ED following an acute assault. Sometimes the abuse is ongoing or even temporally distant. On other occasions, it is ED personnel who suspect abuse based on a child's complaints, physical examination, or behavior. The examiner's approach, including reporting, extent of examination, and collection of evidence, will vary with the presentation and age of the victim. The evaluation of the adolescent victim generally mimics that of the adult (see Chap. 33). This chapter focuses on the emergency department assessment of the prepubertal child.

DEFINITIONS

According to a 1996 survey, sexual abuse accounts for 9 percent of substantiated cases of child maltreatment in the United States.[1] Exact prevalence rates are difficult to assign, but estimates range from 12 to 25 percent for girls and 8 to 10 percent for boys.[2] Sexual abuse encompasses a broad spectrum of activities and occurs when a child under the age of 18 is engaged in sexual acts that he or she cannot understand or that violate the laws and mores of a society. Sexual abuse may include oral-genital, genital, and anal contact, as well as activities in which no physical contact occurs, such as exhibitionism or exposure of a child to pornography.[3] The precise definition of abuse varies with jurisdiction and the practitioner should thus be familiar with the laws of his or her state or locale. Abuse may or may not involve overt physical or psychological coercion. The perpetrator knows the victim in 70 to 90 percent of pediatric cases and half involve a relative.[4]

Health care personnel are "mandated reporters" under the laws of every state and as such are required to report a "reasonable suspicion" of child abuse encountered within the scope of their employment. "Reasonable suspicion" is, of course, an inexact term but is generally interpreted to arise when a "reasonable person" under similar circumstances could suspect abuse. *The practitioner may face civil or criminal liability for failure to report suspected abuse.* At the same time, most states protect the provider against false reporting suits as long as the report is made in good faith.

EMERGENCY DEPARTMENT EVALUATION

History

Assessment of the suspected victim of abuse demands sensitivity by all personnel involved. If possible an interdisciplinary team, including a health care provider, nurse, and social worker, should be available in the ED. The first priority of the staff must be the well-being of the child with attention to both medical and emotional needs.

In situations in which the child is brought to the emergency department specifically for evaluation of alleged abuse, it is best to leave investigative interviews to the appropriate agency in order to minimize repetitive questioning. Nonetheless, the practitioner must obtain sufficient history to guide the examination and provide a general picture of the child's health. When possible, it is best to take a separate history from the parents or guardians and the child. Most experts do not question children under the age of 3 years.

The question of when to suspect abuse when it is not an overt complaint is one of the most difficult that the pediatric practitioner can face. A wide variety of complaints, such as vaginal discharge, anogenital bleeding, encopresis, sleep disorders, and sexualized behavior should raise the possibility of sexual abuse, but it is important to realize that such signs and symptoms are common in the absence of molestation.[5] Accordingly, while such features should prompt an inquiry regarding abuse, they should rarely be used alone to support a report of suspected abuse.

When a history is obtained in the ED, the practitioner should follow the general rules for interviewing any patient. Language should be appropriate for the child's developmental status and leading questions avoided. Questions should be open-ended, beginning with general inquiries and moving to the more specific. For example, appropriate questions might include: "Do you know why you are here today?" "Can you tell me what happened?" "And then what happened?" Responses should be recorded in the patient's own words. The use of props such as anatomically correct dolls is best left to professionals trained in interviewing young children.

Physical Examination

The physical examination of the suspected victim of abuse consists of evidence collection, visual inspection, and assessment for sexually transmitted diseases.

Evidence Collection

The American Academy of Pediatrics (AAP) suggests immediate examination and collection of forensic evidence if abuse is alleged to have occurred within 72 hours, or if there is bleeding or acute injury.[6] If no acute injuries are present or if more than 72 hours have elapsed, the AAP states that an emergency evaluation is not necessary. Instead, assessment by a team trained in such investigations should be scheduled as soon as possible. These recommendations conform to protocols developed for adult rape victims and are based, at least in part, on the amount of time sperm can be expected to be recoverable from the mature vagina.[7]

While there is no doubt that such protocols are applicable to the adolescent victim, the utility of such potentially embarrassing and invasive procedures in the prepubertal child has been hotly debated. In 2000, Christian and colleagues performed a retrospective review of the results of forensic examinations of 273 children under 10 years old seen in three emergency departments in Philadelphia. Forensic evidence was recovered in 25 percent of patients, all of whom were seen within 44 hours of the alleged assault, with 90 percent examined within 24 hours. After 24 hours, all useful evidence had been found on clothing or linens, not the child's body, with the exception of a single pubic hair. Based on these findings, Christian and her coworkers propose modifying the "72 hour rule" for prepubertal children, suggesting that swabbing the body be omitted for children evaluated more than 24 hours after the alleged event. Collection of clothing and linens should be emphasized.[8] Recent evidence has shown little value to use of a Wood's lamp on a victim's body to identify seminal fluid versus products commonly found in the pediatric perineum, such as ointments or emollients.[9] Accordingly, if utilized at all, the Wood's lamp should only be used to locate suspicious areas or specimens for more definitive testing.

When evidence is collected, it is important that the examiner follow the protocol of the appropriate jurisdiction, with close attention to maintaining the chain of evidence. Thus, the practitioner must be familiar with the evidentiary forms provided by local law enforcement agencies.

Visual Inspection

Despite Christian and colleagues' admonitions regarding collection of forensic evidence, this does not imply that a physical examination should not occur as quickly as possible following an alleged incident. Physical findings may provide important corroborative evidence of a child's story and genital injuries heal notoriously rapidly.[10,11] Thus a prompt assessment may be crucial. At the same time, it is essential to realize that physical findings are rare even in cases of penetration. At a minimum, the genital examination is normal in more than two-thirds of victims of abuse.[12] In the study by Christian and associates, for example, only 24 percent of children had physical findings.[8] Accordingly, a lack of abnormalities should not be used to refute allegations of abuse. As one author eloquently concluded, "Its normal to be normal."[12]

If the child is old enough to understand, the practitioner should describe the examination before beginning and throughout the assessment. A chaperone may be helpful in easing anxiety. In the rare situation in which a child

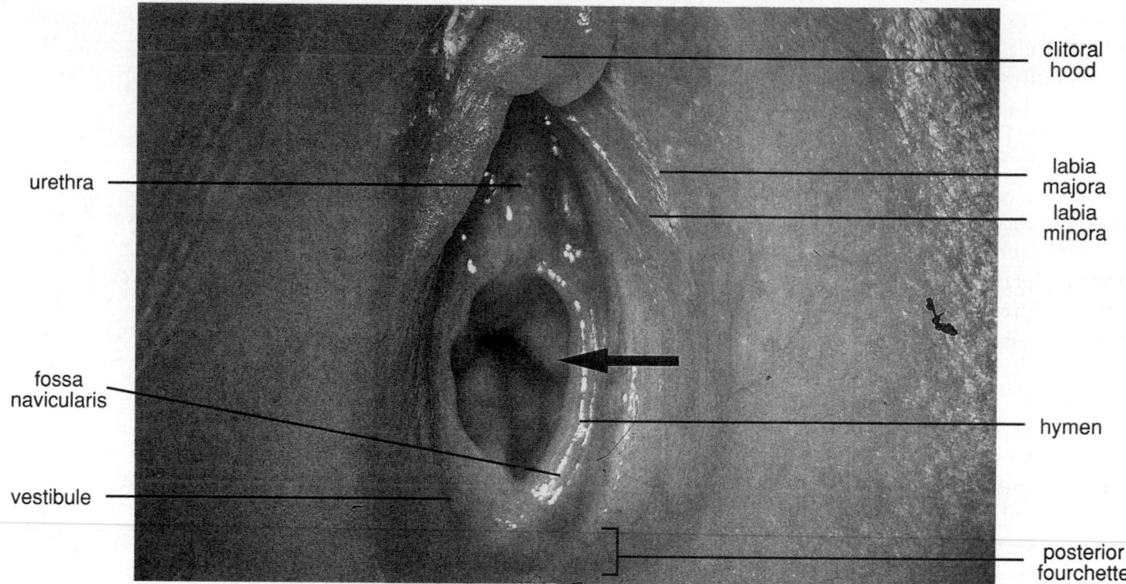

Fig. 25-1. Normal anatomy of the female genital area. Arrow points to vaginal oriface.

is unable to cooperate and an immediate examination is needed because of a high likelihood of injury, infection, or forensic evidence, the practitioner may consider the use of sedation. Physical force should not be used to restrain a reluctant or frightened child. Sometimes an examination must be delayed until the child is more comfortable with the procedure.

Most authorities recommend starting with a brief general pediatric examination, focusing on overall health, development, and emotional status before moving to the sexual abuse assessment. An adequate anogenital examination requires magnification and illumination. A colposcope is the best way to visualize the area, but in the absence of such equipment, an otoscope can be employed.

The evaluation should, of course, be based on the alleged events. In females, the examination includes inspection of the medial thighs, the labia major and minora, clitoris, urethra, periurethral tissues, hymen and hymenal opening, fossa navicularis, and posterior fourchette (Fig. 25-1). The child may be examined in the supine frog-leg and/or prone knee-chest position (see Figs. 23-2A-D) with some examiners routinely recommending both positions. If a child is reluctant, it is sometimes helpful to allow the child to lean back on a parent or chaperone's lap. Labial separation and traction are valuable in optimizing visualization of the genital area.

In viewing the hymen, imagine it as a clock face with the urethra at 12 o'clock. Focus on the area below 3 o'clock to 9 o'clock (the lower half), where trauma from sexual abuse is most often seen.[12] It may be necessary to squirt a small amount of water or saline in the area or use a moistened cotton swab to better define the edges. Because this is a well-innervated area, it may be helpful to apply lidocaine to the swab. Another method for examining the hymen is insertion of a Foley catheter, which is inflated after insertion in the vagina, and the balloon is then pulled outward to the hymenal border. A speculum exam is rarely, if ever, indicated in the prepubertal patient. In males, the medial thighs, penis, and scrotum must be examined. In both sexes, the anal area should be visualized in the supine, knee-chest, or lateral recumbent position.

Again, it must be emphasized that most examinations will be normal, even in the face of genital penetration. The central question, of course, is "What is abnormal?" It is critical that the examiner be familiar with the broad spectrum of "normal" before attempting to label any findings as suspicious. Research over the last several years has elucidated the great array of normal variants in hymenal shape and size of opening (see Fig. 23-3).[13–16] The definition of abnormal has evolved significantly, with findings previously identified as evidence of sexual abuse now recognized as normal variants (Figure 25-2A-C). Venous engorgement of the perianal area is also a normal variant. The size of the hymenal opening, once used as a marker for penetration, has since been found to vary widely among both abused and nonabused children and

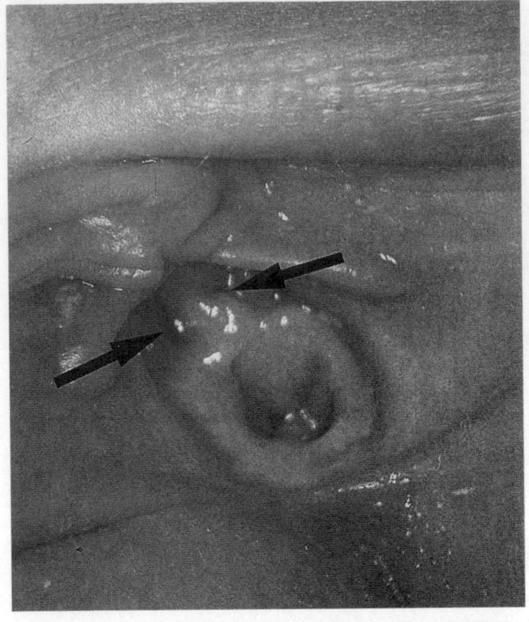

A

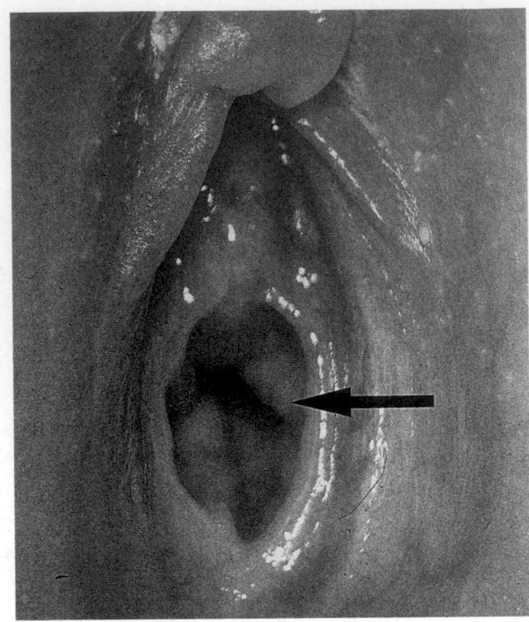

C

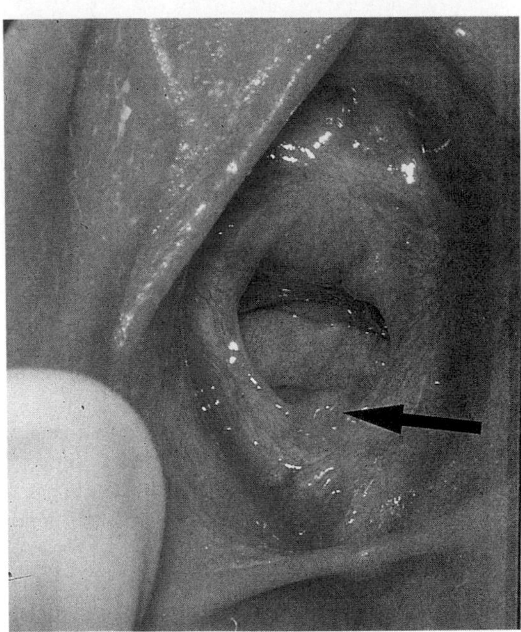

B

Fig. 25-2. Normal perineal variants: A. Periurethral bands (*arrows*), B. Hymenal notch at 6 o'clock (*arrow*), C. Intravaginal ridge (*arrow*).

is thus of limited utility.[17] Medical conditions have often been misinterpreted as signs of abuse. For example, the erythema associated with perianal and vaginal streptococcal infections has been misidentified as evidence of trauma. Lichen sclerosus et atrophicus is a dermatologic condition affecting the perineal skin marked by hypopigmentation and superficial ulceration. Urethral prolapse is also commonly mistaken as evidence of abuse.

Some physical findings are best thought of as nonspecific, because they are present in cases of abuse, but are also widely seen in nonabused children (Table 25-1). In 1999, the AAP published guidelines classifying findings as "concerning for abuse but in isolation not diagnostic," "more concerning for abuse," and "diagnostic for abuse with medical certainty" (Table 25-2).[6] At the same time, it is important to realize that even experienced examiners may disagree about the existence of such findings in a particular case.[12]

Besides a complete anogenital examination, it is important to look for injuries to other parts of the body such as the breasts or oropharynx. Any evidence of trauma or other abnormality in the genital area or elsewhere should be carefully documented with diagrams and/or photographs. In cases in which the ED examiner is unsure of the significance of findings, photographs and careful documentation can be invaluable for later review by experts and to limit the need for repeated examinations.

Table 25-1. Nonspecific Genital Findings

Nonspecific findings

(Findings which may be the result of sexual abuse but which may also be normal variants)

- Erythema of the vestibule or perianal tissues
- Increased vascularity of the vestibule
- Labial adhesions (Fig. 25-3)
- Vaginal discharge
- Friability of the posterior fourchette
- Thickened hymen
- Anal fissures (Fig. 25-4)
- Apparent genital warts
- Flattened anal folds
- Vaginal bleeding

Evaluation for Sexually Transmitted Diseases

The prevalence of sexually transmitted diseases (STDs) in children who have been sexually abused ranges from 2 to 7 percent in girls and 0 to 5 percent in boys.[18,19] These relatively low rates have led to recommendations by the AAP and Centers for Disease Control (CDC) to test only children with clear risk factors for acquiring STDs.[20,21] These include a history of genital penetration or signs and symptoms consistent with a STD (Table 25-3).

Multiple studies have validated the utility of such algorithms in determining who should undergo testing. In 1995, for example, Siegel and associates[22] looked at 855 victims of abuse (704 girls and 151 boys) between the ages

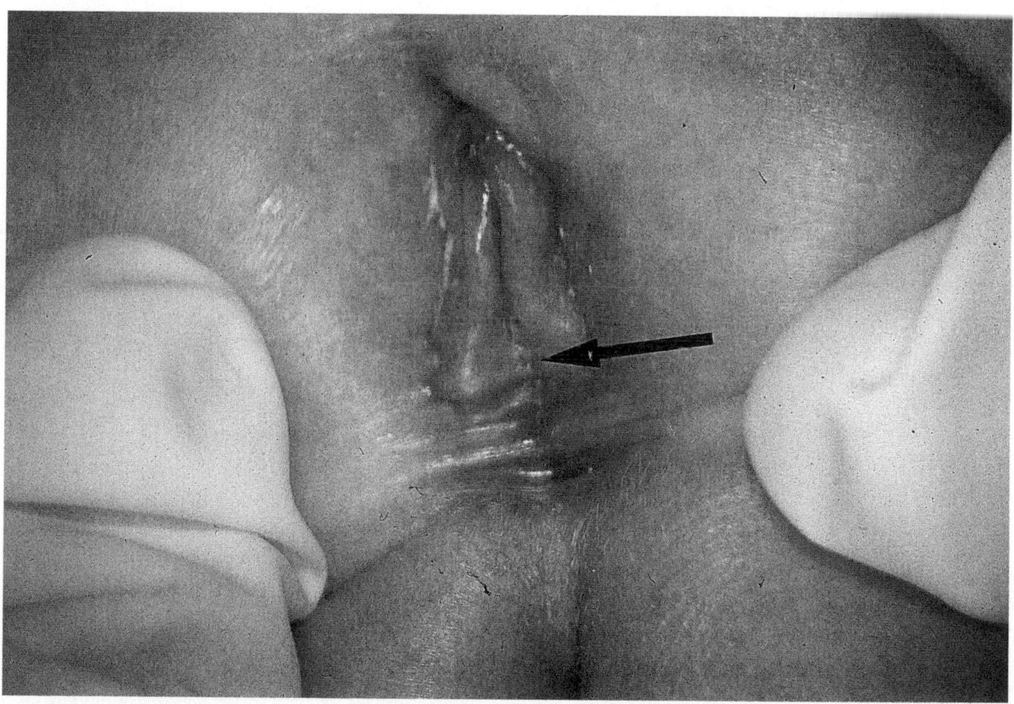

Fig. 25-3. Labial adhesion (*arrow*).

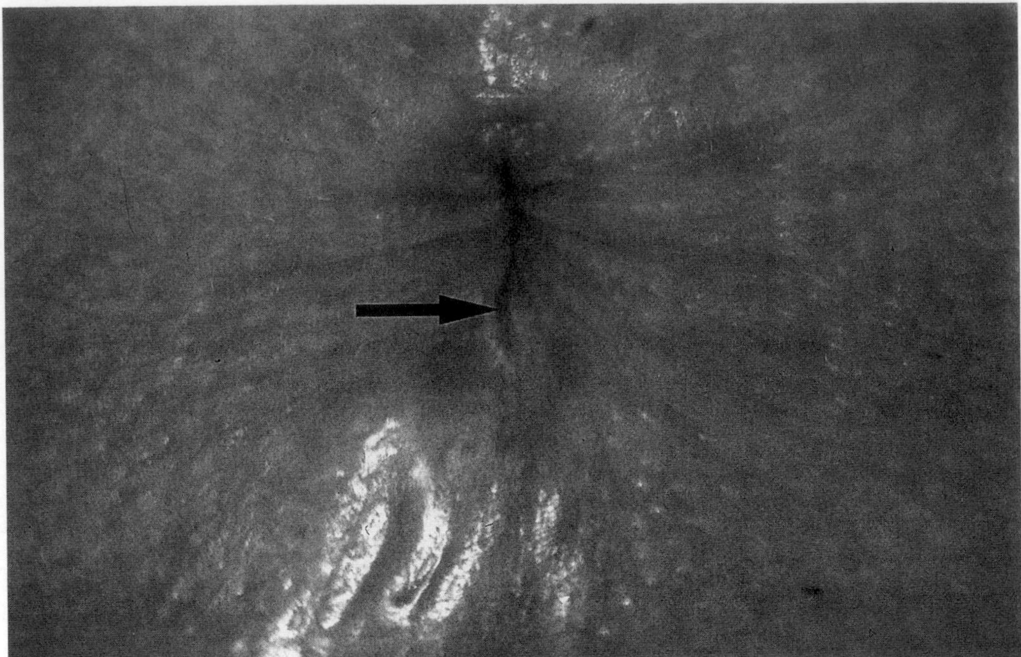

Fig. 25-4. Anal fissure (*arrow*).

Table 25-2. AAP Guidelines for Classifying Potential Signs of Abuse

Findings concerning for abuse, but in isolation not diagnostic
• Abrasions or bruising of the inner thighs and genitalia
• Scarring or tears of the labia minora
• Enlargement of the hymenal opening
Findings more concerning for abuse
• Scarring, tears, or distortion of the hymen (Fig. 25-5)
• Decreased amount of or absent hymenal tissue (Fig. 25-6)
• Scarring of the fossa navicularis
• Injury to or scarring of the posterior fourchette
• Perianal scarring (Fig. 25-7)
• Anal laceration
Findings diagnostic for abuse with medical certainty
• Presence of semen, sperm, or acid phosphatase
• Positive culture for gonorrhea[a]
• Positive serologies for syphilis or HIV infection[a]

[a]Provided congenital or transfusion-acquired disease is ruled-out.

of 3 and 18 years, comparing results of STD evaluation in children who did and did not meet screening criteria. In this group 63 percent of patients met the AAP screening criteria, with 85 percent of these undergoing STD testing; 50 percent of the children who did not satisfy screening criteria also underwent testing. While STDs were identified in 5.7 percent of patients who met screening requirements, no STDs were found in the children who did not fulfill the criteria.

Recent literature suggests that even more limited screening criteria may be useful in decreasing cost and minimizing invasive procedures. In 2001, Ingram and colleagues devised a screening tool, which they retrospectively applied to 3040 children aged 0 to 12 years, 1.2 percent of whom had cultures positive for gonorrhea, and 0.8 percent of whom were infected with chlamydia.[23] By assigning points to historical features presumed to be strongly associated with contracting an STD and testing only those children with a score of 2 or higher, he reported that all infected children would have been identified while reducing the number of cultures obtained by 45 percent (Table 25-4).

Both the CDC and AAP recommend with vaginal and rectal cultures for chlamydia and gonorrhea, as well as

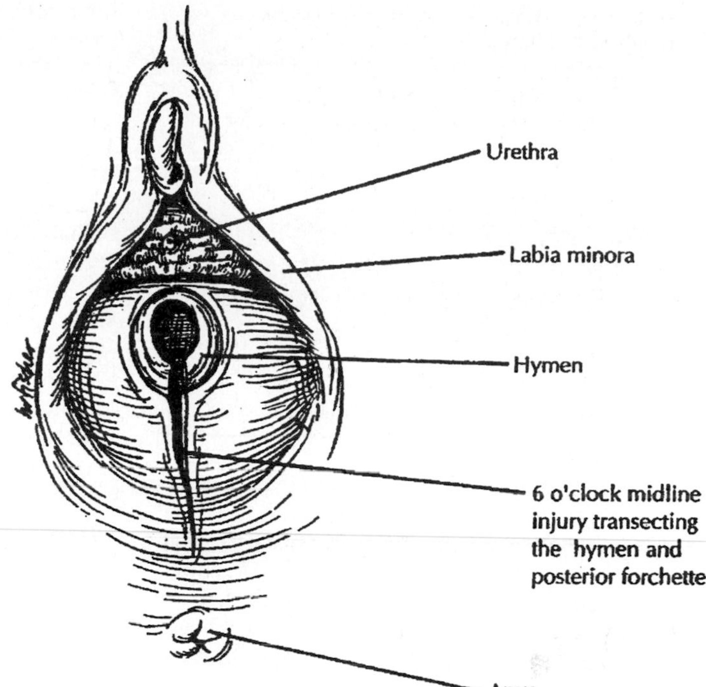

Fig. 25-5. Midline perineal lacerations, common in childhood sexual assault.

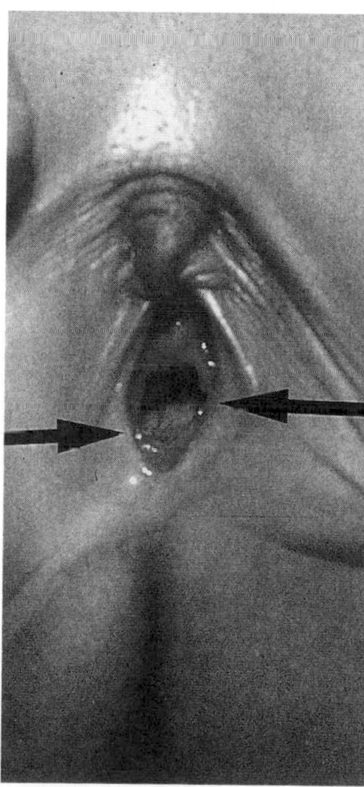

Fig. 25-6. Decreased hymenal tissue at the 7 o'clock and 3 o'clock positions (*arrows*).

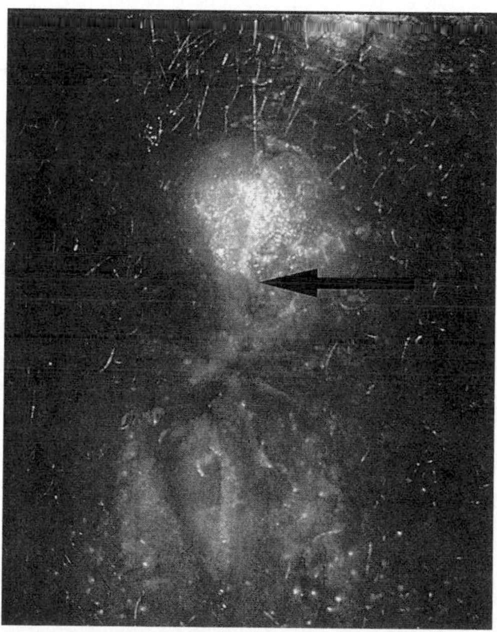

Fig. 25-7. Perianal scarring (*arrow*). Visualization enhanced by toluidine dye application. (Photo courtesy of Robert Morris, MD.)

Table 25-3. Screening Criteria for STD Testing in Prepubertal Children

Screening criteria for STD testing

- The perpetrator has a known STD or is at risk for having an STD
  - Multiple partners
  - History of STD
  - History of IV drug use
- Multiple perpetrators
- Child with signs or symptoms of a STD (e.g., vaginal discharge)
- Child has a sibling with a STD
- History of penetration or ejaculation
- High prevalence of STDs in the community

a throat culture for gonorrhea. Although urine PCRs are available for both organisms, cultures remain the gold standard for legal purposes and no studies have yet evaluated the reliability of PCRs in children.

Besides attempting to establish limited screening criteria, Ingram et al also questioned the yield of throat and rectal cultures.[23] All of the children in his study underwent genital, oral, and rectal cultures for both chlamydia and gonorrhea, and only 58 of 3040 children had infections (37 with gonorrhea; 25 with chlamydia; 4 with both). The one child who had a positive rectal culture for gonorrhea without a concurrent genital gonorrhea infection also had a positive genital culture for chlamydia. No oral infections were found. Accordingly, these researchers concluded that genital cultures alone would have identified 100 percent of infections while obtaining 85 percent fewer cultures. However previous reviews showed higher rates of oral and rectal infection than found by Ingram et al,[24–26] with one study finding that 5 percent of children infected with gonorrhea had the organism isolated only from the rectum.[19]

Most experts also obtain serologies for syphilis, hepatitis B, and HIV, although the possibility of vertical transmission must be considered and addressed at the time of evaluation. In cases of vaginal discharge, a wet mount for *Trichomonas vaginalis* and a general bacterial culture are also worthwhile, and cultures for HSV should be sent of any suspicious lesions. The significance of potentially sexually transmitted diseases varies with the disease, ranging from possible to definite evidence of sexual contact (Table 25-5).[12]

Table 25-4. Factors Strongly Associated with Contracting Gonorrhea or Chlamydia

- Genital-genital, genital-anal contact (2)
- Contact with a person who may have an STD (3)
- Suspicious physical findings (2)
- Abuse of a sibling (1)
- Vaginitis (1)
- Genital discharge (2)

Source: Adapted from Ingram et al.[23]

Numbers in parentheses indicate points assigned to feature, with 2 or more points total considered strongly associated with acquiring STD.

Table 25-5. Significance of Potentially Sexually Transmitted Diseases

Possible abuse

- Herpes simplex type 1 anogenital lesions in a prepubertal child
- Condyloma acuminata in a child with no other sexually transmitted diseases

Probable abuse

- Positive culture for *Chlamydia trachomatis* from the genital area[a]
- Positive culture for herpes type 2 from anogenital lesions[a]
- Trichomonas infection diagnosed by wet mount or culture from vaginal swab[a]

Definite evidence of abuse or sexual conduct

- Positive culture for *N. gonorrhoeae* from vaginal, urethral, anal, or pharyngeal source
- Evidence of syphilis[a]
- HIV infection[a]

[a]Not perinatally acquired.

Table 25-6. Differential Diagnosis of Vulvovaginitis

- Poor hygiene
- Chemical irritation
  - Bubble baths
  - Soap
  - Creams or lotions
- Foreign body (Fig. 25-8)
- Infection
  - Sexually transmitted diseases (e.g., gonorrhea, chlamydia, trichomonas)
  - Nonsexually acquired bacteria (e.g., streptococci, staphylococci)
  - Yeast
  - Other (e.g., pinworms)

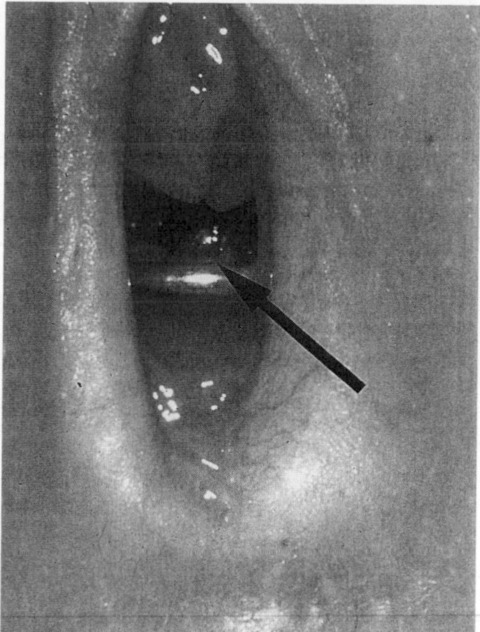

Fig. 25-8. Paper clip (*arrow*) found in a prepubertal girl with vaginal discharge. (Photo courtesy of Robert Morris, MD.)

Table 25-7. Differential Diagnosis of Anogenital Bleeding

- Infection
  - Vulvovaginitis
  - Group A streptococci
  - *Shigella*
  - *Yersinia*
- Endocrine
  - Neonatal estrogen withdrawal
  - Precocious puberty
- Local irritation
  - Accidental injury
  - Foreign body
- Dermatologic disorders
  - Atopic dermatitis
  - Contact dermatitis
  - Seborrheic dermatitis
  - Lichen sclerosus
- Miscellaneous
  - Vaginal polyp
  - Vulvar hemangioma
  - Sarcoma botryoides

Table 25-8. CDC Recommendations for Treatment of Sexually Transmitted Diseases[21]

STD	Preadolescent	Adolescent
Gonorrhea	Children weighing <45 kg Ceftriaxone 125 mg IM single dose Children weighing ≥45 kg Adolescent/adult regimen	Cefixime 400 mg PO single dose OR Ceftriaxone 125 mg IM single dose OR alternatives Ciprofloxacin 500 mg PO single dose OR Ofloxacin 400 mg PO single dose OR Levofloxacin 250 mg PO single dose
Chlamydia trachomatis	Children weighing ≤45 kg Erythromycin 50 mg/kg/day PO divided qid × 14 days Children weighing ≥45 kg but who are aged < 8 years Azithromycin 1 g PO single dose Children ≥8 years Azithromycin 1 g PO single dose OR Doxycycline 100 mg PO BID × 7 days	Azithromycin 1 g PO single dose OR Doxycycline 100 mg PO BID × 7 days
Trichomoniasis or bacterial vaginitis	Metronidazole 15 mg/kg/day PO TID × 7 days	Metronidazole 2 g PO single dose OR Metronidazole 500 mg PO BID × 7 days

The presence of a vaginal discharge warrants special mention. In 1999, Shapiro and associates[24] assessed the prevalence of gonorrhea in girls less than 12 years of age seen for vaginitis and in whom sexual abuse was not initially suspected. While group A *Streptococcus* was the most commonly isolated pathogen in the 43 girls with discharge at the time of examination, 4 (9 percent) had gonorrhea. Conversely, none of the 44 girls without discharge had gonorrhea. While recognizing that vulvovaginitis, vaginal discharge, and anogenital bleeding may have multiple nonabusive causes (Tables 25-6 and 25-7), Shapiro et al recommended that cultures be obtained in all girls with significant vaginal discharge, whether or not sexual contact is acknowledged.

Treatment of Sexually Transmitted Diseases

Because of the low incidence of STDs in prepubertal children,[18] prophylactic treatment is not routinely recommended. However, any unimmunized child should receive a hepatitis B vaccine series. Adolescent patients, on the other hand, should be treated prophylactically. The CDC treatment recommendations are reproduced in Table 25-8.

REFERENCES

1. Wang CT, Daro D: *Current Trends in Child Abuse Reporting and Fatalities: The Results of the 1996 Annual Fifty State Survey*. Chicago: National Committee to Prevent Child Abuse, 1997.
2. Finkelhor D: *Sourcebook on Child Sexual Abuse*. Thousand Oaks, CA: Sage Publications, 1986.
3. Kempe CH: Sexual abuse, another hidden pediatric problem. The 1977 C. Anderson Aldrich lecture. *Pediatrics* 62:382–389, 1978.
4. Finkelhor D: Current information on the scope and nature of child sexual abuse. *Future Child* 4:31, 1994.
5. Krugman R: Recognition of sexual abuse in children. *Pediatr Rev* 8:28, 1986.
6. American Academy of Pediatrics Committee on Child Abuse and Neglect: Guidelines for the evaluation of sexual abuse in children. *Pediatrics* 103:186–191, 1999.
7. American Academy of Pediatrics Committee on Adolescence: Sexual assault and the adolescent. *Pediatrics* 94:761–765, 1994.
8. Christian CW, Lavelle JM, DeJong AR: Forensic evidence findings in prepubertal victims of sexual assault. *Pediatrics* 106:100–104, 2000.
9. Santucci KA, Kennedy DM, Duffy ST: Wood's lamp utilization and the differentiation between semen and commonly applied medicaments. *Pediatrics* 102(Suppl.):718, 1998.
10. McCann J, Voris J, Simon M: Genital injuries resulting from sexual abuse: A longitudinal study. *Pediatrics* 89:307–317, 1992.
11. McCann J, Voris J: Perianal injuries resulting from sexual abuse: A longitudinal study. *Pediatrics* 91:390–397, 1993.
12. Adams JA, Harper K, Knudson S: Examination findings in legally confirmed child sexual abuse: It's normal to be normal. *Pediatrics* 94:310–317, 1994.
13. Berenson AB, Heger AH, Hayes JM. Appearance of hymen in prepubertal girls. *Pediatrics* 89:387–394, 1992.
14. McCann J, Wells R, Simon M: Genital findings in prepubertal girls selected for nonabuse: A descriptive study. *Pediatrics* 86:428–438, 1990.
15. Gardener JT: Descriptive study of genital variations in healthy, nonabused premenarchal girls. *J Pediatr* 120:251–257, 1992.
16. Seifer H: Adhesions of the labia minora in infants and children. *Int Pediatr* 6:347–353, 1991.
17. Berenson AB, Chacko MR, Wiemann CM, et al: Use of hymenal measurements in the diagnosis of previous penetration. *Pediatrics* 109(2):228–35, 2002.
18. Muram D, Speck PM, Dockler MJ: Child sexual abuse examinations: Is there a need for routine screening for *N. gonorrhoeae? Pediatr Adolesc Gynecol* 9:79–80, 1996.
19. Giedinghagen DH, Hoff JL, Biery RM: Gonorrhea in childrens' epidiologic unit analysis. *Pediatr Infect Dis J* 11:973–974, 1992.
20. American Academy of Pediatrics: Report of the Committee on Infectious Diseases. Sexually transmitted diseases. 2000 Redbook, 25th ed, pp 138–147.
21. Centers for Disease Control and Prevention: Guidelines for treatment of sexually transmitted diseases. *MMWR Morb Mortal Wkly Rep* 51:6, 2002.
22. Siegal RM, Schubert CT, Myers PA: The prevalence of sexually transmitted diseases in children and adolescents evaluated for sexual abuse in Cincinnati: Rationale for limited STD testing in prepubertal girls. *Pediatrics* 96:1090–1094, 1995.
23. Ingram DM, Miller WC, Schoenbach VJ, Everett VD, Ingram DL: Risk assessment for gonococcal and chlamydial infections in young children undergoing evaluation for sexual abuse. *Pediatrics* 107:e73, 2001.
24. Shapiro RA, Schubert CJ, Siegel RM: *Neisseria gonorrhoeae* in girls younger than 12 years of age evaluated for vaginitis. *Pediatrics* 104:e72, 1999.
25. Sirotnak AP: Testing sexually abused children for sexually transmitted diseases: Who to test, when to test, and why. *Pediatr Ann* 23:370–374, 1994.
26. Sicoli RA, Losek JD, Hudlett JM: Indicators for *Neisseria gonorrhoeae* cultures in children with suspected sexual abuse. *Arch Pediatr Adolesc Med* 149:86–89, 1995.

Section VII
The Reproductive Age and Older Women

26

Breast Disorders

Janet Simmons Young

KEY POINTS

- Breast Cancer
  - Women less than age 20:
    Rare
    Childhood malignancy
    Chest irradiation
    BRCA1 or *BRCA2* gene
  - Women less than age 30:
    About 1 percent of cases
  - Women over age 65:
    Over 50 percent of all cases
- Puerperal Mastitis Treatment:
  - Antistaphylococcal antibiotics
  - Continue breast feeding and emptying

INTRODUCTION

The most common breast problems in the emergency setting usually involve breast pain, breast mass, nipple discharge, or breast infection. Breast tenderness and abnormalities in texture or contour are quite common during normal breast development and response to hormonal cycling. A large number of breast complaints arise during lactation, as stasis of milk ducts and the presence of infant oral flora increase the likelihood of infection. Not uncommonly, though not usually severe, breast trauma can be seen in patients presenting with blunt thoracic trauma. Postsurgical complications of the breast also prompt women to seek emergency care, so estimates that approximately one of every four women in the United States sees a physician with a chief complaint relating to their breasts are not surprising.[1] Recent prevention services campaigns have increased public awareness of the importance of early detection of breast cancer. Concerns about the potential for cancer contributes to the anxiety experienced by the patient when presenting with an acute breast problem.

This chapter focuses on the evaluation and treatment of breast problems that may be encountered in the emergency department and urgent care settings.

ADULT ANATOMY

Normal breast tissue is a circular mass of glandular tissue located on the anterior chest wall, extending from the sternocostal junction medially to the midaxillary line laterally and from the second to the sixth ribs in the midclavicular line. The axillary tail of Spence, a lateral extension of breast tissue into the armpit, gives the breast a teardrop shape. The areola is a relatively flat area of pigmented skin that is usually well demarcated from the surrounding breast skin. Montgomery's tubercles, the numerous small protuberances on the areola, are the openings of sebaceous glands that lubricate the nipple during breast-feeding.

The breast is suspended from the chest wall and pectoralis muscle by fibrous mammary septations, also called the suspensory ligaments of Cooper.

The breast is richly innervated by sensory nerves along a dermatomal distribution. The arterial supply to the breast arises from branches off the internal mammary, lateral thoracic, thoracodorsal, and subscapular arteries. Venous drainage is accomplished by a plexus of veins that begins in the subareolar region and drains into the intercostal, internal mammary, and axillary veins. The lymphatic drainage of the breast is primarily to the axilla, with a small portion going to internal mammary lymph nodes. Lymph flow is not regionally distributed; lymphatic drainage to either the axilla or to the internal mammary chain can originate from any quadrant of the breast.

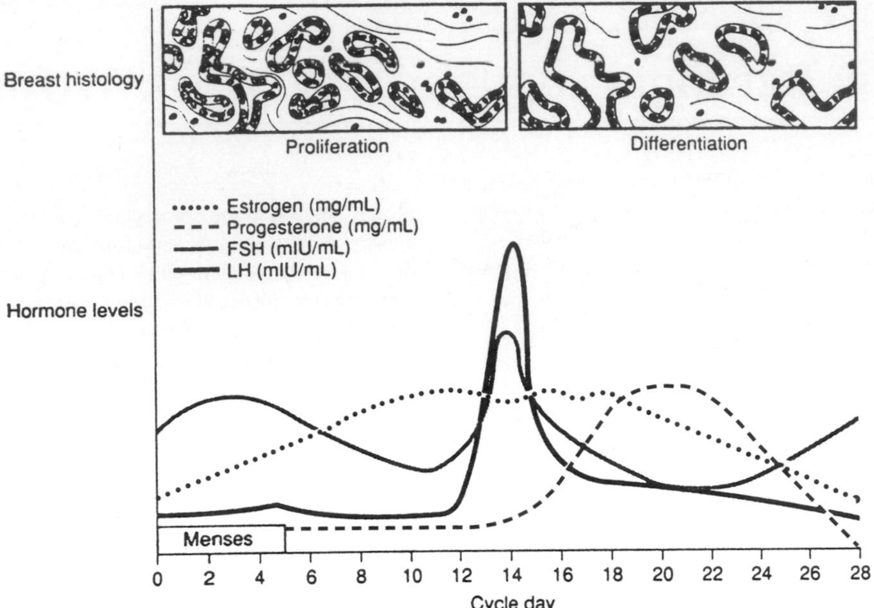

Fig. 26-1. The influence of menstrual variations in sex hormones on breast glandular histology. (From August DA, Sondak VK: Breast disease, in Greenfield LJ (ed): *Surgery: Scientific Principles and Practice*. Philadelphia: Lippincott, 1996, pp 1357–1415, with permission.)

BREAST PHYSIOLOGY

Cyclic changes in pituitary trophic factors, androgens, and estrogens influence both the menstrual cycle and breast physiology (Fig. 26-1). Breast tissue volume and tenderness are at a minimum 5 to 7 days after menstruation due to the relative lack of circulating progesterone, allowing for an examination that is both sensitive for detecting masses and comfortable for the patient. Due to the effects of rising circulating progesterone and a small peak in estrogen levels, the resulting interlobular edema causes the breast swelling, engorgement, and tenderness associated with the premenstrual phase. The average increase in breast volume is approximately 25 to 30 mL.[2] At the onset of menstruation, the rapid decline in estrogen and progesterone levels leads to ductal involution. In contrast, breast changes occurring with menopause involve actual loss of glandular tissue secondary to the gradual loss of estrogen and progesterone synthesis. Atrophy of glandular epithelium and loss of subcutaneous fat, along with replacement of stromal components with fibrous tissue, account for the characteristic wrinkled appearance of the postmenopausal breast. The resulting postmenopausal breast consists predominantly of prepectoral fat, connective tissue, mammary ducts, and minimal lobular elements.

HISTORY AND PHYSICAL EXAMINATION

Most patients seek medical attention because of breast pain, infection, nipple discharge, or mass. The differential diagnosis of breast disorders varies depending on the age and reproductive and physiologic status of the patient. History and physical examination are the first steps in establishing a diagnosis.

A routine breast examination can be a significant source of anxiety for the female patient seeking evaluation of a breast problem in an emergent setting. The examination should be as private, comfortable, and reassuring as possible and should be followed by a discussion in which the diagnosis and treatment strategy are both understandable and acceptable to the patient.

History

Breast cancer is rare in patients less than 20 years old and uncommon in women less than 30.[3] Risk factors for breast cancer in the younger age group include patients who carry the *BRCA1* or *BRCA2* gene, those with a history of childhood malignancy, or those with a history of chest irradiation.[4]

The history should elicit the onset of pain, approximate date of mass presentation, location of the affected area, and duration of the symptoms. Related symptoms, including alleviating and exacerbating conditions, should be explored. Complaints that vary with menses suggest a benign cause, whereas cancers are often asymptomatic. Radiation of the pain to any other body site is particularly important when a malignancy is suspected. The presence of symptoms in the contralateral breast parenchyma is also more reassuring for a benign diagnosis. The color and consistency of a nipple discharge, if present, should be elicited. The color of the discharge does not differentiate a benign from a malignant process.[5,6]

The relation of worsening symptoms to the menstrual cycle or hormonal therapy should be queried. Changes that the patient notes on breast self-examination may be significant and should be correlated with the menstrual cycle. Family history, specifically inquiring about the presence of a first-degree relative with breast cancer, increased exposure to endogenous estrogens (nulliparity or delayed childbearing), or biopsy confirmation of atypical hyperplasia should be obtained. An estimated 6 to 19 percent of all patients with breast cancer have a family history of breast carcinoma.[7] However, it must also be remembered that most women who develop breast cancer have no obvious risk factors beyond the two strongest, female gender and age. More than 50 percent of breast cancers occur in women 65 years of age or older, and women under age 30 make up fewer than 1 percent of all breast cancer patients.[8] Additional information regarding menstrual and reproductive histories, radiation exposure, and current or prior hormone use may also be relevant.

Physical Examination

Physical examination of the breasts is relatively comfortable for the patient during the week after menses, when breast tenderness and engorgement are at a minimum. With the patient fully disrobed from the waist up, the breasts are observed and compared (Fig. 26-2*A*). Minor size differences are common and of no significance. Note should be made of skin changes, dimpling, or nipple abnormalities. Subtle abnormalities in the lower quadrants may be accentuated by having the patient raise her arms above her head (Fig. 26-2*B*) or by pectoral muscle contraction. The axillae, including lymph nodes and the mammary tissue in the axillary tail, are best examined in the sitting position (Fig. 26-2*C*, *D*). Note should be made of the number, size, consistency, and mobility of any palpable lymph nodes. The supraclavicular spaces and the anterior and posterior cervical lymph node chains should be palpated routinely as part of the breast examination.

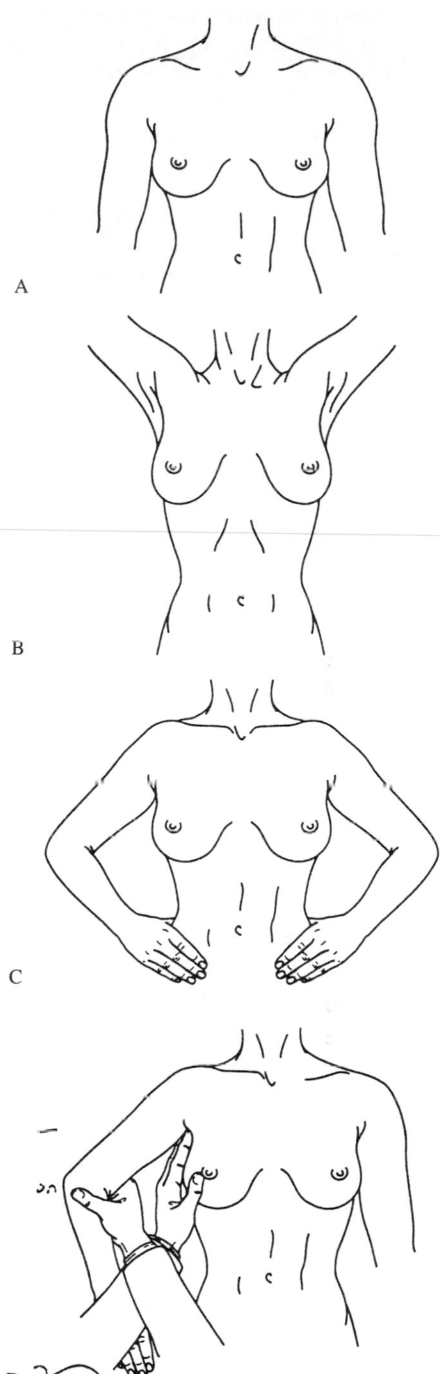

Fig. 26-2. Positioning for examination of the breasts. (From August DA, Sondak VK: Breast disease, in Greenfield LJ (ed): *Surgery: Scientific Principles and Practice*. Philadelphia: Lippincott, 1996, pp 1357–1415, with permission.)

The breast tissue examination is best performed with the patient supine. Placement of the patient's ipsilateral hand behind her head pulls the lateral quadrants and tail of the breast onto the chest wall, facilitating compression on the thoracic cage. Palpation must proceed in an orderly fashion, usually circular, to ensure that the entire breast is evaluated. The upper outer quadrant of each breast should be examined with extra care: approximately half of breast carcinomas originate in that area.[9–11] Additionally, recent data have shown that breast cancer in the U.S. has a greater propensity for left-sided breast involvement.[12] Asymmetry in glandular consistency between breasts should be noted. Discrete or dominant nodules and thickenings should be described by their location (clock-face position and distance from nipple), consistency, borders, and size.

Palpation is completed by gently squeezing the nipple-areolar complex to detect subareolar masses and latent nipple discharge. Although bloody discharge result can from a benign intraductal papilloma, it may mark an underlying cancer and should be evaluated further.[6]

DEVELOPMENTAL AND PHYSIOLOGIC ABNORMALITIES

Asymmetry of the breasts is often seen in the adolescent female, as a result of asynchronous breast development that results in one breast being noticeably larger than the other. The pubertal breast can be somewhat lumpy due to the fibrous stromal growth throughout the ductal tissue accentuating the disparity, but normally the smaller breast will eventually grow to a complementary size, usually within 1 year. If significant differences remain after complete breast development, surgical reduction or augmentation may be beneficial intervention in order to avoid further psychological sequelae.[13]

Breast atrophy may occur secondary to significant weight loss, either from crash dieting or an eating disorder. The patient presents with symmetric, fully developed breasts most notable for the appearance of sagging or elderly-appearing skin overlying a small breast. Emergent presentation of this entity should prompt the clinician to further investigate the underlying causes of acute weight loss. An urgent psychiatric consultation may be required.

Juvenile hypertrophy of the breast, a severe form of macromastia, presents near the time of menarche and is characterized by significant enlargement, either with unilateral or bilateral involvement, of the breast. The patient often presents with firm, pendulous, and very heavy breasts, usually causing musculoskeletal neck and back complaints. The exact mechanism of hypertrophic breast growth is unknown, but an abnormal response to trophic factors may play a role, as macromastia can develop in association with pregnancy. Treatment focused on the presenting complaint, such as nonsteroidal antiinflammatory medications for the relief of musculoskeletal pain, is indicated. Reduction mammoplasty may be an appropriate therapeutic intervention to prevent further somatic and psychiatric sequelae.

Puerperal Mastitis

During pregnancy, marked glandular growth occurs under the influence of estrogen, progesterone, placental lactogen, prolactin, and chorionic gonadotropin. These changes, which begin early in the first trimester, prepare the breasts for milk production at parturition. By parturition, the combined effects of vascular engorgement, epithelial proliferation, and colostrum accumulation may triple the size of the breast. The abrupt fall of progesterone, human placental lactogen (hPL) and estrogen that occurs with delivery leads to the secretion of colostrum and the removal of milk production inhibition. Within 3 to 4 days, milk rich in lipid, protein, carbohydrate, and immunoglobulin is produced. The nursing infant's tactile stimulation of the nipple-areolar complex provides a neurogenic signal to maintain milk production. Throughout lactation, the breasts remain engorged and nodular, sometimes making examination and assessment difficult. Severe engorgement usually presents on the third to fifth postpartum day, with symptoms of painful, hard and enlarged bilateral breasts. Pumping the breasts usually alleviates the pain and allows for decompression of the nipple-areolar complex, facilitating effective breast-feeding. The presence of nutrient-rich milk during lactation facilitates bacterial overgrowth in the breast should obstruction to flow from any of the major ducts occur.

Puerperal mastitis most often occurs secondary to areolar inflammation and glandular obstruction, creating an increased susceptibility to suppurative mastitis during nursing. Puerperal mastitis, or endemic mastitis, has a poorly defined constellation of symptoms, and patients often present with nonfocal symptoms, usually during the first 2 to 8 weeks postpartum. Nursing women are most vulnerable to infection when beginning breast-feeding, when the skin of the nipples is most easily damaged, and much later, when the child has teeth that may traumatize the nipples. The patient may report fever, chills, myalgias, or flu-like symptoms, and examination of the breast reveals an erythematous, localized area of pain. It is most commonly caused by *Staphylococcus aureus*, though *Escherichia coli* and streptococci are also occasional pathogens.[3,14]

Treatment requires breast emptying, skin cleansing, analgesia and staphylococcal resistant penicillins (dicloxacillin or oxacillin) or cephalosporins. There is no current evidence-based recommendation for the interruption of breast feeding with endemic or puerperal mastitis. However, if the infection fails to respond rapidly to antibiotics, a polymicrobial infection or abscess should be suspected.

Differentiation between mastitis, with limited involvement of the superficial dermis, and an abscess that is typically accompanied by palpable fluctuance, is usually straightforward. However, an abscess may present with the signs and symptoms of mastitis or may demonstrate only focal reaction to the underlying purulent collection and may be difficult to diagnose at times. Ultrasound is helpful to diagnose an abscess, as a fluid collection will be demonstrated. Interruption of breast-feeding, to prevent neonatal infection, and immediate surgical drainage of the abscess is required. An excisional biopsy of tissue may be performed by the surgeon to rule out an inflammatory carcinoma.[15]

Nonpuerperal Breast Infections

Breast Cellulitis and Mastitis

Inflammatory and infectious processes involving the nonlactating breast represent a frequent cause of acute care visits. Acute infections of the breast generally present with erythema, edema, tenderness, malaise, and fever. Mastitis, or superficial cellulitis of the breast, is usually treated with antibiotics. Breast cellulitis, if recognized early, responds to oral antibiotic treatment with an antistaphylococcal penicillin (e.g., dicloxacillin 250 mg qid for 7 days) or a first-generation cephalosporin (e.g., as cephalexin 500 qid for 7 days). If the patient is allergic to penicillin, then either clindamycin (300 mg qid) or erythromycin (500 mg qid) is appropriate. The infection should respond rapidly to therapy, demonstrating at least partial resolution within 48 hours. Repeat clinical evaluation is recommended at 48 to 72 hours.

Small, periareolar abscesses may often simply be incised and drained if there is no associated generalized erythema or tenderness. However, most breast abscesses require surgical drainage and antibiotics, depending on the extent of breast involvement and the degree of systemic illness. If the presence of an abscess is suspected, it can be confirmed with the use of breast ultrasound or percutaneous aspiration of the fluctuant area. A large-bore needle, usually 16 gauge or larger, may be necessary to aspirate purulent material under local anesthesia. Aspiration may be adequate management for very small fluid collections with limited breast involvement. However, open surgical drainage is recommended as the most effective treatment. Generally, due to the significant inflammation and the sensitivity of the breast, adequate open drainage and biopsy require general anesthesia. Immediate referral to a surgeon is often preferable to attempting drainage or aspiration under local anesthesia.

Whenever infectious mastitis or a breast abscess is suspected clinically, the possibility of an inflammatory carcinoma or squamous cell carcinoma must also be entertained.[16] Inflammatory breast cancer accounts for approximately 1 to 2 percent of all breast cancers.[17] As the diagnostic name suggests, early inflammatory breast cancer is often erroneously treated as cellulitis due to the benign appearance of the disease. However, more advanced forms of the disease, while still erythematous, may appear clearly ominous. Any inflammatory process, even one that responds quickly or completely to antibiotics, or that requires surgical drainage should be referred to a breast specialist for biopsy to rule out malignancy.

Occasionally, either abscess or simple mastitis may present with obvious signs of regional or systemic toxicity. General indications for admission and immediate surgical consultation are patients with obvious sepsis or hemodynamic compromise, immunosuppressed or immunocompromised hosts (e.g., diabetics), rapidly progressive infection, or failure of outpatient antibiotics. Complications include necrotizing soft tissue infections, bacteremia, or sepsis. Current recommendations for parenteral antibiotics are cefazolin 2 g IV q8h or nafcillin 2 g IV q4h. In penicillin-allergic patients, fluoroquinolones, rifampin, or vancomycin should be considered, though multiple-drug-resistant *Staphylococus* species have been reported.[18]

Periductal Mastitis (Mammary Duct Ectasia)

Periductal mastitis, also called *plasma cell mastitis* or *mammary duct ectasia,* is an uncommon benign disorder characterized by ectatic, or dilated, mammary ducts with retained secretions surrounded by significant inflammation. It generally presents as constant mastalgia, is associated with nipple retraction or discharge, and can (in severe cases) exhibit mammary duct fistulas at the areolar border. Younger women tend to present with inflammatory and infectious processes, such as recurrent subareolar abscesses, while perimenopausal and postmenopausal women are more likely to present with nipple discharge and retraction or sterile subareolar masses.

For older women who present with a thick, white, creamy nipple discharge, follow-up is necessary to exclude a malignancy. Regardless of the patient's age, other presentations (bloody discharge, nipple retraction, mammary duct fistula, or recurrent abscesses) should prompt referral to a specialist for differentiation from a malignant entity, and for definitive treatment.

Hydradenitis Suppurativa

Hydradenitis suppurativa frequently presents with recurrent multiple cutaneous abscesses, sinus tracts, and scarring of the breast folds, axillae, and groin and perineum. It is a chronic inflammatory disease involving the obstruction of sweat glands associated with polymicrobial colonization, with staphylococcal and streptococcal species implicated in the pathogenesis of infection.[19] Frequently, patients present with painful, sebaceous abscesses along the inferior, pendulous surface of the breast, requesting incisional drainage for pain relief. Incision and drainage is usually adequate therapy for a limited area of abscess formation. Antibiotics are rarely used for outpatient management of simple abscesses in immunocompetent patients, though antibiotic suppression therapy is used to decrease the frequency and severity of the disease. There is no cure for the disease except extensive surgical excision of the apocrine tissue, which often results in higher recurrence rates at the excisional sites.

Other Breast Infections

Other spontaneous or chronic breast infections can occur secondary to unusual pathogens, such as actinomycosis, tuberculosis, *Brucella*, syphilis, or even cutaneous mycotic pathogens.[14,20,21] Acute noninfectious mastitis can be seen secondary to a variety of inflammatory processes, such as systemic lupus erythematosus, granulomatous mastitis, calcium deposition secondary to end-stage renal disease, or fibrocystic changes of the breast.[22–24]

BREAST PAIN

One of the most common urgent presentations for women is breast pain, also termed mastalgia or mastodynia. The discomfort is usually cyclical, waxing or waning with the menstrual cycle in up to 80 percent of cases.[25,26] Cyclical breast pain is generally secondary to hormonally-induced changes in the breast tissue (fibrocystic changes). Cyclical mastalgia is usually most severe in the days leading up to the menstrual period and decreases or resolves completely following menstruation. Pain is bilateral, and is usually most severe in the upper, outer breast tissue and may be referred to the axilla, medial arms, or scapulae. Treatment is symptomatic.

Breast pain that is not related to the menstrual cycle (noncyclic) can be a result of infection, cyst, or can be musculoskeletal or cardiac in origin. The breast examination should verify that the pain is in fact originating in the breast. Careful evaluation is necessary to evaluate for breast masses or abscess. At times the examination reveals tender, nodular breasts, suggesting a diagnosis of a cyst or fibrocystic changes.[27] Although less likely, a cancer in association with fibrocystic changes may also present as a tender mass. Patients with breast pain should be referred to their primary care physician for follow-up and for definitive diagnosis. The evaluation of a discrete breast mass is described later in this chapter.

Axillary Lymphadenopathy and Pain

In women with axillary adenopathy, the possibility of breast cancer metastatic to axillary nodes must be considered. This is true even if careful physical examination does not reveal a palpable breast abnormality. Referral to a breast specialist for bilateral mammograms is indicated. Unless there is good evidence that the adenopathy is associated with an infectious or other benign etiology, palpable nodes should prompt a referral to a breast specialist.

NIPPLE DISCHARGE AND IRRITATION

Nipple Discharge

Table 26-1 lists some common causes of discharge. All women with discharge require follow up to ensure there is no malignancy.[3,28]

Intraductal papillomas can present with a bloody nipple discharge. They are most common in 20- to 40-year-old women, and are uncommon in adolescents. Intraductal papillomas arise from abnormal, highly vascular ducts that are susceptible to trauma, resulting in a bloody discharge with or without a palpable mass.

Pregnant women may lactate as early as the second trimester, and milk production may occur for a time after cessation of breast-feeding.[29] Fluctuating hormone levels associated with the menarche or menopause can cause transient lactation.

Bilateral, spontaneous milky nipple discharge can be indicative of hyperprolactinemia resulting from medication use, a pituitary adenoma, or a thyroid disorder. Measurement of serum prolactin level is appropriate in women with onset of new, bilateral galactorrhea who have not lactated within the prior year. Evaluation by a specialist is indicated when cessation of postweaning milk production

Table 26-1. Potential Causes of Nipple Discharge

Discharge	Possible Causes
Purulent	Infection
Milky	Pregnancy Prolactinoma Pituitary adenoma Drugs (phenothiazines, H_2 blockers)
Serous or serosanguineous	Intraductal papilloma Fibrocystic changes Duct ectasia Cancer
Watery	Intraductal papilloma Cancer

Source: Adapted from Neinstein.[3]

fails to occur, or in women with spontaneous development of persistent, bilateral milky discharge.

Unilateral nipple discharges that contain blood and are associated with a palpable mass are often caused by a benign intraductal papilloma. In one study of over 9000 patients, a frequent cause of nipple discharge in patients receiving biopsy was intraductal papilloma (47.8 percent).[30] However, unilateral nipple discharge may also be an early sign of breast cancer, requiring an urgent referral for evaluation.

Nipple Irritation

Nipple irritation may be caused by repeated vigorous friction or abrasion with clothing or by overexposure to the sun (sunburn). The nipples are easily protected from chronic abrasion by application of a small dab of petroleum jelly or use of protective pads inserted into the cups of a well-fitting sports bra. Paget's disease can also present as severe nipple irritation, which is heralded by the appearance of a weeping, eczematoid lesion of the nipple. Clinically there may be accompanying edema and inflammation of the nipple-areolar complex. Nipple biopsy reveals malignant cells within the milk ducts, and a positive diagnosis prompts the search for an underlying carcinoma by the breast specialist. Because these changes may transiently respond to topical treatments, there is often delay of 6 to 12 months prior to biopsy and diagnosis.[31] When Paget's disease is suspected, referral to a specialist is indicated. Bilateral mammography may facilitate subsequent work-up.

TRAUMA

Isolated blunt trauma to the breast is uncommon but most often occurs during motor vehicle crashes when the breast is injured upon contact with restraint devices or the interior of the automobile. Blunt trauma to the breast can be seen in association with multiple thoracic injuries, including rib fractures, and is often accompanied by extensive ecchymoses. The widespread use of shoulder restraints has resulted in an increased incidence of these compressive breast injuries resulting in the often-used term "seat belt sign" to describe the area of localized bruising across the anterior chest.[32] Trauma to both normal and augmented breast tissue can result in significant disruption of native tissue or rupture of a prosthetic implant. Detection of implant rupture is rarely indicated emergently, but ultrasonography may be the most accessible imaging modality in the acute setting with a characteristic "snowstorm" appearance of the area of silicone extrusion or loss of the echo-free space in saline implants.[33,34]

Traumatic breast injuries, whether isolated or associated with multiple trauma, rarely necessitate specific therapy unless there is significant avulsion of breast tissue or an expanding hematoma, both of which require immediate surgical intervention. However, in the absence of a history of trauma, the presence of a significant isolated breast injury should raise the possibility of abuse or cancer. Most of the signs and symptoms of chest wall and breast contusions resolve within weeks of the injury. Long-term sequelae of breast trauma include fat necrosis, Mondor's disease (see below), architectural distortions of the breast, and persistent microcalcification observed on mammography.[32] Persistent abnormalities beyond that time or the presence of a mass after minimal trauma without accompanying ecchymosis must be raise the question of underlying pathology or malignancy.

Fat Necrosis

Trauma to fatty components of the breast can incite an inflammatory cascade. During remodeling, the repair process may result in scarring of normal breast parenchyma or deposition of microcalcifications or even degenerative fatty cysts in the area of injury.[35] Early presentations can include subcutaneous hemorrhage or induration, while later findings can include firm, well circumscribed masses. Fat necrosis can easily be confused with carcinoma, as it can present with a palpable mass and even skin dimpling and retraction. Radiographic examination can reveal mild to moderate scarring years after trauma, biopsy, or breast augmentation (Fig. 26-3). While no spe-

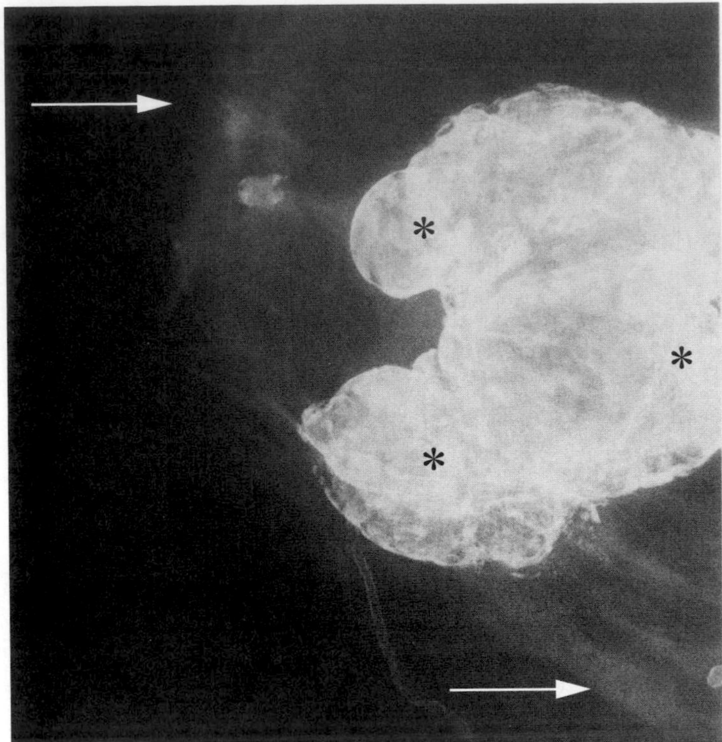

Fig. 26-3. Mammogram demonstrating fat necrosis after reduction mammoplasty. Note the extensive fat necrosis (*arrows*) and the numerous enlarged fatty cysts (*asterisks*). (Courtesy of the University of North Carolina Department of Radiology.)

cific treatment is required for fat necrosis, the presence of cancer must be excluded. Referral to a breast specialist is indicated for persistent or new masses, even when the patient is able to clearly recall a history of significant trauma.

Mondor's Disease

Thrombophlebitis of the superficial thoracoepigastric vein, or Mondor's disease, results in a cord-like mass in the breast, sometimes associated with skin retraction or dimpling.[36] Most cases have no identifiable cause, but localized trauma or an inflammatory process are usually causative. Patients with Mondor's disease may complain of burning breast pain. Physical examination reveals a characteristic cord-like mass in the superficial subcutaneous tissue of the breast, most commonly in the lower breast. Skin changes may be present and patients are often concerned about malignancy. Mondor's disease can be mistaken for cancer; therefore mammography and referral to a breast specialist will confirm the diagnosis. Mondor's disease is benign and usually self-limited, so no specific treatment is required beyond nonsteroidal antiinflammatory medications for symptomatic relief.

PERIOPERATIVE COMPLICATIONS

Complications that may present following breast surgery include hemorrhage or hematoma, wound infection, and seroma formation.

Hemorrhage and Hematoma

Immediate postoperative hemorrhage is best evaluated and treated by the operating surgeon. Exsanguinating hemorrhage is rare, but the presentation is usually straightforward. Expanding hematomas may occur but can usually be controlled with direct pressure until definitive care can be provided by the breast surgeon.

Hematomas occur most commonly following breast biopsy, surgical procedure, or local trauma. They usually present as ecchymotic, painful, and tender masses that generally resolve over a period of several weeks. Fortunately, progressive hematomas sufficiently large to require intervention are very rare and are usually associated with coagulation abnormalities, such as hemophilia or warfarin therapy. Rarely, breast hematomas can be seen in the absence of a history of trauma or coagulopathy due to hemorrhage into a breast cyst. Emergent evaluation

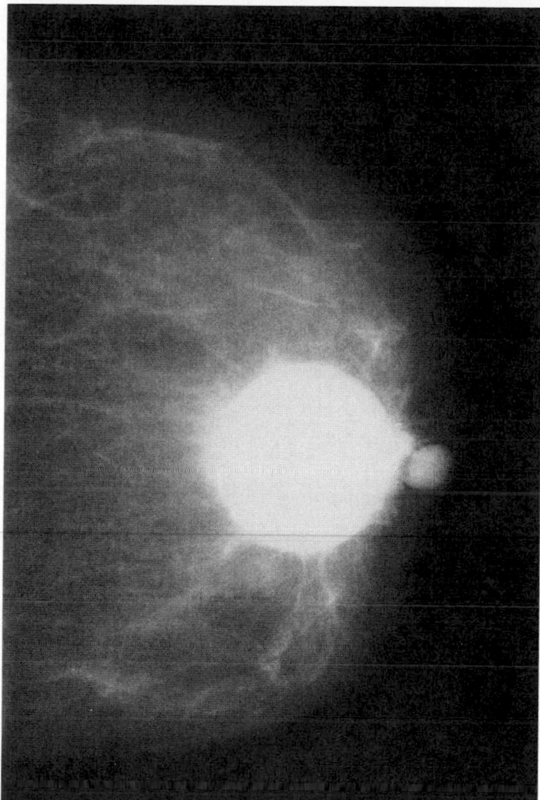

Fig. 26-4. Mammogram of retroareolar hematoma after biopsy. (Courtesy of University of North Carolina Department of Radiology.)

of a breast hematoma requires the clinician to determine whether the hematoma is expanding, tensely distended, or stable. Expanding hematomas, especially those occurring within the first few postoperative days, may signify the presence of ongoing bleeding and usually require surgical evaluation for evacuation of the hematoma or ligation of bleeding vessels. Tense, painful hematomas occurring outside the immediate postoperative period are less likely to be associated with a discrete bleeding vessel and are more difficult to visualize due to surrounding parenchymal clot. Therefore, later presentations of breast hematoma are usually managed conservatively, with analgesics, a compressive bra, and the correction of any coagulopathy. On the radiograph a stable hematoma may appear as a well circumscribed density (Fig. 26-4) that can be confirmed by ultrasonography if the diagnosis is in doubt (Fig. 26-5). Aspiration of the hematoma in the emergency department is generally not effective. An in-

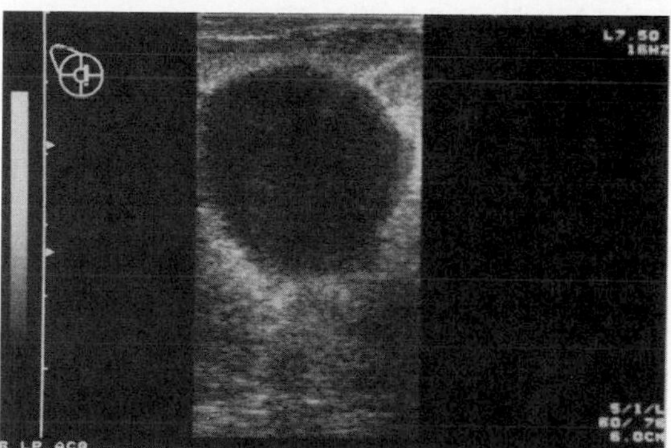

Fig. 26-5. Ultrasonographic evaluation of same patient as seen in Fig 26-4. Note the well-circumscribed, hypoechoic fluid collection of the hematoma. (Courtesy of University of North Carolina Department of Radiology.)

fected hematoma require inpatient management, as percutaneous drainage or open drainage and packing along with parenteral antibiotics are generally indicated.

Wound Infection

Postoperative wound infections may be treated with an oral first-generation cephalosporin on an outpatient basis if there is no abscess, there are no systemic signs of toxicity, and the patient is not immunocompromised. Daily follow-up is necessary to assess response to treatment.

Worsening signs of cellulitis or systemic response to infection, development of purulence, or failure to improve after 48 hours suggest a need for admission and referral to a breast specialist for evaluation. Postsurgical abscesses are treated in much the same way as spontaneous abscesses, as discussed previously.

Seroma

Postoperative seroma formation after major breast surgery can be prevented by suction drain placement to drain serous fluid accumulation in the axillary space and beneath chest wall skin flaps. Postoperative drain infection generally requires drain removal and antibiotic therapy. Any fluid collections that subsequently develop usually require drainage either by repeated aspiration or incision. Malfunction of suction drains usually results in the leakage of serous fluid around the drain with repeated soakings of the overlying dressing. The operating surgeon should be consulted for any of these complications.

PALPABLE BREAST MASS

The American Cancer Society estimates that 203,500 new cases of female breast cancer will be diagnosed and 39,600 women will die from the disease in the United States in 2002.[37] Despite the importance of mammography in the screening and diagnosis of breast cancer, the majority of breast cancers present as a palpable mass. As with any presenting complaint, the emergency evaluation of a breast mass includes careful history and an appropriate medical screening examination. Breast masses should be referred to a breast specialist for diagnosis and management. Because of the likelihood of cancer in postmenopausal women, evaluation of masses in this group is straightforward. Any discrete mass or thickening in a postmenopausal woman that is not well documented in prior exams must be assumed to be cancer until proved otherwise. Urgent outpatient management consists of bilateral mammograms and tissue sampling by means of fine-needle aspiration biopsy (FNAB), core needle biopsy (CNB), or open surgical biopsy.

Appropriate referral can ensure that the clinician will avoid a failure to diagnose a breast cancer. Breast cancer can mimic acute or subacute conditions. Abnormal response to therapy, persistent lesions or symptoms, or diagnostic uncertainty despite thorough history, physical examination, and simple laboratory and radiographic studies should prompt urgent referral.

Chart Documentation

Meticulous documentation is important to facilitate continuity of care, assure appropriate follow-up, and minimize risk of medicolegal liability. Special attention should be given to documenting the pertinent positive and negative findings in the history and physical examination. Breast cancer risk factors (age, menopausal status, reproductive history, family history, history of prior breast problems, and breast cancer risk factors) should be documented. The record should document the general physical examination as well as the important elements of a breast examination: breast appearance, presence of adenopathy, breast contour or position change, nipple discharge, and findings on breast palpation with quality and location documented either by a diagram or using clock-face terms in the written narrative.

Discussions with the patient should be noted, including specific instructions for follow-up action required by the patient.

Characteristics associated with a delayed diagnosis of breast cancer include: nonwhite race, lower socioeconomic status, normal or false-negative mammogram, presentation with nipple lesions or axillary mass, or inadequate biopsy technique.[38,39]

For the emergency physician, when evaluating any woman presenting with a breast problem, a diagnosis of cancer must be considered regardless of patient age. The physical examination and breast imaging studies are complementary; a normal mammogram in the presence of a palpable breast mass does not rule out the possibility of cancer. Referral to a specialist for tissue diagnosis is imperative. Tissue diagnosis is the only definitive means of ruling in or out the possibility of breast cancer. Finally, when either the clinician or the patient is in doubt, referral to a specialist is always the safest course of action.

FIBROCYSTIC BREAST DISEASE

The most common cause of benign breast masses in premenopausal women is fibrocycstic breast disease, which is not a pathologic process but a constellation of breast problems linked by the common pathognomonic finding of breast cysts. The nodularity and tenderness experienced by all women during their reproductive years, as a result of cyclic glandular responses to the hormonal variations of the menstrual cycle, are referred to as fibrocystic or benign breast changes.[3] Many women present for evaluation if these symptoms or masses become more pronounced or lead to anxiety over the possibility of breast cancer. If the history and physical examination in patients presenting with these complaints does not suggest infection, abscess, or another emergency condition, patients should be referred to their primary care physician for follow-up. Written discharge instructions should be clear about the need for follow-up care to confirm the diagnosis.

If a woman under age 30 has a well-circumscribed breast mass, fibrocystic changes or a fibroadenoma should be suspected. Outpatient breast ultrasound may confirm the presence of a simple cyst, whereas fine-needle aspiration may also confirm a simple cyst or demonstrate cells diagnostic of a fibroadenoma. Patients with solid masses on radiologic or tissue biopsy, even those with cytologically-proved fibroadenomas, should be referred to a specialist for further evaluation and follow-up.

ABNORMAL MAMMOGRAM

Patients may present to the emergency department after undergoing screening mammography that reveals an abnormality. When patients seek emergency evaluation for mammographic abnormalities, a thorough medical screening examination should be performed. If possible, the imaging may be reviewed by a qualified radiologist in order to facilitate follow-up imaging or urgent breast specialist referral. These additional steps may assist a specialist in a timely work-up if they are feasible in the emergent clinical setting.

INFLAMMATORY BREAST CANCER

Of all of the potential presentations of a breast malignancy, *inflammatory breast cancer* is the entity associated with the greatest mortality and longest interval from initial presentation to definitive diagnosis and treatment. The clinical presentation is often composed of extensive pain and breast inflammation, sometimes indistinguishable from an infectious etiology, due to the permeation of dermal lymphatics by tumor that leads to edema and erythema of the breast. Specifically, patients present with a clinical syndrome that includes breast warmth, tenderness, edema, and erythema. The combination of swelling and redness can result in an orange-peel appearance of the overlying skin (peau d'orange). The absence of an underlying mass or palpable axillary lymph nodes does not rule out the diagnosis. The signs of inflammatory breast cancer must not be mistaken for indicators of a benign infectious or inflammatory process; prompt mammography, and then biopsy of the palpable or radiographic breast lesions are required by the follow-up physician. Similarly, any diagnosis of an infectious breast condition must be promptly reconsidered if there is not an initial good response to antibiotics or if there is persistence despite apparently good treatment.

Other physical signs of invasive cancer that should prompt immediate surgical referral are the presence of any mass, with or without axillary lymphadenopathy or skin ulceration, fixation of the mass to the chest wall, fixed axillary nodes, or the presence of ipsilateral arm edema. Treatment of patients with locally advanced breast cancer generally involves initial systemic chemotherapy followed by surgery and/or radiation therapy.[40] Immediate recognition of locally advanced breast cancer and prompt referral to a specialist is mandatory.

BREAST DISEASES OF EXTRAMAMMARY ORIGIN

A variety of problems may arise in the nonglandular portions of the breast. Diseases of the skin overlying the breast should be treated as dermatologic problems, not breast disorders. A variety of neoplasms of mesenchymal origin may arise in the breast. Fibromatosis (desmoid tumors), fat necrosis, foreign-body reactions, sarcoidosis, lymphoma, and various infections (including those of mycobacterial and mycotic origin) have also been described.

BREAST IMAGING

Breast imaging techniques are most often used for breast cancer screening and to look for synchronous, clinically occult disease when a patient presents with a palpable breast abnormality. Because these indications are rarely pressing, the role of breast imaging in the emergency department is limited. However, appropriate use of breast ultrasound can occasionally provide diagnostic clues that can facilitate emergent management of traumatic or postoperative complications. In some instances they may even provide diagnostic certainty. Breast imaging methods are complements to, but not substitutes for, a thorough history and physical examination.

Mammography is most helpful in women over age 40, when the incidence of breast cancer begins to rise sharply and the sensitivity of the test increases as the dense parenchymal tissue of young women is progressively replaced by fatty tissue. In the urgent evaluation of a woman presenting with a palpable mass or other clinical abnormality, mammography may help establish a diagnosis for the breast specialist (Fig. 26-6). Mammography should be performed before biopsy in all women over the age of 30 years to detect synchronous, nonpalpable ipsilateral or contralateral disease. Otherwise mammography is rarely indicated in the emergency setting. Currently, the American Cancer Society (ACS) recommends that mammographic screening begin at age 40.[37] The National Cancer Institute (NCI) has taken a more individualized approach, suggesting that women age 39 or younger discuss the indications for mammography with their primary health care provider, and that women 40 and older should receive screening mammography every 1 to 2 years.[41] Table 26-2 compares the current ACS and NCI guidelines for screening.

Ultrasonography uses high-resolution, 1- to 10-MHz acoustic waves to image the breast. The most important feature of ultrasound is its ability to distinguish between cystic and solid masses. It is not an effective screening test for breast cancer. Clinically, emergency breast ultrasound is most helpful in evaluating the presence of a fluid collection in order to more accurately diagnose breast abscess or hematoma. In the outpatient setting, ultrasound is used to confirm the diagnosis of a cyst, or in women under age 30 to support a clinical impression of fibroadenoma. Breast MRI offers a detail evaluation of breast structure and may play a future role in evaluating breast trauma in augmented breasts.

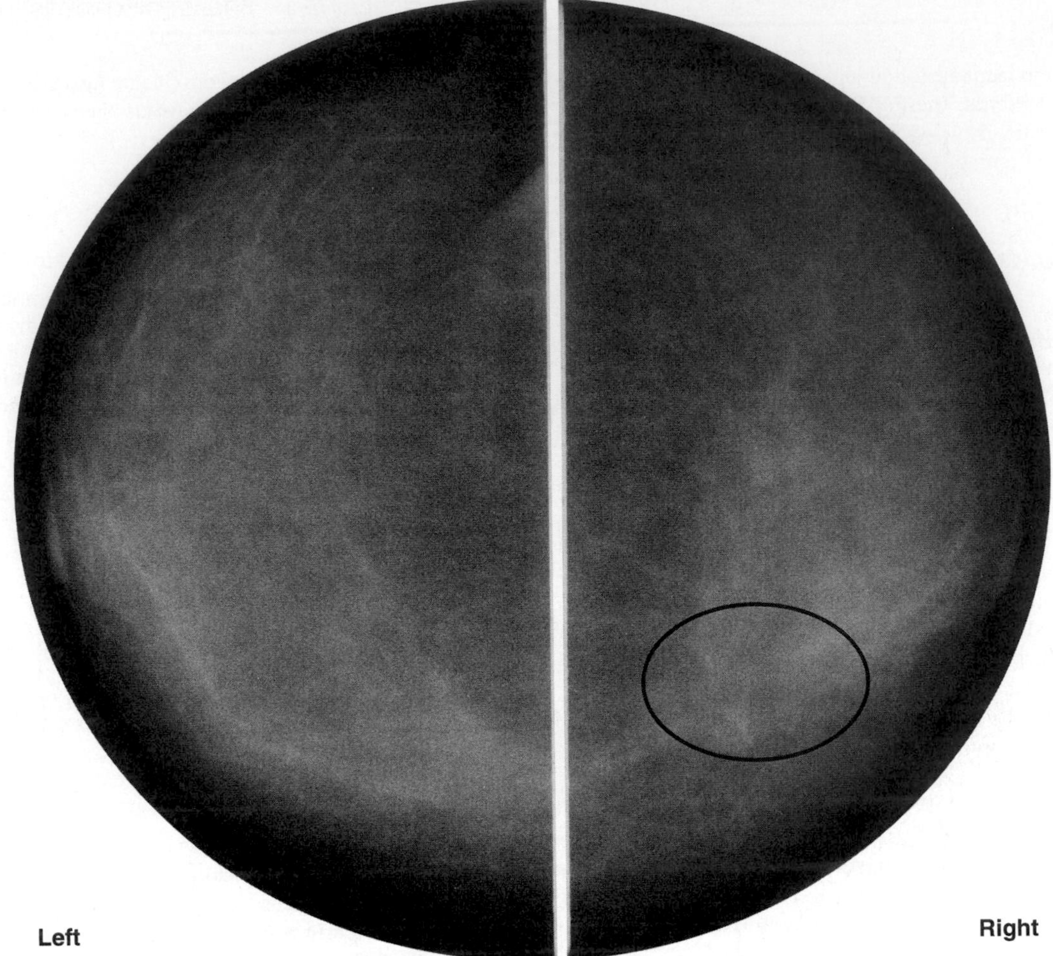

Fig. 26-6. Screening mammogram. Note the subtle, spiculated right inferior mass (*circled*), which was demonstrated on biopsy to be invasive lobular breast cancer. (Courtesy of University of North Carolina Department of Radiology.)

Table 26-2. Recommendations for Breast Cancer Screening

American Cancer Society	National Cancer Institute
Ages 20-39 Clinical exam every 3 years Monthly breast self-examination	Medical consultation with physician
Ages 40-50 Annual mammogram Annual clinical exam Monthly breast self-examination	Mammogram every 1-2 years
Ages 50-69 Annual mammogram Annual clinical exam Monthly breast self-examination	Mammogram every 1-2 years

Source: American Cancer Society: Breast Cancer Facts & Figures 2001–2002, and National Institutes of Health: Update on NCI Statement on Mammography Screening, February 21, 2002.

REFERENCES

1. American College of Obstetrics and Gynecology: *Precis V: An Update in Obstetrics and Gynecology*. Washington: ACOG, 1994, p 75.
2. Droegemueller W, Valea FA: Breast diseases, in Stenchever MA, Droegemueller W, Herbst AL, Mishell DR (eds): *Comprehensive Gynecology*, 4th ed. St. Louis: Mosby, 2001, pp 359–398.
3. Neinstein LS: Breast diseases in adolescents and young women. *Pediatr Clin North Am* 46:607–629, 1999.
4. Templeman C, Hertweck S: Breast disorders in the pediatric and adolescent patient. *Obstet Gynecol Clin North Am* 27:19–34, 2000.
5. Scott S: Breast cancer. Making the diagnosis. *Surg Clin North Am* 79:991–1005, 1999.
6. Morrow M: The evaluation of common breast problems. *Am Fam Physician* 61:2371–2378, 2385, 2000.
7. Fiorica J: Prevention and treatment of breast cancer. *Obstet Gynecol Clin North Am* 28:711–726, 2000.
8. Henderson IC: Breast cancer, in Murphy GP, Lawrence W, Lenhard RE (eds): *American Cancer Society Textbook of Clinical Oncology*. Atlanta, GA: American Cancer Society, 1995, pp 198–219.
9. McMasters KM, Wong SL, Chao C, et al: Defining the optimal surgeon experience for breast cancer sentinel lymph node biopsy: A model for implementation of new surgical techniques. *Ann Surg* 234:292–299, 2001.
10. Hill AD: Lessons learned from 500 cases of lymphatic mapping for breast cancer. *Ann Surg* 229:528–535, 1999.
11. Borgstein PJ: Functional lymphatic anatomy for sentinel node biopsy in breast cancer: echoes from the past and the periareolar blue method. *Ann Surg* 232:81–89, 2000.
12. Weiss HA, Devesa SS: Laterality of breast cancer is the United States. *Cancer Causes Control* 7:539–543, 1996.
13. Kuzbari R, Deutinger M: Surgical treatment of developmental asymmetry of the breast. *Scand J Plast Reconstr Hand Surg* 27:203–207, 1993.
14. Whitaker-Worth DL: Dermatologic diseases of the breast and nipple. *J Am Acad Dermatol* 43(5 Pt 1):733–751, 2000.
15. Scott-Conner CE: The diagnosis and management of breast problems during pregnancy and lactation. *Am J Surg* 170: 401–405, 1995.
16. Wrightson WR: Primary squamous cell carcinoma of the breast presenting as a breast abscess. *Am Surg* 65:1153–1155, 1999.
17. Lopez MJ: Inflammatory breast cancer. *Surg Clin North Am* 76:411–429, 1996.
18. Paradisi F: Antistaphylococcal (MSSA, MRSA, MSSE, MRSE) antibiotics. *Med Clin North Am* 85:1–17, 2001.
19. Jemec GB: The bacteriology of hidradenitis suppurativa. *Dermatology* 193:203–206, 1996.
20. Lemons-Estes FM: Unusual cutaneous infectious and parasitic diseases. *Dermatol Clin* 17:151–185, ix, 1999.
21. Memish ZA, Alazzawi M: Unusual complications of breast implants: *Brucella* infection. *Infection* 29:291–292, 2001.
22. Cernea SS: Lupus mastitis. *J Am Acad Dermatol* 29(2 Pt 2): 343–346, 1993.
23. Pouchot J: Granulomatous mastitis: an uncommon cause of breast abscess. *Arch Intern Med* 161:611–612, 2001.
24. Robinson-Bostom L: Cutaneous manifestations of end-stage renal disease. *J Am Acad Dermatol* 43:975–986, 2000.
25. Goodwin PJ: Breast health and associated premenstrual symptoms in women with severe cyclic mastopathy. *Am J Obstet Gynecol* 176:998–1005, 1997.
26. Ader DN: Prevalence and impact of cyclic mastalgia in a United States clinic-based sample. *Am J Obstet Gynecol* 177:126–132, 1997.
27. Hansen N: Breast disease. *Med Clin North Am* 82:203–222, 1998.
28. Bachman JW, Neinstein LS: Breast disease in adolescents and young women. *Pediatr Clin North Am* 46:607–629, 1999.
29. Peña KS: Evaluation and treatment of galactorrhea. *Am Fam Physician* 63:1763–1770, 2001.
30. Gülay H: Management of nipple discharge. *J Am Coll Surg* 178:471–474, 1994.
31. Rosen PP (ed): Paget's disease of the nipple, in *Rosen's Breast Pathology*, 2d ed. Philadelphia: Lippincott, Williams & Wilkins, 2001, pp 565–579.
32. Majeski J: Shoulder restraint injury to the female breast: a crush injury with long-lasting consequences. *J Trauma* 50:336–338, 2001.
33. Brown SL: Rupture of silicone gel breast implants: causes, sequelae, and diagnosis. *Lancet* 350:1531–1537, 1997.
34. Palmon LU: Ruptured or intact: what can linear echoes within silicone breast implants tell us? *AJR Am J Roentgenol* 168:1595–1598, 1997.
35. Rosen PP (ed): Inflammatory and reactive tumors, in *Rosen's Breast Pathology*, 2d ed. Philadelphia: Lippincott, Williams & Wilkins, 2001, pp 29–63.
36. Pugh CM, DeWitty RL: Mondor's disease. *J Nat Med Assoc* 88:359–363, 1996.
37. American Cancer Society: Cancer facts and figures, 2002. Atlanta, GA: American Cancer Society (www.cancer.org), accessed March 2002.
38. Tartter PI: Delay in diagnosis of breast cancer. *Ann Surg* 229:91–96, 1999.
39. Simon MS: Racial differences in breast cancer survival: the interaction of socioeconomic status and tumor biology. *Am J Obstet Gynecol* 176:S233–S239, 1997.
40. Veronesi U: Conservation surgery after primary chemotherapy in large carcinomas of the breast. *Ann Surg* 222:612–618, 1995.
41. National Cancer Institute: NCI statement on mammography screening, February 21, 2002 update. National Cancer Institute: Bethesda, MD, (www.nci.nih.gov), accessed March 2002.

27

Abnormal Uterine Bleeding

Rita Oregón
Malcolm G. Munro

KEY POINTS

- Dysfunctional uterine bleeding (DUB) is a subset of abnormal uterine bleeding (AUB), and is defined as abnormal bleeding unrelated to pregnancy, exogenous gonadal steroids, intrauterine contraceptive devices (IUDs), or structural uterine pathology.
- The acute care provider must attempt to narrow the differential diagnosis of AUB using history, physical examination, and judiciously selected diagnostic tests in order to initiate appropriate interventions and expedite referral to a specialist, if needed.
- There are two types of DUB unrelated to structural pathology of the genital tract—ovulatory DUB, characterized by cyclical menorrhagia or heavy menstrual bleeding, and anovulatory DUB, which is typically unpredictable in timing and volume of flow.
- Endometrial sampling is used to detect endometrial neoplasia, and should be considered in any woman with chronic abnormal uterine bleeding, particularly above the age of 40.

INTRODUCTION

In the reproductive years, abnormal uterine bleeding (AUB) is defined as bleeding from the uterus that is irregular in amount, timing, or duration. Prior to menarche or following menopause, any uterine bleeding is considered abnormal. The role of the acute care practitioner is to stabilize the patient and assess need for immediate intervention. Diagnosis and ultimate treatment may be left to the specialty practitioner (i.e., gynecologist), but the acute care practitioner should have an understanding of what are believed to be the causes of AUB so that the acute intervention offered is appropriate. In this chapter the physiology of menstruation, the pathogenesis of AUB in the nonpregnant female, and the appropriate evaluation and treatment of affected women are discussed. Dysfunctional uterine bleeding (DUB) is a subset of AUB, and is defined as abnormal bleeding unrelated to pregnancy, exogenous gonadal steroids, intrauterine contraceptive devices (IUDs), or structural uterine pathology, and is estimated to affect up to 20 percent of reproductive-aged women.[1]

PHYSIOLOGY OF MENSTRUATION

Normal menstrual bleeding is orchestrated by cyclical withdrawal of estrogens, largely 17-β estradiol and progesterone, that in the absence of pregnancy, occurs on average 14 days following ovulation. Menses typically last 4 or 5 days, with a normal range of 2 to 7 days. Flow is usually heaviest in the first 2 to 3 days and tapers to spotting in the last 2 to 3 days. The normal volume of blood lost in a single menses averages 30 to 40 mL. Greater than 80 mL is considered excessive, but for the average reproductive-aged North American woman, depletion of iron stores occurs when the monthly blood loss exceeds 60 mL. Menses are normally predictable, with a cycle (first day of one menses to the first day of the next) that ranges from 21 to 35 days. The regulation of menses is dependent upon a number of factors that result in the process of ovulation. Following ovulation, the follicle changes into the corpus luteum, which produces abundant estradiol and progesterone which together exert profound effects on the endometrium. In the absence of pregnancy the demise of the corpus luteum results in withdrawal of the effects of estradiol and progesterone on the endometrium, and culminates in the sloughing and bleeding that comprises menstrual flow.

The normal endometrium has two layers. The *basalis* layer is deep, adjacent to the myometrium, and permanent. The *functionalis* layer comprises the upper two-thirds, and dynamically responds to the sequential effects of ovarian gonadal steroidogenesis. If fertilization and subsequent implantation do not occur, hormonal support from the corpus luteum gradually wanes, leading to a biochemically complex series of endometrial events that result in menstruation (Fig. 27-1).

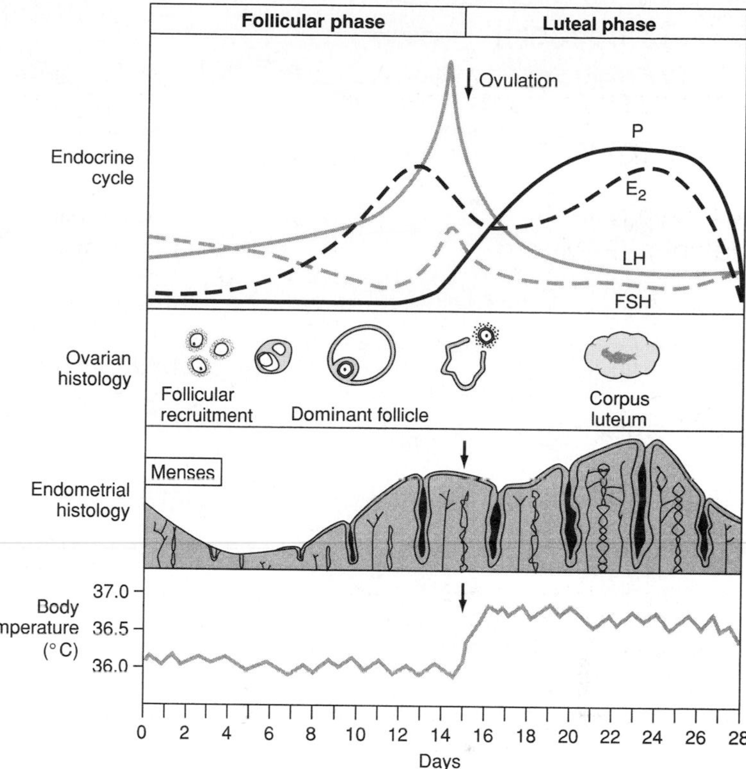

Fig. 27-1. The hormonal, ovarian, endometrial, and basal body temperature changes and relationships throughout the normal menstrual cycle. E_2, estradiol; FSH, follicle-stimulating hormone; LH, luteinizing hormone; P, progesterone. (From Carr BR, Wilson JD: Disorders of the ovary and female reproductive tract, in Isselbacher KJ, Braunwald E, Wilson JD, et al (eds): *Harrison's Principles of Internal Medicine,* 15th ed. New York: McGraw-Hill, 2001, p 2158.)

Knowledge of endometrial physiology is important to understanding the genesis and treatment of many of the causes of AUB. The events immediately leading to menstruation likely commence with ischemia of the functionalis layer, caused by spiral artery vasoconstriction believed to be initiated by the local release of potent vasoconstrictors such as prostaglandin ($PGF_{2\alpha}$) and endothelin-1 (ET-1), which are produced as a result of progestogenic stimulation of an estrogen-primed endometrium. The other important process that contributes to the breakdown of functionalis structure appears to be proteolysis of the extracellular matrix and basement membranes that is initiated by agents such as matrix metalloproteinases (MMPs) and tissue plasminogen activator (tPA).[2,3] The combination of ischemic and proteolytic effects result in breaks in the superficial capillaries and arterioles and destabilization of the weakened functionalis, which finally collapses and sloughs, leaving the basalis intact.

The next steps in the menstrual process are all oriented toward establishing hemostasis and subsequent regeneration of the functionalis layer of the endometrium. The endometrium is unique in that platelets have relatively little role in the process of hemostasis.[4] Instead, endometrial hemostasis relies first upon the presence of local vasoconstrictors, and then on the factors of the extrinsic and intrinsic clotting cascades that result in the formation of a vascular clot.

Once hemostasis has been achieved, the processes of endometrial angiogenesis and reepithelialization must begin to rebuild the functionalis layer, thereby preparing again for implantation should a pregnancy occur. The factors involved in the initiation of angiogenesis are unclear, but appear to be associated with rising estrogen levels as well as local thrombin, tPA, and various subtypes of plasminogen activator.[5,6] Fig. 27-2 is a schematic representation of the endometrium that summarizes the biochemical events that affect it during a menstrual cycle.

ETIOLOGIES OF ABNORMAL UTERINE BLEEDING

Given the variety of medical and structural conditions that result in AUB (Fig. 27-3), it is important for the acute care provider to be able to narrow the differential diagnosis

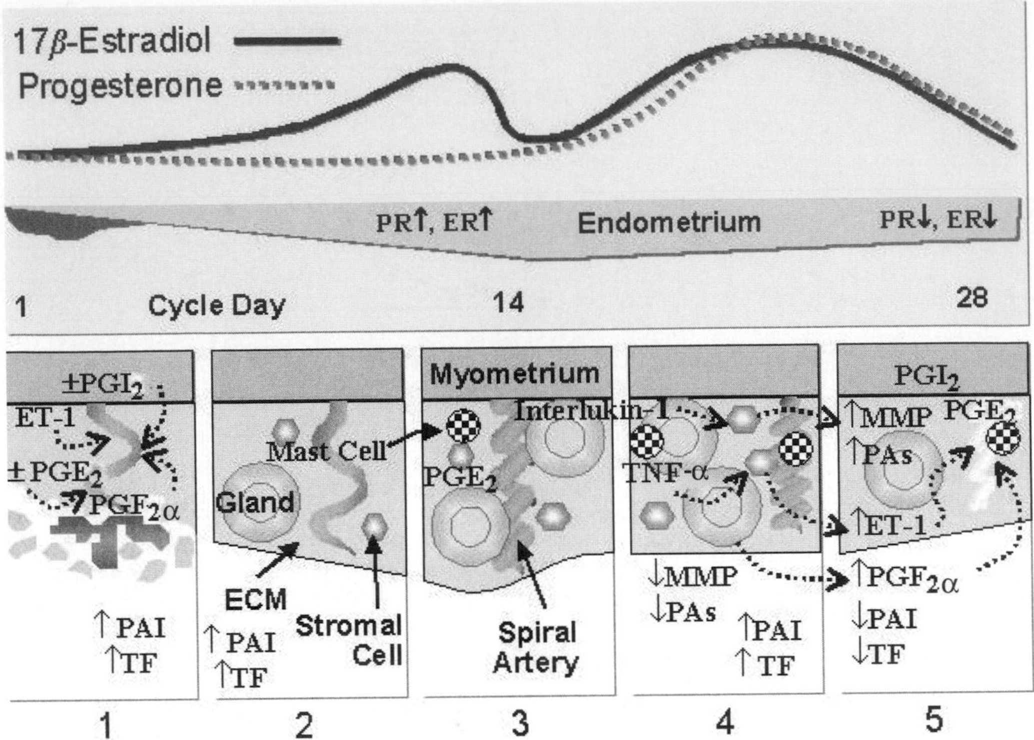

Fig. 27-2. The top panel depicts the systemic production of 17 β-estradiol and progesterone over a stylized endometrium that first responds to unopposed estrogens with growth, and then stabilizes under the influence of the combination of estrogens and progestins from the corpus luteum. While both estrogen (ER) and progesterone (PR) endometrial receptors rise in the proliferative phase of the cycle, the progestagenic influence results in a decrease in both by the later parts of the luteal phase. The bottom five panels depict various endomyometrial biochemical events in the cycle. Panel 1 portrays menstruation. Bleeding volume depends upon primary hemostasis provided by vasoconstrictors like $PGF_{2\alpha}$ and endothelin-1 (ET-1), which is antagonized by endometrial PGE_2, and myometrial PGI_2. Estradiol, plasminogen activator inhibitor (PAI), and tissue factor (TF) promote secondary hemostasis, angiogenesis, and reepithelialization. Panel 2 demonstrates the hemostatic midfollicular endometrium with continuing angiogenesis and growth of glands, stroma, and the extracellular matrix (ECM). In panel 3, the transition from follicular to luteal phase occurs, with increased coiling of the spiral arteries, the continued production of stromal PGE_2, and the appearance of migratory cells including mast cells. The midluteal endometrium depicted in panel 4 is prepared for implantation, but in the absence of conception, the pieces are in place for the induction of endometrial regression and menstruation, shown in panel 5. With the reduction in progestagenic influence, the cytokines interlukin-1 and tumor necrosis factor-α (TNF-α) induce decidualized endometrial stromal cells to produce matrix metalloproteinases (MMP). The levels of plasminogen activator inhibitor and tissue factor decrease in association with rising levels of plasminogen activators (PAs). Collectively, PAs and MMPs break down the components of the ECM, including blood vessels. Vasoconstriction of the spiral arteries is induced by ET-1 from the stromal cells and $PGF_{2\alpha}$, predominantly from endometrial glands, and results in ischemia, necrosis, and sloughing of the components of the functional layer of the endometrium. Bleeding results from a combination of the effects of free radicals, MMPs, and vasodilating agents such as PGE_2 and PGI_2.

to determine and obtain the appropriate diagnostic tests acutely and initiate proper management.

Dysfunctional Uterine Bleeding

Dysfunctional uterine bleeding (DUB) is abnormal bleeding unrelated to pregnancy, exogenous gonadal steroids, an IUD, or structural uterine pathology, and is estimated to affect up to 20 percent of reproductive-aged women.[1] The disorder can be classified as *ovulatory* if bleeding is cyclic and predictable, suggesting that the heavy menstrual flow is occurring despite endometrial exposure to cyclical endogenous progesterone. It is postulated that ovulatory DUB is caused by alterations in one or more of the local mechanisms involved in endometrial hemosta-

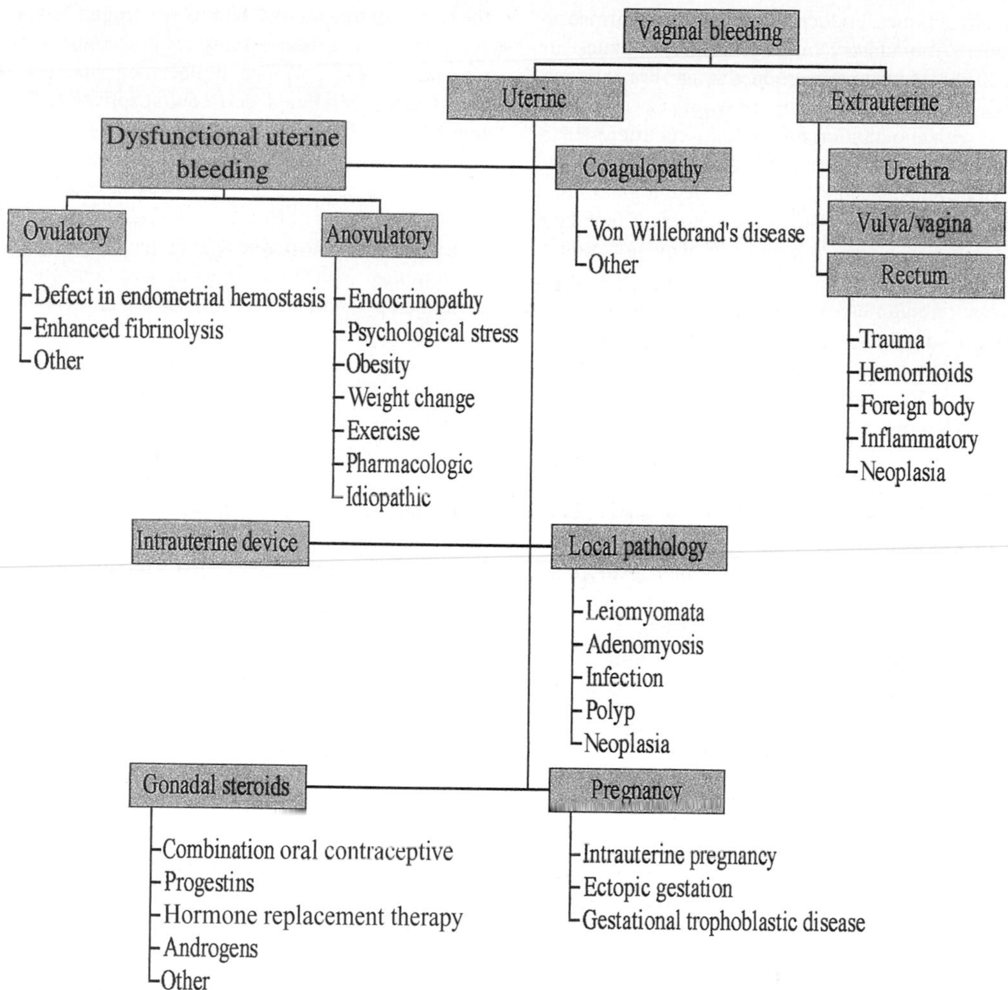

Fig. 27-3. Algorithm of the pathogenesis of abnormal uterine bleeding.

sis. Many authors from other countries, particularly those in Europe, New Zealand, and Australia, use other nomenclature for heavy bleeding in the context of presumed ovulatory cycles, including heavy menstrual bleeding (HMB) or menorrhagia. The latter is a term used by many to define a symptom, not a condition, thereby making the literature on this subject very confusing.

Anovulatory DUB is thought to be estrogen-related bleeding (i.e., bleeding associated with unopposed endogenously-produced estrogens). The bleeding is characteristically irregular in timing and in quantity, including frequent bleeding, episodes of oligomenorrhea (menstrual intervals >35 days), or even amenorrhea (no menses for 6 months). In these instances, the progesterone secreted by the corpus luteum after ovulation does not counter the proliferative effect of estrogen on the endometrium. The endometrial lining then becomes thickened with crowded glands, increased vascularity, and lack of stromal support, and thus sloughs at unpredictable intervals. The absence of locally produced substances that enhance hemostasis (e.g., endothelin-1 and $PGF_{2\alpha}$), which are dependent in large part upon the presence of progesterone, may add to the symptoms by facilitating heavy flow. It should be noted that many women alternate between ovulatory and anovulatory states and are often characterized as oligo-ovulatory.

There are many possible reasons for a woman to be anovulatory, including those related to psychological stress, lifestyle issues, endocrinopathies, and pharmaceutical agents. Anovulatory or oligo-ovulatory states are common at the extremes of reproductive age. For example, in teenagers, an immature pituitary-ovarian axis may be associated with anovulation for the first year after menarche, and women in their 40s and 50s frequently experience anovulatory cycles. Acute or chronic psychological stress can induce anovulatory dysfunctional uterine bleeding, and if isolated to a transient episode, may not require chronic therapy. Lifestyle factors such as weight gain, weight loss, or endurance training are frequently associated with anovulation and resultant amenorrhea or ovulatory dysfunctional uterine bleeding. Clinical or subclinical hypothyroidism may impact ovulation via increased levels of thyrotropin-releasing hormone (TRH), which increases the production of prolactin from the anterior pituitary gland.[7,8] Hyperprolactinemia itself is also known to impact the pituitary-ovarian axis and cause anovulation. Hyperandrogenic insulin-resistant states such as polycystic ovarian syndrome (PCOS) often have high levels of unopposed systemic estrogen and are commonly associated with anovulation.[9] Obesity is associated with increased peripheral conversion of androgens from both the ovary and the adrenal gland to estrone, thereby increasing the amount of circulating estrogens. Insulin resistance may also play a role in obesity-associated anovulation.[10]

There are a number of pharmaceutical agents that are known or suspected to affect ovulation. These include gonadal steroids (estrogens, progestins, and androgens), and drugs known to affect dopamine metabolism such as tricyclic antidepressants and phenothiazines. It is unclear how homeopathic drugs may affect ovulatory function, but many contain elements of gonadal steroids or other substances that may have an effect on the normal function of the pituitary-hypothalamic-ovarian axis.

Coagulopathies

Coagulopathies need to be considered in the differential diagnosis of both adolescent and adult women with heavy menstrual bleeding.[11] The prevalence of occult bleeding disorders (e.g., von Willebrand's disease [vWD], factor deficiency, or platelet abnormality) was estimated to be 10.7 to 20 percent of women with menorrhagia in one series of patients referred to hematology.[12]

Bleeding Secondary to Exogenous Gonadal Steroids

Women who are being treated with exogenous gonadal steroids (estrogens, progestins, and/or androgens) may experience uterine bleeding at some point, usually early in the course of treatment. Combined estrogen and progestin formulations are used extensively for contraception and postmenopausal hormone replacement therapy (HRT). Those using combined oral contraceptives (COC) have breakthrough bleeding 30 to 40 percent of the time in the first 3 cycles of use, which is a nuisance that fortunately tends to decrease in quantity with each subsequent month of exposure.[13] However, women who use COCs inconsistently may experience irregular bleeding that does not diminish with time. Conventional hormone replacement therapy combines a continuous estrogen with either a continuous or cyclical progestin. Cyclical progestins generally result in predictable and cyclical withdrawal bleeding that starts near the end of the progestin phase, or shortly after it is discontinued. However, continuous progestagen regimens such as the common North American formulation of conjugated equine estrogen and medroxyprogesterone acetate (CEE/MPA) are associated with bleeding in 60 percent of women and bleeding and/or spotting in 83 percent in the first 3 months of use.[14] Most women (approximately 90 percent) using these regimens become amenorrheic at 1 year.[15]

Progestin-only contraceptive therapeutic regimens, such as injectable depo-medroxyprogesterone acetate (DMPA), oral progestins, and subdermal progestin implants, are notorious for causing AUB.

Postcoital or emergency contraception may comprise either a combined estrogen-progestin formulation or a progestin-only regimen, and is also associated with AUB. Usually the patient experiences a delay of menses, but one study showed that up to 70 percent of women complained of short-term menstrual irregularities.[16]

Intrauterine Contraceptive Devices

Use of non-hormone-containing intrauterine devices (IUDs) is known to frequently result in increased menstrual bleeding and irregular spotting or bleeding between menses. The cause may be related to one or a combination of local inflammatory reaction and foreign body-induced enhancement of endometrial fibrinolytic activity.[6] An increase of menstrual flow of anywhere from 30 to 55 percent has been seen with the copper-containing or inert IUD.[5,17] Approximately 15 percent of IUDs are removed because of excessive bleeding. Despite these observations, intermenstrual spotting or bleeding may still reflect a pathologic process such as chlamydial cervicitis or an ectopic pregnancy, and consequently should be investigated as if no IUD were present.

The levonorgestrel intrauterine system (LNG-IUS) is a progestin-impregnated IUD that is associated with an initial increase in the mean number of bleeding and spotting days, but in 3 to 6 months the number of bleeding and spotting days is the same as seen in copper IUD users. Additionally, during the first year of use, 20 percent of women become amenorrheic, which is a potentially beneficial side effect in some women with dysfunctional uterine bleeding (see therapy section, below).[18]

Abnormal Bleeding Secondary to Local Pathology

Some women who experience abnormal vaginal bleeding may be experiencing a symptom that originates from lower in the genital tract than the uterine corpus. Vaginal trauma from lacerations or foreign bodies may be associated with bleeding. Vaginitis, particularly when associated with pruritus, irritation, and excoriation, can provoke some vaginal spotting either with or without contact. Cervicitis, particularly when secondary to chlamydial infection, can be associated with cervical friability and subsequent vaginal bleeding, either spontaneously or following contact such as that which occurs with intercourse or the insertion of a contraceptive diaphragm.[19,20]

Endometritis, be it acute or chronic in nature, is frequently associated with abnormal bleeding. Endometrial hyperplasia and carcinomas of the vulva, vagina, cervix, and endometrium are other important local causes that must be considered when evaluating an individual with abnormal bleeding or spotting.

Within the uterine corpus, leiomyomata (especially submucous leiomyomas) are suspected to cause heavy menstrual bleeding by interfering with the normal hemostatic mechanisms of the endometrium. Postmenopausal women rarely manifest abnormal bleeding related to myomas unless they are using HRT. Intracavitary endometrial polyps or polyps of the cervical canal typically cause unpredictable bleeding, and may produce symptoms in both premenopausal and postmenopausal women.

Adenomyosis is a somewhat enigmatic disorder characterized by the presence of endometrial glands deep in the stroma of the myometrium. It is generally associated with heavy menstrual bleeding secondary to altered angiogenesis and subsequent deficient hemostatic mechanisms in the abnormal vessels.[21] There may be a history of severe dysmenorrhea, and on physical examination the uterus is symmetric and globular. If examined at the time of menses, the uterus is diffusely tender.

CLINICAL ASSESSMENT

Even in the reproductive years, the elements of the clinical assessment vary somewhat with the age of the patient. Obviously, in any age group assessment of volume status is the first priority. Bleeding to the point of hypovolemia will require that appropriate steps are taken to establish one or more intravenous lines, restore circulating blood volume, and monitor the response to therapy appropriately. Such circumstances require that blood products be made available and immediate consultation with a gynecologist be obtained. Fortunately, in most instances the patient does not present in such an acute condition, and the clinician may take the time to pursue the investigation in a more circumspect fashion. In the reproductive years, regardless of the age of the patient, it is important to evaluate for pregnancy with a urine or serum assay of β-human chorionic gonadotropin (β-hCG). This includes adolescents, many of whom will not readily admit to sexual activity, especially in the presence of their parent or guardian.

Presentation, History, and Physical Findings

Adolescent

Given the frequency of anovulation or oligo-ovulation in this age group, questions that will help determine the patient's ovulatory status should be asked. This can be difficult depending on the maturity of the patient, and it may be necessary to involve the parent or guardian in the process. Details are very important, and provide information that cannot be ascertained from laboratory investigation. The age of menarche (onset of menses), and menstrual history, including the interval, predictability, and duration of bleeding, in addition to the presence or absence of symptoms of ovulation should be elicited. Any history of easy bruising or bleeding should also be specifically asked about because heavy menstrual bleeding may be the presenting sign of an otherwise occult systemic coagulopathy, particularly in adolescents.

On physical examination, one should look for obesity, evidence of eating disorders such as anorexia or bulimia, and signs of anemia such as pale conjunctiva or mucus membranes or delayed capillary refill. One should note secondary sexual characteristics and look for evidence of androgen excess, such as severe acne or hirsutism. The pelvic examination is one element that must be considered carefully in this age group. See Chap. 23 for discussion of techniques for examining the pelvis in adolescents. The goals of the examination should be to detect lower genital tract pathology that would explain the abnormal uterine bleeding. Many will not have had such an examination before, and some may still be virginal. Consequently, an individual with appropriate training and experience in the assessment of adolescents should perform the examination carefully and gently.

Reproductive-Age Women

In the nonpregnant reproductive-age female, the menstrual history should be taken as described above for adolescents, and the possibility of a congenital coagulopathy should also be considered. The clinician should also diligently search for evidence of endocrinopathies with symptoms such as galactorrhea, evolving hirsutism, or symptoms of thyroid disease. The past medical history may be important in this regard, and the psychiatric history is relevant both as a de novo cause for anovulation, and because therapy with tricyclic antidepressants or phenothiazines may directly contribute to anovulation. The surgical history may be significant, because recent surgery on the reproductive tract may contribute to uterine bleeding, either in an expected fashion or because of a complication. It is important to inquire about the use of other medications suspected to interfere with ovulatory function, including herbal medicine and contraceptives. A sexual history should be taken and the risk for STDs assessed, because infections with *Chlamydia trachomatis* may cause abnormal uterine bleeding from either the cervix or endometrial cavity.

On physical examination, one should note potential contributors to anovulation, including anorexia or obesity, acne, hirsutism, or thyromegaly. A speculum examination, Pap smear (if it has been longer than 1 year since her last smear and there is a mechanism for obtaining results and ensuring follow-up in case of abnormal findings), and swabs for chlamydial antigen should be obtained. A careful inspection of the lower tract and cervix should be performed to search for focal lesions such as polyps or neoplasms, as well as evidence of trauma. The bimanual examination is of limited utility when searching for causes of abnormal uterine bleeding, as lesions within the endometrial cavity cannot be palpated, and frequently, palpable lesions of the uterus may be asymptomatic and not contributing to the bleeding itself. Nevertheless, it is prudent to conduct a careful bimanual examination, noting any uterine enlargement (often the first clue that a patient's symptoms are due to fibroids), or tenderness of the cervix, uterus, or adnexa. A rectovaginal examination may be useful, particularly to delineate findings in the posterior pelvis.

Postmenopausal Patients

Some aspects of the assessment of the postmenopausal female are distinctly different from those of adolescents and other women in their reproductive years. Clearly, there is no current "normal" menstrual function, although it is important to discern the age of menopause, in addition to the features of the presenting problem, including the onset and duration of the bleeding, as well as factors that may have exacerbated it. Given that neoplastic disease is a very common cause of bleeding in this age group, a history of constitutional symptoms should be noted. In this age group, the use of exogenous gonadal steroids is frequently associated with abnormal bleeding, but should not be presumed to be the cause until an appropriate evaluation is undertaken. Note that psychotropic medications are not likely contributors to abnormal uterine bleeding in this population, for there is no normal pituitary-hypothalamic-ovarian axis with which to interfere. Postmenopausal women are more likely to have medical disorders that may contribute to abnormal uterine bleeding. One example is breast cancer, for which many take tamoxifen, an agent with estrogenic activity that frequently contributes to abnormal uterine bleeding and which is occasionally associated with endometrial neoplasia. Postmenopausal women are not exempt from the acquisition of STDs, and the patient should also be questioned and evaluated accordingly.

In addition to urine or serum assay for β-hCG, the basic laboratory investigation should include a hematocrit and a platelet count. Consider sending coagulation studies if the patient's history warrants. A prolactin level and thyroid function tests might be appropriate to send to begin the outpatient work-up.

Endometrial sampling is used to detect endometrial neoplasia, and should be considered in any woman age $\geq$40 years with chronic AUB, because of the increased risk of endometrial hyperplasia and carcinoma. For women with postmenopausal bleeding, endometrial sampling remains a standard approach. However, for postmenopausal women who are not using HRT, the use of transvaginal ultrasound (TVUS) to measure the thickness of the endometrial echo complex (EEC) is an equally effective and less invasive technique. An EEC <4 mm can reliably exclude endometrial neoplasia (Fig. 27-4).[22,23]

Neither physical examination nor endometrial sampling will allow for structural evaluation of the uterus and uterine cavity. Hysteroscopy has generally been considered the gold standard for the structural assessment of the endometrial cavity;[24–27] however, similarly accurate data can be obtained with TVUS that is performed simultaneously with the instillation of saline into the endometrial cavity, a process that allows for contrast imaging (Fig. 27-5 and Fig. 27-6). This process is known by a number of synonymous terms, including sonohysterography (SHG), hysterosonography, and saline infusion sonography (SIS).[28,29] Some have shown that TVUS is also an effective screening technique for structural anomalies involving the endometrial cavity, such as polyps and

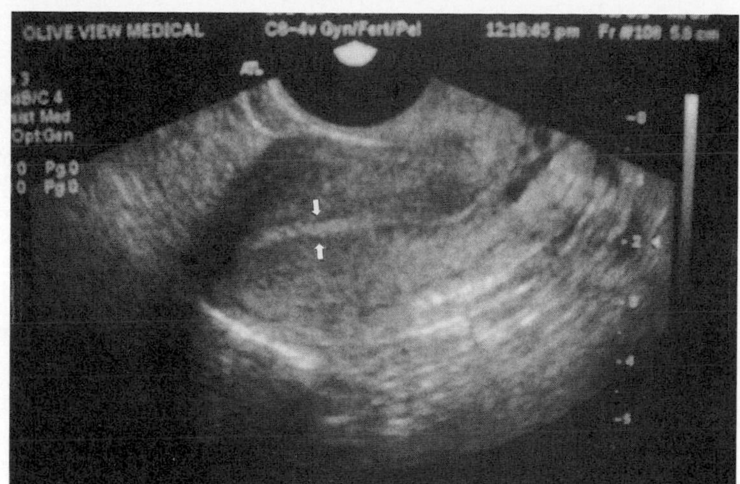

Fig. 27-4. Transvaginal ultrasound showing a thin endometrial stripe (*between arrows*). (Courtesy Gail C. Hansen, MD, Olive View-UCLA Medical Center Department of Radiology.)

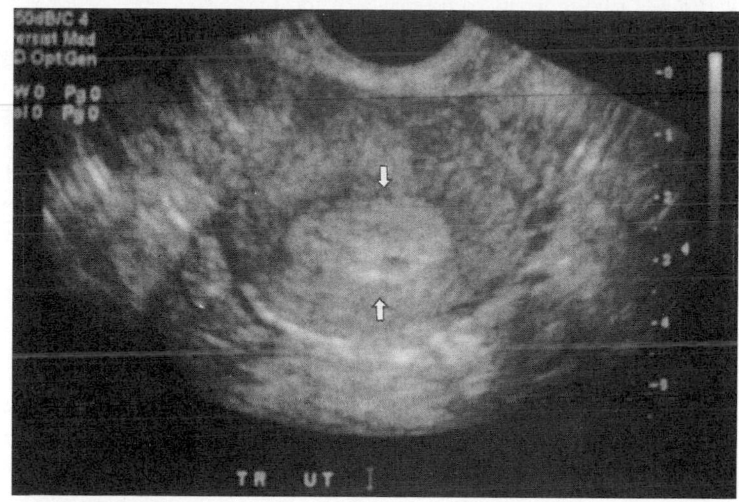

Fig. 27-5. Transvaginal ultrasound showing a thickened endometrial stripe (*between arrows*). (Courtesy Gail C. Hansen, MD, Olive View-UCLA Medical Center Department of Radiology.)

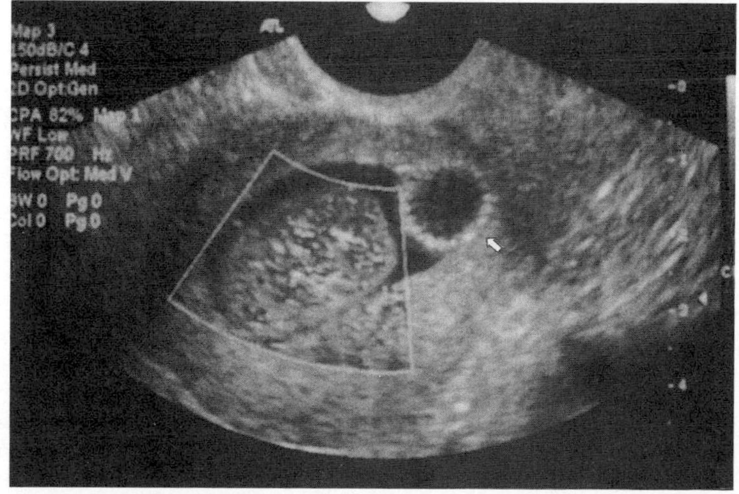

Fig. 27-6. Saline infusion sonogram in the same patient as in Fig. 27-5, showing an intracavitary myoma (*outlined*). The catheter bulb sits adjacent to the myoma (*arrow*). (Courtesy Gail C. Hansen, MD, Olive View-UCLA Medical Center Department of Radiology.)

leiomyomas, especially in postmenopausal women not on HRT.[30]

THERAPY

Acute Episode

When a patient presents to an emergency department or urgent care center for abnormal uterine bleeding, it is usually because of excessive bleeding or symptoms secondary to anemia. When the patient appears hypovolemic, the most important first steps are to stabilize the patient and assess if her blood loss warrants immediate transfusion and inpatient care, or if her anemia is less severe and she is a candidate for outpatient management. If the bleeding is not secondary to pregnancy, if focal lesions such as lacerations are not determined to be the cause of the bleeding, and if the bleeding is determined to emanate from the endometrial cavity, attempts are made to stop the bleeding by medical or mechanical means.

Gonadal Steroids

Estrogens

Immediate therapy for severe symptomatic bleeding may consist of high-dose conjugated equine estrogens given intravenously. Although the mechanism of action of this approach is unclear, there is evidence of its effectiveness from one high-quality trial.[31] The usual dosage is 25 mg IV every 4 hours for no longer than 48 hours. Typical responses are demonstrated by 5 hours following the initiation of treatment. Although there is no evidence that such short-term therapy increases thrombotic risk, it may be prudent to consider a patient's smoking history and other factors that may increase the risk of thromboembolic phenomena.

Progestins

In adolescent girls with menorrhagia, treatment with medroxyprogesterone acetate (MPA) at 60 mg orally on day 1, followed by 20 mg orally daily for 10 days has been shown to be effective. However, luteal phase MPA (i.e. 10 mg orally for 10 days) has not been found to be effective management of menorrhagia.

Combined Estrogens and Progestins

Combined oral contraceptive pills (OCPs) have long been one of the mainstays of therapy for menorrhagia in North America. One suggested regimen uses 2 tablets of a low-dose (less than 50 mcg of ethinyl estradiol) monophasic (constant dosages of estrogen and progestin in each active pill) OCP daily for 1 week, and then decreasing to 1 tablet daily for successive cycles of therapy.[5] Although there are no studies that have subjected such an approach to the rigorous evaluation of a clinical trial,[32] there is a large amount of level 3 (expert opinion) data that support combined OCP use.

Mechanical Therapy

Acute treatment of AUB may also consist of mechanical tamponade with balloon catheters. There are many reports in the literature of using either large Foley catheter balloons or the Sengstaken-Blakemore tube (a 300-mL gastric tube) for obstetric or postpartum hemorrhage[33–36] and for gynecologic hemorrhage.[37] Packing the uterus or vagina with long packing gauze is also a consideration in cases of acute hemorrhage, regardless of the etiology. Packing has become less popular due to the increasingly diverse options for therapy, but it may still be utilized—even if only as a temporary measure until the patient is stabilized or other therapies can be administered. These procedures are simple to perform and the materials needed are usually accessible in the emergency department or urgent care center.

Vascular Occlusion

Successful treatment of gynecologic and obstetric hemorrhage has been reported with selective uterine artery occlusion by interventional radiologic techniques. For treatment of hemorrhage associated with fibroids, success rates of 82 to 92 percent have been cited.[38] Of course, this requires that there be interventional radiologists available, and that they are experienced in performing these procedures.

Chronic Management by Diagnosis

Bleeding secondary to coagulopathies such as vWD has been shown to respond to treatment with combined oral contraceptive therapy.[39] The American College of Obstetricians and Gynecologists suggests that even hormonally-induced amenorrhea may be appropriate in these patients.[11] Desmopressin acetate via intranasal spray is the preferred treatment for patients with type I disease if they do not desire contraception. They may use the spray either just prior to or with the onset of menses.[40]

Bleeding secondary to gonadal steroid administration requires investigation into the medication used, the dosage, and the compliance of the patient with the regimen that was prescribed. If the patient is found to be compliant, it may be necessary to adjust the dosages of estrogen or progestin in a regimen, or add estrogen or progestin to a single-agent regimen. For example, a woman having prolonged spotting while using an oral contraceptive pill with a very low dose of estrogen (e.g., 20 mcg ethinyl estradiol) may benefit by simply switching to a 35 mcg ethinyl estradiol pill. On the other hand, abnormal uterine bleeding in women using long-acting injectable progestin contraceptives (i.e., DMPA) has not been shown to be significantly or consistently improved by exogenous estrogen administration.[41] In these patients, careful counseling and reassurance may be necessary.

IUD users experiencing AUB may find nonsteroidal antiinflammatory drugs (NSAIDs) to be effective in treating bleeding. Ibuprofen and naproxen have both been shown effective in small studies.[42,43]

Bleeding caused by local pathology likely requires therapy specific to the pathology, some of which may be diagnosed in the ED. Other entities require follow-up with a primary care physician or specialist. Vaginal or vulvar lesions may require resection or cauterization to control bleeding and/or for histologic investigation. Lacerations may require surgical repair. Vaginitis, cervicitis, and endometritis should be treated with the appropriate antibiotic therapy, and further investigation should be performed to look for other STDs. Vulvar, vaginal, cervical, or endometrial carcinomas should be referred to a gynecologic oncologist. Endometrial hyperplasia may be treated with any one of several regimens that include a progestational agent. Leiomyomas will require different therapy depending on their location. When leiomyomas are intramural or subserosal in location, it is unlikely that they contribute to AUB. Consequently, and regardless of the presence or absence of such myomas, AUB without intracavitary pathology must be considered to be dysfunctional and appropriate treatment options should be offered (see below). Endocervical polyps may be removed easily in the emergency department by twisting or cutting them off. However, if they are particularly broad-based they may require operative resection. An endometrial polyp that is prolapsing through the cervix may be twisted off, but if it is not visible, or if emergent removal is otherwise not possible, it will require either hysteroscopic resection or manual extraction with polyp forceps after cervical dilatation. Adenomyosis may respond to NSAID therapy alone, possibly combined with oral contraceptive therapy. If refractory, such bleeding may require GnRH-agonist therapy (e.g., leuprolide acetate) for at least temporary relief.[44] However, women with recalcitrant adenomyosis frequently require hysterectomy.

If a patient is deemed to suffer from DUB, it is preferable to make a determination regarding the ovulatory status. Ovulatory DUB (synonymous with HMB or menorrhagia) may be approached as follows:

- Nonsteroidal antiinflammatory agents (e.g., mefenamic acid, naproxen, ibuprofen) started either at or just before the start of the menstrual period and continued for its duration can decrease menstrual blood loss by 25 to 35 percent.[45,46] There is no evidence that one NSAID is superior to another.
- Combined oral contraceptive pills are effective in at least 50 percent of women with ovulatory DUB. Although there is no evidence that one type of product is superior to another, a monophasic formulation with abundant progestogenic activity would be preferable.
- A regimen of long-course or high-dose norethisterone (norethindrone) 10 to 15 mg daily for 21 days of each cycle is effective.[47] Whereas cyclical luteal phase progestins have been demonstrated to be ineffective for the treatment of chronic ovulatory DUB, administration of high doses of progestins for the majority of the cycle is effective. This is most likely because ovulation is suppressed and the direct effects of the progestin on the endometrium are profound.
- The levonorgestrel intrauterine system (LNG-IUS)[48] has been shown to be one of the most effective newer approaches to therapy for women with ovulatory DUB. This 5-year intrauterine system, though originally developed for contraception, decreases menstrual bleeding by 80 percent at 3 months, and by more than 95 percent by 12 months after insertion.[49] Women were also more likely to continue treatment and be satisfied with the LNG-IUS than with norethisterone therapy. In one study, 64.3 percent of women who were scheduled for hysterectomy cancelled their surgery after agreeing to use the LNG-IUS.[50]
- Antifibrinolytic agents (e.g., tranexamic acid) have been shown to significantly decrease menstrual blood loss by approximately 50 percent, without nuisance or serious side effects.[51,52] The typical dosage is 1 mg four times per day during the menstrual period. However, these agents are not available in the U.S.
- Danazol in doses of 50 to 200 mg per day has been found to be highly effective in decreasing HMB, but the side effects are unacceptable to most women.[53]

Patients who fail to respond to first-line therapy should be referred for further evaluation, including assessment of the endometrial cavity with one or a combination of TVUS, SIS, and hysteroscopy. D& C is thought not to be effective in the chronic treatment of menorrhagia.

REFERENCES

1. Hallberg L, Hogdahl A, Nilsson L, Rybo G: Menstrual blood loss—a population study. *Acta Obstet Gynecol Scand* 45:320–351, 1966.
2. Littlefield BA: Plasminogen activators in endometrial physiology and embryo implantation: a review. *Ann N Y Acad Sci* 622:167–175, 1991.
3. Gleeson NC: Cyclic changes in endometrial tissue plasminogen activator and plasminogen activator inhibitor type 1 in women with normal menstruation and essential menorrhagia. *Am J Obstet Gynecol* 171:178–183, 1994.
4. Gelety TJ, Chaudhuri G: Homeostatic mechanism in the endometrium: role of cyclo-oxygenase products and coagulation factors. *Br J Pharmacol* 114:975–980, 1995.
5. Speroff L, Glass RH, Kase NG: *Clinical Gynecologic Endocrinology and Infertility*, 6th ed. Baltimore, MD: Lippincott Williams & Wilkins, 1999.
6. Munro MG: Abnormal uterine bleeding in the reproductive years: Part I, Pathogenesis and clinical investigation. *J Am Assoc Gynecol Laparosc* 6:393–416, 1999.
7. Koutras DA: Disturbances of menstruation in thyroid disease. *Ann NY Acad Sci.* 816:280–284, 1997.
8. Eskildsen PC, Kirkegaard CB: The influence of thyroid disorders on the dopaminergic regulation of prolactin, thyrotropin and growth hormone. *J Endocrinol Invest* 8:427–431 1985.
9. Rajkhowa M, Bicknell J, Jones M, Clayton RN: Insulin sensitivity in women with polycystic ovary syndrome: relationship to hyperandrogenemia. *Fertil Steril* 61:605–612, 1994.
10. Moran C, Hernandez E, Ruiz JE, et al: Upper body obesity and hyperinsulinemia are associated with anovulation. *Gynecol Obstet Invest* 47:1–5, 1999.
11. American College of Obstetricians and Gynecologists: Von Willebrand's disease in gynecologic practice. ACOG committee opinion no. 263. *Obstet Gynecol* 98:1185–1186, 2001.
12. Edlund M, Blomback M, von Schoultz B, Andersson O: On the value of menorrhagia as a predictor for coagulation disorders. *Am J Hematol* 53:234–238, 1996.
13. Rosenberg MJ, Long SC: Oral contraceptives and cycle control: a critical review of the literature. *Adv Contracept* 8:35–45, 1992.
14. Johnson JV, Davidson M, Archer D, Bachmann G: Postmenopausal uterine bleeding profiles with two forms of continuous combined hormone replacement therapy. *Menopause* 9:16–22, 2002.
15. Archer DF, Pickar JH: Hormone replacement therapy: effect of progestin dose and time since menopause on endometrial bleeding. *Obstet Gynecol* 96:899–905, 2000.
16. Efficacy and side effects of immediate postcoital levonorgestrel used repeatedly for contraception. United Nations Development Programme/United Nations Population Fund/World Health Organization/World Bank Special Programme of Research, Development and Research Training in Human Reproduction, Task Force on Post-Ovulatory Methods of Fertility Regulation. *Contraception* 61:303–308, 2000.
17. Nelson AL: The intrauterine contraceptive device. *Obstet Gynecol Clin North Am* 27:723–740, 2000.
18. Lahteenmaki P, Rauramo I, Backman T: The levonorgestrel intrauterine system in contraception. *Steroids* 65:693–697, 2000.
19. Brenner PF: Differential diagnosis of abnormal uterine bleeding. *Am J Obstet Gynecol* 175(3 pt 2):766–769, 1996.
20. French JI: Abnormal bleeding associated with reproductive tract infection. *NAACOGS Clin Issu Perinat Womens Health Nurs.* 2:313–321, 1991.
21. Hickey M, Fraser IS: Clinical implications of disturbances of uterine vascular morphology and function. *Baillieres Best Pract Res Clin Obstet Gynaecol* 14:937–951, 2000.
22. Ferrazzi E, Torri V, Trio D, et al: Sonographic endometrial thickness: a useful test to predict atrophy in patients with postmenopausal bleeding. An Italian multicenter study. *Ultrasound Obstet Gynecol* 7:315–321, 1996.
23. Gull B, Carlsson S, Karlsson B, et al: Transvaginal ultrasonography of the endometrium in women with postmenopausal bleeding: is it always necessary to perform an endometrial biopsy? *Am J Obstet Gynecol* 182:509–515, 2000.
24. Epstein E, Ramirez A, Skoog L, Valentin L: Dilatation and curettage fails to detect most focal lesions in the uterine cavity in women with postmenopausal bleeding. *Acta Obstet Gynecol Scand* 80:1131–1136, 2001.
25. Valle RF: Hysteroscopic evaluation of patients with abnormal uterine bleeding. *Surg Gynecol Obstet* 153:521–526, 1981.
26. Gimpleson RJ, Rappold HO: A comparative study between panoramic hysteroscopy with directed biopsies and dilatation and curettage. A review of 276 cases. *Am J Obstet Gynecol* 158:489–492, 1988.
27. Loffer FD: Hysteroscopy with selective endometrial sampling compared with D& C for abnormal uterine bleeding: the value of a negative hysteroscopic view. *Obstet Gynecol* 73:16–20, 1989.
28. Widrich T, Bradley LD, Mitchinson AR, Collinc RL: Comparison of saline infusion sonography with office hysteroscopy for the evaluation of the endometrium. *Am J Obstet Gynecol* 174:1327–1334, 1996.
29. Saidi MH, Sadler RK, Theis VD, et al: Comparison of sonography, sonohysterography, and hysteroscopy for evaluation of abnormal uterine bleeding. *J Ultrasound Med* 16:587–591, 1997.
30. Emanuel MH, Verdel MJ, Wamsteker K, Lammes FB: A prospective comparison of transvaginal ultrasonography and diagnostic hysteroscopy in the evaluation of patients with abnormal uterine bleeding: clinical implications. *Am J Obstet Gynecol* 172:547–552, 1995.
31. DeVore GR, Owens O, Kase N: Use of intravenous Premarin in the treatment of dysfunctional uterine bleeding—a double-blind randomized control study. *Obstet Gynecol* 59: 285–291, 1982.

32. Nelson L, Rybo G: Treatment of menorrhagia. *Am J Obstet Gynecol* 110:713, 1971.
33. Bowen LW, Beeson JH: Use of a large Foley catheter balloon to control postpartum hemorrhage resulting from a low placental implantation. *J Reprod Med* 30:623–625, 1985.
34. Bakri YN, Amri A, Abdul Jabbar F: Tamponade-balloon for obstetrical bleeding. *Int J Gynaecol Obstet* 74:139–142, 2001.
35. Katesmark M, Brown R, Raju KS: Successful use of a Sengstaken-Blakemore tube to control massive postpartum hemorrhage. *Br J Obstet Gynaecol* 101:1023–1024, 1993.
36. Johanson R, Kumar M, Obhrai M, Young P: Management of massive postpartum haemorrhage: use of a hydrostatic balloon catheter to avoid laparotomy. *Br J Obstet Gynaecol* 108:420–422, 2001.
37. DeLoor JA, van Dam PA: Foley catheters for uncontrollable obstetric or gynecologic hemorrhage. *Obstet Gynecol* 88(4 pt 2):737, 1996.
38. Pelage JP, LeDref O, Soyer P, et al: Fibroid-related menorrhagia: treatment with superselective embolization of the uterine arteries and midterm follow-up. *Radiology* 215:428–431, 2000.
39. *Foster PA*: The reproductive health of women with von Willebrand disease unresponsive to DDAVP: results of an international survey. On behalf of the Subcommittee on von Willebrand Factor of the Scientific and Standardization Committee of the ISTH. *Thromb Haemost* 74:784–790, 1995.
40. Lethagen S: Desmopressin in the treatment of women's bleeding disorders. *Haemophilia* 5:233–237, 1994.
41. Fraser IS: A survey of different approaches to management of menstrual disturbances in women using injectable contraceptives. *Contraception* 28:385–397, 1983.
42. Roy S, Shaw ST: Role of prostaglandins in IUD-associated uterine bleeding—effect of a prostaglandin synthetase inhibitor (ibuprofen). *Obstet Gynecol* 58:101–106, 1981.
43. Davies AJ, Anderson AB, Turnbull AC: Reduction of excessive menstrual bleeding in women using intrauterine devices. *Obstet Gynecol* 57:74–78, 1981.
44. Nelson JR, Corson SL: Long-term management of adenomyosis with a gonadotropin-releasing hormone agonist: a case report. *Fertil Steril* 59:441, 1993.
45. Lethaby A, Augood C, Duckitt K: Nonsteroidal anti-inflammatory drugs for heavy menstrual bleeding (Cochrane Review), in: The Cochrane Library, 1. Oxford: Update Software, 2002.
46. Shaw RW: Assessment of medical treatments for menorrhagia. *Br J Obstet Gynaecol* 101(suppl)11:15–18, 1994.
47. Fraser IS: Treatment of ovulatory and anovulatory dysfunctional uterine bleeding with oral progestogens. *Aust N Z J Obstet Gynaecol* 30:353–356, 1990.
48. Irvine GA, Campbell-Brown MB, Lumsden MA, et al: Randomised comparative trial of the levonorgestrel intrauterine system and norethisterone for the treatment of idiopathic menorrhagia. *Br J Obstet Gynaecol* 105:592–598, 1998.
49. Lethaby A, Cooke I, Rees M: Progesterone/progestogen releasing intrauterine systems versus either placebo or any other medication for heavy menstrual bleeding (Cochrane Review), in: The Cochrane Library, 1. Oxford: Update Software, 2002.
50. Lahteenmaki P, Haukkamaa M, Puolakka J, et al: Open randomised study of use of levonorgestrel releasing intrauterine system as alternative to hysterectomy. *BMJ* 316 (7138):1122–6, 1998.
51. Royal College of Obstetricians and Gynaecologists: The Initial Management of Menorrhagia (Guideline no. 1). Feb 1998.
52. Lethaby A, Farquhar C, Cooke I: Antifibrinolytics for heavy menstrual bleeding (Cochrane Review), in: The Cochrane Library, 1. Oxford: Update Software, 2002.
53. Need JA, Forbes KL, Milazzo L, McKenzie E: Danazol in the treatment of menorrhagia: the effect of a 1 month induction dose (200 mg) and a 2 month's maintenance therapy (200 mg, 100 mg, 50 mg, or placebo). *Aust N Z J Obstet Gynaecol* 32:346–352, 1992.

28

Acute Abdominal Pain in Women of Childbearing Age

Reb Close
Judith E. Tintinalli

KEY POINTS

- For any woman of childbearing age with a presumptive diagnosis of PID or UTI, always consider appendicitis.
- Conversely, in women of childbearing age, clinical diagnosis of appendicitis is inaccurate in up to 45 percent of cases.
- Periappendiceal inflammation may result in both red and white blood cells seen on urinalysis, mimicking UTI or nephrolithiasis.
- Pelvic examination is helpful in women with lower abdominal pain, vaginal bleeding or discharge, to identify masses, cervical and vaginal lesions, obtain specimens for culture, and to identify sources of bleeding.
- All women of childbearing age are suspected to be pregnant until proven otherwise.

The goal of this chapter is to provide an approach to the diagnosis of acute abdominal pain in the woman of childbearing age, and to provide discussion on the most important gastrointestinal, genitourinary and gynecologic causes of acute abdominal pain in women. The reader is directed to standard references, for more specific discussion on disorders which can cause acute abdominal pain.

Understanding the types and etiology of abdominal pain helps the examiner use information obtained through the history and physical examination to narrow the differential diagnosis.

TYPES AND ETIOLOGY OF ABDOMINAL PAIN

Visceral Pain

Obstruction of a hollow organ results in stretching of the smooth muscle wall. Stretching and associated inflammation or ischemia stimulate autonomic nerve fibers, resulting in diffuse, cramping, poorly localized pain. Pain is typically midline and difficult for the patient to describe. Visceral pain is common in early appendicitis, bowel obstruction, renal colic, cholecystitis and early pelvic inflammatory disease (PID).[1–4]

Somatic Pain

Somatic pain fibers are found in the skin, abdominal wall, and musculature, and in the parietal peritoneum. Inflammation or irritation in these areas can be from direct injury, or bacterial or chemical contact. The resulting pain is typically well localized, sharp, and constant. Tenderness is elicited at the area of peritoneal inflammation. Somatic pain is seen with appendicitis, pancreatitis, cholecystitis, and pelvic inflammatory disease (PID).[1–4] Contamination of the peritoneal cavity by blood, urine, pus, or cystic or gastric fluid also results in somatic pain, which can be diffuse in nature.

Referred Pain

Referred pain describes pain that originates in an organ, but is described by the patient as located in a distant area. Visceral nerve fibers that innervate the diseased organ enter the spinal cord at the same level as somatic nerve fibers that innervate the areas of referred pain. As somatic pain is better localized than visceral pain, the patient may emphasize the area of referred pain. Typical examples are shoulder pain with cholecystitis, inner thigh pain seen with appendicitis or PID, or groin and labial pain with renal colic.[1–3,5]

Etiology

There are diverse differential diagnoses for acute abdominal pain in women of childbearing age. Subdividing the diagnostic possibilities into primary location (diffuse, upper abdomen, or lower abdomen) and by organ system can be very helpful. However, these are general guidelines and individual patient presentation may differ.[1,2,6] Table 28-1 lists common gastrointestinal, urologic, and

Table 28-1. Common Causes of Acute Abdominal Pain by Location and Organ System

	Generalized Pain	Upper Abdomen	Lower Abdomen
Gastrointestinal	Bowel obstruction Ulcerative colitis Gastroenteritis Inflammatory bowel disease Irritable bowel syndrome Perforated viscus Constipation	Gastritis Pancreatitis Gastroesophageal reflux disease Dyspepsia Peptic ulcer disease Cholecystitis Biliary colic Hepatitis	Appendicitis Incarcerated hernia Diverticulitis
Genitourinary		Renal colic Pyelonephritis	Cystitis Pyelonephritis
Obstetric/gynecologic			Ectopic pregnancy Mittelschmerz Ovarian cysts Adnexal torsion Pelvic inflammatory disease Dysmenorrhea Endometriosis Degenerating uterine myomas

gynecologic causes of abdominal pain by location and organ system.

HISTORY

The aim of history taking is to identify risk factors for specific disease processes, focus symptomatology on one or two organ systems, and formulate a differential diagnosis.

A standard history regarding the pain characteristics (location, migration, radiation, quality, onset, severity, and exacerbating and relieving factors) and associated symptoms should be followed by a complete gynecologic, obstetric, and sexual history. The examiner must keep in mind that a negative history for pregnancy is unreliable. In one study of patients who stated that their last menstrual period was entirely normal and who denied any chance of pregnancy, over 7 percent were indeed pregnant.[7] Past medical history (sexually transmitted diseases, gallstones, kidney stones), surgical history, history of trauma, and history of similar episodes are important and often narrow the differential diagnosis. Specific risk factors should be ascertained for PID and ectopic pregnancy (Tables 28-2 and 28-3). Recent and current medications and allergies should be documented. Family history of breast or ovarian neoplasms should be identified, as patients with such a family history may have unspoken anxieties about these disorders that can bias or confound the evaluation of acute abdominal pain. Screening for domestic violence or sexual assault should also be part of the history taking.

Pain Characteristics

Ask about the location of primary pain and migration of pain (Table 28-1). The location of pain coupled with a description of its migration and radiation patterns helps to make a diagnosis. Pain moving from the epigastrium or umbilicus to the right lower quadrant suggests appendicitis. Pain in the epigastrium that radiates to the back is often seen with pancreatitis. Pain originating in the flank that radiates to the lower abdomen or groin suggests renal colic or pyelonephritis. Pain encircling the waist or moving to the right or left subscapular area suggests cholecystitis. Pain that is unilateral and stops abruptly at the midline, radiating along a dermatome, should raise the suspicion of herpes zoster.[1,2]

Table 28-2. Risk Factors for Ectopic Pregnancy

Infertility patient: assisted reproduction, in vitro fertilization
Prior PID or tubo-ovarian abscess
History of STD—possible subclinical PID
Prior ectopic pregnancy
Tubal reconstructive surgery and conservative management of tubal pregnancy
Tubal ligation
Intrauterine device (IUD) in place
DES exposure in utero
Prior dilation and evacuation
Smoking
Douching

Note that only ~50% of patients with ectopic pregnancy have at least one risk factor and ~25% of patients with spontaneous abortions have at least one risk factor.[8,9,10,11]

Questions about the quality of the pain can be helpful. True colicky pain is of a visceral origin and is associated with stretching of hollow organs. Bowel obstruction, biliary colic, renal colic, and fallopian tube obstruction due to ectopic pregnancy or ovarian torsion are examples. Renal colic represents an atypical presentation of colicky pain in that one wave of pain has typically not resolved before the next wave begins.[5] This pattern of atypical colicky pain may also be seen with obstruction of other hollow organs. Burning epigastric pain is seen with pancreatitis, dyspepsia, gastroesophageal reflux disease, and ulcer disease. Sharp, well-localized pain indicates peritoneal inflammation and can be a late finding seen with appendicitis, PID, and ectopic pregnancy.[1–3]

The severity and onset of pain can guide the differential diagnosis. Pain that awakens a patient from sleep is generally associated with acute obstruction, ischemia, inflammation, or perforation of an organ. This can be seen with perforation of gastric ulcers, obstruction of the biliary or renal tract by stones, ovarian torsion, or fallopian tube rupture. Severe, sudden-onset pain may be associated with life-threatening pathology (e.g., with organ rupture), but there are instances in which severe pain may have a typically benign etiology as seen with nephrolithiasis.[5,14]

Table 28-3. Risk Factors for PID

Age: late adolescence to early adulthood
Multiple sexual partners
Douching
Recent IUD insertion
Prior episodes of PID
Cigarette smoking

Source: Dart et al,[12] McCormack.[13]

Factors that exacerbate and relieve the pain can provide information about the etiology of the pain. Pain with movement or elicited by tapping the heel suggests peritonitis. Pain that changes with eating, vomiting, or belching suggests gastrointestinal etiology.

Associated gastrointestinal symptoms such as nausea, vomiting, anorexia, diarrhea, or constipation are often nonspecific as they can coexist with genitourinary and gynecologic disorders as well. Genitourinary symptoms such as dysuria, frequency, urgency, and hematuria suggest urinary tract infection or renal stone. However, dysuria and lower abdominal pain radiating to the groin can also be present with gynecologic disorders and gastrointestinal pathology such as appendicitis. Vaginal discharge, irregular bleeding, and dyspareunia are more common with gynecologic disorders, but can also be seen with other pathology. Over 20 percent of women with proven ectopic pregnancy have no history of vaginal bleeding.[12]

PHYSICAL EXAMINATION

Obtaining vital signs, including orthostatic signs to detect hypovolemia, is the first step in examination.

A patient may have normal vital signs early in the course of very serious disease, and the presence or absence of fever has never been shown to aid in the delineation of medical versus surgical pathology.

Focused General Examination

A systematic approach that is used for all patients will help the examiner avoid missing important information.

The patient's general appearance (toxic, nontoxic) and position of comfort should be noted. A patient with peritoneal irritation tends to lie perfectly still as movement exacerbates the pain. The knees may be drawn toward the abdomen in an attempt to reduce intraabdominal pressure. A patient with renal colic or other visceral pain may writhe about searching for a comfortable position. Mucous membranes should be examined to assess hydration status, pallor, or jaundice. The skin should be examined for spider angiomas that may be seen in cirrhosis, pregnancy, and collagen vascular disorders. Crackles or diminished breath sounds could indicate pulmonary pathology.

Abdominal Examination

The patient should be lying flat with the entire abdomen exposed and the extremities extended. Inspect the abdominal wall for contour, asymmetry, distension, scars, masses, or visible peristaltic waves or pulsations. Asking the patient to cough or bear down to increase intraabdominal pressure may demonstrate surgical, inguinal, umbilical, or femoral hernias.

Auscultation of the abdomen may suggest obstruction if there are rushes of high-pitched bowel sounds or absent bowel sounds. Evaluation of a fluid wave or shifting dullness can be performed in the patient with suspected ascites. In a woman with new-onset ascites, ovarian malignancy should be suspected. Abdominal wall metastases have occurred at puncture sites when laparoscopy and paracentesis have been performed in patients with ovarian malignancy.[15,16] Data regarding incidence is lacking, but in a woman with new-onset ascites, ovarian malignancy should be suspected and ruled out before searching for a gastrointestinal cause.

Prior to palpation of the abdomen, it is important to have the patient indicate the point of maximal pain. This area should be palpated last in an attempt to decrease voluntary guarding. Relaxation of the abdominal musculature facilitates palpation. Flexing the knees will relax the abdominal wall. The abdomen should be palpated gently with specific attention to individual organ assessment, identification of masses, and location of tenderness, guarding, and rebound. Voluntary guarding occurs when the patient contracts the abdominal wall musculature in an attempt to protect against the pain elicited by palpation. Involuntary guarding is a reflex contraction of the abdominal wall musculature. This is also known as abdominal wall rigidity. Rebound tenderness is evaluated by palpating deeply and slowly in an area of the abdomen distant from the area of maximal tenderness and pain. With release of the examining hand, the patient experiences severe pain. Other methods of evaluating for rebound tenderness include percussion of the abdomen and heel percussion. Significant pain elicited by any of these methods of assessing rebound tenderness indicates peritoneal inflammation.[1,2] Absence of rebound tenderness should not be used as evidence that the patient is free of a medical or surgical emergency. Early torsion and PID are both diagnoses in which rebound tenderness is unlikely, but in which early surgical or medical treatment is critical to preserve fertility.[3]

There are many signs that have been used to help identify specific disease processes, and these can be useful in discussions with consultants. Murphy's sign is inspiratory arrest during palpation under the right costal margin and is an indicator of cholecystitis. During deep inspiration, the inflamed gallbladder descends against the palpating hand, causing pain and reflex inspiratory arrest. Rovsing's sign is the development of right lower quadrant pain upon palpation of the left lower quadrant. This is often seen with appendicitis. The psoas sign is pain with passive extension of the hip, and the obturator sign is pain with passive internal rotation of the flexed right hip. Both of these are indicative of appendicitis.[4]

Rectal Examination

Perirectal abscesses and fistulae are often seen with inflammatory bowel disease. Stool that is grossly bloody, melanotic, or positive for occult blood strongly suggests gastrointestinal pathology. Tenderness in the right lower quadrant elicited by rectal examination can be seen in appendicitis, PID, and ectopic pregnancy, but the overall sensitivity of the rectal examination for diagnosing pathology is low.[4,8,17]

Pelvic Examination

Indications for Pelvic Examination

There is insufficient evidence published to determine which patients require pelvic examination in the emergency department evaluation of abdominal pain.[6] American College of Emergency Physicians (ACEP) guidelines state that women with signs and symptoms that clearly suggest a nongynecologic disorder, such acute gastroenteritis, cholecystitis, pancreatitis, or pyelonephritis, do not require a pelvic examination. However, if a gynecologic disorder is in the differential diagnosis, pelvic examination is important to identify masses or tenderness, vaginal bleeding or discharge, vaginal or cervical lesions, and to obtain specimens for culture or microscopic examination.

Reliability and Validity of Pelvic Examination

Despite the common performance of the pelvic examination and the historical use of the results for making clinical decisions, few studies have addressed its reliability and validity. Close and colleagues found that bimanual pelvic examinations performed by experienced emergency physicians in the emergency department had poor interobserver agreement for the evaluation of uterine size, uterine tenderness, adnexal tenderness or masses, and cervical motion tenderness.[18] Padilla and associates found bimanual examinations performed under general anesthesia by medical students, gynecology residents, and attending gynecologists to be inaccurate for detecting adnexal masses confirmed surgically. They also found no statistically significant difference in accuracy between the medical students, residents, and attending physicians.[19] Several studies that have compared bimanual pelvic examination to pelvic ultrasonography and laparotomy have shown accuracy of pelvic examination to be poor, especially when pelvic examination is felt to be "normal."[20–22] Many texts and articles cite pelvic examination findings that confirm disease states (e.g., cervical motion tenderness confirming a diagnosis of PID). If the reliability of this examination is poor, then its positive or negative findings should not be the sole criterion for diagnosis.[18]

As evidenced by the currently available data, findings on pelvic examination appear related to examiner experience, patient cooperation, patient body habitus, prior abdominal surgery, and the limitations of the examination itself. Furthermore, criteria have not been standardized for the production of, or scoring of, cervical motion or adnexal tenderness. In addition, infection or inflammation of the peritoneum and urologic, pelvic, or gastrointestinal organs can cause pelvic tenderness.

Therefore, while pelvic examination is necessary to identify bleeding, lesions, tenderness, and to obtain specimens, given the current uncertainty about the validity and reliability of the pelvic examination, further diagnostic testing is often necessary for more precision in diagnosis. There are no validated clinical decision pathways for acute abdominal pain in women, and clinical decisions depend upon results from history, physical examination, age, and risk factors for specific disease processes. Burstin and coworkers published consensus guidelines for the evaluation of abdominal pain, but these are one-step guidelines based upon clinical context, and have not been validated.[23]

Repeat Evaluation

Very often the etiology of abdominal pain will not be clear on initial evaluation. Progression or resolution of pathology can dramatically change the examination findings. Serial examinations can be instrumental in the ultimate diagnosis of abdominal pain. Observation units or scheduled 12-hour re-evaluations are sometimes needed to make a diagnosis.

DIAGNOSTIC TESTING

Diagnostic modalities for the diagnosis of acute abdominal pain include laboratory and radiologic studies. Common laboratory studies include the urine and serum pregnancy test, complete blood count, hepatic enzymes, lipase, urinalysis, serum electrolytes, BUN and creatinine, urinalysis, and cervical cultures. An electrocardiogram can be helpful in older women or in those with risk factors for coronary artery disease. Radiographic studies useful for diagnosis include noncontrast helical CT scan, focused and nonfocused abdominal and pelvic CT scanning, and ultrasonography. These will briefly be discussed in turn.

Laboratory Evaluation

Urine and Serum Pregnancy Tests

A quantitative urine ELISA pregnancy test will detect β-hCG at levels greater than 20 mIU/mL,[8,24,25] and will detect urine β-hCG at about day 21 of the menstrual cycle.[24] If point-of-care testing is done in the emergency department, the manufacturer's recommendations for test performance, including time to read test results, must be exact or false negative results can occur. A screening urine pregnancy test should be performed on all women of childbearing age with abdominal pain because a positive result will change the differential diagnosis and management options (e.g., medications, radiologic procedures).

A serum quantitative β-hCG test should be performed if the patient has a positive urine pregnancy test and either pain or vaginal bleeding. Both ectopic and intrauterine pregnancies produce β-hCG, although there is typically a difference in the rate of production. Ectopic pregnancies and abnormal intrauterine pregnancies tend to have lower quantitative levels of β-hCG than normal intrauterine pregnancies for the same gestational age.[26] Quantitative β-hCG levels typically increase in a linear fashion by $\geq$66 percent every 48 hours for the first 38 days after ovulation in normal first-trimester pregnancies.[27,28] Abnormal increase (<66 percent over 48 hours) is 75 percent sensitive and 93 percent specific for an abnormal gestation.[27] β-hCG levels that are decreasing indicate nonviability of the pregnancy, either intrauterine or ectopic.[28] The rate of β-hCG decline is significantly different for intrauterine gestations and ectopic pregnancies. The half-life of β-hCG for ectopic pregnancy is approximately 7 days, while the half-life for aborting intrauterine pregnancy is approximately 1.4 days.[28]

The sensitivity of ultrasound for detecting ectopic pregnancy when the β-hCG is less than 1000 is ~17 percent.[29] Therefore, there is no true minimum value of β-hCG for which ultrasound is not indicated in a patient with suspected ectopic pregnancy. However, β-hCG levels >50,000 mIU/mL are rarely seen with ectopic pregnancies.[30,31]

Complete Blood Count

An elevated WBC count is neither sensitive nor specific for the diagnosis of an acute surgical condition. At least 11 percent of patients with pathologically-proven appendicitis and up to 40 percent of patients with pathologically-proven cholecystitis had normal white blood cell counts.[32,33,34] Hematocrit may not accurately reflect acute blood loss, although serial determinations of the hematocrit can be of value.

Hepatic Enzymes and Lipase

These tests are useful for the evaluation of possible hepatitis and pancreatitis. Enzymes may be normal in chronic hepatitis, cirrhosis, or cholecystitis in which the obstruction does not involve the common bile duct. Low sensitivities and specificities for gallbladder pathology are reported.[35]

Urinalysis

Positive findings can be used to guide diagnosis and work-up, but have variable sensitivity and are not specific for urinary pathology. Urinalysis has been shown to be falsely positive with hematuria or evidence of infection in ~30 percent of patients with appendicitis, likely due to periappendiceal inflammation.[5,14] Positive urinalysis can similarly be seen with gynecologic infections. The sensitivity of urinalysis for hematuria varies depending on the pathology and on the definition of positive results (≥1 RBC/hpf or ≥5 RBC/hpf considered positive). Up to 20 percent of patients with documented nephrolithiasis do not have hematuria on urinalysis as defined as >1 RBC/hpf.[5] In a study performed by Bove and associates, 51 percent of patients without nephrolithiasis as documented by CT scan had at least 1 RBC/hpf on microscopic urinalysis.[36]

Depending on the criteria used for diagnosis of UTI (nitrite-positive, leukocyte esterase-positive, and/or positive microscopic evaluation for bacteria and WBC), the sensitivity of urine reagent strip test results varies.[37–40] In a study by Lammers and colleagues, if urine reagent strip results are defined as positive when leukocyte esterase or nitrite is positive or blood is more than trace, the overtreatment rate is 47 percent and the undertreatment rate is 13 percent, when compared to the results of urine culture. If the results are considered positive when WBCs are >3/hpf or RBCs are >5/hpf, the overtreatment rate is 44 percent and the undertreatment rate is 11 percent.[38] Also, since infection is a risk factor for nephrolithiasis, both conditions may coexist.[5] Urine culture and sensitivities should therefore be obtained to confirm the diagnosis when there is a moderate to high pretest probability of UTI.

Testing for Gonorrhea and Chlamydia

Refer to Chaps. 29 and 30 for a detailed discussion.

Positive test results have public health implications and increase patient risk for future infertility and ectopic pregnancy.[13] Many studies have shown a very high rate of asymptomatic infection in ED patients, especially teenagers and young adults.[41] Newer modalities of testing include first-catch urine (not practical in the ED, as many patients void their first daily urine before entering the ED), random urine sampling, and patient-obtained vaginal swabs. Each of these has been shown to have high accuracy when compared to the gold standard of culture and are better tolerated by the asymptomatic patient.[42–46] Individual laboratory capabilities vary by institution.

Serum Chemistries

Serum electrolytes and BUN/creatinine can be useful in the evaluation of hydration status in the patient with vomiting and diarrhea. Glucose and bicarbonate are necessary for the evaluation of DKA. In patients under the age of 60 without known diabetes, hypertension, coronary artery disease, collagen-vascular disease, hepatic disease, and/or congestive heart failure, the likelihood of an elevated creatinine (1.6 mg/dL) is approximately 1 percent. In patients with an elevated creatinine there is a potential risk of contrast-induced nephropathy.[47] This potential risk can be reduced by administration of intravenous fluids.

Electrocardiogram

Any woman with risk factors for coronary artery disease, or with epigastric pain that could be cardiac in etiology, should have an ECG as part of the ED evaluation.

Radiologic Evaluation

Abdominal Series

A three-view abdominal series (upright, supine, and upright chest or lateral decubitus) is useful for detecting air-fluid levels, free air, and foreign bodies, and is therefore useful for bowel obstruction, gastrointestinal foreign body, or viscus perforation. Plain films are no longer considered useful for the evaluation of renal stones or gallstones.[5,48]

Abdominal and Pelvic Ultrasonography

RUQ ultrasonography can be used to evaluate for gallstones and evidence of acute cholecystitis (pericholecystic fluid, thickened gallbladder wall, common bile duct dilation).[49] The liver may be evaluated for masses, consistency, and congestion. Pancreatic masses may also be seen.

Renal ultrasonography is useful for the detection of renal calculi and hydronephrosis that may result from a ureteral obstruction, and is safe in pregnancy.[50] However, mild to moderate hydronephrosis can be a normal finding in pregnancy (typically right greater than left), and can also be seen with vigorous hydration.[51]

The ED focused abdominal sonography in trauma (FAST) exam can be used for the evaluation of hemoperitoneum in trauma patients. Bedside ultrasonography is rapid, noninvasive, repeatable, and highly accurate for assessing abdominal injury. Speed and accuracy increase with operator experience.[52–57]

Finally, pelvic ultrasonography is essential for the evaluation of first-trimester vaginal bleeding with or without pain. This rapid examination can be performed at the bedside for an immediate determination of the presence or absence of an intrauterine pregnancy. Presence of a complex adnexal mass and the absence of an intrauterine pregnancy are highly suggestive of ectopic pregnancy in a patient with a positive pregnancy test.[58] Complete pelvic ultrasonography with Doppler flow analysis can be utilized in the evaluation of a patient with lower abdominal pain in whom PID, torsion, and appendicitis are all possible diagnoses.[59] Ultrasonography has been shown to have high sensitivity and specificity for evaluation of surgically-confirmed pelvic masses and is routinely the test of choice for evaluating suspected pelvic and gynecologic pathology.[60,61] Comparison with CT for accuracy in the evaluation of pelvic organs has not yet been performed.

Abdominal and Pelvic Computed Tomography

Abdominal and pelvic computed tomography is becoming the test of choice for diagnosis of undifferentiated abdominal pain or suspected acute appendicitis in nonpregnant patients.[8] Noncontrast abdominal CT using 5-mm slices is the diagnostic procedure of choice for suspected renal colic in nonpregnant patients. Using intravenous, oral, and rectal contrast (if indicated), many abdominal organs and potential pathologies can be evaluated simultaneously. CT compared to 3-view abdominal series in the evaluation of small bowel obstruction showed similar sensitivity, specificity, and positive predictive values, with CT having the added value of revealing the cause of the obstruction.[8,48] CT is superior to ultrasonography for visualizing the common bile duct and demonstrating choledocholithiasis.[8] CT has become the test of choice for the diagnosis of appendicitis. The use of focused contrast technique for the diagnosis of acute appendicitis has been supported by some, but many prefer the nonfocused technique with oral and intravenous contrast material, because it is more sensitive for appendicitis than the focused technique and can detect alternative diagnoses as well.[62–65] Noncontrast CT can also be performed if the pretest probability for renal colic is high. CT has been compared to IVP and to stone retrieval or removal with very high accuracy in the diagnosis of renal calculi. CT scan without contrast does not evaluate renal function.[5] Typically the increased information obtained by CT makes it a more desirable test than IVP.[66,67]

While there are no guidelines or recommendations to suggest which women with acute abdominal pain should undergo pelvic ultrasonography, given the poor reliability and validity of pelvic examination, a logical approach is to obtain pelvic ultrasound if the diagnosis is unclear but the clinician suspects a gynecologic cause of pain. If the pretest probability favors a gastrointestinal disorder, an abdominal/pelvic CT scan should be done first. Rao and associates recently evaluated the use of CT for differentiating appendicitis and acute gynecologic conditions (ovarian cyst rupture, PID, ovarian torsion, ovarian dermoid, hematometra) and found sensitivities of 100 percent and 87 percent and specificities of 97 percent and 100 percent for appendicitis and acute gynecologic conditions, respectively.[68]

There is concern regarding ovarian exposure to radiation incurred during abdominal and pelvic CT. The radiation dose is dependent on several factors, including patient body habitus, the specific scan performed, and scanner characteristics, but the approximate radiation dose delivered is 1-4 rad (10–40 mGy), with a surface dose of approximately 100 mrad (1 mGy) for the scout study.[69] Oocytes in growing follicles are more susceptible to the effects of radiation and the number of oocytes affected is dose-related. Any radiation dose given over a larger number of fractions will cause less oocyte damage than the same dose given over fewer exposures. Information obtained from patients who were exposed to large doses of radiation in the treatment of malignancy and menorrhagia estimate the LD_{50} for oocytes to be 600 to 1800 rads (6 to 18 Gy).[70,71]

Laparoscopy

The utility of laparoscopy for the diagnosis of acute abdominal pain in women has been evaluated. Borgstein and associates examined 161 patients with a clinical diagnosis of appendicitis who underwent diagnostic laparoscopy.[72] Fifty-five percent had an inflamed appendix identified laparoscopically that was subsequently removed. Twenty-three percent had evidence of gynecologic pathology, and 14 percent had a negative laparoscopy. There were 2 false-positives and no false-negatives as shown by clinical follow-up. Of 42 similar patients who did not undergo diagnostic laparoscopy, there was a 38 percent false-positive appendectomy rate.[72] Cox and colleagues performed a similar study on 107 women that showed similar results, with the majority of appendectomies able to be performed laparoscopically.[73] Laparoscopy is the gold standard for diagnosing PID, and has been shown to aid in the diagnosis and surgical treatment if necessary for ovarian torsion, tubo-ovarian abscess, and ectopic pregnancy.[13,74]

TREATMENT OPTIONS

Pain management is one of the most important cornerstones in patient care. Treating pain is humane, safe, and aids in patient evaluation. Patients with surgical conditions are easier to evaluate when their pain is at least partially controlled, and short-acting parenteral narcotic analgesics can be used to decrease pain and anxiety and to facilitate abdominal examination.[8,75] Agreements should be made between emergency services and gynecologic and surgical consultants regarding the need for acute pain management. If the surgeon believes that the narcotic has altered the examination to the point that it is useless, the analgesic will only be effective for only a few hours.

For patients who are unlikely to have surgical conditions, many other analgesics may be used in the treatment of pain. Response to some of the medications may aid in narrowing the differential diagnosis. NSAIDs are typically very helpful with visceral pain and pain associated with inflammation, but should be used with caution in the elderly, the diabetic, those with renal dysfunction, and those taking ACE inhibitors. Ketorolac has been shown to be very effective in treating the pain associated with renal colic.[67,76] A GI cocktail (Mylanta® and viscous lidocaine) may be used in the treatment of dyspepsia, GERD, and peptic ulcer disease. Response to the cocktail can aid in the diagnosis, but should not be the sole determinant of seriousness of disease, as it is well documented that some patients with acute myocardial infarction have a reduction in their pain after a GI cocktail.

DISPOSITION

Patients with a diagnosis that requires surgical or medical intervention obviously need admission. Patients with severe pain uncontrolled with oral medications must be admitted for pain control and further diagnostic evaluation. Patients with persistent dehydration or vomiting unresponsive to the administration of antiemetics and fluids must also be admitted. With thorough history, physical examination, laboratory and radiologic evaluation, and a period of observation, a diagnosis can usually be made for most women with acute abdominal pain. In some the cause of abdominal pain will not be established, and in others the diagnosis may be incorrect. For this reason, patients not being admitted to the hospital must have follow-up arranged in 12 to 24 hours, and the discharge instructions should include clear signs or symptoms that require immediate return to the emergency department.

SPECIFIC COMMON DIAGNOSES

Gastrointestinal

Acute Appendicitis

Acute appendicitis continues to be a difficult diagnosis in women of reproductive age, children, the immunocompromised, and the elderly. Rothrock showed that 33 percent of women of childbearing age who were ultimately diagnosed with appendicitis were initially misdiagnosed with PID, gastroenteritis, or UTI.[77] Newer methods of diagnosis including CT and laparoscopy may decrease the incidence of misdiagnosis. Institution-specific agreements should be developed between emergency physicians, gynecologists, and surgeons in order to optimize the care of women with abdominal pain. It is reasonable to perform pelvic ultrasonography and CT of the abdomen and pelvis, and then consult both services, and if the diagnosis is still unclear, admit the patient for observation. As more institutions become experienced with laparoscopy, future management strategies may change.

Appendicitis remains the most common extrauterine indication for surgery during pregnancy. The long held belief that as pregnancy progresses the appendix migrates from the RLQ to the RUQ has recently been challenged in a large case study performed by Mourad and colleagues. Their findings were that the majority of patients in all trimesters of pregnancy with pathologically proven appendicitis had a complaint of RLQ pain. It is also interesting to note that patients with false-positive appendectomies also complained predominantly of RLQ pain.[78] This reinforces the difficulty in making this diagnosis.

Biliary Tract Disease

The prevalence of gallbladder disease increases with age and it involves a spectrum of pathology from the relatively benign biliary colic to the potentially life-threatening ascending cholangitis. Differentiating biliary colic from cholecystitis is accomplished using clinical and radiographic techniques. By clinical convention, biliary colic is defined as temporary or transient RUQ abdominal pain due to cystic duct obstruction typically caused by passage of a gallstone. The pain can initially be severe but is typically well controlled with moderate amounts of analgesics. The diagnosis of biliary colic is confirmed by ultrasonography, which demonstrates gallstones or sludge with normal gallbladder wall thickness, lack of pericholecystic fluid, and the lack of abnormal biliary duct dilation. Women with biliary colic should be treated with analgesics, instructions to avoid any agents that precipitate attacks (for some patients a fatty meal), and outpatient surgical referral. Any patient with first episode of colicky RUQ pain should have an ultrasound performed to evaluate for the presence of stones and evidence of cholecystitis. Ultrasound is also indicated in any patient with known cholelithiasis whose pain is atypical for gallstones or cannot be controlled with analgesics, or who has evidence of infection.[79]

Ultrasonography is very sensitive for the detection of cholelithiasis and can aid in the diagnosis of cholecystitis (gallbladder wall thickening, pericholecystic fluid, dilation of the common bile duct, and sonographic Murphy's sign). Autopsy reports and imaging studies performed in the evaluation of other pathology have shown that ~20 percent of women have asymptomatic gallstones. Alternatively, ~10 percent of patients with pathologically proven cholecystitis do not have stones.[79] This is known as acalculous cholecystitis, and ultrasound would be expected to show evidence of inflammation but no stones. The HIDA scan is a functional radioisotope test that is the gold standard for diagnosis of cholecystitis, and it should be employed when the diagnosis is still unclear after clinical and ultrasound evaluation. The HIDA scan is positive when the gallbladder is unable to be visualized due to obstruction of the cystic duct.[49] Fever, elevated WBC count, and elevated bilirubin are variably seen with cholecystitis and cannot be relied upon to make the diagnosis. Patients with cholecystitis require surgical admission and cholecystectomy.[1,79]

Choledocholithiasis results from a stone in the common bile duct. Ultrasonography may show the stone or associated dilation of the common bile duct. Admission and surgical consultation are indicated as there is risk of cholangitis.[1,79]

Cholangitis results from biliary tract obstruction and associated bacterial infection. This is a true emergency as sepsis can occur rapidly and the untreated mortality approaches 100 percent. Charcot's triad (RUQ tenderness, jaundice, and fever) is variably seen, but when the patient has systemic infection as indicated by shock and altered mental status (Reynold's pentad), treatment must be initiated immediately with fluid resuscitation, broad-spectrum antibiotics, and early surgical or ERCP decompression.[1,79]

A small percentage of patients with cholecystitis will have severe, life-threatening complications requiring emergent surgery. These complications include empyema, gangrene, and perforation, and are more common in diabetics and patients with sickle cell disease or other immunocompromised states. Empyema is abscess formation in the gallbladder wall as a result of complete cystic duct obstruction. Gangrene of the gallbladder may be localized or diffuse and results from distension, empyema, arterial compromise (torsion) or vasculitis. Gallbladder perforation can occur as a result of empyema or gangrene, and may be locally contained or result in a diffuse peritonitis. All of these conditions are associated with severe systemic toxicity and require fluid resuscitation, broad-spectrum antibiotics and emergent surgical evaluation.[1,79]

Hepatitis

The most common causes of hepatic inflammation and necrosis are infection, toxin ingestion, and cholestasis. Hepatitis may be acute or chronic and the presentation ranges from asymptomatic to fulminant hepatic failure. Patients typically present with RUQ or epigastric pain, fever, malaise, nausea, and vomiting. Risk factors for viral hepatitis (IVDU, history of blood transfusion, sexual or household contact with an infected individual, foreign travel), toxin ingestion (most commonly alcohol, acetaminophen, isoniazid, or phenytoin), and cholestatic hepatitis (oral contraceptive pills, phenothiazines, and anabolic steroid use) should be ascertained. Liver enzymes, alkaline phosphatase, direct and indirect bilirubin, serum chemistries, and tests of hepatic function (glucose, albumin, prothrombin time (PT)) should be performed. A serum ammonia level may be useful in a patient with suspected hepatic encephalopathy, particularly if a premorbid ammonia level is known. Complications of hepatitis include cirrhosis, GI bleeding, encephalitis, ascites and bacterial peritonitis, and hepatorenal syndrome. Without these associated complications, most patients can be treated with supportive care and withdrawal of the offending toxin if possible. Patients who are febrile, or have intractable vomiting or prolongation of the PT, or who are encephalopathic or have evidence of renal failure require admission.

Pancreatitis

Inflammation of the pancreas can be acute or chronic and is associated with alcohol use or gallstones in the majority of patients. The typical presentation is epigastric pain that radiates to the back and is associated with nausea and vomiting. Pancreatitis can be a life-threatening condition requiring aggressive fluid resuscitation and correction of electrolyte abnormalities. Diagnosis is confirmed by an elevated lipase and CT or ultrasound evidence of pancreatic inflammation. Admission is required. Patients with gallstone pancreatitis are typically admitted to a surgical service, while other causes of pancreatitis are best treated with a medical admission. Treatment is mainly supportive and includes bowel rest, replacement of fluids and electrolytes, and pain management.[79]

Small Bowel Obstruction

Patients typically present with abdominal distension, pain, and vomiting. The most common causes for small bowel obstruction include previous abdominal surgery, hernia, and malignancy. For a patient with one of these risk factors with abdominal distension, pain, or vomiting, a 3-view abdominal series demonstrating air-fluid levels and dilated loops of bowel indicate obstruction. CT scan may also be performed, as it is equally sensitive for obstruction and can often reveal the etiology. Patients with small bowel obstruction require gastric decompression, IV fluids, and prompt surgical evaluation.[80]

Urologic

Urinary Tract Infection

The typical patient presents with dysuria, frequency, and urgency, without fever or signs of systemic infection. Suprapubic pain and tenderness are common findings as is low back pain. Urinalysis may show leukocytes, bacteria, or be positive for nitrite or leukocyte esterase. The most common pathogen cultured is *E. coli*. Patients at high risk are those with urinary retention, recent instrumentation, pregnancy, anatomic abnormalities, or immunosuppression, but UTI is a very common diagnosis that may be seen without any apparent risk factors. Fluoroquinolones are commonly prescribed for the nonpregnant patient, and cefalosporins or nitrofurantoin can be used in pregnancy.

Pyelonephritis

Patients are systemically ill with fever, nausea, vomiting, and flank pain. Symptoms of UTI (cystitis) may or may not be present. Tenderness on percussion of the costovertebral angle is suggestive of pyelonephritis. The WBC is typically elevated with a left shift, and urinalysis may be positive for WBC, bacteria, nitrite, or leukocyte esterase. Urine culture and sensitivity can be used to aid the clinician in refining antibiotic therapy, although in vitro sensitivities do not necessarily correlate well with clinical response. BUN and creatinine may be useful in a patient with suspected renal insufficiency. Current recommendations include outpatient therapy for otherwise healthy young patients who are not toxic, not pregnant, and can tolerate oral fluids. Admission is required for patients who are pregnant, unable to tolerate fluids, appear toxic, or who have failed outpatient therapy. Current recommendations include 14 days of fluoroquinolone therapy.

Nephrolithiasis

Patients with nephrolithiasis generally present with severe, colicky flank pain that radiates to the ipsilateral groin or thigh. Hematuria, either gross or microscopic, is commonly seen. Fever is not present unless concomitant infection exists. The patient typically writhes about in severe pain, but other physical findings are few. Without coexisting infection, abdominal tenderness and costovertebral angle tenderness are uncommon. Noncontrast CT is very useful in the evaluation of nephrolithiasis and can provide information regarding stone size, location, and associated hydronephrosis. Urologic consultation and admission are required for high-grade obstruction, stones larger than 5 mm (unlikely to pass spontaneously), patients with associated infection, renal transplant patients, and patients with a single functioning kidney or in whom emesis and pain are unable to be controlled. Fluids and analgesics are the mainstay of ED treatment for patients not requiring admission. Straining the urine to retrieve the stone for pathologic evaluation can be useful for further work-up.[5,67]

Gynecologic

Pelvic Inflammatory Disease

The diagnosis of PID should be considered in any woman of reproductive age who presents with lower abdominal pain. The presentation of bilateral pelvic pain, fever, and vaginal discharge is unfortunately rare and many patients may have subtle and atypical symptoms. McCormick found that up to 30 to 80 percent of women with infertility related to fallopian tube obstruction have positive antibody tests for *Chlamydia,* but report no clinically apparent infection. Clinical diagnosis for PID has an accuracy of 66 percent when compared to laparoscopy.[13] Common misdiagnoses include appendicitis and urinary tract infection.

Ovarian Cyst

Ovarian cyst rupture, hemorrhage, or torsion, results in the typical presentation of sudden onset of unilateral pelvic pain. Pain may be preceded by exercise, intercourse, or trauma. Tenderness may be elicited on the side of the cyst, and peritoneal signs may be present if the cyst has ruptured or is causing peritoneal inflammation. Hemorrhage may be significant. A patient may or may not give a history of ovarian cysts. Ultrasonography aids in the diagnosis and helps quantitate blood loss in the acutely ill patient. As patients with cyst pain may present very similarly to the patient with an ectopic pregnancy, rapid determination of pregnancy status is critical. Ovarian cysts that are less than 8 cm, unilocular, and unilateral are generally observed. The natural history of functional cysts is generally spontaneous resolution within two cycles, with or without hormone administration. Multiloculated, solid, or large cysts (>8 cm) should be considered ovarian endometriomas, dermoid cysts, or potentially neoplastic until proven otherwise.[60,81] Because of the lack of sensitivity and specificity of the pelvic examination, women with acute abdominal pain and a negative pregnancy test should have ultrasonography to confirm the diagnosis of a functional ovarian cyst. Whether this is accomplished in the emergency department or during outpatient gynecologic follow-up depends on a number of factors, including the degree of patient discomfort, the physician's comfort with the diagnostic pretest probability of a functional cyst, and the emergency availability of high-quality pelvic ultrasonography.

Adnexal Torsion

Adnexal torsion is a surgical emergency, both for relief of pain and to preserve ovarian function. Ischemia results from twisting of the vascular pedicle. Patients can either present with sudden onset of severe, unilateral pelvic pain or present with dull, aching pain with acute and sharp exacerbations if the torsion is intermittent. Patients with ovarian masses (cysts or tumors) are at increased risk for torsion as are patients with pelvic adhesions. The onset of pain may occur after trauma, intercourse, or exercise. Tenderness may be elicited on the side of the affected adnexa, with rebound and guarding. Ultrasound with Doppler flow evaluation is used for diagnosis. Early gynecologic consultation and preparation for surgery are important for adnexal salvage. In a 15-year retrospective chart review of ovarian torsion, only 25 percent of patients had a history of an ovarian cyst, pain characteristics were variable, and objective findings on pelvic examination were uncommon.[82] These features confirm the difficulty in making the diagnosis.

Ectopic Pregnancy

Ectopic pregnancy is still the leading cause of death for women during the first trimester of pregnancy. Risk factors are listed in Table 28-2. When evaluating a patient with first-trimester bleeding or pain, ectopic pregnancy is a potentially life-threatening disorder that needs to be considered (for full discussion of ectopic pregnancy, see Chap. 5).

Mittelschmerz

Mittelschmerz is acute, unilateral, lower abdominal or pelvic pain associated with ovulation. It is related to the rupture of the follicular cyst and is the result of a small amount of intraperitoneal fluid.[1,2] Treatment is symptomatic.

REFERENCES

1. Tintinalli JE, Stapczynski, S, Kelen G (eds): *Emergency Medicine: A Comprehensive Study Guide* (American College of Emergency Physicians), 5th ed. New York: McGraw-Hill, 2000.
2. Swartz MH: *Textbook of Physical Diagnosis: History and Examination,* 2d ed. Philadelphia: WB Saunders, 1994.
3. Abbott J: Pelvic pain: Lessons from anatomy and physiology. *J Emerg Med* 8:441–447, 1990.
4. Wagner J, McKinney W, Carpenter J: Does this patient have appendicitis? *JAMA* 276:1589–1594, 1996.

5. Manthey DE, Teichman J: Nephrolithiasis. *Emerg Clin North Am* 19:633–654, 2001.
6. American College of Emergency Physicians: Clinical policy: Critical issues for the initial evaluation and management of patients presenting with a chief complaint of nontraumatic acute abdominal pain. *Ann Emerg Med* 36:406–413, 2000.
7. Ramosa EA, Sacchetti AD, Nepp M: Reliability of patient history in determining the possibility of pregnancy. *Ann Emerg Med* 18:48–50, 1989.
8. Tenore JL: Problem-oriented diagnosis: ectopic pregnancy. *Am Fam Physician* 61:1080–1088, 2000.
9. Kaplan BC, Dart RG, Moskos M, Kuligowska E, et al: General clinical investigation. Ectopic pregnancy: Prospective study with improved diagnostic accuracy. *Ann Emerg Med* 28:10–17, 1996.
10. Kendrick JS, Atrash HK, Strauss LT, et al: Vaginal douching and the risk of ectopic pregnancy among black women. *Am J Obstet Gynecol* 176:991–997, 1997.
11. Kendrick JS, Merritt RK: Women and smoking: An update for the 1990s. *Am J Obstet Gynecol* 175:528–535, 1996.
12. Dart RG, Kaplan B, Varaklis K: Predictive value of history and physical examination in patients with suspected ectopic pregnancy. *Ann Emerg Med* 33:283–290, 1999.
13. McCormack WM: Pelvic inflammatory disease. *N Engl J Med* 330:115–119, 1994.
14. Graff IV LG, Robinson D: Abdominal pain and emergency department evaluation. *Emerg Med Clin North Am* 19:123–136, 2001.
15. Kruitwagen RF, Swinkels BM, Keyser KG, et al: Incidence and effect on survival of abdominal wall metastases at trocar or puncture sites following laparoscopy or paracentesis in women with ovarian cancer. *Gynecol Oncol* 62:322–324, 1996.
16. La Fianza A, Di Maggio EM, Preda L, et al: Infiltrative subcutaneous metastases from ovarian carcinoma after paracentesis: CT findings. *Abdom Imaging* 22:522–523, 1997.
17. Dixon JM, Elton RA, Rainey JB, Macleod DA: Rectal examination in patients with pain in the right lower quadrant of the abdomen. *BMJ* 302:386–388, 1991.
18. Close R, Sachs C, Dyne P: Reliability of bimanual pelvic examinations performed in emergency departments. *West J Med* 175:240–244, 2001.
19. Padilla L, Radosevich DM, Milad MP: Accuracy of the pelvic examination in detecting adnexal masses. *Obstet Gynecol* 96:593–598, 2000.
20. Carter J, Fowler J, Carson L. How accurate is the pelvic examination as compared to transvaginal sonography? *J Reprod Med* 39:32–34, 1994.
21. Voss SC, Lacey CG, Pupkin M, Degefu S: Ultrasound and the pelvic mass. *J Reprod Med* 28:833–837, 1983.
22. Andolf E, Jorgensen C: Prospective comparison of clinical ultrasound and operative examination of the female pelvis. *J Ultrasound Med* 7:617–620, 1988.
23. Burstin HR, Conn A, Setnik G, et al: Benchmarking and quality improvement: The Harvard Emergency Department Quality Study. *Am J Med* 107:437–449, 1999.
24. Gennis P, Hain L, Andersen HF, et al: Utility of a sensitive bedside serum pregnancy test. *Ann Emerg Med* 16:659–661, 1987.
25. Lipscomb GH, Spellman JR, Ling FW: The effect of same-day pregnancy testing on the incidence of luteal phase pregnancy. *Obstet Gynecol* 82:411–413, 1993.
26. Cartwright PS: Diagnosis of ectopic pregnancy. *Obstet Gynecol Clin North Am* 18:19–37, 1991.
27. Pittaway DE: Beta-hCG dynamics in ectopic pregnancy. *Clin Obstet Gynecol* 30:130–135, 1987.
28. Kadar N, Romero R: Further observations on serial human chorionic gonadotropin patterns in ectopic pregnancies and spontaneous abortions. *Fertil Steril* 50:367–370, 1988.
29. Dart RG, Kaplan B, Cox C: Transvaginal ultrasound in patients with low beta-human chorionic gonadotropin values: How often is the study diagnostic? *Ann Emerg Med* 30:135–140, 1997.
30. Emerson DS, McCord ML: Clinician's approach to ectopic pregnancy. *Clin Obstet Gynecol* 39:199–222, 1996.
31. Ling FW, Duff R, eds: *Obstetrics and Gynecology. Principles for Practice*. New York: McGraw Hill, 2001.
32. Coleman C, Thompson JE Jr, Bennion RS, Schmit PJ: White blood cell count is a poor predictor of severity of disease in the diagnosis of appendicitis. *Am Surg* 64:983–985, 1998.
33. Singer AJ, McCracken G, Henry MD, et al: Correlation among clinical, laboratory, and hepatobiliary scanning findings in patients with suspected acute cholecystitis. *Ann Emerg Med* 28:267–272, 1996.
34. Gruber PH, Silverman RA, Gottesfeld S, Flaster E: Presence of fever and leukocytosis in acute cholecystitis. *Ann Emerg Med* 28:273–277, 1996.
35. Geraghty JM, Goldin RD: Liver changes associated with cholecystitis. *J Clin Pathol* 47:457–460, 1994.
36. Bove P, Kaplan D, Dalrymple N, et al: Reexamining the value of hematuria testing in patients with acute flank pain. J Urol 162:165–167, 1999.
37. Bailey BL Jr: Urinalysis predictive of urine culture results. *J Fam Pract* 40:45–50, 1995.
38. Lammers RL, Gibson S, Kovacs D, et al: Comparison of test characteristics of urine dipstick and urinalysis at various test cutoff points. *Ann Emerg Med* 38:505–512, 2001.
39. Van Nostrand JD, Junkins AD, Bartholdi RK: Poor predictive ability of urinalysis and microscopic examination to detect urinary tract infection. *Am J Clin Pathol* 113:709–713, 2000.
40. Sultana RV, Zalstein S, Cameron P, Campbell D: Dipstick urinalysis and the accuracy of the clinical diagnosis of urinary tract infection. *J Emerg Med* 20:13–19, 2001.
41. Mehta SD, Rothman RE, Kelen GD, et al: Unsuspected gonorrhea and chlamydia in patients of an urban adult emergency department: A critical population for STD control intervention. *Sex Transm Dis* 28:33–39, 2001
42. Oh MK, Smith KR, O'Cain M, et al: Urine-based screening of adolescents in detention to guide treatment for gono-

coccal and chlamydial infections. Translating research into intervention. *Arch Pediatr Adolesc Med* 152:53–56, 1998.

43. Hook EW 3rd, Smith K, Mullen C, et al: Diagnosis of genitourinary *Chlamydia trachomatis* infections by using the ligase chain reaction on patient-obtained vaginal swabs. *J Clin Microbiol* 35:2133–2135, 1997.
44. Hook EW 3rd, Ching SF, Stephens J, et al: Diagnosis of *Neisseria gonorrhoeae* infections by using the ligase chain reaction on patient-obtained vaginal swabs. *J Clin Microbiol* 35:2129–2132, 1997.
45. Embling ML, Monroe KW, Oh MK, Hook EW 3rd: Opportunistic urine ligase chain reaction screening for sexually transmitted diseases in adolescents seeking care in an urban emergency department. *Ann Emerg Med* 36:28–32, 2000.
46. Oh MK, Richey CM, Pate MS, et al: High Prevalence of *Chlamydia trachomatis* infections in adolescent females not having pelvic examinations: utility of PCR-based urine screening in urban adolescent clinic setting. *J Adolesc Health* 21:80–86, 1997.
47. Olsen JC, Salomon B: Utility of the creatinine prior to intravenous contrast studies in the emergency department. *J Emerg Med* 14:543–546, 1996.
48. Maglinte DD, Reyes BL, Harmon BH, et al: Reliability and role of plain film radiography and JCT in the diagnosis of small-bowel obstruction. *Am J Roentgenol* 167:1451–1455, 1996.
49. Shea JA, Berlin JA, Escarce JJ, et al: Revised estimates of diagnostic test sensitivity and specificity in suspected biliary tract disease. *Arch Intern Med* 154:2573–2581, 1994.
50. Sinclair D, Wilson S, Toi A, Greenspan L: The evaluation of suspected renal colic: Ultrasound scan versus excretory urography. *Ann Emerg Med* 18:556–559, 1989.
51. Morse JW, Hill R, Greissinger WJ, et al: Rapid oral hydration results in hydronephrosis as demonstrated by bedside ultrasound. *Ann Emerg Med* 34:134–140, 1999.
52. Melanson SW, Heller M: Contemporary issues in trauma: the emerging role of bedside ultrasonography in trauma care. *Emerg Clin North Am* 16:165–189, 1998.
53. Yoshii H, Sato M, Yamamoto S, Motegi M, et al: Usefulness and limitations of ultrasonography in the initial evaluation of blunt abdominal trauma. *J Trauma* 45:45–50, 1998.
54. Richards JR, Schleper NH, Woo BD, Bohnen PA et al: Sonographic assessment of blunt abdominal trauma: a 4–year prospective study. *J Clin Ultrasound* 30:59–67, 2002.
55. Lingawi SS, Buckley AR: Focused abdominal US in patients with trauma. *Radiology* 217:426–429, 2000.
56. Nunes LW, Simmons S, Hallowell MJ, Kinback R: Diagnostic performance of trauma US in identifying abdominal or pelvic free fluid and serious abdominal or pelvic injury. *Acad Radiol* 8:128–136, 2001.
57. Sirlin CB, Casola G, Brown MA, et al: US of blunt abdominal trauma: importance of free pelvic fluid in women of reproductive age. *Radiology* 219:229–235, 2001.
58. Brafman BH, Coleman BG, Ramchandani P: Emergency department screening for ectopic pregnancy: a prospective US study. *Radiology* 190:797–802, 1994.
59. Cacciatore B, Leminen A, Ingman-Friberg S: Transvaginal sonographic findings in ambulatory patients with suspected pelvic inflammatory disease. *Obstet Gynecol* 80:912–916, 1992.
60. Jermy K, Luise C, Bourne T: The characterization of common ovarian cysts in premenopausal women. *Ultrasound Obstet Gynecol* 17:140–144, 2001.
61. Mikkelsen AL, Felding C: Laparoscopy and ultrasound examination in women with acute pelvic pain. *Gynecol Obstet Invest* 30:162–164, 1990.
62. Balthazar EJ, Rofsky NM, Zucker R: Appendicitis: The impact of computed tomography imaging on negative appendectomy and perforation rates. *Am J Gastroenterol* 93:768–771, 1998.
63. Rao PM, Rhea JT, Novelline RA, et al: Helical CT combined with contrast material administered only through the colon for imaging of suspected appendicitis. *Am J Roentgenol* 169:1275–1280, 1997.
64. Rao PM, Rhea JT, Novelline RA, et al: Helical CT technique for the diagnosis of appendicitis: prospective evaluation of a focused appendix CT examination. *Radiology* 202:139–144, 1997.
65. Jacobs JE, Birnbaum BA, Macari M, et al: Acute appendicitis: Comparison of helical CT diagnosis-focused technique with oral contrast material versus nonfocused technique with oral and intravenous contrast material. *Radiology* 220:683–690, 2001.
66. Fielding JR, Steele G, Fox LA, et al: Spiral computerized tomography in the evaluation of acute flank pain: a replacement for excretory urography. *J Urol* 157:2071–2073, 1997.
67. Portis AJ, Sandaram CP: Diagnosis and initial management of kidney stones. *Am Fam Phys* 63:2001, 63(7): 1329–38.
68. Rao PM, Feltmate CM, Rhea JT, et al: Helical computed tomography in differentiating appendicitis and acute gynecologic conditions. *Obstet Gynecol* 93:417–421, 1999.
69. Parry RA, Glaze SA, Archer BR: The AAPM/RSNA physics tutorial for residents. Typical patient radiation doses in diagnostic radiology. *Radiographics* 19:1289–1302, 1999.
70. Ogilvy-Stuart AL, Shalet SM: Effect of radiation on the human reproductive system. *Environ Health Perspect* 101(Suppl 2):109–116, 1993.
71. Wallace HB, Shalet SM, Hendry JH, et al: Ovarian failure following abdominal irradiation in childhood: The radiosensitivity of the human oocyte. *Br J Radiol* 62:995–998, 1989.
72. Borgstein PJ, Gordijn RV, Eijsbouts QA, Cuesta MA: Acute appendicitis—a clear-cut case in men, a guessing game in young women. A prospective study on the role of laparoscopy. *Surg Endosc* 11:923–927, 1997.
73. Cox MR, McCall JL, Padbury RT, et al: Laparoscopic surgery in women with a clinical diagnosis of acute appendicitis. *Med J Aust* 162:130–132, 1995.

74. Porpora MG, Gomel V: The role of laparoscopy in the management of pelvic pain in women of reproductive age. *Fertil Steril* 70:592–594, 1998.
75. Brewster GS, Herbert ME, Hoffman JR. Medical myth: Analgesia should not be given to patients with an acute abdomen because it obscures the diagnosis. *Western Journal of Medicine* 172:209–210, 2000.
76. Cordell WH, Wright SW, Wolfson AB, et al: Comparison of intravenous ketorolac, meperidine, and both (balanced analgesia) for renal colic. *Ann Emerg Med* 28:151–158, 1996.
77. Rothrock SG: Misdiagnosis of appendicitis in nonpregnant women of childbearing age. *J Emerg Med* 13:1–8, 1995.
78. Mourad J, Elliott J, Erickson L: Appendicitis in pregnancy: New information that contradicts long-held clinical beliefs. *Am J Obstet Gynecol* 182:1027–1029, 2000.
79. Moscati RM: Cholelithiasis, cholecystitis, and pancreatitis. *Emerg Med Clin North Am* 14:719–737, 1996.
80. Eskelinen M, Ikonen J, Lipponen P: Contributions of history-taking, physical examination, and computer assistance to diagnosis of acute small-bowel obstruction. A prospective study of 1333 patients with acute abdominal pain. *Scand J Gastroenterol* 29:715–721, 1994.
81. MacKenna A, Fabres C, Alam V, Morales V: Clinical management of functional ovarian cysts: a prospective and randomized study. *Hum Reprod* 15:2567–2569, 2000.
82. Houry D, Abbott JT: Ovarian torsion: A fifteen-year review. *Ann Emerg Med* 38:156–159, 2001.

29

Sexually Transmitted Diseases and Pelvic Inflammatory Disease

Sebastian Faro
Mark D. Pearlman

KEY POINTS

- A careful sexual history is important to identify high-risk individuals who should be tested for STDs because most who are infected are asymptomatic.
- STDs leading to genital ulcers may result from herpes simplex virus (painful) chancroid infection (painful) or syphilis (nonpainful).
- Treatment for pelvic inflammatory disease should be considered in sexually active women with lower abdominal pain, cervical motion tenderness, and adnexal tenderness in the absence of another attributable cause.
- The specificity of clinical diagnosis of PID is approximately 67 percent. While various positive tests can improve specificity (e.g., positive gonorrhea or chlamydial test, elevated white blood cell count), requiring positive test results will substantially reduce the sensitivity of clinical diagnosis.

Sexually transmitted diseases (STDs) constitute one of the largest groups of infectious diseases in the world. The ease of travel from one continent to another facilitates the spread of STDs, including those previously confined to subtropical and tropical areas (e.g., chancroid and lymphogranuloma venereum). All sexually active women are potentially at risk for contracting an STD if they participate in high-risk sexual behavior. Transmission of STDs is best controlled through prevention. The most logical approach to prevention is through education, a process that requires the participation of physicians, nurses, educators, and parents. Unfortunately, education efforts are frequently blocked or inhibited because there is a lack of understanding by community leaders. These individuals often misconstrue the effort and interpret the educational process as fostering sexual activity. Treatment programs directed against acute infection to eradicate the offending organisms are already in place. New antimicrobial agents that have a broader spectrum of activity, have longer half-lives, and achieve high concentrations in tissues when taken orally continue to be developed. In addition, agents such as metronidazole, ofloxacin, and lomefloxacin are available for parenteral and oral use. The administration of these antibiotics is cost effective because a change in administration from intravenous to oral agents can be made without reducing the serum and tissue concentration of the antibiotic.

Physicians, nurse practitioners, and other health care providers should become familiar with the epidemiology of sexually transmitted diseases and the sequelae of these infections. They should be able to determine, through a careful history, who is at risk for contracting a sexually transmitted disease. When treating a patient for a sexually transmitted disease, the physician must remember that the infected woman may have transmitted the infection to all those who have had intimate contact with her. The goals of treating a woman with a sexually transmitted disease are to eradicate the offending organisms and prevent damage to her reproductive organs. In turn, this will reduce her risk of developing infertility, or if she should conceive, ectopic pregnancy.[1] Within every community there is a pool of individuals who are infected with organisms that cause sexually transmitted diseases, and these individuals serve as reservoirs for the dissemination of STDs. This pool of individuals tends to remain constant because they are asymptomatic; some fail to seek treatment because their symptoms abate and they believe they are no longer infected; while others just refuse to be treated or become repeatedly reinfected. This pool serves as the community reservoir and individuals who are not members of this pool, but may have been exposed, serve as vectors to those outside the pool of infected individuals. Thus an individual who is not involved in a truly monogamous relationship may well be an unsuspecting victim of high-risk sexual behavior. Individuals who are highly mobile, traveling to other parts of the world, can also transmit infections that are uncommon in a given region (e.g., lymphogranuloma venereum in the United States).

STDs that are concomitant with pregnancy can have severe and detrimental effects on pregnant women, their partners, and their fetuses. In addition to the effect of STDs on the pregnant woman, many of these organisms can be transmitted to the fetus, causing a myriad of adverse effects, including congenital anomalies, mental retardation, blindness, preterm birth, and intrauterine fetal demise.

DIAGNOSIS OF SEXUALLY TRANSMITTED DISEASES

The initial step in the management of any STD is to obtain a detailed history to determine the degree of risk and the type of infections to which the individual has most likely been exposed. The interview does not have to be long but should be thorough. Typically, women who may have an STD seek medical attention for one of the following reasons: the presence of lower abdominal pain, irregular vaginal bleeding, abnormal vaginal discharge, vulvar or vaginal discomfort, or the fear that they have been exposed to an STD. The patient with an abnormal vaginal discharge may think she has a yeast infection, which is not an STD. One important mistake that the patient may make is to use an over-the-counter antifungal preparation that may mask symptoms or delay treatment of a cervical STD or vaginal trichomoniasis. The latter may serve as an indicator for the presence of another STD such as *Neisseria gonorrhoeae* or *Chlamydia trachomatis* because it is common for a patient to be infected by more than one STD. For example, between 30 and 50 percent of women infected with gonorrhea will also be infected with *Chlamydia.*

The patient should be asked questions that permit the physician or nurse to determine the degree of risk, the extent of symptoms, and possibly the time elapsed since exposure. Questions may be posed as follows:

1. Are you sexually active?
2. At what age did you first experience sexual intercourse?
3. How many sexual partners have you had in your lifetime?
4. How many sexual partners have you had in the last year?
5. Do you believe that your current partner is having sex with any other partners?
6. Do you suspect or know if your current partner is bisexual?
7. Do you live with your current partner?
8. Do you use drugs, including alcohol?
9. Do you have lower abdominal pain, cramping, or discomfort?
10. Do you have bleeding or spotting associated with sexual intercourse?
11. Do you have vaginal bleeding or spotting at any time other than at the time of your menses?
12. Have you had a recent Pap smear that was abnormal?
13. Have you ever had gonorrhea, chlamydia, syphilis, herpes, genital warts, HPV, HIV, or hepatitis?
14. Have you ever been treated for an infection in your fallopian tubes or been told you had pelvic inflammatory disease (PID)?
15. Have you ever been exposed to anyone who had an STD?
16. Have you ever been treated for an STD?
17. Do you practice anal intercourse?

Questions such as those listed above will facilitate in determining the patient's risk for STD. Once the interview is concluded, the patient should be prepared for the examination. If the patient participates in oral-genital contact, specimens from the posterior pharynx should be obtained for the detection of *N. gonorrhoeae* and *C. trachomatis.* If one or more oral ulcerations are found, specimens should be obtained for the detection of herpes simplex virus. If the patient does practice anal intercourse, specimens should be obtained from the rectum for the detection of *N. gonorrhoeae* and *C. trachomatis.*

The pelvic examination begins with a thorough examination of the external genitalia. Specifically, the examiner should check for fissures, ulcerations, blisters, and exophytic lesions. The lesions produced by herpes simplex virus can vary from tiny fissure-like lesions to frank ulcerations. The presence of ulcerated lesions should spark further examination for the possible presence of a variety of STDs as well as non-STDs (e.g., Crohn's disease or lichen sclerosus). The presence of exophytic lesions, pyriform and moist, or flat, dry, and rough, indicates the probable presence of human papillomavirus (condylomata acuminata). Flat and waxy lesions (condylomata lata) indicate the probable presence of syphilis. A speculum is then inserted into the vagina and the vaginal epithelium should be examined for the presence of erythema, ulcerations, and exophytic lesions. The vaginal discharge should also be evaluated by determining the pH, reaction with potassium hydroxide (whiff test), color, and microscopic analysis; see also Chap. 30).

The cervix should be closely inspected for the presence of infection and/or inflammation. The portio of the cervix should be pink and smooth. The presence of petechial hemorrhages indicates the possible presence of trichomoniasis. The presence of shallow ulcerations suggests herpes simplex, syphilis, or chancroid. If the endocervical

Table 29-1. Diagnostic Features of Infectious Vaginitis

	Normal	Candidal Vaginitis	Bacterial Vaginosis	Trichomonas Vaginitis
Symptoms	None or physiologic leukorrhea	Vulvar pruritus, soreness, increased discharge, dysuria, dyspareunia	Malodorous moderate discharge	Profuse purulent discharge, offensive odor, pruritus, and dyspareunia
Discharge				
Amount	Variable, scant to moderate	Scant to moderate	Moderate	Profuse
Color	Clear or white	White	White/gray	Yellow
Consistency	Floccular nonhomogeneous	Clumped but variable	Homogeneous, uniformly coating walls	Homogeneous
"Bubbles"	Absent	Absent	Present	Present
Appearance of vulva and vagina	Normal	Introital and vulvar erythema, edema and occasional pustules, vaginal erythma	No inflammation	Erythema and swelling of vulvar and vaginal epithelium ("strawberry cervix")
pH of vaginal fluid	<4.5	<4.5	>4.5	5-6.0
Amine test (10% KOH)	Negative	Negative	Positive	Occasionally positive
Saline microscopy	Normal epithelial cell Lactobacilli predominate	Normal flora, blastospores (yeast), 40-50% pseudohyphae	Clue cells, coccobacillary flora predominates, absence of leukocytes, motile curved rods	PMNs + + + Motile trichomonads (80-90%), no clue cells, abnormal flora
10% KOH microscopy	Negative	Positive (60-90%)	Negative (except in mixed infections)	Negative

columnar epithelium appears to be everting and is slightly erythematous, this may be nothing more than an eversion commonly seen in teenagers, pregnant women and women taking oral contraceptive pills. The presence of markedly erythematous and edematous columnar epithelium is highly suggestive of inflammation (cervicitis).

A cotton- or Dacron-tipped swab should be inserted into the endocervical canal and gently rotated several times. The swab is then withdrawn and examined for the presence of mucopus, which suggests infection and requires testing for both *N. gonorrhoeae* and *C. trachomatis.* The cervix should be examined for the presence of white lesions, either flat or exophytic, indicating the presence of human papillomavirus (condylomata acuminatum). If the cervix bleeds briskly following cotton swab examination, this is suggestive of inflammation and possible infection.

The speculum is withdrawn and a bimanual examination should always follow. The cervix should be palpated and should be firm, and not tender to palpation or gentle motion. A tender cervix indicates the possibility of infection. If the cervix is soft, the possibility of pregnancy should be entertained. The uterus should be palpated for consistency, size, symmetry, and pain or tenderness. Pain on palpation and motion of the uterus is suggestive of infection (endometritis). Patients with endometritis may present with lower abdominal pain, described as crampy, dull, or sharp. It is not uncommon for these patients to present with irregular uterine bleeding. A pregnancy test should be performed to rule out pregnancy. If the pregnancy test is positive in a patient who is bleeding, the differential diagnosis includes threatened, missed, incomplete or complete abortion, and ectopic pregnancy. Patients fewer than 12 weeks pregnant (with an intrauterine pregnancy) can develop salpingitis (PID), though PID is much less common during pregnancy. The patient with an early intrauterine pregnancy presenting with pain and vaginal bleeding may also have a septic abortion (see Chap. 6)

Palpation of the adnexa should be performed gently; exerting too much pressure will cause pain for the patient, even the healthy one. The presence of pain on palpation and motion of the adnexa is suggestive of inflammation and infection. Only one-third of patients with demonstrable pelvic pain actually have pelvic inflammatory disease. Two-thirds of these patients will have no adnexal pathology, endometriosis or other pelvic processes.

SYPHILIS

The rates of primary and secondary syphilis have progressively declined in the United States since 1990.[2] The CDC reported that there were 6993 cases of primary and secondary syphilis (2.6 cases/100,000 population) in 1998. The highest incidence was in the South (5.1 cases/100,000), followed by the Midwest (1.9 cases/100,000), the West (1.0 cases/100,000), and the Northeast (0.8 cases/100,000). In 1999 the CDC reported that there were 6657 cases of primary and secondary syphilis in the United States.[3] The South continued to have the highest incidence (4.5 cases/100,000), and the Midwest reported an increase from 1.9 to 2.2 cases/100,000.

The etiologic agent of syphilis is the spirochete *Treponema pallidum.* Transmission of *Treponema pallidum* is primarily by mucosal contact with a lesion during sexual activity. Acquisition of syphilis can also occur via contact between a lesion and a break in the dermis, or via contact with infected blood during transfusion, delivery of an infant by a patient infected with *T. pallidum,* or through sharing needles among drug users. Transmission can also occur via oral contact, either through fellatio, cunnilingus, or kissing if one of the partners has an oral lesion. Perinatal transmission occurs through hematogenous spread and should be screened for and treated during pregnancy.

Syphilis is divided into the following stages:

1. Primary syphilis: This may last up to 3 months and is usually undetected in the female patient because the ulcer or chancre is asymptomatic. Women typically do not examine their genitalia; therefore unless the ulcer is on the vulva it will not be noticed.
2. Secondary syphilis: This begins approximately 3 to 6 weeks after the primary chancre appears and is highly infectious. Secondary syphilis is divided into two phases: (a) *early latent phase:* This phase can be asymptomatic or symptomatic, it lasts up to 1 year, and the patient can easily transmit the disease to others; and (b) *late latent phase:* This begins after the disease has been present for >1 year. Typically the patient is asymptomatic and this phase can last for up to 10 years. Pregnant women can transmit the disease to the fetus, but women who have the disease for >4 years and subsequently become pregnant are not likely to transmit the disease to their fetus.
3. Tertiary (late) syphilis: This includes benign tertiary syphilis and the involvement of the cardiovascular and central nervous systems.

All patients who have a positive test for syphilis should have an HIV test performed.

Primary Syphilis

Primary syphilis is characterized by the presence of an asymptomatic chancre. The chancre or ulcer is usually a solitary lesion with a bright erythematous base that may be indurated and has a raised margin. The lesion can become secondarily infected, and in this case it will have a purulent base that can be painful.

Chancres can be found anywhere on the body, but are typically found on the labia majora, labia minora, the vestibule, the vaginal walls, the cervix, and the perianal area. Inguinal lymphadenopathy is usually present and is bilateral.[4]

The diagnosis of primary syphilis is made either by darkfield microscopy or serology. Darkfield microscopy can also be used on lesions associated with early latent secondary syphilis (e.g., the chancre, maculopapular skin rash, and condylomata lata). Serology should be obtained for all individuals suspected of having syphilis. Antibodies to nonspecific (VDRL, RPR) and specific tests (MHA-TP, FTA-ABS) will be positive in 75 percent of infected individuals approximately 3 weeks after infection. If the initial serology is negative, the tests should be repeated in 1 month if there is concern about recent exposure. The initial tests for syphilis are nonspecific screening tests; the rapid plasma reagin (RPR) or Venereal Disease Research Laboratory (VDRL) are the most common tests used.[5] If the nonspecific test is positive, confirmatory testing is usually automatically performed via the fluorescent treponemal antibody absorbed (FTA-ABS) test or the microhemagglutination assay for antibodies to *T. pallidum* (MHA-TP). The FTA-ABS and MHA-TP are highly specific and tend to remain positive for life. Therefore these tests are only of value to rule out a false-positive nonspecific test in individuals who have not already had syphilis.[6,7] However, 15 to 25 percent of treated individuals will revert to being serologically nonreactive after 2 to 3 years.

Individuals suspected of having early primary syphilis should be screened with a nontreponemal serum test (e.g., VDRL); of those infected, 70 percent will be found to be positive. Individuals suspected of having syphilis who have a nonreactive nontreponemal test should be retested in 1 to 3 months to ensure that they remain negative. The repeat testing is necessary because if the individual is found to be positive at any of the testing times, treatment can be instituted, the infection eradicated, and potential transmission of the disease can be curtailed.

If the individual's specific and nonspecific test returns positive, the titer is >1:16, and there are no visible lesions, the patient should be considered to have secondary syphilis and not primary syphilis. If the individual is known to have had a nonreactive nontreponemal test in the previous year, then the patient should be considered to have early latent syphilis. If this information is not known, the patient should be considered to have late latent syphilis. Some experts recommend that individuals with late latent syphilis and a nontreponemal serolic test less than 1:32 should be evaluated for neurosyphilis. Approximately 20 percent of individuals with late latent syphilis will have a nonreactive nontreponemal test (RPR or VDRL). Therefore, an individual with a positive FTA-ABS or MHA-TP should have a spinal tap and a VDRL performed on the spinal fluid. If the VDRL is positive the presence of neurosyphilis is confirmed. If the VDRL is negative, however, the presence of neurosyphilis is not ruled out. A CSF with increased lymphocytes (>5/mm^3) and an elevated total protein (>45 mg/dL) are highly suggestive of central nervous system involvement.[8]

The nonspecific nontreponemal screening tests are also used to follow the efficacy of treatment for both primary and secondary disease. The VDRL or RPR should be obtained 3 to 4 months following therapy, via follow-up with their ongoing care provider, and there should be a fourfold decline in titer. Six to eight months following the completion of therapy there should be an eightfold decline in the titer.[8,9] Patients with early syphilis who have been successfully treated will generally have a negative titer after 1 year, whereas latent syphilis patients will have a slower rate of decline in titer.[9] Approximately 50 percent will have a lower titer 2 years after treatment. A fourfold rise in titer is an indication that the patient has been reinfected.

False-positive nontreponemal tests may occur following a viral infection, bacterial infections, fever, recent immunization, pregnancy, and with other treponemal infections (e.g., Lyme disease). Patients with early human immunodeficiency virus (HIV) infection may yield a false-positive test for syphilis. Individuals with an autoimmune disease, narcotic addiction, or chronic bacterial infection may also yield a false-positive RPR, VDRL, or automated regain test (ART). Although specific tests for *T. pallidum* (FTA-ABS or MHA-TP) are highly specific, there is a 1 percent false-positive rate.[9–12]

Diagnosis

The differential diagnosis of a patient with a genital ulcer includes:

Herpes simplex
Chancroid
Lymphogranuloma venereum
Granuloma inguinale
Traumatic lesion
Furuncles
Drug eruptions
Beçhet's disease
Carcinoma

The approach to the patient with a genital ulcer can be as follows:

Nonpainful and not secondarily infected:

1. If it is not painful, there is a higher probability that it is a syphilitic chancre.
2. The surface of the ulcer should be gently scraped to produce a serous exudate.
3. A drop or two of serum can be placed on a slide, covered with a glass coverslip, and examined by darkfield microscopy for the presence of spirochetes. An alternative to darkfield microscopy is direct fluorescent an-

tibody test for *T. pallidum* (DFA-TP). The sensitivity and specificity for DFA-TP are 86 percent and 100 percent, respectively.[13]

4. Draw venous blood for a nonspecific nontreponemal screening test (i.e., VDRL or RPR) and if positive, an FTA-ABS or MHA-TP should be performed.
5. Screen patient for *Neisseria gonorrhoeae* and *Chlamydia trachomatis.*
6. If the test for *T. pallidum* is positive, screen patient for hepatitis B and C and HIV.

Treatment

Treatment of primary syphilis is benzathine penicillin G, 2.4 million units IM in a single dose or 1.2 million units in each buttock.[14]

Nonpregnant patients who are allergic to penicillin can be treated with tetracycline 500 mg PO two times a day for 14 days, or doxycycline 100 mg PO four times a day for 14 days. Pregnant patients allergic to penicillin should be hospitalized and desensitized.[14]

Secondary Syphilis

Early secondary syphilis is characterized by a variety of clinical manifestations: chancre, condylomata lata, maculopapular rash, inguinal lymphadenopathy, fever, and alopecia. However, the individual may also be asymptomatic. Pregnant patients are likely to be asymptomatic and detected only by a reactive RPR that is routinely performed as part of the prenatal blood tests. Pregnant patients with primary and early secondary syphilis can easily transmit the infection transplacentally, even during the asymptomatic phase.

Diagnosis

The diagnosis in women, especially during pregnancy, is made by positive serology. Patients presenting with a genital ulcer, raised, flat, or waxy-appearing lesions (condylomata lata), or a maculopapular rash distributed over their body, including the palms of their hands and soles of their feet, should be tested for syphilis. The condylomatous lesions usually are found on the vulva and perirectal areas. These lesions, like the maculopapular rash and all lesions of early latent secondary syphilis, are infectious and can therefore transmit the infection. The patient may not have any lesions, but present with fever, headache, malaise, myalgias, or pharyngitis (i.e., a typical flu-like syndrome). The patient may also present with hepatosplenomegaly and hepatitis. The patient may report spontaneous alopecia. The differential diagnosis for a patient with a clinical presentation suggesting secondary syphilis is as follows:

Rubella
Measles
Rash associated with medications
Erythema multiforme
Early Kaposi's sarcoma
Condylomata acuminata

Treatment

Treatment of early latent secondary syphilis (<1 year) is benzathine penicillin G 2.4 million units IM in a single dose, or 1.2 million units in each buttock.

The treatment for late latent secondary syphilis is benzathine penicillin G 7.2 million units. The regimen is 2.4 million units administered IM weekly for 3 weeks.

Other Management Issues

Patients with syphilis and any of the following should be evaluated for neurosyphilis.

- Neurologic or opthalmic signs or symptoms
- Evidence of tertriary syphilis (e.g., gumma, aortitis)
- Treatment failure, or
- Late latent syphilis plus HIV infection

Treatment

Penicillin G 18–24 million units per day administered as 3–4 million units every 4 hours for 10–14 days.

Jarisch-Herxheimer Reaction

The Jarisch-Herxheimer reaction may occur within a few hours of the administration of penicillin. It is characterized by rapid development of fever and skin and mucosal lesions. It is thought to be the result of the patient's response to treatment by producing cytokines and tumor necrosis factor-α (TNF-α). Pregnant patients who are treated for syphilis with penicillin while carrying a viable fetus should be monitored in a labor and delivery setting for up to 12 hours, as intrauterine death has been reported following treatment and the occurrence of the Jarisch-Herxheimer reaction.[15,16]

HERPES SIMPLEX

Occasionally, an initial primary herpes infection will cause the patient such discomfort that she will require immediate evaluation and treatment. The type 2 herpes simplex virus (HSV-2) is usually transmitted by direct sexual contact, and the symptoms associated with an initial primary infection usually develop between 3 and 7 days after contact with the virus. Approximately 80–85 percent of genital herpes are caused by HSV-2; the remainder result from HSV-1 infections. Often, an initial infection may be mild or even completely asymptomatic, but occasionally patients develop severe, disabling symptoms. The patient may complain of severe vulvar pain and tenderness. She may also experience severe dysuria and urinary retention. Inguinal and pelvic pain related to lymphadenopathy is frequently observed with primary infection. Systemic symptoms of headache, generalized aching, and malaise with fever are also common.

The lesions seen in a primary herpes infection are frequently extensive and involve the labia majora, labia minora, perianal skin, vestibule of the vulva, and possibly the vaginal as well as the cervical mucosa. Profuse watery discharge can also be present with primary infection. Early in the course of the disease, multiple vesicles on an erythematous base may be scattered over these areas, but they rapidly rupture and leave shallow ulcerated areas (Fig. 29-1). Lesions may coalesce to form large bullae that subsequently lead to the development of large ulcers. Superficial ulcerations may be seen in the ectocervix and within the vagina. Occasionally, a fungating necrotic mass may be seen covering the ectocervix. The latter can easily be confused with invasive cervical carcinoma. Under these circumstances, the cervix may be exquisitely tender, may bleed easily, and when manipulated can provoke severe pelvic pain. Inguinal lymphadenopathy is usually present. The primary lesions may persist for 2 to 6 weeks without treatment.

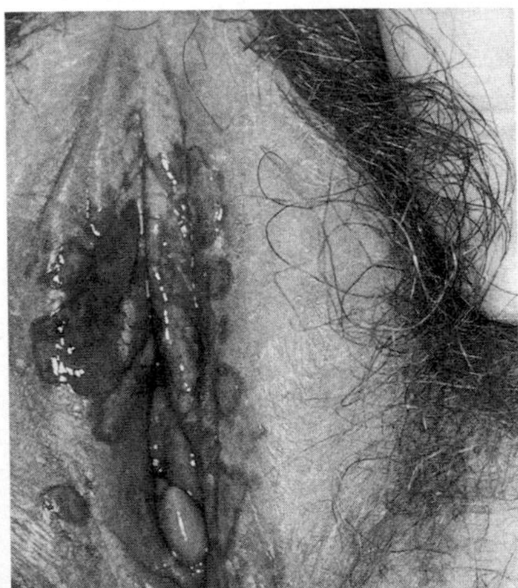

Fig. 29-1. Primary herpes genitalis. One week after the development of herpes genitalis, multiple painful, shallow ulcers are seen. (From Kaufman RH, Gardner HL, Rawls WE, Dixon RE, Young RL: Clinical features of herpes genitalis. *Cancer Res* 33:1446–51, 1973, with permission.)

Occasionally, meningitis may be seen in association with a primary infection. Under these circumstances, the patient usually complains of severe headache, neck stiffness, and/or blurring of vision. Rarely, encephalitis can develop during a primary infection. If the sacral plexus is involved, acute urinary retention can result. However, the most common reason for urinary retention is infection involving the urethra and bladder.

Diagnosis

The disease is usually diagnosed on the basis of clinical findings. However, the diagnosis should be confirmed by culture and the identification of the virus, antigen detection, immunofluorescence, or enzyme-linked immunosorbent assay (ELISA).[17,18,19] Patients should not be told they have a sexually transmitted disease unless confirmed by a specific test. As with all STDs, when given to the patient, this information can have significant deleterious effects on her relationships, and also can have a significant impact on the future delivery of her children. Although the clinical presentation of genital herpes is quite distinctive, it can be confused with other genital diseases. It is also important to determine whether the current infection is the result of HSV-1 or HSV-2, as this will have bearing on the potential for recurrent episodes.

Herpes simplex infection may present as any of the following:

Oral lesions (cold sores, fever blisters)
Pharyngitis
Gastrointestinal lesions
Pneumonia
Hepatitis
Herpetic whitlow
Keratitis
Eczema herpeticum
Genital lesions
Disseminated infection

Encephalitis

Newborn infection

Patients presenting with fever, cognitive or emotional changes, seizures, and an altered sensorium should be considered to possibly have herpetic meningoencephalitis and should have a lumbar puncture. The central spinal fluid in these cases will reveal a WBC count of 5 to 1000, mostly PMNs early in the disease, but later they are replaced by monocytes. Glucose is typically normal (40 to 80 mg or at least 40 percent of the blood sugar), and the protein content is less than 100 mg (normal is less than 50 mg).[19] Meningoencephalitis caused by HSV-2 is milder than that caused by HSV-1. Thus patients complaining of photophobia or headache should be evaluated for meningeal irritation and the possibility of HSV meningoencephalitis. Prompt initiation of parenteral acyclovir is imperative.

Treatment

Primary Herpetic Infection

Treat with one of the following:

- Acyclovir 200 mg five times a day for 10 days or 400 mg twice a day for 10 days; or
- Valacyclovir 1000 mg twice a day for 10 days; or
- Famciclovir 250 mg three times a day for 10 days.

Recurrent Herpes Treatment

Treat with one of the following:

- Acyclovir 400 mg three times a day for 5 days; or 800 mg twice a day for 5 days.
- Valacyclovir 500 mg twice a day for 3 to 5 days;
- Famciclovir 125 mg twice a day for 5 days.

Suppressive Therapy

Treat with one of the following:

- Acyclovir 400 mg twice a day;
- Valacyclovir 1000 mg once a day; or
- Famciclovir 250 mg twice a day for 1 year.

Treatment for disseminated herpetic infection including pneumonia, hepatitis, or CNS complications (e.g., meningitis or encephalitis): acyclovir 5 to 10 mg/kg of body weight administered intravenously every 8 hours until clinical resolution is obtained.

Follow-Up

Patients should be advised that there is up to a 90 percent chance that they will have recurrent episodes of genital herpes virus infections if due to HSV-2. If recurrences occur frequently, they can be controlled by the use of suppressive therapy with acyclovir, valacyclovir, or famciclovir. In addition, the patient should be counseled regarding the possible risks associated with vaginal delivery in the presence of an active herpesvirus infection.

All patients should be counseled about the sexual transmission of HSV including the possibility of transmission even when a lesion is not present.

LYMPHOGRANULOMA VENEREUM

The etiologic agent is *Chlamydia trachomatis,* serovars L1, L2, and L3, and it is very rare in the United States. These should not be confused with the serovars responsible for cervicitis, endometritis, and salpingitis (PID). *Chlamydia trachomatis* is a true bacterium and a parasite because it requires an exogenous source of adenosine triphosphate (ATP), which is derived from the host. *Chlamydia trachomatis* also utilizes amino acids derived from the host. It has a unique life cycle consisting of two stages: an extracellular stage known as the infectious phase and an intracellular phase known as the metabolic phase.

The diagnosis of lymphogranuloma venereum (LGV) can be established by clinical findings combined with the use of specific laboratory tests that include the complement fixation tests, the microimmunofluorescent test with a titer >1:512, and the isolation of the organism in tissue culture.[20]

Clinically, LGV presents in one of three stages: primary, secondary, and tertiary. Primary LGV is characterized by the development of an ulcer or chancre, which appears approximately 1 to 3 weeks after inoculation.[21,22] The ulcer, unlike that seen with syphilis, lasts for only a few days and is painful. The lesion may initially develop as a small papule or may appear herpetiform and be confused with herpes.

Secondary LGV is characterized by the development of unilateral inguinal lymphadenopathy. The femoral lymph nodes may also become involved. Poupart's ligament separates these two groups of lymph nodes, creating the characteristic "groove sign." The lymph nodes may become large and tender and can often be extremely painful. They become soft and are referred to as buboes. The lymphatics of the vulva may become involved, giving rise to significant edema. Sclerosing ulcerations may also form and are typically painful. This condition is known as esthiomene, tertiary or late-stage LGV; it is characterized by vulvar elephantiasis. Ulcerations of the urethra may occur, disrupting its integrity; this may result in incontinence. Rectovaginal fistulas also develop and strictures may form in the pelvis along with significant granulation tissue resembling a "frozen pelvis."[23]

Diagnosis

The differential diagnosis includes the following:

- Syphilis
- Chancroid
- Genital ulcers
- Granuloma inguinale
- Cat-scratch fever
- Filariasis
- Incarcerated inguinal hernia
- Inguinal lymphadenitis secondary to a septic lesion of the lower extremity
- Anorectal syndrome
- Malignancy
- Trauma
- Tuberculosis
- Schistosomiasis
- Fungal infection
- Parasites

The diagnosis of LGV is usually made serologically with complement fixation titers $\geq$1:64.

Treatment

Treatment is with doxycycline 100 mg orally twice a day for 21 days.[14]

Alternative regimens include:

- Erythromycin 500 mg orally four times a day for 21 days (recommended regimen for pregnant patients)
- Sulfisoxazole 500 mg orally four times a day for 21 days.

CHANCROID

The etiologic agent is *Haemophilus ducreyi,* a gram-negative bacillus. The organism is transmitted by mucosal contact with a lesion and should be isolated by culture to establish the diagnosis. The incubation period following contact is 7 days or longer in women. The lesion begins as a papule, that develops into a pustule, and then forms a well-circumscribed ulcer.[24] The edges are irregular, undermined, and surrounded by an erythematous halo. The lesion is typically painful, but in women the chancre can be asymptomatic and not easily differentiated from a syphilitic chancre. The patient may develop unilateral inguinal lymphadenopathy, which is often painful. The enlarged lymph node appears erythematous; after 1 to 2 weeks, the center becomes fluctuant and ulcerates.

Diagnosis

The organism can be cultured directly from a lesion and the specimen should be obtained by directly swabbing it. The laboratory should be contacted prior to receiving the specimen to ensure that proper preparations are made for its handling. A special medium is required for the growth and isolation of *H. ducreyi,* such as Sheffield's medium or two different types of media.[25,26] A probable diagnosis can be made if all of the following are present: 1. One or more painful genital ulcers; 2. No evidence of syphilis (i.e., negative darkfield exam); 3. Lesion is consistent with chanerdid; and 4. Negative test for HSV.

Treatment

Treatment consists of any of the following:[14]

- Azithromycin 1 g orally in a single dose; or
- Erythromycin 500 mg orally three times a day for 7 days; or
- Ceftriaxone 250 mg IM in a single dose
  or
- Ciprofloxacin 500 mg orally twice a day for 3 days

GRANULOMA INGUINALE

The etiologic agent is *Calymmatobacterium granulomatis,* which belongs to the family Brucellaceae. This disease is also known by the name donovanosis, because upon staining, the material from a lesion reveals elliptical structures referred to as Donovan bodies within mononuclear cells and polymorphonuclear leukocytes.[27]

Typically, Giemsa and Wright stains are utilized and reveal characteristically stained bacilli within the host cells. The bacteria are deeply stained along the lateral edges and at each end, giving the organism an appearance resembling a safety pin.[28] When stained with Gram reagents, the organism is gram-negative.

The organism is endemic to southern India, western Australia, and tropical regions of Africa, Vietnam, Indonesia, Papua New Guinea, and the West Indies. It has also been reported in the southern part of the United States.[29] It is a known co-factor for HIV infection.

Clinically, ulcerative lesions appear on the external genitalia. The lesions are usually multiple, rupture spontaneously, and form round, elevated, velvety granulomatous ulcers that bleed easily and are infectious. As subsequent lesions develop secondary to autoinoculation, involvement of regional lymph nodes occurs. Indolent masses may form in the inguinal area, forming granulomatous lesions in the subcutaneous tissue. This may lead to scarring adjacent to the lymphatics, causing strictures and obstruction resulting in pseudoelephantiasis.

Diagnosis

The diagnosis is made by the identification of Donovan bodies in clinical specimens obtained from a chancre. An immunofluorescent antibody test using Donovan bodies as the antigen has been developed.[29] The differential diagnosis includes syphilis, LGV, chancroid, and anogenital amebiasis.

Treatment

Treat with any of the following regimens:

- Doxycycline 100 mg orally twice a day for at least 3 weeks; or
- Trimethoprim-sulfamethoxazole 1 DS (800 mg/160 mg) tablet orally twice a day for at least 3 weeks; or
- Erythromycin base 500 mg orally four times a day for 14 days.

Follow-Up

Patients should be followed clinically until signs and symptoms have resolved.

GONORRHEA AND CHLAMYDIA

The etiologic agent of gonorrhea is *Neisseria gonorrhoeae,* a gram-negative diplococcus typically seen within polymorphonuclear leukocytes in clinical specimens. When this observation is made, infection can be assumed to be present and treatment initiated. The organism is predominantly transmitted through sexual contact.

Infection of the cervix tends to be asymptomatic, whereas infection of the urethra and Skene's and Bartholin's glands tends to be symptomatic (e.g., purulent discharge, associated cellulitis, swelling, and frequently abscess of the gland). Unlike the case with *C. trachomatis* infection, salpingitis secondary to *N. gonorrhoeae* tends to be symptomatic. It is common to find these two organisms as coinfecting agents. Individuals who complain of symptoms of acute cystitis and are not found to be bacteriuric should be evaluated for the possible existence of the acute urethral syndrome. This is seen in women with dysuria, presence of WBCs in the urine, and a negative culture for typical uropathogens. A urethral swab culture for *N. gonorrhoeae, C. trachomatis, Mycoplasma hominis,* and *Ureaplasma urealyticum* will often identify the etiologic agent. This is important, because except for ofloxacin, antibiotics typically employed to treat cystitis may not be effective against these STD organisms.

Chlamydia trachomatis appears to be more prevalent in certain regions of the United States (Northeast, Northwest, and Midwest), while *N. gonorrhoeae* appears to be prevalent in the southern regions. The significant difference between the two STDs is that *C. trachomatis* tends to cause asymptomatic disease and is probably responsible for the greatest number of cases of fallopian tube damage resulting in unsuspected infertility. Therefore when patients are screened for any STD, they should be screened for both *C. trachomatis* and *N. gonorrhoeae*. Treatment should always be directed against the probability that both bacteria are present. Treatment regimens are discussed in detail below.

Chlamydia trachomatis is diagnosed either by culture, DNA recognition tests, ELISA, or direct fluorescent antibody test. When specimens are collected, they should be taken with a Dacron applicator on a plastic shaft to avoid potential exposure of toxic substances found in the adhesive used in cotton-tipped applicators. Specimens for either antigen detection or nucleic acid analysis are usually fixed when placed in the specific transport system.

CERVICITIS

Gonococcal or chlamydial cervicitis is typically asymptomatic, but may present with subtle signs of infection. The patient may note a sudden onset of postcoital bleeding, dyspareunia, or increased yellowish vaginal discharge. Examination may reveal the presence of endocervical mucopus or hypertrophy of the endocervical epithelium.[31] Gentle palpation of the endocervix with a sterile cotton- or Dacron-tipped applicator may precipitate brisk bleeding. Palpation and motion of the cervix may result in patient complaints of tenderness or pain. Specimens from the endocervix should be obtained with a Dacron-tipped applicator for the isolation of *N. gonorrhoeae* and *C. trachomatis.*

TREATMENT OF GONOCOCCAL AND CHLAMYDIAL INFECTIONS

Treatment is guided by the principle that one must always administer an antibiotic regimen that is effective against both *N. gonorrhoeae* and *C. trachomatis.*[14]

Urethritis and Cervicitis

Neisseria gonorrhoeae

The following antibiotics are administered in a *single dose:*

- Ceftriaxone 125 mg IM; or
- Cefixime 400 mg PO; or
- Ciprofloxacin 500 mg PO; or
- Ofloxacin 400 mg PO.
- Spectinomycin 2 grams IM

Chlamydia trachomatis

Administer doxycycline 100 mg PO twice a day for 7 days. Alternatives include:

- Azithromycin 1 g in a single dose; or
- Ofloxacin 300 mg twice a day for 7 days; or
- Erythromycin base 500 mg four times a day for 7 days; or
- Amoxicillin 500 mg three times a day for 7 days.

If gonococcal cervicitis is documented, 25 to 50 percent of patients will be coinfected with chlamydia.[32] As such, a presumptive diagnosis of chlamydial infection should be made and the patient treated unless a documented negative chlamydia test is confirmed. Sexual partners of these women should be referred for treatment.

Table 29-2. Common Sequelae of Pelvic Inflammatory Disease

Sequelae	Approximate Incidence after a Single Episode of PID
Infertility	20-25%
Chronic pelvic pain/dyspareunia	15-20%
Ectopic pregnancy	6-10%
Tuboovarian abscess	2-5% (of patients hospitalized for PID)
Need for surgery	15%
Any of the above	≥25%

PELVIC INFLAMMATORY DISEASE

Pelvic inflammatory disease (PID) is the clinical syndrome resulting from infection of the female upper genital tract and can include any combination of endometritis, salpingitis, pelvic peritonitis, or tuboovarian abscess.[14] Pelvic inflammatory disease is the most frequent cause of hospitalization for gynecologic disorders in reproductive-age women. According to the National Hospital Discharge Survey (1988–1990), the average annual hospitalization rate for women aged 15 to 28 for pelvic inflammatory disease was 49.3 per 10,000 (range, 31.4 to 48.6 for ages 15 to 19 and 25 to 29, respectively). When hospitalization rates were stratified by races other than white, the average annual hospitalization rate was 75.5 per 10,000 women (range, 58.3 to 88.3 for ages 15 to 19 and 25 to 29, respectively). More than 40 percent of women diagnosed with PID are between the ages of 15 and 24, and over half are nulliparous. Of all women hospitalized with PID, about one-third had a surgical procedure during the admission, and in one-third of those having surgery, the procedure was a hysterectomy.[33] Of women hospitalized with chronic PID, 90 percent underwent an operation during that admission.[34] Other consequences of PID include recurrent infection, formation of pelvic adhesions, development of tuboovarian abscess (TOA), chronic pelvic pain, infertility, and ectopic pregnancy (Table 29-2). The estimated annual cost for PID ranges from $800 million to $3 billion in the United States.

Pathophysiology and Microbiology

The most common mechanism of infection is a sexually acquired organism (e.g., *Chlamydia trachomatis* or *Neisseria gonorrhoeae*), leading to the ascending spread of microorganisms from the vagina and endocervix to the normally sterile upper reproductive tract. Other much less common mechanisms include spread from adjacent infection, such as appendicitis or diverticulitis; hematogenous dissemination from a distant focus, such as in tuberculosis; and transuterine spread, as from iatrogenic instrumentation (dilatation and curettage or abortion) or the placement of an intrauterine device. Bacteria attach to the ciliated tubal epithelium and invade the tubal muscularis. An intense inflammatory reaction results in the adherence of tubal surfaces, which may result in occlusion of the lumen, destruction of the cilia and microvilli on the mucosal surface of the lumen, or the formation of blind pouches, all of which can predispose to ectopic pregnancy or infertility. Pyosalpinx or TOA may form, and rupture of the abscess can result in intraperitoneal dissemination of infection.[35] Although most cases of PID are polymicrobial, it has no typical microbiologic profile. Aerobic and anaerobic bacteria such as streptococci, staphylococci, *Gardnerella vaginalis,* peptostreptococci, *Bacteroides* spp., *Escherichia coli, N. gonorrhoeae, C. trachomatis,* and genital mycoplasmas have all been cultured from the genital tracts of women with documented PID.[35] In about half of the cases of PID, *N. gonorrhoeae* and *C. trachomatis* are isolated from the upper genital tract, with a variety of nongonococcal and nonchlamydial organisms isolated in 60 to 85 percent.[36] *Chlamydia* and *N. gonorrhoeae* are the primary pathogens of the endocervix and cause a mucopurulent endocervicitis. The endocervical canal and its mucous plug are thought to provide a mechanical barrier, protecting the endometrium and upper genital tract from the vaginal flora. The most likely mechanism of disease development is through cervical infection with chlamydial or gonococcal organisms, which interfere with these barriers and permit ascending infection from a variety of pathogenic and endogenous vaginal flora.[37]

A relationship exists between the onset of PID and the time of menses, such that two-thirds to three-quarters of women with PID present during or just after their menses. This relationship may be due to the fact that normal menses brings about changes in the cervical mucus, permitting passage of organisms to the upper genital tract.

Diagnosis

The clinical diagnosis of PID can be difficult. Its presentation and severity vary widely, and there is no single historical, physical, or laboratory finding that is both sensitive and specific for PID.[38] Common historical findings in women with laparoscopically confirmed PID include lower abdominal pain (94 percent), subjective increase in vaginal discharge (55 percent), history of fever and/or chills (41 percent), irregular bleeding (35 percent), and urinary or GI symptoms (19 and 10 percent, respectively). Objective findings in this same group of women have included adnexal tenderness in 97 percent, visually abnormal vaginal discharge in 64 percent, and fever in one-third.[39] However, many women with these findings were subsequently shown to have other pathology (e.g., appendicitis, endometriosis, ruptured ovarian cysts, or normal pelvis), demonstrating the nonspecificity or poor positive predictive value of clinical diagnosis. In fact, 20 to 25 percent of women given a diagnosis of PID will have a normal pelvis on laparoscopic examination, and another 10 to 15 percent will have another attributable cause of lower abdominal pain. A list of other disease processes with similar symptoms is provided in Table 29-3.

Table 29-3. Differential Diagnosis of Acute Pelvic Inflammatory Disease

Adnexal torsion with or without neoplasm
Appendicitis
Diverticulitis
Ectopic pregnancy
Endometriosis
Gastroenteritis
Lower genital tract infection (cervicitis)
Normal pelvis (20-25%)
Ruptured ovarian cyst (mittelschmerz, hemorrhagic corpus luteum)
Septic abortion
Urinary tract pathology (pyelonephritis, low ureteral calculus)

The accurate clinical diagnosis of PID is often dependent upon and improved by evaluating the epidemiologic characteristics and clinical setting of the patient. Women presenting with signs and symptoms of PID who are sexually active, are in their teens, are attending an STD clinic, have a prior history of PID, or belong to a socioeconomic group with a high incidence of gonorrhea or chlamydial infections are more likely to have PID compared to women who do not have these characteristics.[14] Other factors associated with PID include douching, bacterial vaginosis, recent IUD insertion or uterine manipulation (e.g., dilatation and curettage), and presentation during or following the bleeding phase of the menstrual cycle.[40] A list of risk factors for PID is given in Table 29-4.

The accurate diagnosis of PID on the basis of clinical signs and symptoms is a challenging task since the positive predictive value of clinical diagnosis is only slightly bet-

Table 29-4. Risk Factors for Pelvic Inflammatory Disease

- Prior episodes of PID
- Multiple sexual patterns (more than two partners in the past 30 days)
- Exposure to gonorrhea or chlamydial infection
- Recent IUD insertion (within 4 months) or IUD use with multiple sexual partners
- Sexually active adolescents
- Douching

ter than two-thirds, using laparoscopy as the standard.[39] The Centers for Disease Control and Prevention (CDC) developed guidelines for the diagnosis of PID.[14] Because a delay in the diagnosis of PID can result in substantial tubal damage, an effort was made to make these diagnostic criteria as sensitive as possible. These criteria (Table 29-5) were established knowing that the specificity and hence positive predictive value of the diagnostic criteria would not be as high as more rigorous criteria. Simply put, the use of these criteria will likely overdiagnose PID, resulting in an effort to treat as many women as possible who actually have PID. Recognizing this, one must be aware of the social implications of these diagnostic criteria, which are likely to be inaccurate one-third of the time. Counseling patients (couples) about the imprecision of diagnosis is a good policy. Although prior PID is a risk factor for future episodes of PID, caution should be exercised in simply rediagnosing PID each time a woman presents again with lower abdominal pain, as recurrent pelvic pain can have many other causes (e.g., endometriosis, adenomyosis, ovarian cysts). Of course, should cervical specimens tested for *N. gonorrhoeae* or *C. trachomatis* return positive, the definite sexually-acquired nature of this infection must be discussed to prevent further spread. It is important to inform women diagnosed with PID of the possibility of a STD, the need for treatment or testing of sexual partners, and the need for condom use if sexual activity occurs before laboratory results return. It is also important to recommend screening for other STDs in these women (e.g., human immunodeficiency virus [HIV], syphilis, hepatitis B). Women who are HIV-positive are more likely to fail antimicrobial therapy and to require operative intervention.[41]

The physical examination of women with PID can be quite variable. Fever is likely to be present in only one-third of these women. Unless a ruptured TOA is present (rare), vital signs are usually stable, with only mild tachycardia being common. The lower abdomen is virtually always tender, ranging from mild to severe. The finding of peritoneal signs (involuntary guarding, rebound tenderness) may simply reflect the presence of purulent material in the peritoneal cavity from an otherwise uncomplicated PID, but should raise some suspicion about a more

Table 29-5. Criteria for the Diagnosis of Pelvic Inflammatory Disease

Empiric treatment of PID should be initiated in sexually active young women and other women at risk for STD, if the following minimum criteria are present and no other cause(s) for the illness can be identified:

Lower abdominal tenderness
Adnexal tenderness
Cervical motion tenderness

Additional criteria (improve specificity):

Temperature >38°C (100.9°F)
Abnormal cervical or vaginal discharge
Elevated erythrocyte sedimentation rate
Elevated C-reactive protein
Cervical culture positive for *N. gonorrorhoeae* or *C. trachomatis*

Most specific criteria:

Endometritis on endometrial biopsy
Transvaginal ultrasound demonstrating thickened, fluid-filled tubes with or without free fluid or a tuboovarian complex may also be seen on MRI, though this is not a typical initial test for PID
Demonstration of findings consistent with PID by laparoscopy

Source: Adapted from Centers for Disease Control and Prevention,[14] with permission.

complicated process, such as a ruptured appendicitis or a tuboovarian mass. The presence of fever and lower abdominal tenderness and signs of peritoneal irritation in a woman with unstable vital signs (tachycardia, hypotension, tachypnea) should raise the specter of a ruptured tuboovarian abscess—a true surgical emergency.

On speculum examination, an inflamed cervix with mucopurulent discharge supports the diagnosis, but its absence does not eliminate the possibility of PID. Adnexal tenderness (usually bilateral) and cervical motion tenderness are almost always present, but in varying degrees of severity. Physical evaluation of cervical motion tenderness (CMT) should be performed with care, as it can be elicited in women without pelvic pathology if excessive or rapid lateral displacement of the cervix is used. In patients with PID, CMT results from stretching of the inflamed parametrial structures, including the fallopian tube as well as the broad ligament and its contents. Gentle, limited lateral movement of the cervix (2 to 3 cm) is sufficient to elicit CMT if it is present. Adequate examination of the adnexal structures is frequently compromised by tenderness. If the examination is inadequate because of tenderness or if a mass is palpable, pelvic ultrasound should be obtained (see section on imaging studies, below). Although the clinical criteria for diagnosing PID are listed in Table 29-5, the gold standard for the diagnosis of PID is laparoscopy with demonstration of tubal edema, erythema, and purulent exudate. Laparoscopy is usually reserved for women with an uncertain diagnosis, particularly if there is concern over the need for surgical intervention (e.g., differentiating PID from appendicitis or adnexal torsion). Laparoscopy is not the panacea for diagnosis, however, as it will not always detect endometriosis and may not detect subtle inflammation of the fallopian tubes.

Routine laboratory studies are not necessary (except cervical cultures for gonorrhea and chlamydia) for the diagnosis of PID; however, their use can help to improve the specificity (and hence the positive predictive value) of the diagnosis. Cultures (or other methods of identification) of *N. gonorrhoeae* and *Chlamydia* from the cervix should be routinely performed. Determination of the WBC count, sedimentation rate, or level of C-reactive protein may be helpful in supporting the diagnosis.[43] Most women with PID have either abnormal numbers of WBCs on saline microscopy ("wet prep") or evidence of vaginal mucopurulent discharge. If the cervical discharge appears normal and there is no evidence of WBCs on saline microscopy, the diagnosis of PID is less likely and alternative causes of lower abdominal pain should be considered. Pregnancy should be excluded using a sensitive pregnancy test. Screening for other STDs including HIV, syphilis, and hepatitis B is appropriate. Screening for other, more uncommon STDs may also be performed if clinical signs and symptoms are present. These women are also more likely to have Pap smear abnormalities. Pap smears, if not obtained within the prior year, should either be performed in the ED or the patient should be referred for follow-up.

Treatment

Treatment can be accomplished as an inpatient or outpatient, depending on the clinical status of the patient. There are recent efficacy data suggesting that parenteral to oral regimens may be comparable in women with mild to moderate PID.[43] Despite early data suggesting women with HIV and PID have a greater risk of TOA, greater need for surgical intervention, and a higher failure rate, there are no direct data indicating a higher failure rate of HIV-infected women presenting with mild PID. Until further studies are available, it may be prudent to admit those patients for parenteral therapy. Tables 29-6, 29-7, and 29-8 list the CDC's guidelines for hospitalization as well as inpatient and outpatient treatment regimens. There is no single antimicrobial agent that both provides adequate antibiotic coverage and that has been evaluated sufficiently in this setting. Some practitioners consider providing empiric treatment of the patient's sexual partner(s) for both gonorrhea and chlamydial infection, whether or not cultures from the partner have been obtained and whether or not they are positive. An algorithm for the diagnosis and management of PID is shown in Fig. 29-2.

Women with an intrauterine device and suspected PID may recover from the initial infection with the IUD remaining in place, but such women are at high risk for recurrence. Therefore most experts advise removal of an IUD in the presence of PID. If the IUD is to be removed, intravenous antibiotics should be administered before IUD removal to prevent bacteremia or septic shock.[44]

Table 29-6. Indications for Hospitalization for Pelvic Inflammatory Disease

1. Uncertain diagnosis, especially if appendicitis or ectopic pregnancy is in the differential diagnosis
2. Pelvic abscess (tuboovarian abscess)
3. Concomitant pregnancy
4. Adolescence
5. Severe illness, nausea or vomiting, or high fever
6. Inability to manage outpatient therapy
7. Failure to respond to outpatient management

Source: Adapted from Centers for Disease Control and Prevention,[14] with permission.

Table 29-7. Recommendations for Inpatient Therapy

Regimen A[a]

Cefoxitin 2 g IV every 6 hours

OR

Cefotetan 2 g IV every 12 hours **PLUS**

Doxycycline 100 mg IV or PO every 12 hours

(Oral doxycyline is preferred due to pain associated with infusion and similar bioavailability between oral and parenteral administration.)

Regimen B[b]

Clindamycin 900 mg IV every 8 hours

AND

Gentamicin 2 mg/kg loading dose, followed by 1.5 mg/kg IV every 8 hours

[a]This regimen should be continued for at least 24 hours after a patient improves clinically. After termination of intravenous therapy, doxycycline should be continued at a dose of 100 mg PO twice a day to a total 14 days of treatment.

[b]Preferred for tuboovarian abscess. Although use of a single dose of gentamicin has not been evaluated for the treatment of PID, it is efficacious in other analogous situations. Parenteral therapy can be discontinued 24 hours after a patient improves clinically; continuing oral therapy should consist of doxycycline 100 mg orally twice a day or clindamycin 450 mg orally four times a day to complete a total of 14 days of therapy. When tuboovarian abscess is present, many health care providers use clindamycin for continued therapy rather than doxycycline, because clindamycin provides more effective anaerobic coverage.

Source: Adapted from Centers for Disease Control and Prevention,[14] with permission.

Table 29-8. Outpatient Treatment of Pelvic Inflammatory Disease[a]

Regimen A

Ofloxacin 400 mg orally twice a day for 14 days

OR

Clindamycin 450 mg PO qid for 14 days

OR

Levofloxacin 500 mg orally once daily for 14 days

WITH OR WITHOUT

Metronidazole 500 mg orally twice a day for 14 days

Regimen B

Cefoxitin 2 g IM in a single dose plus 1 g of probenecid orally administered concurrently in a single dose

OR

Ceftriaxone 250 mg IM in a single dose

OR

Other parenteral third-generation cephalosporin (e.g., ceftizoxime or cefotaxime)

AND

Doxycycline 100 mg orally twice a day for 14 days

WITH OR WITHOUT

Metronidazole 500 mg orally twice a day for 14 days.

[a]Follow-up in 72 hours. Patients who do not respond in 72 hours should be re-evaluated to confirm the diagnosis and should be administered parenteral therapy on an inpatient or outpatient basis.

Source: Adapted from Centers for Disease Control and Prevention,[14] with permission.

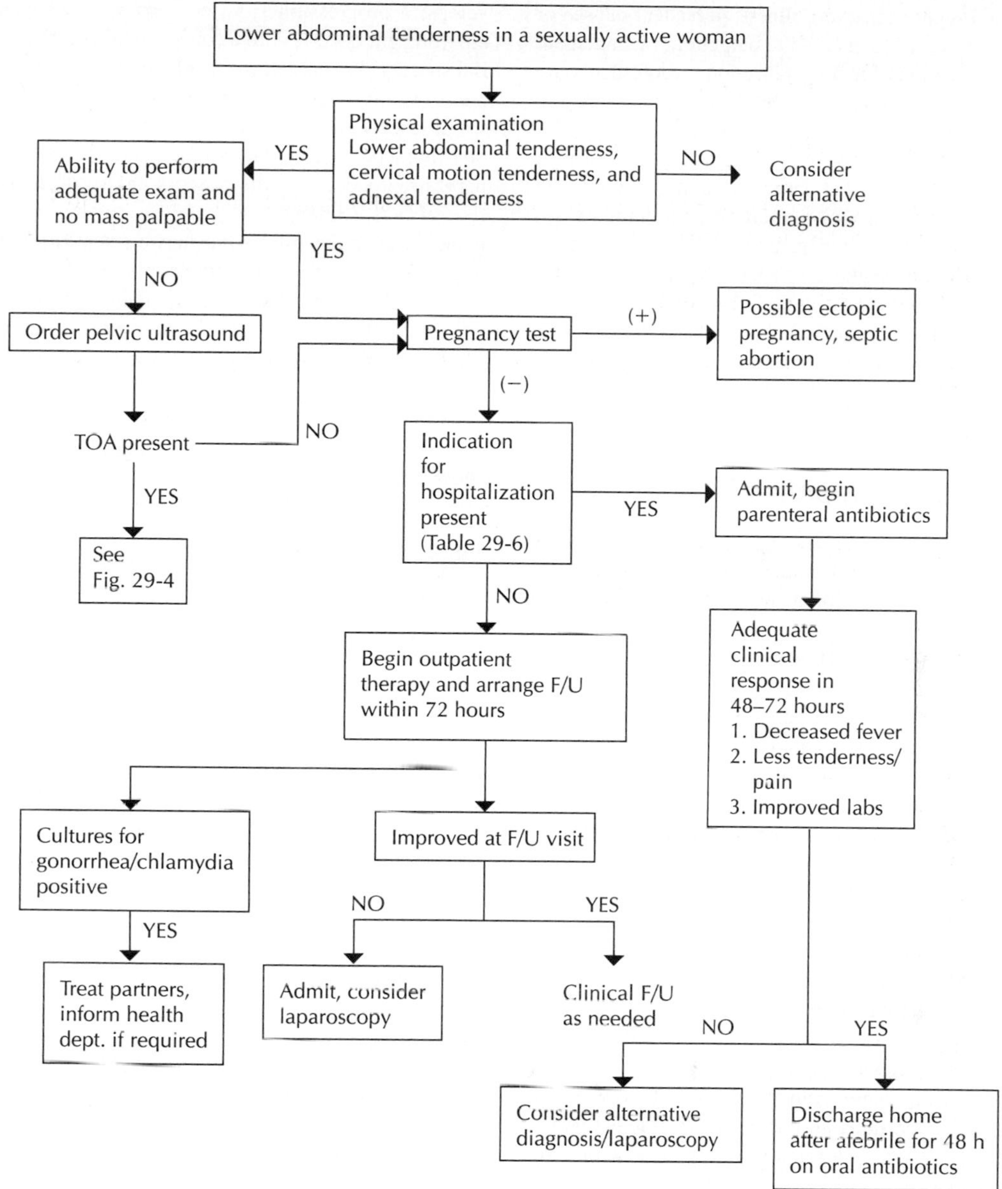

Fig. 29-2. Algorithm for the diagnosis and treatment of pelvic inflammatory disease. F/U = follow-up.

Indications for Specialty Consultation and Follow-Up

Any of the indications for hospitalization (Table 29-6) should initiate a consultation with a practitioner familiar with the inpatient management of PID. When the diagnosis is not certain and there is a reasonable possibility of the need for surgical intervention (e.g., lower abdominal tenderness and signs of peritoneal irritation), consultation with a gynecologist or surgeon is appropriate. If outpatient therapy is chosen, follow-up should be arranged within 72 hours to assess adequate response to therapy. Inability to arrange follow-up is a reason to consider hospitalization. Pregnancy, severe illness, persistent nausea or vomiting or failure to respond to outpatient management are also indications for hospitalization. Adolescents are known to be less compliant with completing medication, though there are no data that directly indicate that adolescent women benefit from hospitalization for treatment of PID. There are data that demonstrate that women ≥ 35 years of age have a more complex clinical course when treated for PID, although data are lacking to demonstrate improved outcome if they are routinely hospitalized for treatment of PID. Finally, patients must be informed of their gonorrheal and chlamydial culture results and state or county health departments should also be informed of positive cultures, as required by local ordinance.

TUBOOVARIAN ABSCESS

Tuboovarian abscess (TOA) occurs in approximately 5 percent of women hospitalized for PID, though estimates of up to one-third of hospitalized women with PID have been reported. Interestingly, 30 to 40 percent of women diagnosed with TOA will have no preceding diagnosis of PID and may present with a variety of findings, including an asymptomatic pelvic mass.

Women presenting with symptomatic TOA have a constellation of findings similar to those of PID. Therefore lower abdominal pain, cervical motion tenderness, adnexal tenderness, and the presence of an inflammatory adnexal mass is the most predictable combination of findings. However, pelvic tenderness may preclude the performance of an adequate exam, and reliance on imaging techniques, particularly ultrasound, becomes important in establishing the diagnosis. In a large series of patients with TOA, a history of fever and chills was present in half, whereas abnormal vaginal discharge, nausea, and abnormal bleeding were found in 25 percent or fewer.[45] On physical examination, only two-thirds of women have documented fever, and a similar frequency of leukocytosis was seen. Therefore one cannot rely on absence of fever or leukocytosis to rule out a TOA.

Pathophysiology and Microbiology

The basic cause of TOA is similar to that of PID cervicitis: an ascending migration of bacteria from the lower genital tract, resulting in tubal infection with erythema, edema, and the production of purulent fluid. Though the process is usually initiated via an STD, genital tract or colon malignancy and diverticulitis are important causes of TOAs in older, particularly menopausal women. As a TOA develops, a progression from an aerobic to an anaerobic environment occurs, with a concomitant change in bacterial species. As such, primary infecting organisms, which are typically facultative anaerobes (*Escherichia coli*, streptococci), are gradually replaced by obligate anaerobic organisms (e.g., *Bacteroides* spp., *Prevotella* spp., peptostreptococci) as the abscess cavity develops over several days. Although many of these organisms originate in the lower genital tract, some may originate in the bowel, migrating across the inflamed bowel wall. Both the small and large bowel can be primarily involved as part of the abscess wall. While *N. gonorrhoeae* and *C. trachomatis* can frequently be isolated from the cervix of women with TOA, it is unusual to isolate either organism from the abscess cavity itself (<5 percent). *Actinomyces* may also be isolated from the abscess, particularly in women with IUDs.

Imaging Studies

Ultrasound is the primary imaging procedure used in the diagnosis of adnexal masses, including inflammatory complexes. While alternative modalities like computed tomography (CT), magnetic resonance imaging, and radionuclide scanning can also demonstrate TOAs, their expense, radiation exposure, or general inability to produce fine resolution make them less desirable as primary imaging modalities. Ultrasound is helpful for primary diagnosis and is a useful method of following response to therapy through serial examinations. The characteristic appearance of a TOA on ultrasound is a thick-walled, multiseptate mass that has layered sediment or debris in the most dependent portion (Fig. 29-3). Similar findings can be seen on CT.

Treatment

Rupture of a TOA is a true surgical emergency. Hemodynamic stabilization and initial administration of a broad-spectrum antibiotic followed by prompt surgical intervention with removal of the involved pelvic organs is necessary. Delay in diagnosis and surgical management results in increased mortality. Untreated mortality rates of up to 100 percent have been reported.

Unlike abscesses elsewhere in the body, many unruptured TOAs can be successfully managed with antibiotics alone, without the need for drainage or surgical removal.[36,45] The use of antibiotics without surgery or drainage is associated with a 60 to 80 percent likelihood of clinical improvement and hospital discharge. One of the key factors in obtaining an adequate response to

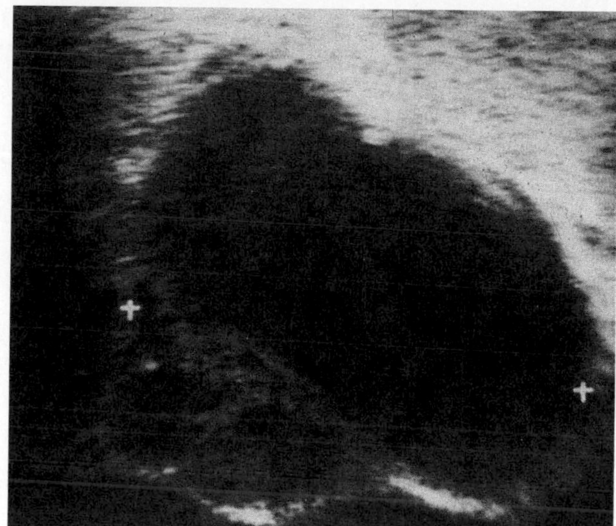

Fig. 29-3. Ultrasound of tuboovarian abscess demonstrating thick-walled, multiseptate adnexal abscess with dependent layering of inflammatory debris. (From Sweet RL, Gibbs RS: *Infectious Diseases of the Female Genital Tract,* 3d ed. Baltimore: Williams & Wilkins, 1996, with permission.)

Suspected TOA

Signs or symptoms of rupture

YES

1. Stabilize
2. Begin broad-spectrum antibiotics
3. Immediate surgical consultation with laparotomy

NO

Menopausal

NO

Begin broad-spectrum antibiotic therapy (see Table 29-8)

YES

1. Stabilize
2. Antibiotics
3. CT
4. Consult gynecology and/or surgery for a laparotomy

Favorable response in 48–72 h?

1. Improved fever
2. Decreased tenderness
3. Less pain
4. Improvement in labs (CBC, C-reactive protein, sedimentation rate)

YES

Continue antibiotics until afebrile for 48 h, discharge home on oral antibiotics for a minimum of 14 days

Continued improvement?

YES

Cure

NO

Consider surgery

NO

Surgical intervention or drainage procedure

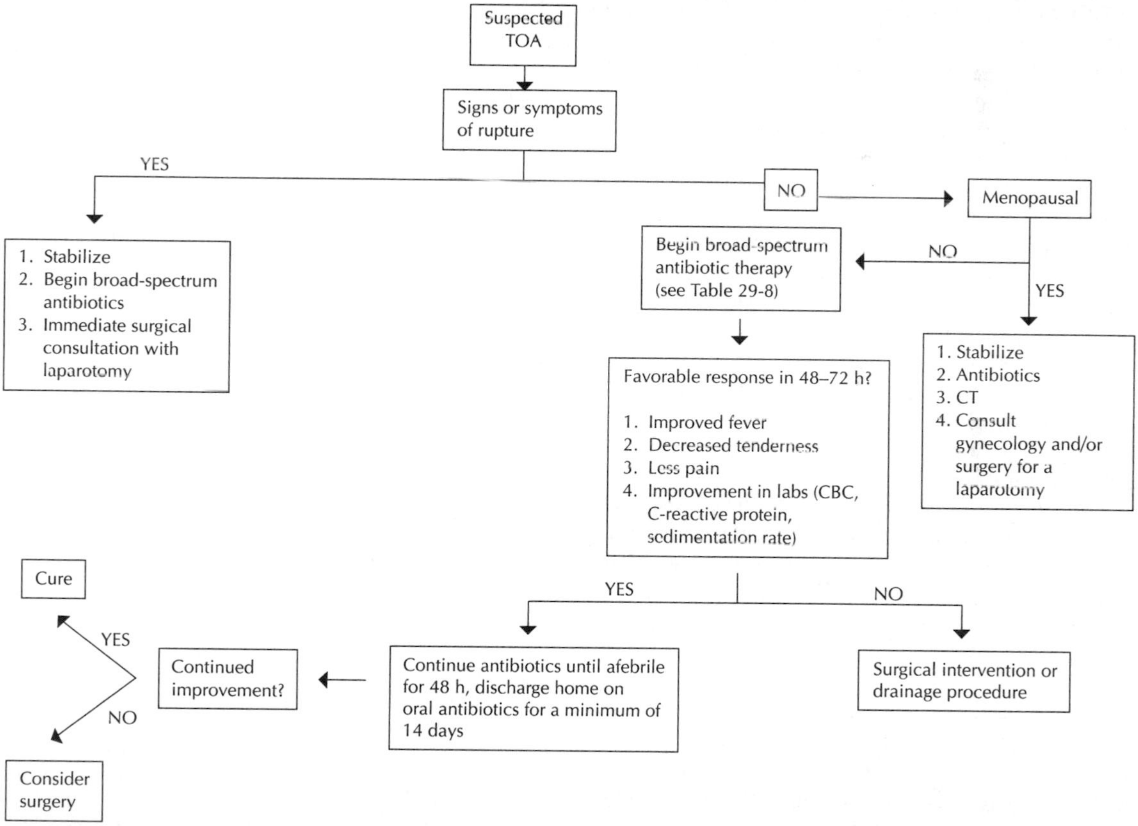

Fig. 29-4. Algorithm for the management of tuboovarian abscess. (From Sweet RL, Gibbs RS: *Infectious Diseases of the Female Genital Tract,* 3d ed. Baltimore: Williams & Wilkins, 1996, with permission.)

antibiotics is the utilization of agents with a sufficiently wide antimicrobial spectrum to cover the bacteria typically seen in TOAs (Table 29-7). One large observational study demonstrated an 81 percent response rate (175 of 217) with the use of clindamycin and gentamicin.[45] In a similar population, the same investigators reported that the use of antibiotics with poor anaerobic coverage (e.g., penicillin and gentamicin) resulted in a failure rate of two-thirds. However, long-term success of antibiotics without surgery is less than the quoted 60 to 80 percent, as some of these initial responders (perhaps 20 to 30 percent) will eventually require an operation because of continued or recurrent pain. *Bacteroides fragilis,* a common isolate, has shown increasing resistance to clindamycin in the last 5 to 10 years, and metronidazole-containing regimens (e.g., ampicillin, metronidazole, and gentamicin) or broad-spectrum single agents with good anaerobic coverage (e.g., ampicillin-sulbactam) are being used with success comparable to that of clindamycin-containing regimens reported in the 1980s, albeit with a more limited experience.[36]

Clinical response to antibiotic therapy is usually demonstrated in 48 to 72 hours, with reduction in fever, pain, abdominal tenderness, and laboratory markers of inflammation (e.g., WBC count, C-reactive protein, sedimentation rate). Failures are more commonly seen in TOAs larger than 8 cm in diameter or when there is bilateral adnexal involvement.

Failure of TOA to respond to initial medical management indicates a need for surgical intervention. A variety of treatment modalities—ranging from drainage procedures under imaging guidance to hysterectomy with bilateral salpingo-oophorectomy—have been successfully used. There are increasing reports of successful series of ultrasound- or CT-guided drainage.[46] However, in general the experience is limited, and clear recommendations for patient selection are lacking.

Total abdominal hysterectomy with bilateral salpingo-oophorectomy results in the highest rate of successful resolution of symptoms, but is less desirable in some women, as it leaves them menopausal and infertile. Unilateral involvement has been treated successfully with unilateral adnexectomy. An algorithm for management of TOA is shown in Fig. 29-4.

Tuboovarian abscess in the older ($\geq$35 years old) and menopausal age group represents a special circumstance, since there is a significant association between TOAs and gastrointestinal or genitourinary malignancy[47,48] (colon, endometrial, cervical, and ovarian cancer). Diverticular abscess is also seen as a cause of TOAs in this group of women. Because of the high incidence of malignancy, stabilization, antibiotics, and gynecologic or other surgical referral is recommended in menopausal women with a pelvic abscess.

REFERENCES

1. Faro S: Quinolones for the treatment of *Neisseria gonorrhoeae* and *Chlamydia trachomatis. Infect Dis Obstet Gynecol* 1:108, 1993.
2. Centers for Disease Control and Prevention: Primary and secondary syphilis—United States, 1998. *MMWR Morb Mortal Wkly Rep* 48:873–878, 1999.
3. Centers for Disease Control and Prevention: Primary and secondary syphilis—United States, 1999. *MMWR Morb Mortal Wkly Rep* 50:113–117, 2001.
4. Csonka GW, Oates JK: Syphilis, in Csonka GW, Oates JK (eds): *Sexually Transmitted Diseases.* Philadelphia: Bailliere Tindall: 1990, pp 227–276.
5. March RW, Stiles GE: The reagin screen test: A new reagin card test for syphilis. *Sex Transm Dis* 7:66, 1980.
6. Hunter EF, McKinney RM, Maddison SE, Cruce DD: Double staining procedure for fluorescent treponemal antibody-absorption (FTA-ABS) test. *Br J Venereal Dis* 55:105, 1979.
7. Coffey EM, Braford LL, Naritomi LS, Wood RM: Evaluation of the qualitative and automated quantitative microhemagglutination assay for antibodies to *Treponema pallidum. Appl Microbiol* 24:26, 1972.
8. Lukehart SA, Hook FW, Baker-Zander SA, et al: Invasion of the central nervous system by *Treponema pallidum:* Implications for diagnosis and therapy. *Ann Intern Med* 109:855, 1988.
9. Jaffe HW, Larsen SA, Jones OG, Dans PE: Hemagglutination tests for syphilis antibody. *Am J Clin Pathol* 78:230, 1978.
10. Goldman JN, Lantz MA: FTA-ABS and VDRL slide test reactivity in a population of nuns. *JAMA* 217:53, 1971.
11. Buchanan CS, Haserick JR: FTA-ABS test in pregnancy: A probable false-positive reaction. *Arch Dermatol* 102:322, 1970.
12. Kraus SJ, Haserick JR, Lantz MA: Fluorescent treponemal antibody-absorption test reactions in lupus erythematosus. *N Engl J Med* 282:1287, 1970.
13. Daniels KC, Ferneyhough HS: Specific direct fluorescent antibody detection of *Treponema pallidum. Health Lab Sci* 14:164–171, 1977.
14. Centers for Disease Control and Prevention: Sexually transmitted diseases—Treatment guidelines. *MMWR Morb Mortal Wkly Rep* 51:RR-6, 2002.
15. Negussie Y, Remick DG, DeForge LE, et al: Detection of plasma tumor necrosis factor, interleukins 6 and 8 during the Jarisch-Herxheimer reaction of relapsing fever. *J Exp Med* 175:1207, 1992.
16. Fekade D, Knox K, Hussein K, et al: Prevention of Jarisch-Herxheimer reaction by treatment with antibodies against tumor necrosis factor-α. *N Engl J Med* 335:311, 1996.

17. Yolken RH: Enzyme immunoassays for the detection of infectious antigens in body fluids: Current limitations and future prospects. *Rev Infect Dis* 146:35, 1982.
18. Vestergaard BF, Jensen O: Diagnosis and typing of herpes simplex virus in clinical specimens by the enzyme-linked immunosorbent assay (ELISA), in Nahmias AJ, Dowdle WR, Schniazi RF (eds): *The Human Herpesviruses.* New York: Elsevier-North Holland, 1981, pp 343–349.
19. Schlossberg D, Shulman JA: *Differential Diagnosis of Infectious Diseases.* Baltimore: Williams & Wilkins, 1996, p 56.
20. Wang SP: A simplified method for immunological typing of trachoma-inclusion conjunctivitis-lymphogranuloma venereum organism. *Infect Immun* 7:356, 1973.
21. Abrams AJ: Lymphogranuloma venereum. *JAMA*. 205:59, 1968.
22. Coutts WE: Lymphogranuloma venereum: A general review. *WHO Bull* 2:545, 1950.
23. Dan M, Rotmench HH, Eylan E, et al: A case of lymphogranuloma venereum of 20 years duration: Isolation of *Chlamydia trachomatis* from perianal tissue. *Br J Venereal Dis* 56:344, 1980.
24. Hammond GW, Slutchuk V, Scatliff J, et al: Epidemiology, clinical, laboratory and therapeutic features of an urban outbreak of chancroid in North America. *Rev Infect Dis* 1:867, 1980.
25. Hafiz S, Kinghorn GR, McEntegart MG: Sheffield medium for *Haemophilus ducreyi. Br J Venereal Dis* 60:196, 1984.
26. Nsanze H, Plummer FA, Magwa A, et al: Comparison of media for the primary isolation of *Haemophilus ducreyi. Sex Transm Dis* 11:6, 1984.
27. Kuberski T: Granuloma inguinale (donovanosis). *Sex Transm Dis* 7:26, 1980.
28. Rosen T, Tschen JA, Ramsell W, et al: Granuloma inguinale. *J Am Acad Dermatol* 11:433, 1984.
29. Sehgal VN, Shyamprasad AL, Bechar PC: The histopathological diagnosis of donovanosis. *Br J Venereal Dis* 60:45, 1984.
30. Westrom L, Joesoef J, Reynolds G, et al: Pelvic inflammatory disease and fertility. *Sex Transm Dis* 19:185, 1992.
31. Brunham RC, Paavonen J, Stevens CE, et al: Mucopurulent cervicitis: The ignored counterpart in women of urethritis in men. *N Engl J Med* 311:1, 1984.
32. Centers for Disease Control and Prevention: Recommendations for the prevention and management of *Chlamydia trachomatis* infections. *MMWR Morb Mortal Wkly Rep* 42:(RR-12), 1993.
33. Velebil P, Wingo P, Zhisen X, et al: Rate of hospitalization for gynecologic disorders among reproductive age women in the United States. *Obstet Gynecol* 86:764, 1995.
34. Rolfs RT, Galaid EL, Zaida AA: Pelvic inflammatory disease: Trends in hospitalization and office visits, 1979 through 1988. *Am J Obstet Gynecol* 166:983, 1992.
35. Rice P, Schachter J: Pathogenesis of pelvic inflammatory disease. *JAMA* 266:2587, 1991.
36. Sweet RL: Pelvic inflammatory disease and infertility in women. *Infect Dis Clin North Am* 1:199, 1987.
37. Pastorek JG: Pelvic inflammatory disease and tubo-ovarian abscess. *Obstet Gynecol Clin North Am* 16:347, 1989.
38. Kahn J, Walker C, Washington AE, et al: Diagnosing pelvic inflammatory disease. *JAMA* 266:2594, 1991.
39. Jacobsen L, Westrom L: Objectivized diagnosis of acute pelvic inflammatory disease. *Am J Obstet Gynecol* 105:1088, 1969.
40. Washington AE, Aral SO, Wolner-Hanssen PW, et al: Assessing risk for pelvic inflammatory disease and its sequelae. *JAMA* 266:2581, 1991.
41. Korn AP, Landers DV, Green JR, Sweet RL: Pelvic inflammatory disease in HIV infected women. *Obstet Gynecol* 82:765, 1993.
42. Piepert JF, Boardman L, Hogan JW, et al: Laboratory evaluation of acute upper genital tract infection. *Obstet Gynecol* 87:730, 1996.
43. Ness RB, Soper DE, Holley RL, et al: Effectiveness of inpatient and outpatient treatment strategies for women with pelvic inflammatory disease. *Am J Obstet Gynecol* 186:929, 2002.
44. Peterson HB, Walker CK, Kahn JG, et al: Pelvic inflammatory disease. *JAMA* 266:2605, 1991.
45. Landers DV, Sweet RL: Tubo-ovarian abscess: Contemporary approach to management. *Rev Infect Dis* 5(Suppl.):876, 1983.
46. Aboulghar MA, Mansour RT, Serour GI: Ultrasonographically guided transvaginal aspirations of tuboovarian abscess and pyosalpinges: An optional treatment for acute pelvic inflammatory disease. *Am J Obstet Gynecol* 172:1501, 1995.
47. Hoffman M, Molpus K, Roberts WS, et al: Tuboovarian abscess in postmenopausal women. *J Reprod Med* 35:525, 1990.
48. Barton DP, Fiorica JV, Hoffman MS, et al: Cervical cancer and tuboovarian abscesses: A report of three cases. *J Reprod Med* 38:561, 1993.

30

Vulvar Disease

Sebastian Faro
Raymond H. Kaufman

KEY POINTS

- Vulvar pruritus is a common presenting complaint and may be due to (in order of decreasing frequency): vulvovaginal candidiasis; nonneoplastic epithelial disorders (e.g., contact dermatitis, lichen sclerosus); and rarely vulvar cancer.
- Acute vulvar pain may be due to Bartholin's duct abscess, necrotizing fasciitis (rare, but life-threatening), genital herpes, imperforate hymen (in teenagers), and complications of trauma (e.g., hematoma).
- Vulvar manifestations of disease are commonly caused by vaginitis (see Chap. 31) and STDs (see Chap. 29).

A basic tenet in the management of women with vulvar disease is that a correct diagnosis must be established before treatment is instituted. A careful history and physical examination is paramount in making this diagnosis. However, unless the diagnosis is clear-cut, in many instances vulvar biopsy is required before a diagnosis can be established. But in dealing with acute emergencies involving the vulva, a biopsy will shed little light to clarify the management plan necessary to deal with the emergency. Nevertheless, certain laboratory tests can be of value in the emergency department setting. The simplest and the one used most often is a wet-mount preparation using saline and potassium hydroxide mounts to exclude various vaginitides as a cause of the vulvar symptoms. In addition, a scraping taken from a vulvar lesion that is then placed in potassium hydroxide solution can be of value in excluding fungal infection as the source of the vulvar symptoms. When the latter is performed, the scraping is easily taken using the edge of a scalpel blade. The material obtained is then placed on a glass slide, to which 15 to 20 percent potassium hydroxide is added. Gently heating the slide over a flame helps dissolve keratinized material. The specimen is then cover-slipped and examined under the microscope using both low- and high-power magnification.

PRURITUS

The most common cause of acute vulvar pruritus is related to either vaginal candidiasis or trichomoniasis. This subject is discussed in Chap. 31. The nonneoplastic epithelial disorders which include lichen simplex chronicus, lichen sclerosus, and other dermatoses such as eczema, psoriasis, and sebhorreic dermatitis are common causes of vulvar pruritus. Rarely, however, will the pruritus be so severe that it requires emergency treatment. However, a patient will occasionally have such intense and persistent pruritus that she will seek emergency care in the ED for relief of this symptom. The nonneoplastic epithelial disorders are classified on the basis of gross and histopathologic changes, as follows: (1) squamous cell hyperplasia (formerly hyperplastic dystrophy), including lichen simplex chronicus; (2) lichen sclerosus; and (3) contact and allergic dermatoses.

Squamous Cell Hyperplasia

Frequently, areas of squamous cell hyperplasia are localized, elevated, and well delineated, but more often these changes are quite diffuse, resulting in significant thickening, lichenification, and both red and white appearance of the vulvar tissues (Fig. 30-1). If the condition has been chronic the tissue becomes thick, often taking on a rough texture and a gray color. Fissures and excoriations are quite common secondary to chronic scratching. Scrapings for the presence of fungi should be taken from such lesions to exclude fungal infection as the underlying cause of the patient's symptoms. The differential diagnosis includes contact allergic and irritant dermatitis, lichen sclerosus, and fungal infections involving the vulvar tissue.

Treatment

If an eczematous type of vulvitis is present as the result of infected excoriations or irritants in previously used medications, wet dressings with an agent such as aluminum acetate (Burow's solution) applied to the vulva three or four times daily will be beneficial. Topical application of corticosteroids is also effective in alleviating pruritus. The high- or medium-potency glucocorticoids such as 0.025 or 0.01 percent fluocinolone acetonide or 0.01 percent triamcinolone acetonide are effective in relieving pruritus.

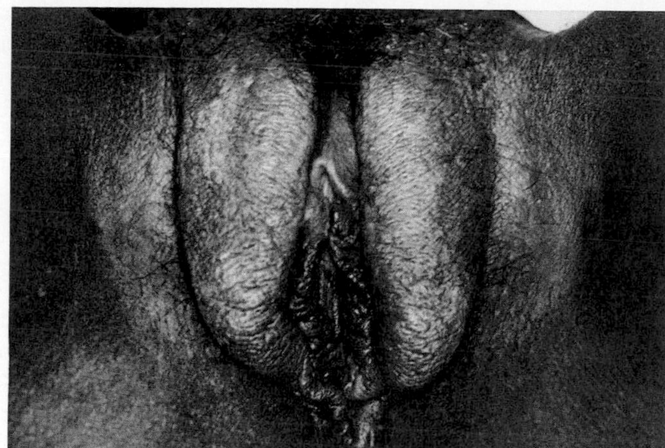

Fig. 30-1. Squamous cell hyperplasia. This patient had experienced vulvar pruritus for many years. Thickening, lichenification, and whitening of the tissue are evident. The patient presented with acute exacerbation of the pruritus.

The drug should be applied two or three times daily; however, it should not be used on a continuous basis for more than several weeks, since secondary changes may develop or the patients may experience a "rebound" effect when the medication is discontinued. If a fungal infection is found involving the vulva, it should be treated separately with one of the antifungal agents such as clotrimazole 1 percent cream or ketoconazole 2 percent cream twice daily for a period of 1 to 2 weeks. Warm sitz-baths are also extremely effective in alleviating pruritus. It is generally advisable for the patient to take a warm sitz-bath, adequately dry the vulva, and then apply a topical agent for relief of pruritus.

Lichen Sclerosus

The gross appearance of lichen sclerosus is often characteristic. In well developed and classic lesions, the skin has a crinkled, "cigarette paper" or parchment-like appearance (Fig. 30-2). The changes commonly extend around the anus in a figure-eight configuration. Often, there is edema of the clitoral foreskin, which completely hides the clitoris. Phimosis of the clitoris may be seen late in the course of the disease. The labia minora often fuse with the labia majora and are not identifiable as such. Splitting of the skin in the midline is often observed. Fissures may also develop in the natural folds of the skin and in the posterior fourchette. Small ecchymotic areas and areas of telangiectasia may be noted within the skin and mucosa. The diagnosis of lichen sclerosus is best confirmed on vulvar biopsy; however, the patient should be referred to her primary care physician for this procedure.

Treatment

Clobetasol 0.05 percent ointment is effective in alleviating the symptoms of pruritus as well as causing regression of the lichen sclerosus. Of interest is the fact that relatively long-term use of this potent steroid usually does not result in some of the secondary changes seen when other glucocorticoids are used for a long period of time on the vulva. When used, clobetasol should be applied twice daily for 1 month, at bedtime for 2 months, and then twice weekly for 3 months. Follow-up examination should be carried out after 1 month of therapy. The patient should also be referred to her primary-care physician for vulvar biopsy to confirm the diagnosis. Patients should be cautioned not to discontinue potent steroids suddenly to avoid an Addisonion type reaction.

Contact Irritant and Allergic Dermatitis

Contact dermatitis is an inflammatory reaction of the skin to a primary irritant or an allergenic substance. It is often difficult to distinguish the two. Many individuals reporting that they are allergic to a substance have really had contact irritant reactions.

Most instances of contact dermatitis involving the vulva are truly primary irritant responses. Patients usually complain of marked irritation, itching, and burning. Significant edema, formation of vesicles, and even bullae are often seen (Fig. 30-3). Contact dermatitis should not be confused with a primary herpes infection. Often the reaction is so severe that the patient finds the symptoms to be intolerable and requires immediate attention. Vesiculation and ulceration are most often induced by primary irritants

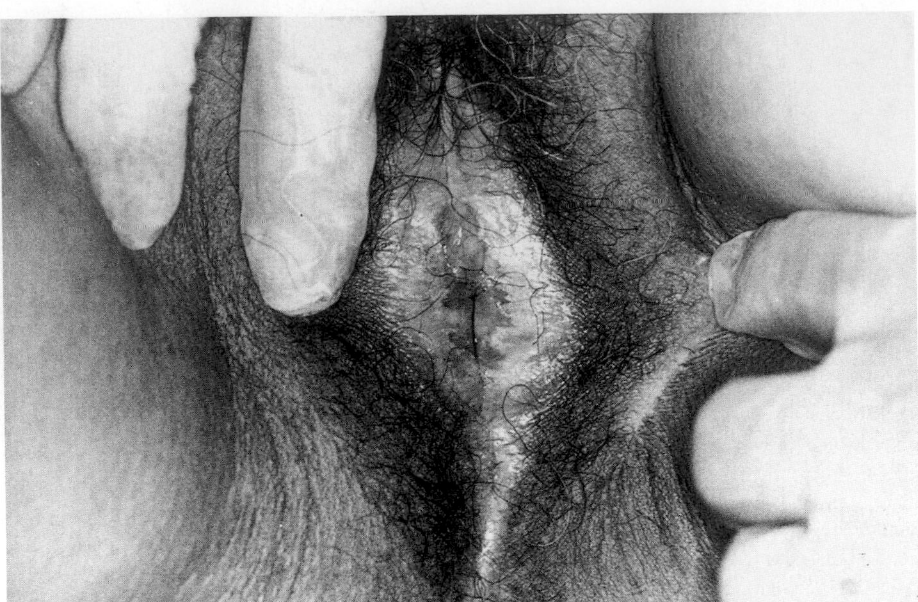

Fig. 30-2. Lichen sclerosus with introital stricture. This patient had long-standing vulvar pruritus. She presented in the emergency department complaining of severe pain when coitus was attempted, which was a result of the marked introital stenosis.

used in strong substances over a prolonged period or by allergenic substances. The severity of the reaction is influenced by the sensitivity of the patient to the substance with which she has come into contact. Occasionally, urinary retention may develop in association with a severe reaction, and infrequently painful regional lymphadenitis may be experienced.

Diagnosis

A careful history is often of help in establishing the diagnosis. Have the patient's vulvar tissues been in contact with any chemicals or medications? Have they been exposed, as occasionally happens, to poison oak or poison ivy? The oleoresins produced by poison ivy and poison oak result in classic allergic contact dermatitis. The allergen is usually transmitted to the vulvar tissues by contaminated hands and less often by direct contact. The period between contact with the allergen and the eruption varies from several hours to several days. The symptoms and findings are similar for this type of reaction and for contact irritant reactions. Contact and allergic vulvitis must be differentiated from a variety of eruptions including squamous cell hyperplasia, acute candidiasis, trichomoniasis, tinea cruris, and herpes simplex virus infections. Diagnostic tests such as microscopic examination of a scraping of involved skin and vaginal discharge to rule out candidiasis and trichomoniasis should be performed. If vesicles are present they should be unroofed and a specimen obtained for the detection of herpes simplex (HSV-1 and HSV-2). If tinea cruris is suspected, skin scrapings are collected and used to inoculate Sabouraud's agar to isolate yeast. If the patient has a vaginal discharge suggestive of trichomoniasis, but no trichomonads are identified on microscopic examination of the vaginal discharge, a drop or two of the vaginal discharge can be used to inoculate Diamond's medium in an attempt to isolate *T. vaginalis.*

Treatment

Mild reactions often subside rapidly after the causative agent is withdrawn, so aggressive therapy is not necessary. When the patient has a severe, painful reaction, immediate institution of therapy is usually indicated after a diagnosis of contact vulvovaginitis is established and an infectious cause for the problem is eliminated. Wet compresses of aluminum acetate (Burow's solution 1:20) may provide rapid relief of symptoms. After 1 or 2 days of wet compresses, a previously weeping, tender lesion may become dry, clean, and less painful. Then, the topical application of a corticosteroid cream or lotion will often relieve the patient's symptoms and bring about rapid improvement in the lesions. Allergic reactions respond more rapidly to corticosteroids than to any other therapeutic agent. Sys-

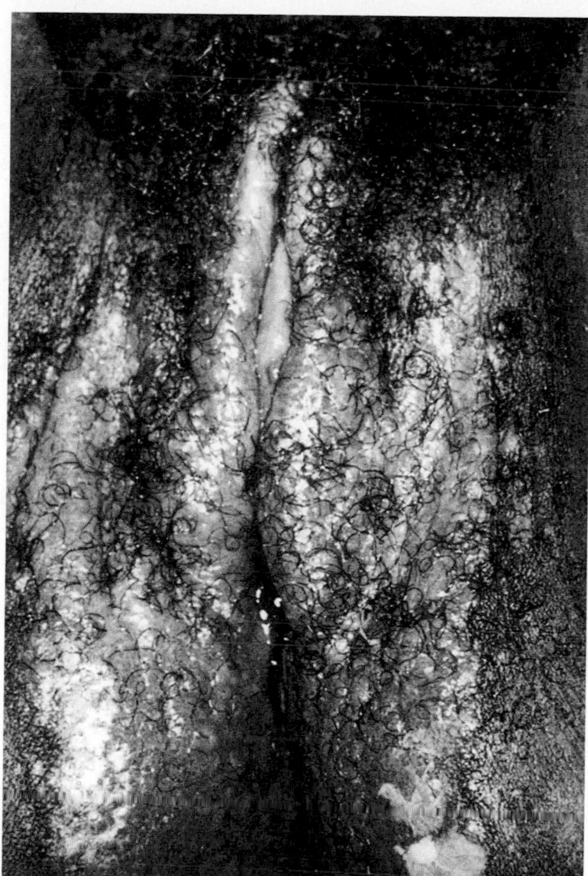

Fig. 30-3. Severe contact vulvitis. This severe reaction developed 4 days after injudicious use of podophyllin. (From Kaufman R, Faro S: *Benign Diseases of the Vulva and Vagina.* St Louis: Mosby-Year Book, 1994, with permission.)

temic glucocorticoids are often necessary and are quite effective in the presence of a severe allergic reaction, such as is seen with poison ivy or poison oak. They are best administered in diminishing doses over a 2- or 3-week period.

ACUTE VULVAR PAIN

Bartholin's and Skene's Gland Abscess

Skene's and Bartholin's gland abscesses typically present with a clinical picture of swelling, erythema, and pain. The area overlying the gland may be indurated with no evidence of spontaneous drainage. This is usually due to the fact that the duct draining the gland has become occluded and thus blocked. The duct continues to expand, causing the tissue and skin overlying the abscess to become inflamed and indurated and eventually to thin out.

Contrary to common teaching, most Bartholin abscesses result from a nongonococcal infection of Bartholin duct cysts. Culture taken from the abscess contents usually reveals a wide spectrum of organisms. *Escherichia coli* is the organism found most often. Bartholin abscesses often develop in preexisting duct cysts, but can occur in the absence of a cyst. It is possible that obstruction of the Bartholin duct, possibly due to inspissated mucus, may lead to the development of bartholinitis and subsequent abscess. Bartholin abscesses generally develop in women of reproductive age. In older women, associated cellulitis, necrotizing fasciitis, or rarely tumor, should be ruled out.

Symptoms

Exquisite pain and tenderness are the primary symptoms seen in the presence of a Bartholin abscess. Some abscesses develop slowly, occasionally over a week or longer, and give rise only to mild symptoms as they

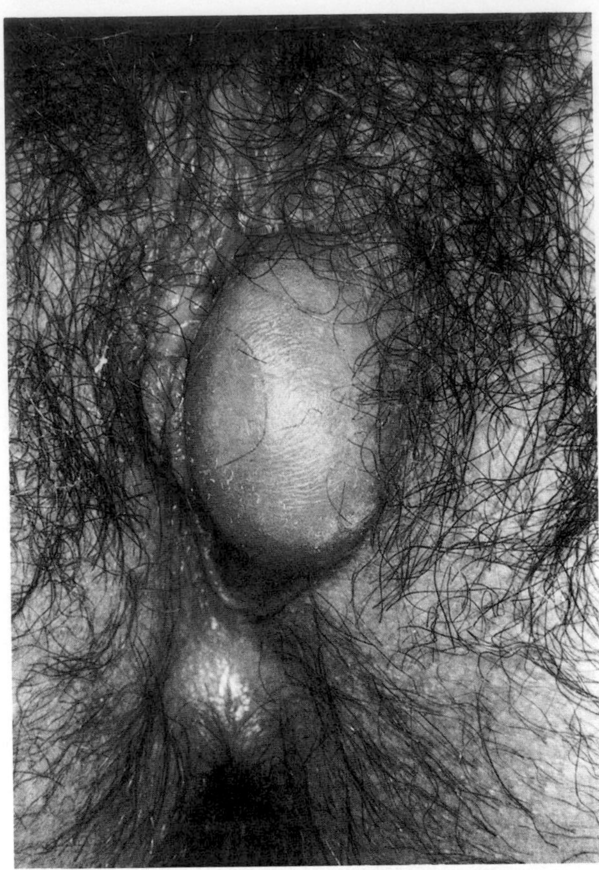

Fig. 30-4. Abscess of Bartholin gland. Marked swelling and redness is noted on the left side of the patient's vulva. This encompasses the region of the Bartholin gland and extends up the entire side of the labia. (From Kaufman R, Faro S: *Benign Diseases of the Vulva and Vagina.* St Louis: Mosby-Year Book, 1994, with permission.)

slowly develop. Occasionally, this type of abscess may spontaneously regress, although usually it will continue to enlarge and spontaneously drain. Most commonly, the Bartholin abscess develops rapidly; within 2 or 3 days marked edema, swelling, pain and tenderness become evident (Fig. 30-4). These abscesses may undergo spontaneous rupture within 72 hours if they are not surgically drained. Swelling and redness over the site of the affected gland is usually obvious. Associated severe lateral edema may also be present. The abscess is usually palpable as an exquisitely tender, fluctuant mass.

Treatment

Occasionally, the early treatment of bartholinitis with broad-spectrum antibiotics may prevent abscess formation. However, the typical infected Bartholin gland is usually not seen at this stage of development. Most often, patients will present with an exquisitely tender, hyperemic, fluctuant mass. Under these circumstances, incision and drainage is necessary and can easily be performed in an outpatient setting. Prior to making the incision, the point of planned entry into the abscess may be infiltrated with 1 to 2 mL of 1 percent lidocaine, although usually this is not required. Ethyl chloride spray can be used over the puncture site for local anesthesia. Systemic analgesia may also provide additional comfort. A 20-gauge needle on a 5-mL syringe should be inserted into the abscess at the site of the planned incision. The aspirated fluid should be sent to the laboratory for Gram staining, and cultured for *Neisseria gonorrhoeae, Chlamydia trachomatis,* aerobic, facultative, and obligate anaerobic bacteria. If no fluid is aspirated, consider that this may not be a cystic mass. The incision into the abscess should be made along the medial aspect of the fluctuant mass. If one traces the labium minus into the swelling, it will be noted that the swelling is equally distributed lateral and medial to the plane of the labium minus. The incision should be made just lateral to the hymenal ring in the region where the Bartholin duct orifice is found. Care should be taken not to make the incision over the keratinized labial skin as a chronic, externally draining Bartholin gland may result. A stab incision

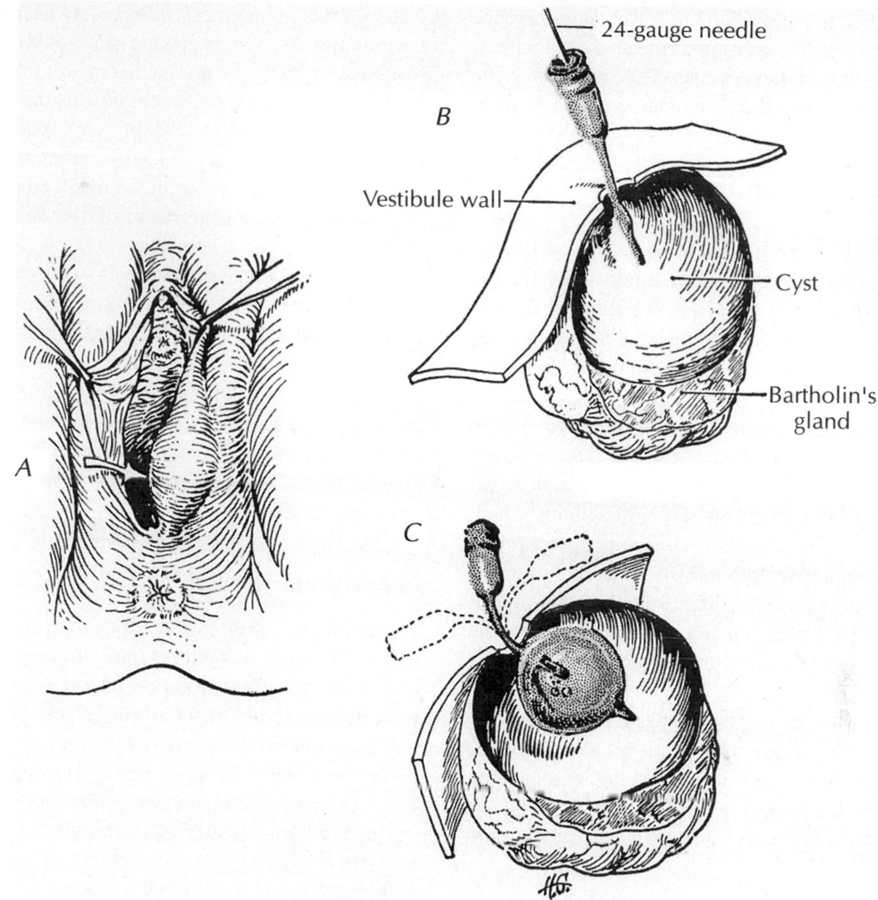

Fig. 30-5. Inflatable bulb-tipped (Word) catheter used in the treatment of Bartholin abscess. *A*. Stab wound in the abscess (*arrow*). It should be made just lateral to the region of the hymenal ring on the medial aspect of the mass. *B*. Insertion of the catheter into the stab wound. *C*. Inserted catheter inflated with 2 to 4 mL of water. (From Word B: New instrument for office treatment of cysts and abscesses of Bartholin's gland. *JAMA* 190:777, 1964, with permission.)

is made into the abscess cavity with a #11 blade and extended for several millimeters in each direction, allowing drainage of the purulent material. Cultures may be useful, especially if there is extensive cellulitis. Two sterile swabs can also be inserted into the cavity and the material obtained can be sent to the laboratory for Gram staining and culture of both aerobic and anaerobic bacteria as well as *N. gonorrhoeae* and *C. trachomatis.* Once the purulent material has drained, a small, curved clamp (e.g., hemostat) should be inserted into the abscess cavity and any loculations still present should be broken up. Failure to break up areas of loculation will result in treatment failure. The abscess cavity should be copiously irrigated with sterile saline to ensure all purulent material has been evacuated. Suture marsupialization of the abscess cavity at this time is not recommended because the tissue is friable, inflamed, and edematous, and the suture cuts through this tissue very easily, making repair difficult. However, the insertion of a Word catheter (Fig. 30-5) into the cavity will often result in a functional marsupialization, resulting in the development of a new orifice from the Bartholin gland. The Word catheter is the size of a #10 Foley catheter with a stem 1 inch long and a single barrel. A solid stopper is attached to one end and a 5-mL latex inflatable balloon is attached to the other. The catheter is inserted into the abscess cavity and the bulb is inflated with 2 to 4 mL of water. It is important to distend the balloon with sterile water or saline; if air is used the balloon will deflate rapidly and the catheter will fall out. If the catheter falls out too soon, the incision will close and the cyst or abscess can reform. The end of the catheter is then tucked up into the lower vagina, where it can be left in place. Usually, the catheter should remain in place for a period of 4 to 6 weeks. The patient may engage in all activities, including intercourse, with the catheter in place.

Postprocedure Care

The patient should be instructed to take warm sitz-baths for 15 to 20 minutes three or four times a day for the next 72 hours. If there is extensive cellulitis, or the patient is at increased risk for complicated infection (e.g., diabetes mellitus or immunosuppression) she should be started on antibiotics and continue them until the edema and erythema have disappeared. Therapy with amoxicillin clavulanate 500 mg every 8 hours or lomefloxacin 400 mg orally every 24 hours for 7 days should be initiated. All of these agents have a broad spectrum of activity, which includes coverage for *N. gonorrhoeae* and *C. trachomatis,* as well as facultative and obligate anaerobic bacteria. If the microbiology report indicates that another antibiotic should be administered based on identification of the bacterium and sensitivities, alterations in therapy can be made.

Skene's gland abscess can be managed in a fashion similar to that described above for Bartholin's gland abscess. Aspirating its contents, incising, irrigating, and packing with gauze is all that may be needed. In incising a Skene's gland, care should be taken not to enter the urethra and disrupt its integrity.

Necrotizing Fasciitis

Necrotizing fasciitis of the vulva is a rare but severe soft tissue infection that has high morbidity and mortality if not recognized early (see also Chap. 22). Prompt recognition and immediate debridement in the operating room are critical aspects of care that reduce mortality. This infection is uncommon, can be difficult to recognize, and can progress insidiously or rapidly. Although most commonly affecting diabetics, necrotizing fasciitis must also be suspected in postmenopausal women with abscesses involving the vulva or Bartholin glands.[1–3] Other risk factors include vascular insufficiency, immunocompromised states, surgical incisions, cutaneous trauma, and decubitus ulcers. Necrotizing fasciitis is a polymicrobial infection. Aerobic organisms consume oxygen in the infected tissue, providing a more desirable environment for anaerobic organisms to proliferate.

Necrotizing fasciitis is an infection of the subcutaneous tissues that spreads along fascial planes. It is characterized by severe tenderness, edema, and necrosis of subcutaneous tissues. The overlying skin may not be initially involved, or it may be erythematous or violaceous. As infection progresses and nutrient vessels thrombose, bullae and cutaneous necrosis develop. Purulent exudate or pustules are usually not present, and crepitance is a late finding. Numbness may occur in the involved area secondary to infarction of cutaneous nerves. Fever, leukocytosis, and systemic toxicity are late signs.

Once the clinical diagnosis is suspected, antibiotics should be given and the gynecologist consulted urgently for aggressive surgical debridement. Antibiotics alone are insufficient without debridement. A comprehensive antibiotic regimen should be given that provides coverage against mixed anaerobes, enterococci, and group A streptococci. It should include the use of expanded-spectrum penicillins and clindamycin, plus metronidazole and an aminoglycoside.

Imperforate Hymen

Typically, an imperforate hymen (also covered in Chap. 24) is not recognized until after puberty, when retention of menstrual blood becomes troublesome. As the child menstruates each month, larger amounts of blood accumulate within the vagina, which slowly becomes distended to form a hematocolpos. Eventually, the cervix may become dilated with the accumulation of blood, giving rise to hematometra and hematosalpinx. The patient will often complain of increasingly severe cyclic lower abdominal pain; occasionally, a large, tender mass will be palpated arising from the pelvis. Associated bladder pressure, frequency, and urinary retention may develop. The diagnosis can be made if an imperforate hymen is found (Fig. 30-6). A history of cyclic lower abdominal cramping pain not associated with menses in a young woman in the pubertal age range should make the examining physician suspicious of such a problem. Associated amenorrhea, urinary retention, lower abdominal pain, and a palpable pelvic mass should prompt the examiner to do a careful examination of the external genitalia as well as a rectal examination. Ultrasonography will be of considerable help in establishing the diagnosis of hematocolpos and the possible presence of a hematometra. Usually, examination will reveal an intact hymen that is bulging outward. Occasionally, if the hymen is firm and fibrotic, this will not be observed. However, rectal examination should help to confirm the diagnosis of a hematocolpos. A very thick septum can be a result of a transverse vaginal septum. This condition is not easily corrected with a simple incision, and caution should be exercised when

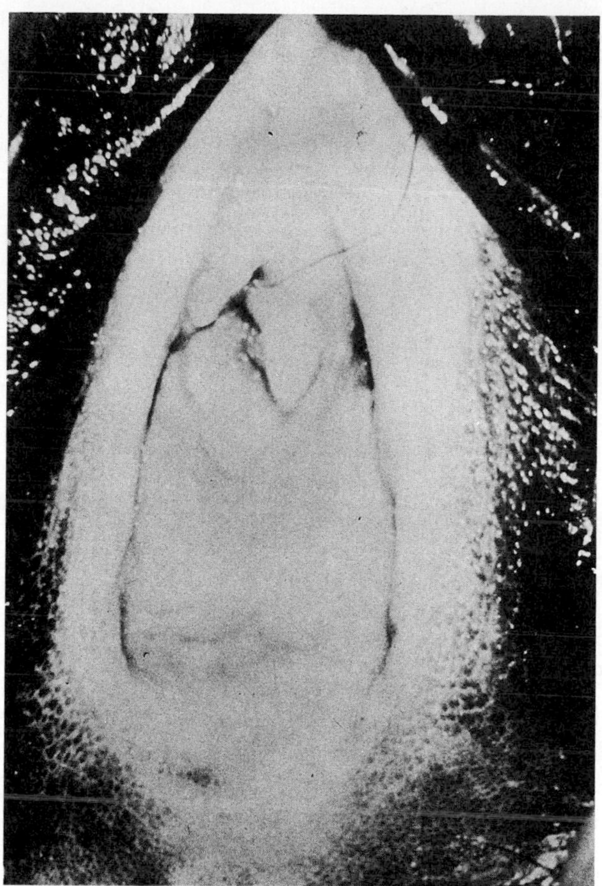

Fig. 30-6. Imperforate hymen in a 14-year-old girl. She had been having increasingly severe lower abdominal pain for several months.

contemplating hymenectomy for a presumed inperforate hymen. Imperforate hymen is typically characterized by a convexity (outward bulging) and a purplish or bluish coloration from the visible hematocolpos. In the absence of these findings, referral to an experienced gynecologist for examination is prudent.

Treatment

If a bulging intact hymen is present, a cruciate incision should be made at the introitus through the hymen. Consultation with a practitioner experienced with this procedure (e.g., gynecologist) is appropriate. If significant bleeding is noted coming from the edges of the hymen, the edges can be oversewn with a fine absorbable suture. Because the external and internal genitalia of these patients are susceptible to infection in the presence of old blood, strict aseptic conditions should be maintained and prophylactic antibiotics (cefazolin 1 g, cefoxitin 2 g, or cefotetan 1 to 2 g) given prior to starting the operative procedure. A specimen of the fluid should be obtained either via aspiration or by sterile swab for the culture of bacteria, especially facultative and obligate anaerobes. Following drainage of the hematocolpos, a bimanual examination should be avoided because of the risk of infection, and should be delayed until the follow-up visit.

ACUTE VULVAR EDEMA

Acute vulvar edema is a rare occurrence, with multiple causes. In the postpartum patient, the sudden occurrence of unilateral vulvar edema associated with a significantly elevated white blood cell count may foreshadow the development of necrotizing fasciitis. Prompt diagnosis and radical surgical excision are necessary if due to nerotizing fasciitis. Significant bilateral labial edema occurring during the third trimester of pregnancy or in the postpartum period is occasionally associated with a hypertensive disorder of pregnancy. Bed rest and appropriate management of preeclampsia is the recommended treatment.

Seasonal edema of the vulva may occur in some individuals with hay fever. It may also be seen in association with peritoneal dialysis, as well as in patients who have had intraperitoneal installation of dextran 70. The latter is still used by some gynecologic surgeons following pelvic surgery in the belief that it may be of some benefit in preventing postoperative adhesions. This edema will slowly resolve as the dextran is absorbed. Severe cutaneous edema is also occasionally seen in association with vulvovaginal candidiasis. This is often associated with physical findings suggesting an intravaginal candidal infection causing a white, cheesy discharge. Saline and potassium hydroxide wet-mount preparations will be of help in establishing the diagnosis. Regardless of the cause of the acute vulvar edema, bed rest and perineal ice packs are useful therapeutic measures. Once the specific etiology is established, it will require treatment (i.e., for acute candidiasis, an oral antifungal agent or the intravaginal instillation of an antifungal agent, plus the topical application of an antifungal agent).

NONTRAUMATIC VULVAR HEMORRHAGE

Acute hemorrhage arising from the vulva is most unusual; however, it is occasionally seen in association with vulvar carcinoma. A tumor large enough to result in acute hemorrhage will usually be obvious on physical examination. However, a thorough pelvic examination should still be performed to exclude the possibility of bleeding from the vagina, cervix or uterine corpus. If obvious bleeding is seen coming from the carcinoma, the bleeding site should be identified and the bleeding controlled either by coagulation or a figure-eight suture. The direct application of silver nitrate or ferrous subsulfate (Monsel's solution) are usually effective for slow, oozing bleeding. Unfortunately, if there is significant tumor necrosis, it may be difficult to place a suture that will provide hemostasis.

On rare occasions, a large varicose vein may rupture, with subsequent hemorrhage. This is most likely to occur after acute trauma to the vulva. When this occurs, the bleeding vessels need to be identified and a suture ligature placed around the bleeding site. If extensive, management in an operating room setting may be necessary.

TRAUMA

Because of its location, the vulva is seldom injured accidentally. The injuries most commonly seen are in the prepubertal female and usually result from straddling injuries. Sexual assault is also a common cause of acute trauma to the vulvovaginal tissues (see Chap. 33). Traumatic injuries in the adult are occasionally seen following an automobile, bicycle, or motorcycle accident and are usually associated with trauma elsewhere, such as pelvic fractures. Pelvic examination should be done in women with severe multisystem trauma, particularly if there has been a pelvic fracture, to identify potential vaginal, vulvar, or perineal injury.

Occasionally, injuries occur following insertion of a foreign body into the vagina by the patient or a second party. Injuries to the vulva are usually manifest as hematomata and/or lacerations.

Laceration

Laceration of the vulva and vagina is likely to occur after a violent fall onto a slender object such as a stake or by impalement on the handlebars of a motorcycle or bicycle. Such injuries may extend through the vagina into adjacent organs such as the rectum, bladder, urethra, and cul-de-sac. When this occurs, hemorrhage may be severe. When multiple lacerations are seen primarily within the vagina, a foreign body should be sought as the cause. Commonly, remnants of metal, glass, or plastic objects may be found within the vagina as well as in the paravaginal tissues. Anterorposterior and lateral x-rays should be taken to locate any radiopaque object. In most instances, when hemorrhage is severe, control of the hemorrhage and repair of the defects should be performed in the operating room under appropriate anesthesia. If a vaginal laceration is bleeding profusely, the vagina can temporarily be packed with sterile plain gauze. The surgical treatment of these lacerations should be directed toward restoration of normal anatomy. The bleeding blood vessels should be ligated and the tissue edges carefully approximated. In the presence of severe traumatic injuries involving the vulva and vagina, careful evaluation of the rectum and bladder for injury should also be carried out. If the injury extends through the cul-de-sac, a laparotomy will be required, since injury to the small or large intestine may well have occurred and will require appropriate repair.

Lacerations involving the vulva and vagina of a child require special consideration. Forcible examination of a child should never be attempted. In the presence of

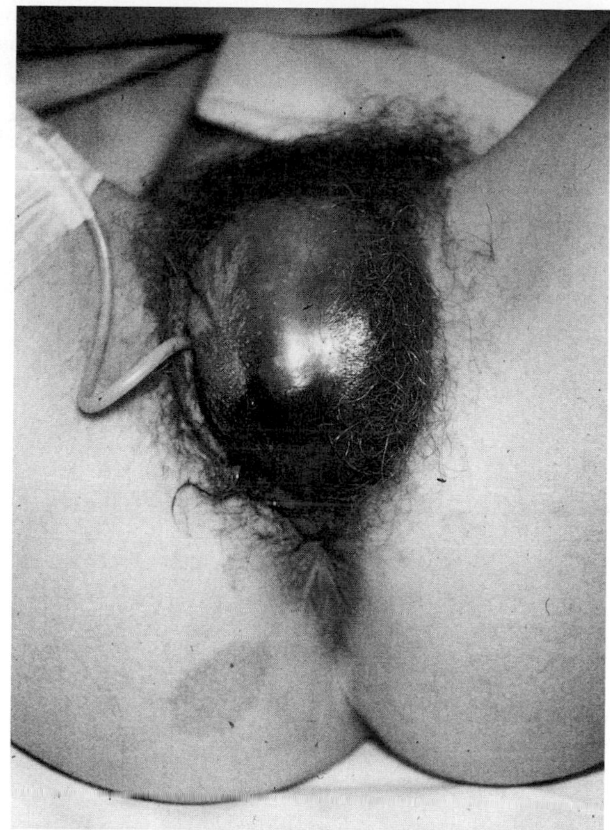

Fig. 30-7. Vulvar hematoma.

pain, significant bleeding, or evident laceration, the child should be examined in the operating room under anesthesia. Lacerations should be repaired by careful approximation of the tissue edges.

HEMATOMA

Hematomas of the vulva most commonly occur during childbirth and occasionally secondary to retracted blood vessels following an episiotomy. They usually become clinically manifest after the patient has been discharged from the hospital following delivery. This is especially true because of the short postpartum stay allowed to most women today. The hematoma is manifest by swelling and tenderness, and if it is large, by significant pain. Usually such hematomas are small, although occasionally they may become extensive and extend from the vulva through the paravaginal tissues and into the broad ligament. The skin over a large hematoma is often black, shiny, and edematous (Fig. 30-7). When there is extensive extravasation into the tissue spaces, the blood loss may be significant enough to result in hemorrhagic shock. Nonpuerperal hematomas are almost invariably secondary to trauma, and these patients will usually present with such a history.

Treatment

Small hematomas with an intact surface can usually be managed by careful observation for evidence of continued enlargement. Bed rest with the application of an ice pack for 12 to 24 hours is advisable. If the hematoma continues to enlarge, it will then be necessary to incise the mass, evacuate the blood clot, find the bleeding blood vessels, and ligate them. This is best performed in the operating room by an obstetrician/gynecologist. Occasionally, bleeding is diffuse and obvious vessels causing the hematoma cannot be identified. Under these circumstances, the cavity of the hematoma should be carefully packed. Appropriate antibiotic coverage should be given (e.g., cefotetan, ampicillin-sulbactam, or clindamycin and gentamicin), since infection will often develop. Large hematomas should be evacuated. As a general rule, a hematomas larger than 5 to 10 cm in diameter should be evacuated, since the risk of complications in such patients is greater than when the hematomas are smaller. Conservative management of large vulvar hematomas often results in the need for subsequent operative intervention because of secondary infection; it may also require transfusions that are unnecessary when they are managed surgically.

REFERENCES

1. Stephenson H, Dotters DJ, Katz V, et al: Necrotizing fasciitis of the vulva. *Am J Obstet Gynecol* 166:1324, 1992.
2. Addison WA, Livengood CH III, Hill GB, et al: Necrotizing fasciitis of vulvar origin in diabetic patients. *Obstet Gynecol* 63:473, 1984.
3. Roberts DB: Necrotizing fasciitis of the vulva. *Am J Obstet Gynecol* 157:568, 1987.

31

Vaginitis

Jack D. Sobel

KEY POINTS

- Vulvovaginal symptoms are extremely common, but symptoms and signs are nonspecific. Neither self-diagnosis nor diagnosis by a physician is reliable without laboratory confirmation.
- Vulvovaginal symptoms, even when severe and seen in the ED setting, are as likely to be caused by noninfectious causes as by infectious agents.
- Vulvovestibular symptoms and signs of inflammation are rare in uncomplicated bacterial vaginosis.
- Bacterial vaginosis (BV) is no longer simply viewed as a nuisance infection with malodorous discharge, but is now thought to be responsible for multiple serious obstetric and gynecologic complications including increased risk of HIV transmission.
- Resistant trichomoniasis is fortunately rare, but it can be effectively eradicated with oral and vaginal tinidazole.
- Vulvar pruritus, although the dominant feature of vulvovaginal candidiasis, is frequently caused by noninfectious causes (i.e., contact dermatitis or allergies).

Vaginal symptoms are extremely common; they are responsible for millions of visits annually to gynecologists' offices. Vaginal discharge is among the 25 most common reasons for consulting physicians in private office practice in the United States.[1] It is found in more than 25 percent of women attending sexually transmitted disease (STD) clinics. Not all women with vaginal symptoms have vaginitis; however, approximately 40 percent of those with vaginal symptoms will have some type of vaginitis.

With 40 million uninsured individuals in the United States combined with the fact that millions of Americans lack a regular primary care physician mean that there are millions of visits each year to emergency departments. Such visits are of two varieties: (1) those women with severe symptoms who are unable to wait the several hours needed to see their practitioners; and (2) women with less acute symptoms who utilize EDs as their primary site of health care delivery.

Vaginitis is rarely if ever associated with mortality or even with hospitalization; accordingly, there is a marked tendency to trivialize this entity. The most obvious manifestation of this is the practice of diagnosing the cause of vulvovaginal symptoms inaccurately without an examination. Accurate diagnosis is the foundation of effective management so thorough examination is crucial.

A major error in medical education has been to equate vulvovaginal symptoms with vaginitis. This is compounded by a tendency to equate vaginitis with infectious vaginitis. Of the infectious causes of vaginitis, three common entities—bacterial vaginosis (BV), vulvovaginal candidiasis (VVC), and trichomoniasis—are responsible for over 90 percent of vaginal infections (Table 31-1). This chapter emphasizes the provision of a rational diagnostic management approach to the symptomatic patient instead of the traditional approach found in most textbooks that deals only with candidal vaginitis, bacterial vaginosis, and trichomonal vaginitis. The recent availability of over-the-counter antimycotics has confounded the accurate diagnosis of candidal vaginitis. For example, only 33 percent of women purchasing OTC antifungals for personal treatment of presumed VVC actually have VVC.[2]

Readers are referred also to the chapters on STDs and vulvar disease (Chaps. 29 and 30), since there is considerable overlap in symptomatology.

APPROACH TO THE PATIENT WITH VAGINAL SYMPTOMS

Symptoms related to vaginitis include vaginal discharge, pruritus, and a variety of manifestations of inflammation of the vagina, introitus, and vulva, depending on the extent and severity of the inflammatory reaction (Table 31-2). These symptoms include soreness, irritation, discomfort, dysuria, and dyspareunia. Physicians frequently fail to inquire about the association of these symptoms with sexual activity and thus lose valuable insight into the chronicity and cause of symptoms. Coitus constitutes a nonspecific but useful "stress test" in establishing the presence, site, and extent of vaginal and introital inflammation.

A thorough history should be obtained, including a detailed description of the symptoms and their duration;

Table 31-1. Causes of Vaginitis in Adult Women

Infectious vaginitis
Bacterial vaginosis (40–50%)
Vulvovaginal candidiasis (20–25%)
Trichomonal vaginitis (15–20%)
Less common
Foreign body with secondary infection
Desquamative inflammatory vaginitis (clindamycin-responsive)
Streptococcal vaginitis (group A)
Ulcerative vaginitis associated with *Staphylococcus aureus* and toxic shock syndrome
Idiopathic vulvovaginal ulceration associated with HIV
Noninfectious vaginitis
Chemical/irritant
Allergic, hypersensitivity, and contact dermatitis (lichen simplex)
Traumatic
Atrophic vaginitis
Postpuerperal atrophic vaginitis
Desquamative inflammatory vaginitis (glucocorticoid-responsive)
Erosive lichen planus
Collagen vascular disease, Behçet's syndrome, pemphigus syndromes
Idiopathic

sexual history, including recent change of sexual partner; past therapy; and response to therapy. Specific details include a description of the vaginal discharge—its color and consistency and, most importantly, the presence or absence of an offensive odor. Although the odor associated with VVC is absent, minimal, or nonoffensive, most women will describe it as unpleasant. However, women with BV or trichomoniasis have little hesitation in mentioning the offensive, embarrassing nature of the discharge, which characteristically increases in severity immediately after unprotected coitus.

Physical examination includes careful inspection and palpation (with a cotton swab) of the vulva as well as the vaginal vestibule. The latter area is frequently ignored; as a result, the diagnosis of vulvar vulvitis (vulvar vestibulodynia or vestibulitis), is frequently missed. Inspection with a vaginal speculum includes examination of the vaginal mucosa for erythema, petechiae, ulceration, edema, atrophy, and adherent discharge. The pooled vaginal secretions are also assessed with regard to color, consistency, and volume. Finally, as mentioned previously, no vaginal examination is complete without evaluation of the cervix and bimanual digital pelvic examination.

Vaginal discharge can also be caused by mucopurulent cervicitis (MPC) and endometritis; therefore, it is essential to evaluate the cervix in all patients with vulvovaginal complaints. Caused by *Chlamydia trachomatis* and *Neisseria gonorrhoeae,* MPC is characterized by a yellow endocervical exudate and confirmed by the simple identification of yellow exudate on a white cotton-tipped swab specimen of endocervical secretions. The cervix is frequently friable, edematous, and bleeds easily on physical contact. Mucopurulent cervicitis must be differentiated from cervicitis caused by herpes simplex virus (HSV), inflammatory vaginitis, and ectropion of the cervix (ectopy). The latter is a normal finding without a mucopurulent exudate, although ectopy is associated with increased numbers of polymorphonuclear leukocytes (PMNs) in the vaginal discharge as determined by microscopy.

After inspection, the middle third of the vagina is swabbed to obtain a valid specimen of secretions suitable for rapid pH estimation. Swabs of mucosal secretions are then obtained for saline and 10 percent potassium hydroxide (KOH) microscopic examination. Bacterial and fungal cultures are not routinely required. An additional swab is obtained for the immediate performance of a 10 percent KOH amine elaboration test (whiff test). In the presence of suspected cervicitis, cervical specimens should also be obtained for identification of *C. trachomatis, N. gonorrhoeae,* and HSV.

The saline microscopy examination has many purposes, including identification of clue cells, trichomonads, yeast or hyphae, and estimation of whether PMNs are present and/or increased. Most investigators consider a ratio of PMNs to epithelial cells of one or less as within

Table 31-2. Diagnostic Features of Infectious Vaginitis

	Normal	Candidal Vaginitis	Bacterial Vaginosis	Trichomonas Vaginitis
Symptoms	None or physiologic leukorrhea	Vulvar pruritus, soreness, increased discharge, dysuria, dyspareunia	Malodorous moderate discharge	Profuse purulent discharge, offensive odor, pruritus, and dyspareunia
Discharge				
Amount	Variable, scant to moderate	Scant to moderate	Moderate	Profuse
Color	Clear or white	White	White/gray	Yellow
Consistency	Floccular, nonhomogeneous	Clumped but variable	Homogeneous, uniformly coating walls	Homogeneous
"Bubbles"	Absent	Absent	Present	Present
Appearance of vulva and vagina	Normal	Introital and vulvar erythema, edema and occasional pustules, vaginal erythma	No inflammation	Erythema and swelling of vulvar and vaginal epithelium ("strawberry cervix")
pH of vaginal fluid	<4.5	<4.5	>4.5	5-6.0
Amine test (10% KOH)	Negative	Negative	Positive	Occasionally positive
Saline microscopy	Normal epithelial cell Lactobacilli predominate	Normal flora, blastospores (yeast), 40–50% pseudohyphae	Clue cells, coccobacillary flora predominates, absence of leukocytes, motile curved rods	Motile trichomonads (80–90%), no clue cells, abnormal flora
10% KOH microscopy	Negative	Positive (60–90%)	Negative (except in mixed infections)	Negative

normal limits. Likewise, exfoliated vaginal epithelial cells are studied in order to identify an increase in basal or parabasal cells, which may indicate a relative estrogen deficiency or reflect a desquamating inflammatory reaction in the wall of the vagina. The final useful component of saline microscopy includes examination of the vaginal flora, particularly as evident in the intercellular spaces (i.e., those not adherent to epithelial cells). The normal appearance of the vaginal flora consists of rod-like organisms that are unclumped. This description is preserved in VVC, but it dramatically changes in both trichomoniasis and BV, in which the normal flora is lost and replaced by larger numbers of coccobacillary microorganisms that are often clumped. Gram-stain examination of vaginal secretions, although a useful research and epidemiologic tool, is not required on a routine basis and adds little to a properly performed saline wet-mount examination. Given the low sensitivity of the saline examination in detecting *Candida* species, a 10 percent KOH microscopic examination should always be performed, even if the saline wet mount identifies other causes of vaginitis, because mixed infections are common.

In the majority of symptomatic women, a thorough history, careful physical examination, and the aforementioned rapid laboratory tests should provide an immediate and reliable clinical diagnosis. In a small percentage of women, the diagnosis will be deferred pending the availability, within a few days, of results of additional studies, especially cultures. Each of the previously described tests has variable sensitivity and specificity depending on the

Table 31-3. Some Pitfalls in the Diagnosis and Treatment of Vaginitis: Causes of Treatment Failure

Failure to see and examine patient (telephone diagnosis)
Assuming diagnosis in previous attack is same as in present episode
Patient interviewed but not examined
Patient manually examined but no speculum inserted
Speculum examination but no laboratory tests performed
Failure to examine introitus and missing diagnosis of vestibulitis
Limiting differential diagnosis to BV, VVC, and trichomoniasis
Assuming that positive culture for *Gardnerella vaginalis* implies presence of BV
Treating *Escherichia coli,* enterococcus, and other normal flora as pathogens
Relying on Pap smear to make diagnosis
Use of "shotgun" polypharmacy
Selecting therapy on the basis of odds and statistics
Use of topical glucocorticoids for all vulvar symptoms
Failure to recognize that topical therapy may exacerbate symptoms

specific clinical entity in question, and each test is discussed below. Nevertheless, as outlined in Table 31-2, an accurate reliable diagnosis can be reached within a few minutes utilizing the stated guidelines. The fact that the patient may be seen under urgent circumstances in no way nullifies this principle. Physicians should recognize that diagnostic algorithms for vaginitis are designed to facilitate the diagnosis of BV, VVC, or trichomoniasis, whereas the vaginal symptoms of many women will not be due to these three most common causes of infectious vaginitis. When no specific etiologic agent has been identified, physicians should not feel obliged to prescribe antimicrobial agents routinely. If no diagnosis is forthcoming, a variety of effective, nonspecific palliative measures can be prescribed. Nevertheless, practitioners too often rely on the clinical response to empirically selected antimicrobial therapy and polypharmacy, exploiting the safety and potency of most therapeutic agents and the relatively narrow differential diagnosis. Common pitfalls of diagnosis and management are listed in Table 31-3.

INFECTIOUS VAGINITIS

Bacterial Vaginosis

Epidemiology

Bacterial vaginosis is the most common cause of vaginitis in women of childbearing age. It has been diagnosed in 17 to 19 percent of women seeking gynecologic care in family practice or student health care settings. The prevalence increases considerably in symptomatic women in STD clinics, reaching 24 to 37 percent. Bacterial vaginosis has been observed in 16 to 29 percent of pregnant women, the lowest figures being found among private patients and the highest in STD and university clinics. Evaluation of epidemiologic factors has revealed few clues as to the cause of BV. Use of an intrauterine device and douching were found to be more common among women with BV. It is significantly more common in African-Americans and sexually active women, including lesbians.

Pathogenesis

Bacterial vaginosis is the result of a massive overgrowth of mixed flora, including peptostreptococci, *Bacteroides* spp., *Prevotella* spp., *Porphyromonas* spp.,*G. vaginalis, Mobiluncus* spp., and genital mycoplasmas.[3] There is little inflammation, and the disorder represents a disturbance of the vaginal microbial ecosystem rather than a true infection of tissues. The overgrowth of mixed flora is associated with a loss of the normal *Lactobacillus*-dominated vaginal flora. It is apparent that no single recognized bacterial species is responsible for BV. Experimental studies in human volunteers and animal studies indicate that inoculation of the vagina with individual species of bacteria associated with BV (e.g., *G. vaginalis*) rarely results in

BV. The role of sexual transmission, however, remains controversial.

The cause for the massive overgrowth of anaerobes and *Gardnerella, Mycoplasma,* and *Mobiluncus* spp. is unknown. Theories include increased substrate availability, increased pH, and loss of the restraining effects of the normally dominant *Lactobacillus* flora that act to inhibit the aforementioned bacteria. Moreover, Eschenbach and colleagues reported that although women without BV are colonized by H_2O_2-producing strains of lactobacilli, women with BV have reduced overall population numbers of lactobacilli, and the *Lactobacillus* species that are present lack the ability to produce H_2O_2.[4] The H_2O_2 produced by lactobacilli may inhibit the pathogens associated with BV, either directly by the toxicity of H_2O_2 or as a result of the production of H_2O_2-halide complex catalyzed by natural cervical peroxidase.

Accompanying the bacterial overgrowth in BV is the increased production of amines by anaerobes, facilitated by microbial decarboxylases. Amines in the presence of increased vaginal pH volatilize to produce the typical abnormal fishy odor, which is also produced when 10 percent KOH is added to vaginal secretions. The aromatic amines responsible for the characteristic odor were originally thought to be putrescine and cadaverine; however, trimethylamine is the dominant abnormal amine in BV. It is likely that bacterial polyamines produced together with the organic acids found in the vagina in BV (acetic and succinic acids) are cytotoxic, resulting in exfoliation of vaginal epithelial cells and creating the vaginal discharge. *Gardnerella vaginalis* attaches avidly to exfoliated epithelial cells, especially at the alkaline pH found in BV. The adherence of *Gardnerella* organisms results in the formation of the pathognomonic clue cells.

Clinical Features

As many as 50 percent of women with BV may be asymptomatic. The cardinal symptom is that of vaginal malodor, often described as fishy and frequently manifesting after unprotected coitus. An abnormal vaginal discharge, which is rarely profuse, is usually described. Pruritus, dysuria, abdominal pain, and dyspareunia are *not* manifestations of BV. Examination reveals a nonviscous, grayish-white adherent discharge, often visible on the labia and introital area. Apart from the discharge, no other abnormalities are apparent on examination.

Bacterial vaginosis was once thought to be a disorder that was primarily a nuisance. However, there is now considerable evidence that BV may have serious obstetric and gynecologic complications. Obstetric complications include chorioamnionitis, preterm labor, prematurity, and postpartum fever.[5] Gynecologic sequelae are postabortion fever, posthysterectomy fever, cuff infection, and chronic mast-cell endometritis. More recently, an association was reported of untreated BV with cervical inflammation and low-grade dysplasia. BV is a risk factor for HIV infection.[6]

Diagnosis

As with all forms of vaginitis, signs and symptoms alone are unreliable in establishing the diagnosis of BV. The clinical diagnosis can be made reliably in the presence of at least three of the following objective criteria: (1) adherent, white, nonfloccular homogenous discharge; (2) positive amine test, with release of fishy odor on addition of 10 percent KOH to vaginal secretions; (3) vaginal pH >4.5; and, (4) presence of clue cells on light microscopy. These clinical signs are simple and reliable, and testing is easy to perform. Of the four cardinal clinical signs, abnormal discharge has the least specificity. The presence of clue cells is the single most reliable predictor of BV. Clue cells are exfoliated vaginal squamous epithelial cells covered with *G. vaginalis,* giving the cells a granular or stippled appearance with characteristic loss of clear cell borders. At least 20 percent of observed epithelial cells should be clue cells if they are to be of diagnostic significance. Occasionally, clue cells consisting exclusively of curved gram-negative rods belonging to *Mobiluncus* spp. can be demonstrated. The offensive fishy odor may be apparent during the physical examination or may become apparent only during the amine test. Several investigators consider the positive amine test the least sensitive of the four clinical tests, especially compared with the Gram stain. Of the various signs, the pH of the vaginal fluid has the greatest sensitivity but the lowest specificity. A pH of >4.7 increases the specificity of BV diagnosis.

The wet-mount examination is critical, not only because it allows detection of clue cells and exclusion of trichomoniasis, but because the diagnosis of BV is supported by the absence of PMNs and the characteristic appearance of the background bacterial flora with the dominance of the coccobacillary organisms. Similar information may also be obtained with the use of Gram stain. This test has a sensitivity of 93 percent and a specificity of 70 percent.

Finally, although cultures for *G. vaginalis* are positive in almost all cases of BV, *G. vaginalis* may be detected in 50 to 60 percent of women who do not meet the diagnostic criteria for BV. Accordingly, vaginal culture has no role in the diagnosis of BV. DNA probes for *G. vaginalis* are available but expensive and suffer from the same limitations as culture. More recently, diagnostic cards have become available, and although useful, they have only modest sensitivity (87 percent) and specificity (92 percent).

Treatment

Poor efficacy has been observed with triple sulfa creams, erythromycin, tetracycline, acetic acid gel, and povidone-iodine vaginal douches.

Only moderate cure rates have been obtained with ampicillin (mean, 66 percent) and amoxicillin. The most successful oral therapy remains oral metronidazole. Most studies using multiple divided-dose regimens of 800 to 1200 mg/d for 1 week achieved clinical cure rates in excess of 90 percent immediately and of approximately 80 percent at 4 weeks (i.e., 10 percent recur by 4 weeks). The usual treatment is metronidazole 500 mg orally twice a day for 7 days. Although single-dose therapy with 2 g of metronidazole achieves comparable immediate clinical response rates, higher recurrence rates have been reported. The beneficial effect of metronidazole results predominantly from its antianaerobic activity and because *G. vaginalis* is susceptible to the hydroxymetabolites of metronidazole. Although *Mycoplasma hominis* is resistant to metronidazole, the organisms are usually not detected at follow-up visits of successfully treated patients. Similarly, *Mobiluncus curtisii* is resistant to metronidazole but usually disappears after therapy.

Topical therapy with 2 percent clindamycin once daily for 7 days or metronidazole gel 0.75 percent administered daily for 5 days has been shown to be as effective as oral metronidazole, without any of the latter's side effects. More recently, a 3-day regimen of clindamycin vaginal ovules has been shown to be as effective as 7 days of clindamycin cream. Thus the practitioner has several therapeutic options, and the topical clindamycin regimen is particularly useful for women who are allergic to or cannot tolerate oral metronidazole.

In the past, asymptomatic BV was generally not treated, especially since patients often improve spontaneously over several months. However, the growing evidence linking asymptomatic BV with numerous obstetric and gynecologic upper tract complications has brought a reassessment of this policy, especially with the available additional convenient topical therapies. Asymptomatic BV should be treated prior to pregnancy, in women with cervical abnormalities, and prior to elective gynecologic surgery. Screening and treatment of asymptomatic BV in pregnancy remains controversial pending the outcome of studies proving that treatment reduces preterm delivery.

Treatment of male sexual partners remains controversial despite indirect evidence of sexual transmission. No study has documented reduced recurrence rates of BV in women whose partners have been treated with a variety of regimens, including metronidazole. Accordingly, most clinicians do not routinely treat male partners.

Within 3 months after successful clinical therapy over 7 days with metronidazole, approximately 30 percent of patients who respond initially experience a recurrence of identical signs and symptoms. Recurrence rates in as many as 80 percent of patients within 9 months have been reported. The reasons for recurrence are unclear; they include the possibility of reinfection, but recurrence more likely reflects vaginal relapse with failure to eradicate the offending organisms at the same time that the normally protective *Lactobacillus*-dominant vaginal flora fails to reestablish itself. Management of acute BV symptoms during relapse once more includes oral or vaginal metronidazole or topical clindamycin, usually prescribed for a longer treatment period of 10 to 14 days. Maintenance antibiotic regimens have largely been disappointing and new approaches including exogenous *Lactobacillus* recolonization by use of suppositories containing selected bacteria are being studied.

Asymptomatic BV has typically not been treated since patients often have spontaneous improvement over several months. Therapy is recommended when asymptomatic women are scheduled for elective abortions or gynecologic surgery.

Treatment is indicated for pregnant women with symptomatic BV. The Centers for Disease Control and Prevention recommendations are for oral metronidazole, avoiding use of intravaginal topical antibiotics. Screening and treatment for asymptomatic disease is controversial. Although 15 to 20 percent of pregnant women in the United States have BV (most of which are asymptomatic), the benefits of screening all pregnant women for BV and treatment thereof have not been substantiated. Even though antibiotic therapy is highly effective in eradicating BV, one study did not a significant reduction in the rate of preterm birth.[7] Accordingly, screening all pregnant women and treating all with asymptomatic BV to prevent chorioamnionitis and prematurity is not recommended, except in a subgroup of women at high risk for preterm birth because of at least one prior preterm birth. In this latter group, a significant reduction in preterm delivery was evident when asymptomatic BV was treated. The optimal time for screening and the optimal treatment regimens are unknown. In studies demonstrating therapeutic benefit, patients were screened in the second trimester and treated with oral metronidazole or oral metronidazole and erythromycin.[8]

Trichomoniasis

Epidemiology

Studies estimate that 2 to 3 million American women contract trichomoniasis annually, with a worldwide distribution of approximately 180 million annual cases of trichomonal vaginitis. The prevalence of trichomoniasis correlates with the overall level of sexual activity of the specific group of women under study. Thus trichomoniasis has been diagnosed in about 5 percent of women in family-planning clinics, 13 to 25 percent of women attending gynecology clinics, 50 to 75 percent of prostitutes, and 7 to 35 percent of women in STD clinics. In many countries, recent epidemiologic surveys indicate a decline in the prevalence of trichomoniasis.

Pathophysiology

Sexual transmission is undoubtedly the dominant method of introduction of *Trichomonas vaginalis* into the vagina. The organism is identified in 30 to 40 percent of male sexual partners of infected women, with identification of urethral isolates rapidly decreasing over a period of days. A prevalence of 70 percent was found among men who had had sexual contact with infected women within the previous 48 hours. Trichomoniasis can be documented in at least 85 percent of female partners of infected men. Several studies have demonstrated an increased cure rate in women after treatment of their male sexual partners. There is also a high prevalence of gonorrhea in women with trichomoniasis, and both infections are significantly associated with use of nonbarrier methods of contraception. Oral contraceptives may decrease the prevalence of trichomoniasis; moreover, spermicidal agents such as nonoxynol 9 reduce transmission.

Repeated trichomonal infections are common; therefore, clinically-significant protective immunity does not appear to occur. Nevertheless, an immune response to *Trichomonas* does develop, as indicated by low titers of serum antibody. The latter response is insufficient to permit diagnostic use of serology. The predominant host-defense response is provided by the numerous PMNs, which respond to chemotactic substances released by trichomonads, and without ingesting trichomonads are capable of killing *T. vaginalis.* The exact mechanisms by which *T. vaginalis* induces disease remain to be determined. It is thought that *T. vaginalis* destroys epithelial cells by direct cell contact and cytoxicity. Within the vagina, only areas covered by squamous (not columnar) epithelium are involved. The urethra and Skene's glands are infected in the majority of patients, and organisms are occasionally isolated from bladder urine.

Clinical Features

Trichomonas infection in women ranges from an asymptomatic carrier state to severe, acute inflammatory disease. Approximately one-third of asymptomatic infected women become symptomatic within 6 months.

Vaginal discharge is reported by 50 to 70 percent of women diagnosed with trichomoniasis; however, the discharge is not always described as malodorous.[9,10] Pruritus occurs in 25 to 50 percent of patients and is often severe. As many as half of infected women admit to some degree of dyspareunia. Other infrequent symptoms include vulvovaginal burning, dysuria and rarely, frequent micturition. Lower abdominal pain has been described in fewer than 10 percent of patients and should alert the physician to the possibility of concomitant salpingitis due to other organisms. Symptoms of acute trichomoniasis often appear during or immediately after menstruation. The incubation period has been estimated to range from 3 to 28 days, although this is controversial.

Physical findings represent a spectrum depending on the severity of disease. Vulvar findings may be absent but are typically characterized in severe cases by diffuse erythema (10 to 33 percent) and a profuse vaginal discharge. Edema of the labia may occasionally be present in severe cases. Although the typical discharge of trichomoniasis is often described as being yellow-green and frothy, such a discharge is seen in only a minority of patients. The discharge is gray in about 75 percent; likewise, frothiness is seen in a minority of patients and is more commonly seen in BV.

The vaginal walls are typically erythematous and in severe cases may be granular in appearance. Punctate hemorrhages (colpitis macularis) of the cervix may result in a strawberry-like appearance that, although apparent to the naked eye in only about 1 to 2 percent of patients, is present in 45 percent on colposcopy.

The clinical course of trichomoniasis in pregnancy is identical to that seen in the nonpregnant state, and untreated trichomoniasis is associated with premature rupture of membranes and prematurity. Trichomoniasis is also reported to facilitate the transmission of human immunodeficiency virus (HIV).

Diagnosis

None of the clinical features of *Trichomonas* vaginitis are sufficiently specific to allow a reliable diagnosis of trichomonal infection based on signs and symptoms alone.[9,10] Definitive diagnosis requires the demonstration of the organism. Vaginal pH is markedly elevated, almost always above 5.0, and sometimes above 6.0. On saline microscopy, an increase in PMNs is almost invariably present, although an absence of PMNs does not exclude trichomoniasis. The ovoid parasites are slightly larger than PMNs and are best recognized by their mobility. The wet-mount is positive in only 40 to 80 percent of cases. Gram stain is of little value because of its inability to differentiate PMNs and nonmotile trichomonads, and use of Giemsa, acridine orange, and other stains has no advantage over saline preparation. Although trichomonads are often seen on Pap smears, this method has a sensitivity of only 60 to 70 percent compared with saline preparation microscopy, and false-positive results are not uncommon.

Several culture-medium methods are available and are probably equivalent. Cultures on Diamond's medium should be incubated anaerobically, and growth is usually detected within 48 hours. Culture is now recognized as the most sensitive method for detecting the presence of trichomonads (95 percent sensitivity) and should be considered in patients with vaginitis in whom there is a markedly elevated pH, PMN excess, absence of motile trichomonads, and presence of clue cells. Several new rapid diagnostic kits using DNA probes are under investigation.

Treatment

The cornerstone of therapy remains the 5-nitroimidazole group of drugs—metronidazole, tinidazole, and ornidazole—which are all of similar efficacy. Only metronidazole is available in the United States. Oral therapy, as opposed to topical vaginal therapy, is generally preferred, primarily because of the frequency of infection of the urethra and periurethral glands, which provide sources for endogenous reinfection.

Treatment consists of oral metronidazole, 500 mg twice a day for 7 days, with a cure rate of 95 percent. Comparable results, however, have also been obtained with a single oral dose of 2 g, achieving cure rates in the range of 82 to 88 percent. The latter cure rate increases to >90 percent when sexual partners are treated simultaneously. The advantages of single-dose therapy include better patient compliance, lower total dose, a shorter period of alcohol avoidance, and possibly decreased subsequent candidal vaginitis. A disadvantage of single-dose therapy is the need to insist on simultaneous treatment of sexual partners.

Most strains of *T. vaginalis* are highly susceptible to metronidazole with minimal inhibitory concentrations of 1 μg/mL. Patients not responding to an initial course often respond to an additional standard course of 7-day therapy. Some patients are refractory to repeated courses of therapy, even when compliance is assured and sexual partners are known to have been treated. If reinfection is excluded, these rare patients may have strains of *T. vaginalis* genuinely resistant to metronidazole. The isolates can be shown in vitro to have metronidazole resistance. Increased doses of metronidazole and longer duration of therapy are necessary to cure these refractory patients. The patients should be given maximal tolerated doses of oral metronidazole of 2 to 4 grams/day for 10 to 14 days. Rarely, high-dose intravenous metronidazole in dosages as high as 2 to 4 grams daily may be necessary, with careful monitoring for drug toxicity.

Considerable success has been observed in treating resistant infections with oral tinidazole; however, the drug is not readily available and the optimal dose is unknown. Most investigators use high-dose tinidazole 1 to 4 grams daily for 14 days.[11] Rare patients not responding to nitroimidazoles can be treated with topical paramomycin.

Side effects of metronidazole include an unpleasant metallic taste. Other common side effects include nausea (10 percent), transient neutropenia (7.5 percent), and a disulfiram-like effect when alcohol is ingested. Caution should be observed when 5-nitroimidazoles are used in patients taking warfarin. Long-term and high-dose therapy increases the risk of neutropenia and peripheral neuropathy. In experimental studies, metronidazole has been shown to be mutagenic for certain bacteria, indicating a carcinogenic potential, although cohort studies have not established an increase in cancer morbidity. Thus the risk to humans of short-term low-dose metronidazole treatment is extremely small. Superinfection with *Candida* is by no means uncommon.

Treatment of trichomoniasis in pregnancy consists of oral metronidazole. Metronidazole readily crosses the placenta, and because of concern for teratogenicity, some have considered it prudent to avoid its use in the first trimester of pregnancy. More recently, investigators have become more comfortable using metronidazole throughout pregnancy and there is no evidence of fetal harm when used at any time during pregnancy. Topical clotrimazole and povidone-iodine jelly may offer some benefit, although sound evidence for their efficacy is lacking. Treatment of asymptomatic vaginal trichomoniasis is not recommended because it does not prevent and may even increase the risk of preterm delivery.

Vulvovaginal Candidiasis

Epidemiology

There are no reliable figures defining the incidence of vulvovaginal candidiasis (VVC) in the United States, mainly because VVC is not reportable. Data from Great Britain reveal a sharp increase in the incidence of VVC. In the United States, *Candida* is now the second most common cause of vaginal infections.

It is estimated that 75 percent of women experience at least one episode of VVC during their childbearing years, and approximately 40 to 50 percent of them experience a second attack.[12] A small subpopulation of women, probably less than 5 percent of the adult female population, suffers from repeated, recurrent, often intractable episodes of candidal vaginitis.

Point-prevalence studies indicate that *Candida* may be isolated from the genital tract of approximately 20 percent of asymptomatic, healthy women of childbearing age. The natural history of asymptomatic colonization is unknown, although both animal and human studies suggest that vaginal carriage may continue for several months and perhaps years. Several factors are associated with increased rates of asymptomatic vaginal colonization with *Candida,* including pregnancy (30 to 40 percent), use of oral contraceptives, uncontrolled diabetes mellitus, and frequent visits to STD clinics (Table 31-4). The rarity of candidal isolation in premenarchal girls, the lower prevalence of candidal vaginitis after menopause, and the possible association of this condition with hormone replacement therapy (HRT) emphasize the hormonal dependence of VVC.

Table 31-4. Factors Associated with Increased Asymptomatic Vaginal Colonization with *Candida* and Candidal Vaginitis

Factors
Genetic
Blood-group antigen/secretor status
Acquired
Pregnancy
Uncontrolled diabetes mellitus
High refined sugar consumption
Corticosteroids/immunosuppressives
Antimicrobial therapy (systemic, topical)
HIV infection
Hormone replacement therapy
Vulvar dermatosis
Behavioral (sexual)
Oral contraceptives
Intrauterine device
Nonoxynol 9 spermicide
High-risk sexual behavior
Frequent visits to STD clinics
Receptive oral-genital sex
Coital frequency (?)

Pathogenesis

The Organism

Between 85 and 90 percent of yeasts isolated from the vagina are *Candida albicans* strains.[13] The remainder represent other species, the most common being *C. glabrata* and *C. tropicalis*. Non-albicans *Candida* spp. are capable of inducing vaginitis and are often more resistant to conventional therapy. Although more than two hundred strains of *C. albicans* have been identified by typing, there is no evidence of strain tropism selecting for strains with a predilection to colonize the vagina or to cause vaginitis. Recent surveys indicate an increase in VVC due to non-albicans *Candida* spp., particularly C. *glabrata.*

For candidal organisms to colonize the vaginal mucosa, they must first adhere to the vaginal epithelial cells. *Candida* albicans adheres in significantly higher numbers to vaginal epithelial cells than do non-albicans *Candida* spp. This may explain the relative infrequency of the latter strains in vaginitis. There is considerable person-to-person variation in terms of vaginal cell receptivity to candidal organisms in adherence assays. Nevertheless, vaginal cells from women with recurrent VVC do not show increased in vitro cell avidity or affinity kinetics for *Candida*.

Germination of *Candida* enhances colonization and facilitates tissue invasion. Factors that enhance or facilitate germination (e.g., estrogen therapy and pregnancy) tend to precipitate symptomatic vaginitis, whereas measures that inhibit germination (e.g., bacterial flora and local mucosal cell-mediated immunity) may prevent acute vaginitis in women who are asymptomatic carriers of yeast.

Candidal organisms gain access to the vaginal lumen and secretions predominantly from the adjacent perianal area. This finding is borne out by several epidemiologic and typing studies. Candidal vaginitis is seen predominantly in women of childbearing age, and only in a minority of cases can a precipitating factor be identified to explain the transformation from asymptomatic carriage to symptomatic vaginitis in individual patients.

Host Factors

During pregnancy, the vagina is more susceptible to vaginal infection, resulting in a higher incidence of vaginal colonization and vaginitis and lower cure rates. The clinical attack rate is maximal in the third trimester, and symptomatic recurrences are also more common throughout pregnancy. By providing a higher glycogen content in the vaginal environment, the high levels of reproductive hormones provide an excellent source of carbon for the growth and germination of *Candida*. Several studies have shown increased vaginal colonization rates with *Candida* after the use of estrogen oral contraceptives. Vaginal colonization with *Candida* is more common in diabetic women, and uncontrolled diabetes predisposes to symptomatic vaginitis. Glucose tolerance tests have been recommended for women with recurrent VVC; however, the yield is low, and testing is not justified in otherwise healthy premenopausal women.

Symptomatic VVC is frequently observed during or after courses of systemic antibiotics. Although no antimicrobial agent is free of this complication, broad-spectrum antibiotics such as tetracycline, ampicillin, and cephalosporins are mainly responsible and are thought to act by eliminating the normally protective vaginal bacterial flora. The natural flora provides a colonization-resistance mechanism and prevents germination of *Candida. Lactobacillus* spp. have been singled out as providing this protective function. *Lactobacillus-Candida* interaction includes competition for nutrients, stearic interference with the adherence of *Candida,* and elaboration of bacteriocins that inhibit yeast proliferation and germination.

Other factors that contribute to the increased incidence of candidal vaginitis include the use of tight, poorly ventilated clothing and nylon underclothing, which increases perineal moisture and temperature. Chemical contact, local allergy, and hypersensitivity reactions may also predispose to symptomatic vaginitis (see section on other noninfectious forms of vaginitis, below).

During the phase of asymptomatic carriage, candidal organisms exist predominantly in the nonfilamentous form and are found in relatively low numbers. There is a delicate equilibrium among *Candida,* the resident protective bacterial flora, and other local vaginal defense mechanisms. Symptomatic vaginitis develops in the presence of factors that enhance candidal virulence factors or as a result of loss of local defense mechanisms.

Candida may cause cell damage and resulting inflammation by direct hyphal invasion of epithelial tissue. It is possible that proteases and other hydrolytic enzymes facilitate cell penetration, with resultant inflammation, mucosal swelling, erythema, and exfoliation of vaginal epithelial cells. The characteristic nonhomogenous vaginal discharge consists of a conglomerate of hyphal elements and exfoliated nonviable epithelial cells with few PMNs. *Candida* may also induce symptoms by hypersensitivity or allergic reaction, particularly in women with idiopathic recurrent VVC (see section on other noninfectious forms of vaginitis, below).

Oral and vaginal thrush correlates well with depressed cell-mediated immunity in debilitated or immunosuppressed patients. This is particularly evident in patients with chronic mucocutaneous candidiasis and acquired immunodeficiency syndrome.

Pathogenesis of Recurrent and Chronic Candidal Vaginitis

Women who are HIV-seropositive have higher vaginal colonization rates than do seronegative women, but the attack rate of symptomatic VVC appears only slightly increased. Reports of chronic, severe, poorly responsive recurrent vulvovaginal candidiasis (RVVC) have been given much media attention but remain largely unsubstantiated. In the absence of other risk factors for HIV, RVVC is not an indication for HIV testing.

Clinical Manifestations

The most frequent symptom is vulvar pruritus, since vaginal discharge is not invariably present and is frequently minimal. Although described as typically cottage cheese-like in character, the discharge may vary from watery to homogenously thick. Vaginal soreness and irritation, vulvar burning, dyspareunia, and external dysuria are commonly present. If present, odor is minimal and nonoffensive. Examination frequently reveals erythema and swelling of the labia and vulva, often with discrete pustulopapular peripheral lesions. The cervix is normal, and vaginal mucosal erythema with adherent whitish discharge is present. Characteristically, symptoms are exacerbated in the week before the onset of menses, with some relief upon the onset of menstrual flow (Table 31-5).

Diagnosis

The relative lack of specificity of symptoms and signs precludes a diagnosis that is based only on history and physical examination. Most patients with symptomatic VVC may be readily diagnosed on the basis of simple microscopic examination of vaginal secretions (Fig. 31-1). A wet-mount or saline preparation has a sensitivity of 40 to 60 percent. The 10 percent KOH preparation is even more sensitive in diagnosing the presence of germinated yeast. A normal vaginal pH (4.0 to 4.5) is found in candidal vaginitis; the finding of a pH in excess of 4.5 should suggest the possibility of BV, trichomoniasis, or a mixed infection.

Table 31-5. Clinical Clues in History Useful in Diagnosis of Vulvovaginal Candidiasis

Abdominal pain (suggestive of cystitis or pelvic inflammatory diseases) is extremely rare with vaginitis
Exposure to a new sexual partner (suggestive of sexually transmitted diseases such as trichomonas, chlamydia or cervicitis)
Timing of symptom onset (*Candida* often flares premenstrually, trichomonas often during and bacterial vaginosis immediately after menses)
Medication use (antibiotics, high-estrogen oral contraceptives, and vaginal topical estrogen may predispose to candida/vulvovaginitis; increased physiologic discharge can occur with oral contraceptives, pregnancy, and hormone replacement therapy)

Although routine fungal cultures are unnecessary, vaginal culture should be performed in the presence of suggestive symptoms and negative microscopy. The Pap smear is unreliable, being positive in only about 25 percent of cases. There is no reliable serologic technique for the diagnosis of symptomatic candidal vaginitis.

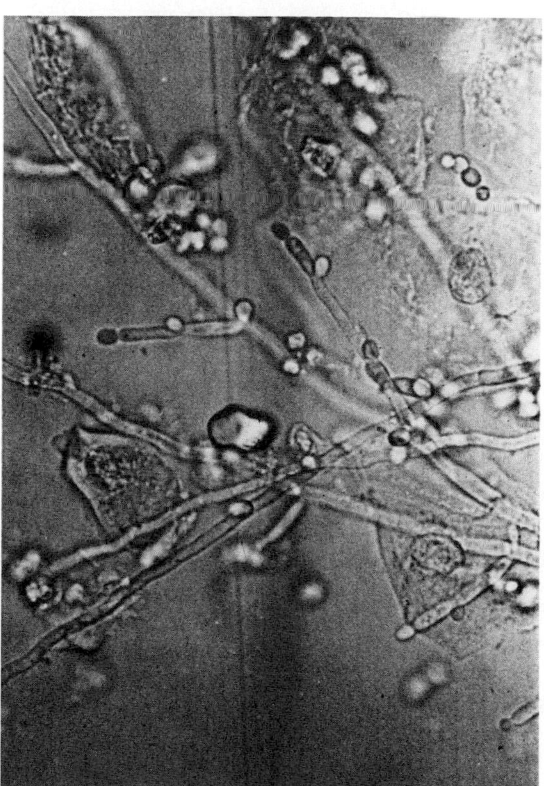

Fig. 31-1. Hyphal elements of *C. albicans* seen on high power magnification during saline microscopy. Patient had florid candidal vaginitis.

Treatment

Topical Agents for Acute Candidal Vaginitis

Antimycotics are available for local use as creams, lotions, aerosol sprays, vaginal tablets, suppositories, and coated tampons. There is little to suggest that formulation of the topical antimycotic influences clinical efficacy; in most cases, the patient's preference should dictate which vehicle is used to deliver the local therapy. Extensive vulvar inflammation dictates local application of antifungal cream. Antifungal agents that have been used in the topical treatment of candidal vaginitis are listed in Table 31-6.

Nystatin creams and vaginal suppositories have been used extensively for almost three decades. The average mycologic cure rate of 7- and 14-day courses is approximately 75 to 80 percent. Azole derivatives appear to achieve slightly higher clinical mycologic cure rates than do the polyenes (nystatin), approximately 85 to 90 percent. Although many studies have compared the clinical efficacy of the various azoles, there is little evidence that any one azole agent is superior to others.

Topical azoles are remarkably free of local and systemic side effects; nevertheless, the initial application of topical agents is sometimes accompanied by local burning and discomfort.

There has been a major trend toward shorter treatment courses with progressively higher antifungal doses, culminating in highly effective single-dose topical regimens. Although short-course regimens are effective for mild and moderate vaginitis, cure rates for severe, complicated and recurrent vaginitis are lower.[13]

Over-the-counter (OTC) topical antimycotics, although highly effective for VVC, are frequently abused because of poor self-diagnosis by women. More than 40 percent of women who use OTC medications do not suffer from VVC, but have an alternative diagnosis.

Oral systemic azoles are now available for the treatment of VVC, including ketoconazole 200 mg twice a

Table 31-6. Therapy for Vaginal Candidiasis—Topical Agents

Drug	Formulation	Dosage Regimen
[a]Butoconazole	2% cream	5 g/d for 3 days
	2% sustained release	5 g single application
[a]Clotrimazole	1% cream	5 g/d for 7–14 days
	100-mg vaginal tablet	1 tablet per day for 7 days
	100 mg vaginal tablet	2 tablets per day for 3 days
	500 mg vaginal tablet	1 tablet (single dose)
[a]Miconazole	2% cream	5 g/d for 7 days
	100 mg vaginal suppository	1 suppository per day for 7 days
	200 mg vaginal suppository	1 suppository per day for 3 days
	1200 mg vaginal suppository	1 suppository (single dose)
Econazole	150 mg vaginal tablet	1 tablet per day for 3 days
Fenticonazole	2% cream	5 g/d for 7 days
[a]Tioconazole	2% cream	5 g/d for 3 days
	6.5% cream	5 g (single dose)
Terconazole	0.4% cream	5 g/d for 7 days
	0.8% cream	5 g/d for 3 days
	80 mg vaginal suppository	80 mg/d for 3 days
Nystatin	100,000-U vaginal tablet	1 tablet/day for 14 days

[a]Available over the counter (OTC).

day for 5 days, itraconazole 200 mg daily for 3 days (or a 200-mg twice a day single-day regimen), and finally fluconazole 150 mg in a single dose.[13] All the oral regimens achieve clinical cure rates in excess of 80 percent; however, only fluconazole is approved for use for VVC in the United States. Oral regimens are generally preferred by women because of their convenience and lack of local side effects. None of the systemic regimens should be prescribed during pregnancy and, as with all oral agents, the potential for systemic side effects and toxicity exists. In particular, hepatotoxicity with ketoconazole precludes its widespread use in VVC.

A useful guide to selecting antifungals for VVC is provided in Table 31-6. Vulvovaginal candidiasis is classified as uncomplicated or complicated on the basis of the likelihood of achieving clinical and mycologic cure with short-course therapy. Uncomplicated VVC represents by far the most common form of vaginitis seen, is caused by highly sensitive *C. albicans,* and provided that the severity is mild to moderate, patients respond well to all topical or oral antimycotics including single-dose therapy. In contrast, patients with complicated VVC have either an organism, host factor, or severity of infection that dictates more intensive and prolonged therapy lasting 7 to 14 days.[14] Non-albicans *Candida* infections often respond to conventional topical or oral antifungals, provided they are administered long enough. Vaginitis caused by *C. glabrata* often fails to respond to azoles and may require treatment with vaginal capsules of boric acid 600 mg/day for 14 days. Recurrent VVC due to *C. glabrata* mandates referral to a vaginitis specialist.

Treatment of Recurrent Vulvovaginal Candidiasis

The management of women with RVVC aims at control rather than cure. The clinician should first confirm the diagnosis of RVVC. Uncontrolled diabetes must be controlled if there is to be any chance of clinical success. Similarly, the use of corticosteroids, other immunosuppressive agents, and hormones such as estrogen should be discontinued when possible. Unfortunately, in the majority of women with RVVC, no underlying or predisposing factor can be identified.

Recurrent VVC requires long-term maintenance with a suppressive prophylactic regimen. Several studies have confirmed the success of maintenance regimens in reducing the frequency of symptomatic episodes of VVC during long-term prophylactic therapy. Because of the chronicity of therapy, the convenience of oral treatment is apparent, and the best suppressive prophylaxis has been achieved with weekly fluconazole orally at a dose of 100 mg. An effective topical prophylactic regimen consists of weekly vaginal suppositories of clotrimazole 500 mg. Treatment of male partners of women with RVVC is rarely of benefit.

ATROPHIC VAGINITIS

It is important to distinguish between the symptomatic patient with an inflamed atrophic vagina and the patient with simple atrophy who has no symptoms other than dryness and no specific inflammation. Clinically significant atrophic vaginitis is actually quite rare, and the majority of women with an atrophic vagina are asymptomatic. Because of reduced endogenous estrogen, the epithelium becomes thin and lacking in glycogen, which contributes to a reduction in lactic acid production and an increase in vaginal pH. This change in the environment encourages the overgrowth of nonacidophilic coliform organisms and the disappearance of *Lactobacillus* spp. Despite these major but usually gradual changes, symptoms are usually absent, especially in the absence of coitus.

Typical symptoms include vaginal soreness, dyspareunia, and occasional spotting or discharge. Burning is a frequent complaint and is often precipitated by intercourse. The vaginal mucosa is thin, with diffuse redness, occasional petechiae, or ecchymoses with few or no vaginal folds. Vulvar atrophy may also be present; discharge, if present, may be blood-like, thick, or watery, and the pH of the vaginal secretions ranges from 5.5 to 7.0. The wet smear frequently shows increased PMNs associated with small, round epithelial cells. The latter parabasal cells represent immature squamous cells that have not been exposed to sufficient estrogen. The *Lactobacillus*-dominated flora is replaced by a mixed flora of gram-negative rods. Bacteriologic cultures in these patients are not unnecessary and can be misleading.

The treatment of atrophic vaginitis consists primarily of topical vaginal estrogen, especially in the absence of systemic symptoms. Nightly use of half or all the contents of an applicator for 1 to 2 weeks is usually sufficient to alleviate the atrophic vaginitis. Oral treatment with the usual doses of estrogen replacement therapy (e.g., 0.625 mg of conjugated estrogen) is also effective.

OTHER NONINFECTIOUS VAGINITIS

Women frequently present with chronic or acute vulvovaginal symptoms due to noninfectious etiologies. Symptoms are indistinguishable from those of infectious syndromes, but are most commonly confused with acute candidal vaginitis, as these patients present with pruritus, irritation, burning, soreness, and variable discharge. Noninfectious causes have been poorly studied and their true prevalence is largely unknown. Such causes include (1) irritants, physical (e.g., minipads) or chemical (e.g., spermicides, povidone-iodine, topical antimycotics, soaps and perfumes); and (2) allergens, responsible for immunologic acute and chronic hypersensitivity reactions including contact dermatitis (e.g., latex condoms, antimycotic creams). There is an endless list of topical factors responsible for local inflammatory reactions and symptoms and many more have yet to be defined. Depending on the site of contact, symptoms may be vaginal or vulvar. Sometimes a noninfectious mechanism may coexist with an infectious process or may follow it.

A noninfectious cause should be considered in patients when the three common infectious causes are excluded and in the presence of normal vaginal pH, normal saline, KOH microscopy, and ultimately a negative yeast culture. Unfortunately, given the anticipated 20 percent colonization rate in normal, asymptomatic patients, a positive yeast culture will occasionally reflect the presence of an innocent bystander and not the putative cause of the vulvovaginal symptoms. The only logical way of establishing the role of *Candida* in this context is to treat with an oral antifungal agent and assess the clinical response.

Once a local chemical, irritant, or allergic reaction is suspected, the practitioner is required to initiate a detailed inquiry into possible causal factors. Offending agents or behaviors should be eliminated wherever possible. In addition, patients should generally be advised to avoid chemical irritants and allergens (e.g., soaps, detergents, etc.). The immediate management of severe vulvovaginal symptoms of noninfectious etiology remains a challenge and does not consist of topical corticosteroids, which are rarely the solution; moreover, high-potency steroid creams frequently cause intense burning. Avoidance of the offending agent, if identified, will usually result in improvement or resolution of the symptoms. Local relief measures include sodium bicarbonate sitz-baths or oral antihistamines.

Some investigators have described a syndrome of hyperacidity of the vagina due to overgrowth of lactobacilli. Rebound increase in the *Lactobacillus*-dominant vaginal flora occurs after completion of topical antimycotics, which may suppress the population of healthy resident flora. This proposed syndrome of cytolytic vaginosis is characterized clinically by vulvovaginal burning, irritation, soreness, and dyspareunia and is usually incorrectly diagnosed as VVC. The finding of large numbers of lactobacilli on wet mount together with extensive cytolysis of squamous epithelial cells is said to confirm the diagnosis. Recommended therapy for cytolytic vaginosis is daily al-

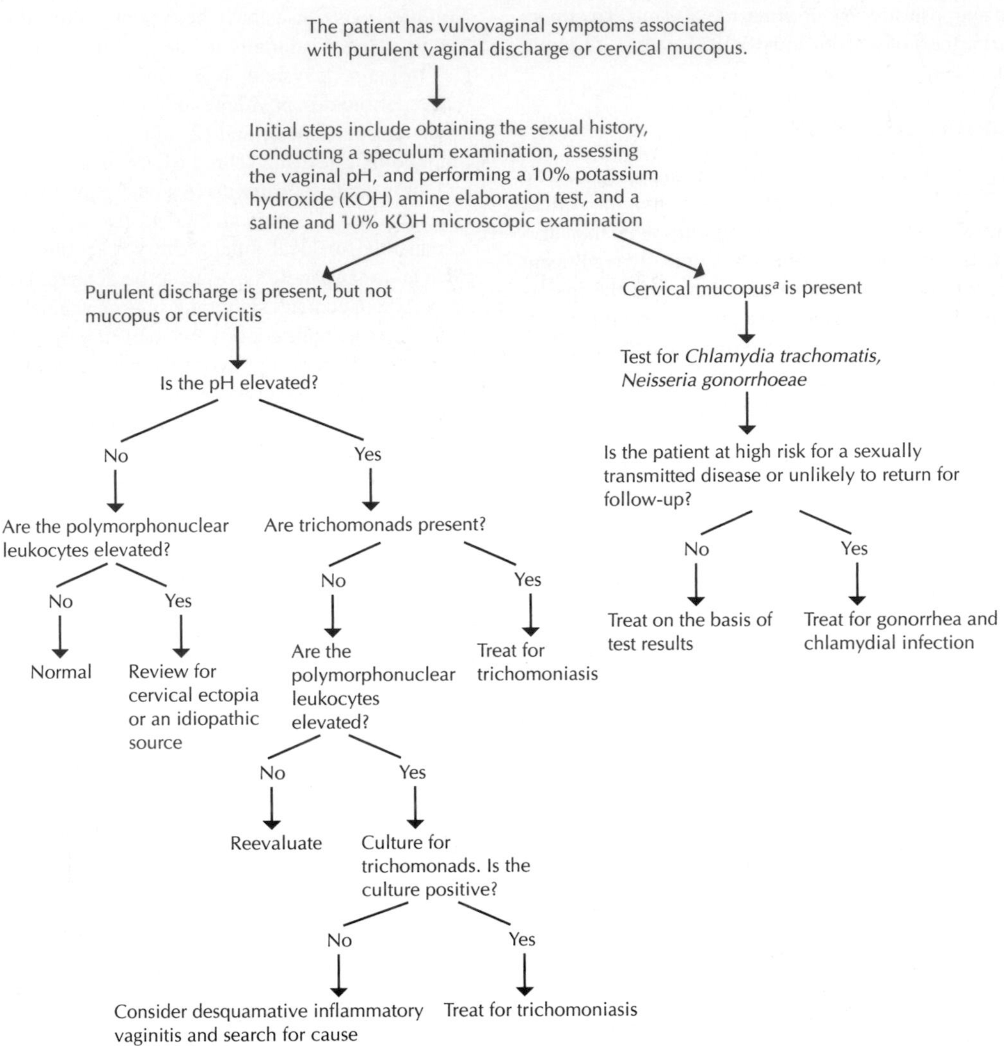

Fig. 31-2. The algorithm summarizes initial management of a patient with vulvovaginal symptoms that include either purulent vaginal discharge or the presence of cervical mucopus. Mixed infections are possible.

kaline douching using sodium bicarbonate to elevate the low vaginal pH and suppress growth of lactobacilli.

ALGORITHMS IN THE MANAGEMENT OF ACUTE VAGINITIS

Several algorithms have recently been published that base diagnosis entirely on symptoms, without performing a physical examination or any laboratory tests. These algorithms, although useful in the developing world where the lack of medical care precludes accurate diagnosis, are to be condemned and not applied in the United States. All courses of management should avoid guesswork and empiricism. Figures 31-2 and 31-3 outline a rational approach to the management of women with symptomatic vulvovaginal disease. These pathways are not empiric, but

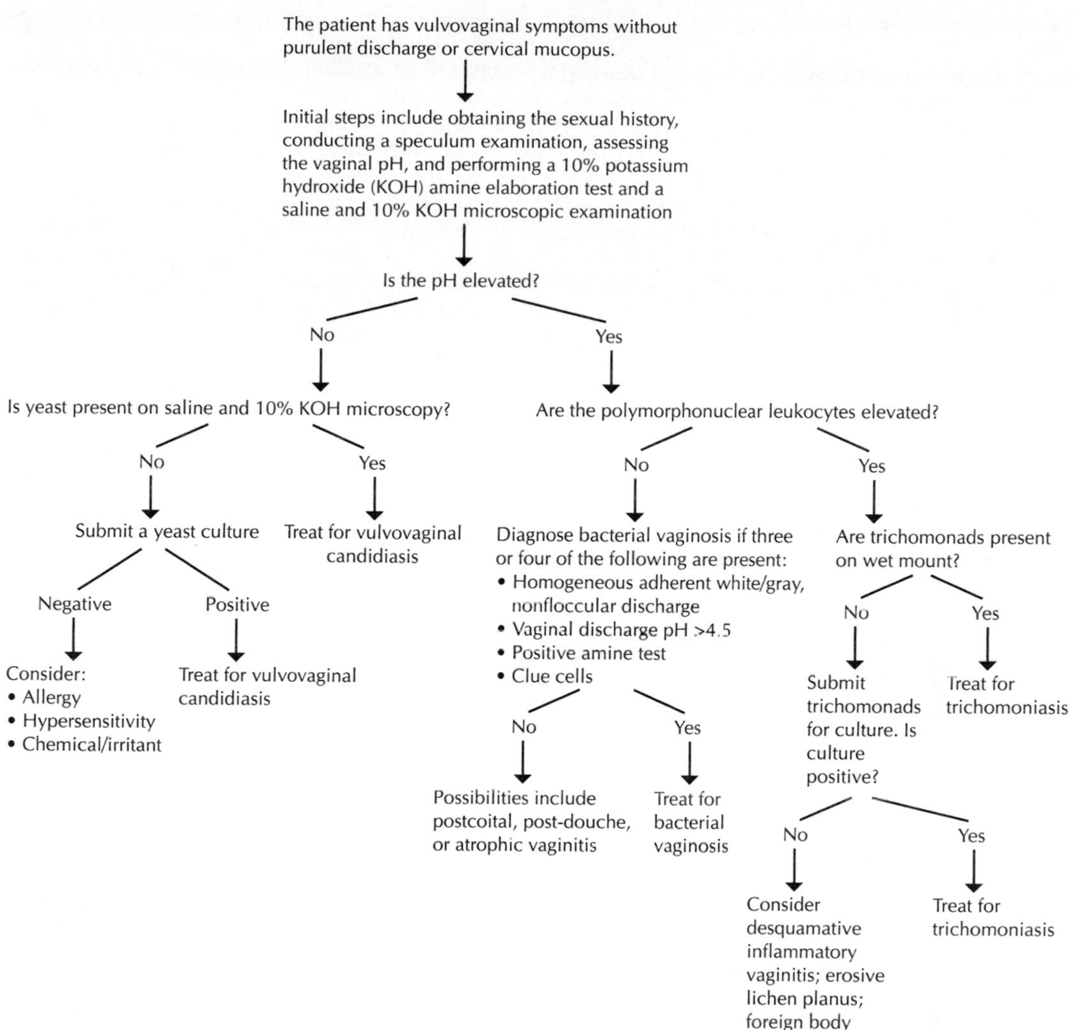

Fig. 31-3. The algorithm summarizes initial management of a patient with vulvovaginal symptoms that *do not* include either purulent vaginal discharge or the presence of cervical mucopus. Mixed infections are possible.

are based on easily measurable objective findings (e.g., pH and microscopy of vaginal secretions).

REFERENCES

1. Kent HL: Epidemiology of vaginitis. *Am J Obstet Gynecol* 165(4 Pt 2):1168, 1991.
2. Ferris DG, Nyirjesy P, Sobel JD, et al: Over-the-counter antifungal drug misuse with patient diagnosed vulvovaginal candidiasis. *Obstet Gynecol* 99:419, 2002.
3. Hill GB: Microbiology of bacterial vaginosis. *Am J Obstet Gynecol* 169:450, 1969.
4. Eschenbach DA, Davick PR, Williams BL, et al: Prevalence of hydrogen peroxide producing *Lactobacillus* species in normal women and women with bacterial vaginosis. *J Clin Microbiol* 27:251, 1989.
5. Hillier SL, Krohn MA, Cassen E, et al: The role of bacterial vaginosis and vaginal bacteria in amniotic fluid infection in women in preterm labor with intact fetal membranes. *Clin Infect Dis* 20(Suppl 2):276, 1995.
6. Tana TE, Hoover DR, Dallabetta GA, et al: Bacterial vaginosis and disturbances of vaginal flora: Association with increased acquisition of HIV. *AIDS* 12:1699, 1998.
7. Carey JC, Klebanoff MA, Hauth JC, et al: Metronidazole to prevent preterm delivery in pregnant women with

asymptomatic bacterial vaginosis. *N Engl J Med* 342:534, 2000.

8. Hauth JC, Goldenberg DL, Andrews WW, et al: Reduced incidence of preterm delivery with metronidazole and erythromycin in women with bacterial vaginosis. *N Engl J Med* 333:1732, 1995.
9. Wolner-Hanssen P, Krieger JN, Stevens CE, et al: Clinical manifestations of vaginal trichomoniasis. *JAMA* 261:571, 1989.
10. Spence MR, Hollander DH, Smith J, et al: The clinical and laboratory diagnosis of *Trichomonas vaginalis* infection. *Sex Transm Dis* 7:168, 1980.
11. Sobel JD, Nyirjesy P, Brown W: Tinidazole therapy for metronidazole-resistant vaginal trichomoniasis. *Clin Infect Dis* 33:1341 2001.
12. Sobel JD: Candidal vulvovaginitis. *Clin Obstet Gynecol* 36:153, 1993.
13. Sobel JD, Brooker D, Stein GE, et al: Single oral dose fluconazole compared with clotrimazole topical therapy of *Candida* vaginitis: Fluconazole Vaginitis Study Group. *Am J Obstet Gynecol* 172:1263, 1955.
14. Sobel JD, Kapernick PS, Zervos M, et al: Treatment of complicated *Candida* vaginitis: Comparison of single and sequential classes of fluconazole. *Am J Obstet Gynecol* 185:363, 2001.

32

Complications of Gynecologic Procedures

William W. Hurd
Sheela M. Barhan
Jean A. Hurteau

KEY POINTS

- Patients are often discharged within 12 to 24 hours of abdominal surgery. The unavoidable result is the increased presentation of postoperative complications to the emergency department (ED).
- Gynecologic surgery, whether approached abdominally or vaginally, carries a risk of postoperative complications in the range of 1 to 4 percent.[1,2] Most commonly, these complications involve the abdominal incision, the urinary tract, or the gastrointestinal tract, and rarely vascular or nerve injuries.
- In general, pain improves daily following laparoscopic procedures. Worsening pain is a worrisome sign and should prompt a timely and appropriate evaluation.
- A clinical presentation of ascites or a watery vaginal discharge following a pelvic surgery should always raise suspicion of ureteral or bladder injury.
- Thermal injury of the colon may characteristically be delayed in presentation for 1 to 5 days or more, until bowel wall necrosis results in intraperitoneal infection.

Gynecologic procedures are among the most common surgical procedures performed in the United States today. In the past, all abdominal surgical procedures were followed by close hospital observation until complete recovery was assured. Today, in part because of fiscal considerations, patients are often sent home within 12 to 24 hours of abdominal surgery. The unavoidable result is the increased presentation of postoperative complications to the emergency department (ED) and other ambulatory settings that only a generation ago would have rarely been seen outside an inpatient hospital environment. In contrast to the hospital setting, where trained observers can often detect and treat a complication at its earliest stage, a patient may not return for evaluation until the complication has progressed significantly. The result is that complications seen in the ED may be further advanced than those seen in an inpatient setting.

After any gynecologic surgery, a progressive resolution of postoperative symptoms during the first week is to be expected. With abdominal procedures, slow return to normal bowel function may take several days. For any procedure, pain may be perceived as slightly worse on the day following the procedure, but it should only improve after that. Likewise, the incision should appear healthy (skin edges well opposed, minimal to no erythema and no drainage) and should become almost painless within the first week.

Patients should be clearly counseled on the natural postoperative course of events at the time of discharge, and any deviation from this course should lead the patient to seek medical advice. A natural tendency may be to reassure the patient that her postoperative discomfort is within the normal range. However, delay of appropriate care can often compound the effects of complications and may potentially be fatal. If a patient who calls cannot be assured with absolute certainty that she is not experiencing surgical complications, the patient should be advised to come in for an evaluation by a practitioner experienced in recognizing them.

PATHOPHYSIOLOGY

Incision/Wound Complications

Gynecologic surgery, whether approached abdominally or vaginally, carries a risk of postoperative complications in the range of 1 to 4 percent.[1,2] Most commonly, these complications involve the abdominal incision, the urinary tract, or the gastrointestinal tract, and rarely vascular or nerve injuries. Because of the unique nature of both laparoscopic and vaginal surgery, the seriousness of the complication may have no relationship to the size (or even presence) of an abdominal incision.

Complications related to abdominal incisions may result from operative procedures involving either laparotomy or laparoscopy. Wound infections are among the most common complications after laparotomy, but they are relatively infrequent with laparoscopy.[3] In either case, infection will most commonly develop within 3 to 5 days of surgery, with erythema and tenderness and, in some cases, purulent discharge along all or part of the incision. This complication is most commonly related to bacterial contamination of the wound at the time of surgery or colonization shortly after surgery by skin flora. It is extremely important to determine the extent of the infection, since superficial infections are safely treated in an outpatient setting, whereas extensive cellulitis and necrotizing fasciitis are almost always treated in an inpatient setting. Gynecologic surgeries that involve entry into the vagina such as hysterectomy and cervical conizations are classified as clean-contaminated procedures and carry a significant risk of postoperative infection. Since the introduction of routine use of intravenous antibiotic prophylaxis in clean-contaminated procedures, the risk of pelvic infection in abdominal and vaginal hysterectomy has decreased from 25 to approximately 5 percent.[1]

With laparoscopy, wound infections are relatively rare. However, laparoscopy more commonly results in the formation of a hematoma beneath the incision site. This is because laparoscopic trocar insertion can result in occult injury to vessels in the abdominal wall, in some cases with little external bleeding. This problem is much more likely to arise when large trocars ($\geq$10 mm in diameter) are placed lateral to the midline. In most cases, problems of this nature appear within hours of surgery.

Incisional drainage may sometimes be encountered after laparotomy or laparoscopy. When significant drainage originates from an incision immediately above the symphysis, bladder injury should always be suspected, as this may be the first indication of such a problem. Bladder injury may be more common in cases in which the patient has undergone a previous laparotomy that resulted in displacement of the bladder above the symphysis. Bowel injuries may occasionally present as incisional drainage from a enterocutaneous fistula. Wound dehiscence can also present as a serosanguineous discharge; thus the integrity of the fascia should be verified. Finally, a seroma, or subcutaneous collection of serous fluid, which may occur as part of the normal healing process, may present as wound discharge. However, the possibility of a more serious underlying condition should always be ruled out before making this diagnosis.

Abdominal pain may be the most common presenting symptom after gynecologic surgery. In some cases, this pain may represent an incisional complication (e.g., wound infection or hematoma). A special case may be entrapped incisional hernias that occur after laparoscopy. Herniation is a rare complication that occurs at the site where the laparoscope is placed through the umbilicus. However, bowel herniation has been reported to occur when large trocars ($\geq$10 mm) are used in locations lateral to the midline. Apparently, this is not related to herniation through a fascial defect, but rather to entrapment of bowel that has herniated through the peritoneum into the preperitoneal space. This appears to be a different process from that of an incisional hernia occurring after laparotomy, in which a palpable bulge is the most common presenting symptom and entrapment is uncommon. After laparoscopy, herniation may present as severe abdominal cramping accompanied by signs of bowel obstruction without any perceptible bulge on exam. Although incisional hernias should always be considered as a possible cause of abdominal pain after laparoscopic surgery, they are relatively infrequent. Thus other intraabdominal processes (e.g., ileus, bowel injury) should also be considered.

Urinary Tract Complications

Abdominal pain may be related to problems involving the urinary tract. A common complaint within the first 24 hours after laparoscopy is urinary retention. Even if no surgery has been performed around the bladder, some patients find it difficult to void immediately after receiving general anesthesia for surgery.[4] Whether this is an anesthetic effect or the result of the inability to relax the pelvic floor muscles because of incisional pain is debatable. Whatever the cause, increasing lower abdominal discomfort associated with a midline suprapubic mass should suggest this easily treatable possibility.

Occasionally postoperative abdominal pain may result from a urinary tract infection (UTI). Prior to most gynecologic procedures, most patients are catheterized to minimize the risk of bladder injury during trocar placement. For laparoscopy, an indwelling catheter is not commonly used. For laparotomy, an indwelling bladder catheter is used in most cases. In either case, catheterization is associated with the risk of UTI regardless of the sterile precautions taken. The result can be symptomatic cystitis or pyelonephritis that may not manifest until days after the original surgery.

Ureteral injury is another complication that may be seen after hysterectomy or any surgery requiring dissection or ligation of side-wall vessels, such as removal of an adnexum or at the time of a hysterectomy. It has also been reported after fulguration of endometriosis on the pelvic side wall. Ureteral injuries—including complete ligation, transection, partial resection, or thermal injuries—will usually manifest within hours to days of surgery. With shorter periods of hospitalization after surgery, this may be more commonly diagnosed in an outpatient. Complete obstruction will usually result in severe flank pain and fever, whereas transection may manifest with symptoms of intraabdominal irritation caused by urine leakage. A clinical presentation of ascites or a watery vaginal discharge following a pelvic surgery should always raise suspicion of ureteral or bladder injury. Transperitoneal thermal injuries resulting from fulguration of endometriosis may be similar to those seen after transection, but the appearance of symptoms may be delayed for several days until tissue necrosis occurs.

Intraabdominal/Hemorrhage

Although incisional or urinary tract problems can result in postoperative abdominal pain, this symptom may represent a more serious intraabdominal complication. When extensive intraabdominal surgery has been performed by laparotomy, by laparoscopy, or via the vagina, the risk of a major complication is increased. Intraabdominal hemorrhage, while not the most common complication, is probably the most serious. Postoperative hemorrhage is a risk after any gynecologic surgery, which usually manifests within 24 hours of surgery. In rare cases, hemorrhage may take several days to become apparent. From an ED perspective, this complication may be of increased importance after operative laparoscopy, since laparoscopic procedures are almost always performed on an outpatient basis. Blood usually causes peritoneal irritation; thus most patients will present with abdominal pain with or without signs of hemodynamic compromise. In other patients, dizziness or syncope may be the earliest signs of a significant intraabdominal hemorrhage. Abdominal distention is a late finding consistent with massive intraabdominal hemorrhage.

Vaginal Cuff Infection

Infection at the site of surgery is the most common complication following hysterectomy or vaginal procedures.[1] It is not uncommon to see surgical site infections develop in patients who had a postoperative fever that resolved with or without antibiotic treatment. Such indolent infections can manifest as a pelvic abscess or cellulitis at the vaginal cuff after hysterectomy. The presenting symptom may be pain and fever, abnormal vaginal discharge, or abdominal distention due to functional ileus related to bowel irritation. Presentation of this problem to the ED may be more common when patients are discharged within 24 hours of surgery after laparoscopically assisted vaginal hysterectomy or vaginal hysterectomy, since the first signs of infection may appear after the patient has been discharged. After vaginal hysterectomy, no special precautions are needed for a speculum examination Vaginal cuff disruptions are rare and impossible to cause by routine vaginal examination.

Bowel Injuries

A potentially catastrophic complication of gynecologic surgery is bowel injury. During laparotomy, this is usually recognized immediately and repaired because there is more complete visualization of the surgical field. During laparoscopic or vaginal surgery, bowel injuries may be more difficult to recognize and thus may go undiagnosed until secondary symptoms develop. The potential for this problem to go unrecognized is increased by the brief hospitalizations associated with these procedures.

With vaginal hysterectomy, the peritoneal cavity is never completely visualized. Bowel injuries may result from blunt lysis of unseen adhesions between the reproductive organs and bowel or by the inadvertent inclusion of a section of bowel in a uterine pedicle above the view of the operator. Bowel injuries of this nature will often manifest with peritonitis or signs of bowel obstruction several days after surgery.

Laparoscopic surgery may result in injuries to either the small or large intestine by several mechanisms. An unrecognized bowel injury may occur at the time of trocar insertion (e.g., a "through and through" injury). Thermal bowel injuries may also occur during laparoscopy, since power sources such as electrocautery and laser are commonly used during these procedures. Major bowel injuries usually become obvious during surgery. However, because of the limited field of view, some major bowel injuries and many smaller ones may not be seen during surgery. These injuries usually manifest themselves 1 to 3 days after surgery, well after the patient has been released following these primarily outpatient procedures. Perforations of the large intestine resulting from direct injury usually present as an intraabdominal infectious process within the first 24 hours after surgery because of the resulting bacterial contamination of the peritoneal cavity. Thermal injury of the colon may characteristically be delayed in presentation for 1 to 5 days or more, until bowel wall necrosis results in intraperitoneal infection. Thermal injuries are more common when monopolar electrical energy sources are used during laparoscopy. Injuries of the small intestine are often more subtle in presentation. Apparently normal postoperative discomfort may progress to signs of peritonitis with eventual abdominal distention as the sterile contents of the small intestine leak from the bowel. Because of the lack of signs of infection in many cases, this diagnosis may be more difficult to make.

Vaginal Bleeding and Discharge

Another presentation of complications following gynecologic surgery is vaginal bleeding or discharge. After hysterectomy, a minimal amount of bleeding commonly occurs within the first 2 to 3 weeks as the sutures at the top of the vagina (the cuff) dissolve and loosen, exposing healing tissue that can ooze. During the first few days after hysterectomy, profuse vaginal bleeding may occur if a suture has loosened from a vascular pedicle. After a cone biopsy of the cervix, in which the center of the cervix is removed and hemostasis is obtained by a combination of cauterization and suturing, significant bleeding will occur within the first 6 weeks (usually within the first 10 days) in approximately 10 percent of patients.[5] After vaginal reconstructive surgery, bleeding may be the only sign of a vaginal hematoma that can form underneath the repair.

Significant vaginal discharge, especially that associated with fever or pain, may indicate infection at the site of the surgery. After minor gynecologic surgery, such as dilatation and curettage or laparoscopic tubal surgery, endometritis or cervicitis may manifest as a purulent discharge associated with pelvic tenderness. Even though minor procedures performed through the vagina have a low risk of infection and do not require antibiotic prophylaxis, a patient with an untreated sexually transmitted disease or bacterial vaginosis can develop a clinical presentation of pelvic inflammatory disease in the week following the surgery. After hysterectomy, a similar presentation may represent localized cuff cellulitis or a cuff abscess. Less commonly after hysterectomy, a bowel or bladder injury with resultant fistula formation may present as vaginal discharge.

DIAGNOSIS AND DIFFERENTIAL DIAGNOSIS

Incisional Pain

In general, the diagnosis of infection or hematoma is made by inspection and palpation of the incision. Localized erythema and induration suggest a superficial infection. Fluctuance indicates a possible subcutaneous abscess. A deeper mass suggests a subfascial hematoma or abscess, although bowel herniation should also be considered (Fig. 32-1).

If cellulitis is present, the extent of the infection must be determined accurately. One of the most important differential diagnoses to make in this situation is that of necrotizing fasciitis. This rare complication may present similar to a wound abscess; however, erythema and induration with ecchymosis may be relatively more widespread and the wound is usually extremely painful. Comorbidities such as diabetes or immunosuppression are frequently present. Fascial and subcutaneous necrosis may manifest as a relative lack of resistance to probing of these tissue planes. Late signs of necrotizing fasciitis are tissue crepitus and decreased sensation at the incision site. This surgical emergency requires immediate hospitalization with high-dose antibiotics and surgical debridement in an effort to treat this condition effectively, as it is associated with a 20 to 30 percent mortality rate.[6]

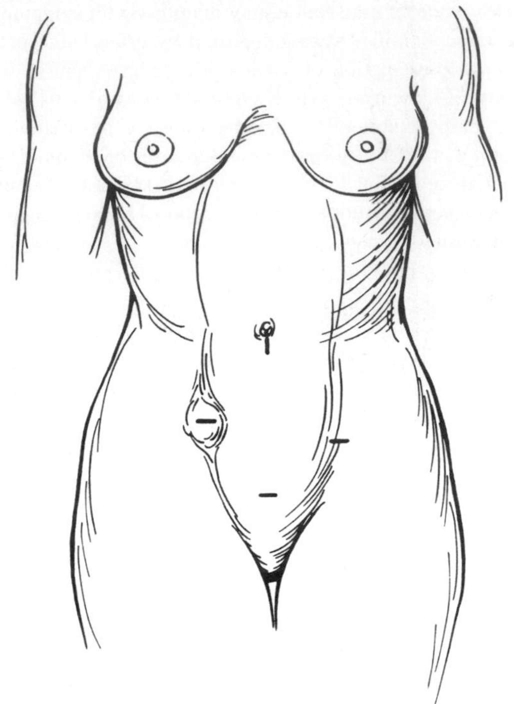

Fig. 32-1. The differential diagnosis for a bulging mass underlying a surgical incision after laparoscopy should include hematoma, abscess, and bowel herniation.

Incisional drainage of clear fluid can be the sign of something as innocuous as a subcutaneous seroma. However, it must be verified that this is not the symptom of something more serious, such as a fascial dehiscence or injury of bladder or bowel. Initial evaluation should be probing of the wound with a sterile, cotton-tipped applicator to verify that the fascial layer is intact. If the wound drainage is significant in quantity or resembles urine, indigo carmine or methylene blue can be used to check for bladder or ureter injuries. These dyes can be either given intravenously, or diluted with normal saline and instilled into the bladder via an indwelling catheter. A sponge placed in the vagina will be stained blue if a vesicovaginal or uterovaginal fistula is present. Bowel injuries that present as wound drainage are usually associated with hypoactive bowel function. However, if bowel contents drain only transcutaneously and do not spill intraperitoneally, diffuse abdominal signs may be absent. Oral charcoal has been used as a simple method to determine the presence of an enterocutaneous fistula of the small bowel.

Abdominal Pain

Abdominal pain, probably the most common presenting symptom to the ED after gynecologic surgery, can be of multiple etiologies. One common cause in the first 24 hours postoperatively is urinary retention. Severe pain with a midline mass in a woman who has not voided recently suggests this diagnosis. A more common condition that may manifest postoperatively is UTI, either cystitis or pyelonephritis. With cystitis, suprapubic tenderness, dysuria, with or without urgency or frequency may be the presenting symptom. With pyelonephritis, costovertebral angle tenderness, usually associated with fever and leukocytosis, may be accompanied by abdominal pain or other symptoms of cystitis. Urinalysis will usually reveal bacteriuria, pyuria, leukocyte esterase activity, and occasion ally hematuria.

The rest of the problems that may cause postoperative abdominal pain originate intraabdominally and may be difficult to differentiate. Intraabdominal hemorrhage may present with peritoneal signs and is further supported by a decreased hemoglobin. Usually some degree of hemodynamic instability will also be apparent, ranging from tachycardia and orthostatic hypotension to hypovolemic shock.

Operative site infection (i.e., intrapelvic or vaginal cuff infection) may also present with localized peritoneal signs associated with fever and leukocytosis. Although generalized peritonitis may be present, discrete tenderness to deep palpation over the site of surgery is more common.

Abdominal pain may also result from a bladder or ureteral injury. Intraabdominal leakage of urine will result in peritoneal signs and leukocytosis. Fever is usually not present unless the injury has resulted in the development of a concomitant urinary tract infection. In contrast, occlusion of the ureter will result in flank pain without any peritoneal signs. On urinalysis, hematuria alone is suggestive of a urinary tract injury. Hematuria with bacteriuria and pyuria may indicate either injury with a superimposed infection, or more commonly infection alone. Conversely, the absence of hematuria can be seen in the complete occlusion of a ureter.

Bowel problems usually present as signs of obstruction, such as cramping associated with nausea, vomiting, and abdominal distention. When bowel herniation at a laparoscopic trocar site leads to mechanical obstruction, there may be tenderness and a mass at the incision as well. With perforating injuries of the colon, signs of bowel obstruction are usually associated with peritonitis, functional bowel obstruction, and possibly signs of sepsis. In contrast, perforating injuries of the small intestines may be associated with functional bowel obstruction because of chemical irritation, but signs of infection are less common.

Vaginal Symptoms

Vaginal bleeding or discharge may occur after minor vaginal surgery or hysterectomy. Vaginal bleeding is the most common symptom. After cone biopsy of the cervix, approximately 10 percent of patients will have significant enough bleeding (usually occurs between 7 and 10 days) to seek medical attention.[5] Speculum examination will usually reveal a discrete bleeding site on the cervix. After uterine curettage or hysteroscopy, subsequent heavy bleeding originating from the uterine cavity is uncommon. However, after hysterectomy performed either vaginally or abdominally, vaginal bleeding may occasionally occur within the first week. In the presence of bright red vaginal bleeding, inspection of the highly vascular vaginal apex where the cervix has been excised may reveal an active bleeding site. If dark, sanguineous discharge is coming from the vaginal cuff, this may be the manifestation of a cuff hematoma that is draining vaginally.

Surgical manipulation and suture placement leads invariably to some change in the bacterial flora of the vagina. This in itself is a localized problem of the vaginal vault and does not indicate infection of the pelvic tissues. A finding of significant pelvic tenderness associated with an elevated serum white blood cell count does confirm the diagnosis of pelvic infection. Vaginal drainage of purulent discharge indicates infection of the surgical site. Purulence can be confirmed by wet prep microscopic findings of an overabundance of white blood cells. After minor gynecologic surgery, cervicitis may present as inflammation and cervical discharge associated with cervical tenderness. Endometritis and parametritis may appear similar, but may be associated with uterine or ovarian tenderness as well. Advanced cases of parametritis may result in more generalized peritoneal signs as well as fever and chills.

After hysterectomy, significant malodorous discharge usually indicates an infection at the vaginal cuff. Cuff

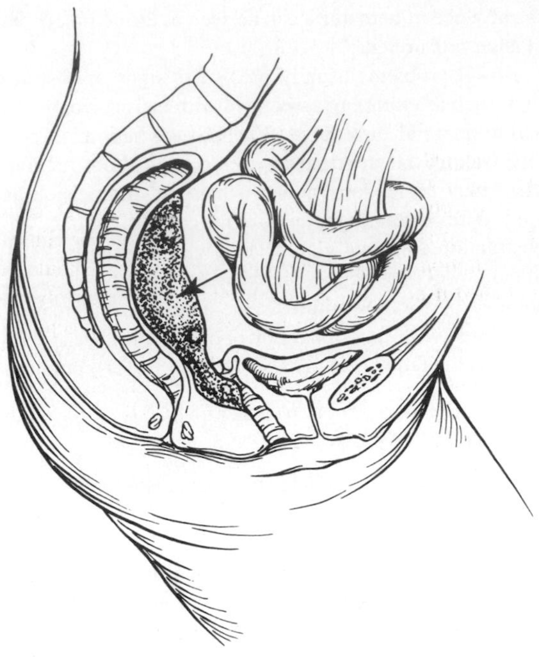

Fig. 32-2. A cuff abscess after hysterectomy will present as a discrete mass at the apex that is either palpable or visible by ultrasound (*arrow*).

cellulitis is characterized by induration and tenderness at the vaginal apex. In addition, a cuff abscess will have a discrete mass at the apex that is either palpable or visible by ultrasound (Fig. 32-2). Both of these conditions are usually associated with fever and leukocytosis.

When excessive vaginal discharge after hysterectomy is noted, a fistula between the vagina and either the bladder or bowel should be considered. A vesicovaginal fistula is associated with leaking of clear fluid (urine) vaginally that the patient cannot control. This condition is usually associated with recurrent urinary tract infections. An enterovaginal fistula is associated with the passage of intestinal contents, which may vary depending on the level of the fistula. A fistula involving the rectosigmoid is associated with passage of malodorous fecal material. In contrast, a fistula involving the small intestines will be associated with significant vaginal and vulvar inflammation, resulting from the irritating nature of the small bowel contents.

Laboratory Tests

In almost every case in which a woman presents to the ED after gynecologic surgery, a complete blood count and urinalysis will be helpful. Leukocytosis or anemia may be one of the earliest signs of several postoperative complications, as noted above. The urinalysis will help to detect urinary tract injuries or infections, both of which are common problems after gynecologic procedures. Although hematuria as an isolated finding suggests a urinary tract injury, hematuria with pyuria and bacteriuria may represent either a urinary tract infection or a urinary tract injury with a superimposed infection.

Radiologic examinations are often helpful. If an intraabdominal process is suspected, flat and upright abdominal examinations that include the diaphragm are helpful. Free air under the diaphragm more than 2 days after laparoscopy or more than a week after open abdominal surgery suggests a bowel injury. A much less common cause is a fistula between the vaginal cuff and the peritoneal cavity. Although gas under the diaphragm can be seen the same day as laparoscopy because of the gas used for insufflation of the peritoneal cavity, the carbon dioxide that is used for this purpose is quickly absorbed. If any air is seen under the diaphragm more than 48 hours after laparoscopy, bowel perforation must be strongly considered.

Pelvic ultrasound can also be very helpful in the presence of a fever or pain after hysterectomy. The presence of a loculated fluid collection in this case is suggestive of a cuff abscess, which may be drained transvaginally. In some cases, computed tomography may be necessary to locate abscesses distant from the vaginal cuff.

TREATMENT

Relatively few postoperative complications will be treated in the ED without gynecologic consultation (Fig. 32-3). Many serious complications first appear with very subtle findings that can mimic normal postoperative discomfort. The most common problems that can be treated without gynecologic consultation are superficial wound infections and urinary tract problems after injury has been ruled out.

Superficial wound infections are examined carefully to rule out deep tissue involvement, and then gently explored to determine if an abscess or fascial defect exists. If an abscess is discovered but the fascia is intact, the wound should be opened completely, thoroughly irrigated, and packed with iodoform gauze. If the surrounding inflammation is limited and the patient does not appear toxic, she may be treated as an outpatient with daily dressing changes. Systemic antibiotics are often given but may be of limited benefit in a well-localized wound infection. If there is any indication of a fascial defect or a surrounding cellulitis or fasciitis, gynecologic evaluation is required for possible inpatient therapy with appropriate antibiotic coverage and surgical treatment.

Vaginal bleeding after cervical cone biopsy can often be effectively treated in the ED. In the presence of a discrete bleeding site, hemostasis can usually be obtained by suturing the site. If more widespread oozing is present, packing the operative site with a hemostatic material such as oxidized cellulose may be effective.

Many urinary tract problems that occur after gynecologic surgery can also be treated effectively in the ED. Urinary retention after laparoscopy is treated by draining the bladder with a catheter. If the urinalysis is completely normal, the patient can be observed until she voids spontaneously. If the postvoid residual is low (i.e., <100 mL), she can be sent home with instructions to return if further problems with voiding arise. However, if the residual is more than 100 mL, she should be sent home with an indwelling catheter connected to a collection bag for follow-up the following day. This problem almost always resolves spontaneously within 24 hours. Medications that may contribute to urinary retention, such as narcotics, may need to be discontinued until normal bladder function resumes.

In the absence of hematuria or significant abdominal tenderness, cystitis and pyelonephritis can also be treated appropriately in the ED. However, in the presence of flank tenderness after pelvic surgery, intravenous pyelography or renal ultrasonography should be performed to investigate the possibility of ureteral injury or obstruction. In the presence of hematuria or any intraabdominal symptoms, gynecologic evaluation may be required.

DISCHARGE INSTRUCTIONS AND FOLLOW-UP INTERVAL

For any postoperative problem treated in the ED, close follow-up is extremely important. Telephone or clinical consultation with the operating gynecologist should be obtained if possible. What appears to be a relatively minor problem may be the first symptom of a potentially serious postoperative complication. Follow-up within 24 to 48 hours is appropriate in most cases, usually with the operating gynecologist. Wound infection, urinary retention, and urinary tract infection should respond quickly with appropriate treatment. If the symptoms do not resolve or are worsening, the possibility of a more serious complication must be considered.

INDICATIONS FOR SPECIALTY CONSULTATION AND HOSPITALIZATION

Because of the risk of serious postoperative complications, the vast majority of postoperative complications will require gynecologic evaluation in the ED. Even after diagnosis and treatment of a relatively minor problem, close follow-up by the operating gynecologist is important. Complications after gynecologic surgery are inevitable. However, failure to recognize the complication or inappropriate treatment or follow-up can significantly compound the problem.

If there is any concern that a wound infection is more than superficial, gynecologic evaluation is required to rule out dehiscence, cellulitis, or fasciitis. If an apparent UTI is associated with hematuria or signs and symptoms of an intraabdominal process, gynecologic evaluation is warranted to rule out ureteral or bladder injury. In the presence of localized abdominal pain or more widespread peritonitis, gynecologic evaluation is always required.

In the case of significant vaginal bleeding after gynecologic surgery, gynecologic evaluation is usually required. When significant vaginal discharge indicates a postoperative infection, the need for gynecologic evaluation is determined by the type of surgery and the degree of infection.

After minor surgery, mild infections confined to the cervix and uterus (i.e., without abdominal manifestations) can often be treated with oral antibiotics. However, if infection is accompanied by temperature elevation or leuko-

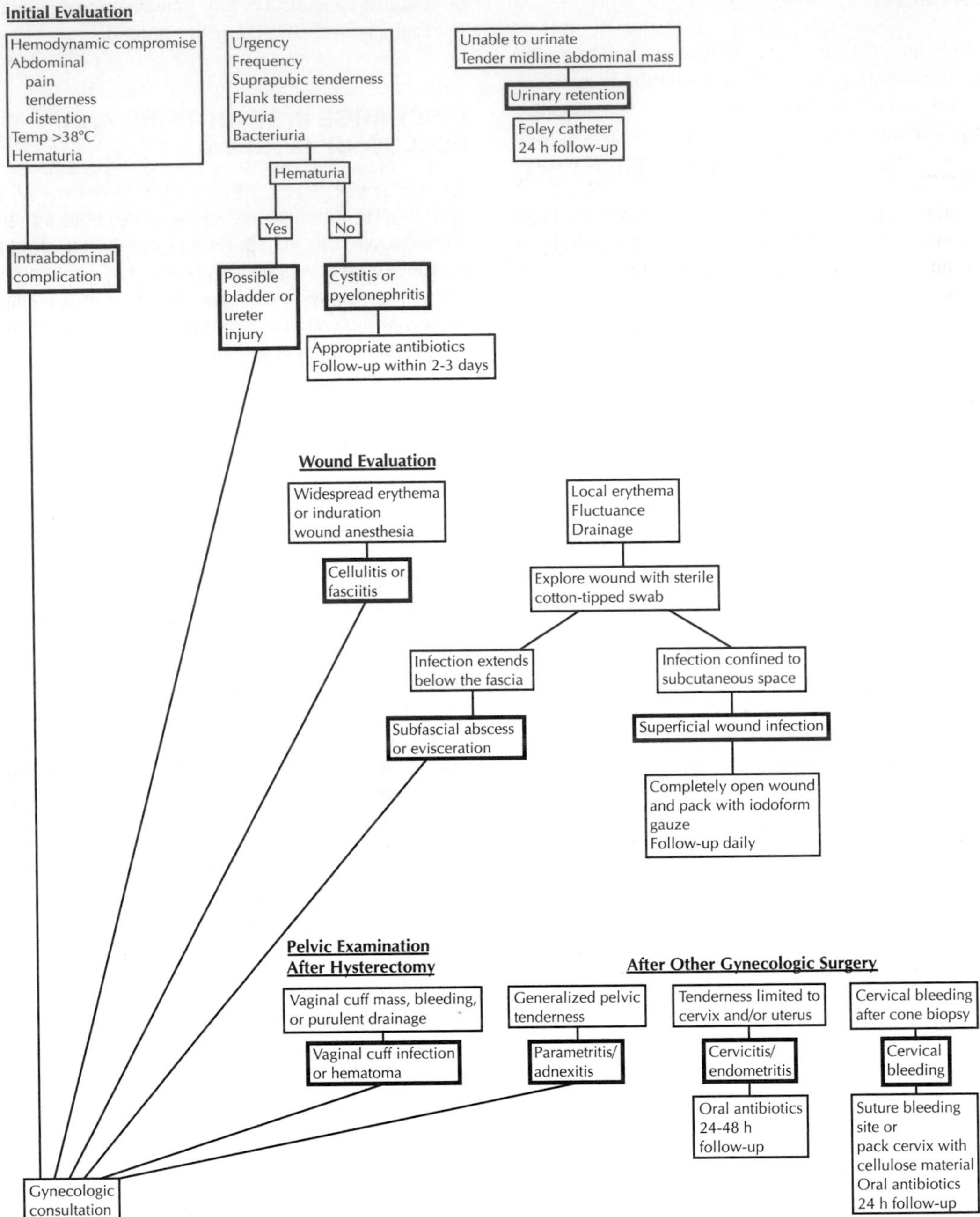

Fig. 32-3. Algorithm for evaluation and treatment of postoperative complications.

cytosis after minor surgery, or in the presence of any sign of infection after hysterectomy, gynecologic consultation is usually required.

PROCEDURES

Exploration and Packing of Infected Wounds

The patient is placed in a supine position and the area of the wound is prepped and draped. A sterile, cotton-tipped applicator is used to gently probe along the incision until the wound is entered. If purulent discharge is encountered, the wound is opened gently along its entire course if possible. The base of the wound is probed for defects in the fascial layer. If none are encountered, the entire wound is copiously irrigated with a solution of half normal saline and half hydrogen peroxide (5 percent solution). After appropriate irrigation, the wound should appear clean and the edges slightly bloody. If the wound is surrounded by necrotic tissue, it should be lightly dressed and the gynecologist called to evaluate the wound for possible surgical debridement. If the wound appears to be surrounded by viable tissue, it should be packed with gauze to the level of the skin. A large dressing is then placed over the packing. The patient is instructed to return for follow-up at frequent intervals until the base of the wound shows signs of granulation.

Evaluation for Bladder Injuries with Indigo Carmine

In the presence of a copious amount of watery discharge after gynecologic surgery from either a suprapubic incision or from the vagina, the possibility of a bladder injury should be investigated by dyeing the urine. One simple technique is to use a balloon catheter to instill a dilute solution of indigo carmine or methylene blue in normal saline (2 mL in 200 mL of normal saline) directly into the bladder. If a gauze pad placed over the wound is dyed blue within 10 to 20 minutes, bladder involvement is verified. For a vaginal discharge after hysterectomy, a tampon can be placed in the vagina and removed after 20 to 30 minutes. A blue stain on the tampon indicates bladder involvement. An alternate approach is to inject 5 mL of indigo carmine intravenously. Methylene blue should not be given intravenously because of the risk of hemolytic anemia associated with this drug.

REFERENCES

1. Harris WJ: Complications of hysterectomy. *Clin Obstet Gynecol* 40:928–938, 1997.
2. Mintz M: Risks and prophylaxis in laparoscopy: A survey of 100,000 cases. *J Reprod Med* 18:269, 1977.
3. Taylor G, Herrick T, Mah M: Wound infections after hysterectomy: opportunities for practice improvement. *Am J Infect Control* 26:254–257, 1998.
4. Frazee RC, Thames T, Appel M, et al: Laparoscopic cholecystectomy: A multicenter study. *J Laparoendosc Surg* 1:157, 1991.
5. Duggan BD, Felix JC, Muderspach LI, et al: Cold-knife conization versus conization by the loop electrosurgical excision procedure: a randomized, prospective study. *Am J Obstet Gynecol* 180:276–282, 1999.
6. File TM Jr, Tan JS: Treatment of skin and soft-tissue infections. *Am J Surg* 169:27S, 1995.

33

Sexual Assault

Ritu Malik
Carolyn Sachs

KEY POINTS

- Advanced physician and emergency department preparation for evaluation and treatment of sexual assault victims will eliminate much of staff members' anxiety and hesitation, and allow them to spend their time and energy making the patient feel more comfortable.
- Treatment of the victim of sexual assault includes referral to counseling and postexposure prophylaxis for pregnancy, STDs, hepatitis B, and HIV.
- Even if a patient does not plan to pursue prosecution at the time of medical evaluation, physicians should encourage a complete forensic examination as a victim may change her mind.
- Sexual assault response teams (SARTs) are multidisciplinary specialty services that assist patients and practitioners with evaluation and treatment.
- It is not the physician's responsibility to decide whether or not a crime has occurred. Physicians are advised to avoid legal conclusions in their documentation because usually it cannot be determined with certainty whether consent for the sexual act was given.

INTRODUCTION

The term *sexual assault* includes several types of forced or inappropriate sexual activity. State laws define sexual assault in various separate statutes. These may include sexual contact with or without penetration with force or coercion,[1] such as rape, oral copulation, sodomy, intercourse with a minor, sexual abuse, and sexual misconduct.[2] Although sexual assault victims can be men, women, or children, this chapter will cover the crime of sexual assault against women.

Sexual assault is very common in the United States and has grave personal consequences for the survivor as well as serious costs to society. The 2001 Uniform Crime Report indicates that 90,186 forcible rapes were reported to law enforcement agencies in the United States in 2000. Though this represents a 6 percent decline since 1996, the rate is still very high. This rate means that yearly 63 of every 100,000 women in the U.S. are the victims of a forcible rape and report the crime to the police.[3] The actual rate of sexual assault is unknown due to underreporting. A recent study from the University of Denver randomly surveyed their emergency department female patients and estimated that fewer than half of sexual assault victims report the assault to the police or seek medical care.[4] Estimates of the number of women who are actually raped range from an additional four to nine victims for every one that reports it.[2]

These violent crimes are underreported in part because of societal misconceptions about the victims regarding provocative clothing and behavior. It is important to understand that sexual assault is a crime of violence and power, and that no behavior of the victim encourages or justifies such an act. Underreporting also occurs because of fear of retaliation and embarrassment.[5] Improving our social climate through education about these misconceptions may increase the reporting of these crimes and the prosecution of perpetrators.

Emergency medical personnel need to be well equipped to handle victims of sexual assault. Preparation will eliminate much of the anxiety and hesitation on the part of medical care personnel and allow them to spend their energy on making the patient feel more comfortable.

Patients may self-refer after an assault or may be brought by law enforcement officials to the ED for evaluation. Some may not present reporting assault, but may have a related physical complaint, such as abdominal pain or vaginal discharge. The emergency physician should be aware of the various presentations of such patients and maintain a high index of suspicion to pursue a more detailed history.

Many emergency health care providers lack formal training in treatment of the sexual assault survivor and have limited experience with such patients. Physicians may be apprehensive about providing care for sexual assault victims because they view these evaluations as time-consuming; others fear the potential need to testify in court. In many areas across the country, sexual assault response teams (SART) have been established with well-trained practitioners, social workers, and counselors to assist with such patients. When available, sexual assault victims preferentially receive evaluation and treatment in these centers. These multidisciplinary specialty centers may even be staffed by mobile personnel who work out of more than one medical center. Coordinating medical care, forensics, and victim advocacy is the expertise of a SANE (sexual assault nurse examiner). These nurses are specifically trained to care for the victim in the acute environment and are usually the individuals who complete the initial examination. Other core members of the team include medical experts, law enforcement officers, patient advocates, prosecutors, and forensic lab personnel.[2] SARTs have the potential to enhance public safety by increasing public awareness, increase reporting, and facilitating investigation.[2] The guiding principle behind SARTs is joining medicine, law enforcement, and victim advocacy in a coordinated effort to ensure that rape survivors receive comprehensive medical attention, evidentiary examinations, emotional support, and referral information.[6]

On occasion, sexual assault victims present themselves or are brought to emergency departments that are not specifically set up to provide these services. In these cases, the role of the emergency physician is to be a patient's advocate, care for her medical needs, gather medicolegal evidence, and facilitate appropriate follow-up. If this is not done properly, there can be adverse long-term emotional, physical, and legal consequences for the patient. Hence the physician evaluation must be done thoroughly and sensitively.

THE MEDICAL EVALUATION

To prepare for such circumstances, it is important for emergency medical personnel to become familiar with the state and local laws regarding reporting sexual assault. In addition, the physician should review the contents of the evidence collection kit, and learn about local support services for sexual assault survivors. Preparation will prevent mistakes and allow for information to be obtained in a standardized fashion. Some jurisdictions provide examination kits and forms to be completed. In other areas, emergency departments must devise their own kit or buy commercially available kits (Table 33-1).

Care for the sexual assault survivor in the ED involves informed consent, a detailed history of the event, past medical history including relevant gynecologic history, physical examination including gynecologic examination, laboratory and radiographic data, notation of the chain of evidence, medical treatment of injuries, prophylaxis for STDs and pregnancy, and coordination of future care.

Table 33-1. Contents of a Sexual Assault Examination Kit

Medical report form
Labeled envelopes for each specimen
Bags for clothing
Blood collecting tubes
Card for dried blood sample
Urine specimen containers
Fingernail file for scraping
Combs for pubic and head hair
Cotton swabs for oral, vaginal, skin, and anal samples
Toluidine dye
Fluid specimen containers for rectal and vaginal washings

Preparation

Before the evaluation is started the patient should be taken to a private, quiet area in the ED to help the patient feel as safe and as comfortable as possible. The patient should be offered an opportunity to call any friends or family to accompany her and support her through the process of evaluation and evidence collection. The entire process should be explained to the victim in detail so that she understands what to expect.

Informed Consent

Consent for medical evaluation, treatment, evidence collection, and photography must be obtained. An informed consent form is often included as the first page of the state evidentiary documentation packets. Each part of the evaluation should be explained to the patient in advance. The patient should be reminded that anytime during the history and exam she can refuse all or any part of the evaluation. She also has the right to have an advocate, friend, or family member present to provide support for all or any part of the history and physical examination. The experience of informed consent should empower the survivor and give her the feeling of ultimate control. During the assault, the patient's power was taken away. Obtaining informed consent is required by law, and is also just the beginning of a long road to recovery. In order to be considered legal the informed consent must be signed and witnessed by a third party.

Occasionally, practitioners may be unsure about a patient's ability to reliably give informed consent. Such a patient's mental capacity should be noted during the initial history and physical examination and should be included in the report. Special attention should be given to describing any mental handicaps, and the appearance of any substances that may be affecting the victim, such as drugs or alcohol.

Reporting of the Crime

Most jurisdictions require reporting of sexual assault crimes to law enforcement. In these areas, the patient should be informed of this law, but should understand that though the physician is required to report the event to the local authorities, the victim is not obligated to speak with law enforcement officials who may attempt to question her.

Whether law enforcement officials have already been notified or if the health care professionals are the first to report the event, the names and identification of the officers involved must be documented as part of the sexual forensic medical report.

History

Questions should be asked to the victim in a nonthreatening, nonaccusatory manner. Patients should feel comfortable and safe enough to recount the entire event. Questions should be open ended to allow the patient to be as descriptive as possible. Very specific details of the event, such as the exact location and precise time line of events should not be documented. These should be avoided because any discrepancies between the history obtained by medical personnel and law enforcement officials may later be used against the victim in court.[7] However, practitioners should document time, date, and location; the use of force (weapons, drugs, or other means of coercion); and whether penetration occurred or was attempted, which body part was penetrated, and what was used for penetration. The position of both the victim and the assailant and the use of any weapons or restraints should be documented. Practitioners need to ask about and document areas that were touched, licked, bitten, or ejaculated on, and any areas that could have physical evidence of the assailant's contact with the victim. It is also important to determine whether the victim may have voluntarily or involuntarily taken mind-altering substances that may have facilitated the act, or if the patient lost consciousness at any time. Any use of contraception by the assailant is important and will suggest to the examiner what sort of physical findings to expect. What the patient did since the assault, such as showering, brushing teeth, douching, urinating, eating, drinking, changing clothes, or engaging in consensual sex must also be noted. This is referred to as the postassault history. The patient's relevant medical and gynecologic history should also be obtained. This includes allergies, medications, and immunizations, relevant past medical history, use of contraceptives, last consensual sexual activity (if less than 72 hours earlier), and menstrual history. It should also include any history of recent anogenital trauma or surgeries. This information should guide the physical examination and provide clues to the examiner of what sort of injuries to look for, what parts of the victim's body need to be more carefully examined, and where samples need to be taken.

Before moving on to the physical examination, the medical examiner should make sure that all the questions needed to complete the legal forms have been asked and documented. Meticulous documentation is important, as medical records may be used as legal evidence during case prosecution.

It is important to remember that it is not the physician's responsibility to decide whether or not a crime has been committed. Physicians should not document conclusions such as "rape" because they can rarely determine whether consent for the sexual act was given. They should use the patient's descriptive words in quotes to detail events and record the physical findings that may allow the legal system to establish perpetrator guilt or innocence.

Table 33-2. Sexual Assault History

Date and time
Patient demographics
Law enforcement officer identification
Physical surroundings
Number, relationship and brief description of assailants
Use of force, trauma, or coercion
Weapons used
Sexual acts performed
Penetration
Ejaculation
Medical history
Gynecologic history
Postassault history

To summarize, the history should include the patient's demographics, the law enforcement officer's identification, the informed consent, and the patient's history. The patient's history must include her relevant medical and gynecologic history, as well as the assault and postassault history (Table 33-2).

Physical Examination of the Sexual Assault Victim

The General Examination

Before the evidence collection examination, all injuries that require acute treatment and stabilization must be addressed. The treatment of any unstable condition should never be delayed for the sake of forensic evidence collection.

The purpose of the examination is to detect and treat any physical injuries, and to collect forensic evidence to aid in the identification and prosecution of the assailant.[8] Even if the patient does not plan to pursue prosecution at the time of the medical evaluation, it is important to complete a thorough examination. A victim may change her mind and decide to proceed with prosecution once the acute emotional shock has passed.[9] Medical practitioners must keep in mind that the victim has just been through a highly traumatic experience, and they should be as patient and understanding as possible while obtaining all the necessary information to complete the examination. Again, completion of every aspect of the forensic examination is extremely important. This is the only opportunity to collect this evidence that may have life-altering consequences to the patient.[2]

Evidence collection may vary based on the time of presentation after the assault has occurred and what the patient has done since the event. Usually any presentation within 72 hours enables a complete examination as detailed below. If a patient presents after 72 hours has passed, or if she has completed specific postassault activities, the examination may be modified based on the likelihood of finding evidence of the assault. The modifications most often pertain to vaginal and skin specimens that may initially have had potential DNA evidence identifying the assailant. If a patient has bathed, for example, the chance that any foreign secretions such as semen will be collectable from the victim's skin and hair is quite remote.

Although the presence of bodily injuries has been shown to correlate positively with successful prosecution, it is important to note that sexual assault may have occurred despite a lack of evidence of injury.[10,11] It is also important to recognize that injuries occur and have been documented in cases of consensual intercourse.[12] It is because of these confusing facts that physicians are not asked to establish legal blame and to restrict their involvement to describing and treating injuries and to the collection of forensic evidence. Having said that, evidence that supports the assertion that force was used in a sexual encounter can aid a victim in court in the event the perpetrator alleges that the act was consensual. This is very important, as recent studies have shown that over 75 percent of all rapes and sexual assaults are committed by persons known to the victim.[13]

The sexual assault evidence collection procedures detailed below are based on guidelines distributed by the American College of Emergency Physicians. The full report may be obtained by contacting the organization via the Internet at www.acep.org.

Collection of physical evidence needs to be completed in a fashion that prevents cross-contamination of evidence, so gloves should be worn at all times, and they should be changed when moving from one part of the body or article of clothing to the next. Clothes often contain valuable DNA evidence.Before the patient is asked to disrobe, a clothed photograph should be taken for identification and to document general appearance.

The patient's general appearance, vital signs, and clothing should be described in detail. If the patient presents immediately after the event before bathing and changing clothes, a sheet is placed on the floor, a large piece of paper is placed on top of it, and the patient should be asked to undress on the paper. Each piece of clothing and any fallen debris should be placed in a separate paper bag. As foreign material or biological evidence is found, each item should be collected and bagged separately, and the location from which it was collected described in detail. All injuries and debris, large and small, should be described in detail, and for each item its size, color, and location should be noted on a body diagram. Special attention should be given to evaluating the back, thighs, breasts, wrists, and ankles. Any areas of bruising, biting, or tenderness should be documented. If any bite marks are present, they should be described in detail including their location, shape, color, and size.[2] Photographs should be taken and the area should be swabbed for possible salivary evidence. Examiners must be careful to use a ruler or other item to indicate scale when photographing bite marks in case a forensic dentist needs to match up a given bite mark to a potential suspect. Moist secretions should be collected on dry swabs and then air dried. Dry secretions and debris should be removed with a moist swab and air dried. These secretions may be better identified by shining an ultraviolet Wood's lamp on the patient's body in a darkened room. Although semen may fluoresce under UV light, many other substances such as urine, cream, and soap also fluoresce. An alternative light source, one that emits a shorter wavelength of light than the Wood's lamp, may provide better detection of semen; however, only crime labs currently have ready access to this type of equipment.

Fingernail scrapings may be helpful for identifying the perpetrator and may be collected by cleaning debris from under the nail with a toothpick or by cutting the nails. Some jurisdictions may require reference samples such as buccal sampling, blood, and hair specimens from the victim. The examiner should learn about such local requirements in advance.

The Genital Examination of the Assaulted Woman

Genital injuries have been reported in 5 to 30 percent of sexual assault victims. Frequently these are minor and may be asymptomatic,[14] but occasionally an injury may require a major intervention.

The External Examination

The examiner should remember that the genital examination of an assault victim is different than the usual pelvic examination. A great deal of attention is given to the examination of the external genitalia. The patient should be placed in the lithotomy position and the surrounding area including the abdomen, thighs, buttocks, anal region, and perineum should be examined. Signs of trauma and stains should be noted. A Wood's lamp may be used again to inspect this area and aid in collecting samples of suspicious matter. Despite the limitations of Wood's lamp detection, most experts recommend collection of Wood's lamp positive secretions.[15] Examiners should label them appropriately for the examination kit, and send them to the lab for definitive forensic analysis. These secretions can be analyzed for seminal fluid components and for DNA analysis. Even when no suspicious areas are noted, two swabs of the external area should be collected and smeared onto glass slides. The slides and the swabs should be dried and stored in an appropriately labeled envelope. This external genital examination should be completed before the speculum examination because of concern that trauma may result from insertion of the vaginal speculum, and such trauma might make the forensic detection of injury more difficult. The most common sites of external injury in these crimes are the posterior fourchette, fossa navicularis, the hymen, and the labia.[16] Special attention should be paid to these regions of the external genitalia. From the time of presentation, delay of examination should be minimized because a shorter period between the assault and the examination is strongly correlated with the degree of injury noted.[17]

Toluidine Blue Dye Staining

Toluidine blue dye may be applied to the external genital and anal area to make more apparent perineal lacerations not normally visible to the naked eye. This agent adheres to the nuclei of deeper dermal cells that may be exposed when the skin is broken by superficial trauma. One small study evaluating the efficacy of toluidine dye in sexual assault examinations showed its use increased detection of posterior fourchette lacerations from 16 to 40 percent in adult rape victims.[18] Although it does not interfere with DNA analysis, the dye may have spermicidal activity, so some recommend that suspected seminal secretions be collected from the perineum before its application.[19] The dye is usually applied carefully with a cotton applicator and the excess is removed with a piece of gauze that has been moistened with lubricating jelly or acetic acid. Many practitioners may prefer to use lubricating jelly as acetic acid will irritate injured skin. After all the excess dye is removed, lacerations should be very obviously visualized in blue (Fig. 33-1). The folds in the perineum should be gently separated with traction and all areas should be thoroughly inspected for injury. Effective separation and traction of the perineal and labial folds is important to ensure adequate visualization of potential injuries. Striations and abrasions stained with the toluidine are consistent with injury and should be photographed and described in detail.[14]

The Internal Examination

Preferably, the speculum examination should be conducted using warm water rather than other lubricating substances. Some lubricants may decrease sperm motility.[16] The vagina should be inspected for signs of trauma such as erythema or lacerations. Next, vaginal specimens should be collected. Secretions in the vaginal vault can be collected with a dry cotton-tipped swab. Some jurisdictions also request collection of vaginal washings. This is done by introducing 3 to 5 mL of normal saline into the vaginal vault and then aspirating this fluid into a catheter-tipped syringe and placing it in a collection vial that is then sealed. A cervical specimen may also be of benefit in a case in which the examination is made more than 24 hours after the event. Immotile sperm have been noted in

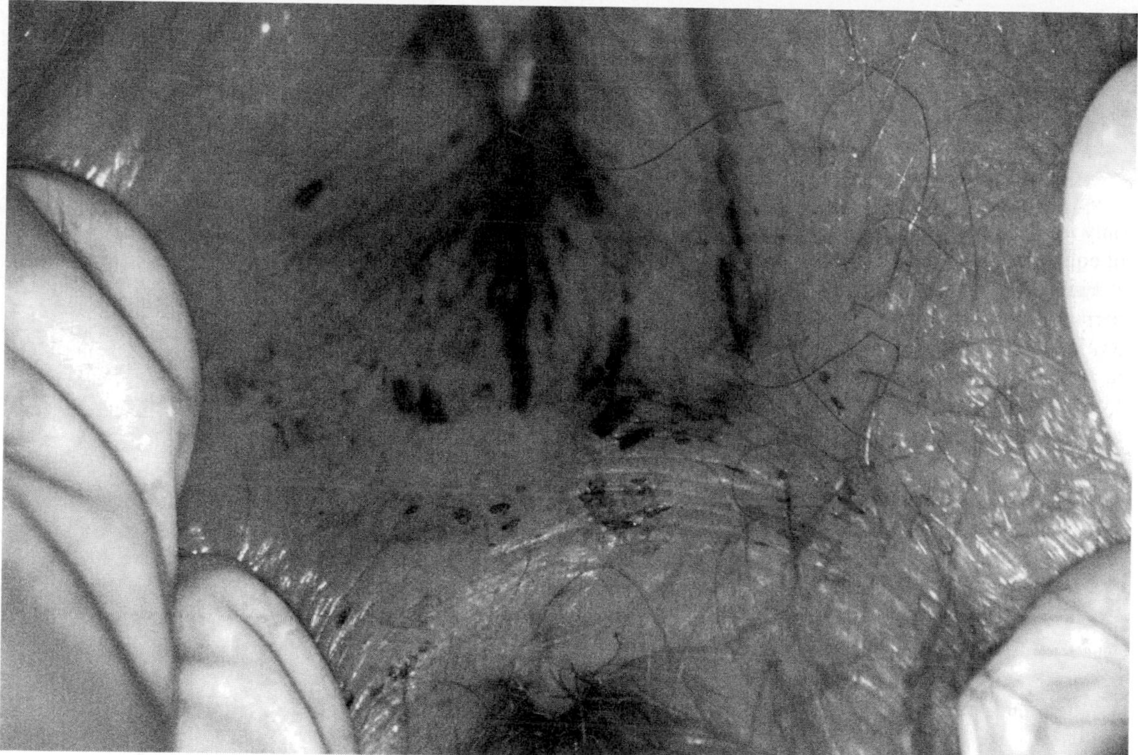

Fig. 33-1. Toluidine blue dye staining of perineal abrasion.

the cervix up to 17 days after coitus and in the vagina for up to 9 days.[20]

Colposcopy

A colposcope is a device used routinely by gynecologists for the detection of cervical lesions. The colposcope provides a magnified view of the vagina and cervix, with excellent lighting. Since its introduction for use in forensic examinations by Teixeira in the early 1980s, colposcopy has become a critical component of the sexual assault examination and has revolutionized documentation of injuries.[21] The addition of colposcopy to routine sexual assault examination has been shown to dramatically improve detection of genital trauma.[22] With a camera attached, photographic documentation can be used to prevent the need for repeat examinations and provide evidence that can be used in court. McGregor and colleagues have showed that prosecution is more likely to be successful with such documentation of trauma and other physical findings.[23]

The Anal Examination

Many patients find it difficult and embarrassing to report anal trauma and/or penetration. This reluctance makes the history of whether it occurred unreliable. In a recent study analyzing over 1000 individual cases of sexual assault, 17 percent of cases involved anal penetration;[24] therefore examiners should routinely examine the anus for signs of trauma. The anal cavity and surrounding area should be swabbed separately and collected routinely. If any evidence of trauma is noted, examiners should also collect rectal washing. Just as in vaginal washings, 5 mL of normal saline can be instilled into the rectal vault, the fluid collected through a plastic catheter connected to a syringe, and the fluid placed in a vial for analysis.

Oral Sample

If oral penetration may have occurred, the oral cavity should be examined carefully. Lacerations and abrasions seen on the palate, buccal mucosa, tongue, and posterior oropharyngeal wall should be documented. Samples from the buccal mucosa should be taken if the patient presents within 12 hours of the assault. Usually, seminal fluid traces are destroyed and undetectable after 12 hours due to the enzymatic action of the saliva in the oral cavity. Sampling of buccal mucosa is done by swabbing the entire oral cavity with two cotton swabs. Samples should include wipes of the buccal gingiva and under the tongue. As with all wet swabs, the samples should be air dried and submitted with the kit. Some jurisdictions may request a separate reference buccal-salivary sample.

Hair Sample

Either the patient or examiner must comb the patient's pubic hair while she is lying on a clean piece of paper to collect any potential hairs from the perpetrator. Any hair removed should fall on the paper, which is then folded closed. The folded paper and the comb are placed into an envelope and submitted as evidence. If the hair is matted because of blood or other secretions, it should be cut and placed in an envelope for analysis. In some cases, the patient should be asked to comb her head hair onto a piece of paper that is then folded and placed in the collection kit. Again, if hair is matted with dried secretions, it should be cut and collected. The comb should also be included in the envelope.[2]

Plucked head hair and pubic hair may be requested in certain jurisdictions to provide a reference sample from the victim. If this is needed, its collection can be delayed and it does not usually need to be done at the time of the initial assault examination. Again, knowledge of the requirements of the local jurisdiction is important.

PHOTOGRAPHS

When possible, the examiner should photographically document all visible bodily and genital injuries. Consent for photography must first be obtained from the victim, and this is usually covered during the initial consent process. Before starting to take photos or video, the victim's name, the date, and examiner's name should be written on a piece of paper and a photo or video should be made of this note to identify the roll of film or videotape. Photos should be taken both from a distance and up close, so the viewer can gain perspective. As mentioned above, photos of injuries should include a ruler or common object placed next to the lesion for scale.[2]

LABORATORY ANALYSIS

Blood and urine samples for toxicology analysis should be collected from patients as soon as possible, often even before the physical examination is done because this is important evidence with a small window of opportunity for collection (as short as 12 hours). Flunitrazepam (Rohypnol®), GHB (gamma hydroxybutyrate), ketamine, benzodiazepines, ethanol, cocaine, methamphetamine, and marijuana are the most common substances associated with date rape.[25] Several of these agents have extremely rapid clearance from the body and are thus ideal choices for an assailant to use to temporarily alter a victim's level of consciousness. For this reason, in cases in which drugs or alcohol may have been used to facilitate the attack, urine should be collected within 72 hours and blood within 13 hours for the best chance of detection of these substances.[26] These blood and urine samples should be sent with the sexual assault examination kit for toxicology and DNA analysis to the forensics lab. The urine collected should also routinely be tested to detect pregnancy to assist in choosing needed postassault medications.

In some areas, a dry blood sample may be requested as a reference sample. This is obtained by pricking the patient's finger with a lancet, milking the digit for blood, and then carefully dropping 1 to 2 drops onto the collection card. There are usually four sites on each card, and each spot must be filled with the blood. A lavender-topped tube containing EDTA is used when a whole blood sample is requested by the crime lab for DNA analysis.

Reference samples are used to differentiate the bodily secretions of the victim from those of the assailant. The crime lab may detect seminal fluid in samples from the body, anus, and vagina; this may provide key data that can assure successful prosecution. Motile and immotile spermatozoa may be noted in these samples, and DNA analysis may allow identification of the assailant. The forensic lab may also utilize testing for prostate acid phosphatase and p30, which are both protein components of seminal fluid. These tests may indicate transfer of seminal fluid from perpetrator to victim, even in cases of an azoospermic perpetrator. The p30 Antigen has become the preferred test in most crime labs because of its greater sensitivity and specificity.[27]

Although recommended in some jurisdictions, many emergency physicians are unfamiliar with the microscopic identification of motile and immotile sperm in wet mounts of vaginal, rectal, and oral samples. If this is the case, the examiner may choose to bypass this step on the forms as it is unlikely to yield any valuable information.

Any miscellaneous items found on the scene or within the patient, such as tampons or condoms, should also be collected separately in paper bags after they are swabbed and the swab's source is appropriately labeled. These items must be packaged in a way that prevents bacterial contamination. It is recommended that examiners dry all wet items before packaging. However, a lack of time may prevent drying of some items (e.g., extremely wet tampons or tissues) and alternative arrangements for preservation (e.g., freezing) must be secured with law enforcement officials.

CHAIN OF EVIDENCE

Before the patient leaves the ED, the medical report should be completed and all the samples should be double checked for proper labeling and placement into envelopes. All the seals should be double checked, and the examiner should initial the sealed envelope over the seal. A list of all the enclosures should be placed in a larger envelope and all the evidence should be placed inside and handed over to law enforcement officials (Table 33-3).

Table 33-3. Contents of Completed Evidence Collection Kit

Clothing
Swabs of dried secretions on skin
Buccal swab
Head hair combing and comb
Pubic hair combing and comb
External genital swab
Vaginal sample swab
Vaginal washings
Vaginal sample slide
Rectal and anal swab
Rectal washing
Fingernail scrapings
Blood specimens for toxicological, DNA, and blood type analysis
Urine specimens for toxicology and pregnancy
Pulled head and pubic hair (optional)
Photographs, including those made colposcopically, those made with toluidine dye, any injuries on the victim, and full-body and close-up photos of the victim
Completed medical report

Another copy of all the enclosures should be saved and made part of the medical record. As evidence is transferred from the initial examiner to the law enforcement officer, and each time the evidence changes hands, each new recipient of the evidence must sign their name and write the date on a list on the outside of the sealed envelope.[2] In this way, a precise record is made of each person who handles the evidence and when they received it. This is known as the *chain of evidence*. Any photographic and videotape evidence must also undergo the same strict documentation of each individual who handles it.

TREATMENT

Any unstable medical conditions should be initially addressed, and then any other injuries sustained should be treated appropriately. Once this is complete, the physician should consider HIV, STD, hepatitis, tetanus, and pregnancy prophylaxis.

Pregnancy Prevention

Pregnancy occurs as a result of sexual assault in 1 percent of all victims.[28] Emergency physicians need to reduce the risk of pregnancy in women who were not adequately protected at the time of the assault.[29] Urine pregnancy tests are sufficient to detect preexisting pregnancy. Emergency contraception (the "morning-after" pill) works by inhibiting ovulation, fertilization, or implantation. Hence it will be ineffective for any patients who were previously pregnant,[30] because it cannot cause abortions in previously implanted pregnancies. For all nonpregnant survivors, postcoital contraception should be routinely offered up to 72 hours after the assault. It has been found that the earlier the treatment is given, the more effective it is,[31] therefore it should be given as soon as practically possible. Levonorgestrel (a synthetic progestogen) 0.75 mg followed with a second dose 12 hours later is the most efficacious hormonal postcoital contraception currently available.[32] Known as Plan B®, this regimen is the first progestin-only FDA-approved emergency contraceptive kit. Other progestin-only medications may be equally effective. Since the early 1970s, combined estrogen-progestin regimens (the Yuzpe method) have been the mainstay of postcoital contraception. The Yuzpe method utilizes widely available combination oral contraceptive pills that include at least 50 mcg of ethinyl estradiol in combination with a progestin, given as two pills by mouth every 12 hours for 2 doses. The progestin-only regimen is slightly more efficacious than the combination regimen and is better tolerated.[33] The main side effects of both regimens include nausea and vomiting, although they occur much less with the progestin-only regimen. If vomiting occurs, antiemetics may be recommended. Some practitioners routinely offer antiemetics to prevent nausea and vomiting; in fact, both the Plan B and Preven® (the Yuzpe regimen in a prepackaged kit) kits include antiemetic medications. Other side effects include lower abdominal pain, fatigue, headache, dizziness, breast tenderness, and menstrual changes. Patients should be advised about these potential side effects to reduce patient anxiety and increase tolerance.

STD Prevention

Following sexual assault, victims are often concerned about possible contraction of sexually transmitted diseases from the assailant.[34]

The most common STDs contracted during a sexual assault are bacterial vaginosis, trichomoniasis, gonorrhea, and chlamydia; less common diseases include syphilis, herpes, and HIV.[33] Most practitioners offer prophylactic antibiotics to prevent STD transmission after sexual assault rather than relying on follow-up cultures. The Centers for Disease Control and Prevention recommends coverage against the most common organisms mentioned above. A single dose of IM ceftriaxone 125 mg will treat gonorrhea and incubating syphilis (but not active syphilis). Oral 4 mg may be given as an oral choice though it is no longer available from the manufacturer at the time of this publication. Additionally, ciprofloxacin 500 mg or ofloxacin 400 mg may be given to treat gonorrhea as a substitute oral choice and in cephalosporin-allergic patients, but these agents have not been shown to have activity against syphilis or resistant gonorrhea. In addition, a one-time dose of azithromycin 1 g orally or doxycycline 100 mg twice a day orally for a week can be used against chlamydia. These two drugs are also thought to have some activity in reducing the likelihood of syphilis.[35] For the prevention of bacterial vaginosis and trichomoniasis, one dose of metronidazole 2 g may be given orally. However, metronidazole does cause significant nausea, vomiting, and diarrhea. Many practitioners choose to forgo this component of the STD treatment as bacterial vaginosis and trichomoniasis rarely cause significant morbidity (Table 33-4).

Table 33-4. Postassault STD Regimens

For gonorrhea
Ceftriaxone 125 mg IM (also covers most incubating syphilis)
or a single dose of ciprofloxacin 500 mg, **or** ofloxacin 400 mg, **or** cefixime 400 mg PO
For chlamydia
Azithromycin 1 g PO
or doxycycline 100 mg, PO bid for 7 days **or** erythromycin 500 mg PO tid for 7 days (if pregnant)
For bacterial vaginosis and trichomoniasis (optional)
Metronidazole 2 g PO (not in pregnancy)
For hepatitis B prophylaxis
HBV vaccine: first of 3 total doses.
If perpetrator is known to be hepatitis B-positive and victim is not immune, add HBIG

Source: Recommendations from the Centers of Disease Control and Prevention.[36]

Hepatitis B Prevention

Patients with a history of hepatitis B vaccination or positive antibody titers are considered protected against hepatitis B. Patients who have not completed a hepatitis B immunization course that are assaulted by an individual with an *unknown* hepatitis B status should be given the first dose of the HBV vaccination series. The second and third doses should be followed at 1 to 2 months and 4 to 6 months, respectively. Individuals assaulted by a *known* hepatitis B-positive person are recommended by the CDC to receive the vaccination series, as well as hepatitis B immune globulin for passive protection.[36] It is important that these patients be reminded of the need for retesting and follow-up at a later date. Further details and recommendations are available on the Internet at www.cdc.gov or by telephone at (888) 448-4911.

HIV Prevention

Although few cases of HIV seroconversion after sexual assault have been documented, the exact risk of transmission is unknown and may vary depending on the nature of the exposure; however, the overall rate of transmission is estimated to be less than 1 to 2 percent.[37] The probability of HIV transmission following a single exposure depends on many variables, including the likelihood that the assailant is infected with HIV, the viral load of the infected person, the route and number of exposures, the body fluids contacted, and the presence of breaks in skin or mucosa.[36] Despite the lack of direct evidence that postexposure prophylaxis (PEP) prevents HIV infection after sexual exposure, it may be reasonable to assume that the risk can be reduced, given the efficacy of treatment

Table 33-5. HIV Exposure Risk Categories

Measurable Risk	Possible Risk	No Risk
Anal penetration	Oral penetration with ejaculation	Kissing
Vaginal penetration	Unknown acts	Digital penetration
Injection with contaminated needle	Contact with other mucous membranes	Ejaculation on intact skin

after occupational exposure.[36] The risks and benefits of PEP must be weighed at the time of counseling the often-distraught patient in the ED. Because we lack definitive evidence that HIV prophylaxis prevents transmission of the virus post-sexual exposure, counseling by different health care workers may be in conflict. In response to the lack of information and uniform counseling standards, the state of California has published guidelines to clarify recommendations for prophylaxis of post-sexual assault patients and to help develop statewide standards. The following recommendations are based on those published for the State of California by Myles and Bamberger of Urban Community Health of the San Francisco Department of Public Health and The California HIV PEP after Sexual Assault Task Force in conjunction with The California State Office of AIDS.[34]

PEP is recommended for appropriate patients who present within the first 72 hours after the assault. Although the best risk reduction of HIV seroconversion for occupational exposures has been shown to occur within the first 4 hours after exposure, it is offered for assault victims presenting up to 72 hours after exposure. For patients who present after 72 hours, HIV testing with pre- and posttest counseling is recommended.

The specific acts of sexual assault should also be taken into consideration when considering PEP. Different acts have been attributed differing risk categories. Acts that are considered to be *measurable risk* include anal and vaginal penetration. Acts with *possible risk* include oral penetration with ejaculation, unknown acts, contact with other mucous membranes, and the victim biting the assailant. Acts that are considered *no risk* include kissing, digital or object penetration, and ejaculation onto intact skin (Table 33-5).

In addition, the assailant's HIV status must be considered. In some cases it is known, but most often it is unknown. Any known or suspected risk factors in the assailant should also be considered in cases of an assailant of unknown HIV status.

The decision of whether to offer PEP to the survivor should take into consideration all of the above factors, in addition to other extenuating circumstances that may not have been mentioned. If the decision is made to either offer or recommend prophylaxis, the medical provider should explain the possible benefits and side effects of the medications, in addition to explaining the lack of definitive data on the efficacy of these medications in preventing HIV transmission. When a survivor is unable to make a decision, the provider should encourage the initiation of the medications, as the survivor may later choose to discontinue them at any time.

If the decision is made to treat, zidovudine 300 mg and lamivudine 150 mg taken in a combination pill (Combivir®) twice a day is a logical choice. In cases in which an assailant is known to be HIV-negative no PEP should be offered. Finally, in cases in which the assailant is known to be HIV positive, a specialist should be consulted to determine the best regimen.

These medications are known to cause various side effects that may be difficult to tolerate, including nausea, vomiting, and diarrhea. Patients should be counseled about what to expect and should also be advised on the most common presentation of primary HIV infection such as fever, fatigue, sore throat, rash, and lymphadenopathy.

FOLLOW-UP

After the examination, evidence collection, and treatment are complete, the patient should be advised regarding the necessity for follow-up and psychological counseling, and be given a list of community resources that offer further help. Initially, all sexual assault survivors should receive medical follow-up at 1 to 2 weeks. Longer-term follow-up should include HIV antibody testing, other indicated serologic testing (i.e., hepatitis B, hepatitis C, VDRL), and the remaining hepatitis vaccinations when indicated.

Ideally, all victims should have advocate services offered at the time of initial contact with the health care professional. In fact, some SARTs prefer to have the advocate be the first person to greet a victim at the ED. After the examination, survivors should be referred to local rape crisis centers for follow-up counseling in 1 to 2 days. This criminal act has serious life-altering effects on the victims, and patients often choose to isolate themselves. Depression and posttraumatic stress disorder are frequent sequelae. The goal of immediate advocate counseling is to decrease the long-term effects of the assault on the health and well-being of survivors.[38]

REFERENCES

1. American Academy of Pediatrics, Committee on Adolescence: Sexual assault and the adolescent. *Pediatrics* 107:761–765, 2001.
2. American College of Emergency Physicians: *Evaluation and Management of the Sexually Assaulted or Sexually Abused Patient*. Produced by ACEP under contract with the U.S. Department of Health and Human Services, 1999. (Copies are available from ACEP by calling 1-800-798-1822.)
3. U.S. Department of Justice, Federal Bureau of Investigation: *Crime in the United States, 2000*. Washington, DC: FBI National Press Office, 2001.
4. Feldhaus KM, Houry D, Kaminsky R: Lifetime sexual assault prevalence rates and reporting practices in an emergency department population. *Ann Emerg Med* 36:23–27, 2001.
5. Braen GR: Examination of the sexual assault victim, in Roberts JR, Hedges JR (eds): *Clinical Procedures in Emergency Medicine,* 3d ed. Philadelphia: WB Saunders, 1998, p 1022.
6. Voelker R: Experts hope team approach will improve the quality of rape exams. *JAMA* 275:973–974, 1996.
7. Young WW, Bracken AC, Goddard MA, et al: Sexual assault: Review of a national model protocol for forensic and medical evaluation, *Obstet Gynecol* 80:878, 1992.
8. Gold CR: Sexual assault, in Rosen R, Barkin R (eds.): *Emergency Medicine Concepts and Clinical Practice*, 4th ed. St. Louis: Mosby, 1998, p 2321.
9. Dunn SF, Gilchrist VJ: Sexual assault. *Primary Care* 20:359–373, 1993.
10. Gray-Eurom K, Seaberg DC, Wears RL: The prosecution of sexual assault cases: correlation with forensic evidence. *Ann Emerg Med* 39:39–46, 2002.
11. Bowyer L, Dalton ME: Female victims of rape and their genital injuries. *Br J Obstet Gynaecol* 104:617–620, 1997.
12. Norvell MK, Benrubi GI, Thompson RJ: Investigation of microtrauma after sexual intercourse. *J Reproduct Med* 29:269–271, 1984.
13. Bachman RB, Saltzman LE: Bureau of Justice Statistics Special Report, National Crime Victimization Survey, Violence against women: Estimates from the redesigned survey. US Department of Justice, 1995, NC 154348, p 6.
14. Geist RF: Sexually related trauma. *Emerg Med Clin North Am* 6:439–466, 1988.
15. Santucci KA, Nelson DG, McQuillen KK, et al: Wood's lamp utility in the identification of semen. *Pediatrics* 104, 1342–1344, 1999.
16. Slaughter L, Brown CV, Crowley S, et al: Patterns of genital injury in female assault victims. *Am J Obstet Gynecol* 176:609–616, 1997.
17. Adams JA, Giardin B, Faugno D: Adolescent sexual assault: documentation of acute injuries using photo-colposcopy. *J Pediatr Adolesc Med* 150:850–857, 1996.
18. Hochmeister MN, Whelan M, Borer UV, et al: Effects of toluidine blue and destaining reagents used in sexual assault examinations on the ability to obtain DNA profiles from post coital vaginal swabs. *J Forensic Sci* 42:316–319, 1997.
19. McCauley J, Guzinski G, Welch R, et al: Toluidine blue in the corroboration of rape in the adult victim. *Am J Emerg Med* 5:105–108, 1987.
20. Davies A, Wilson E: The persistence of seminal constituents in the human vagina. *Forensic Sci* 3:45–55, 1974.
21. Teixeira WR: Hymenal colposcopic examination in sexual offenses. *Am J Forensic Med Pathol* 2:209–215, 1981.
22. Lenahan LC, Ernst A, Johnson B: Colposcopy in evaluation of the adult sexual assault victim. *Am J Emerg Med* 16: 183–184, 1998.
23. McGregor MJ, Du Mont J, Myhr TL: Sexual assault forensic medical examination: is evidence related to successful prosecution? *Ann Emerg Med* 39:639–647, 2002.
24. Riggs N, Houry D, Long G, et al: Analysis of 1076 cases of sexual assault. *Ann Emerg Med* 35:358–362, 2000.
25. Slaughter L: Involvement of drugs in sexual assault. *J Reprod Med* 45:425–430, 2000.
26. Le Beau M, Andollo W, Hearn WL, et al: Recommendations for toxicological investigations of drug-facilitated sexual assaults. *J Forensic Sci* 44:227–230, 1999.
27. Graves HC, Sensabaugh GF, Blake ET: Postcoital detection of a male specific protein. Application to the investigation of rape. *N Engl J Med* 312:338–343, 1985.
28. Blackmoore CA, Keegan RA, Cates W: Diagnosis and treatment of sexually transmitted diseases in rape victims. *Rev Infect Dis* 4(Suppl):S877–S882, 1982.
29. Atabaki S, Paradise JE: The medical evaluation of the sexually abused child: Lessons from a decade of research. *Pediatrics* 104:178–186, 1999.
30. Glasier A: Emergency post coital contraception. *N Engl J Med* 337:1058–1079, 1997.
31. Trussell J, Rodriguez G, Ellerston G: Updated estimates of the effectiveness of the Yuzpe regimen of emergency contraception. *Contraception* 59:147–151, 1999.
32. Task Force on Postovulatory Methods of Fertility Regulation: Randomized controlled trial of levonorgestrel versus the Yuzpe regimen of combined oral contraceptives for emergency contraception. *Lancet* 352:428–433, 1998.
33. Hooton TM, Bowers A, Copass MK, et al: Sexually transmitted diseases in victims of rape. *N Engl J Med* 322: 713–716, 1990.
34. Myles JE, Bamberger J: Urban Community Health of the San Francisco Department of Public Health and The

California HIV PEP after Sexual Assault Task Force in conjunction with The California State Office of AIDS, Offering HIV Prophylaxis Following Sexual Assault: Recommendations for the State of California, August 2000.

35. Moran GJ: Pharmacologic management of HIV/STD exposure. *Emerg Med Clin North Am* 18:829–842, 2000.
36. Centers for Disease Control and Prevention: 1998 Guidelines for treatment of sexually transmitted diseases. *MMWR Morb Mortal Wkly Rep* 47:RR-1, 1998.
37. Gostin LO, Lazzarini Z, Alexander D, et al: HIV testing, counseling, and prophylaxis after sexual assault. *JAMA* 271:1436–1444, 1994.
38. Linden JA: Sexual assault. *Emerg Med Clin North Am* 17:685–697, 1999.

34

Intimate Partner Violence

Deirdre Anglin
Connie Mitchell

KEY POINTS

- Due to the varied presentations of patients victimized by intimate partner violence (IPV) in the health care setting, it is recommended that at a minimum, all adult and adolescent female patients be routinely screened for IPV at all ED visits.
- The evaluation and management of a patient who may be the victim of a crime requires additional attention to the forensic needs of the patient.
- IPV is a complex problem that will require a multidisciplinary approach to intervention in the ED, the health care institution, and the community.
- Health care providers need to recognize their liability if the health and safety needs of the patient who is a victim of IPV are not addressed.
- Health care providers should be aware of IPV screening and reporting requirements in the state in which they practice.
- Adult Maltreatment Syndrome is the ICD-9 diagnosis that should be used for adult patients who have been abused or neglected by another person.

INTRODUCTION

Since the early 1970s, intimate partner violence (IPV) has been recognized as a serious multifaceted issue that interfaces the social service and criminal justice systems. Now, it is also recognized as a significant health care issue and a serious and recurrent public health problem. Therefore, emergency health care providers need to become comfortable and competent in addressing the health and safety issues of IPV patients so their care is not overlooked in the demanding practice of emergency medicine.

Victims of IPV frequently present to the emergency department (ED) to access health care services. Therefore it is imperative that health care providers, in particular those in emergency services, be able to identify these patients so they may intervene on their behalf. At least 85 percent of victims of IPV are females, with the overwhelming majority abused by male partners.[1] According to the National Crime Victimization Survey, only about half the victims of IPV assaults report the violence to law enforcement officials.[2] As many as 43 percent of victims of IPV seek assistance for the abuse primarily from health care providers.[3] Approximately 75 percent of women who are first identified in the health care setting as being victims of IPV go on to suffer repeated abuse.[4] Two studies revealed that as many as 43 percent of female IPV homicide victims were seen in an ED within the 2 years prior to being killed.[5,6] Victims of IPV have been documented to have increased health care utilization,[7] and they report poorer health status compared to those who are not victims of IPV.[7] They also have increased health care costs.[8] It has been estimated that IPV has an annual medical and societal cost of $67 billion in the United States.[9]

DEFINITION

Intimate partner violence is defined by the Centers for Disease Control and Prevention (CDC) as the threat or infliction of physical or sexual abuse by adults or adolescents against their intimate partners. The physical abuse is frequently associated with psychological abuse.[10] It is a pattern of assaultive and coercive behaviors (Table 34-1).

The definition of intimate partner violence that is used in state penal codes may vary from that of the CDC in terms of the relationship between the two individuals and the type(s) of abuse that has occurred.

Many terms have been previously used to refer to intimate partner violence. These have included: domestic violence, spouse abuse, battered woman, wife beating, battering, and wife abuse. However, the term *intimate partner violence* is more inclusive, and applies equally to adolescents or adults, same- or opposite-sex intimate partners, current or previous intimate partners, and intimate partners who have and have not been married.

EPIDEMIOLOGY

Numerous studies have been conducted in the ED to determine the prevalence of IPV among ED patients. There

Table 34-1. Patterns of Abuse in Intimate Partner Violence.

Physical abuse	Hitting, slapping, pushing, punching, kicking, beating, biting, strangulation, burning, involving the use of weapons or household objects; controlling access to medications and health care
Sexual abuse	Forced sex, coerced sex by manipulation or threat, sexual assault with violence, refusing to use condoms (in association with sexually transmitted disease or HIV disease)
Psychological abuse	Threats of violence against the victim or others; intimidation, humiliation, degradation, isolation, attacks against pets or property, stalking; controlling the victim's access to food, clothing, shelter, transportation, money, medications and health care; controlling the victim's activities.

is some difficulty in comparing the results due to differences among the studies in the definitions of IPV used, the types of abuse measured, the population studied (i.e., gender, age), and the ED setting (i.e., trauma center, inner city ED, community hospital ED). In addition, there is no gold standard test for the identification of IPV among ED patients.

The results of the ED-based studies are reported as the incidence of acute abuse, 1-year prevalence, and lifetime prevalence. Summarizing several ED-based studies, 1 to 7 percent of all adult and adolescent females who presented to the ED did so due to an acute episode of physical abuse.[11–14] Further, of all female patients who presented to the ED, 14 to 22 percent had experienced IPV during the previous year,[13,15] and up to 54 percent had experienced IPV sometime during their lifetime (lifetime prevalence).[16]

Few studies have been conducted on the incidence and prevalence of IPV among males who present to the ED. Those that have been done did not assess for the severity of injury (i.e., defensive injuries such as scratches), or determine who was the primary aggressor in the relationship (i.e., perpetrator).[17] It appears that the prevalence of IPV in same-sex couples may be 25 to 33 percent,[18] although in some studies of lesbian couples, the violence was actually perpetrated by a former male intimate partner.[19]

Results of studies of IPV among pregnant women have shown that they are at increased risk for IPV. In a meta-analysis of 13 studies of pregnancy and IPV, it was found that between 1 and 20 percent of patients had experienced IPV during their pregnancy.[20] The higher prevalence of abuse during pregnancy was detected with verbal questioning, questioning later during the pregnancy, and questioning on multiple visits. In addition, up to one-quarter of patients had experienced IPV during the previous year, and the lifetime prevalence was as high as 30 percent.[20] Homicide was found to be the leading cause of maternal mortality in one study.[21]

There are other populations who frequently seek medical care in the ED who are often victims of IPV. Women who attempt suicide are frequently victims of IPV. Among all women who attempted suicide, 29 percent were victims of IPV, and in one study of African-American women who had attempted suicide, 50 percent were victims of IPV.[22,23] Further, Abbott and colleagues found that 81 percent of female patients with a history of suicide attempts also had a history of IPV.[16] IPV is also prevalent among HIV-positive women. Between 67 and 83 percent of HIV-positive female patients in one clinic had been in abusive relationships with men who had refused to use condoms.[24] Between one- and two-thirds of homelessness of women is attributed to IPV.[25,26] Abbott and associates found that 71 percent of women with a positive screen for alcoholism also had a history of IPV.[16]

Homicide victims may also be transported to the ED. The relationship of the perpetrator to the victim is sometimes unknown at the time the patient is transported to the ED, and in some cases is never known. However, 30 percent or more of adult female homicide victims are murdered by their current or former intimate partner.[27] Homicide is the most common cause of death in the workplace for women.[28]

IPV is underreported by patients for several reasons, including fear of the abuser; economic dependency; poor self esteem; fear of losing the children; fear of the health care provider's response; cultural and religious reasons; and at times, fear of being deported.[29] IPV is underrecognized by health care providers for reasons that include lack of understanding of the populations at risk and prevalence of IPV; fear of opening Pandora's box (fear of problems for the health care provider instigated by reporting or pursuing claims of IPV); fear that it will take too much time; belief that IPV is not a medical issue; belief that IPV is a private matter; conservative attitudes; and lack of knowledge of how to intervene with patients victimized by IPV.[30]

DYNAMICS OF INTIMATE PARTNER VIOLENCE

In order to understand the perspective of patients who are victims of IPV, it is necessary for health care providers to understand the complexities of abusive intimate relationships. Several theories have been postulated to explain the dynamics of abusive intimate relationships, such as biologic-based theories, family-centered theories, or sociocultural models. Multidimensional theories arose out of the inability of any single theory to explain the dynamics of IPV. The Social Ecology Model,[31] an example of a multidimensional theory, takes into account the multidisciplinary nature of IPV. The Social Ecology Model identifies numerous factors in an individual's life that may singly or in combination precipitate IPV. These factors include personal history (e.g., persons impacted as a child by IPV); family dynamics (e.g., male dominance, marital conflict, alcohol and drug abuse); community structure (e.g., socioeconomic status, isolation); and cultural values and beliefs (e.g., male entitlement, acceptance of interpersonal violence).

Partner violence may have different patterns of interaction that can be identified in the abusive relationship. Researchers have proposed three patterns: (1) a pattern of increasing control; (2) a cycle of violence; and (3) a pattern of escalating mutual attacks.[32]

For some couples, the need for power and control in the relationship can lead to violence. Higher levels of dominance (i.e., the need for one person to dominate another within a couple) have been associated with higher levels of violence. Other studies have shown that men who had more aggressive or assaultive-type behaviors also demonstrated higher needs for power than nonassaultive men.[33,34] The Power and Control Wheel was also developed to help understand abusive, violent relationships.[35] It describes abusive behaviors frequently used by perpetrators to exert power and control over their intimate partners. The clinician who cares for a victim of partner violence may need to identify multiple ways in which the patient is victimized and subjugated to her partner's need for power and control.

The Cycle of Violence was first described by Lenore Walker in 1979, and has been used to describe the sometimes cyclical nature of IPV.[36,37] The cycle consists of 3 phases: a tension-building phase; a violent episode; and a reconciliation phase. A violent assault is followed by a period of remorse and a return to hopefulness that it will not occur again. A violence-free period ensues and may even predominate for a significant period of time. Gradually, tensions and stressors within the relationship escalate, culminating in another act or threat of violence. This pattern of abuse may gradually escalate in frequency and intensity or remain stable and intermittent for a long period of time. The periods of calm and hopefulness may become shorter and less influential, and the violence may become more deliberate, dangerous, and premeditated. The health care practitioner may see the victim in the ED during the recovery phase, and without an understanding of the cycle of violence, may wonder how the victim can deny abuse and return again and again to the dangerous environment.

A common dynamic in many relationships with a high degree of conflict is that the couple is unable to communicate or negotiate in rational, nonjudgmental ways. In 1995, Johnson[38] described a type of "couple violence," in which there is less severe violence than in the pattern of increasing control. During verbal arguments partners attack each other "in ways that diminish self-esteem, create feelings of vulnerability, and activate fears of rejection and abandonment."[38] Either partner may escalate the attacks until one partner feels so vulnerable that he or she reacts violently. The pattern of escalating mutual attacks is believed to have less severe consequences, in terms of physical and psychological injury, than the pattern of increasing control. However, it is still abuse even though there is reciprocity of assaults between partners.

During the assessment phase of partner abuse, the provider may need to ask about the victim's own violent acts and attempt to characterize those acts as primary, retaliatory, or defensive. Regardless of reciprocity, women are six times more likely than men to require medical attention for injuries sustained in family violence.[39] In addition, criminal justice reports indicate that 93 percent of female assault victims have a male perpetrator.[40]

There are many associated conditions that coexist with IPV, and these must be differentiated from actual causes. Some may allege that IPV is due to batterers having anger management problems, or to the fact that they are abusing alcohol or illegal drugs. While IPV perpetrators often have a history of other violent criminality, anger does not appear to be the precipitating cause of most IPV.[41] Further, though alcohol and drugs may lower the threshold at which violence occurs, they have not been shown to cause IPV. Studies have shown, however, that alcohol and drug use by the perpetrator is frequently associated with physical IPV assaults.[42] Alcohol and drug abuse are commonly viewed by the perpetrator as an excuse, while by the victim they are viewed as a reason or cause of a physical assault.

Children Impacted by Intimate Partner Violence

There is a large overlap of IPV and child abuse, with 30 to 60 percent of abused women reporting that their children had also been abused.[43] Children who live in homes where there is ongoing IPV may be physically abused, neglected, endangered, or impacted as witnesses to violence. While children are more likely to be physically abused by the batterer, studies have shown that at times the abused parent may also abuse the children.[44–47] Children may be endangered during the course of a violent assault, either if they get caught in the crossfire, or if they attempt to intervene on behalf of their mother.[48] Even children who are not directly abused or neglected can suffer serious sequelae as a result of witnessing IPV (Table 34-2).[49]

Table 34-2. Behaviors of Children Who Witness Intimate Partner Violence

Infants	Crying and irritability Sleep disturbances Digestive problems
Toddlers/preschool	More aggressive or more withdrawn than other children Impaired cognitive abilities Delays in verbal or motor development Sleep disturbances Delays in bowel or bladder control
School-age	Declining academic performance Poor social skills Low self-esteem Increased aggressiveness Digestive problems Headaches
Adolescents/teens	Declining academic performance Low self-esteem Isolation from friends or family Running away Violent behavior or vandalism Digestive problems Headaches

While screening children and adolescents for violence and abuse is recommended, interventions must be designed to provide for the health and safety of adult and child victims of abuse. The American Academy of Pediatrics Committee on Child Abuse and Neglect recognizes that intervention on behalf of battered women is an active form of child abuse prevention.[50] It is the responsibility of the emergency department personnel to assess the well-being of children or other dependents of their adult IPV victims and to assess the well-being and safety of mothers of children whom they suspect have been abused.[51]

Teen Dating Violence

Teen dating violence is more complicated than adult IPV because teens are so immersed in developmental tasks, they are often more vulnerable to abuse, and are less able to seek help. Teens need to work though issues of intimacy and independence, and when their dating relationships are hurtful, they experience a "double whammy" of having been hurt and perceiving failure to complete a developmental step.[32]

Teen physical dating violence was reported in 8.8 percent of high school students, with 12.5 percent of females and 5.2 percent of males reporting forced intercourse by a date.[52] About 38 percent of eighth- and ninth-grade boys and 34 percent of girls reported being a victim of physical dating violence. Surprisingly, 27 percent of girls and 13 percent of boys admitted to perpetrating physical violence, although other studies indicate girls have lower thresholds for defining violent acts than boys do.[53]

Females reporting dating violence are more likely than those who did not to have attempted suicide, engaged in high HIV-risk behaviors, been pregnant, experienced forced sex, and have ridden in a car with a drunk driver. Males reporting dating violence are more likely to have a same gender sex partner, to have experienced forced sex, and to have been threatened with further physical violence.[54] Dating violence against adolescent girls is associated with an increased risk of substance abuse, unhealthy weight control behaviors, sexual risk behaviors, pregnancy, and suicidality.[55] Pregnant adolescents who have been assaulted by an intimate partner appear to have significantly more exposures to other forms of violence than non-IPV pregnant adolescents.[56]

Without a doubt, because of the prevalence of IPV, emergency physicians and nurses are treating injuries and illnesses in teens without identifying the primary cause as abuse by someone close to that teenager.

IDENTIFICATION

Over the past decade, there has been increasing pressure for health care providers to identify IPV among patients in the ED. Since victims of IPV frequently present to the ED for medical care, emergency physicians are ideally suited to take the lead in identification of these patients. There are two clinical approaches to identifying IPV among patients: screening and pattern recognition.[57]

Screening

Screening is the process of inquiry (verbal or written) about a specific history of abuse. In the ED, the clinical goal is to identify patients who have presented for acute injuries or illnesses related to abuse, as well as those patients who are not suffering from an acute episode of abuse, but are in abusive or violent intimate relationships, so they may be referred for appropriate interventions. Numerous professional health care organizations, including the American Medical Association,[4] the American College of Emergency Physicians,[58] American College of Obstetricians and Gynecologists,[59] American Academy of Family Practice,[60] American Academy of Nurse Practitioners,[61] and the Emergency Nurses Association,[62] have officially supported routine screening of patients for IPV. Research has shown that victims of IPV have stated they believe that health care providers should ask their patients about IPV. In one study, 78 percent of patients favored universal inquiry about physical abuse and 65 percent of patients favored universal inquiry about sexual assault.[63] In addition, women have reported feeling comfortable about being asked about IPV by health care providers.[63] Screening has been hypothesized by experts as being the best way to begin to validate and assist victims of IPV. However, more research is needed to confirm whether this is actually true.

Most screening research has been conducted in populations of adult or adolescent females. Further research is needed about how to safely and effectively screen children and men. The American Medical Association has recommended that all female patients be routinely screened for IPV by all health care providers.[4] Some health care providers advocate screening a subgroup of patients (i.e., patients with injuries). However, due to the varied presentations of patients in the health care setting who are victimized by IPV, it is recommended that at a minimum, all adult and adolescent female patients be routinely screened for IPV at all ED visits.

Screening may be carried out using a verbal screen, a written questionnaire, or a computer-based questionnaire.[64] Patients may feel more comfortable responding to verbal questions, resulting in a higher positive response. If written questions are to be used, it is important that assistance be available for patients who are unable to read or need translation.

There are a number of verbal screening tools available. However, for use in the ED it is important that the screening tool be brief. The Partner Violence Screen (Table 34-3), which consists of 3 questions, was tested among female ED patients.[11] If the Partner Violence Screen were to be used, it would be advisable to add two additional questions concerning sexual abuse and strangulation, as this tool does not specifically address these forms of abuse. Patients are often reticent to talk about sexual abuse voluntarily. Yet 33 to 46 percent of women who are physically abused by their partners are also sexually abused by them.[65] In addition, IPV patients often do not realize the clinical or legal significance of strangulation, therefore a specific question about strangulation may be helpful.[66] When questioning patients about strangulation, the term "choked" should be used as it is likely to be better understood by patients. The Abuse Assessment Screen (Table 34-3), which consists of 4 questions (5 for pregnant patients), was validated among pregnant non-ED patients.[67] As this screening tool does not address strangulation either, an additional question could be asked to make a more comprehensive screen.

It is suggested that prior to screening patients for IPV, a framing statement be used, such as "I ask all my female patients these questions routinely." This may make the patient as well as the health care provider more comfortable when screening for IPV as the question appears routine and nonprejudicial in its administration. When asking a woman questions about her intimate partner, be sure to use all-inclusive phrases such as "boyfriend, husband, or partner," in the event that she has a partner of the same sex. Screening questions should be asked in a nonjudgmental manner. Prior to being screened, patients should be informed of the limits of confidentiality if the health care provider has a legal responsibility to report abuse if it is disclosed.

When screening patients for IPV, screening should be carried out in as private a location as possible. Relatives or friends at the bedside can bias a response. Likewise, patients should be provided with a safe private location to complete written health questionnaires. At times, the patient's partner may be reluctant to leave the examination room, such as in the case of a controlling batterer. In these cases the health care provider may have to be creative, and find an opportunity to question the patient in private, such as after escorting the patient to radiology without their partner. If a translator is required to assist in screening

Table 34-3. Screening Tools for the Identification of Intimate Partner Violence among Female Patients

Partner Violence Screen

1. Have you been hit, kicked, punched or otherwise hurt by someone within the past year? If so, by whom?
2. Do you feel safe in your current relationship?
3. Is there a partner from a previous relationship who is making you feel unsafe now?

Abuse Assessment Screen

1. Have you ever been emotionally or physically abused by your partner or someone important to you?
   Yes No
2. Within the last year, have you been hit, slapped, kicked, or otherwise physically hurt by someone?
   Yes No
   If yes, by whom? (circle all that apply)
   Husband Ex-husband Boyfriend Ex-boyfriend Partner Stranger Other
   How many times? ———
   Mark the area of injury on the body map.
   Score the most severe incident according to the following scale:
   1 = Threats of abuse, including use of weapon
   2 = Slapping, pushing; no injuries but lasting pain
   3 = Punching, kicking, bruises, cuts or continuing pain
   4 = Heat up, severe contusions, burns, broken bones
   5 = Head, internal or permanent injury
   6 = Use of weapon; wound from weapon
3. Within the last year has anyone forced you to have sexual activites? Yes No
   If yes, by whom?
   Husband Ex-husband Boyfriend Ex-boyfriend Partner Stranger Other
   How many times? ———
4. Are you afraid of your partner or anyone listed above? Yes No

Source: From Feldhaus et al[11] and Soeleen et al.[67]

patients, someone other than a friend, family member, child, or the potential batterer should translate.

Although screening is being described here as a process of identification, it is also a form of prevention. Screening is a form of primary prevention, in that it may increase awareness about the health risks of IPV among women who have never been abused. Screening may function as secondary prevention among women currently in abusive relationships presenting to the ED for reasons other than acute abuse. Identification of these patients as victims of IPV and making the appropriate referrals and interventions will help prevent further episodes of violence. Lastly, screening for IPV may be a form of tertiary prevention by identifying women who are suffering the consequences and complications of IPV, by enabling them to be referred to health care and mental health resources and interventions, thereby assisting them to recover from the abuse. Talking about abuse with patients may provide them with validation. Research indicates that this may help victims.[23]

Pattern Recognition

Pattern recognition refers to a cognitive process of sorting historical clues, physical findings, and patient presentations into a diagnosis, based on the research of clinical findings for that particular health problem. IPV research also suggests some diagnostic patterns the health care provider should recognize.

Medical History

When obtaining a medical history from a patient, the health care provider should be alert to responses that may be indicative of IPV (Table 34-4). If IPV is suspected, the patient should be questioned further regarding the possibility of abuse. If a history of abuse is obtained, further details should be elicited. In addition, the patient should be questioned about their past medical history, use of alcohol or illegal drugs, and the availability of a firearm to the batterer.

Table 34-4. Factors in the Medical History that May Be Indicative of Intimate Partner Violence

Changing history
A history that is inconsistent with the injuries
A delay in seeking medical care
Previous injuries
Frequent visits to the ED
"Accident prone" or "clumsy"
Alcohol or substance abuse
Noncompliance with medications or medical appointments
Use of alcohol or illegal drugs

Physical Examination

The physical examination may reveal inconsistencies with the history or physical findings, suggestive of IPV (Table 34-5). Most patients do not seek medical care for IPV injuries. However, injuries due to IPV may be detected in the course of the physical examination for other complaints.

Injuries of the head, face, and neck are the most commonly seen injuries in IPV and should prompt further inquiry as to the nature of the precipitating event.[68] These injuries include contusions and fractures, as well as ocular, ear, and dental trauma. Specific types of injuries commonly seen as a result of IPV assaults should alert the health care provider to the possibility of IPV as the underlying etiology (Table 34-6). Injuries should be assessed in a systematic manner, assessing each one for the presence or absence of tenderness, swelling, evidence of healing, and coloration. These characteristics may assist in determining the timing of the injury. Health care providers should avoid documenting specific ages of injuries based on coloration, as it is not possible to determine the exact age of an ecchymosis based on its color. The location of each injury and whether or not it is a patterned injury should also be noted.

Table 34-5. Physical Examination Findings That May Be Indicative of Intimate Partner Violence

Multiple injuries
Injuries in different stages of healing
Multiple contusions of different ages
Injuries to the head, face, and neck
Bilateral injuries
Central injuries
Injuries that are not consistent with stated mechanism of injury
Defensive injuries (i.e., nightstick fracture of the ulna)
Bite marks
Patterned injuries
Genital injuries
Stab wounds or gunshot wounds

Table 34-6. Common Injuries in Intimate Partner Violence

Head, face and neck
Facial contusions
Facial fractures
Facial petechiae
Traumatic alopecia
Concussion
Basilar skull fractures
Intracranial hemorrhages
Ocular injuries
Subconjunctival hemorrhages
Conjunctival abrasions and lacerations
Hyphema
Retinal detachment
Orbital floor fractures
Ruptured globe
Traumatic iritis
Otic trauma
Ruptured tympanic membranes
Hearing loss
Dental/oral trauma
Fractured, chipped, or avulsed teeth
Ecchymoses and lacerations of the mucosa and tongue
Neck trauma
Erythema, contusions, scratches, abrasions
Ligature marks
Fractured hyoid
Subcutaneous emphysema
Voice changes
Stridor
Extremity injuries
Contusions, lacerations, abrasions
"Grab" marks of upper arms
Fractures, dislocations
Other
Genital injuries
Burns
Blunt abdominal trauma in pregnancy

Strangulation is a form of asphyxia due to compression of the arteries or veins in the neck, or compression of the trachea. It is more common among women than among men as a cause of homicide. Patients may complain of a change in their voice, dysphagia, shortness of breath, confusion, and anxiety. Physical findings as a result of strangulation include erythema, facial petechiae, subconjunctival hemorrhage, ligature marks on the neck, ecchymoses on the neck, voice changes (e.g., hoarseness, aphonia), altered mental status, laryngeal fracture, and stridor. The patient may also have a completely normal examination. Direct laryngoscopy, computed tomography (CT), or magnetic resonance imaging (MRI) may further elucidate the degree of injury following strangulation.[69–71]

Other Health Care Conditions

Victims of IPV present to the ED with a variety of complaints. They present due to trauma, obstetric and gynecologic problems, nonspecific medical complaints, gastrointestinal disorders, mental health problems, and alcohol and substance abuse issues. There are also a number of adverse outcomes that should raise the health care provider's suspicion of abuse during pregnancy. These include a delay in seeking prenatal care, preterm labor, miscarriage, abruption of the placenta, and low birth weight babies.[72,73] Patients may also present with gynecologic problems such as chronic pelvic pain, sexually transmitted diseases, and frequent urinary tract infections. Nonspecific medical complaints may include fatigue, dizziness, lethargy, atypical chest pain, chronic headaches, insomnia, and palpitations. Gastrointestinal disorders, such as irritable bowel syndrome, have been well documented in victims of IPV.[74] Patients may experience mental health problems such as depression, suicidal and homicidal ideation and attempts, anxiety disorders, panic attacks, and posttraumatic stress disorder.

Mental Status Examination

The health care provider should assess the patient's mental status during the ED evaluation. It should be assessed for the possibility of neurologic injury due to repetitive blunt head trauma or hypoxia secondary to strangulation from IPV. The patient should also be assessed for signs of depression, posttraumatic stress disorder, and suicidal and homicidal ideation. If a patient expresses homicidal ideation related to a specific individual, the health care provider has a duty to warn that individual under the Tarasoff vs University of California Regents decision.[75,76]

DOCUMENTATION

In cases of IPV, documentation by health care providers has three main purposes. First, it helps fulfill the requirements for documentation in the medical record, and of having a complete record of the patient's ED visit. Second, it may be required to comply with legal requirements health care providers may have in some states regarding screening of patients for IPV and reporting of IPV to law enforcement or other agencies. Third, documentation, whether performed by the ED health care provider or a forensic examiner, may serve as forensic evidence in the course of a criminal or civil trial.

Medical Record

When completing the medical record of a patient who presents for IPV, use clear, legible, and thorough documentation (Table 34-7). If a health care provider has a concern or suspicion that a patient is a victim of IPV based on pattern recognition, even if it is denied by the patient, document in the medical record that referrals (e.g., victim service hotline number) and interventions were offered to the patient. In the event of an adverse outcome for the patient, and in the absence of adequate documentation, the health care provider may be liable.[77]

ICD-9 diagnostic codes are used to describe primary and secondary diagnoses. Diagnostic codes exist for IPV, and are listed under Adult Maltreatment and Abuse.[78] The American Medical Association has recommended that physicians use the diagnostic codes in their practice (Table

Table 34-7. Critical Documentation Elements in Intimate Partner Violence

Date and time of assessment
History in the patient's own words
Identity of perpetrator
Results of screen for IPV
Past history of IPV
Past medical history and any sequelae of IPV assaults
Physical examination findings
Body map or photographs
Laboratory results
Radiographic results
Consultations
Interventions
Referrals to advocacy programs
Badge number and name of officer(s) to whom report was made

Table 34-8. General Diagnostic Codes for Intimate Partner Violence

Adult Maltreatment and Abuse (995.8)

- 995.81: Physically abused person, battered person, spouse or woman
- 995.82: Adult emotional/psychological abuse
- 995.83: Adult sexual abuse
- 995.84: Adult neglect (nutritional)
- 995.85: Other adult abuse and neglect (multiple forms)

34-8). In 1998, the Health Care Financing Administrator proposed a new severity-adjusted weighting system that would increase the reimbursement for domestic violence, but this proposal has not been implemented at the time of this writing.

Forensic Documentation

Whenever a patient is also a victim of a crime, the medical record becomes part of the forensic record. (In this context, *forensic* simply means pertaining to the law.) A patient who is also the victim of a crime has additional forensic care needs. A well-documented case helps the practitioner prepare for accurate verbal testimony in a court of law, especially when elapsed time results in blurred details and forgotten facts. The medical record is a critical element in successful prosecution and stricter sentencing of perpetrators of violence.[79]

Good documentation does not have to take a lot of time if one knows what to note and it is done consistently. Here are a few general guidelines to follow in making forensically defensible notes that will stand up in court:[57]

- Each page must have proper patient identification and pagination such as "Jane Doe, page 2/5."
- Wherever possible, use the patient's own words to describe a discrete event or a history of abuse and its health impact. Use quotation marks for key phrases. For example: "He came at me with a knife and I pushed him away."
- In cases of IPV, the health care provider is considered to be an objective source. Therefore notations about what an injured patient said, such as " . . . my husband slapped me and I fell to the floor," are admissible in court as an exception to the hearsay rule, which usually prohibits a witness from describing what another person said.
- "Excitable utterances" are spontaneous phrases or statements blurted out when the speaker is in an agitated state. These are particularly important to note in IPV cases because the victim often is under extreme pressure to recant or change testimony after the abuse has occurred. Excitable utterances can also be admitted as an exception to the hearsay rule.
- Do not be tempted to change a patient's word use or word order. If the changes appear inconsistent with what the patient may actually have said, the physician's objectivity could be challenged in court, ultimately compromising the entire medical record. Long patient descriptions may be paraphrased, but critical elements should be recorded verbatim or in quotation marks.
- Try to avoid passive reporting such as "Patient struck in face by fist." Instead, ask (and note) "*Whose* fist?" Passive reporting has traditionally been taught in medical schools. It focuses on the type and force of the trauma so the health care provider can subsequently assess what kind and degree of injuries to anticipate. In passive reporting, the focus has been on *tertiary prevention,* (i.e., on caring for an injury and *thereby preventing further harm from this injury*). Health care providers now need to shift the focus to *secondary prevention,* which means asking, "Whose fist?" "Whose bat?" Secondary prevention means *preventing the injury from happening again.* In the case of IPV, secondary prevention includes identifying the perpetrator(s).
- Identify the abuser by his or her full name and relationship to the patient, and note the abuser's whereabouts when the victim provides this information in order to address safety needs of the patient and staff.
- Avoid pejorative comments, such as, "Patient rambling and not making sense" or "Patient uncooperative" or "Patient refuses care." Instead, use words that describe the patient's state "agitated, nervous, speaking rapidly," or "Patient chooses to do . . . at this time." Even the phrase "patient alleges" casts doubt on the reliability of the statements. Use the phrase "Patient states . . . " instead.

In addition to written documentation of the physical examination, IPV patients may have injuries that need to be accurately depicted. Detailed body diagrams are essential, but photographic documentation is probably the best means of documenting injuries. In this age of height-

Table 34-9. Tips for Photographic Documentation

First image is an identifier
• Photo of chart with name and medical record number or an identification plate
Include a whole body image
• Distant image of victim's entire clothed body, including face
• Insert a color bar so developer can adjust color appropriately for the roll of film
Each injury requires two images
• Geographic photo of body part with the injury (i.e., arm, face, thigh)
• Close-up photos of injury from at least two different, (usually perpendicular) angles to demonstrate depth and swelling
Arrange for serial imaging over time
• 2 day follow-up should be arranged for victims for re-evaluation of their injuries and further photodocumentation
• Follow-up visit should be at a facility with available legal resources, community advocates, and social service professionals

Source: From Mitchell and Kuelbs.[57]

ened concern about privacy issues, a separate consent for photo documentation should be obtained. In urgent care settings and in EDs where injury documentation is done routinely, a camera should be readily available. Training in the use of the camera and effective photographic techniques is essential for ED personnel. A protocol for safe storage and retrieval of images should be established that preserves a legal chain of evidence. It is helpful to think about photodocumentation as a series of photos. Table 34-9 provides useful tips for photographic documentation.

Patients who are victims of IPV may be pursuing criminal investigation, so there may be other evidence to collect. Local law enforcement officials may have guidelines about how to proceed. Here are some general procedures to follow:[57]

- Collect or photograph torn or bloody clothing.
- Collect debris found on the body or in wounds.
- Swab bite marks with saline-soaked cotton swabs for saliva analysis.
- Collect scrapings under fingernails when victim or perpetrator is scratched.
- Consider further imaging or laryngoscopic evaluation when strangulation is involved.
- Refer to sexual assault protocols if victims have been sexually assaulted by their partners. These patients usually require additional forensic evidence collection (see Chap. 33).

Thorough forensic care of a patient requires precise documentation of what the patient says happened, including the name(s) of the assailant(s), detailed diagrammatic or photodocumentation of injuries, and further collection of physical evidence per protocols of local law enforcement.

Legal Requirements

During the past decade, some states have enacted laws mandating health care providers in the areas of screening and reporting IPV.[80] Screening laws have been enacted in three states as of 2001 (California, Pennsylvania, New York), mandating health care providers to screen patients for the purposes of identifying IPV.[80] It is hoped that through screening and identification, larger numbers of patients will be referred for appropriate interventions. Laws have also been enacted mandating that health care providers in certain professions report injuries due to assaultive behavior to law enforcement.[80,81] There are 42 states that mandate that health care providers report injuries from firearms, knives, or other weapons. Twenty-three states have reporting requirements for health care providers treating assaultive injuries, and seven states have laws that require health care providers to specifically report injuries resulting from IPV. Five states have no reporting requirements. Emergency physicians and other health care providers are advised to check their local and state laws for specific reporting requirements.

All states have laws mandating the reporting of child abuse and elder or dependent adult abuse by health care providers. In cases of IPV in which the health care provider suspects there is also ongoing child abuse or child

Table 34-10. Intimate Partner Violence Screening and Intervention Guidelines

Steps	Level I	Level II	Level III	
			Recent or present history of abuse	
			Without injuries and Danger Assessment[a] (–)	With injuries OR Danger Assessment[a] (+)
SCREEN	• No history or present threat of abuse	• Past history of abuse		
INTERVENE	• Provide patient education about IPV • Give information regarding community resources	• Assess for sequelae of past abuse • Provide patient education about IPV and information regarding community resources	• Comprehensive assessment • Individual counseling • Assist patient in contacting community IPV, safety planning • Arrange follow-up visit	• Crisis intervention • Notify police if required by state law • Consider protective orders • Contact IPV services and request advocate to see or talk to patient in ED • Arrange follow-up visit
DOCUMENT	• Statement of no abuse or threat of abuse • Handouts/educational materials given to patient	• Statement of past abuse and sequelae • Education/resources given to patient • Add IPV to problem list and address periodically at subsequent visits	• Describe present or recent abuse and any sequelae • Counsel patient • Resources given, safety planning done • Add IPV to problem list and indicate next follow-up visit	• Complete forensic exam and body diagram or photo documentation • If required by law, complete injury report form and forward to law enforcement or designated agency • Describe law enforcement intervention • Describe advocacy intervention • Add IPV to problem list

[a] See Figure 34-1
Adapted from Lazzaro MV and McFarlanc J.[91]
Adapted by C. Mitchell, California Medical Training Center, University of California Davis.

endangerment, child protective services must be contacted and a report made. In cases of IPV in which an elderly or dependent adult is involved, the health care provider must report to adult protective services.

INTERVENTIONS AND REFERRALS

The majority of the time, the emergency medicine practitioner will be screening for IPV and maintaining a heightened suspicion for IPV in the diagnostic process. But once identified, a protocol for interventions should be well established. The National Health Resource Center on Domestic Violence at the Family Violence Prevention Fund can provide resources to help emergency health care providers develop IPV protocols (phone: 1-888-Rx-Abuse; Internet: www.endabuse.org). Table 34-10 is an example of a protocol for screening and interventions.

Upon identifying a patient as being a victim of IPV, the health care provider should tell the patient that they believe her, that she does not deserve the abuse, that she is not alone, that it is not her fault, and that there are options and resources available to her. Her immediate safety needs should also be addressed. She should be asked about the whereabouts of her partner, if she has any children, and about their whereabouts and safety.

IPV is a potentially life-threatening condition. Much like other life-threatening conditions managed in the ED, the IPV patient should be given careful directions for follow-up care and appropriate referrals. The patient's acute and chronic medical and mental health needs should be addressed. Laboratory and radiographic studies should be obtained as appropriate. In addition, patients and their children should be referred for medical, surgical, and psychiatric consultations as necessary. When requesting a psychiatric consultation it is important to specify the reason for the consultation (i.e., anxiety due to IPV). Many women have lost custody of their children when they were made to appear as though they had psychiatric illnesses.

The ultimate goal in IPV interventions is for the victim and her children to be safer, and not necessarily for them to leave the abuser. Leaving an abusive relationship is one of the most difficult steps for a victim to take. While most victims do eventually leave, there are numerous barriers for them to overcome. These barriers include fear of their abusive partner; fear of losing the children; believing that it is better for the children to have a father in the home; isolation from outside support; family pressures to try to make their marriage work; religious beliefs; immigration issues; and financial reasons.[29]

There are also reasons why victims do leave their abusive relationships. These include escalating violence; fear that they will be killed; abuse of the children; and intervention by others outside of the family. The Process of Change was theorized by Prochaska and associates in 1992.[82] It was later applied to IPV and the five stages a victim in an abusive relationship may experience when making changes.[83] These stages begin with *precontemplation,* a time in which the victim does not even see change as an option. The second stage is *contemplation,* a phase when the victim begins to consider the possibility of leaving her abusive relationship. The *preparation* stage follows, with the victim resolving to leave her abusive partner. The *action* stage occurs when the victim is ready to leave and tries to improve their situation. Last, the *maintenance* stage is a stage of healing. The Stages of Change can be very useful to health care providers in helping them understand why one patient doesn't perceive her situation as dangerous or unhealthy, while another patient actively seeks help from law enforcement or counselors.

Safety Planning

Health care providers need to address the safety needs of a victim of IPV. Patients should be assisted to plan for their safety and that of their children in a variety of circumstances (e.g., leaving temporarily, recurring violence if she decides to return to her abusive partner, recurring violence if her abusive partner returns, and violence at work). Numerous tools have been used to assess a victim's risk for injury and death from IPV, but to date none are reliably predictive of IPV homicide. The Danger Assessment instrument, developed by Jacqueline Campbell, was intended for use in the clinical setting with victims of IPV.[84] It has undergone substantial validity testing and is often used to assess the degree of peril a victim is in.[85] The revised Danger Assessment (Fig. 34-1) is still not predictive of outcome with its current scoring system, but each item is strongly associated with IPV homicide.[86] Research is ongoing to attempt to develop a scoring system that would determine a cutoff level with high sensitivity and specificity for IPV homicide.

Emergency protective orders (EPOs) may be obtained by law enforcement 24 hours a day. Health care providers may request that law enforcement obtain an EPO for a patient. If a patient does not feel safe to go home, such as when the batterer has not been arrested, and she does not have friends or family with whom she can stay, then emergency shelter will be necessary. Community advocacy programs that have emergency shelters should be contacted in order to find available space. In many places the demand for emergency shelter exceeds the number of shelter beds available. On occasion, it may be necessary to admit a patient to the hospital for health and safety reasons, or hold her overnight in the ED so she has a safe place to stay. When admitting an IPV patient to the hospital, if safety is a concern, the patient should be admitted as a "Jane Doe."

Additional Victim Services

Increasingly, EDs are partnering with community programs to provide services to ED patients who are victims of IPV. In addition, there are a few hospital-based victim service programs in the country. These programs offer crisis intervention to patients in the ED, either at the bedside or on the telephone. Trained counselors can come to the ED and provide crisis care or supportive counseling to patients during their ED stay. They assess safety needs including shelter needs, and can arrange for food and transportation. They also provide referrals for follow-up mental health counseling (multilingual or culturally-specific, depending on the community) for victims and their children. Counselors can also provide referrals to legal resources, inform patients about immigrants' legal rights, assist in obtaining protective orders, and help prepare for court hearings. Counselors can assist patients to access victim restitution funds and other victims of crime programs. The National Domestic Violence Hotline may be contacted if local resources are not available, by calling 1-800-799-7233 (TTY: 1-800-787-3224).

Few longitudinal studies have been done to determine the outcome of referring victims of IPV to victim services programs. However, some studies have shown that there is a tendency toward improved outcomes for victims of IPV who have followed-up with these programs.[87–89] Further research is needed to determine the effectiveness of available interventions.

THE ROLE OF CULTURE OR ETHNICITY

Culture refers to the shared experiences or other commonalities of groups of individuals, based on factors of identification such as race, ethnicity, gender, sexuality, class, disability status, religion, age, military experience, immigration status, nationality, regionality, and language. The term *cultural competence* refers to a set of attitudes, knowledge, and behaviors on the part of the health care professional that reflect openness and understanding about differences and power differentials.[90]

In addition to demonstrating cultural competency, cultural considerations should guide a care plan that is devel-

Danger Assessment

Several risk factors have been associated with homicides (murders) of both batterers and battered women in research conducted after the murders have taken place. We cannot predict what will happen in your case, but we would like you to be aware of the danger of homicide in situations of severe battering and for you to see how many of the risk factors apply to your situation.

Mark **Yes** or **No** for each of the following. ("He" refers to your husband, partner, ex-husband, ex-partner, or whoever is currently physically hurting you.)

____ 1. Has the physical violence increased in severity or frequency over the past year?
____ 2. Has he ever used a weapon against you or threatened you with a weapon?
____ 3. Does he ever try to choke you?
____ 4. Does he own a gun?
____ 5. Has he ever forced you to have sex when you did not wish to do so?
____ 6. Does he use drugs? By drugs, I mean "uppers" or amphetamines, speed, angel dust, cocaine, "crack," street drugs,or mixtures.
____ 7. Does he threaten to kill you and/or do you believe he is capable of killing you?
____ 8. Is he drunk every day or almost every day? (in terms of quantity of alcohol-consumed)
____ 9. Does he control most or all of your daily activities? For instance: does he tell you who you can be friends with, when you can see your family, how much money you can use, or when you can take the car? (If he tries, but you do not let him, check here: ____)
____ 10. Have you ever been beaten by him while you were pregnant? (If you have never been pregnant by him, check here: ____)
____ 11. Is he violently and constantly jealous of you? (For instance, does he say "If I can't have you, no one can"?)
____ 12. Have you ever threatened or tried to commit suicide?
____ 13. Has he ever threatened or tried to commit suicide?
____ 14. Does he threaten to harm your children?
____ 15. Do you have a child that is not his?
____ 16. Is he unemployed?
____ 17. Have you left him during the past year? (If have *never* lived with him, check here:___)
____ 18. Do you currently have another (different) intimate partner?
____ 19. Does he follow or spy on you, leave threatening notes, destroy your property, or call you when you don't want him to?

_____ Total "Yes" Answers

Thank you. Please talk to your nurse, advocate, or counselor about what the Danger Assessment means in terms of your situation.

Fig. 34-1. Danger assessment instrument. (From Campbell.[86] Copyright 1985, 1988, 2001. Permission to use this instrument in clinical settings has been universally granted by its creator. Dr. Campbell requests notification if the instrument is used in formal research studies.)

oped with the IPV patient. Some of these considerations are:

- To promote disclosure, protect confidentiality, and avoid unintended bias, it is critical that translators not be family members or friends.
- Patients who are immigrants may have fears and anxieties about the involvement of the Immigration and Naturalization Service (INS). Although there are some protections in place for victims of IPV, nonnaturalized citizens who are arrested for a crime can be deported. That threat may severely restrict a victim's willingness to talk about IPV.
- Gay and lesbian patients may experience additional threats of being "outed" by their batterer.
- Gay male victims often lack shelter resources in their community. Some gays and lesbians are unwilling to disclose their sexual preferences because of fear of homophobia.
- Physically disabled victims lack shelter resources, particularly if they are wheelchair-dependent. Their increased dependency may drastically impede their ability to change their living situation.
- Some victims of color are reluctant to contact law enforcement due to a history of racism. Although they want the violence to stop, they also have concerns about the treatment of their partners by law enforcement.
- Native American patients may be reluctant to disclose IPV because it may also mean disclosure to a tribal council.
- Patients from rural or close-knit communities may be hesitant to use local IPV resources and may need referrals outside of the area where the patient is known.

Different cultures and communities can also have strengths that can support intervention and provide additional resources. These are important considerations that need to be addressed when providing care to IPV victims. Local victim advocacy programs can offer assistance to identify the culture-specific services and resources available in the local community.

REFERENCES

1. Bureau of Justice Statistics: Bureau of Justice Statistics Special Report, Intimate Partner Violence and Age of Victim, 1993–99. 2001.
2. Bachman R, Saltzman L: Violence against women: Estimates from the redesigned survey. U.S. Department of Justice: Office of Justice Programs Document NCJ-154348, 1995.
3. Bowker LH, Maurer L: The medical treatment of battered wives. *Women's Health* 12:25–45, 1987.
4. American Medical Association: *Diagnostic and Treatment Guidelines on Domestic Violence*. American Medical Association, 1992.
5. Wadman MC, Muelleman RL: Domestic violence homicides: ED use before victimization. *Am J Emerg Med* 17:689–691, 1999.
6. Sharps PW, Koziol-McLain J, Campbell J, et al: Health care providers' missed opportunities for preventing femicide. *Preventive Med* 33:373–380, 2001.
7. Plichta SB: Violence, health and the use of health services, in *Women's Health: Health and Care Seeking Behavior*. Baltimore: Johns Hopkins University Press, 1997.
8. Wisner CL, Gilmer TP, Saltzman LE, et al: Intimate partner violence against women: Do victims cost health plans more? *J Fam Pract* 48:439–443, 1999.
9. National Institute of Justice: *Victims Costs and Consequences: A New Look*. Washington: 1996.
10. Saltzman LE, Fanslow JL, McMahon PM, et al: Intimate Partner Violence Surveillance—Uniform Definitions and Recommended Data Elements Version 1.0. Atlanta, GA: National Center for Injury Prevention and Control, Centers for Disease Control and Prevention, 1999.
11. Feldhaus KM, Koziol-McLain J, Amsbury HL, et al: Accuracy of 3 brief screening questions for detecting partner violence in the emergency department. *JAMA* 277:1357–1361, 1997.
12. Fanslow JL, Norton RN, Robinson EM: Outcome evaluation of an emergency department protocol of care on partner abuse. *Aust NZ J Public Health* 22:598–603, 1998.
13. Dearwater SR, Coben JH, Campbell JC, et al. Prevalence of intimate partner abuse in women treated at community hospital emergency departments. *JAMA* 280:433–438, 1998.
14. Olson L, Anctil C, Fullerton L, et al: Increasing emergency physician recognition of domestic violence. *Ann Emerg Med* 27:741–746, 1996.
15. McFarlane J, Greenberg L, Weltege A, et al. Identification of abuse in emergency departments: Effectiveness of a two-question screening tool. *J Emerg Nurs* 21:391–394, 1995.
16. Abbott J, Johnson R, Koziol-McLain J, et al: Domestic violence against women—Incidence and prevalence in an emergency department population. *JAMA* 273:1763–1767, 1995.
17. Ernst AA, Nick TG, Weiss SJ, et al: Domestic violence in an inner-city ED. *Ann Emerg Med* 30:190–197, 1997.
18. National Coalition of Anti-Violence Programs (NCAVP): NCAVP Report on Lesbian, Gay, Bisexual, Transgender Domestic Violence. National Coalition of Anti-Violence Programs, 1998.
19. Pitt EL: Domestic violence in gay and lesbian relationships. *J Gay Lesbian Med Assn* 4:195–196, 2000.

20. Gazmararian JA, Lazorick S, Spitz AM, et al: Prevalence of violence against pregnant women. *JAMA* 275:1915–1920, 1996.
21. Horon IL, Cheng D: Enhanced surveillance for pregnancy-associated mortality—Maryland, 1993–1998. *JAMA* 285: 1455–1459, 2001.
22. Stark E, Flitcraft A: Killing the beast within: Woman battering and female suicidality. *Int J Health Serv* 25:43–64, 1995.
23. Stark E, Flitcraft A, Frazier W: Medicine and patriarchal violence: The social construction of a "private" event. *Int J Health Serv* 9:461–492, 1979.
24. Warshaw C: Identification, assessment and intervention with victims of domestic violence, in Lee D, Durborow N, Salber PR (eds): *Improving the Health Care Response to Domestic Violence: A Resource Manual for Health Care Providers*. Family Violence Prevention Fund: 1995, pp 49–86.
25. Knickman JR: Forecasting Models to Target Families at High Risk of Homelessness. New York Health Research Program, Graduate School of Public Administration. New York University, 1989.
26. D'Ercole A, Struening E: Victimization among homeless women: Implications for service delivery. *J Comm Psychol* 18:141–152, 1990.
27. Federal Bureau of Investigation: Crime in the United States 1998—Uniform Crime Report. Washington: Federal Bureau of Investigation, 1998.
28. Jenkins EL: Occupational injury deaths among females—The U.S. experience from the decade 1980 to 1989. *Ann Epidemiol* 4:146–151, 1994.
29. Ganley AL: Understanding domestic violence, in Lee D, Durborow N, Salber PR (eds): *Improving the Health Care Response to Domestic Violence: A Resource Manual for Health Care Providers*. Family Violence Prevention Fund: 1995, pp 15–45.
30. Waalen J, Goodwin MM, Spitz AM, et al: Screening for intimate partner violence by health care providers—Barriers and interventions. *Am J Preventive Med* 19:230–237, 2000.
31. Heise LL: Violence against women: An integrated, ecological framework. *Violence Against Women* 4:262–290, 1998.
32. Mitchell C: Guidelines for the Health Care of Partner Violence. Office of Criminal Justice Planning and California Medical Training Center, University of California Davis, Sacramento. In press.
33. Dutton DG, Strachan CE: Motivational needs for power and spouse-specific assertiveness in assaultive and nonassaultive men. *Violence Vict* 2:145–146, 1987.
34. Prince JE, Arias I: The role of perceived control and the desirability of control among abusive and nonabusive husbands. *Am J Fam Ther* 22:126–134, 1994.
35. Pence E, Paymar M: Power and Control. Domestic Abuse Intervention Project, Duluth, MN.
36. Walker LE: *The Battered Woman*. New York: Harper & Row, 1979.
37. Walker LE. *The Battered Woman Syndrome*. New York: Springer, 2000.
38. Johnson MP: Patriarchal terrorism and common couple violence: Two forms of violence against women. *J Marriage Fam* 57:283–297, 1995.
39. Langhinrichsen-Rohling J, Smutzler N, Vivian D: Positivity in marriage: The role of discord and physical aggression against wives. *J Marriage Fam* 56:69–79, 1994.
40. Tjaden P, Thoennes N: Prevalence, incidence, and consequences of violence against women: Findings from the National Violence Against Women Survey. National Institute of Justice, Centers of Disease Control and Prevention, NCJ-172837, 1998.
41. Moffitt TE, Caspi A: Findings About Partner Violence from the Dunnedin Multidisciplinary Health and Development Study. National Institute of Justice, 1999.
42. Kyriacou DN, Anglin D, Taliaferro E, et al: Risk factors for injury to women from domestic violence. *N Engl J Med* 341:1892–1898, 1999.
43. Wright RJ, Wright RO, Isaac NE: Response to battered mothers in the pediatric emergency department: A call for an interdisciplinary approach to family violence. *Pediatrics* 99: 186–192, 1997.
44. Stark E, Flitcraft AH: Women and children at risk: A feminist perspective on child abuse. *Int J Health Serv* 18:97–118, 1988.
45. Bowker L, Arbetel M, McFerron J: On the relationship between wife beating and child abuse, in: Yllo K, Bograd M (eds): *Feminist Perspectives on Wife Abuse*. Newbury Park, CA: Sage Publications, 1988.
46. Ross S: Risk of physical abuse to children of spouse abusing parents. *Child Abuse Neglect* 20:589–598, 1996.
47. Strauss MA, Gelles RJ: Societal change and change in family violence from 1975 to 1985 as revealed by two national surveys. *J Marriage Fam* 48:465–479, 1986.
48. Christian CW, Scribano P, Seidl T, et al: Pediatric injury resulting from family violence. *Pediatrics* 99:E8, 1997.
49. Edelson JL: Children's witnessing of adult domestic violence. *J Interpersonal Violence* 14:839–970, 1999.
50. Committee on Child Abuse and Neglect: The role of the pediatrician in recognizing and intervening on behalf of abused women. *Pediatrics* 101:1091–1092, 1998.
51. Duffy SJ, McGrath ME, Becker BM, et al: Mothers with histories of DV in a pediatric emergency department. *Pediatrics* 103:1007–1013, 1999.
52. Kann L, Kinchen SA, Williams BL, et al: Youth risk behavior surveillance—United States, 1999. *CDC Surveillance Summaries* 49:7–104, 2000.
53. Foshee V: Gender differences in adolescent dating abuse prevalence, types, and injuries. *Health Education Res* 11:275–286, 1996.
54. Kreiter SR, Krowchuk DP, Woods CR, et al: Gender differences in risk behaviors among adolescents who experience date fighting. *Pediatrics* 104:1286–1292, 1999.
55. Silverman JG, Raj A, Mucci LA, et al: Dating violence against adolescent girls and associated substance use, unhealthy weight control, sexual risk behavior, pregnancy, and suicidality. *JAMA* 286:572–579, 2001.
56. Wiemann CM, Agurcia CA, Berenson AB, et al: Pregnant adolescents: Experiences and behaviors associated with

physical assault by an intimate partner. *Maternal Child Health J* 4:93–101, 2000.

57. Mitchell C, Kuelbs C: Advanced Training in Domestic Violence for Health Care Providers. Office of Criminal Justice Planning and California Medical Training Center, University of California Davis, Sacramento, 2001.
58. American College of Emergency Physicians: Emergency medicine and domestic violence. *Ann Emerg Med* 25:442–443, 1995.
59. American College of Obstetrics and Gynecologists: Domestic violence. ACOG technical bulletin no. 209. *Int J Gynaecol Obstet* 51:161–170, 1995.
60. American Academy of Family Practice: Family violence. *Am Fam Physician* 50:1636–1646, 1994.
61. Quillian JP: Screening for spousal abuse in a community health setting. *J Am Acad Nurse Pract* 8:155–160, 1996.
62. Emergency Nurses Association: Position statement: Domestic violence. Park Ridge, IL: Emergency Nurses Association, 1996.
63. Friedman LS, Samet JG, Roberts MS: Inquiry about victimization experiences: A survey of patient preferences. *Arch Intern Med* 152:1186–1190, 1992.
64. Rhodes K, Lauderdale DS, Stocking CB, et al: Better health while you wait: A controlled trial of a computer-based intervention for screening and health promotion in the emergency department. *Ann Emerg Med* 37:284–291, 2001.
65. Campbell JC: Women's responses to sexual abuse in intimate relationships. *Women's Health Care Int* 8:335–347, 1989.
66. Wilbur L, Higley M, Hatfield J, et al: Survey results of women who have been strangled while in an abusive relationship. *J Emerg Med* 21:297–302, 2001.
67. Soeken KL, McFarlane J, Parker B, et al: The abuse assessment screen, in: Campbell JC (ed): *Empowering Survivors of Abuse*. Thousand Oaks CA, Sage Publications, 1998.
68. Muelleman RL, Lenaghan PA, Pakieser RA: Battered women: Injury locations and types. *Ann Emerg Med* 28:486–492, 1996.
69. McClane GE, Strack GB, Hawley DA: A review of 300 attempted strangulation cases. Part II: Clinical evaluation of the surviving victim. *J Emerg Med* 21:311–315, 2001.
70. Hawley DA, McClane GE, Strack GB: A review of 300 attempted strangulation cases. Part III: Injuries in fatal cases. *J Emerg Med* 21:317–322, 2001.
71. Smith DJ, Mills T, Taliaferro EH: Frequency and relationship of reported symptomatology in victims or intimate partner violence: The effect of multiple strangulation attacks. *J Emerg Med* 21:323–329, 2001.
72. McFarlane J, Parker B, Soeken K, et al: Assessing for abuse during pregnancy—Severity and frequency of injuries and associated entry into prenatal care. *JAMA* 267:3176–3178, 1992.
73. Berenson AB, Wiemann CM, Wilkinson GS, et al: Perinatal morbidity associated with violence experienced by pregnant women [see comments]. *Am J Obstet Gynecol* 170:1760–1766, discussion 1766–1769, 1994.
74. Drossman DA, Leserman J, Nachman G, et al: Sexual and physical abuse in women with functional or organic gastrointestinal disorders. *Ann Intern Med* 113:828–933, 1990.
75. Bloom JD, Rogers JL: The duty to protect others from your patients—Tarasoff spreads to the northwest. *West J Med* 148:231–234, 1988.
76. Oppenheimer K, Swanson G: Duty to warn: When should confidentiality be breached? *J Fam Pract* 30:179–184, 1990.
77. Brown-Cranstoun J: Kringen v. Boslaugh and Saint Vincent Hospital: A new trend for healthcare professionals who treat victims of domestic violence? *J Health Law* 33:97–118, 2000.
78. Rudman WJ: *Coding and Documentation of Domestic Violence*. San Francisco: Family Violence Prevention Fund, 2000.
79. Belknap J, Graham DLR, Allan PG, et al: Predicting court outcomes in intimate partner violence cases: Preliminary findings. *Domestic Violence Rep* 5:1–10, 1999.
80. Family Violence Prevention Fund: State-by-state report card on health care laws and domestic violence. August 2001, http://endabuse.org/statereport/list.php3.
81. Houry D, Sachs CJ, Feldhaus KM, et al: Violence-inflicted injuries: Reporting laws in the fifty states. *Ann Emerg Med* 39:56–60, 2002.
82. Prochaska JO, DiClemente CC, Norcross JC: In search of how people change: Applications to addictive behaviors. *Am Psychologist* 47:1102–1114, 1992.
83. Brown J: Working toward freedom from violence. *Violence Against Women* 3:5–26, 1997.
84. Campbell J: Nursing assessment for risk of homicide with battered women. *Adv Nurs Sci* 8:36–51, 1986.
85. Campbell JC, Sharps P, Glass NE: Risk assessment for intimate partner homicide, in Pinard G, Pagani L (eds): *Clinical Assessment of Dangerousness: Empirical Contributions*. New York: Cambridge University Press, 2001, pp 136–157.
86. Campbell JC: Danger Assessment. 2001 www.son.jhmi.edu/research/CNR/homicide/DANGER.htm
87. Muelleman RL, Feighny KM: Effects of an emergency department-based advocacy program for battered women on community resource utilization. *Ann Emerg Med* 33:62–66, 1999.
88. McFarlane J, Soeken K, Reel S, et al: Resource use by abused women following an intervention program: Associated severity of abuse and reports of abuse ending. *Pub Health Nurs* 14:244–250, 1997.
89. Sullivan CM, Bybee DI: Reducing violence using community-based advocacy for women with abusive partners. *J Consult Clin Psychol* 67:43–53, 1999.
90. Warrier S, Brainin-Rodriquez J: *Sensitivity to Competency: Clinical and Departmental Guidelines to Achieving Cultural Competency*. San Francisco: Family Violence Prevention Fund, 1998.
91. Lazzaro MV, McFarlane J: Establishing a screening program for abused women. *Journal of Nursing Administration* 21:24–29, 1991.

35

Ultrasound in Obstetrics and Gynecology

Christine H. Comstock

KEY POINTS

- Ultrasound transducers are fragile, cannot be repaired, and are expensive to replace.
- The incidence of both an intrauterine pregnancy and an ectopic (heterotopic pregnancy) is high in women with assisted reproduction.
- Ultrasound is not of benefit in bleeding in third-trimester pregnancies known to not have placenta previa and is not a sensitive test for placental abruption.
- A diagnosis of placenta previa cannot be made until the third trimester.
- A pregnant woman with urinary retention may have an incarcerated uterus.
- Fibroids in pregnancy may cause pain, particularly at 15 to 20 weeks; the site of tenderness usually corresponds to visualized fibroids.

ULTRASOUND AS A DIAGNOSTIC MODALITY

In pregnancy there are two patients—the mother and her fetus. Ultrasound has revolutionized obstetrics because it shows us the "other patient." The emergency physician may be ordering a scan, and therefore needs to understand the indications and sensitivity of ultrasound for varying entities. In addition, in limited circumstances, ultrasound scans of early pregnancies by ED physicians may expedite decision-making and care.

What is Ultrasound?

Ultrasound means "beyond sound"—i.e., frequencies greater than 20,000 Hz (cycles per second), above which sound is not audible to the human ear. Ultrasound frequencies used in obstetrics are extremely high—usually 3,500,000 Hz and above or 3.5 to 7 MHz. Consequently, this sound is not audible to either the fetus or the mother.

Ultrasound is generated by passing an electric current through special crystals (piezoelectric), causing them to expand. As the faces of the crystals expand, molecules in front of them are pushed away, creating a sound wave. These crystals are located in the transducer, which in turn is connected to the computer and controls.

The sound wave travels through the patient's skin and is reflected back when it encounters the dividing line between two substances of different acoustic impedance; the greater the difference in acoustic impedance, the greater the amount of reflection. The transducer, which is both the sending and listening device, is deformed by the returning sound wave, setting up an electric current in the piezoelectric crystal, thus reversing the process used in producing sound initially. This current is transformed into a signal, which is displayed on the ultrasound monitor. The computer constructs an ever-changing two-dimensional image while the transducer is moved across the patient's skin.

Doppler Ultrasound

The portable fetal heart monitor used to hear the fetus's heart beat relies on the Doppler effect, which describes the change in the frequency of sound when it is reflected from a moving object. The portable monitors send sound toward the fetal heart and its valves, and since those objects are moving, the returned sound is of a different frequency. The difference in those two frequencies is amplified so the human ear can clearly hear it.

Care of Transducers

The piezoelectric crystals in the ultrasound transducer are very delicate. They break if dropped, and if broken, the transducer usually cannot be repaired—a new one must be purchased. Hence, great care must be taken in the handling and storage of transducers. A special gel is used to obliterate the air interface between the transducer and the skin surface. It is formulated to transmit sound completely and to not damage the face of the transducer. The special ultrasound gel is water-based and will not damage clothing, although it will leave a white powder when it dries. The use of lanolin-based creams (hand cream, for example) will dissolve the latex on most transducer faces.

Frequencies of Transducers

Transducers send different frequencies of sound; there are, for example, 2.5-, 3.0-, and 5.0-mHz transducers, among others. *The rule of thumb is the higher the frequency, the better the resolution, but the poorer the penetration.* Consequently, a 5-MHz transducer would be selected for a thin woman and a 2.5- or 3-MHz transducer would be used for a heavy woman or for a term pregnancy, where increased depth of penetration was needed. If a patient is extremely obese, it may not be possible to get much useful information even with an abdominal or transvaginal transducer because fat (subcutaneous or omental) is highly reflective of sound.

Types of Transducers

The shape of the image is determined by the array pattern of the piezoelectric crystals. If they are lined up in a row (curved or straight), the transducer is termed *linear.* If they are arranged and the beam is steered so that the image is wedge-shaped, the transducer is called a *sector transducer.*

A real advance was made with the introduction of long, narrow transducers that could be inserted into the vagina (Fig. 35-1), because the pelvic contents could be visualized without sound first traversing the skin, muscle, and fat of the anterior abdominal wall. A full bladder is not needed (and actually hinders the exam) and gas in the bowel is not a problem. This is the most common type of transducer used in early pregnancy in the emergency department.

Abdominal versus Transvaginal Scanning

For a complete scan, in which visualization of the ovaries is essential, an abdominal scan should be done first. The high-frequency transducers used for pelvic sonography are designed to reveal excellent detail, but the trade off is that they do not penetrate long distances well. The transvaginal transducer often cannot be used to visualize the adnexa since they may be too high in the pelvis. Hence it is standard to first look abdominally, if possible. For this exam, a full bladder is needed to push bowel out of the pelvis (air does not transmit sound well) and to provide an acoustic window. This full bladder does not need to be achieved by drinking fluids. The best way to achieve this is by not urinating until after the abdominal scan is completed. It should not be necessary to introduce a catheter. If the uterine contents are well seen, a heart beat is identified, the fetus measured, and the adnexa seen, it is not necessary to proceed to a transvaginal scan.

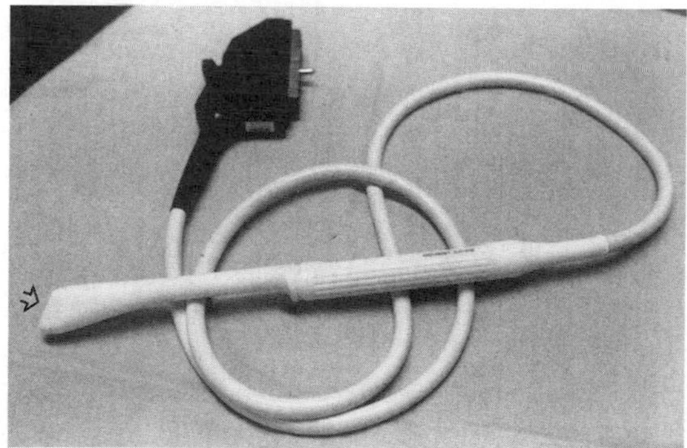

Fig. 35-1. Transvaginal transducer. The transducer face (*arrow*) is linear. A special covering must be used before this is inserted into the vagina.

A full bladder interferes with the transvaginal scan, so first do an abdominal scan, have the patient urinate, and then do the transvaginal scan. Beware that obesity and fat make both types of scans more difficult; the abdominal fat scatters the beam when doing an abdominal scan and mesenteric fat scatters it when doing a vaginal scan.

The Use and Care of a Transvaginal Transducer

Since the vaginal transducer is placed into a body cavity, it must be covered with a sterile cover. This can be a specially-made endovaginal transducer cover or a high-quality condom. Ultrasound gel is placed on the tip of the transducer and then the cover is placed on it and secured, usually with a rubber band that sits in a groove near the examiner's hand. These should be put on without touching anything but the cuff. Sterile ultrasound gel is then placed on the covered tip.

Before covering the transducer, be sure to inquire about latex allergies. The use of a latex cover inserted into the vagina can induce an allergic reaction, including anaphylaxis. If the patient is allergic to latex, use a vinyl cover. These can be obtained from medical supply houses. *Do not secure with a rubber band,* which always contains latex. Just hold the cover on with the hand holding the transducer.

Once the exam is over the probe must be cleansed according to a certain protocol; this should be done in a "dirty" utility room. Remove the cover, rinse the probe under running water, and then soak it in a commercial glutaraldehyde soaking solution for 12 minutes. The fumes of glutaraldehyde are toxic, so this soaking thus must be done in a very well ventilated area. If possible, a special ventilation system should be used to carry the fumes away. A recent alternative is to use Cidex-OPA, the fumes of

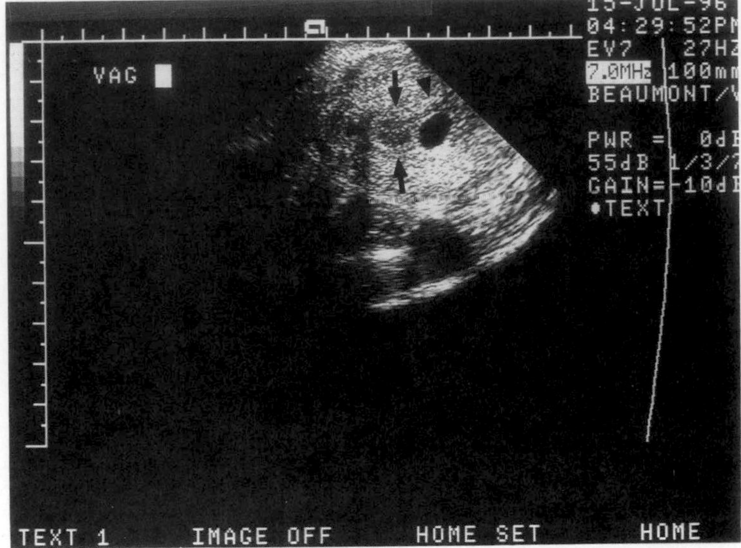

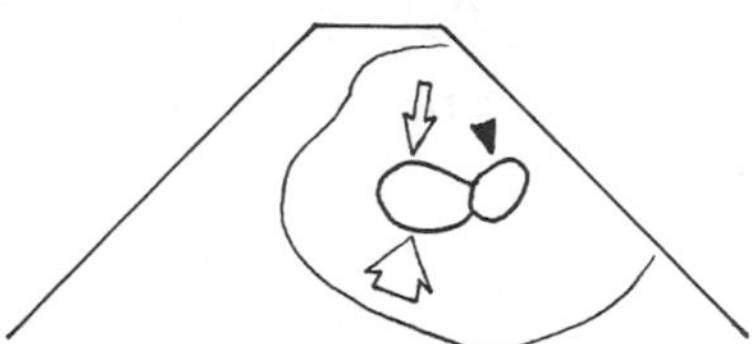

Fig. 35-2. Vaginal scan, transverse plane. An early gestational sac appears as a black circle (*arrowhead*). Note that it is eccentrically placed in relation to the uterine cavity (*arrows*). This is an important point in differentiating a true gestational sac from a pseudosac of an ectopic pregnancy, which is centrally placed.

which are not toxic. This is more expensive, but does not require a ventilation system. The soaking system should be away from the reach of children, preferably on the wall or on a counter. Soaking should not be done in the exam room itself. Only the part of the probe which extends up to the rubber band line should be soaked; soaking anything higher may damage the cord or its connection to the probe. When soaking, the probe should be suspended in the solution so the tip of the probe is not damaged, since the covering of the end is very delicate.

When the timer for soaking has gone off, remove the probe, run under running water to get the glutaraldehyde off, and dry. Hang in a clean utility room or back in the exam room. Once they have been cleaned, the probes need to be covered. This can be done by storing in a cupboard or covering the tip with a clean dry cloth such as a washcloth.

The concentration of the glutaraldehyde solution must be checked once a day since it is possible that the solution will become diluted and ineffective. Testing strips are available and a written record must be kept of this testing. Every 2 weeks a fresh solution must be made up and the old solution discarded. The latter can be poured down a drain or flushed down a toilet.

How to Order an Ultrasound Examination

Often a clinician will not provide clinical information to the imaging department in the hope of having them take a fresh unbiased look. However, this is fallacious thinking for the same reason that no other physician would see a patient without a clinical history. The clinical context is very helpful to the interpreting radiologists in providing the most accurate reading.

THE FIRST 20 WEEKS OF PREGNANCY

Normal Development

An intrauterine sac can first be seen by ultrasound with a transvaginal transducer at about 5 weeks (Fig. 35-2) or when the β-human chorionic gonadotropin (β-hCG) level is above the discriminatory zone. The discriminatory zone is defined as the level of β-hCG above which an intrauterine gestational sac should always be seen. There is some debate as to what this level is with many sources using 1500 mIU/mL, though there is a range in the literature of 1000 to 3000 mIU/mL.[1–4] This range likely is the result of differences in skill and experience of the sonographer, the equipment utilized in performing the ultrasound and making measurements, as well as the incidence of multiple gestations in the populations studied. On an abdominal scan, the sac may not be visible until the β-hCG is about 6000 mIU/mL.[1] The next development in sonoembryology is a doughnut-shaped structure called the yolk sac (Fig. 35-3). At about $5\frac{1}{2}$ weeks (menstrual age), a faint flickering can be seen along one of the surfaces of the yolk sac; this means that the embryonic

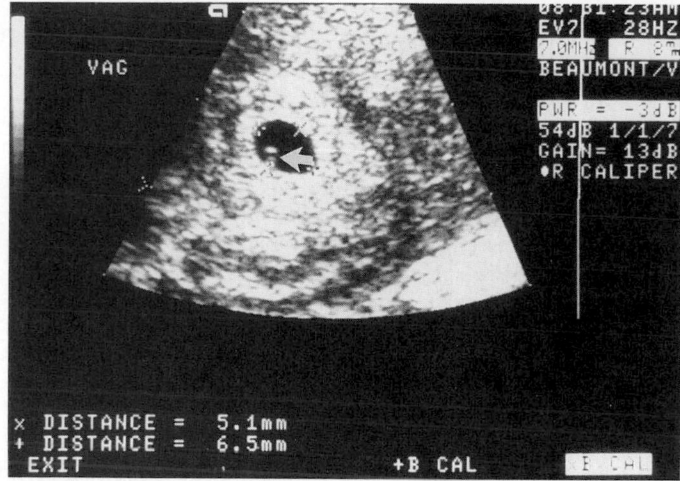

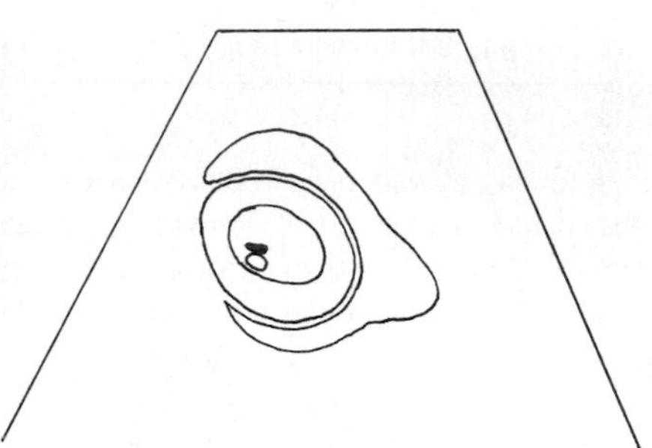

Fig. 35-3. Yolk sac. This can be detected by ultrasound at about $5^1/_2$ weeks (menstrual dates). It is a round, doughnut-shaped structure (*arrow*), on the surface of which the embryo will appear (*white "dash" just above tip of arrow*).

heart tube has started to contract. The fetal heart rate is almost always over 100 bpm. If a slower rate is observed, this may be due to maternal blood being pumped into vasculature of the sac, or may indicate a nonviable pregnancy.

Next, an embryonic pole appears (Fig. 35-4). It may be as small as 1 to 2 mm if transvaginal scanning is being used. The crown-rump length (CRL) is usually the most reliable way to establish gestational age because there is little variation in size for each gestational week (i.e., all fetuses 3 mm long are 6 weeks of age, with a variation of only ±3 days). By the time the pole measures 4 to 5 mm (6 to 6.5 weeks), it will be visible by transabdominal scanning in most patients. From 6.5 to 11 weeks, fetal age will be measured by a crown-rump length (CRL).

The Abnormal Intrauterine Pregnancy

If no sac can be seen even when the β-hCG is 1500 mlU/mL or higher (or the level reaches the designated descriminatory zone for the institution), the following possibilities should be considered; the patient has more than two sacs (e.g., triplets),[1] the sac is outside the uterus (ectopic pregnancy), or the patient has had an intrauterine pregnancy (IUP) that she has passed or which has been resorbed (Table 35-1). If there has been no bleeding, the latter is unlikely. If the patient has had any assisted reproduction, the first possibility is likely. A history of previous ectopic pregnancy suggests another. Examination of the cul-de-sac and adnexa will often determine the diagnosis.

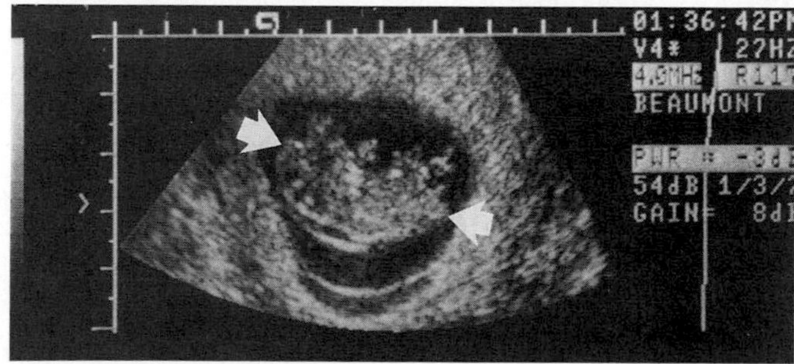

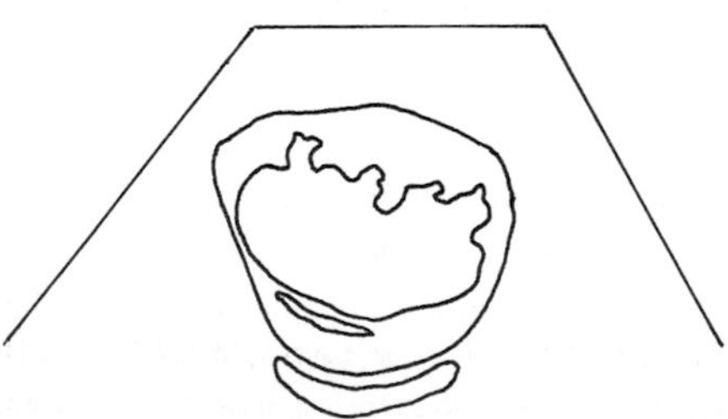

Fig. 35-4. Crown-rump length. From the time the embryo can be seen by ultrasound to 11 weeks (menstrual dates). It is measured from the head to rump (*arrows*).

Table 35-1. Implications of Absent Gestational Sac

No sac on transvaginal ultrasound with β-hCG >1500 mIU/mL:

- Intrauterine pregnancy <5 weeks with 3 or more embryos
- Ectopic pregnancy
- Failing intrauterine pregnancy >5 weeks

A fetal heart rate under 100 is abnormal and should not be considered to be part of a normal pregnancy. Such a low rate should be reported to the patient's primary physician or obstetrician. Although it has been reported that heart motion may not be visible until the embryo is 4 mm long, in our experience, if the equipment is in good working order this is not the case; usually heart motion is visible on the surface of the sac before the embryo is large enough to be measured.

The normal intrauterine sac should be high in the fundus and will expand downward as it grows. If it is located low in the uterus, it may not be well attached. If the patient has a uterine scar, a low implanted sac may be abnormally attached to that scar, a situation in which growth of the placenta into the uterus may occur. Such abnormal adherence results in placenta accreta or cervical pregnancy, both potentially threatening to the mother's life.

Frequently, a sac implants in the uterus and then fails to produce an embryo or the embryo fails to grow. The popular term for the latter is *miscarriage;* a more correct term is *demise of an intrauterine pregnancy* (IUP) or *failed IUP*. The placenta may grow for a while and the β-hCG level may rise appropriately, but eventually the placenta degenerates and the β-hCG level falls.

Often an embryo or yolk sac will altogether fail to appear on ultrasound. While this is another type of failed IUP, the common term for this is *blighted ovum*. In some pregnancies, growth has stopped before the embryo appears or when it is less than 1 mm in length, but more often an embryo has formed and then died and resorbed, leaving only a visible sac. History or previous scans may differentiate this from lagging dates and very early intrauterine pregnancy.

Ectopic Pregnancy

This term means that a pregnancy is developing outside of the uterus—in a fallopian tube, ovary, the cervix, or free in the abdomen. *It is imperative that every woman of reproductive age presenting in an emergency situation be considered pregnant until proven otherwise.* As a corollary to this statement, *it is imperative that every woman of reproductive age presenting in an emergency department with any bleeding, abdominal pain, discomfort, syncope, rapid pulse, or hypotension be suspected of having an ectopic pregnancy until a pregnancy test can be shown to be negative or an intrauterine pregnancy is confirmed.*

Ultrasound has played a large role, along with increasingly sensitive tests for hCG, in cutting the death rate in ectopic pregnancy.[5,6] With a combination of these two modalities, it is possible to detect most ectopics when a high index of suspicion is maintained.

The ultrasound examination of the problematic early pregnancy is the most difficult in pelvic ultrasonography and one that should be entrusted to the most experienced person available; it is not an exam to be left to someone who does not have considerable experience in this diagnosis, as the stakes are too high. A case has been made that it is possible to triage patients by allowing relatively inexperienced physicians to identify heart motion in an intrauterine pregnancy, thereby excluding ectopic pregnancy.[7–10] In the patient without a history of assisted reproduction, tubal disease, tubal surgery, use of an intrauterine device (IUD), or severe pain, this is probably a valid pathway.

The Discriminatory Zone

The gestational sac can be seen at 23 days postconception, but it is unusual to know the exact date of conception unless the patient has been testing for ovulation. The discriminatory zone is an important concept to understand in the patient who does not know when she ovulated, which includes most women. The discriminatory level is defined as the β-hCG level at which a gestational sac is seen in 100 percent of intrauterine pregnancies. For example, a sac should be seen in a singleton pregnancy with a transvaginal transducer in 100 percent of cases by a β-hCG level of 1500 mIU; otherwise the pregnancy is not normal. The discriminatory zone varies depending on whether there is a single or multiple pregnancy. Since the ED physician usually does not know whether there is a singleton or multiple pregnancy the best choice is to use the discriminatory zone for triplets, which is 3372 mIU.[1] Each institution must determine what discriminatory level of β-hCG it will use for this cut-off based on their own experience and patient population.

Extrauterine Findings

The primary use of ultrasound is to positively identify an intrauterine pregnancy. If none can be definitely identi-

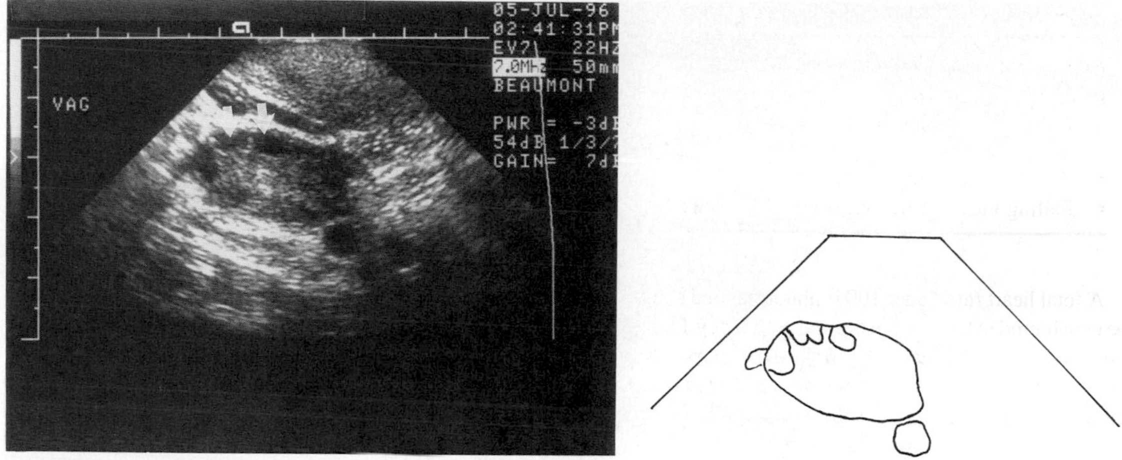

Fig. 35-5. Normal ovary. The ovary is oval with small follicles (*arrows*) arrayed around the outer rim.

fied, experienced examiners will then attempt to identify the ovaries (Fig. 35-5) and search for masses in the area around them. The fallopian tubes are not visible unless they are abnormal.

Often there will be echogenic fluid in the pelvis; if small particles can be seen swirling around within the fluid, it most is likely blood.[11] When present, a mass completely separate from the ovaries can usually be detected by an experienced examiner. Sometimes it appears to be solid and in other instances it may contain just a visible sac within a mass ("bagel sign") (Fig. 35-6). In others an actual embryo with a heartbeat will be seen (Fig. 35-7). The latter is absolutely diagnostic of an ectopic pregnancy. A major difficulty is that the ectopic mass can be hidden behind swirling loops of bowel or can be of such similar acoustic impedance as the ovaries or uterus or in such close approximation to them that it cannot be distinguished as a separate mass. An extra-ovarian mass and an empty uterus are together very sensitive signs for an ectopic pregnancy. An ectopic pregnancy can also occur

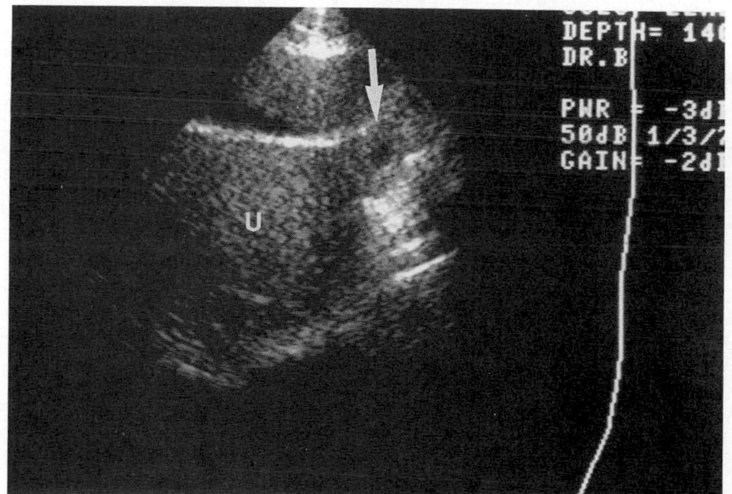

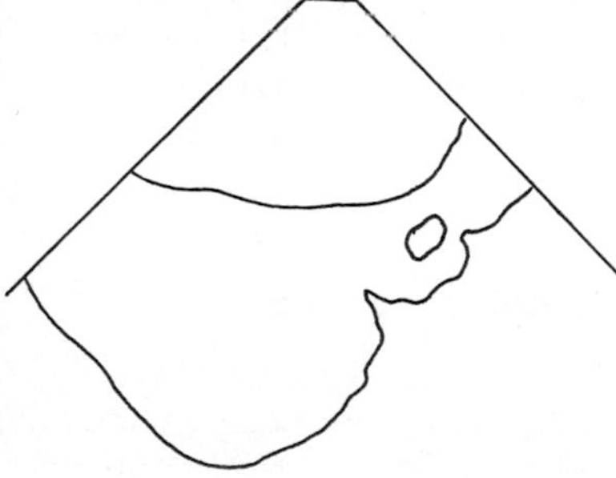

Fig. 35-6. Ectopic pregnancy. An extrauterine mass containing a small gestational sac ("bagel sign") (*arrow*) lies to the right of the top of the uterus (u).

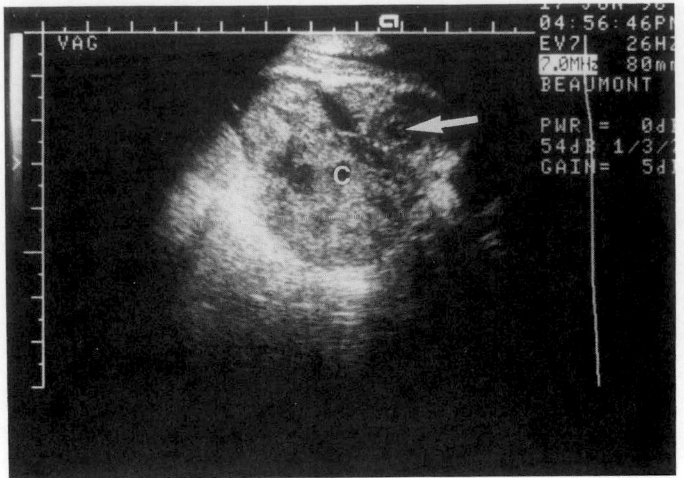

Fig. 35-7. Ectopic pregnancy. A mass containing a gestational sac and small embryo (*arrow*) lies to the right of an intraperitoneal clot (c). Since a heartbeat could be seen in the embryo, this was absolutely diagnostic of an ectopic pregnancy.

within an ovary (Fig. 35-8). The diagnostic challenge is to then distinguish between this and a corpus luteum cyst or other ovarian mass. A pregnancy may also implant in the cervix. This type of ectopic pregnancy is notorious for causing heavy bleeding when it is disturbed.

Intrauterine Findings

Unless there is a heterotopic pregnancy (both in the uterus and ectopic), the uterine cavity will not contain a gestational sac. However, in some ectopics, a pseudogestational sac (a collection of fluid surrounded by uterine lining which mimics a gestational sac) will be seen; these can be notoriously difficult to distinguish from an intrauterine sac (Fig. 35-9). Occasionally a sac will be seen in the uterus but will be markedly eccentric in location. This appearance raises the possibility of an *interstitial pregnancy* (sometimes erroneously termed a *cornual pregnancy*), one that implants in the part of the tube that travels through the myometrium into the uterine cavity. It is

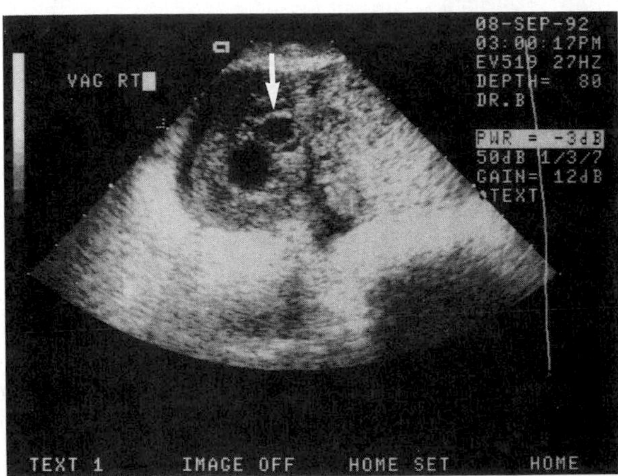

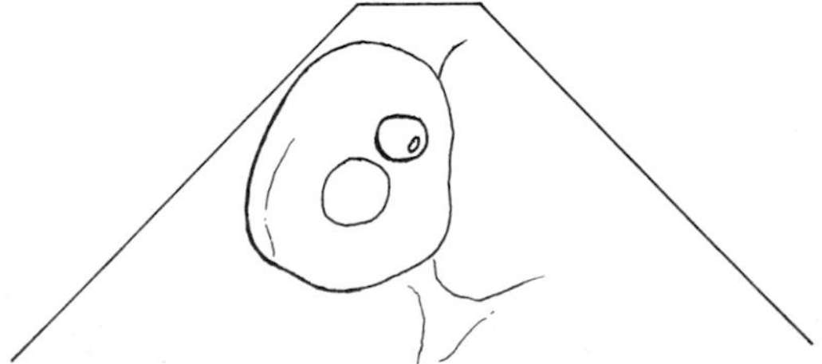

Fig. 35-8. Ovarian ectopic. The sac with the definitive white line around it (*arrow*) proved to be an ovarian ectopic. The diagnosis was made by laparoscopy after a tentative diagnosis of ectopic was made by clinical and ultrasound evidence.

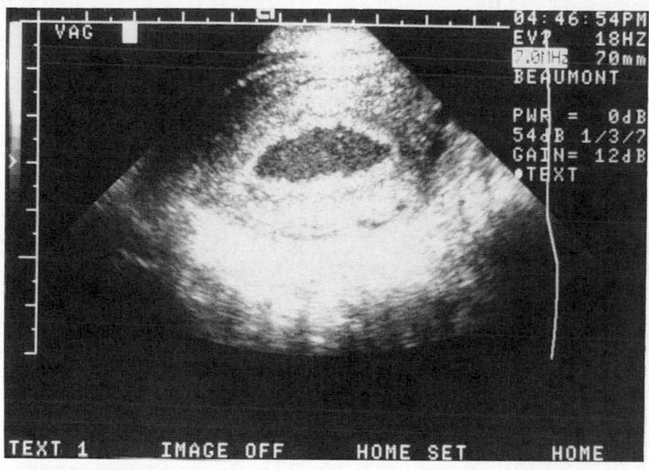

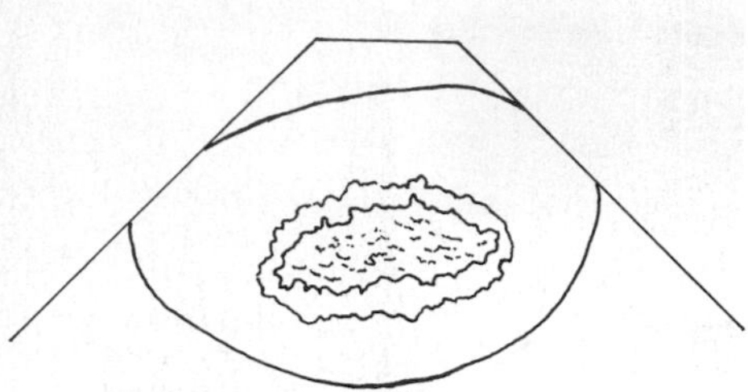

Fig. 35-9. A pseudogestational sac. This sac has a definite border similar to the one found in a true gestational sac. However, note that it is centrally located and contains debris. Compare to Fig. 35-2.

important to make the distinction between an eccentric intrauterine pregnancy and an interstitial pregnancy, because the latter is also notorious for the amount of bleeding that occurs upon rupture. The problem becomes one of determining if it is an ectopic pregnancy in the proximal tube or in the interstitium.[12] In any case, interstitial pregnancies can easily be missed unless the top of the uterus is examined with meticulous care by an experienced examiner.[13]

Heterotopic Pregnancy

The incidence of *heterotopic pregnancies* (simultaneous intrauterine pregnancy and ectopic pregnancy) has increased markedly with the advent of assisted reproduction (the use of ovulation induction, in vitro fertilization, or zygote implantation). Although deaths from ectopic pregnancy have markedly decreased, heterotopic pregnancies are still a cause of maternal death because the intrauterine pregnancy is identified but the ectopic gestation is missed.

Using Ultrasound in the Emergency Department

There are two recognized levels of scans: limited and complete. A limited exam is one which is performed for the purposes of obtaining a specific piece of information. They are not complete scans as defined below. Limited scans in the emergency department have been studied to determine whether or not their performance in the emergency department can speed up the care of the pregnant patient in that setting.[7–10]

Much information can be obtained with a limited scan, performed only to search for a gestational sac. In fact, this one piece of information—the existence of a gestational sac and embryo—excludes an ectopic in all but a few specific patients who are at high risk for a coexisting ectopic pregnancy. This limited scan can be performed by someone who can identify a normal gestational sac. Whether or not time is saved depends upon the response time of the ultrasonographer or the obstetric resident. As would be expected, time savings are greatest at night and when it takes a long time to obtain a scan by a radiology sonographer.

A *complete* gynecologic scan requires all of the following:

- Evaluation of the cervix
- Evaluation of the adnexa
- Evaluation of the uterus (shape and contents)
- Evaluation of the pelvis for abnormal contents such as blood, pelvic kidney, or abnormal bowel

The American Institute of Ultrasound in Medicine (AIUM) is an organization made up of professionals—physicians from all specialties, sonographers, and physicists—that utilize diagnostic ultrasound. The AIUM publishes guidelines for standard obstetric and gynecologic scans. These can be ordered from AIUM or viewed at www.AIUM.org. When doing a full scan, all of the above points must be commented upon. In addition, the scan must be documented and records kept. The American

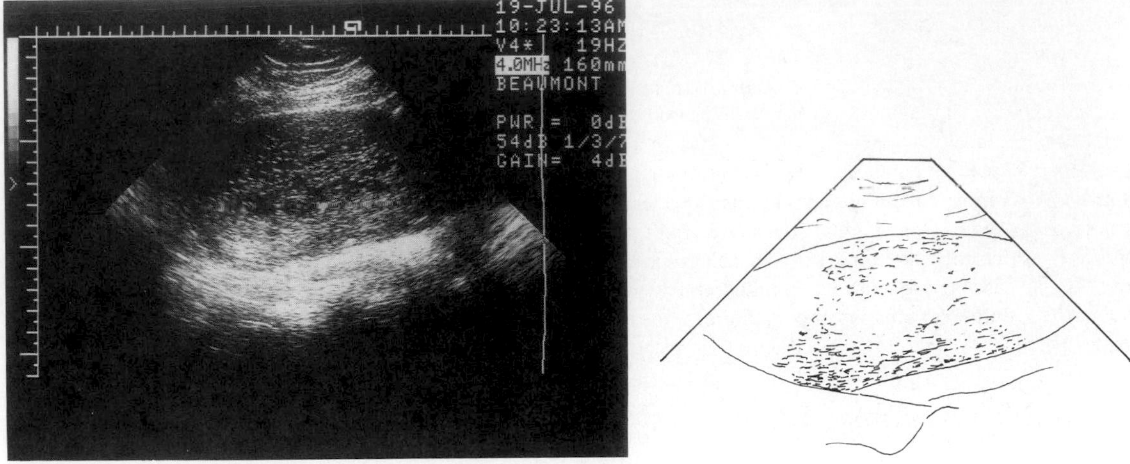

Fig. 35-10. Hydatidiform mole. The uterus is occupied by echogenic material.

College of Obstetricians and Gynecologists (ACOG) also has a set of standards, as does the American College of Radiology (ACR).

Hydatidiform Mole

When the uterus appears to be occupied only by the placenta and there is no fetus, the patient may have a hydatidiform mole. In this entity, the placenta appears very heterogeneous, with many lucent areas interspersed with brighter areas (Fig. 35-10). This brightness is a reflection off the surfaces of the vesicles of the mole. In the older literature, it was referred to as a "snowstorm," but the advent of gray-scale imaging (showing gradations of gray rather than black and white only) has made that term obsolete. This appearance can be mimicked by a degenerating placenta in the demise of an intrauterine pregnancy which occasionally occurs when the fetus is resorbed first and the placenta becomes very heterogeneous in appearance. The actual diagnosis can be determined only by pathologic

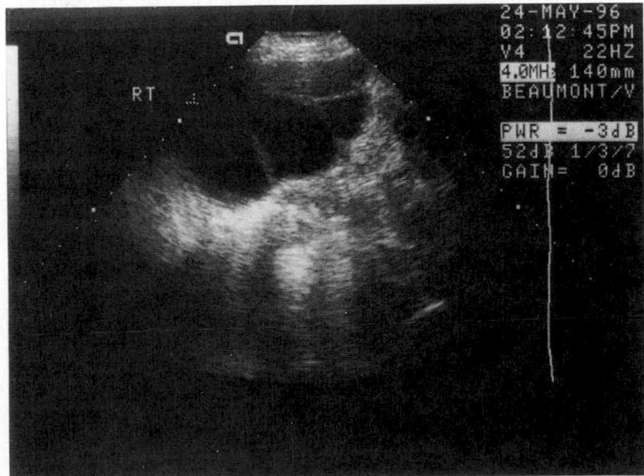

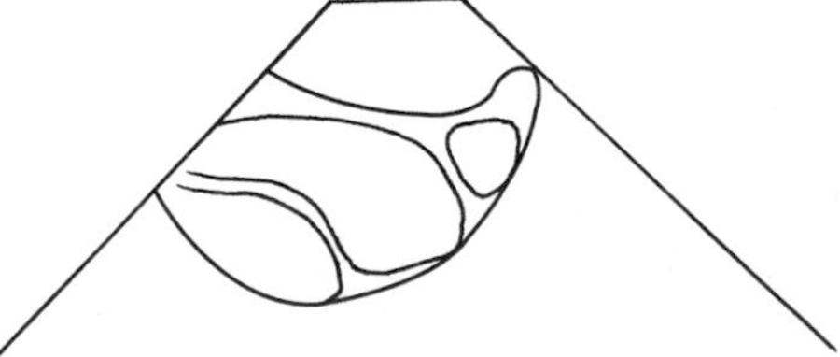

Fig. 35-11. Theca lutein cysts. Both ovaries of a patient with a hydatidiform mole were very enlarged and contained discrete cysts.

examination. However, the sonographic appearance described above and a β-hCG greater than 100,000 mIU/mL is almost always due to hydatidiform mole. The ovaries sometimes contain theca lutein cysts, which result from stimulation from the large amount of hCG produced by the mole (Fig. 35-11).

Occasionally, part of the placenta appears normal, but part resembles a mole and an abnormal fetus is present; this is termed a *partial mole* and is usually a result of *triploidy,* in which there are three sets of each chromosome. These fetuses usually have very small abdomens and abnormal central nervous systems, and almost never reach term.

Incarceration of the Uterus

Occasionally a patient with an early pregnancy will present with acute urinary retention and abdominal pain. If the patient is more than 11 weeks pregnant and the fundus is still in the pelvis with nothing palpable over the symphysis, it is possible that she has an incarcerated uterus. In this entity a sharply retroflexed uterus does not straighten out and rise into the abdomen; instead, the fundus becomes wedged on the sacrum, forcing the cervix up against the symphysis and compressing the urethra between the fundus and symphysis. This entity is seen in patients with very "tipped" or retroflexed uteri and is even more likely in patients with uterine malformations such as uterine didelphia. This diagnosis can be made clinically and confirmed by ultrasound, which shows the fundus wedged in the pelvis and the cervix immediately under the symphysis (Fig. 35-12).

Determining Fetal Age

At 11 weeks it becomes possible to measure the width of the head; this is measured from leading edge to leading edge and is known as the biparietal diameter (BPD) (Fig. 35-13). The mandible, maxilla, cranium, spine, and long bones are calcified enough to provide strong reflections of sound back to the transducer, allowing measurement of calcified bones such as the femur (Fig. 35-14). These measurements are more accurate than crown-rump length (CRL) at this age, because the fetus is curling and uncurling, making a CRL measurement variable. Measurements at 11 to 20 weeks of gestation will provide a very accurate estimate of dates, with only a slightly greater variation ($\pm$1 week) than a CRL performed at 6 to 11 weeks. In addition, it is now possible to identify some major organs: the bladder and stomach are seen as dark (echolucent) areas within the fetus. The placenta is homogeneous at this point and fluid is plentiful. If the placenta is heterogeneous or there is little fluid, referral to an obstetrician should be made.

THE SECOND 20 WEEKS OF PREGNANCY

Bleeding in Later Pregnancy

Bleeding in the first half of pregnancy is usually a variation of normal or related to failure of the pregnancy. In the late second and all of the third trimester placental causes are more common (Table 35-2).

Placenta Previa

The placenta frequently lies over the internal os in the first and second trimesters of pregnancy, but as the lower uterine segment elongates in the second and third trimesters, the edge becomes farther and farther from the uterine os. If it still covers the internal os in the third trimester, this is termed *placenta previa* (Fig. 35-15). If the margin of the placenta comes just up to, but not over, the internal os, this is termed a *marginal previa.*

If the placenta is centrally implanted so that its center is somewhere overlying the internal os, abdominal ultrasound is quite accurate. However, if the edge of the placenta appears to be just up to or over the internal os on abdominal scan, it is useful to perform a vaginal scan. Bladder filling so influences the appearance of the lower uterine segment that vaginal scanning not only gives better definition, but obviates the need for a full bladder. Transvaginal scanning will not cause additional bleeding when properly done, since usually only 2.5 to 5 centimeters of the probe are inserted and its tip is nowhere near the internal os.

Low-Lying Placenta

In the third trimester, if the edge of the placenta is within 2 centimeters of the internal os but its edge is not up to

Table 35-2. Bleeding in the Third Trimester

Placenta previa
Abruptio placentae
Vasa previa
Low-lying placenta
Polyp

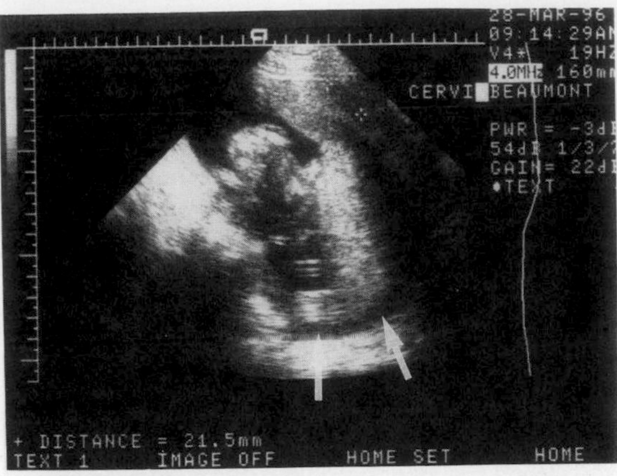

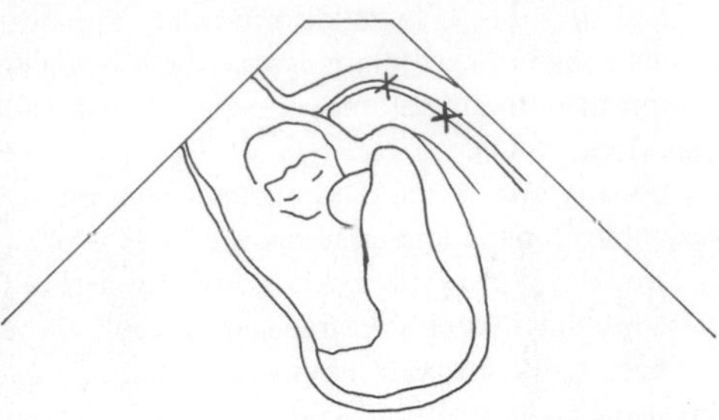

Fig. 35-12. Incarcerated uterus. The fundus (*arrows*) is trapped between the sacrum and the symphysis pubis (at the apex of this sector scan). This patient presented with acute urinary retention because the urethra (*above crosshairs on cervix*) was compressed between the symphysis and cervix.

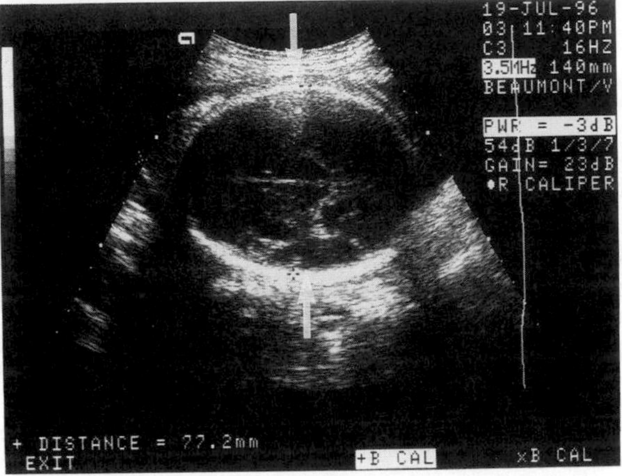

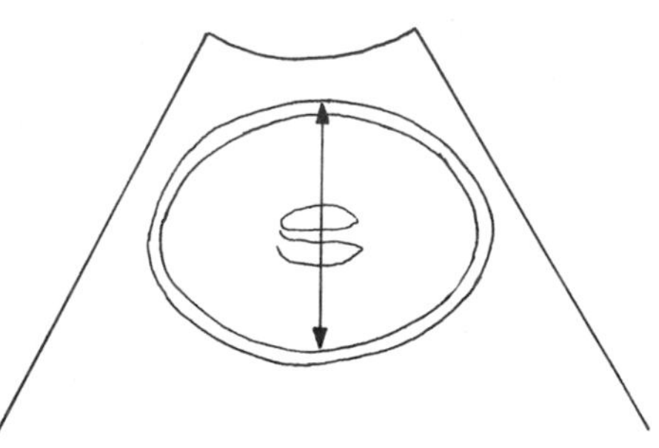

Fig. 35-13. Biparietal diameter. The measurement across the widest part of the fetal head in this axial (transverse) scan (*arrows*) is a reliable measure of gestational age from 11 weeks upward.

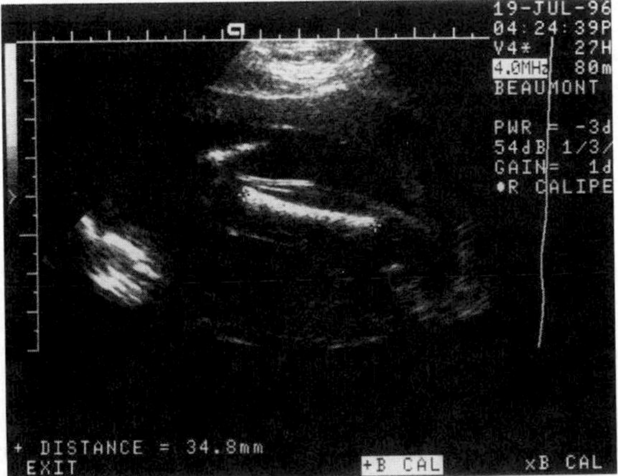

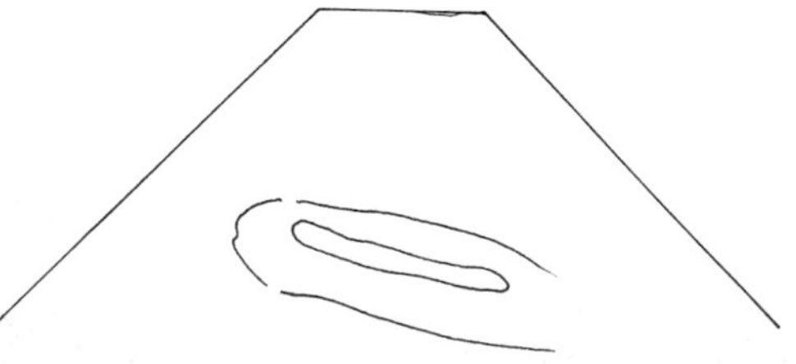

Fig. 35-14. Femur length. The measurement of the calcified part of the femur from metaphysis to lesser trochanter is also a reliable measurement of gestational age.

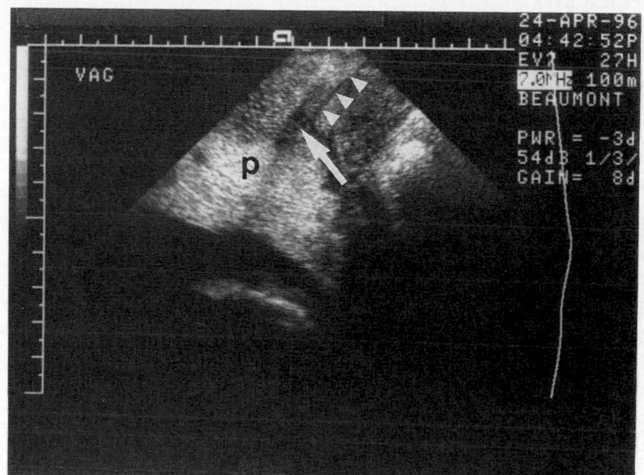

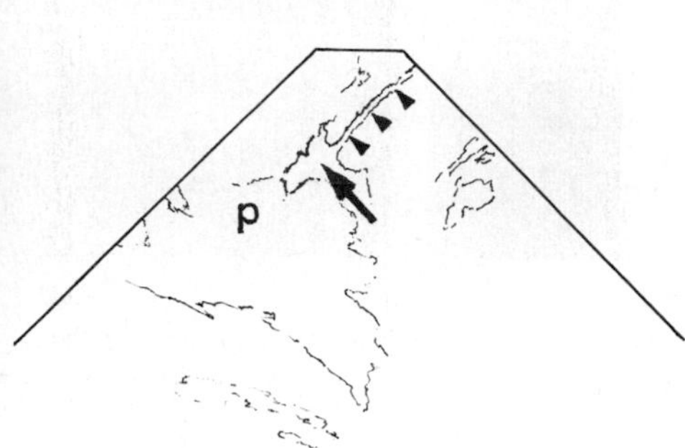

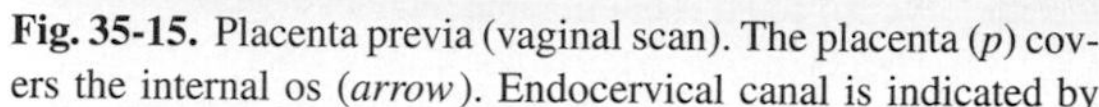
Fig. 35-15. Placenta previa (vaginal scan). The placenta (*p*) covers the internal os (*arrow*). Endocervical canal is indicated by arrowheads.

the os itself, this is termed a *low-lying* placenta. Although it is not a placenta previa, some bleeding may occur since the lower edge is not well attached.

Placental Abruption

If the patient has had a scan by a reliable source and is known to not have a placenta previa, it is not necessary to obtain a scan to exclude abruption. Abruption is a clinical diagnosis made when a patient known to not have a previa has pain, tenderness, bleeding, and uterine contractions. *Ultrasound is not a sensitive test for abruption.* These patients need continuous fetal monitoring and should not be sent to be scanned unless the value of the clinical information provided outweighs the risk of sending the patient away from a monitored bed. An abruption may appear as a collection of fluid behind the placenta or at its edge, but usually the scan is entirely normal. Occasionally a patient will have unusual pain or contractions, the source of which cannot be identified, and she will be found to have an abruption on ultrasound. In cases in which the clinical picture is not diagnostic, ultrasound may be of value.

Vasa Previa

Vasa previa describes the condition in which fetal cord vessels cross the internal os of the cervix. The vessels lead from one lobe of the placenta to the other or from the cord, which inserts into the membranes (velamentous insertion) to the placenta (Fig. 35-16). If these vessels cross the internal os, vasa previa occurs. When ruptured, those vessels may tear, allowing the fetus to quickly exsanguinate. Vasa previa is sometimes, but not always, detectable by ultrasound. Its detection depends upon the identification of vessels crossing the internal os (something which generally requires color flow doppler ultrasound). Conditions which can produce vasa previa are either an extra lobe of the placenta (succenturiate) or a velamentous insertion of the cord.[14]

Placenta Accreta

Occasionally the normal separation of the placenta and uterine wall by decidua is not present and the trophoblast of the placenta actually grows into the myometrium (placenta accreta) (Fig. 35-17) and even through it (placenta percreta) and occasionally into the bladder (Fig. 35-18). At delivery, the uterus cannot contract; continuous uncontrollable bleeding results, usually necessitating cesarean hysterectomy. Although the latter may be unavoidable, it is sometimes possible, if the condition is identified beforehand, to plan for appropriate blood replacement and cardiovascular support.

There are some clues on ultrasound that may strongly suggest placenta accreta.[15] In a patient with a previous cesarean section, the normal clear space between the placenta and uterine wall should be evaluated on any second- or third-trimester scan. If this is absent, there may be a placenta accreta. Numerous clear spaces in the placenta and increased blood flow also suggest it. The loss of bladder

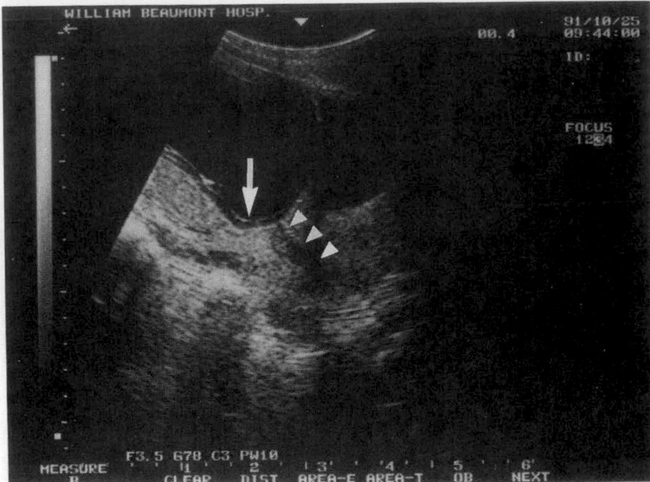

Fig. 35-16. Vasa previa. A vessel (*arrow*) traverses the area of the internal os (*cervical canal—arrowheads*) from placenta to a succenturiate lobe. Rupture of this vessel could result in rapid fetal loss.

wall definition suggests that the placenta may have grown through the bladder wall.

Abdominal Pregnancy

Occasionally a pregnancy develops outside the uterus. Its placenta implants on the bowel, abdominal wall, or mesentery. Clues are a relative lack of amniotic fluid, unusual lie (e.g., persistent transverse), and no uterine wall seen under the surface of the placenta.[16] These pregnancies can reach term.

Fibroids

Fibroids are benign overgrowths of uterine muscle that can be located in the submucosal or subserosal areas or in the wall of the uterus (intramural) (Fig. 35-19), or they may be on a pedicle either within the cavity or outside of the uterus. Not all fibroids increase in size in pregnancy. If they do, however, they are susceptible to infarction due to an insufficient blood supply. This causes exquisite site tenderness and considerable pain. The most frequent time for infarction is between 16 to 20 weeks. A good question to pose when ordering a scan in cases of abdominal pain

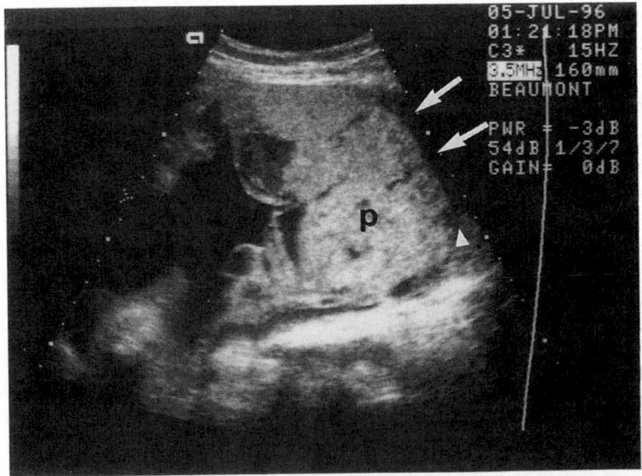

Fig. 35-17. Placenta accreta. The internal os (*arrowhead*) is covered by placenta (*p*). It contains many more lakes (*clear spaces*) than usual. The normal clear space (*arrows*) between the placenta and uterus does not extend upward.

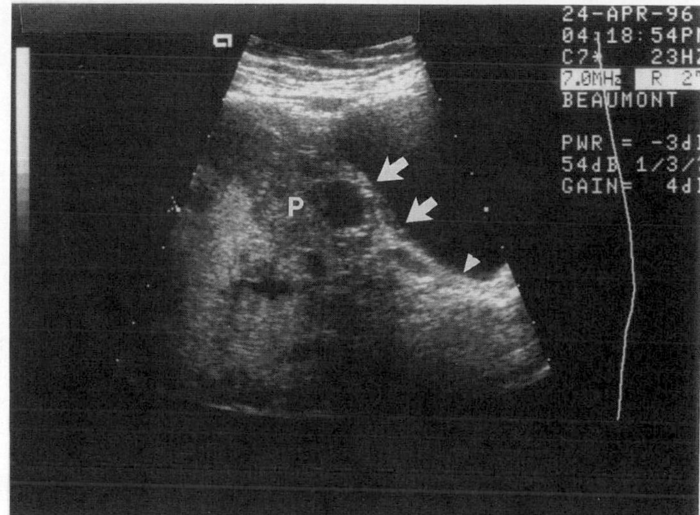

Fig. 35-18. Placenta percreta. The normal smooth white line of the bladder wall (*arrowhead*) is interrupted (*arrows*) by placenta (*p*), which has grown through it.

is whether or not the painful or tender area appears to be at the site of a fibroid.

The Ovary in Pregnancy

As the uterus enlarges, the ovaries, which are not closely attached to the pelvic side wall, but rather are tethered by ligaments, rise into the abdomen like sandbags attached to a hot-air balloon. This is one of the reasons the entire abdomen should be scanned in pregnancy; the appendix and ovaries can be located at a very high point. All of the ovarian conditions described later in the chapter can be found in pregnancy, but functional cysts are particularly common.

Fetal Size and Weight

Fetal weight can be determined by measuring the size of the head, femur, and abdomen (Fig. 35-20) and using one of several formulas to determine weight.[17] Actual fetal length cannot be determined. The accuracy of these estimates depends upon several factors, primary among

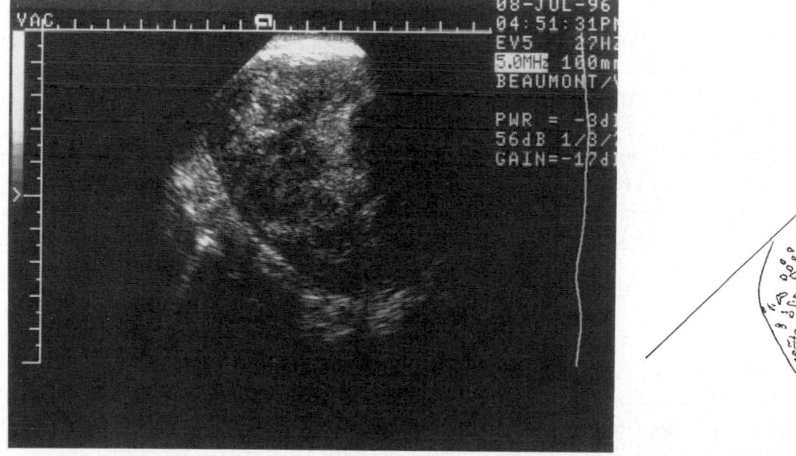

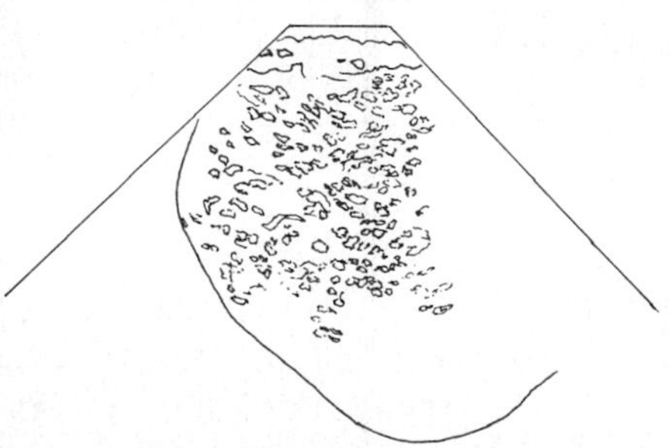

Fig. 35-19. Uterine fibroid. These usually have a whorled appearance but can occasionally mimic cysts.

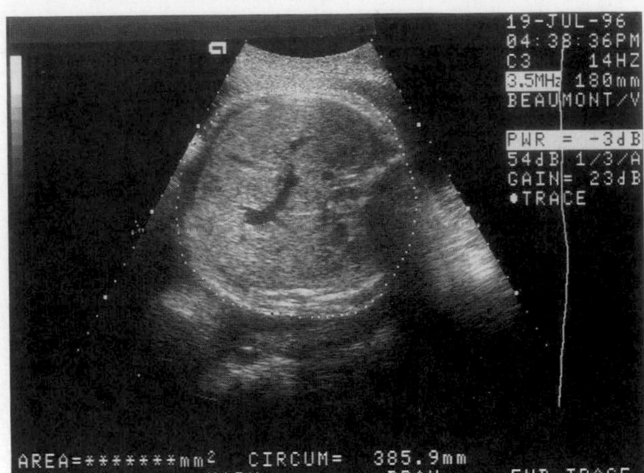

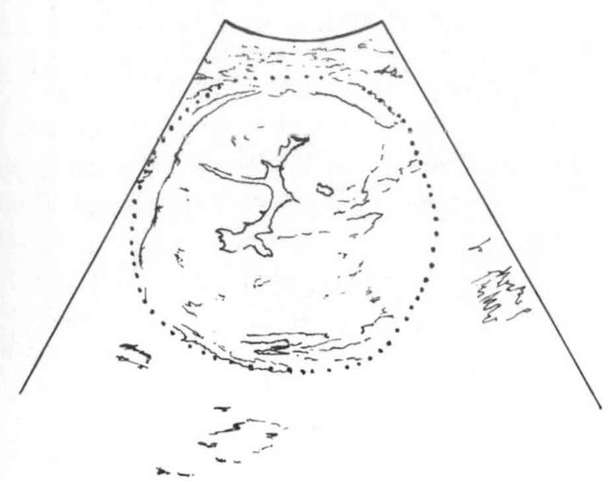

Fig. 35-20. Abdominal circumference. This measurement is traced around the skin of the fetal abdomen scanned transversely at a certain level. It reflects gestational age, liver size, and subcutaneous fat.

which is the accuracy of the measurements of the femur, abdomen, and head. There are many instances in which these cannot be obtained. The abdominal measurement is particularly difficult to obtain when the fetus is lying against the abdominal wall, is large, or there is little fluid. The estimates are more accurate in the lower weight categories and become less accurate, particularly in the 4000-g range and above.

All fetuses have similar growth patterns in early pregnancy. It is only later that they express their genetic variability (family, racial), influence of environment (social, economic status, and smoking), and influence of medical factors such as glucose intolerance and hypertension. As mentioned previously, CRL is used to express the size of a fetus until 11 weeks. Crown-rump length is quite accurate and can establish dates to within ±4 days. At 11 weeks and beyond, the usual measurements of head, femur, and abdomen are used. From that point up to about 20 weeks, fetal size predicts gestational age ±1 week. Later, as fetal size variability increases, measurements are less accurate in predicting gestational age than before 20 weeks.

Amniotic Fluid

In the second trimester, amniotic fluid is essentially fetal urine. It can be decreased for no obvious cause, because of rupture of membranes, obstruction of the fetal urinary tract, or due to decreased fetal glomerular filtration. Causes of complete absence are rupture, failed fetal kidneys (dysplasia), urinary obstruction, or more frequently, absence of fetal kidneys. The latter is incompatible with life but is a difficult diagnosis best left to experienced individuals. Rupture of membranes is a known complication of genetic amniocentesis, fortunately with usual re-accumulation of fluid and a good outcome. It is also related to chorioamnionitis.

Multiple Gestations

Ultrasound is very important in identifying multiple pregnancies and following growth, because in these instances the tape measure fails us and does not reflect what is occurring in the uterus. Twins normally follow along singleton growth curves. In the older literature, there was frequent mention of growth discordance or a size difference between twins. This has given way to an evaluation of each twin's growth potential and growth between exams (Fig. 35-21). In fraternal (dichorionic) twins, particularly of different sexes, there may be significant size differences at each point, but neither should drop below the tenth percentile in weight at any time. Besides evaluation of the growth of twins, it is imperative to establish amnionicity as early as possible. At the first exam, amnionicity should be established without a doubt and the presence or absence of a dividing membrane should be documented (Fig. 35-22). If no dividing membrane is seen on an exam by an experienced operator and there is no great disparity of size, the twins are probably *monoamniotic* and the pregnancy will need special care.

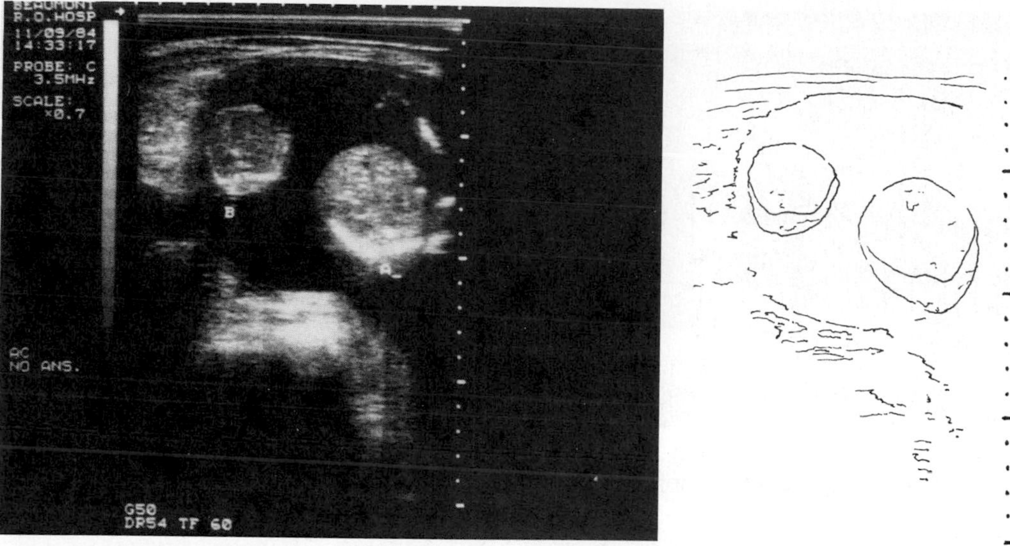

Fig. 35-21. Growth restriction of one twin. Transverse scans through both abdomens show that twin B is markedly smaller than twin A (which has grown at a normal rate).

Sometimes the placentas appear to be one but are actually just fused. Placental tissue between these placentas will indicate that they are actually dichorionic (Fig. 35-22).

It twins are facing each other and are in the same presentation (e.g., vertex-vertex), it is important to make sure they are completely separated. Conjoined twins are an obstetric as well as a pediatric problem (Fig. 35-23).

Fetal Cardiac Arrhythmias

Both auscultation with a stethoscope and Doppler devices detect the fetal ventricular cardiac rate which should be between 120 to 180 bpm. Does a heart rate of 80 beats per minute mean that the fetus 24 weeks or more is in distress? Not necessarily. If a slow heart rate is heard with a Doppler device, stethoscope auscultation will often detect the true fetal rate and show that the slow rate detected with

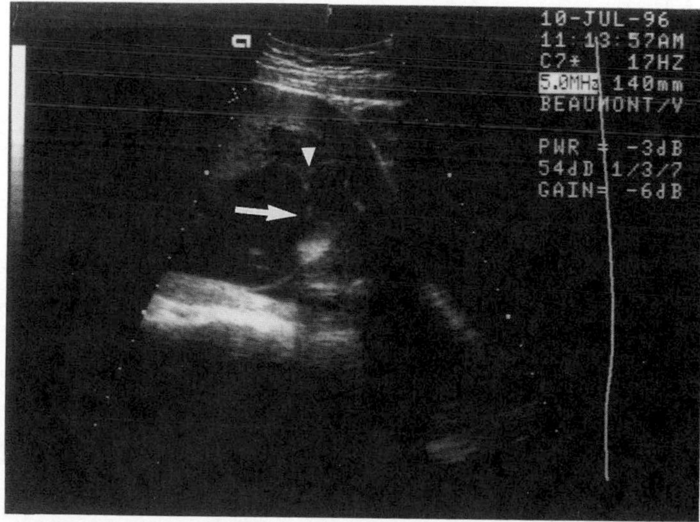

Fig. 35-22. Twins—dividing membrane (*arrow*). This should be documented early, since management will be changed if it is not present. In monochorionic (identical) twins, it will contain two layers; in dichorionic twins, four layers. A placental peak (*arrowhead*) reliably establishes dichorionicity in this pregnancy.

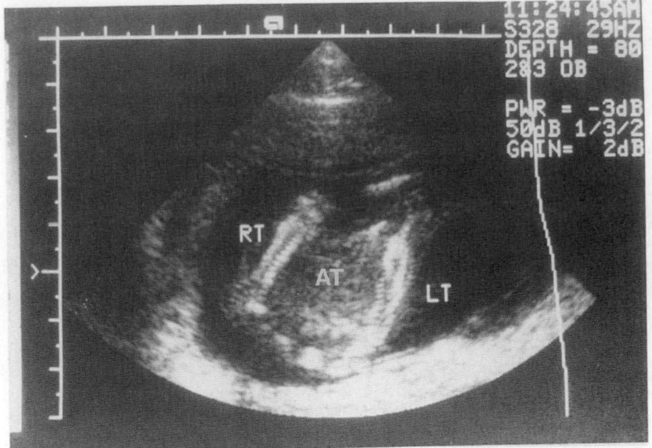

Fig. 35-23. Conjoined twins. The spines of these conjoined twins are echogenic (*white*). They are facing each other and joined by a common abdomen and thorax (*AT*).

Doppler was that of the mother's aorta. The reason for this is that anything in the path of the ultrasound beam will be reflected back to the transducer, including the maternal aorta.

If a normal rate cannot be detected, real-time ultrasound should be used to find the fetal heart. If the fetal heart is truly beating at 80 beats per minute, there may be normal slowing and speeding up of the fetal heart when the mother is in the recumbent position (only before 30 weeks). Turning the mother on her side or supporting the transducer's weight with the operator's hand will usually result in a rapid return to normal sinus rhythm. An alternative possibility is that there is fetal heart block due to antibodies to the fetal conducting system, as found in lupus, or to disruption of the conduction system by severe structural anomalies. Heart block can be distinguished by M-mode scanning; the atrial rate will be normal but the ventricular rate will be disparate and invariably slower (Fig. 35-24). Fetal bradycardia is usually constant or disappears and returns with the next contraction. A rate of over 200 beats per minute may reflect supraventricular tachycardia, in which the atrium is beating at that rate; the ventricular rate may be the same or, if the heart has trouble conducting from the atrium to the ventricle at this fast rate, some

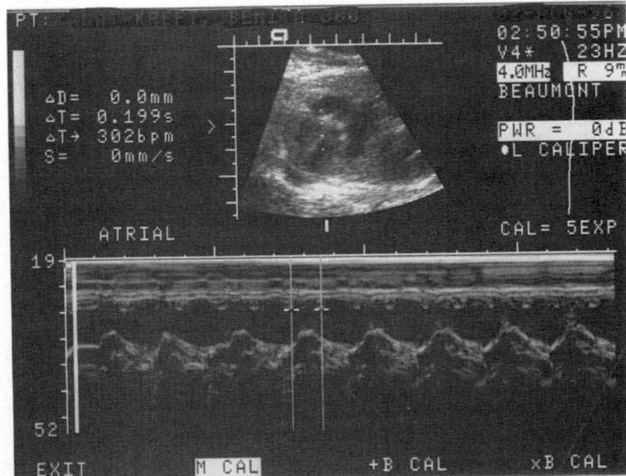

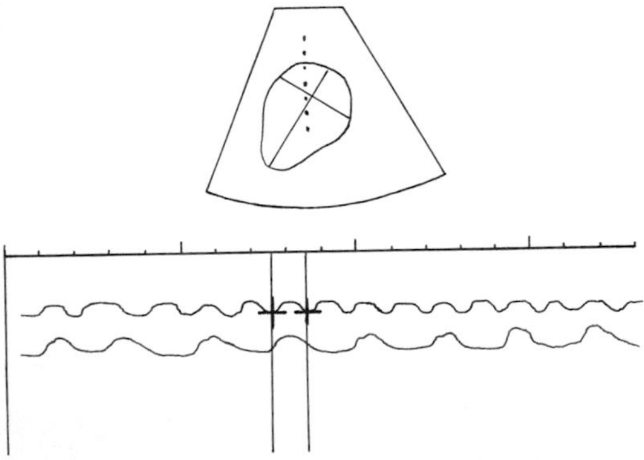

Fig. 35-24. A B-mode image of the fetal heart is at the top. The dotted line through it defines the line along which the M-mode (*bottom*) image will be produced. The M-mode shows rapid motion (302 beats per minute) of the atrial wall (one cycle is between the cursors) and a ventricular rate of 150 beats per minute. This is supraventricular tachycardia with a 2:1 block. It may be auscultated as an irregular heartbeat as the degree of block changes.

beats may be dropped and a slow or irregular ventricle rate will be heard.

ULTRASONOGRAPHY OF GYNECOLOGIC DISORDERS

An emergency setting in gynecology almost always involves pain or profuse bleeding. Before working up a patient for the usual causes of pelvic pain, it must be remembered that *a woman of reproductive age is considered pregnant until proven otherwise* (despite a history of regular menses, tubal ligation, or even of "no intercourse ever, at all"). There are many causes of pelvic pain in the pregnant woman, the most threatening of which is an ectopic pregnancy (Table 35-3). As in the pregnant patient, in the nonpregnant woman the differential diagnosis revolves around all the organs of the pelvis—not just the uterus and ovaries, but also the bowel and urinary system.

Ultrasound is not a substitute for a pelvic exam. A thorough history and physical exam, including a pelvic exam, will help interpret the results of the pelvic ultrasound. Has the patient had a history of endometriosis? Renal stones? Has the patient ever menstruated at all? Has she ever had an ultrasound exam of the pelvis, and if so what did it show?

Ultrasound of a pelvic mass may be nonspecific unless the mass has very unique ultrasound characteristics. Benign masses have thin exterior walls, no septae or thin, smooth septae and little if any solid material within them. Doppler of supplying arteries occasionally can aid in the differentiation of benign and malignant masses, but is by no means foolproof. It is based upon the fact that there is little resistance to flow in tumor vessels because they contain no smooth muscles in their walls.

There are some artifacts and pitfalls in pelvic ultrasound that can lead to the discovery of a normal pelvis at laparotomy or laparoscopy. The usual problem is that bowel can simulate or hide a mass. In addition, in some institutions, only a pelvic scan is performed when ultrasound of the pelvis is ordered. With a proper history and physical, it may be appropriate to extend that exam to the appendix, kidneys, and even the gallbladder.

Table 35-3. Pelvic Pain in Early Pregnancy

Failing IUP (contractions)
Ectopic pregnancy
Ovarian cyst—torsion, rupture, pressure
Incarceration of the uterus
Stretching of the round ligament
Ureteral stones
Appendicitis

The pelvic scan is not complete unless the uterus, ovaries, and cul-de-sac are visualized. This is usually accomplished first by abdominal scan with a partially filled bladder and then, when necessary, by a transvaginal scan after the bladder is emptied. As in all imaging, "the most commonly missed abnormality is the second"; an ovarian mass or enlarged uterus may not be the reason for the patient's pain.

Intrauterine Devices

There are occasions when an ultrasound examination is necessary to find an intrauterine device (IUD). Usually this occurs when the string is not visible. Because IUDs are reflective, they can usually be located with ultrasound (Fig. 35-25), unless they are outside the uterus. Whether or not they are entirely in the uterine cavity or partially embedded in the uterine wall can often be determined by ultrasound. If they are not visible in the uterus, a plain film of the pelvis will reveal whether or not the IUD is in the body at all or has been expelled.

Functional Cysts

The term *functional cysts* refers to enlarged follicles or corpora luteia. The ultrasound appearance is usually that of a cyst completely filled with clear or nonechoic fluid (Fig. 35-26). However, bleeding into this cyst may produce some solid material, which can then mimic cysts of different origin. These cysts have smooth, thin walls if any internal septations are present. Pain occurs when they are very large, have internal bleeding, have ruptured, or have caused torsion of the ovary. Considerable bleeding can occur upon rupture.

Ovarian Remnant

Occasionally, when an ovary is removed, a microscopic part of it is left behind, particularly if there were intraabdominal adhesions. This tiny piece of ovary, often invisible to the human eye, can produce functional cysts and resulting pain (Fig. 35-27). These can produce a confusing clinical picture in the patient who claims to have had an oophorectomy.

Mucinous Cystadenomas

These benign masses are the largest of the ovarian neoplasms. They can grow so large that they occupy most of the abdomen, making the patient look pregnant. They

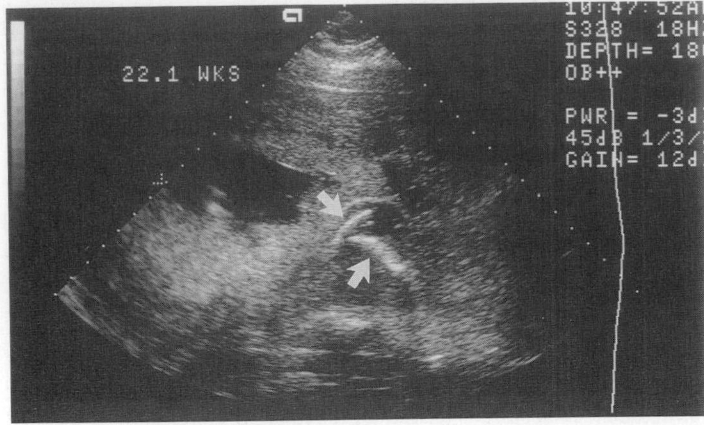

Fig. 35-25. Intrauterine device. A copper 7 IUD (*arrows*) lies below an intrauterine pregnancy (the cervix lies to the right).

are filled with a mucinous material that produces an ultrasound picture of many small white dots (Fig. 35-28). They have little if any solid material within.

Serous Cystadenomas

These contain serous fluid and are generally not as large as mucinous cystadenomas. The more septations they have, the thicker the wall and the more solid material they contain, the more likely it is that they are malignant (serous cystadenocarcinoma).

Endometriomas

These ovarian masses are lined with endometrium-like tissue (uterine gland tissue) and contain old blood, hence the name *chocolate cysts*. They are found in patients with a history of endometriosis. Their ultrasound appearance is quite variable, but normally they appear almost semisolid with considerable echoic material within them (Fig. 35-29). Although endometrial tissue can be implanted on any of the surfaces of the pelvis, usually only those contained in the ovary are visible on ultrasound.

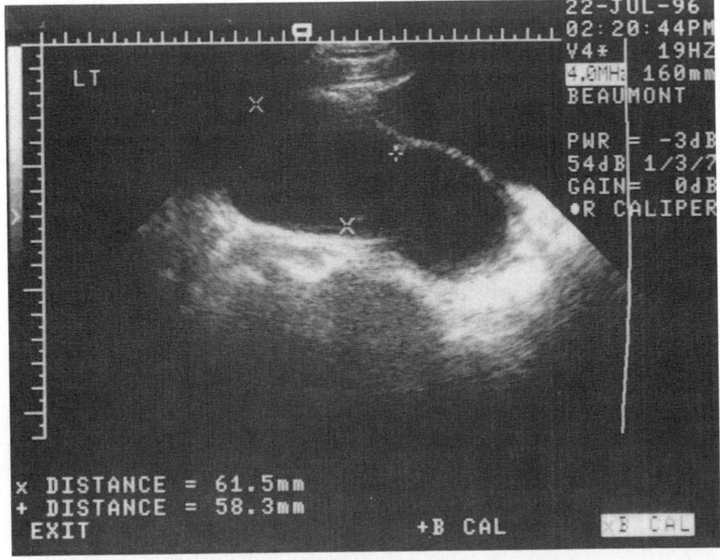

Fig. 35-26. Functional cysts. Two follicular cysts are shown here. Note the lack of internal material or septations.

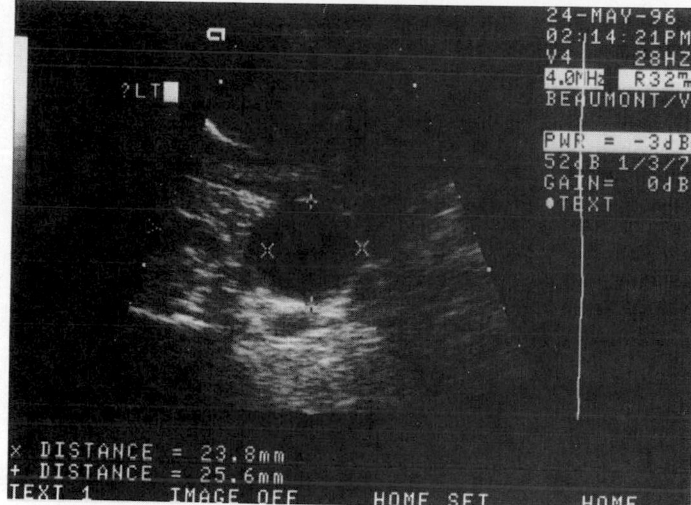

Fig. 35-27. Ovarian remnant. A functional cyst has formed in a microscopic ovarian remnant left behind after removal of an ovary.

Dermoids

Other than functional cysts, these are the most common ovarian masses in the younger woman. They contain elements of fat, cartilage, teeth, and hair, which give a very characteristic appearance: hair and fat provide a strong acoustic interface that strongly reflects sound (Fig. 35-30). Fat may layer out on surrounding fluid. Calcified areas produce a sound shadow behind them by reflecting sound completely. Dermoids may be the cause of ovarian torsion in younger women, a condition that produces severe pain and occasionally an acute abdomen. If present, the contained teeth can be seen on a plain film of the pelvis. Occasionally these tumors are a part of a complex ovarian mass.

Torsion of an Ovary

The ovary is a rather loosely tethered structure. The most striking example of this mobility is its frequent location in pregnancy above the uterus. When an ovary enlarges (due to dermoid, corpus luteum, or any of the previous dis-

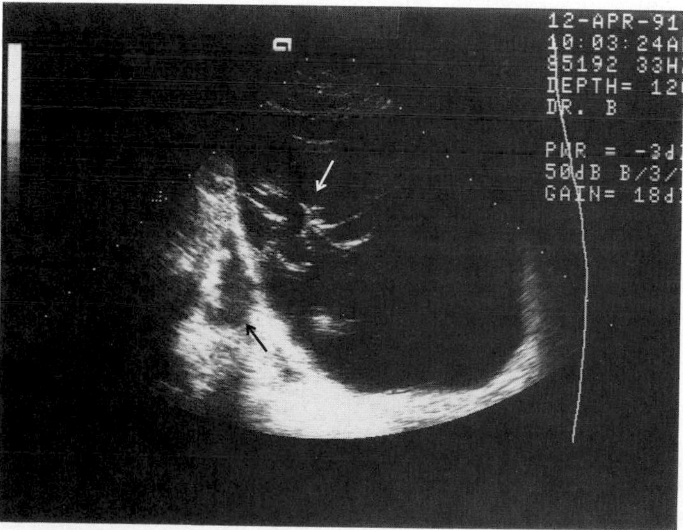

Fig. 35-28. Mucinous cystadenoma. This large mass (*black arrow*) contains faintly echogenic material and "daughter cysts" (*white arrow*).

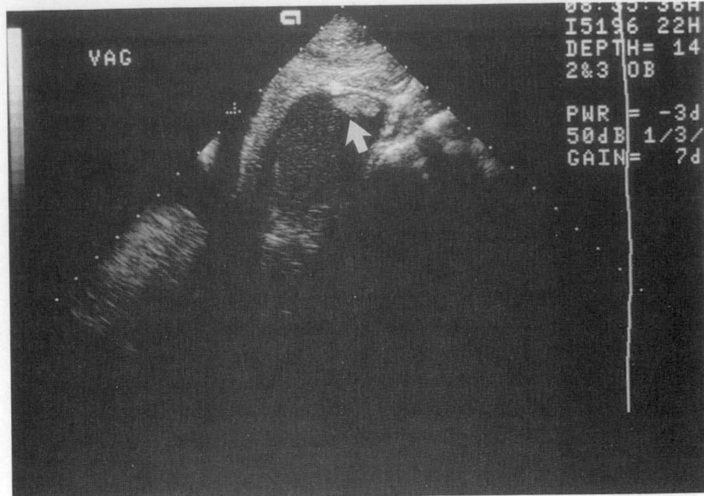

Fig. 35-29. Endometrioma. The content (old blood) is quite echogenic, giving a "salt and pepper" appearance. There is a small amount of solid material (*arrow*).

cussed ovarian masses), its weight may cause its pedicle to turn and torse. Acute pain is the result. The adnexa on the affected side are tender and there are usually signs of peritoneal irritation. Occasionally there is free peritoneal fluid. Like abruption in pregnancy, this is a diagnosis best made clinically since the ultrasound findings are usually not specific. A very experienced examiner may be able to show impeded or no arterial and venous flow along the ovarian and/or infundibulopelvic ligaments. However presence of normal flow does not rule out the diagnosis of adnexal torsion. Most importantly, the same symptoms can be produced by an ectopic pregnancy or fibroid in pregnancy, and therefore it is important to remember the maxim that *any woman of reproductive age is pregnant until proven otherwise.*

Uterine Anomalies

Rarely, there can be a blind horn of a uterus that acts like an endometrioma. The patient experiences severe pain during menses and can present with a tender pelvic mass. A careful ultrasound examination will show that the mass is separate from the ovary on that side. Alternatively, there may be a high vaginal septum that impedes the exit of

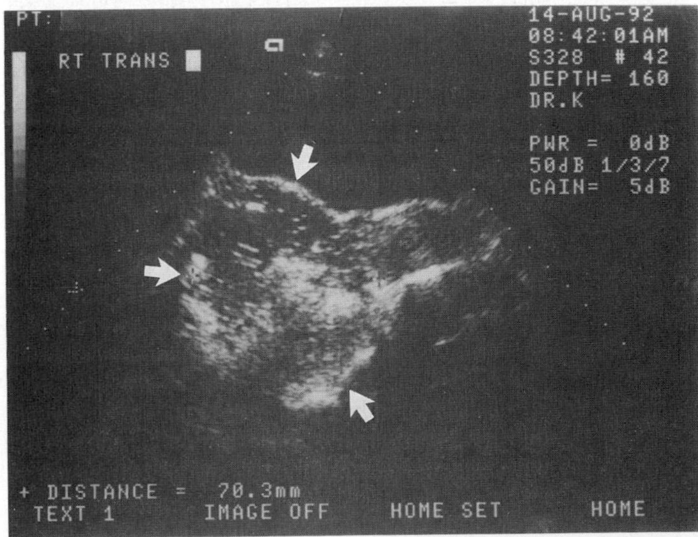

Fig. 35-30. Dermoid. A mass of fat and hair produce heterogeneously echogenic areas in this dermoid (*arrows*).

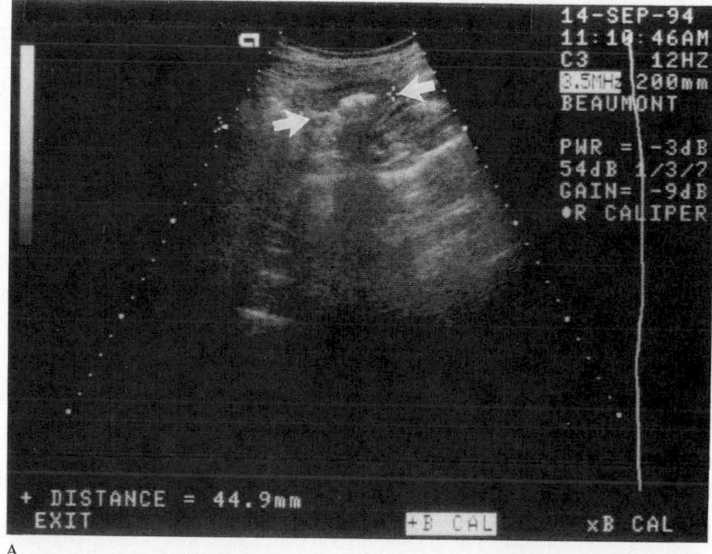

A

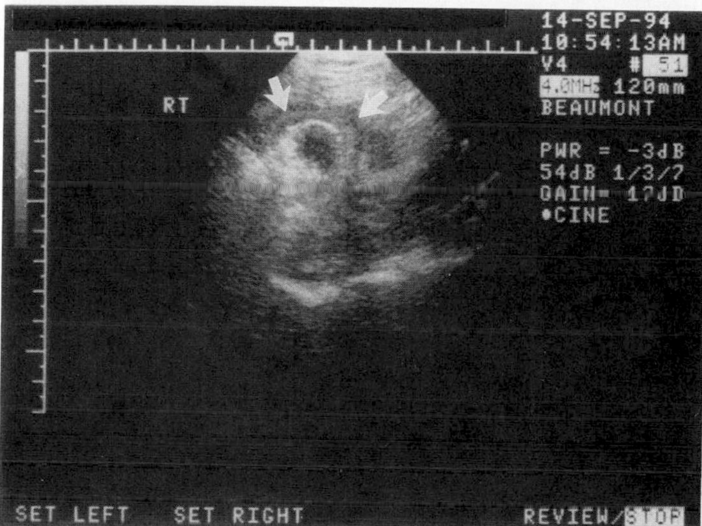

B

Fig. 35-31. Appendicitis. *A*. The length of the appendix is bracketed by arrows. Note the linear echo within the appendix. *B*. The appendix wall (*arrows*) is thickened and the interior contains an echogenic ring. This appearance can be mimicked by an inflamed fallopian tube.

menstrual flow or normal mucus, causing the uterus to become larger and larger. Again, physical examination and history are key, since an ultrasound examination may be confusing.

Fibroids may be single or multiple and are usually easily identified by ultrasound (see Fig. 35-19).

Nongynecologic Causes of Pelvic Pain

Conditions such as appendicitis, diverticulitis, a pelvic kidney, or a ureterovesical stone may cause acute pelvic pain, simulating pain from a gynecologic source. Again, careful bimanual and abdominal examinations will usually point to the correct diagnosis. If the bimanual examination is unrevealing, a pelvic ultrasound may be of help. Its first use is to show a normal uterus and ovaries and no free intraperitoneal fluid. After looking at the uterus and ovaries, it is useful to determine if there is unilateral hydronephrosis. If the pain is in the midline or to the right of midline, an attempt should be made to visualize the appendix. When the appendix is inflamed and swollen, its wall is thickened and echoic areas may be seen within it (air or a fecalith) (Fig. 35-31 *A* and *B*). Diverticulitis may produce a mass as well, but again, it will be separate from the ovaries. It is important to inspect a pelvic ultrasound report for identification of the ovaries and to ask whether a described mass could be definitely seen to be separate from the ovaries.

REFERENCES

1. Keith SC, London SN, Weitzman GA, et al: Serial transvaginal ultrasound scans and β-human chorionic gonadotropin levels in early singleton and multiple pregnancies. *Fertil Steril* 59:1007, 1993.
2. Kadar N, Bohrer M, Kemmann E, et al: The discriminatory human chorionic gonadotropin zone for endovaginal sonography: a prospective randomized study. *Fertil Steril* 61:1016–1020, 1994.
3. Cacciatore B, Stenman U, Ylostalo P: Diagnosis of ectopic pregnancy by vaginal ultrasonography in combination with a discriminatory serum hCG level of 1000 IU/L (IRP). *Brit J Obstet Gynecol* 97:904–908, 1990.
4. Dart R, Kaplan B, Ortiz L: Normal intrauterine pregnancy is unlikely in emergency department patients with either menstrual days >38 days or β-hCG >3,000, but without a gestational sac on ultrasonography. *Acad Emerg Med* 4:967–971, 1997.
5. Cacciatore B: Can the status of tubal pregnancy be predicted with transvaginal sonography? A prospective comparison of sonographic, surgical, and serum HCG findings. *Genitourin Radiol* 177:481, 1990.
6. Frates MC, Laing FC: Sonographic evaluation of ectopic pregnancy: An update. *AJR* 165:251, 1995.
7. Braffman BH, Coleman BG, Ramchandani P, et al: Emergency department screening for ectopic pregnancy: A prospective U.S. study. *Genitourin Radiol* 190:797, 1994.
8. Blaivas M, Sierzenski P, Plecque D, et al: Do emergency physicians save time when locating a live intrauterine pregnancy with bedside ultrasonography? *Acad Emerg Med* 7:988, 2000.
9. Burgher SW, Tandy TK, Dawdy MR: Transvaginal ultrasonography by emergency physicians decreases patient time in the emergency department. *Acad Emerg Med* 5:802, 1998.
10. Shih CH: Effect of emergency physician-performed pelvic sonography on length of stay in the emergency department. *Ann Emerg Med* 29:348, 1997.
11. Nyberg DA, Hughes MP, Mack LA, Wang KY: Extrauterine findings of ectopic pregnancy of transvaginal US: Importance of echogenic fluid. *Radiology* 178:823, 1991.
12. Ackerman TE, Levi CS, Dashefsky SM, et al: Interstitial line: Sonographic finding in interstitial (cornual) ectopic pregnancy. *Radiology* 189:83, 1993.
13. Dewitt C, Abbott J: "Interstitial pregnancy: A potential for misdiagnosis with emergency department ultrasonography." *Ann Emerg Med* 40:106–109, 2002.
14. Gianupoulo SJ, Carver T, Tomich PG, et al: Diagnosis of vasa previa with ultrasonography. *Obstet Gynecol* 769:488, 1987.
15. Finberg HJ, Williams JW: Placenta accreta: Prospective sonographic diagnosis in patients with placenta previa and prior cesarean section. *J Ultrasound Med* 11:333, 1992.
16. Hallatt JG, Grove JA: Abdominal pregnancy: a study of twenty-one consecutive cases. *Am J Obstet Gynecol* 152: 444, 1985.
17. Hadlock FP, Harrist RB, Carpenter RJ, et al: Sonographic estimation of fetal weight. *Radiology* 150:535, 1984.

36

Non-Sexually Transmitted Gynecologic Infections: Urinary Tract Infections and Toxic Shock Syndromes

Brian Tiffany

KEY POINTS

- Given that resistance to trimethoprim-sulfamethoxazole (TMP-SMX) in *E. coli* isolates is in excess of 20 percent in some studies,[13] a fluoroquinolone should be the first choice for empiric therapy for all nonpregnant adult women with urinary tract infections (UTIs). In areas where local resistance rates are <10 percent, TMP-SMX is a less costly choice.
- Pyelonephritis is diagnosed by findings consistent with cystitis, with the addition of fever, chills, and either flank pain or costovertebral angle tenderness, often associated with nausea and vomiting. In patients with this diagnosis, a urine culture should be routinely done, but blood cultures are unnecessary.
- Between 2 and 10 percent of pregnancies are complicated by UTIs; left untreated more than 1/4 of these women will develop pyelonephritis with associated morbidities.
- The characteristic rash of staphylococcal toxic shock syndrome (TSS) is a blanching, nonpruritic, macular eruption that has a sunburn-like appearance, a key feature of the disease, and its best diagnostic clue.
- Streptococcal TSS patients frequently present with localized pain out of proportion to examination findings, with a localized area of soft-tissue infection (80 percent) or febrile flu-like illness (20 percent), and are likely to be normotensive at presentation (50 percent). However, most will drop their blood pressure significantly over 4 to 8 hours of observation and require emergent surgical exploration.

INTRODUCTION

This chapter focuses on two main types of infections that affect females: the spectrum of severity of urinary tract infections and toxic shock syndromes. Both of these can occur during pregnancy, but the focus here is on nonpregnant women with these illnesses.

URINARY TRACT INFECTIONS

Epidemiology

Infections of the urinary tract (UTIs) are a major cause of morbidity and health care expenditures. Sexually active young women are disproportionately affected, but these infections may occur in men and women of all ages.

Because UTIs are so common and many go untreated, it is somewhat difficult to estimate the number of infections that occur annually. Self-reporting surveys have found between 40 and 60 percent of all women experience at least one UTI during their lives.[1,2] Office practice surveys and review of hospital admissions suggest that there are approximately 7 million episodes of acute cystitis and 250,000 cases of pyelonephritis each year in the U.S.[3,4] A random-digit dialing survey of women greater than 18 years of age found a 10.8 percent annual incidence of physician-diagnosed UTI, leading to an estimate of 11.3 million cases per year.[2] A survey of sexually active college age women in Seattle found an incidence of 0.7 episodes per person-year, while a similar study in an HMO population found an incidence of 0.5 episodes per person-year.[5] Given that some 50,000,000 women reported being sexually active,[6] these incidence numbers would suggest that many more millions of cases occur each year than the office- and hospital-based surveys demonstrate.

Morbidity from UTI is considerable. Foxman and Frerichs found that the average UTI episode in a woman was associated with 6.1 days of symptoms, 1.2 lost work days, and 0.4 bed days.[7] The total cost of outpatient evaluation and treatment has been estimated at between 1 and 2 billion dollars per year in the United States.[2,8]

Table 36-1. The Spectrum of Acute UTI in Non–Pregnant Women

Diagnosis	Clinical Manifestations	Diagnostic Test	Therapy
Uncomplicated cystitis	Dysuria, frequency, hematuria, urgency, in patient without comorbidities or an indwelling catheter	Empiric vs. urinalysis	Ciprofloxacin 250 mg PO every 12 hours for 3 days **or** Levofloxacin 250 mg PO daily for 3 days
Uncomplicated pyelonephritis	Cystitis, with the addition of fever, chills, and either flank pain or costovertebral angle tenderness, often associated with nausea and vomiting	Urinalysis, urine culture/sensitivities	Ciprofloxacin 400/500 mg IV/PO every 12 hours for 10–14 days **or** Levofloxacin 250 mg IV/PO daily for 10–14 days
Complicated UTI	Host factors such as functional, structural, or metabolic abnormalities of the urinary tract, or a UTI caused by resistant organisms	Urinalysis, urine culture/sensitivities	Ceftriaxone 1–2 g IV every 12–24 hours **or** Ampicillin 1 g IV every 4–6 hours **and** gentamicin 5 mg/kg IV every 24 hours **or** Imipenem 500 mg IV every 6 hours **or** Levofloxacin 500 mg IV/PO daily for 10–14 days **or** Ciprofloxacin 400/500 mg IV/PO every 12 hours for 10–14 days

Classification

The most important classification distinction to be made is between complicated and uncomplicated UTI. Complicated infections are those that occur in a patient who has a functionally, metabolically, or anatomically abnormal urinary tract, or are caused by pathogens that have unusual resistance patterns. Using this distinction, UTI in adult women can be broadly classified as uncomplicated cystitis, recurrent cystitis, uncomplicated pyelonephritis, complicated UTI, and asymptomatic bacteriuria in pregnancy. While this classification has some artificial divisions of what is a continuous spectrum of disease, the microbiology and pathophysiology of these infections are sufficiently different to make these distinctions clinically useful in making diagnostic and therapeutic choices in the emergency department setting (Table 36-1).

Acute Uncomplicated Cystitis

The overwhelming majority of urinary tract infections fall into the category of uncomplicated cystitis. In the population of young women presenting with the classic symptoms of dysuria, frequency, urgency, and/or hematuria, the incidence of structural abnormalities is less than 1 percent, so a work-up for such problems is unwarranted.[9]

A remarkably narrow spectrum of pathogens with predictable antimicrobial susceptibility profiles cause cystitis in young women. *Escherichia coli* is by far the most common organism isolated, comprising 70 to 95 percent of all cases. *Staphylococcus saprophyticus* accounts for 5 to 20 percent, and *Proteus* spp., *Klebsiella* spp., and enterococci each make up 1 to 2 percent of cases.[10]

Diagnosis

The classic criteria for diagnosing UTI, a quantitative urine culture with greater than 100,000 colony-forming units (CFU) per milliliter of urine, has been shown to miss symptomatic UTI in as many as $^{1}/_{3}$ of women.[11,12] Given this fact and the predictable spectrum of pathogens, routine urine culture is no longer advocated for uncomplicated cystitis. Confirmation of clinically suspected cases is accomplished by confirming pyuria, either by means of a traditional urinalysis and/or a dipstick test for leukocyte esterase, or by confirming bacteriuria with a dipstick test for nitrite.

Leukocyte esterase has a reported sensitivity of 75 to 90 percent in detecting pyuria associated with a UTI. Most coliform bacteria reduce nitrate to nitrite, and therefore produce a positive dipstick test for nitrite. However, the enterococci, *S. saprophyticus,* and *Acinetobacter* spp. do not and will therefore yield false negative results.

Management

Because of increasing resistance to trimethoprim-sulfamethoxazole (TMP-SMX) in *E. coli* isolates, in excess of 20 percent in some studies,[13] this longtime mainstay of therapy is no longer recommended as a first-line agent for empiric use. If significant resistance is present in local *E. coli* isolates, then a fluoroquinolone should be the first choice for empiric therapy in nonpregnant women. Where local resistance rates are <10 percent, TMP-SMX remains a less costly choice.

Nitrofurantoin, in general, provides a lower eradication rate than TMP-SMX in head-to-head trials. Because of limited literature on 3-day regimens, nitrofurantoin treatment for uncomplicated cystitis should be for 7 days. Its most important role is in the treatment of asymptomatic bacteriuria and cystitis during pregnancy. The β-lactam antibiotics consistently result in lower eradication and higher recurrence rates in head-to-head studies against fluoroquinolones and TMP-SMX.

Multiple studies have shown that 3 days of treatment with TMP-SMX is equivalent to 7 or 10 days of such treatment, with the trade-off of increased rates of recurrence with the 3-day regimen and a higher rate of adverse effects with the 7- and 10-day courses of therapy.[14] Few head-to-head comparisons of TMP-SMX and fluoroquinolones have been done at the same duration of therapy; those that exist show similar eradication rates at 3 days and similar recurrence rates.

Single-dose treatment is attractive because of improved compliance and a lower likelihood of selecting resistant strains. Unfortunately, single-dose therapy with TMP-SMX is associated with lower bacterial eradication rates and a higher incidence of recurrent infections. Single-dose regimens with the fluoroquinolones appear to be more promising, but an insufficient body of evidence exists to recommend this treatment strategy.

Acute Uncomplicated Pyelonephritis

Pyelonephritis is diagnosed by findings consistent with cystitis, with the addition of fever, chills, and either flank pain or costovertebral angle tenderness. It is often associated with nausea and vomiting. In patients with this diagnosis, a urine culture should routinely be done. While blood cultures are positive in up to 25 percent of cases, there is no association with increased morbidity. Thus there is no need for routine blood cultures in these patients.

Routine work-up for obstruction is not necessary. Risk factors for obstruction include symptoms >48 hours, pyelonephritis in the elderly, and diabetic patients. Imaging should be considered if obstruction is felt to be a clinically significant possibility.

Management

The Infectious Disease Society of America (IDSA) treatment guidelines divide patients into those with mild symptoms, in whom a trial of outpatient therapy is appropriate, and moderately or severely ill patients, who require a course of intravenous antibiotics.[15] Clinical judgement makes the distinction between these two categories, considering factors such as ability to tolerate oral antibiotics and maintain good hydration, evidence of sepsis, and likelihood of compliance. Many patients who appear quite ill on presentation can benefit from a few hours of hydration and observation, allowing a reasonable trial of outpatient management.

Due the increasing prevalence of resistance to TMP-SMX in pyelonephritis isolates (18 percent in 1996 in a Seattle study[13]), IDSA guidelines recommend empiric treatment with a fluoroquinolone as first-line therapy. If sensitivities are known, use the least expensive agent to which the bacterial isolate is sensitive. Historically, pyelonephritis was treated with up to 6 weeks of antibiotics. Numerous studies have proven that 2 weeks of therapy provides an equivalent cure rate to 6 weeks.[16] It is well accepted that 10 to 14 days of therapy is adequate in uncomplicated patients. There is controversy as to whether a shorter course of 5 to 7 days is acceptable, with results of well-designed randomized trials endorsing both sides of the question.[17,18] While the conservative approach would be to treat for a minimum of 10 days, a large, randomized, double-blind trial demonstrated a higher clinical and bacteriologic cure rate for a 7-day course of ciprofloxacin than for 14 days of TMP-SMX.[19]

Pyelonephritis in Pregnancy

Pyelonephritis in the pregnant patient deserves special mention. This diagnosis is associated with an increased incidence of low birth weight infants and prematurity, and an increased risk of perinatal morbidity. There is also an increased incidence of maternal sepsis with multisystem involvement and acute respiratory distress syndrome. Management of these patients therefore mandates obstetric consultation and admission. Recommended antibiotic therapy includes ampicillin plus an aminoglycoside, aztreonam, cefazolin, or TMP-SMX (but not in the third trimester). Due to the increasing incidence of ampicillin resistance, it should not be used as single-agent therapy in this patient population, and the choice of antibiotics for empiric therapy must be guided by knowledge of local resistance patterns. Fluoroquinolones are contraindicated during pregnancy.

Recurrent Cystitis

Recurrent cystitis, in which the patient is reinfected by a new exogenous strain of bacteria, must be distinguished from a relapse of the original infection. Because emergency physicians rarely have consistent follow-up, making this diagnosis requires a careful history.

If this diagnosis is suspected, urine culture is essential to guide therapy and follow-up. Most authors recommend empiric therapy with a fluoroquinolone. Recurrent UTI with the same strain of bacteria in spite of appropriate therapy indicates a need for urologic work-up to look for structural abnormalities. Nonstructural risk factors for recurrent UTI include sexually active women who use spermicides and diaphragms for contraception and postmenopausal women with low estrogen states.[20]

Complicated Urinary Tract Infections

Complicated UTIs are defined by UTI in the presence of host factors such as functional, structural, or metabolic abnormalities of the urinary tract, or a UTI caused by resistant organisms. Specific complicating factors include nephrolithiasis, reduced bladder tone, diabetes, chronic indwelling catheters, immunosuppression, and patients at high risk for resistant pathogens such as those with recent antimicrobial treatment. The clinical spectrum can range from mild cystitis to life-threatening urosepsis. The bacteriology of complicated UTI is broad. Coliforms remain the most common etiology, while *Proteus, Enterococcus, Pseudomonas, Serratia,* and *Enterobacter* species are much more common now than in the past.

While ED therapy is generally empiric by definition, obtaining cultures in these patients prior to initiating therapy is critical to their management. In general, outpatient empiric therapy begins with the fluoroquinolones, and then can be switched based on culture and sensitivity results. Many patients with complicated UTIs will require hospitalization for inability to tolerate oral medications, concomitant medical problems, or for the severity of the UTI itself. In these patients, empiric IV therapy should include an antipseuodomonal penicillin and an aminoglycoside, a third-generation cephalosporin with antipseudomonal activity, or imipenem. The local resistance patterns of the enterococci and *Pseudomonas aeruginosa* must be considered in the choice of antibiotics.

Catheter-associated UTI is an important subset of complicated UTI. There are more than 1 million catheter-associated urinary infections each year in the United States. With the presence of an indwelling catheter, the risk of bacturia is approximately 5 percent per day. Catheter-associated UTIs account for 40 percent of nosocomial infections and are the most common source of gram-negative bacteremia.[21]

The diagnostic criterion is a urine culture showing more than 100 CFU/mL. Since this is not a practical standard for use in the ED, the finding of symptomatic bacteriuria in a catheterized patient merits antibiotic therapy. Polymicrobial UTIs, rare in other settings, are more common with indwelling catheters. Empiric therapy should begin with IV ampicillin plus gentamicin, IV ticarcillin plus clavulanate, or an IV fluoroquinolone. Some patients may be appropriate for oral therapy, in which case fluoroquinolones are the drugs of choice. Most authors recommend a minimum of 14 days of therapy.

Asymptomatic Bacteriuria in Pregnancy

Between 2 and 10 percent of pregnancies are complicated by UTIs; left untreated more than 25 percent of these women will develop pyelonephritis with the associated morbidities previously discussed.[22] Bacteriuria in this patient population should therefore be sought out and treated. A 3- to 7-day course of therapy with TMP-SMX, nitrofurantoin, or cephalexin should be followed by a follow-up test-of-cure urinalysis and culture. TMP-SMX and nitrofurantoin should generally be avoided in the third trimester. With the increasing prevalence of antimicrobial resistance, pretreatment cultures are critical.

TOXIC SHOCK SYNDROME

The toxic shock syndrome (TSS) is a serious and potentially life-threatening medical problem that is easily missed early in its course. In the early 1980s a large number of cases were reported in both the medical literature and the lay press that were either menstrual- or tampon-associated.[23] Later in the 1980s and 1990s, nonmenstrual cases of TSS due to a variety of causes were recognized with much greater frequency.[24] While TSS is thought of as a new disease, it has been recognized and reported in medical history to have been linked to *Staphylococcus aureus* infection since at least 1927.

Toxic shock syndrome is caused by *S. aureus, S. pyogenes* (the group A β-hemolytic *Streptococcus*), and occasionally other gram-positive coccal organisms: *Streptococcus agalactiae* (the group B β-hemolytic *Streptococcus*), certain strains of α-hemolytic streptococci, and on rare occasions, strains of coagulase-negative staphylococci. In contrast to septic shock due to gram-negative rods, which usually occurs as a nosocomial infection or in debilitated, elderly, or immunosuppressed patients, TSS most commonly occurs in otherwise healthy outpatients. The manifestations of TSS may actually be different or atypical in immunosuppressed patients, such as those with acquired immunodeficiency syndrome (AIDS), than in patients who have an intact immune system.[25]

Staphylococcal TSS (versus streptococcal TSS) occurs predominantly in women (over 80 percent), the overwhelming majority occurring in white women between the ages of 15 and 19 years.In the early 1980s, epidemiologic studies linked staphylococcal TSS to young, menstruating women with *S. aureus* vaginal colonization and/or infection sustained while using super absorbent tampons. The isolation and subsequent identification of a new staphylococcal enterotoxin, toxic shock syndrome toxin-1 (TSST-1) from over 90 percent of *S. aureus* strains in patients with menstrual TSS confirmed the etiology of the syndrome.

After the early 1980s, there was a marked decline in the number of cases of staphylococcal TSS, entirely accounted for by a decline in the menstrual cases associated with tampon use.[26] This led many to speculate that Rely® tampons, which had been removed from the market, had in fact been a major cofactor in the expression of the tampon-associated syndrome. In some parts of the U.S., however, menstrual cases of TSS did not decline. Other factors that may have contributed to the overall decline in menstrual cases of TSS include increased public and medical awareness, more aggressive use of antistaphylococcal antibiotics with even the most minor of symptoms associated with menstruation, and underreporting of cases.

Once menstrual cases became less prevalent, the breadth and scope of nonmenstrual cases of staphylococcal TSS were better appreciated. The literature was filled with case reports of TSS associated with postoperative infections and trauma as well as nasal and wound packs. The nonmenstrual TSS cases were as common in men as in women, occurred in any and all ages, were less often associated with different toxins, and were more often associated with staphylococcal enterotoxin B (SEB).

In 1987, Cone and colleagues[27] described their "clinical and bacteriologic observations of a toxic shock-like syndrome due to *Streptococcus pyogenes*." The medical literature began to document increasing numbers of streptococcal TSS infections as well as fulminant, rapidly fatal cases of invasive streptococcal bacteremias, necrotizing fasciitis, myositis, and multiple organ failure. The prevalence has been estimated at approximately 10 to 20 cases per 100,000 population. This syndrome was more fully characterized in a series of 20 patients described by Stevens and coworkers[28] in 1989. The case fatality rate in this series was 30 percent. In some patients, no site of infection was readily identified at the time of presentation, even though the patients progressed rapidly into shock.

Pathophysiology

The major toxins of *S. aureus* can be divided into three groups: enterotoxins, exfoliative toxins, and toxic shock syndrome toxin-1 or TSST-1. The enterotoxins are medium-sized proteins, of which there are seven distinct types, that can cause staphylococcal food poisoning and shock in humans and experimental animals.[29] These toxins are very potent; submicrogram quantities can induce vomiting and diarrhea 1 to 4 hours after ingestion. The exfoliating toxins A and B (EXF-A, EXF-B) that cause the staphylococcal scalded-skin syndrome in children may also cause bullous impetigo in adults as well as in children.

Specific humoral immunity to TSS is confirmed by identifying the antibody to TSST-1. Acquisition of this antibody is age-related, and the great majority of persons who are over age 30 have measurable quantities. Patients with antibody to TSST-1 are still found to be susceptible to nonmenstrual TSS caused by staphylococcal enterotoxin B or other toxins.Most patients with TSS related to menstruation either lack this antibody or have a very low titer. Over 50 percent of recovered patients do not develop anti-TSST-1 antibodies, which may explain the recurrent bouts some individuals experience.

In contrast to staphylococcal TSS, in which *S. aureus* bacteremia is uncommon, streptococcal TSS is associated with bacteremia with *S. pyogenes* in 60 percent of cases.[28] In fact, bacteremia is so rare in staphylococcal TSS that its presence in a TSS-like illness was originally considered an exclusion factor in the early Centers for Disease Control and Prevention (CDC) case definition.

Staphylococcal Toxic Shock Syndrome

Sudden vasomotor collapse in a previously healthy person is a striking and regular feature of toxic shock syndrome.[23] In milder cases, transient hypotension and syncope or near syncope occur. Severe cases are usually marked by a fever of more than 38.9°C (102°F) and diffuse erythroderma. The involvement of multiple body systems and the exclusion of alternative diagnoses help to establish the clinical diagnosis. Some signs and symptoms develop over the first 1 to 3 days. In particular, mucous membrane involvement tends to become most prominent on day 4 or 5 in most patients, and the very characteristic digital desquamation appears at 7 to 14 days.

The skin manifestations cannot be considered parallel to those of septic shock, in which rash is uncommon. The rash of TSS differs from the hemorrhagic changes of meningococcemia and/or DIC, and is a key feature of the disease and the best clue to early diagnosis. Usually a blanching, nonpruritic, macular eruption that has a sunburn-like appearance, the rash is easy to overlook or to ascribe to the flushing associated with a high fever. Although in the U.S. the incidence of TSS seems to be lower in African-Americans than in whites, the rash is extremely difficult to see on darker skin. The mucosal changes in all patients can be dramatic, typically involving the eyes, mouth, tongue, and vagina. The frequently identified "strawberry tongue" is indistinguishable from that of scarlet fever.

Many of the gastrointestinal manifestations of TSS are likely to be direct effects of the staphylococcal toxins as the dramatic secretory diarrhea is not often seen in septic shock. Vomiting usually appears early, while diarrhea often develops 1 to 2 days later. Clinical and histologic changes in the gut mucosa are similar to those seen in association with staphylococcal food poisoning, a disease caused by different staphylococcal enterotoxins.

Nonmenstrual cases of TSS span the spectrum of focal and systemic staphylococcal diseases. Postpartum infections, surgical wound infections, infected sites of trauma, the use of barrier contraception, and various skin, soft tissue, and mucosal abscesses have been implicated.[24] Respiratory infections, including sinusitis, infections behind nasal packs, and postinfluenza bronchitis-pneumonias, are a few selected examples.

Several aspects of postpartum TSS deserve special emphasis. Both staphylococcal and streptococcal TSS cases have been described in the postpartum period. In most such patients, there has been no evidence of preexisting intrauterine infection and no history of postpartum tampon use. Postpartum intrauterine manipulation is documented in some of the staphylococcal TSS cases. Often these patients present with a septic or "toxic" clinical picture, but lack the localizing signs and symptoms of an intrauterine infection, such as pain, tenderness, and abnormal vaginal discharge. Fatal cases of *Clostridium sordelli* infection, a TSS-like syndrome, have been described in the postpartum patient with retained gauze sponges.[30]

Another interesting aspect of postpartum TSS is the occasional description of congenital TSS in infants born to mothers with postpartum TSS. Mahieu and colleagues[31] described such a neonate born to a mother with streptococcal TSS. At presentation, this infant lacked antibodies against streptococcal pyrogenic exotoxins. He responded to treatment with intravenous immune globulin, which was later demonstrated to contain neutralizing antibodies against all three streptococcal pyrogenic exotoxins. Others had previously reported staphylococcal TSS in mother-infant pairs, with suspected intrapartum transmission of the *S. aureus* infection.[31]

Streptococcal Toxic Shock Syndrome

In contrast, patients with streptococcal TSS often present with severe or even excruciating pain of abrupt onset.[32] This pain can be dramatic and quite puzzling to both the patient and the physician, since it often precedes the development of local tenderness and/or physical signs of inflammation. The pain usually begins in an extremity, but it can occur in the head, chest, or abdomen, mimicking such other disorders as sinusitis, myocardial infarction and pericarditis, and peritonitis and pelvic inflammatory disease, respectively.

About 20 percent of patients with streptococcal TSS may first appear with symptoms that suggest a febrile gastroenteritis or an influenza-like illness.[28] Fever, myalgias, nausea, vomiting, and diarrhea are not uncommon in such patients, and they may suspect food poisoning or other gastroenteritides. The onset of the illness may be very subtle in such patients and fulminant in others.

A fever often as high as 40.5 to 41°C (105 to 106°F) is usually the first sign at the onset of streptococcal TSS.[28] Other common clinical features include confusion (50 percent) and soft tissue infection (80 percent). About 70 percent of the patients with focal soft tissue infection will develop necrotizing soft tissue infection, heralded by the appearance of vesicles, bullae, and ultimately necrosis. The ensuing necrotizing fasciitis and/or myositis will require emergent surgical exploration for diagnosis and debridement. Delayed diagnosis and surgery may lead to amputation and death.

Only about 10 percent of patients with streptococcal TSS develop a diffuse faint rash.[32] Localized erythema overlying the site of focal cellulitis is more common. This absence of a generalized diffuse erythema is in distinct contrast to staphylococcal TSS, in which over 80 percent of patients will develop a rash. Nearly half of patients with streptococcal TSS are normotensive at presentation.[28] However, most will manifest a significant drop in blood pressure over 4 to 8 hours of observation.

Laboratory Tests

Mild anemia evolves quickly and probably has several causes. Leukocytosis is universal and often includes immature forms (band forms, or "left shift"), and toxic neutrophilic changes are usually present. In milder cases, a reduction in platelets is an isolated finding, but a decreased platelet count is part of a generalized DIC syndrome in some severe cases. A prolonged prothrombin time (PT), partial thromboplastin time (PTT), and decreased serum fibrinogen will be seen if severe DIC is present. Eosinophils may increase later in the course, sometimes creating diagnostic confusion between an allergic reaction to antibiotics and TSS itself. Liver, pancreatic, and skeletal muscle enzymes may rise quite significantly. Creatine phosphokinase levels are less commonly elevated in staphylococcal TSS than in streptococcal TSS.

Electrolyte abnormalities are also very common and include hypokalemia, hyponatremia, hypocalcemia, hypophosphatemia, and hypomagnesemia. Hypocalcemia is almost universal, is not proportional to mild hypoalbuminemia, and is not explained by the occasional episodes of pancreatitis, renal dysfunction, or hypomagnesemia. It is not due to hypotension or toxic shock alone. The changes are similar to those seen in septic shock but do not occur in otherwise uncomplicated cardiogenic shock. Calcium depression, which can be profound, lasts for 5 to 7 days. The clinical severity of the TSS seems to determine the degree of serum calcium depression.

A positive culture for *S. aureus* from an obviously involved focus (e.g., vagina, tampon materials, an infected postoperative wound, or traumatic injury site) supports the clinical diagnosis. In many patients, the site of infection may be subtle; some of these toxic staphylococcal strains are apparently weakly invasive, eliciting little to no local inflammatory reaction. A high clinical index of suspicion is required in septic patients and wounds that are not obviously infected should therefore be opened and cultured.

Treatment

The most important component of managing TSS is making the diagnosis early. This is best done by maintaining a high index of suspicion and early recognition as the process unfolds. The diagnosis can be quite challenging with an atypical presentation.

Initial steps include early consultation and admission to an ICU, antibiotic therapy, and judicious fluid and electrolyte management. Cardiorespiratory support with mechanical ventilation and vasoactive agents may be needed. Some severely affected patients require as much as 20 L of normal saline or Ringer's lactate in the first 24 hours.

Sources of staphylococcal or streptococcal infection must be searched for assiduously, abscesses should be drained, and wounds need to be explored even if they do not look obviously infected. Any packing must be removed and fasciitis, myositis, or gangrenous areas should be promptly and extensively debrided in an operating room setting.

Antibiotic therapy is mandatory. The antistaphylococcal β-lactams are first-line agents. First-generation cephalosporins, such as cefazolin sodium, are also very effective. The fixed drug combination of ampicillin-sulbactam has appreciable antistaphylococcal, as well as antistreptococcal activity. However, it is not considered effective against methicillin-resistant staphylococci. Ampicillin-sulbactam is an attractive initial antibiotic choice in patients in whom mixed aerobic-anaerobic infections or gas gangrene is part of the differential diagnosis.

Although the prevalence of methicillin-resistant *S. aureus* infection has increased dramatically in the past two decades, TSS-producing strains have rarely been encountered. Nonetheless, in certain high-risk clinical settings—i.e., with intravenous drug abusers and in hospital-acquired infections—initial treatment with intravenous vancomycin is recommended. For the penicillin-allergic patient, vancomycin or clindamycin are appropriate alternatives. Clindamycin may have a unique role in TSS. Laboratory studies have shown that, independent of its antibiotic activity, it can suppress toxin production in the staphylococci. A 5- to 7-day course of antibiotics is reasonable. Longer treatment may be required in severe cases, especially when an infectious focus cannot be found or is not amenable to drainage.

Many textbooks continue to recommend penicillin G, 1 to 2 million units intravenously every 4 hours for severe streptococcal infections. However, accumulating laboratory data, animal studies, and anecdotal clinical reports provide compelling data that favor clindamycin in toxic streptococcal infections. The killing of group A β-hemolytic streptococci (GABS) in the laboratory by penicillin is highly inoculum-dependent, but this inoculum effect does not occur with clindamycin. The inoculum or load of GABS in the blood and tissues of patients with invasive and toxic GABS infections can be very high. This lack of an inoculum effect coupled with the ability of clindamycin to suppress the microorganisms' ability to produce toxins may partly explain its observed clinical superiority. Penicillin remains effective for clostridial soft tissue infections.

More controversial forms of therapy include the use of corticosteroids and intravenous immune globulins. Animal studies and two human studies[33,34] support the administration of corticosteroids if begun as early as possible—no later than the third day of illness in staphylococcal TSS. Since most patients lack anti-TSST-1 antibody and some may be incapable of developing protective antibody, passive immunization with intravenous immune globulin seems rational. Commercial intravenous immune globulin preparations in the United States and Europe contain appreciable quantities of neutralizing antibody to TSST-1. At least two animal studies support this approach, but no controlled studies have been performed in humans.

Some brands and lots of commercial intravenous immune globulin preparations in the U.S. and Europe may also contain appreciable quantities of neutralizing antibodies against the streptococcal enterotoxins. Isolated case studies have described impressive improvements in patients with streptococcal TSS.[31] In one large, uncontrolled study of 15 patients, the mortality was 13 percent in patients given intravenous immune globulin. The expected mortality, based on historic controls, was 66 percent.[35]

REFERENCES

1. Kunin CM: Urinary tract infections in females. *Clin Infect Dis* 18:1–10, 1994.
2. Foxman B, Barlow R, D'Arcy H, Gillespie B, Sobel JD: Urinary tract infection: self-reported incidence and associated costs. *Ann Epidemiol* 10:509–515, 2000.
3. Schappert SM: National ambulatory medical care survey: 1992 summary. Advance data from vital and health statistics. No. 253. Hyattsville, MD: National Center for Health Statistics, 1994.
4. Stamm WE, Hooton TM, Johnson JR, et al: Urinary tract infections: from pathogenesis to treatment. *J Infect Dis* 159:400–406, 1989.
5. Hooton TM, Scholes D, Hughes JP, et al: A prospective study of risk factors for symptomatic urinary tract infection in young women. *N Engl J Med* 335:468–474, 1996.
6. Bureau of the Census: Statistical Abstracts of the United States, 1995, ed 115. National Data Book. Washington: Government Printing Office, 1995, p 82.
7. Foxman B, Frerichs RR: Epidemiology of urinary tract infection: I. Diaphragm use and sexual intercourse. *Am J Public Health* 75:1308–1313, 1985.
8. Johnson JR, Stamm WE: Diagnosis and treatment of acute urinary tract infections. *Infect Dis Clin North Am* 1:773–791, 1987.
9. Orenstein R, Wong ES: Urinary tract infections in adults. *Am Fam Physician* 59:1225–34; 1999.
10. Nicolle LE: A practical guide to the management of complicated urinary tract infection. *Drugs* 53:583–592, 1997.
11. Kunin CM: Guidelines for urinary tract infections. Rationale for a separate strata for patients with "low-count" bacteriuria. *Infection* 22:S38–S40, discussion S41, 1994.
12. Komaroff AL: Urinalysis and urine culture in women with dysuria. *Ann Intern Med* 104:212–218, 1986.
13. Gupta K, Scholes D, Stamm WE: Increasing prevalence of antimicrobial resistance among uropathogens causing acute uncomplicated cystitis. *JAMA* 281:736–738, 1999.
14. Trienekens TA, Stobberingh EE, Winkens RA, Houben AW: Different lengths of treatment with co-trimazole for acute uncomplicated urinary tract infections in women. *Br Med J* 299:1319–1322, 1989.
15. Warren WJ, Abrutyn E, Hebel JR, et al: Guidelines for the antimicrobial treatment of uncomplicated acute bacterial cystitis and acute pyelonephritis in women. *Clin Infect Dis* 29:745–758, 1999.
16. Stamm WE, McKevitt M, Counts GW: Acute renal infection in women: treatment with trimethoprim-sulfamethoxazole or

ampicillin for two to six weeks. *Ann Intern Med* 106:341–345, 1987.

17. Jernelius H, Zbornik J, Bauer CA: One or three weeks' treatment of acute pyelonephritis? A double-blind comparison, using a fixed combination of pivampicillin plus pivmecillinam. *Acta Med Scand* 223:469–477, 1988.
18. Bailey RR, Peddie BA: Treatment of acute urinary tract infection in women. *Ann Intern Med* 107:430, 1987.
19. Talan DA, Stamm WE, Hooton TM, et al: Comparison of ciprofloxacin (7 days) and trimethoprim-sulfamethoxazole (14 days) for acute uncomplicated pyelonephritis in women: a randomized trial. *JAMA* 283:1583–1590, 2000.
20. Staptleton A: Prevention of recurrent urinary tract infections in women. *Lancet* 53:7–8, 1999.
21. Warren WJ: Catheter-associated urinary tract infections. *Infect Dis Clin North Am* 11:609–622, 1997.
22. Patterson TF, Andriole VT: Detection, significance, and therapy of bacteriuria in pregnancy. Update in the managed care era. *Infect Dis Clin North Am* 11:593–608, 1997.
23. Shands KN, Schmidt GP, Dan BB, et al: Toxic shock syndrome in menstruating women. *N Engl J Med* 303:1436–1442, 1980.
24. Garbe PL, Arko RJ, Reingold AL, et al: *Staphylococcus aureus* isolates from patients with non-menstrual toxic shock syndrome. *JAMA* 253:2538–2542, 1985.
25. Cone LA, Woodard DR, Byrd RG, et al: A recalcitrant erythematous desquamating disorder associated with toxin-producing staphylococci in patients with AIDS. *J Infect Dis* 165:638–643, 1992.
26. Jacobson JA, Kasworm E, Daly JA. Risk of developing toxic shock syndrome associated with toxic shock syndrome toxin-1 following non-genital staphylococcal infection. *Rev Infect Dis* 11:S8–S13, 1989.
27. Cone LA, Woodard DR, Schlievert PM, et al: Clinical and bacteriologic observations of a toxic shock-like syndrome due to *Streptococcus pyogenes*. *N Engl J Med* 317:146–149, 1987.
28. Stevens DL, Tanner MH, Winship J, et al: Severe group A streptococcal infections associated with a toxic shock-like syndrome and scarlet fever toxin A. *N Engl J Med* 321:1–7, 1989.
29. Marrack P, Kappler J: The staphylococcal enterotoxins and their relatives. *Science* 1990;248:705–711.
30. McGrego JA, Soper DE, Lovell G, Todd JK: Maternal deaths associated with *Clostridium sordelli* infection. *Am J Obstet Gynecol* 161:987–995, 1989.
31. Mahieu CM, Holm SE, Goossens HJ, et al: Congenital streptococcal toxic shock syndrome with absence of antibodies against streptococcal pyrogenic exotoxins. *J Pediatr* 127:987–989, 1995.
32. Wolf JE, Rabinowitz LG: Streptococcal toxic shock-like syndrome. *Arch Dermatol* 131:73–77, 1995.
33. Todd JK, Ressman M, Caston SA, et al: Corticosteroid therapy for patients with toxic shock syndrome. *JAMA* 252:3399–3402, 1984.
34. Barry W, Hudgins L, Donta ST, et al: Intravenous immunoglobulin therapy for toxic shock syndrome. *JAMA* 267:3315–3316, 1992.
35. Lamothe F, D'Amico P, Ghosn P, et al: Clinical usefulness of intravenous immunoglobulins in invasive group A strep infections. Case report and review. *Clin Infect Dis* 21:1469–1470, 1995.

Appendix 1

Diagnostic Imaging During Pregnancy: Risks to the Fetus

Mitchell M. Goodsitt
Emmanuel G. Christodoulou

KEY POINTS

- Fetal doses for most diagnostic x-ray procedures are less than those that produce statistically significant increases in fetal abnormalities.
- Radiation risks to maternal ovaries

Dose	Effect
10 rads	Delay in menses, reduced ovarian size, no evidence of genetic mutations in ovum
200 rads	Temporary infertility
500 rads	Permanent sterility

- Effects from radiation dose **10–20 rads** to the whole body of the fetus

Age post-conception (weeks)	Effects (dose-dependent)
0–2	Embryo resorption
2–8	Teratogenesis, neuropathology
8–15	Neuropathology, mental retardation, small head size
15–25	If >50 rads, mental retardation, growth retardation, fetal sterility as an adult

Note: Gestation age = conception age + 2 weeks

- Effects from nonionizing imaging

Diagnostic ultrasound	None of clinical significance
MRI	None reported but use with caution, especially in first trimester

- Diagnostic imaging resulting in a fetal dose of 5 rads or more
  - Large numbers of plain radiographs (30 or more) involving abdomen, pelvis, lumbar spine, and hip
  - Multiphase CT examination of the abdomen/pelvis
  - Fluoroscopic examination of abdomen/pelvis lasting several minutes

This appendix can probably be best summarized by a set of guidelines that was recommended in September 1995 by the Committee on Obstetric Practice of the American College of Obstetricians and Gynecologists.[1] They state:

The following guidelines for x-ray examination or exposure during pregnancy are suggested:

1. **Women should be counseled that x-ray exposure from a single diagnostic procedure does not result in harmful effects. Specifically, exposure to less than 5 rads has not been associated with an increase in fetal anomalies or pregnancy loss.**
2. **Concern about possible effects of high-dose ionizing radiation exposure should not prevent medically indicated diagnostic x-ray procedures from being performed on the mother. During pregnancy, other imaging procedures not associated with ionizing radiation (e.g., ultrasonography, MRI) should be considered instead of x-rays when possible.**
3. **Ultrasonography and MRI are not associated with known adverse fetal effects. However, until more information is available, MRI is not recommended for use in the first trimester.**
4. **Consultation with a radiologist may be helpful in calculating estimated fetal dose when multiple diagnostic x-rays are performed on a pregnant patient.**
5. **The use of radioactive isotopes of iodine is contraindicated for therapeutic use during pregnancy.**

When a pregnant woman undergoes a diagnostic x-ray procedure, possible deleterious effects to the fetus are a logical concern. Fortunately, recent analyses have shown that in nearly all cases, the x-ray doses for clinical radiologic examinations are below those at which statistically significant increases in fetal abnormalities arise.[2] This ap-

Table A1-1. Measures of Radiation

Measure	Definition	Unit	SI Unit
Exposure	Ions produced per kilogram of air	Roentgen (R)[a]	Coulomb/kg[a]
Dose	Energy absorbed per kilogram of tissue	Rad (rad)[b]	Gray (Gy)[b]
Equivalent dose	Energy absorbed per kilogram of tissue corrected for biological effect	Rem (rem)[c]	Sievert (Sv)[c]
Effective dose	Energy absorbed per kilogram of tissue corrected for biological effect partial body irradiation, and radiosensitivity of organs	Rem (rem)[c]	Sievert (Sv)[c]

[a] $1\ \text{R} = 2.58 \times 10^{-4}$ C/kg
[b] 1 Gy = 100 rad
[c] 1 Sv = 100 rem
kg = kilogram; C = coulomb

pendix explains the units used to measure x-ray exposure and dose, lists fetal doses for many common procedures, discusses the risks of ionizing and nonionizing radiation to the fetus, gives recommendations concerning alternative imaging modalities such as ultrasound and magnetic resonance imaging, and provides an example of a policy to follow when a pregnant or potentially pregnant patient presents for a possible x-ray procedure.

THE THREE Rs: ROENTGEN, RAD, AND REM

X-rays are a form of electromagnetic radiation, similar to visible light, ultraviolet light, microwaves, and radio waves. The primary distinguishing feature of x-ray photons is that they have much higher energies and can therefore ionize matter. Ionizing radiation is commonly quantified in terms of: *exposure, dose, equivalent dose,* and *effective dose.* The unit of x-ray exposure, the *roentgen* (R), is a specific amount of ions or electric charge per unit mass (or volume) of air. Skin surface exposures are often provided in units of roentgens or milliroentgens (mR), where 1 mR equals 1/1000 R (Table A1-1).

The *dose* is the amount of energy deposited by the x-rays in our tissues and is measured in *rads* (*r*adiation *a*bsorbed *d*ose). One rad is equal to 0.01 joule per kilogram of tissue. At diagnostic x-ray energies, 1 rad is roughly equal to 1 R.

In addition to x-rays, we are exposed to other types of ionizing radiation, such as alpha particles from the decay of radon gas. In contrast to x-rays, which can penetrate our bodies, alpha particles are completely absorbed by less than 1 mm of soft tissue (actually, by just a few hundredths of a millimeter).[3] Consequently, the energy deposition and damage are more localized resulting in greater biological effect. The relative biological effect of the different types of ionizing radiation is accounted for in the quantity termed the *equivalent dose*. The unit for equivalent dose is the *rem.* For diagnostic x-rays, 1 rem equals 1 rad. The rem is also used as the unit for *effective dose*,[4,5] which accounts for the effects of partial rather than whole body irradiation and the radiosensitivity of the specific organs that are exposed.

In summary, *for diagnostic x-rays, 1 R of exposure is equal to approximately 1 rad of absorbed dose in soft tissue, which is equal to approximately 1 rem equivalent dose.*

Recently, the Système International d'Unités (SI) set of units has been established. The SI unit for dose is the *gray* (Gy). One gray is equal to 1 joule (J) of absorbed energy per kilogram of tissue; hence, 1 Gy is equal to 100 rads. The SI unit for equivalent dose and effective dose is the *sievert* (Sv), and 1 Sv is equal to 100 rem.

RISKS OF IONIZATION

The primary risk of ionization is damage to the DNA. Depending upon the extent, location, and timing of the x-ray exposure, the DNA damage may be repaired, or it may result in cell death, rapid cell growth (cancer), abnormal growth (birth defects) in the fetus, and/or genetic mutation. The majority of the damage to DNA from x-ray exposure arises indirectly from interactions with free radicals produced when the x-rays ionize water molecules in our bodies. These free radicals are electrically neutral hydrogen atoms and hydroxyl molecules that have an unpaired electron in the outermost shell and are chemically very reactive. In order to become stable, they rapidly acquire or share electrons with nearby molecules, in the process breaking chemical bonds within those molecules. Furthermore, free radicals can interact with themselves and other molecules to produce toxins such as hydrogen peroxide. Compared with chemical agents, ionizing radiation is particularly effective at damaging DNA because of the ability of ionizing radiation to break chemical bonds and cause defects in the various components of DNA, all within a very small area.[6]

DOSE TO THE FETUS FROM COMMON DIAGNOSTIC X-RAY PROCEDURES

The x-ray dose to the fetus depends upon a number of factors, including the skin surface exposure to the mother, the effective energy of the x-ray beam, the size of the x-ray field, the depth of the fetus, and the size of the patient. Even when the fetus is not located within the x-ray field, it can still receive an x-ray dose due to x-rays scattered within the mother's body. Abdominal shielding can reduce external scatter of radiation and resultant fetal dose, and is advised when the patient is pregnant. However, shielding has little effect on fetal dose once the beam has entered the body (internal scatter). In that case, in addition to the above factors, the dose depends on the distance between the x-ray field and the fetus.[7–18]

Fetal Doses from Radiographic Examinations

There are several techniques that can be used to estimate the dose to the conceptus when it is directly exposed to x-ray radiation from radiographic procedures.[7] These include the normalized depth-dose technique,[15] the percentage depth-dose technique,[8,9] and the tissue-air ratio technique.[10,12] One of the most useful references for calculating doses to the conceptus when it is located either within or outside the x-ray field is the *Handbook of Selected Tissue Doses for Projections Common in Diagnostic Radiology*,[11] published by the Food and Drug Administration (FDA). The organ doses in this pamphlet are based on calculations made with a sophisticated computer simulation method known as the Monte Carlo method. Normalized organ dose (dose divided by free-in-air exposure at the skin surface position) tables are provided for various x-ray beam qualities. Estimated conceptus doses are accurate to the degree that the patient undergoing the study is adequately described by the average female mathematical model used in the simulation method. It is specifically stated in this handbook that "assignment of organ doses to individual patients using the *Handbook* is not recommended." We measured the free-in-air exposures and beam qualities for many common radiographic procedures that women undergo in the emergency department and used the normalized organ dose tables[11] to estimate fetal dose. That dose is actually the dose to the uterus and is valid for fetuses up to the age of 2 months. Beyond 2 months, because of the increased uterine size, other methods must be employed. Table A1-2 lists the estimated doses to the uterus for the various types of examinations. The doses in Table A1-2 represent values for an average-sized patient. The doses are directly proportional to the x-ray tube current (mA) and exposure time (s) product (mAs) employed, and they are fairly strongly dependent upon the x-ray beam's half-value layer (HVL). As long as the HVL, or effective energy, for a particular examination is similar to the one listed, the dose to the conceptus of a specific average-sized patient can be estimated by simply multiplying the dose in the final column of Table A1-2 by the ratio of the actual mAs to the mAs in the table. If the HVL of a particular x-ray unit differs from that listed in Table A1-2 by more than 0.2, the actual dose may differ by more than 20 percent. Under those circumstances, we recommend using the organ dose versus HVL data in the original FDA publication[11] to obtain a more accurate dose estimate. The normalized organ doses are not applicable to individuals whose anthropometric characteristics differ significantly from the reference (average) patient. Hence, the fetal doses listed in the last column of Table A1-2 are not as accurate in very thin or obese patients. Finally, if an average-sized patient has multiple examinations, the total dose to the conceptus is computed by simply summing the doses from each individual examination. Organ doses for common radiographic procedures can also be estimated for the average-sized adult and child using the computer programs XDOSE and CHILDOSE by J.C. Le Heron (email address: John_Le_Heron@nrl.moh.govt.nz located at the National Radiation Laboratory, Ministry of Health, Christchurch, New Zealand). These programs use the normalized organ dose data sets in the reports NRPB-SR262 and NRPB-SR279 (National Radiological Protection Board, UK). These data sets can be purchased from the NRPB (web address: http://www.nrpd.org.uk/services/software).

Fetal Doses from Computed Tomography Examinations

Computed tomography (CT) examinations usually involve higher radiation doses than other radiographic examinations. For an examination of the pelvic region, the conceptus dose will be in the vicinity of 2000 mrad (20 mGy). The dose depends on the position of the

Table A1-2. Estimated Fetal Doses for Common Radiographic Examinations

Examination	kVp	mAs	HVL, mmAI	SID, cm	Field Size at Film, cm-cm	Average Patient Thickness, cm	Exposure in Air at Skin Surface mR	Dose to the Uterus (Fetus) per Film, mrad‡
Chest AP/PA	125	4	5.4	183	35 × 43	22	21	0.1
Chest lateral	125	20	5.4	183	35 × 43	32	121	0.2
Chest AP/PA (portable)	120	4	4.9	122	35 × 43	22	19	0.1
Abdomen AP	70	40	3.0	102	35 × 43	20	272	94.0
Abdomen decub.	70	80	3.0	102	35 × 43	20	544	27.0
Abdomen (portable/grid)	70	64	2.3	102	35 × 43	20	521	135.0
Pelvis AP	75	40	3.2	102	35 × 43	20	308	116.0
Pelvis lateral/grid	75	200	3.2	102	35 × 43	35	1890	107.0
Pelvis (portable/grid)	76	40	2.4	102	35 × 43	20	343	95.0
C-spine AP	75	8	3.2	102	24 × 30	13	51	0.0
C-spine lateral	70	10	3.0	102	24 × 30	17	51	0.0
C-spine lateral/grid	75	16	3.2	102	24 × 30	17	142	0.0
C-spine AP (portable/grid)	70	12	3.0	102	24 × 30	13	77	0.0
C-spine oblique	65	10	2.8	102	24 × 30	13	46	0.0
C-spine odontoid	75	25	3.2	102	24 × 30	13	160	0.0
T-spine AP	75	32	3.2	102	35 × 43	22	261	0.4
T-spine lateral	80	32	3.4	102	35 × 43	32	427	0.2
L-spine AP	75	40	3.2	102	35 × 43	20	308	101.0
L-spine lateral	85	64	3.6	102	35 × 43	32	953	44.0
IVP	65	30	2.8	102	35 × 43	20	167	51.0
Hip AP	75	32	3.2	102	24 × 30	20	247	64.0
Hip lateral	75	32	3.2	102	24 × 30	18	234	10.0
Femur AP	75	12	3.2	102	18 × 43	20	92	0.7
Femur lateral	75	10	3.2	102	18 × 43	20	77	0.2
Shoulder AP	70	8	3.0	102	24 × 30	17	50	0.0
Humerus AP	60	2	2.5	102	18 × 43	17	8	0.0
Orbits AP	70	50	3.0	102	24 × 30	18	322	0.0
Orbits lateral	70	7	3.0	102	24 × 30	18	45	0.0
Skull AP	70	40	3.0	102	24 × 30	18	258	0.0
Skull lateral	70	10	3.0	102	24 × 30	18	64	0.0
Skull townes	70	64	3.0	102	24 × 30	18	412	0.0
Skull waters	70	40	3.0	102	24 × 30	18	258	0.0
Zygoma axial	70	6	3.0	102	24 × 30	18	39	0.0
Soft tissue neck AP	70	10	3.0	102	24 × 30	13	57	0.0
Soft tissue neck lateral	100	2	4.4	102	24 × 30	17	28	0.0
Nuclear Medicine Studies								270*†
Thyroid scan								
Bone, brain, renal, cardiovascular scan								<500[19,20]
Pulmonary Ventilation/perfusion scan								~50[21]

*Per study

kVp = peak kilovoltage (x-ray tube potential); mAs = milliampere·seconds (x-ray tube current exposure time product); HVL = half-valve-layer (thickness of aluminum necessary to reduce x-ray intensity by a factor of 2); SID = source-to-image distance (x-ray tube to film distance).

†*Source:* Husak V. Wiedermann M: Radiation absorbed dose estimates to the embryo from some nuclear medicine procedures. *Eur J Nucl Med* 5:205, 1980.

‡The fetal doses represent values for an average-sized patient.

Table A1-3. Conversion Factors (F)[a] for Radiation Doses to the Uterus for Computed Tomography Examinations of Three Regions

Thorax	Abdomen	Pelvis
7	40	441

[a] mrad to uterus/rad free-in-air kerma at center of gantry.
Source: Mini et al,[22] with permission.

conceptus with respect to the part of the patient's body that is scanned, the beam quality, the examination technique used, and the patient's size and contour. One of the methods for estimating fetal doses from CT examinations was developed by Mini and colleagues.[22] This group used thermoluminescent dosimeters (TLDs) to measure doses at 70 locations inside an anthropomorphic phantom that was scanned using standard CT examination protocols. They determined the typical location and size of several organs of interest in that phantom from CT images of previously examined patients. The dose to the fetus was assumed to be equal to the mean dose to the uterus. In addition, Mini and coworkers established conversion factors that relate measured free-in-air dose (kerma) to organ dose at the rotation axis of any CT scanner. One of the simplest methods to estimate fetal dose from a CT examination is to measure the free-in-air dose for the technique employed and multiply by the appropriate conversion factor. Table A1-3 shows the conversion factors (F) for radiation doses to the uterus for whole-area CT examination of the thorax, abdomen, and pelvis. Our calculated doses to the uterus for the GE HiSpeed® CT/i and GE LightSpeed® (multislice) CT scanners at our institution, and those calculated by Mini and associates for their Siemens Somatom Plus® CT scanner are listed in Table A1-4.

Notice that the dose values for the three CT scanners are similar. Also, the doses quoted by Mini and associates include the dose for the scout (localization) view, whereas ours do not. The doses to the conceptus for the scout views are quite small (<l mrad, 3 mrad, and 31 mrad for the thorax, abdomen, and pelvic regions, respectively).[22] For helical CT scanning, the doses listed in Table A1-4 should be divided by the true pitch factor, which is equal to the table travel per gantry rotation divided by the total slice thickness (number of simultaneous slices times the individual slice thickness). For example, when the GE LightSpeed scanner is operated in the HS mode, the true pitch is 1.5, and all of the axial mode doses for the LightSpeed scanner in the table should be divided by 1.5. Similarly, when the LightSpeed CT scanner is operated in the HQ mode, the true pitch is 0.75, and the axial doses should be divided by 0.75. In general, CT doses are proportional to mAs and independent of slice thickness.

When a more accurate assessment of the fetal dose from a CT examination is required, a method developed by Felmlee and colleagues[23] may be used. This method is especially useful when more detailed information is available concerning the exact locations of the CT slices and/or when slice thicknesses other than the 10 mm assumed by Mini and coworkers are employed.

Felmlee and associates[23] measured fetal doses in an adult anthropomorphic phantom. For these measurements, they used four CT scanners (Picker 1200®, Siemens DRH®, GE 9800®, and GE 8800®), four kilovoltages (100, 120, 130, and 140 kVp), and three radiation scan thicknesses (2, 5, and 10 mm). The fetal dose esti-

Table A1-4. Mean Dose to the Uterus (Conceptus)

CT Scanner	Examination Site		
	Thorax	Abdomen	Pelvis
Siemens Somatom Plus (Mini et al.)	**16 mrad** 120 kVp 150 mAs 10 mm	**150 mrad** 120 kVP 210 mAs 10 mm	**1930 mrad** 120 kVP 340 mAs 10 mm
GE LightSpeed (multislice) (University of Michigan)	**23 mrad** 120 kVp 200 mAs 10 mm	**186 mrad** 120 kVp 280 mAs 10 mm	**2050 mrad** 120 kVp 280 mAs 10 mm
GE Hi Speed CT/i	**25 mrad**	**200 mrad**	**2200 mrad**

mrad = millirad; kVp = peak kilovoltage; mAs = milliampere · second; mm = millimeter.
Source: Mini et al,[22] with permission.

mates are based on the CT dose index (CTDI) measured using a pencil ionization chamber (10 cm long, 3 cm^3) at the center position of a 16-cm diameter cylindrical acrylic phantom.

Other methods for computing fetal doses that have appeared in the literature include those of Panzer and Zankl,[24] who calculated doses with a Monte Carlo method using a "female mathematical reference phantom," and referenced the uterine dose to the free-in-air dose at the rotational axis of the scanner for a 10-mm 360° slice, and Wagner and associates,[21] who measured doses along the central axis and surface of two abdominal phantoms that simulated the female pelvis and derived formulas for computing fetal dose for specific CT scanners from the mAs, number of sections over the conceptus, and total number of sections.

The most recent methods for computing patient organ (including the uterus, or the embryo/fetus) and effective doses from CT examinations include one developed by the ImPACT group (the UK's CT scanner evaluation center), and one described in the book *Radiation Exposure in Computed Tomography*.[19] The ImPACT group method is implemented in a spreadsheet that makes use of the NRPB-SR250 normalized dose data sets. The spreadsheet can be downloaded from the ImPACT group's website: http://www.impactscan.org/ctdosimetry.htm, and the NRPB-SR250 data package that is used by this spreadsheet can be purchased from the NRPB (http:www.nrpd.org.uk/services/software/sr250.htm). The ImPACT method employs a single adult anthropomorphic mathematical model that is both male and female for its dose calculations.

The second method[19] is implemented in a program called CT-Expo V 1.2 (email: stamm.georg@mh-hannover.de), and it makes use of the four anthropomorphic mathematical models,[19,20] "EVA," "ADAM," "CHILD," and "BABY" for its dose calculations.

Fetal Doses from Fluoroscopy Examinations

In general, fluoroscopy examinations, especially those that are long and involved, result in the highest patient doses in radiology departments. The typical skin surface exposure rate is about 3000 mR/min. The dose to the conceptus from fluoroscopic studies can be computed using the normalized-organ-dose tables for corresponding radiographic techniques.[11] To use these tables, one must account for the closer x-ray focus-to-patient distance employed in conventional (x-ray tube under table) fluoroscopy. Usually, this distance is about 50 cm for fluoroscopy units, as compared with about 72 cm for radiography units. Assuming these distances, that the thickness of the mother's body is approximately 20 cm, and that the uterus is located 8 cm from the front surface for the anteroposterior (AP) projection and 12 cm from the rear surface for the posteroanterior (PA) projection,[10] one can estimate that the normalized organ doses (mrad/R free-in-air skin surface exposure) for AP fluoroscopy are about 0.92 times those for AP radiography, and those for PA fluoroscopy are about 0.89 times those for PA radiography. For example, the normalized dose to the uterus (conceptus) for PA fluoroscopy of the abdomen, assuming an x-ray spectrum with a HVL of 4 mm of Al (aluminum), would be 0.89 times the normalized dose from PA radiography (235 mrad/R),[11] (i.e., 209 mrad per 1 R entrance exposure). If a woman undergoes a fluoroscopic procedure that lasts 3 minutes and receives a typical free-in-air skin surface exposure of 3 R/min, her total skin surface exposure is 9 R, and the estimated dose to the fetus is 1881 mrad (18.8 mGy).

Table A1-5. Dose to the Uterus (mrad) per 1 R Free-In-Air Skin Entrance Exposure

	HVL (mmAI)	
Examination	**4.0**	**5.0**
Gastroesophageal junction, LPO	0.2	0.2
Stomach, LPO	2.0	2.0
Duodenum, LPO	1.0	0.9
Gastroesophageal junction, RAO	0.3	0.4
Stomach, RAO	1.0	2.0
Duodenum, RAO	1.0	1.0

mmAI = millimeters of aluminum; LPO = left posterior oblique; RAO = right anterior oblique.

If a pregnant woman undergoes an upper gastrointestinal fluoroscopic examination, in particular an examination using barium as the contrast agent, the dose to the fetus can be estimated using data from another FDA publication.[12] Some examples of normalized doses to the uterus for such examinations are listed in Table A1-5. We have chosen not to list the normalized dose to the uterus for many upper GI examinations such as LPO (left posterior oblique) and RAO (right anterior oblique) projections of the upper, middle, and lower esophagus because those doses are very low (<0.1 mrad). Furthermore, the doses listed in the table are considerably less than those for the lower GI tract and abdomen, where the fetus is directly exposed. In particular, using the same fluoroscopy factors as those used above to estimate the conceptus dose for a fluoroscopy examination of the abdomen, (4 mm HVL and 9 R entrance exposure), one would estimate a conceptus dose of only 9 mrad (0.09 mGy) for an RAO barium study of the stomach. This is about 209 times less than the 1881 mrad dose we estimated for a lower abdomen study. In estimating the dose from fluoroscopy studies, one must consider the fact that the skin surface exposure varies dramatically with patient thickness and fluoroscopic image field of view. In general, higher skin surface exposures are required for thicker patients and smaller fields of view. An increase in patient thickness by only 1 inch typically results in a twofold increase of the skin surface exposure, and changing the field of view from 12 to 6 inches often results in a fourfold increase in the exposure. Federal regulations limit the maximum free-in-air skin surface exposure to 10 R/min under normal fluoroscopic operation and 20 R/min under optional high-dose-level operation.

Dose to the Fetus from Common Nuclear Medicine Procedures

Radioactive isotopes are used in nuclear medicine primarily to image internal organs and to evaluate various physiologic functions and secondarily for therapeutic purposes.[3] During a nuclear medicine study, a chemical agent labeled with a radioactive isotope is introduced into the patient's body and selectively accumulated in the region of interest. For example, radioactive isotopes of iodine accumulate in the thyroid. Iodine is also used to treat hyperthyroidism.

The factors to consider in evaluating fetal doses from nuclear medicine examinations include: the amount of radioactivity administered, the particular types and energies of radiations emitted by the radionuclide, the uptake concentrations of the radioactivity in the various organs of the patient's body, the proximity of each of these organs to the fetus, the effective half-life of the radiopharmaceutical, the amount of radiopharmaceutical that crosses the placenta and enters the embryo/fetus, and the age of the embryo/fetus.[7]

Conceptus dose calculations from nuclear medicine studies are only approximations and may over- or underestimate doses to the embryo/fetus by a large factor.[7]

During pregnancy, the ventilation-perfusion study is very commonly performed for detecting pulmonary embolism. Macroaggregated albumin labeled with technetium 99m (^{99m}Tc), one of the radioactive isotopes used most often in diagnostic procedures, is used for the perfusion portion and inhaled xenon 127 (^{127}Xe) or xenon 133 (^{133}Xe) is used for the ventilation portion. The dose to the fetus from such a study is approximately 50 mrad (0.5 mGy).[25] The doses to the fetus during bone, cardiovascular, brain, and renal imaging procedures with ^{99m}Tc are each less than 500 mrad (5 mGy) (Table A1-2).[26,27]

Radioactive iodine readily crosses the placenta and can affect the fetal thyroid, especially when used after 10 to 12 weeks of pregnancy. If a diagnostic procedure of the thyroid is deemed necessary, iodine 123 (^{123}I) or ^{99m}Tc should be used instead of iodine 131 (^{131}I) because ^{131}I results in a much higher dose per unit activity to the fetal thyroid. **It is highly recommended that therapeutic use of radioactive iodine in the mother be delayed until after the delivery of the baby.**[25]

RISKS TO THE EMBRYO AND FETUS FROM EXPOSURE TO IONIZING RADIATION

Some of the most recent information concerning the risks to the embryo and fetus from exposure to ionizing radiation is contained in the National Council on Radiation Protection (NCRP) commentary number 9, which was published in May 1994;[28] much of what follows is based on the material in that commentary and reference 6. In general, the risks to the embryo and fetus can be classified into two categories: those due to deterministic effects and those due to stochastic effects.

Deterministic Effects

Deterministic effects are those believed to occur only at x-ray doses above certain thresholds. Both the probability of inducing the effect and the severity of the effect increase with dose after the threshold has been exceeded. The probabilities of these effects are strongly related to the stage of pregnancy at which the embryo/fetus is exposed. All of the deterministic effects have been observed after fetal doses of 100 rads (1 Gy) or more. The exact values of the thresholds for the deterministic effects are not known. However, studies to date indicate that for acute exposures of the whole body of the conceptus, the thresholds for malformations and growth retardation may be in the range of 10 to 20 rads (0.1 to 0.2 Gy); for mental retardation, 10 to 20 rads (0.1 to 0.2 Gy), or as high as 40 rads (0.4 Gy) if Down syndrome cases are excluded; for decline in IQ, 10 rads (0.1 Gy); and for small head size, as low as 5 rads (0.05 Gy).

Exposure During the First 2 Weeks of Pregnancy

The predominant deterministic effect due to exposure during the first 2 weeks of pregnancy is resorption of the embryo.

Exposure During Weeks 2 To 8

The second to eighth week postconception is the period of organogenesis. Significant x-ray exposure during this period may result in teratogenesis (birth defects). Examples include gross malformation and growth retardation, the latter of which can occur both at term and later at adulthood. Neuropathology and small head size may also occur as a result of significant exposures during weeks 2 to 8.

Exposures During Weeks 8 To 15

The embryo has developed into a fetus at about the seventh to eighth postconception week, and neurologic development occurs during the next 7 weeks. Significant x-ray exposure at this time (between weeks 8 and 15) may result in mental retardation, small head size, and decreased IQ. Studies to date indicate that for acute exposures of the whole body of the conceptus that **exceed the respective thresholds mentioned above,** the risk for severe mental retardation is 0.04 percent per mGy (0.4 percent per rad). The decrease in IQ is 25 points per Gy (per 100 rads). The risk for small head size is believed to be 0.05 to 0.1 percent per mGy (0.5 to 1 percent per rad). Other possible but less likely effects due to significant exposure during this period include growth retardation as an adult and sterility. Even less likely but still possible are cataracts, neuropathology, and growth retardation at term.

Exposures Beyond Week 15

Most of the deterministic effects mentioned above are either not observed or observed much less frequently when the fetus receives significant radiation dose beyond 15 weeks postconception. Mental retardation has been observed as a result of significant exposure during the eighth to twenty-fifth weeks but not beyond. For exposures during the sixteenth to twenty-fifth week, the risk for severe mental retardation is ~0.02 percent per mGy (0.2 percent per rad) with a threshold at 500 mGy (50 rads). Other effects that have been observed because of exposure after week 15 include sterility and growth retardation as an adult. Less likely effects that have been demonstrated are cataracts, neuropathology, and growth retardation at term.

Risks of Deterministic Effects in Perspective

To better comprehend the actual risks involved with exposure of the conceptus to doses at or above a threshold, consider the case of mental retardation. When the fetus receives an unusually high dose of 100 rads (1 Gy) during the eighth to fifteenth weeks postconception, the frequency of severe mental retardation is 43 percent.[29] This is 100 times greater than the 0.4 percent frequency of severe mental retardation due to natural causes.[30] On the other hand, if the fetus were to receive a dose of 10 rads (0.1 Gy), which is closer to the threshold for severe mental retardation due to radiation exposure during this period, the frequency of severe mental retardation is about 4 percent. While it is true that this frequency is 10 times that due to natural causes, one must also consider that there is about a 96 percent chance that the person will not be severely mentally retarded subsequent to receiving such a dose in utero. Furthermore, had the 10-rad x-ray dose been received 16 to 25 weeks after conception, the relative risk of severe mental retardation due to radiation exposure would have been extremely low because this dose is less than the 50-rad threshold for this time period. Another example is small head size. The natural incidence is about 4 percent.[31] A whole-body dose of 10 rads (0.1 Gy) to a fetus 4 to 7 weeks after conception increases the incidence to about 9 percent (a 91 percent chance of not having a small head size).[32] If this dose is received 9 to 11 weeks postconception, the risk of small head size increases to about 13 percent (an 87 percent chance of not having a small head size).[32] The exact thresholds and risks are still a matter of debate, and the values cited above are not to be taken as absolutes, but as reasonable estimates that may be revised with further studies.

Stochastic Effects

Stochastic effects have no threshold. They occur at random with a probability that increases with radiation dose. Interestingly, the severity of the effect is unrelated to dose, indicating that radiation triggers a disease process "whose ultimate course is determined by other factors in the individual."[6] The most prevalent stochastic effects are induction of cancer and genetic mutations in future generations. The probabilities of these effects are quite low. In fact, the most recent analyses of Japanese A-bomb survivors who were exposed in utero show no significant increase in rates of childhood or adult cancer.[34,35]

Furthermore, no radiation-induced genetic effects have been observed in the births of the Japanese A-bomb survivors. Because of the uncertainties involved in estimating risks, experts believe it is reasonable to assume that "the embryo or fetus is as susceptible to the carcinogenic effects of radiation as the young child . . . viz. 10×10^{-2} Sv^{-1}" or 1/1000 per rem and that "the embryo, fetus and nursing child are as sensitive to induction of hereditary effects as the adult . . . viz. 1×10^{-2} Sv^{-1}"[26] or 1/10,000 per rem.

Risks of Stochastic Effects in Perspective

To put the risks of stochastic effects in perspective, consider the increase in the probability that a fetus exposed to 10 rem (0.1 Sv) will develop cancer in his or her lifetime. This increase is about 0.01. If this increase is added to the normal probability of developing cancer during one's lifetime, which is 0.20, the overall risk increases from 20 to 21 percent, which is relatively insignificant.

Risks to the Ovaries

High x-ray dose to the ovaries is of concern. According to Bushong,[36] the sensitivity of the ovaries to x-ray radiation varies with age. The sensitivity starts out very high during fetal life and early childhood, at which time the irradiation causes the ovaries to reduce in size due to germ cell death. The radiation sensitivity declines to a minimum between the ages of 20 and 30 years old, and subsequently increases. X-ray doses as low as 10 rads to the ovaries of a mature woman can result in a delay in menstruation as well as a reduction in ovary size, and doses of 200 rads can cause temporary infertility. An extremely high dose of 500 rads is required to produce permanent sterility. In addition to infertility, another danger of x-ray dose to the ovaries is genetic mutations. Although such effects have been observed in animal experiments at doses of about 25 to 50 rads, there is little if any evidence of this effect in humans. In fact, the latest analyses of the Hiroshima and Nagasaki data show the genetic risk is measured at approximately 10^{-7}/rad, and the somatic risk is even less when exposure occurs before conception [Stewart C. Bushong, Sc.D., Baylor College of Medicine, personal communication]. Therefore some experts believe there is no reason to abstain from procreation for a period of time after the ovaries are exposed to x-rays. Others, however, choose to err on the side of caution based on animal data that suggest oocytes can repair genetic damage as they mature to ova, and recommend "that 6 months be allowed to elapse between the exposure to radiation and a planned conception, to minimize the genetic consequence." In particular, they state that this "would be good advice to a person accidentally exposed to, say 0.1 Gy (10 rad), to young patients with Hodgkin's disease receiving radiotherapy, or even to patients subjected to diagnostic x-ray procedures involving the lumbar spine or the lower gastrointestinal tract, in which a large exposure is used and the gonads must be included within the radiation field."[37]

BIOLOGICAL RISKS ASSOCIATED WITH NONIONIZING IMAGING MODALITIES

Although the risks to the fetus are relatively small from the ionization produced in diagnostic examinations with x-rays, it is possible to avoid those risks entirely by employing a nonionizing imaging modality such as ultrasound or MRI. These alternative modalities (in particular, ultrasound) have been found to be relatively free of risk. The risks of ultrasound and MRI are described below.

Risks of Ultrasound Examinations

Although no ultrasonically induced adverse bioeffects have been reported during the approximately four decades that ultrasonography has been used clinically, at sufficiently high exposure levels, ultrasound has been demonstrated to produce changes in living systems.

Ultrasonography involves the transmission of high-frequency pressure waves into the body and the reception of echoes (reflections and scatter) from interfaces and regions characterized by variations in compressibility and/or mass density. The interaction of the ultrasonic waves with tissues can produce heating and/or cavitation.

Heating results from the absorption of ultrasound energy by tissues. The absorption is highly dependent upon the tissue type and ultrasonic frequency. For example, fluids such as amniotic fluid, blood, and urine absorb almost no ultrasound energy. Soft tissues attenuate (absorb and scatter) a typical (5-MHz) ultrasound beam by about 50 percent for every centimeter traveled (e.g., intensity is ~50 percent after 1 cm, ~25 percent after 2 cm, etc.). Cartilage absorbs more than soft tissue, and bone is the most absorbing tissue. Fetal bone absorption depends upon the degree of ossification. Ultrasonic absorption and scatter increase in all tissues as the ultrasonic frequency is increased (e.g., greater absorption for 5 MHz than 3.5 MHz). In scanning a pregnant woman, one of the potential concerns is significant temperature rises at or near the fetal bone due to its high absorption coefficient. Indeed, if one neglects the pulsed nature of ultrasound employed in imaging and the cooling effects of local blood flow and assumes an ultrasound power level near the maximum employed clinically, temperature rises of about 4°C (7.2°F) are possible.[38] This is very close to the temperature rise of 5°C (9°F) that has been associated with cell killing. The low duty factor of the pulsed beam (pulses "on" about 0.5 to 1.0 percent of the time) and the local blood flow make such temperature rises extremely unlikely. Cavitation is a general term used to describe the generation, growth, oscillation, and possible collapse of microbubbles in tissues.[38] The generation of new microbubbles and growth of existing microbubbles is due to the negative pressure (rarefaction) part of the ultrasound wave. Cavitation is unlikely to produce a significant adverse biological effect unless the cavitation is widespread over an organ or tissue. To date, there is no evidence that diagnostic ultrasound examinations have resulted in cavitation in humans.[38]

In the interest of keeping the ultrasound exposure to the patient as low as reasonably achievable, manufacturers are now incorporating in diagnostic ultrasound equipment real-time display of indexes related to the potential for bioeffects. Establishment of these indexes is the result of a joint effort by the National Equipment Manufacturers Association (NEMA), the FDA, and the American Institute of Ultrasound in Medicine (AIUM).[39] Two types of indexes may be displayed: a thermal index (TI), which is related to potential temperature increase, and a mechanical index (MI), which is related to potential cavitation. Both types are relative. For example, a thermal index of 2 does not indicate a temperature rise of 2°C. Rather, it indicates a temperature rise twice as great as that for a thermal index of 1.

Furthermore, the fact that an index is displayed does not mean that temperature rise or cavitation is actually occurring. Many other factors such as tissue types, intervening layers of absorbing or nonabsorbing tissues, ultrasound beam focus and tissue perfusion may alter the bioeffects. In terms of official recommendations, in March 1997 the AIUM approved the following official statement on the clinical safety of diagnostic ultrasound:[40]

> **Diagnostic ultrasound has been in use since the late 1950s. Given its known benefits and recognized efficacy for medical diagnosis, including use during human pregnancy, American Institute of Ultrasound in Medicine herein addresses the clinical safety of such use: There are no confirmed biological effects on patients or instrument operators caused by exposures from present diagnostic ultrasound instruments. Although the possibility exists that such biological effects may be identified in the future, current data indicate that the benefits to patients of the prudent use of diagnostic ultrasound outweigh the risks, if any, that may be present.**

The most recent official statements from the AIUM regarding the clinical use of ultrasound can be found at the AIUM website (www.aium.org) in the consumer and provider information section.

Risks of Magnetic Resonance Imaging Examinations

In magnetic resonance imaging, the human body is placed in a strong static magnetic field and exposed to radiofrequency fields as well as static and rapidly switching magnetic field gradients. The purpose of all these is to image the distribution of hydrogen in the body and the rates at which hydrogen atoms perturbed by radiofrequency (RF) pulses at specific locations return to equilibrium (T1 and T2 relaxation times).

The predominant sources of possible bioeffects from MRI are (1) the static magnetic field of the MRI system, (2) the gradient magnetic fields, (3) the RF electromagnetic fields, (4) the combination of the three different electromagnetic fields, and (5) the imaging contrast agents. Effects 1 through 3 have been reviewed comprehensively by Hendee and Ritenour.[6]

The primary effect of the static field is the induction of electrical potentials in the body. These result from blood (a conductor) moving through the magnetic field. The induced potentials are quite small (on the order of millivolts) and do not have any known adverse effects. To ensure that the effects from the static fields are minimal, the FDA has established guidelines that restrict the intensity of the static magnetic fields to less than or equal to 4.0 teslas.

Time-varying gradient fields on the order of 2 teslas per second (T/s) are fairly typical in today's images. Such fields induce currents of about 10 to 30 mA/m^2 in the body. Chronic exposure to currents of this magnitude can result in changes in cell function, including variations in cell growth rate, respiration, and metabolism, immune response, and gene expression. However, patient exposure to time-varying fields in MRI is of an acute nature, and scan duration is orders of magnitude less than that which has been associated with the above-mentioned effects. The FDA guidelines recommend that the time-varying fields be less than or equal to 20 T/s.

The RF pulses of energy to which the patient is exposed during the "transmit" portion of the imaging cycle can cause heating of tissue. The RF pulses induce electrical currents in the tissues, and the resistance of the tissues to these currents result in the conversion of the energy of the currents to heat with an associated temperature rise. While temperature rises of about 5°C (9°F) above body core temperature are known to cause cell killing, typical temperature elevation with clinical MRI is significantly below this. The FDA guidelines require that the specific absorption rate (SAR) from RF pulses be less than 4 W/kg whole body for 15 minutes.

It has been shown that some intravenous MRI contrast agents cross the placenta and circulate through the fetus several times as it swallows and excretes the amniotic fluid. The rates of clearance of these contrast agents from the amniotic fluid and the fetal circulation are unknown. Therefore, some authors recommend against administering any MRI contrast agents to pregnant patients until more data become available.[40]

The issue of the possible adverse bioeffects on pregnant women of the MRI environment is reviewed extensively in a recent book by Shellock and Kanal.[41] They state that there are two facts that make it nearly impossible to prove the safety of MRI for pregnant women: (1) the many possible combinations of the multiple risk factors associated with the MRI environment and (2) the relatively high spontaneous abortion rate in humans (>30 percent) during the first trimester of pregnancy.

Shellock and Kanal reviewed the literature related to MR procedures and pregnancy over a period of 20 years (1973–1993). They point out that the evidence regarding the bioeffects of the electromagnetic fields used in MRI procedures, particularly on developing organisms, is contradictory. At present, there is no conclusive evidence regarding any deleterious effects that MRI may have on the developing fetus. It is well known, though, that cells undergoing division are more susceptible to damage. Also, a number of mechanisms exist with which the electromagnetic radiation used in MRI could be hazardous to the developing fetus. Therefore, until further investigations prove otherwise they recommend that MRI be used with caution during pregnancy, especially during the first trimester.[41]

In terms of official recommendations, the *Policies, Guidelines, and Recommendations for MR Imaging Safety and Patient Management* issued by the Safety Committee of the Society for Magnetic Resonance Imaging[42] states:

> **MR imaging may be used in pregnant women if other nonionizing forms of diagnostic imaging are inadequate or if the examination provides important information that would otherwise require exposure to ionizing radiation (e.g., fluoroscopy, CT, etc.). It is recommended that pregnant patients be informed that, to date, there has been no indication that the use of clinical MR imaging during pregnancy has produced deleterious effects. However, as noted by the FDA, the safety of MR imaging during pregnancy has not been proved.**

Furthermore, the International Non-Ionizing Radiation Committee of the International Radiation Protection Association has issued an article entitled "Protection of the patient undergoing a magnetic resonance examination,"[43] in which the following is stated:

> **There is no firm evidence that mammalian embryos are sensitive to the magnetic fields encountered in magnetic resonance systems. However, pending the accumulation of more data regarding MR in pregnancy, it is recommended that elective examination of pregnant women should be postponed until after the first trimester. Because ultrasound is the modality of choice for fetal and uterine examination during pregnancy, an MR examination should be limited to cases in which unique diagnostic information can be obtained. Exposure duration should be reduced to the minimum consistent with obtaining useful diagnostic information.**

Additional information regarding the safety of MRI procedures can be found at the FDA's web page: http://www.fda.gov/cdrh/, by performing a search using the keywords "MRI" and "safety." Another good reference for MRI safety information is the website http://fmrib.ox.ac.uk/~peterj/safety_docs/.

PREGNANT PATIENT POLICY

It is recommended that all clinics and institutions adopt a policy to follow when a pregnant or potentially pregnant patient presents for a possible x-ray procedure. An example of a step-by-step flowchart section of such a policy is shown in Fig. A1-1.

Most of this flowchart should be self-explanatory. The recommendation to proceed with an elective x-ray procedure when 0 to 28 days have passed since the beginning of the last menstrual period is based on an International Commission on Radiological Protection (ICRP) recommendation,[44] which states in part: "The effects on the conceptus of exposure to radiation depend on when the exposure occurs relative to conception. Exposure of the embryo in the first 3 weeks following conception is not likely to result in deterministic or stochastic effects after birth." Methods that can be employed to reduce x-ray dose include (1) use of a higher x-ray tube voltage (kVp) technique in both radiography and fluoroscopy, (2) employment of a technique without a grid in both fluoroscopy and radiography, (3) employment of a higher-speed screen-film combination in radiography, (4) operation of fluoroscopy equipment in a pulsed mode at a lower pulse rate if available (e.g., the dose for

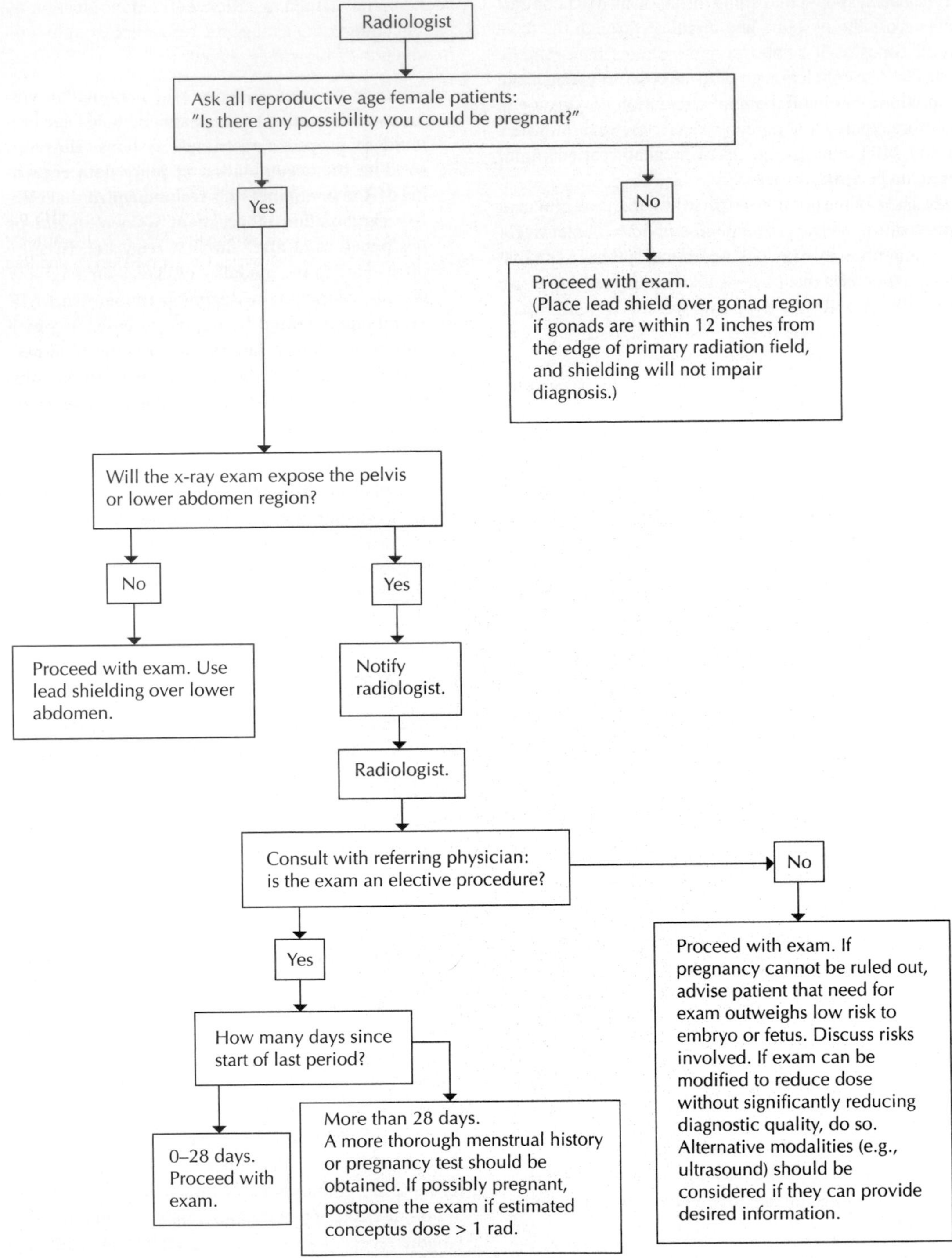

Fig. A1-1. Flowchart for x-ray imaging of reproductive-age women.

7.5 pulses per second is about one-fourth the dose for 30 pulses per second), (5) use of greater TV camera gain in fluoroscopy, and (6) use of larger fields of view in fluoroscopy. All of these methods have disadvantages in terms of reducing image quality. For example, use of higher-kVp techniques, greater fluoroscopic TV camera gain, removal of the scatter-reducing grid, and lower fluoroscopic pulse rates will all result in degraded image contrast. Use of higher-speed screen-film combinations and larger fluoroscopic fields of view will result in degraded spatial resolution. Physicians must decide upon the amount and type of image degradation they are willing to accept before choosing to use one of the dose-reduction techniques.

REFERENCES

1. American College of Obstetricians and Gynecologists, Committee on Obstetric Practice: *Guidelines for Diagnostic Imaging During Pregnancy.* ACOG committee opinion No. 158, September 1995.
2. Brent RL: The effect of embryonic and fetal exposure to x-ray, microwaves, and ultrasound: Counseling the pregnant and nonpregnant patient about these risks. *Semin Oncol* 16:347, 1989.
3. Johns HJ, Cunningham JR: *The Physics of Radiology,* 4th ed. Springfield, IL: Charles C Thomas, 1983.
4. NCRP Report No. 91: *Recommendations on Limits for Exposure to Ionizing Radiation.* Bethesda, MD: National Council on Radiation Protection, 1987.
5. NCRP Report No. 116: *Limitation of Exposure to Ionizing Radiation: Recommendations of the National Council on Radiation Protection and Measurements.* Bethesda, MD: National Council on Radiation Protection, 1993.
6. Hendee WR, Ritenour ER: *Medical Imaging Physics,* 3d ed. St Louis, MO: Mosby-Year Book, 1992, p 649.
7. Wagner LK, Lester RG, Saldana LR: *Exposure of the Pregnant Patient to Diagnostic Radiations: A Guide to Medical Management,* 2d ed. Philadelphia: Lippincott, 1997.
8. Harrison RM: Central axis depth-dose data for diagnostic radiology. *Phys Med Biol* 26:657, 1981.
9. Kelly JP and Trout ED: Physical characteristics of radiation from 2-pulse, 12-pulse, and 1000-pulse x-ray equipment. *Radiology* 100:653, 1971.
10. Schulz RJ and Gignac CE: Application of tissue-air ratios for patient dosage in diagnostic radiology. *Radiology* 120:687, 1976.
11. Rosenstein M: *Organ Doses in Diagnostic Radiology.* HEW publication (FDA) 76-8030. Rockville, MD: U.S. Department of Health and Human Services, Center for Devices and Radiological Health, 1976.
12. Rosenstein M: *Handbook of Selected Tissue Doses for Projections Common in Diagnostic Radiology.* HEW publication (FDA) 89-8031. Rockville, MD: U.S. Department of Health and Human Services, Center for Devices and Radiological Health, 1988.
13. Rosenstein M, Suleman OH, Burkhart RL, et al: *Handbook of Selected Tissue Doses for the Upper Gastrointestinal Fluoroscopic Examination.* HHS publication (FDA) 92-8282. Rockville, MD: U.S. Department of Health and Human Services, Center for Devices and Radiological Health, 1992.
14. Stern SH, Rosenstein M, Renaud L, Zankel M: *Handbook of Selected Tissue Doses for Fluoroscopic and Cineangiographic Examination of the Coronary Arteries.* HHS publication (FDA) 95-8289. Rockville, MD: U.S. Department of Health and Human Services, Center for Devices and Radiological Health, 1995.
15. Ragozzino MW, Gray JE, Burke TM, Van Lysel MS: Estimation and minimization of fetal absorbed dose: Data from common radiographic examination. *AJR* 137:667, 1981.
16. Sabel M, Bednar W, Weishaar J: Investigation of the exposure to radiation of the embryo/fetus in the course of radiographic examinations during pregnancy. First communication: Tissue-air ratios for x-rays with tube voltages between 60 kV and 120 kV. *Strahlentherapie* 156:502, 1980.
17. Glaze S, Schneiders N, Bushong S: A computer-assisted procedure for estimating patient exposure and fetal dose in radiographic examinations. *Radiology* 145:187, 1982.
18. Chapple CL, Faulkner K: Computerized calculation of radiation dose to patients from radiography. *Br J Radiol* 63:801, 1990.
19. Nagel HD, Galanski M, Hidajat N, Maier W, Schmidt TH (eds): *Radiation Exposure in Computed Tomography.* Frankfurt: COCIR, 2000.
20. Zankl M, Panzer W, Drexler G: The calculation of dose from external photon exposures using reference human phantoms and Monte Carlo methods part VI: Organ doses from computed tomographic examinations. GSF report 30/91. Oberschleiβheim: GSF-Forschungszentrum, 1991.
21. Wagner LK, Archer BR, Zeck OF: Conceptus dose from two state-of-the-art CT scanners. *Radiology* 159:787, 1986.
22. Mini RL, Vock P, Mury R, Schneeberger PP: Radiation exposure of patients who undergo CT of the trunk. *Radiology* 195:557, 1995.
23. Felmlee JP, Gray JE, Leetzow ML, Price JC: Estimated fetal radiation dose from multislice CT studies. *AJR* 154:185, 1990.
24. Panzer W, Zankl M: A method for estimating embryo doses resulting from computed tomographic examinations. *Br J Radiol* 62:936, 1989.
25. Zankl M, Panzer W, Drexler G: Tomographic anthropomorphic models part II: Organ doses from computed tomographic examinations in paediatric radiology. GSF report 30/93. Oberschleiβheim: GSF-Forschungszentrum, 1993.
26. Ginsberg JS, Hirsh J, Rainbow AJ, Coates G: Risks to the fetus of radiologic procedures used in the diagnosis of maternal venous thromboembolic disease. *Thromb Haemost* 61:189, 1989.
27. Twickler DM, Clarke G, Cunningham FG: Diagnostic imaging in pregnancy: Supplement, in *Williams Obstetrics,* 18th

ed. Norwalk, CT: Appleton & Lange, June/July 1992, pp 1–15.

28. NCRP Commentary No. 9: *Considerations Regarding the Unintended Radiation Exposure of the Embryo, Fetus or Nursing Child.* Bethesda, MD: National Council on Radiation Protection, 1994.
29. Mettler GA, Guiberteau MJ: *Essentials of Nuclear Medicine Imaging.* Philadelphia: Saunders, 1991, pp 320–321.
30. Committee on Biological Effects of Ionizing Radiation, Board on Radiation Effects Research Commission on Life Sciences, National Research Council: *Health Effects on Exposure to Low Levels of Ionizing Radiation: BEIR V.* Washington, DC: National Academy Press, 1990, pp 352–370.
31. Blot WJ: Growth and development following prenatal and childhood exposure to atomic radiation. *J Radiat Res* 16(Suppl):82–88, 1975.
32. Miller RW, Mulvihill JJ: Small head size after atomic radiation. *Teratology* 14:355, 1976.
33. Otake M, Schull WJ: In utero exposure to A-bomb radiation and mental retardation: A reassessment. *Br J Radiol* 57: 409–414, 1984.
34. UNSCEAR (1994) United Nations Scientific Committee on the Effects of Atomic Radiation, Annex A: Epidemiological studies of radiation carcinogenesis, in *Sources and Effects of Ionizing Radiation*, Publication E.94.IX.11. New York: United Nations Publications, 1994.
35. Yoshimoto Y, Soda M, Schull WJ, et al: Studies of children in utero during atomic bomb detonations, in *Proceedings of the 203rd National Meeting of the American Chemical Society.* San Francisco, CA, April 5–10, 1992.
36. Bushong SC:*Radiologic Science for Technologists,* 7th ed. St Louis, MO: Mosby, Inc., 2001, p 490.
37. Hall EJ: *Radiobiology for the Radiologist*, 5th ed. Philadelphia: Lippincott Williams & Wilkins, 2000, p 173.
38. American Institute of Ultrasound in Medicine: *Medical Ultrasound Safety.* Laurel, MD: AIUM, 1994.
39. National Equipment Manufacturers Association: *Standard for Real-Time Display of Thermal and Mechanical Acoustic Output Indices on Diagnostic Ultrasound Equipment.* NEMA Electrical Standards and Product Guide, Standard ID Number 312, Catalog Number 90252, Standard Designator UD3-1992. Washington, DC: NEMA, 1992.
40. American Institute of Ultrasound in Medicine: *Bioeffects and Safety of Diagnostic Ultrasound.* Laurel, MD: AIUM, 1993 (also approved as an official statement of the AIUM, March 1997).
41. Shellock FG, Kanal E: *Magnetic Resonance: Bioeffects, Safety and Patient Management.* New York: Raven Press, 1994.
42. Shellock FG, Kanal E: Policies, guidelines, and recommendations for MR imaging safety and patient management. *J Magn Reson Imag* 1:97, 1991.
43. IRPA/INIRC: Protection of the patient undergoing a magnetic resonance examination. *Health Phys* 61:923, 1991.
44. ICRP (International Commission on Radiological Protection): *Publication 73. Radiological Protection and Safety in Medicine*. Oxford: Pergamon, 1996.

Appendix 2

Collection and Transport of Gynecologic Microbiologic Specimens

Carl L. Pierson

GENERAL CONSIDERATIONS REGARDING SPECIMEN COLLECTION AND WORKING WITH THE DIAGNOSTIC LABORATORY

Proper collection and handling of microbiology specimens requires the collector to know which infectious agents may be present in the sample, and to have some understanding of the procedures that will be used in the microbiology laboratory to detect these agents once the specimen is received (Table A2-1). Culture continues to be an important method used to detect potential pathogens; therefore, when this method is used, the organism must be received in a viable state. With very few exceptions, specimens consisting of bodily fluids or tissues are superior to swabs for the isolation of infectious agents. As more molecular diagnostic techniques are developed and adapted for clinical laboratory use, the preservation of specific target molecules in the specimen is becoming an important consideration and usually requires that the specimen be placed in a specially designed transport device. These devices frequently are specific for a commercial kit or instrument being used in a laboratory, and a substitute collection device may yield an erroneous test result.

The collector must also be aware of the time it may take a specimen to get from the collection point to the testing laboratory as well as the transport conditions. If the specimen will arrive within 1 to 2 hours, room temperature transport may be satisfactory; however, if the specimen may set overnight or require prolonged transport, cold storage and transport may be required. Specimens sent for wet mount examination (e.g., for *Trichomonas vaginalis*) need to be examined within 30 minutes of collection to detect motility. Information provided on the accompanying requisition is usually the only information that the laboratory will receive prior to processing the sample; therefore, the requisition should be carefully completed and include pertinent clinical information that may assist the technologists. Including a probable diagnosis with a suspected etiologic agent can significantly alter a set-up routine. It also gives the technologist an opportunity to match the requested test with the specimen received for appropriateness. Can the test be done from the sample received? If not, the practitioner should be contacted in a timely manner and specimen requirements discussed so that less time is wasted; there may still be time to take another specimen. When in doubt, it is advisable to contact the laboratory and discuss specimen requirements. This is one of the most underused services provided by laboratory personnel, and such contact can prevent a considerable amount of frustration and unnecessary expenditure of time and effort for all parties. Also, if the exact test desired is not obvious from the requisition, there is usually space available to write in which tests are needed, or to indicate the organism(s) suspected. If the receiving laboratory does not perform the requested test, the specimen should automatically be sent to a certified reference laboratory that does. The Food and Drug Administration (FDA) requires that the actual laboratory performing the test be identified on the issued report.

Most laboratories provide their clients with handbooks or websites that should provide the necessary information and instructions for proper collection and transport of specimens. Having such information available on site can be very helpful and may decrease the frequency of rejected specimens and increase the probability of detecting the etiologic agent.

INFECTIOUS LESIONS OF THE EXTERNAL GENITALIA

Herpes Simplex Virus Types 1 and 2

The most commonly used methods for the laboratory diagnosis of herpetic infections are culture and direct antigen testing. Vesicular or pustular fluid usually contains a high concentration of virus particles that can be collected either with a swab or by needle aspiration. As the lesion ulcerates and then crusts over, the number of viable virions decreases; therefore samples taken from older lesions may result in a false-negative culture (Fig. A2-1).

To send a specimen for culture, the skin covering the vesicle should first be cleaned with water or saline, not with alcohol or iodine compounds that may inhibit viral replication. Vesicular fluid can be aspirated with a tuberculin syringe fitted with a 26-gauge needle. Optimally, the fluid should be placed into viral transport medium and sent to the virology laboratory on ice. Alternatively, the aspirated fluid can be pulled into the syringe barrel, the needle removed and discarded appropriately, and the

Table A2-1. Collection and Transport of Specimens from the Female Genital Tract

Clinical Condition	Probable Organism(s)	Optimal Collection Site	Lab Test Method	Appropriate Collection Method	Transport
External genital lesions	HSV	Vesicle/lesion base	Culture/DFA	Syringe/Dacron swab	On ice
	HPV	Condyloma	DNA hybridization	Biopsy (not usually necessary)	
	T. pallidum	Chancre (soft)	Dark field/DFA	Aspiration/scraping	Saline at RT
	H. ducreyi	Chancre (hard)	Gram stain/culture	Swab of lesion base	Aerobic transport
	LGV	Inguinal node	Culture/DFA	Aspiration of node	Sucrose phosphate medium On ice
	Granuloma inguinale	Lesion	Fixed tissue stains	Biopsy	In formalin
	Molluscum contagiosum	Lesion	Fixed tissue stains or viral culture	Biopsy (not usually necessary)	In formalin Viral transport medium
Bartholinitis	*N. gonorrhoeae* *C. trachomatis* Mixed aerobes/ anaerobes	Drainage from duct or abscessed gland	Culture w/Gram stain Culture/DFA Aerobic culture Anaerobic culture	Collection of exudate with Dacron swab	Aerobic transport at RT Sucrose phosphate medium/kit slide Anaerobic Transport at RT
Vaginitis/vaginosis	Mixed aerobes/ anaerobes (BV)	Vaginal exudate/ discharge	Slide wet mount/ Gram stain	Collection of vaginal exudate	Microscopic examination at point of care
	Yeast Vaginal exudate/ discharge				10% KOH pretreatment
	Trichomonas Vaginal exudate/ discharge		Wet mount/culture	Saline washings	Maintain washings at RT

(*Continues*)

Table A2-1. (*Continued*) Collection and Transport of Specimens from the Female Genital Tract

Clinical Condition	Probable Organism(s)	Optimal Collection Site	Lab Test Method	Appropriate Collection Method	Transport
Toxic shock syndrome	*S. aureus*	Vagina	Culture/toxin test	Swab of exudate	Aerobic transport
Prenatal screening for Group B Strep	Group B Strep	Vagina and perirectal	Culture	Swab of vagina and perirectal area	Send swab in selective Todd-Hewett, broth or aerobic transport
Cervicitis	*N. gonorrhoeae* *C. trachomatis*	Endocervix Endocervix	Culture/DNA probe/EIA/NA amplification	Collect: exudate endocervical cells/urine	Sucrose phosphate medium/kit transport devices
Upper genital tract infection	*N. gonorrhoeae* *C. trachomatis* Mixed aerobes/ anaerobes *Mycoplasma*/ *Ureaplasma*	Collection of tissue &/or fluids from site of infection	Culture/NA amplification	Tissue and/or fluids from site of infection, or Dacron swab	*See* above *Mycoplasma*/ *Ureaplasma;* Send swab in balanced salt with albumin (e.g., M-4 medium)

DFA = Direct fluorescent antibody; EIA = Enzyme immunoassay; NA = nucleic acid; RT = room temperature; BV = bacterial vaginosis.

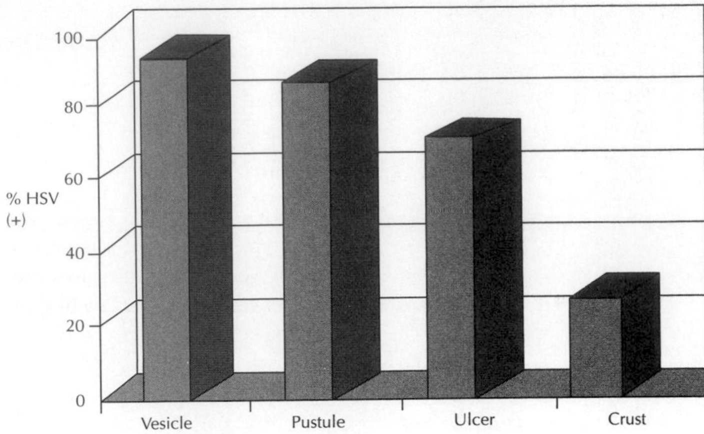

Fig. A2-1. Herpes simplex virus culture by stage of lesion. (Modified from Fife KH, Corey L: Herpes simplex virus, in Holmes KK, Mardh PA, Sparling PF, et al (eds): *Sexually Transmitted Diseases,* 2d ed. New York: McGraw-Hill, 1990, p 942, with permission.)

syringe capped and placed in ice for transport. (Syringes with attached needles are considered a biohazard and are no longer accepted in clinical laboratories.) If a swab is to be used, the skin covering the vesicle must be removed (unroofed). This can be done with a small-gauge needle. A Dacron swab is then used to absorb the vesicular fluid. The swab needs to be placed immediately into a viral transport device that will maintain the specimen in moist condition. The device should be placed on ice for transport to the virology laboratory for culture. Herpes simplex virus can be stored under these conditions for at least 24 hours without significant loss of cell culture infectivity. If an ulcer is present, the base should be swabbed with a Dacron swab and the swab placed in viral transport medium.

Direct antigen test methods are rapid (tests can be completed within 1 to 2 hours following specimen receipt) and do not require viable virions. Vesicular fluid collected either by aspiration or swab can be tested using rapid enzyme-linked antigen-capture methods.[1] Herpes simplex virus antigens can also be detected directly by harvesting cells from the base of the vesicle with a swab and sending it to the laboratory. The technologist will transfer the cells to a slide for special staining with specific fluoroscein-labeled antibody that can differentiate between HSV types 1 and 2.[2] Nucleic acid detection methods using specific probes with or without initial amplification are available, but are usually not required for the detection of HSV in lesions of the skin or mucous membranes; they are also considerably more expensive to use.[3]

Histologic stains (Papanicolaou or Tzanck) can be used, but are both insensitive and less specific. Solomon and colleagues found that only 67 percent of vesicular lesions positive by culture were positive by Tzanck stain.[4]

Herpes simplex virus serology is of limited usefulness for initial diagnosis. Blood collected during the course of the infection may contain elevated IgM-class antibodies that may aid in the diagnosis of a primary infection. Serology is of little value in the diagnosis of recurrent HSV infections. Many of the standard serologic tests available cannot be relied upon to accurately assess whether the infection was caused by HSV type 1 or 2 due to cross-reactivity as a result of shared antigens.[5] Recently, however, serologic tests (immunoblot and ELISA) using specific recombinant antigens have become available that can differentiate between anti-HSV 1 and anti-HSV 2 antibodies.[6]

Human Papillomavirus

The human papillomavirus (HPV) family of viruses are not cultivated in the clinical laboratory and viral antigens may not be detectable in tissues. External genital warts, also known as condyloma acuminata, are one manifestation of HPV that can be readily detected by hybridization assays that use specific nucleotide probes labeled with immunoperoxidases or fluorescent molecules. Probe sets for detecting "high/intermediate risk" and "low-risk" genotypes are available that can be run on urogenital specimens collected by a cervical sampler, biopsy, or by using a liquid technique (e.g., ThinPrep™). Many diagnostic laboratories test for only the "high/intermediate risk" genotypes since it is these types that are more strongly associated with the eventual development of epithelial cell transformation.[7,8] Hybridization techniques can also be used to determine the specific HPV type.[9] Assay sensitivity can be enhanced using nucleic acid amplification methods, such as the polymerase chain reaction (PCR).[10,11]

Cytologic examination for the presence of koilocytes in lesions is also quite specific but insensitive.[12]

Specimens can be collected by biopsy or by scraping the base of the lesion with a scalpel. The tissue should be kept cold and transported to the laboratory in special kit-specific transport fluid. The biopsy can also be frozen and maintained at –70°C (–94°F) during shipment using dry ice.

Syphilis or Soft Chancre

Treponema pallidum is not cultivated in the clinical laboratory. The laboratory diagnosis of *T. pallidum* in lesions of the skin or mucous membranes is made by direct microscopic examination of serous exudate collected from the base of the suspected lesion. Accumulated exudate should be removed to expose the ulcer base prior to scraping. The base is then gently scraped (e.g., with a scalpel blade) to cause serous fluid to collect within the ulcer base. In primary and early secondary syphilitic lesions, this fresh exudate should contain viable treponemes. The exudate is then collected and placed directly onto the surface of a glass slide, covered with a coverslip and examined by dark-field microscopy within minutes of collection for detection of characteristic morphology and motility. The organism is quite thin (~0.2 μm in diameter) and variable in length (6 to 20 μm) with a helical morphology having a wavelength of about 1 μm. Freshly isolated organisms may demonstrate a corkscrew type of motility coupled with an undulating motion. The scrapings can also be suspended in a tube containing a small amount (~0.5 mL) of saline or nutrient broth available from the laboratory and transported immediately to the laboratory at room temperature for immediate dark-field examination. Extreme care should be taken in handling such samples since the spirochetes in this state are highly infectious. A limited number of laboratories have specific fluorescein-conjugated antibody (DFA-TP) that can detect nonviable *T. pallidum* in exudate which has been dried and fixed on a standard microscope slide. The inoculated slide can be transported to the laboratory in a clean, dry container at room temperature.

Serology is the method by which most cases of syphilis are diagnosed.[13] This is discussed in detail in Chap. 29.

Chancroid or Hard Chancre

Chancroid is caused by *Haemophilus ducreyi.* Chancroid ulcers must be cleaned to reduce the amount of necrotic exudate frequently present. A swab is then used to collect residual exudate from the ulcer base or margin. The laboratory will use the swab to prepare a slide for Gram staining and to inoculate enriched, nonselective, and selective blood-containing media.

Lymphogranuloma Venereum

Lymphogranuloma venereum (LGV) is caused by *Chlamydia trachomatis* serotypes L1, 2, or 3. Its prevalence in the United States is very low; most cases are imported. Samples of the ulcer can be obtained by biopsy or swab and transported to the laboratory, preferably in a sucrose phosphate solution, for culture in permissive cell lines (e.g., McCoy or HeLa 229 cells). Calcium alginate-containing swabs may be toxic to *Chlamydia* and should not be used for collection.

Granuloma Inguinale or Donovanosis

Granuloma inguinale is caused by a gram-negative bacillus currently classified as *Calymmatobacterium granulomatis.* Diagnosis is based on the appearance of donovan bodies (bipolar-staining bacilli in tissue macrophages) in Giemsa- or Wright-stained material collected from the lesions. Lesion biopsies can be submitted in a small amount of saline or formalin if available.

Molluscum Contagiosum

Molluscum contagiosum virus is the etiologic agent and it can be cultured; however, this is not attempted in the typical clinical laboratory. The diagnosis is usually made clinically based on the characteristic appearance of the lesion, which presents as a 3- to 5-mm umbilicated, dome-shaped papule. If culture is needed, biopsied tissue should be sent to a special reference laboratory where the characteristic cytopathic effect that occurs in selected cell lines can be recognized.[14] Lesion biopsies should be kept cold in a moist saline environment during transport. No serologic tests are currently available.

Bartholinitis or Infection of the Greater Vestibular Gland or Duct

Since the ducts open onto the inner surface of the labia minora, any organisms colonizing the vaginal mucosa could cause infection of either the duct or the gland. Usually specimens are submitted for detection of *C. trachomatis* or *Neisseria gonorrhoeae,* but other aerobic and anaerobic organisms may be involved.

Table A2-2. Preparation of Vaginal Secretions for Wet Prep Examination

1. Collect vaginal secretions from middle third of the vaginal wall using a swab.
2. Roll swab onto nitrazine paper to obtain pH, then place into test tube with 1-2 mL of saline.
3. Place one drop of fluid from swab onto each end of a clean microscope slide.
4. Add one drop of 10% KOH to one of the two drops on the slide, noting any amine or fishy odor.
5. Coverslip both drops, taking care not to intermix the two drops.
6. Examine both drop areas using the low-power objective, noting:
   a. Appearance of epithelial cells (look for clue cells)
   b. Presence of WBCs
   c. Motile trichomonads
   d. Fungal elements, pseudohyphae (easier to visualize in KOH-treated drop)
   e. Background bacterial morphotypes, e.g., predominant rods, cocci, etc.

To collect exudate from the duct, decontaminate the duct orifice with an iodine solution and collect the expressed exudate on a swab. Place the swab or aspirate in an anaerobic transport medium and instruct the laboratory to perform a Gram stain and process for *C. trachomatis* and *N. gonorrhoeae* only on exudate from the duct. Concurrent endocervical specimens should be collected for *C. trachomatis* and *N. gonorrhoeae* to improve diagnostic sensitivity.

INFECTIONS OF THE VAGINA

Vaginitis/Vaginosis

The three most common infectious agents associated with vaginitis/vaginosis are (1) mixed aerobic and anaerobic bacteria associated with bacterial vaginosis; (2) yeast; and (3) *Trichomonas vaginalis*. Diagnosis and management is discussed in detail in Chap. 31 (see also Tables A2-2 and A2-3).

Toxic Shock Syndrome

Toxic shock is usually caused by the proliferation of *Staphylococcus aureus* in the vaginal mucosa and production of a potent exotoxin designated TSST-1.[15] A Dacron swab can be used to collect vaginal exudate and be sent to a laboratory for culture using an aerobic transport device. The isolated organism can be sent to a reference laboratory that tests for toxigenic isolates. *Streptococcus pyogenes* has proved to be responsible for producing a toxic shock-like syndrome.[16] Isolation of *S. pyogenes* from this body site should be reported to the clinician immediately. Clinical management of toxic shock syndrome is covered in Chap. 36.

Group B *Streptococcus* (*Streptococcus agalactiae*)

Approximately 15 to 20 percent of women are colonized with *S. agalactiae* and remain asymptomatic; therefore, culturing for this organism in normal, nonpregnant women is of little clinical value. However, during pregnancy, urogenital antepartum carriage of *S. agalactiae* may present a significant risk to the fetus during labor and may cause neonatal sepsis, pneumonia, and meningitis as well as postpartum endometritis. Therefore, pre- or intrapartum screening for the presence of this organism in the vagina or anorectal area is recommended.[17]

To screen for *S. agalactiae,* use a single Dacron swab to collect a specimen from the vaginal wall and perirectal area. A speculum should not be used for this collection. For optimal recovery, place the swab directly into a tube of Todd-Hewitt broth or Lim medium.

CERVICITIS

Chlamydia Trachomatis Serotypes D Through K

Chlamydia trachomatis is an obligate intracellular gram-negative bacterium that primarily infects columnar and cuboidal epithelial cells found within the endocervix, urethra, and upper genital tract. Infection may be asymptomatic initially, but they eventually can cause PID and salpingitis, leading to diverse sequelae, including infertility. Several methods are being employed to detect *C. trachomatis,* including cell culture,[18,19] antigen capture enzyme immunoassay (EIA),[20] direct fluorescent monoclonal antibody,[21,22] DNA probe,[22–24] and nucleic acid amplification techniques such as the PCR, the ligase chain

Table A2-3. Diagnostic Features of Infectious Vaginitis

	Normal	Candidal Vaginitis	Bacterial Vaginosis	*Trichomonas* Vaginitis
Symptoms	None or physiologic leukorrhea	Vulvar pruritus, soreness, increased discharge, dysuria, dyspareunia	Malodorous moderate discharge	Profuse purulent discharge, offensive odor, pruritus, and dyspareunia
Discharge				
Amount	Variable, scant to moderate	Scant to moderate	Moderate	Profuse
Color	Clear or white	White	White/gray	Yellow
Consistency	Floccular nonhomogeneous	Clumped but variable	Homogeneous, uniformly coating walls	Homogeneous
"Bubbles"	Absent	Absent	Present	Present
Appearance of vulva and vagina	Normal	Introital and vulvar erythema, edema and occasional pustules, vaginal erythma	No inflammation	Erythema and swelling of vulvar and vaginal epithelium ("strawberry cervix")
pH of vaginal fluid	<4.5:	<4.5	>4.5	5–6.0
Amine test (10% KOH)	Negative	Negative	Positive	Occasionally positive
Saline microscopy	Normal epithelial cell Lactobacilli predominate	Normal flora, blastospores (yeast), 40–50% pseudohyphae	Clue cells, coccobacillary flora predominates, absence of leukocytes, motile curved rods	PMNs+ + + Motile trichomonads (80–90%), no clue cells, abnormal flora
10% KOH microscopy	Negative	Positive (60–90%)	Negative (except in mixed infections)	Negative

reaction,[25] and transcription-mediated amplification. For optimal detection, the specimen must be collected and transported using collection kits that are compatible with the method of detection. Collecting specimens from both endocervical and urethral sites improves diagnostic sensitivity compared with that achieved by sampling either site alone. Avoid sampling in the presence of lubricants, which may cause false-negative test reactions.

For culture, columnar or transitional endocervical cells containing infectious elementary bodies must be collected using a Dacron swab (avoid calcium alginate swabs) and transported in a preservative-free buffered sucrose phosphate solution. M-4 transport medium appears to be a good choice for this purpose and the specimen can be used for most amplification methods as well.

The remaining detection methods do not require viable organisms, but do require the use of special collection and transport materials to preserve either target proteins or nucleic acids. Once the specimen is in the appropriate transport container, it is usually stable for several days—a distinct advantage over culture when the specimen must be sent to a distant reference laboratory. Methods that employ amplification techniques can detect specific nucleotide sequences shed in urine as well as endocervical specimens with increased sensitivity.[25] Collection kits are available for both specimen types and are specific to the manufacturer of the kit (e.g., Roche Diagnostic Systems, Branchburg, NJ, and Abbott Diagnostics, North Chicago, IL).

Neisseria gonorrhoeae

The endocervix is the optimal site to sample for the diagnosis of *N. gonorrhoeae.* Additional sites to consider are the urethra, anorectum, and oropharynx. The most convenient collection method is by swab through a water-lubricated speculum. Other lubricants may be bactericidal. Excess mucus should be removed prior to collection, since organisms in the mucus are frequently nonviable. Microscopic examination of Gram-stained exudate can be useful, but it should be followed up by culture. Errors in interpretation are possible, since other organisms with similar morphology may be present (e.g., other *Neisseria* spp., *Moraxella* spp., and *Acinetobacter* spp.), but if intracellular gram-negative diplococci are seen, a presumptive diagnosis of gonorrhea can be made. *Neisseria gonorrhoeae* is a relatively fastidious bacterium that frequently dies in transport unless it is maintained on nutrient media in an elevated CO_2 atmosphere at room temperature.[26] Endocervical specimens collected by swab, especially cotton-tipped swabs, and transported in the typical aerobic transport devices frequently yield false-negative culture results. Dacron or calcium alginate swabs are preferred. The swabs must be maintained in a moist environment at room temperature and used to inoculate supportive growth media within 12 hours of collection. Commercial nutrient transport devices such as JEMBEC (Ames Co., Elkhart, IN), and Isocult, BioBag, and Gono-Pak (Becton Dickinson Microbiology Systems, Cockeysville, MD) contain selective growth media such as Thayer-Martin or Martin-Lewis formulations, along with a CO_2-generating tablet that can be activated to maintain a favorable atmosphere. These systems can be incubated on site if transport is to be delayed.

Alternative methods for direct detection of specific antigens and nucleic acid sequences in endocervical and urine specimens are now available. They are quite sensitive and highly specific. These methods are similar to those described above for the direct detection of *C. trachomatis* and both agents can usually be detected in a single specimen. Samples are to be collected and transported according to kit instructions using kit-specific materials. Currently these direct, nonculture methods cannot be used if the organism is to be tested for antimicrobial susceptibility. Nonculture based methods may not be acceptable for testing specimens collected from patients who may have suffered sexual abuse. Checking with local or state law enforcement agencies is recommended if nonculture methods are used.

REFERENCES

1. Sewell DH, Horn AS: Evaluation of a commercial enzyme-linked immunosorbent assay for the detection of herpes simplex virus. *J Clin Microbiol* 21:457, 1985.
2. Lafferty WE, Krofft SK, Remington M, et al: Diagnosis of herpes simplex virus by direct immunofluorescence and viral isolation from samples of external genital lesions in a high-prevalence population. *J Clin Microbiol* 25:323, 1987.
3. Nahass GT, Goldstein BA, Zhu WY, et al: Comparison of the Tzanck smear, viral culture, and DNA diagnostic methods in detection of herpes simplex and varicella zoster infection. *JAMA* 268:2541, 1992.
4. Solomon AR, Rasmussen JE, Varaini J, Pierson CL: The Tzanck smear in the diagnosis of cutaneous herpes simplex. *JAMA* 251:633, 1984.
5. Ashley R, Cent A, Maggs V, et al: Inability of enzyme immunoassays to discriminate between infections with herpes simplex virus types 1 and 2. *Ann Intern Med* 115:520, 1991.
6. Ashley RL, Wald A: Genital herpes: Review of the epidemiology and potential use of type-specific serology. *Clin Microbiol Rev* 12:1, 1999.

7. Manos MM, Kinney WK, Hurley LB, et al: Identifying women with cervical neoplasia using HPV DNA testing for equivocal Papanicolaou results. *JAMA* 281:1605, 1999.
8. Wright TC, Lorincz A, Ferris DG, et al: Reflex human papillomavirus deoxyribonucleic acid testing in women with abnormal Papanicolaou smears. *Am J Obstet Gynecol* 178:962, 1998.
9. Wilber DC, Reichman RC, Stoler MH: Detection of infection by human papillomavirus in genital condylomata: A comparison study using immunocytochemistry and in situ nucleic acid hybridization. *Am J Clin Pathol* 89:505, 1988.
10. Bauer HM, Ting Y, Greer CE, et al: Genital human papillomavirus infections in female university students as determined by a PCR-based method. *JAMA* 265:472, 1991.
11. Karlsen F, Kalantari M, Jenkins A, et al: Use of multiple PCR primer sets for optimal detection of human papillomavirus. *J Clin Microbiol* 34:2095, 1996.
12. Bergeron C, Ferenczy A, Shah K-V, Naghashfar Z: Multicentric human papillomavirus infections of the female genital tract: Correlation of viral types with abnormal mitotic figures, colposcopic presentation and localization. *Obstet Gynecol* 69:736, 1987.
13. Larson SA, Steiner BM, Rudolph AH: Laboratory diagnosis and interpretation of tests for syphilis. *Clin Microbiol Rev* 8:1, 1995.
14. Dennis J, Oshiro LS, Bunter JW: Molluscum contagiosum, another sexually transmitted disease: Its impact on the clinical virology laboratory. *J Infect Dis* 151:376, 1985.
15. Shands KN, Schmid GP, Dan BB, et al: Toxic shock syndrome in menstruating women: Association with tampon use and *Staphylococcus aureus* and clinical features in 52 cases. *N Engl J Med* 303:1436, 1980.
16. Musser JM: Clinical relevance of streptococcal pyrogenic exotoxins in streptococcal toxic shock-like syndrome and other severe invasive infections. *Pediatr Ann* 21:821, 1992.
17. Yancey MK, Armer T, Clark P, Duff P: Assessment of rapid identification tests for genital carriage of group B streptococci. *Obstet Gynecol* 80:1038, 1992.
18. Mahoney JB, Phernesky MA: Effect of swab type and storage temperature in the isolation of *Chlamydia trachomatis* from clinical specimens. *J Clin Microbiol* 22:865, 1985.
19. Aarnaes SL, Peterson EM, de la Maza LM: The effect of media and temperature on the storage of *Chlamydia trachomatis*. *Am J Clin Pathol* 81:237, 1984.
20. Forbes BA, Bartholoma N, McMillan J, et al: Evaluation of a monoclonal antibody test to detect *Chlamydia trachomatis* in cervical and urethral specimens. *J Clin Microbiol* 23:1127, 1986.
21. Cheresky MA, Mahoney JB, Castriciano S, et al: Detection of *Chlamydia trachomatis* antigens by enzyme immunoassay and immunofluorescence in genital specimens from symptomatic and asymptomatic men and women. *J Infect Dis* 154:141, 1986.
22. Krepel J, Laur I, Sposton A, et al: PCR and direct fluorescent-antibody staining confirm *Chlamydia trachomatis* antigens in swabs and urine below the detection threshold of Chlamydiazyme Enzyme Immunoassay. *J Clin Microbiol* 33:2847, 1995.
23. Kluytmans JAJW, Niesters HGM, Moulton JW, et al: Performance of a non-isotopic DNA probe for the detection of *Chlamydia trachomatis* in urogenital specimens. *J Clin Microbiol* 29:2685, 1991.
24. Limberger RJ, Biega R, Evancoe A, et al: Evaluation of culture and Gen-Probe Pace 2 assay for the detection of *Neisseria gonorrhoeae* and *Chlamydia trachomatis* in endocervical specimens transported to a state health laboratory *J Clin Microbiol* 30:1161, 1992.
25. Schachter J, Moncada J, Whidden R, et al: Noninvasive tests for diagnosis of *Chlamydia trachomatis* infection: Application of ligase chain reaction to first-catch urine specimens of women. *J Infect Dis* 172:1411, 1995.
26. Spence MR, Guzik DS, Katta LR: The isolation of *Neisseria gonorrhoeae*—A comparison of three culture transport systems. *Sex Transm Dis* 10:138, 1983.

Appendix 3

Dermatologic Problems Associated with Pregnancy

Lisa L. May

KEY POINTS

Avoid these topical dermatologic agents in pregnancy
- Retinoids
- Salicylic Acid
- Tar compounds
- Silver sulfadiazine
- Podophyllin
- Lindane
- Topical fluorinated corticosteroids

Avoid these systemic dermatologic agents in pregnancy
- Tetracyclines
- Sulfonamides
- Retinoids

The cutaneous changes associated with pregnancy can be divided into three major groups: physiologic changes of pregnancy, dermatoses specific to pregnancy, and tumors of pregnancy. Each of these topics is discussed in this chapter.

TOPICAL AND SYSTEMIC DERMATOLOGIC AGENTS IN PREGNANCY

As in the case of any treatment during pregnancy, caution must be used in selecting a medication because of potential teratogenic or perinatal risks. A firm diagnosis must be established and the potential risks of a given therapy weighed carefully against potential benefits. This is especially important in dermatology, where diseases may be short-lived, have minimal morbidity, be cosmetic in nature, or can have treatment delayed until after delivery.

Some of the topical preparations that should be avoided in pregnancy include retinoids, salicylic acid, tar compounds, silver sulfadiazine (to large surface areas), podophyllin, and lindane. Two case reports in the literature suggest topical retinoids can cause the same congenital malformations as those seen with Accutane®.[1] Topical erythromycin and benzoyl peroxide can probably be used safely during pregnancy.

Topical nonfluorinated corticosteroid use during pregnancy has not been associated with unfavorable outcomes. Low-potency nonfluorinated topical corticosteroids are thus considered safe and effective. Concern does exist, however, over the application of fluorinated topical corticosteroids to large surface areas. The fluorinated glucocorticoids more readily cross the placenta and may be associated with a reduction in fetal growth.[2] Oral glucocorticoids like prednisone may be preferred over topical therapy in instances in which large surface areas of skin are involved in the disease process (e.g., extensive allergic contact dermatitis).

Commonly used oral medications that should be avoided include tetracycline and related compounds as well as sulfonamides (near term). Oral retinoids (Accutane®) have devastating teratogenic effects and are contraindicated during pregnancy. Oral antihistamines are probably safe to use during pregnancy.[2]

PHYSIOLOGIC CHANGES OF THE SKIN IN PREGNANCY

Physiologic skin changes are usually only of esthetic concern, tend to resolve postpartum, and rarely require treatment during pregnancy. The three main types of physiologic changes are hyperpigmentation, varicosities, and hair changes (Table A3-1).

Hyperpigmentation is one of the most common findings in pregnancy and is most pronounced on the areola, external genitalia, and linea nigra (Fig. A3-1). Melasma, the "mask of pregnancy," is a specific type of hypermelanosis that occurs as blotchy, irregular pigmentation on the face. Melasma tends to be more pronounced in darker-pigmented skin. It usually regresses by 1 year after delivery. As sunlight may play an etiologic role, sunscreens should be used during pregnancy.[3] Oral contraceptives can exacerbate melasma.[4] Thus patients with pregnancy-associated melasma should be informed of this potential risk, because melasma due to oral contraceptives tends to be more persistent and less responsive to therapy.[5] Melasma that persists after pregnancy can be treated with any one or several of the following therapies: Retin-A®, hydrocortisone, hydroquinones, azelaic acid, chemical peels, or laser therapy.

Table A3-1. Physiologic Skin Changes Associated with Pregnancy

Localized hyperpigmentation
(areola, genitalia, linea nigra)
Melasma
Striae gravidarum
Vascular
Spider angiomas
Palmar erythema
Varicosities
Gingivitis
Hair
Thickening of scalp hair
Hirsutism
Postpartum telogen effluvium

Varicosities of the saphenous, vulval, and hemorrhoidal veins are also quite common. Patients should be counseled on ways to minimize these, including leg elevation, exercise, use of compression stockings, and avoidance of prolonged standing or sitting.

Postpartum hair loss can be alarming. Postpartum alopecia results from a telogen effluvium, which occurs between 1 and 5 months after delivery. Patients should be reassured that hair loss is actually a precursor of new hair growth.

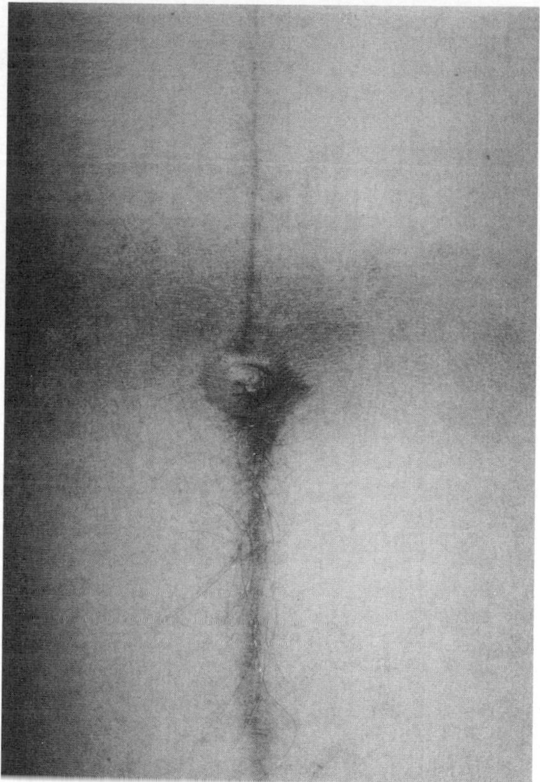

Fig. A3-1. Linea nigra. The linea alba becomes darkened during pregnancy and gradually resolves postpartum.

DERMATOSES SPECIFIC TO PREGNANCY

Herpes Gestationis

Also known as pemphigoid gestationis, herpes gestationis (HG) is a rare vesiculobullous dermatosis of pregnancy sharing many features with bullous pemphigoid (Table A3-2). The incidence is estimated to be between 1 per 1700 and 1 per 5000.[6] It usually develops during the first pregnancy but can begin during any pregnancy. When HG occurs after the first pregnancy, it appears to coincide with a change in sexual partners.[7] Herpes gestationis tends to recur in subsequent pregnancies with an earlier onset and more severe course. Flares with oral contraceptive use and menses also occur.

This disorder typically begins in the second or third trimester. Initially, intensely pruritic urticarial papules and plaques develop. Tense vesicles and bullae form within these plaques or on normal skin (Fig. A3-2). The lesions may be annular or polycyclic or may even resemble erythema multiforme. The majority of cases begin in the periumbilical region, with the abdomen, thighs, palms, and soles most commonly affected. Mucous membranes and the face are generally spared. These lesions will heal without scarring; however, postinflammatory hyperpigmentation is common.

Herpes gestationis is an autoimmune vesiculobullous disease in which antibodies capable of fixing complement are directed against an 180 kDa basement membrane protein known as the *bullous pemphigoid antigen-2*.[8] The inciting event that leads to antibody formation remains unclear, but appears to be hormonally influenced.[9]

Differential Diagnosis

Herpes gestationis is the only pregnancy-associated dermatosis with bulla formation. Other blistering disorders, however, have been reported to begin during pregnancy. These include pemphigus vulgaris, pemphigus foliaceous, bullous drug eruption, and erythema multiforme. Bullous impetigo can certainly occur in pregnancy as well. Bacte-

Table A3-2. Dermatoses Specific to Pregnancy

Disorder	Skin Lesion	Treatment	Maternal Outcome	Fetal Outcome
Herpes gestationis	Bullae	Topical or systemic steroids	Spontaneous clearing after delivery; may reoccur with subsequent pregnancies or oral contraceptives	5% of newborns with lesions
PUPPP	Urticarial papules and plaques	Topical steroids	Clears after delivery	No complications
Impetigo herpetiformis	Erythema and pustules	Systemic steroids and antibiotics	Hypocalcemia, hyperphosphatemia hypoparathyroidism	Fetal morbidity, mortality
Prurigo	Papules	Topical steroids	Clears after delivery; may reoccur with subsequent pregnancies	None
Pruritus gravidarum	None	Antihistamines, cholestyramine	If nausea, vomiting, epigastric discomfort, or abnormal liver enzymes, look for serious hepatobiliary disorders, HELLP syndrome, or preeclampsia	Fetal morbidity, mortality

HELLP syndrome = hemolysis, elevated liver enzymes, and low platelets; PUPPP = Pruritic urticarial papules and plaques of pregnancy.

rial culture can be helpful; however, HG lesions can also become secondarily infected. Thus culture should not be the sole means of differentiating these two entities. Early lesions of HG must also be distinguished from pruritic urticarial papules and plaques of pregnancy (PUPPP). PUPPP tends to appear predominantly in striae and to spare the periumbilical area. There may be vesicles, but bullae do not develop. Herpes gestationis may be differentiated from all of the above-mentioned disorders by skin biopsy for histology and direct immunofluorescence.

Course and Prognosis

Once HG develops, the disease persists throughout the remainder of the pregnancy. Although flaring around the time of delivery is common, clearing of lesions is usually complete by 3 months after delivery. Patients may have long-lasting postinflammatory hyperpigmentation. Exacerbations may occur with menses, oral contraceptive use, and repeat pregnancies. Maternal prognosis is excellent in pemphigoid gestationis.

Less than 5 percent of newborns will develop vesiculobullous lesions, and if they do occur, they are transient. The question of fetal morbidity and mortality has been debated. Although one report by Lawley and associates showed an increase in fetal mortality,[10] no other studies have confirmed this. Other studies have shown an increase in prematurity and infants that are small for gestational age.[11–13] These patients need to be followed closely with antepartum fetal testing. It is not known whether treatment alters prognosis.

Treatment

Mild cases of HG can be treated with antihistamines and topical corticosteroids. Prednisone, 40 to 60 mg/d orally may be required in more severe disease. Complete tapering should not be attempted until after delivery. The patient may also require increased doses of prednisone in the immediate postpartum period to control flaring of the disease after delivery.[5]

Pruritic Urticarial Papules and Plaques of Pregnancy (PUPPP)

Synonyms include *polymorphic eruption of pregnancy, toxemic rash of pregnancy,* and *papular dermatitis of pregnancy.* This skin condition is a benign pruritic skin

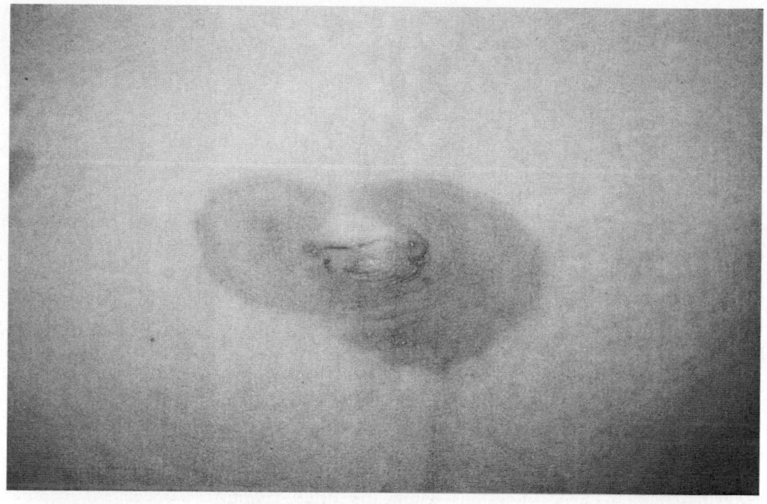

A

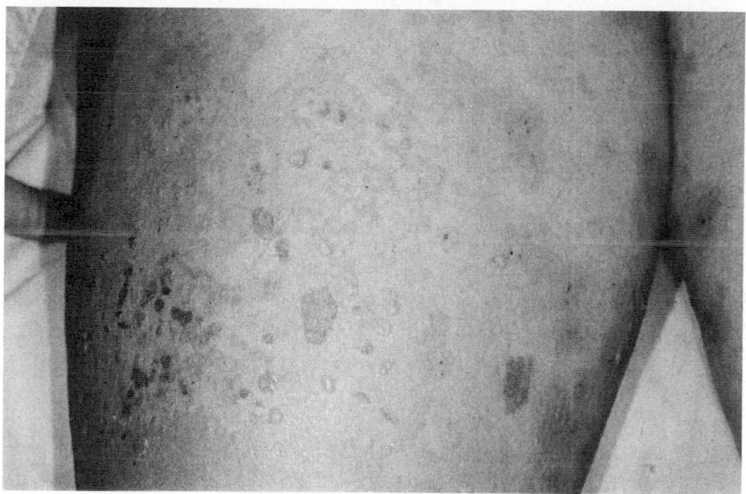

B

Fig. A3-2. Herpes gestationis. *A*. Lesions often begin as urticarial plaques in the periumbilical area. *B*. Bullae and erosions on the thighs.

eruption of variable morphology that develops late in pregnancy. PUPPP constitutes the most common dermatosis specific for pregnancy, with an incidence estimated at 1 in 160.[14] This is a disease primarily of the first pregnancy, and 80 percent of patients with PUPPP are primigravidas.

PUPPP tends to appear in the late third trimester, but can begin any time from the second trimester to 1 week postpartum. Intensely pruritic, blanchable, erythematous papules and urticarial plaques develop acutely. About 40 percent of patients develop papulovesicles, 20 percent have targetoid lesions, and 18 percent develop annular or polycyclic plaques.[14] The eruption is often confined to the striae initially. It commonly extends to the thighs, buttocks, upper arms, and lower thorax (Fig. A3-3). Despite the intense pruritus, excoriations are infrequent. No systemic manifestations have been reported.

No evidence supports an autoimmune or hormonal etiology. One theory is that the eruption is the result of an inflammatory response to damaged connective tissue in striae.[14] This theory is based on the observation that PUPPP is more likely to occur in patients with excessive maternal and fetal weight gain and in twin pregnancies.

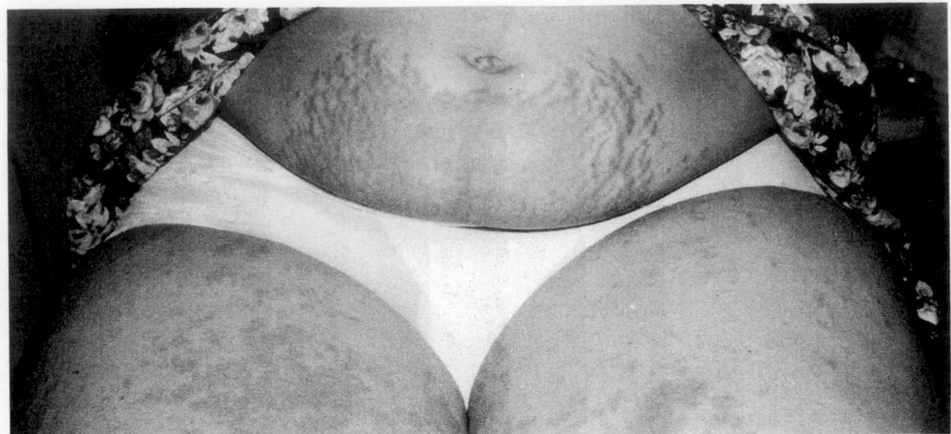

Fig. A3-3. Pruritic urticarial papules and plaques of pregnancy. Note the predominance of lesions within the striae, sparing the periumbilical area in this primigravida. The thighs are also involved.

Differential Diagnosis

Herpes gestationis may initially be urticarial and thus be confused with PUPPP. Another blistering disease, dermatitis herpetiformis, presents as pruritic vesicles and can be excluded by skin biopsy for histology and immunofluorescence. The targetoid lesions of PUPPP may also resemble erythema multiforme. Unlike erythema multiforme, PUPPP tends to spare the palms, soles, and oral mucosa. Skin biopsy can help differentiate between PUPPP, erythema multiforme, HG, and dermatitis herpetiformis. Scabies can also present as itchy papules and vesicles and thus must also be ruled out.

Course and Prognosis

The eruption improves in 2 to 3 weeks after onset and usually clears quickly in the postpartum period. No maternal or fetal complications have been reported.

Treatment

Topical corticosteroids and oral antihistamines are usually sufficient to control symptoms. Occasionally, however, oral prednisone may be required.

Impetigo Herpetiformis (Pustular Psoriasis of Pregnancy)

Also known as *pustular psoriasis of pregnancy*, impetigo herpetiformis (IH) is a rare form of pustular psoriasis with an acute onset without an antecedent history of psoriasis.[5] It may be associated with severe maternal and fetal complications. Impetigo herpetiformis is a misnomer in that it is not related to either a bacterial or a herpesvirus infection. The etiology is unknown.

The onset of IH is usually in the third trimester, but it has been reported to begin as early as the first month.[15] The cutaneous eruption develops acutely and can be accompanied by fever, malaise, nausea, diarrhea, lymphadenopathy, and even tetany secondary to hypocalcemia. Impetigo herpetiformis begins as slightly pruritic erythema that rapidly enlarges and develops rings of pustules at the margins (Fig. A3-4). The pustules break down in the center to leave painful erosions. The eruption initially appears on the thighs, groin, and other intertriginous surfaces and then spreads to other parts of the body. Face, hands, and feet are rarely involved.

Leukocytosis is a common finding. Hypocalcemia, hyperphosphatemia, and hypoparathyroidism have been reported and should be checked in patients suspected of having IH. Bacterial cultures of pustules are initially negative but are susceptible to secondary infection.

Differential Diagnosis

Herpes gestationis, dermatitis herpetiformis, impetigo, and subcorneal pustular dermatosis have a clinical resemblance to IH and must be excluded. A skin biopsy is necessary to make the diagnosis.

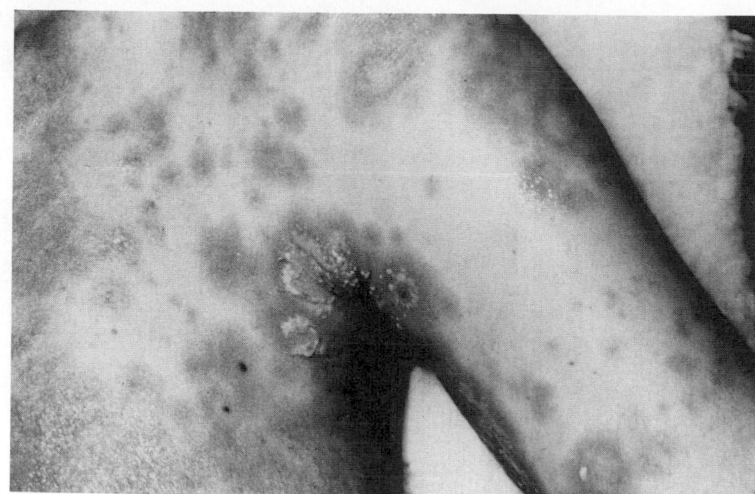

Fig. A3-4. Impetigo herpetiformis. Erythematous plaques with pustules at the periphery.

Course and Prognosis

IH tends to worsen as the pregnancy progresses. Resolution occurs rapidly after delivery or termination of pregnancy.

Prior to corticosteroids and antibiotics, maternal and fetal or neonatal deaths were common. Maternal mortality is now rare; however, fetal mortality may be increased despite control of the disease in the mother.[16] The etiology of the increased fetal mortality is not clear, although placental insufficiency has been suggested.[17]

Treatment

Treatment consists of fluid and electrolyte replacement, corticosteroids, antibiotics if secondary infection occurs, and fetal monitoring. Prednisone, 60 to 80 mg/d orally may be necessary. In severe cases with minimal response to the interventions mentioned above and evidence of maternal compromise or fetal distress, termination of the pregnancy may be indicated.[17]

Prurigo of Pregnancy

Prurigo of pregnancy is another pruritic eruption that typically begins on the extremities in early pregnancy. Early-onset prurigo of pregnancy, prurigo gestationis, papular dermatosis of pregnancy, and pruritic folliculitis of pregnancy are grouped under this diagnosis. Prurigo of pregnancy has been estimated to involve about 1 in every 300 pregnancies.[18] Its onset is usually during the second or third trimester, in contrast to PUPPP, which tends to occur in the last several weeks of pregnancy. The etiology is unknown.

Prurigo of pregnancy usually occurs on the extensor surfaces of the extremities as discrete excoriated or crusted papules (Fig. A3-5). Follicular involvement is variable. Pustules may be seen but vesicles are not.

Differential Diagnosis

An earlier onset with a predilection for the extremities and lack of involvement of the striae favor the diagnosis of prurigo of pregnancy over PUPP. Unlike PUPP, the lesions of prurigo of pregnancy are often excoriated. If primary lesions are not present, these excoriations should be separated from cholestasis of pregnancy. Furthermore, cutaneous disorders not specific to pregnancy also enter into the diagnosis. In particular, scabies, contact dermatitis, and drug eruptions should be excluded.

Course and Prognosis

The eruption may continue for up to 3 months postpartum and may recur during subsequent pregnancies.[3] Prurigo of pregnancy is not associated with an increase in maternal or fetal morbidity or mortality.

Treatment

Treatment is symptomatic and consists of emollients, nonfluorinated topical corticosteroids, and oral antihistamines.

Fig. A3-5. Prurigo of pregnancy. Note the excoriated discrete papules.

Intrahepatic Cholestasis of Pregnancy (Pruritus Gravidarum)

Cholestasis of pregnancy is characterized by onset of generalized pruritus during pregnancy, no primary cutaneous lesions, and can occur with or without jaundice. The anicteric form of cholestasis of pregnancy is often referred to as *pruritus gravidarum*.[19] Jaundice develops in about 20 percent of cases.[20] Cholestasis of pregnancy is thought to result from estrogen and progesterone interference with hepatic conjugation and excretion of bile acids.[20,21] A genetic predisposition appears to exist, and patients often report a family history. It is uncommon in Asians and African-Americans, but very common in Scandinavians and Chileans.[3] Intrahepatic cholestasis is associated with fetal prematurity, fetal distress, and increased perinatal mortality.[20]

Differential Diagnosis

There are no primary cutaneous lesions. Thus if lesions other than excoriations are present, one must search for an alternative diagnosis. If pruritus is associated with nausea,

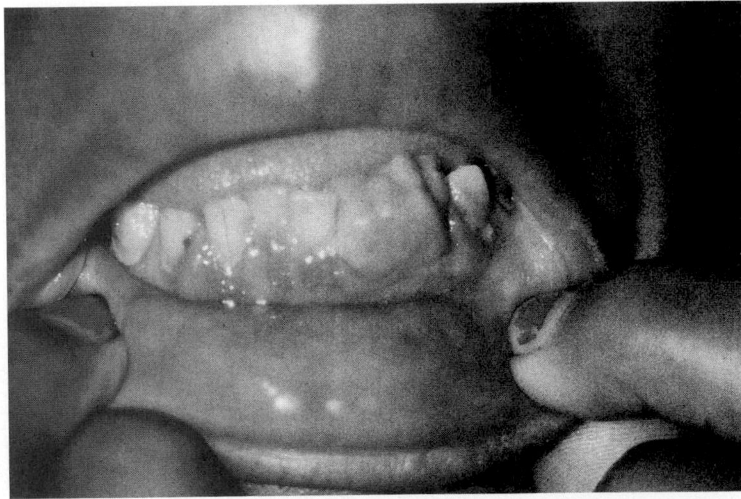

Fig. A3-6. Granuloma gravidarum. Bright red papule located between incisors with background gingivitis.

vomiting, or epigastric distress; or if there are abnormalities of hepatic enzymes, careful evaluation is necessary because serious disorders such as hepatitis, cholecystitis, cholelithiasis, acute fatty liver, HELLP syndrome, and preeclampsia are in the differential diagnosis.[22]

Course and Prognosis

Pruritus gravidarum begins in the second or third trimester and persists until delivery. Maternal complications are low if liver function tests are normal. However, there is increased fetal morbidity and mortality and close fetal surveillance is necessary during pregnancy.[20,23] Maternal symptoms resolve rapidly after delivery; however, abnormal liver function tests may take weeks to return to normal.[19] The condition may recur with subsequent pregnancies and oral contraceptive use.

Treatment

In mild cases, emollients and antihistamines may be helpful. Cholestyramine (12 g/d in 3 to 4 divided doses) may be helpful in some patients.[22] Because it is not absorbed, it is not harmful to the fetus; however, cholestyramine prevents adsorption of fat-soluble vitamins (especially vitamin K), so the prothrombin time should be monitored. If the prothrombin time is prolonged, parenteral vitamin K should be administered. Because of the potential for fetal morbidity and mortality, close fetal surveillance is necessary.

SKIN TUMORS ASSOCIATED WITH PREGNANCY

Granuloma Gravidarum

Granuloma gravidarum is a pyogenic granuloma occurring most commonly in the oral cavity. It typically presents as a friable red papule or nodule on the gingival surface next to a tooth or between two teeth (Fig. A3-6). Gingivitis is often present. The treatment for these lesions is surgical excision. Without treatment, the lesion usually regresses postpartum.

Nevi and Malignant Melanoma

Nevi have been reported to undergo enlargement or color change by patient history in approximately one-third of pregnancies. When skin biopsies were performed on these lesions, there was no statistically significant level of atypia as compared with nonpregnant controls.[24] This finding implies that atypical change during pregnancy is uncommon.[25] Nevertheless, changing pigmented lesions or those with any atypical features should be biopsied to rule out the possibility of malignant melanoma.

The influence of previous, current, and subsequent pregnancies on the prognosis of malignant melanoma has also been debated. Various studies have reported both increases and decreases in maternal survival.[25,26] Because the likelihood of recurrence is greatest during the first 2 years after the diagnosis of melanoma is made, it has been recommended that pregnancy be avoided during this time.[25]

REFERENCES

1. Lipson AH, Collins F, Wester WS: Multiple congenital defects associated with maternal use of topical tretinoin. *Lancet* 314:1382, 1993.
2. Robert E, Scialli AR: Topical medications during pregnancy. *Reprod Toxicol* 8:197, 1994.
3. Demis DJ: *Clinical Dermatology*. New York: Harper & Row, 1997, pp 1–18.
4. Resnick S: Melasma induced by oral contraceptive drugs. *JAMA* 199:95, 1967.
5. Winton GB, Lewis CW: Dermatoses of pregnancy. *J Am Acad Dermatol* 6:977, 1992.
6. Roger D, Vaillant L, Fignon A, et al: Specific pruritic diseases of pregnancy. *Arch Dermatol* 130:734, 1994.
7. Holmes RC, Black MM, Jeurecka W, et al: Clues to the aetiology and pathogenesis of herpes gestationis. *Br J Dermatol* 109:131, 1983.
8. Morrison LH, Labib RS, Zone JJ, et al: Herpes gestationis autoantibody recognize a 180-kD human epidermal antigen. *J Clin Invest* 81:2023, 1988.
9. Lynch FW, Albrecht RJ: Hormonal factors in herpes gestationis. *Arch Dermatol* 93:446, 1966.
10. Lawley TJ, Stingl G, Katz SI: Fetal and maternal risk factors in herpes gestationis. *Arch Dermatol* 114:552, 1978.
11. Holmes RC, Black MM, Dann J, et al: A comparative study of toxic erythema of pregnancy and herpes gestationis. *Br J Dermatol* 106:499, 1982.
12. Shornick JK, Bangert JL, Freeman RG, et al: Herpes gestationis: Clinical and histologic features of twenty-eight cases. *J Am Acad Dermatol* 8:214, 1983.
13. Holmes RC, Black MM: The fetal prognosis in pemphigoid (herpes) gestationis. *Br J Dermatol* 110:67, 1984.
14. Holmes RC: Polymorphic eruption of pregnancy. *Semin Dermatol* 8:18, 1989.
15. Gligora M, Kolacio Z: Hormonal treatment of impetigo herpetiformis. *Br J Dermatol* 107:253, 1982.
16. Beveridge GW, Harkness RA, Livingston JRB: Impetigo

herpetiformis in two successive pregnancies. *Br J Dermatol* 78:106, 1966.

17. Wolf Y, Groutz A, Walmar I, et al: Impetigo herpetiformis during pregnancy: Case report and review of the literature. *Acta Obstet Gynecol Scand* 74:229, 1995.
18. Black MM: Prurigo of pregnancy, papular dermatitis of pregnancy and pruritic folliculitis of pregnancy. *Semin Dermatol* 8:23, 1989.
19. Shanmugan S, Thappa DM, Habeebullah S: Pruritus gravidarum. A clinical and laboratory study. *J Dermatol* 25:582–586, 1998.
20. Davies MH, Ngong JM, Yucesoy M, et al: The adverse effects of pregnancy upon sulphation: a clue to the pathogenesis of intrahepatic cholestasis of pregnancy? *J of Hepatol* 211: 1127–1134, 1994.
21. Riely CA: Hepatic disease in pregnancy. *Am J Med* 96(1A):18S–22S, 1994.
22. Hunt CM, Sharara AI: Liver disease in pregnancy. *Am J Fam Physician* 59:829–836, 1999.
23. Johnson MB, Baskett TF: Obstetric cholestasis: A 14-year review. *Am J Obstet Gynecol* 133:299, 1979.
24. Foucar E, Bentley TJ, Laube DW, Rosai J: A histopathologic evaluation of nevocellular nevi in pregnancy. *Arch Dermatol* 121:350, 1985.
25. Driscoll MS, Grin-Jorgensen GM, Grant-Kels JM: Does pregnancy influence the prognosis of malignant melanoma? *J Am Acad Dermatol* 29:619, 1993.
26. Travers RL, Sober AJ, Berwick M, et al: Increased thickness of pregnancy-associated melanoma. *Br J Dermatol* 132:876, 1995.

Appendix 4

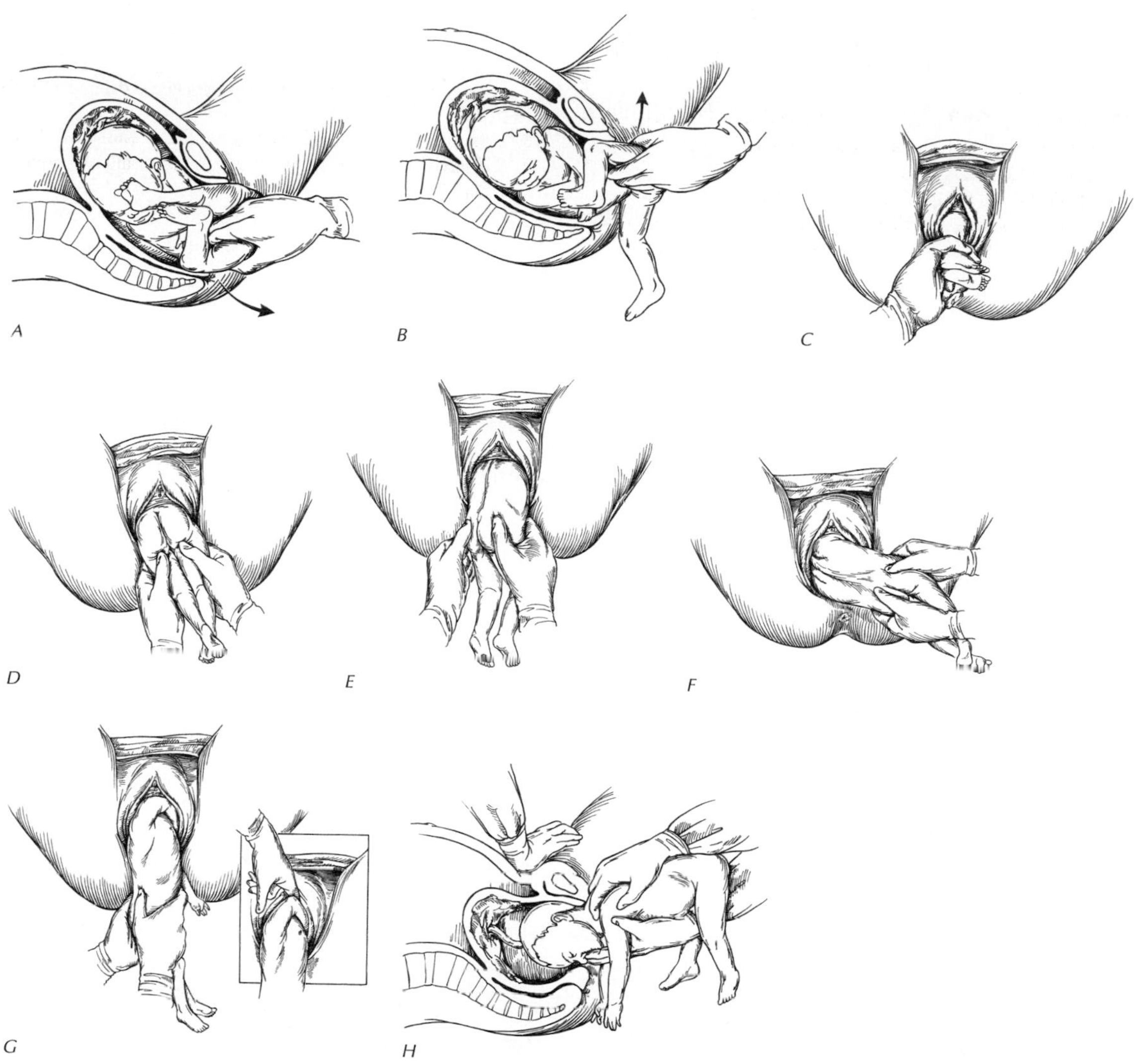

Fig. A4-1. Management of the vaginal breech delivery. *A.* The Pinard maneuver. The operator's hand is placed behind the fetal thigh, putting gentle pressure at the knee and allowing delivery of the leg. *B.* A similar maneuver of the opposite leg. *C.* The feet are grasped with the thumb and third finger over the lateral malleolus and the second finger is placed between the two ankles. *D.* With maternal expulsive efforts, the breech is delivered to the level of the umbilicus. The sacrum should be kept anterior. *E.* Again, with maternal expulsive efforts, the infant is delivered to the level of the clavicles, keeping the sacrum anterior. Excessive outward traction by the operator will frequently result in nuchal arms. *F.* The fetus is rotated 90° allowing visualization of the now anterior right arm. *G.* The arm is well visualized and a single digit is used to deliver it. Delivery of the opposite arm is accomplished by rotating the fetus 180° in a clockwise direction and repeating the maneuver. *H.* Delivery of the fetal vertex is accomplished by placing the operator's fingers over the maxillary processes of the fetus, keeping the body parallel to the floor. The body should never be lifted above parallel to prevent hyperextension of the neck. An assistant applies suprapubic pressure, aiding flexion of the fetal head and accomplishing delivery.

Index

A

D

J

O

P

Q

W

X

Y

Z